2015
Twenty-Seventh Edition

HMO/PPO
Directory®

Detailed Profiles of U.S. Managed Healthcare
Organizations & Key Decision Makers

A SEDGWICK PRESS Book

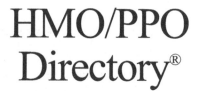

Grey House
Publishing

PUBLISHER: Leslie Mackenzie
EDITORIAL DIRECTOR: Laura Mars

PRODUCTION MANAGER: Kristen Thatcher
COMPOSITION: David Garoogian
MARKETING DIRECTOR: Jessica Moody

A Sedgwick Press Book
Grey House Publishing, Inc.
4919 Route 22
Amenia, NY 12501
518.789.8700
FAX 845.373.6390
www.greyhouse.com
e-mail: books @greyhouse.com

While every effort has been made to ensure the reliability of the information presented in this publication, Grey House Publishing neither guarantees the accuracy of the data contained herein nor assumes any responsibility for errors, omissions or discrepancies. Grey House accepts no payment for listing; inclusion in the publication of any organization, agency, institution, publication, service or individual does not imply endorsement of the editors or publisher.

Errors brought to the attention of the publisher and verified to the satisfaction of the publisher will be corrected in future editions.

First edition published 1987
Twenty-seventh edition published 2015
Printed in Canada

HMO/PPO directory — 1986–
    586 p. 28 cm.
    Annual
    HMO PPO directory
    Includes index.
    ISSN: 0887-4484
1. Health maintenance organizations—United States—Directories. 2. Preferred provider organizations (Medical care)—United States—Directories. I. Title: HMO PPO directory.

RA413.5.U5 H58
362.1'0425—dc21

ISBN: 978-1-61925-283-7 Softcover

Table of Contents

Introduction

This 27th edition of the *HMO/PPO Directory* profiles 1,213 managed care organizations in the United States, and lists important, current, and comprehensive information for HMO, PPO, POS, and Vision & Dental Plans.

In addition to detailed profiles of **Managed Healthcare Organizations,** this edition includes a valuable timeline entitled "Key Features of the Affordable Care Act, by Year." Starting with what has changed since 2010, and ending with a 2015 provision that ties physician payments to the quality of care they provide, this clearly written timeline makes sense of this complex topic. Plus, a **State Statistics and Rankings** section provides state-by-state numbers of individuals covered by type of health plans, and also ranks states by number of individuals enrolled in health plans.

Praise for *HMO/PPO Directory:*

> *"...of a topic that has grown exponentially more complex each year, this well-organized resource tries its best to keep it simple...The detailed user guide and five indexes enhance navigation...Written for both the consumer and the researcher, this work is a vital resource for public, academic and medical libraries."*
> —Library Journal, 2013

> *"...Information is clear, consistently presented, and easily located, making the guide extremely user friendly. Of particular note is the valuable...health care reform time line...A practical addition to public and medical library collections."*
> —Library Journal, 2012

Arrangement of State Chapters

Plan profiles are arranged alphabetically by state. An important feature of each state chapter is the state summary chart of Health Insurance Coverage Status and Type of Coverage by Age. This chart is broken down into 13 categories from "Covered by some type of health insurance" to "Not covered at any time during the year."

Directly following the State Summary, plan listings provide crucial contact information, including key executives, often with direct phones and e-mails, fax numbers, web sites and hundreds of e-mail addresses. Each profile provides a detailed summary of the plan, including the following:

- Type of Plan, including Specialty and Benefits
- Type of Coverage
- Type of Payment Plan
- Subscriber Information
- Financial History
- Average Compensation Information
- Employer References
- Current Member Enrollment
- Hospital Affiliations
- Number of Primary Care and Specialty Physicians
- Federal Qualification Status
- For Profit Status
- Specialty Managed Care Partners
- Regional Business Coalitions
- Employer References
- Peer Review Information
- Accreditation Information

The 1,213 plan profiles, combined, include 5,802 key executives, 639 fax numbers, 1,201 web sites, and 522 emails—8,164 ways to directly access the health care information needed by you and your business.

Additional Features

In addition to the educational material in the front matter, state statistics and detailed plan profiles, *HMO/PPO Directory* includes two Appendices and five Indexes.

- Appendix A: Glossary of Health Insurance Terms—Includes more than 150 terms such as Aggregate Indemnity, Diagnostic Related Groups, Non-participating Provider, and Waiting Period.
- Appendix B: Industry Web Sites—Contains dozens of the most valuable health care web sites and a detailed description, from Alliance of Community Health Plans to National Quality Forum to National Society of Certified Healthcare Business Consultants.
- Plan Index: Alphabetical list of insurance plans by seven plan types: HMO; PPO; HMO/PPO; Dental; Vision; Medicare; and Multiple.
- Personnel Index: Alphabetical list of all executives listed in the directory, with their affiliated organization.
- Membership Enrollment Index: List of organizations in the directory by member enrollment.
- Primary Care Physician Index: List of organizations in the directory by their number of primary care physicians.
- Referral/Specialty Care Physician Index: List of organizations in the directory by their number of referral and specialty care physicians.

To broaden its availability, the *HMO/PPO Directory* is also available for subscription online at http://gold.greyhouse.com. Subscribers can search by plan details, geographic area, number of members, personnel name, title and much more. Users can print out prospect sheets or download data into their own spreadsheet or database. This database is a must for anyone in need of immediate access to contacts in the US managed care marketplace. Plus, buyers of the print directory get a free 30-day trial of the online database. Call (800) 562-2139 x118 to start your trial.

User Guide

Descriptive listings in the *HMO/PPO Directory* are organized by state, then alphabetically by health plan. Each numbered item is described in the User Key on the following pages. Terms are defined in the Glossary.

---

1. → **U Healthcare**
2. → **3000 Riverside Road**
   Sharon, CT 06069
3. → **Toll Free: 060-364-0000**
4. → **Phone: 060-364-0001**
5. → **Fax: 060-364-0002**
6. → Info@uhealth.com
7. → www.uhealth.com
8. → Mailing Address: PO Box 729 Sharon, CT 06069-0729
9. → Subsidiary of: USA Healthcare
10. → For Profit: Yes
11. → Year Founded: 1992
12. → Physician Owned: No
13. → Owned by an IDN: No
14. → Federally Qualified: Yes 08/01/82
15. → Number of Affiliated Hospitals: 2,649
16. → Number of Primary Physicians: 4,892
17. → Number of Referral/Specialty Physicians: 6,246
18. → Current Member Enrollment: 204,000 (as of 7/1/01)
19. → State Member Enrollment: 29,000

Healthplan and Services Defined

20. → Plan Type: HMO
21. → Model Type: Staff, IPA, Group, Network
22. → Plan Specialty: ASO, Chiropractic, Dental, Disease Management, Lab, Vision, Radiology
23. → Benefits Offered: Chiropractic, Dental, Disease Management, Vision, Wellness
24. → Offers a Demand Management Patient Information Service: Yes
    DMPI Services Offered: Vision Works, Medical Imaging Institute

25. → **Type of Coverage**
    Commercial, Medicare, Supplemental Medicare, Medicaid
    Catastrophic Illness Benefit: Varies by case

26. → **Type of Payment Plans Offered**
    POS, Capitated, FFS, Combination FFS & DFFS

27. → **Geographic Areas Served**
    Connecticut, Maryland, New Jersey, Vermont, New York

Subscriber Information

28. → Average Monthly Fee Per Subscriber (Employee & Employer Contribution):
    Employee Only (Self): $8.00
    Employee & 1 Family Member: $10.00
    Employee & 2 Family Members: $15.00
    Medicare: $ 10.00
29. → Average Annual Deductible Per Subscriber:
    Employee Only (Self): $200.00

Employee & 1 Family Member: $250.00
Employee & 2 Family Members: $500.00
Medicare: $200.00

30.➤ Average Subscriber Co-Payment:
Primary Care Physician: $8.00
Non-Network Physician: $10.00
Prescription Drugs: $5.00
Hospital ER: $50.00
Home Health Care: $25.00
Home Health Care Max Days Covered/Visits: 30 days
Nursing Home: $5.00
Nursing Home Max Days/Visits Covered: 365 days

31.➤ **Network Qualifications**
Minimum Years of Practice: 10
Pre-Admission Certification: Yes

32.➤ **Peer Review Type**
Utilization Review: Yes
Second Surgical Opinion: No
Case Management: Yes

33.➤ **Accreditation Certification**
JCAHO, AAHC (formerly URAC), NCQA
Publishes and Distributes a Report Card: Yes

34.➤ **Key Personnel**
CFO...........................David Williams
Marketing.....................Clarence J. Fist
Medical Affairs...............Samantha Johnson, MD
Provider Services.............Laura Falk

Average Claim Compensation
35.➤ Physician's Fee's Charged: 22%
36.➤ Hospital's Fee Charged: 34%

37.➤ **Specialty Managed Care Partners**
AMBI, Pharmaceutical Treatment, OxiTherapy

38.➤ **Enters into Contracts with Regional Business Coalitions: Yes**
New York Healthcare

39.➤ **Employer References**
Life Science Corporation

User Key

1. → **Health Plan:** Formal name of health plan
2. → **Address:** Physical location
3. → **Toll Free:** Toll free number
4. → **Phone:** Main number of organization
5. → **Fax:** Fax number
6. → **E-mail:** Main e-mail address of health plan, if provided
7. → **Website:** Main website address of health plan, if provided
8. → **Mailing Address:** If different from physical address, above.
9. → **Subsidiary of:** Corporation the health plan is legally affiliated with
10. → **For Profit:** Indicates if the organization was formed to make a financial profit. Non-profit organizations can make a profit, but the profits must be used to benefit the organization or purpose the corporation was created to help
11. → **Year Founded:** The year the organization was recognized as a legal entity
12. → **Physician Owned:** Notes if the organization is owned by a group of physicians who are recognized as a legal entity
13. → **Owned by an IDN:** Notes if the organization is owned by an Integrated Delivery Network
14. → **Federally Qualified:** Shows if and when the plan received federally qualified status
15. → **Number of Affiliated Hospitals:** In-network hospitals contracted with the health plans
16. → **Number of Primary Physicians:** In-network primary physicians contracted with the health plan
17. → **Number of Referral/Specialty Physicians:** In-network referral/specialty physicians contracted with the health plan
18. → **Current Member Enrollment:** The number of health plan members or subscribers using health plan benefits, and date of last enrollment count
19. → **State Member Enrollment:** The number of health plan members or subscribers using health plan benefits in that state, and date of last enrollment count
20. → **Plan Type:** Identifies the health plan as an HMO, PPO, Other (neither an HMO or PPO) or Multiple (both an HMO and PPO, or an HMO and TPA or POS; see Glossary for definitions of terms). Note: If a plan is both an HMO and PPO with different product information, i.e. number of hospitals or physicians, the plan is listed as two separate entries
21. → **Model Type:** Describes the relationship between the health plan and its physicians
22. → **Plan Specialty:** Indicates specialized services provided by the plan
23. → **Benefits Offered:** Indicates specialized benefits offered in addition to standard coverage for physician services, hospitalization, diagnostic testing, and prescription drugs
24. → **Offers Demand Management Patient Information Services:** Notes if Triage and other services are offered to help plan members find the most appropriate type and level of care, and what those services are
25. → **Type of Coverage:** Lines of business offered
26. → **Type of Payment Plans Offered:** How the insuror pays its contracted providers
27. → **Geographical Areas Served:** Geographical areas the health plan services
28. → **Average Monthly Fee Per Subscriber:** Monthly premium due to the carrier for each member
29. → **Annual Average Deductible Per Subscriber:** The deductible each member must meet before expenses can be reimbursed
30. → **Average Subscriber Co-Payment:** The co-payment each member must pay at the time services are rendered
31. → **Network Qualifications:** Qualifications a physician must meet to contract with the plan
32. → **Peer Review Type:** The type of on-going peer review process used by the health plan

33. ➤**Accreditation Certification:** Specific certifications the health plan achieved after rigorous review of its policies, procedures, and clinical outcomes

34. ➤**Key Personnel:** Key Executives in the most frequently contacted departments within the plans, with phone and e-mails when provided

35. ➤**Physician's Fees Charged:** The percentage of physicians' billed charges that is actually paid out by the plan

36. ➤**Hospital's Fees Charged:** The percentage of hospitals' billed charges that is actually paid out by the plan

37. ➤**Specialty Managed Care Partners:** Specialty carve-out companies that are contracted with the health plan to offer a broader array of health services to members

38. ➤**Regional Business Coalitions:** Notes if physician or business entities have formed for the sole purpose of achieving economies of scale when purchasing supplies and services, and the names of those businesses

39. ➤**Employer References:** Large employers that have contracted with the health plan and are willing to serve as references for the health plan

Key Features of the Affordable Care Act, By Year

On March 23, 2010, President Obama signed the Affordable Care Act. The law puts in place comprehensive health insurance reforms that will roll out over four years and beyond.

OVERVIEW OF THE HEALTH CARE LAW

2010: A new Patient's Bill of Rights goes into effect, protecting consumers from the worst abuses of the insurance industry. Cost-free preventive services begin for many Americans.

2011: People with Medicare can get key preventive services for free, and also receive a 50% discount on brand-name drugs in the Medicare "donut hole."

2012: Accountable Care Organizations and other programs help doctors and health care providers work together to deliver better care.

2014: All Americans will have access to affordable health insurance options. New Health Insurance Exchanges will allow individuals and small businesses to compare health plans on a level playing field. Middle and low-income families will get tax credits that cover a significant portion of the cost of coverage. And the Medicaid program will be expanded to cover more low-income Americans. All together, these reforms mean that millions of people who were previously uninsured will gain coverage, thanks to the Affordable Care Act.

2010

NEW CONSUMER PROTECTIONS

Putting Information for Consumers Online. The law provides for where consumers can compare health insurance coverage options and pick the coverage that works for them. *Effective July 1, 2010.*

Prohibiting Denying Coverage of Children Based on Pre-Existing Conditions. The health care law includes new rules to prevent insurance companies from denying coverage to children under the age of 19 due to a pre-existing condition. *Effective for health plan years beginning on or after September 23, 2010 for new plans and existing group plans.*

Prohibiting Insurance Companies from Rescinding Coverage. In the past, insurance companies could search for an error, or other technical mistake, on a customer's application and use this error to deny payment for services when he or she got sick. The health care law makes this illegal. After media reports cited incidents of breast cancer patients losing coverage, insurance companies agreed to end this practice immediately. *Effective for health plan years beginning on or after September 23, 2010.*

Eliminating Lifetime Limits on Insurance Coverage. Under the law, insurance companies will be prohibited from imposing lifetime dollar limits on essential benefits, like hospital stays. *Effective for health plan years beginning on or after September 23, 2010.*

Regulating Annual Limits on Insurance Coverage. Under the law, insurance companies' use of annual dollar limits on the amount of insurance coverage a patient may receive will be restricted for new plans in the individual market and all group plans. In 2014, the use of annual dollar limits on essential benefits like hospital stays will be banned for new plans in the individual market and all group plans. *Effective for health plan years beginning on or after September 23, 2010.*

Appealing Insurance Company Decisions. The law provides consumers with a way to appeal coverage determinations or claims to their insurance company, and establishes an external review process. *Effective for new plans beginning on or after September 23, 2010.*

Establishing Consumer Assistance Programs in the States. Under the law, states that apply receive federal grants to help set up or expand independent offices to help consumers navigate the private health insurance system. These programs help consumers file complaints and appeals; enroll in health coverage; and get educated about their rights and responsibilities in group health plans or individual health insurance policies. The programs will also collect data on the types of problems consumers have, and file reports with the U.S. Department of Health and Human Services to identify trouble spots that need further oversight. *Grants Awarded October 2010.*

IMPROVING QUALITY AND LOWERING COSTS

Providing Small Business Health Insurance Tax Credits. Up to 4 million small businesses are eligible for tax credits to help them provide insurance benefits to their workers. The first phase of this provision provides a credit worth up to 35% of the employer's contribution to the employees' health insurance. Small non-profit organizations may receive up to a 25% credit. *Effective now.*

Offering Relief for 4 Million Seniors Who Hit the Medicare Prescription Drug "Donut Hole." An estimated four million seniors will reach the gap in Medicare prescription drug coverage known as the "donut hole" this year. Each eligible senior will receive a one-time, tax free $250 rebate check. *First checks mailed in June, 2010, and will continue monthly throughout 2010 as seniors hit the coverage gap.*

Providing Free Preventive Care. All new plans must cover certain preventive services such as mammograms and colonoscopies without charging a deductible, co-pay or coinsurance. *Effective for health plan years beginning on or after September 23, 2010.*

Preventing Disease and Illness. A new $15 billion Prevention and Public Health Fund will invest in proven prevention and public health programs that can help keep Americans healthy - from smoking cessation to combating obesity. *Funding begins in 2010.*

Cracking Down on Health Care Fraud. Current efforts to fight fraud have returned more than $2.5 billion to the Medicare Trust Fund in fiscal year 2009 alone. The new law invests new resources and requires new screening procedures for health care providers to boost these efforts and reduce fraud and waste in Medicare, Medicaid, and CHIP. *Many provisions effective now.*

INCREASING ACCESS TO AFFORDABLE CARE

Providing Access to Insurance for Uninsured Americans with Pre-Existing Conditions. The Pre-Existing Condition Insurance Plan provides new coverage options to individuals who have been uninsured for at least six months because of a pre-existing condition. States have the option of running this program in their state. If a state chooses not to do so, a plan will be established by the Department of Health and Human Services in that state. *National program effective July 1, 2010.*

Extending Coverage for Young Adults. Under the law, young adults will be allowed to stay on their parents' plan until they turn 26 years old (in the case of existing group health plans, this right does not apply if the young adult is offered insurance at work). Check with your insurance company or employer to see if you qualify. *Effective for health plan years beginning on or after September 23.*

Expanding Coverage for Early Retirees. Too often, Americans who retire without employer-sponsored insurance and before they are eligible for Medicare see their life savings disappear because of high rates in the individual market. To preserve employer coverage for early retirees until more affordable coverage is available through the new Exchanges by 2014, the new law creates a $5 billion program to provide needed financial help for employment-based plans to continue to provide valuable coverage to people who retire between the ages of 55 and 65, as well as their spouses and dependents. *Applications for employers to participate in the program available June 1, 2010.* For more information on the Early Retiree Reinsurance Program, visit www.ERRP.gov.

Rebuilding the Primary Care Workforce. To strengthen the availability of primary care, there are new incentives in the law to expand the number of primary care doctors, nurses and physician assistants. These include funding for scholarships and loan repayments for primary care doctors and nurses working in underserved areas. Doctors and nurses receiving payments made under any state loan repayment or loan forgiveness program intended to increase the availability of health care services in underserved or health professional shortage areas will not have to pay taxes on those payments. *Effective 2010 .*

Holding Insurance Companies Accountable for Unreasonable Rate Hikes. The law allows states that have, or plan to implement, measures that require insurance companies to justify their premium increases will be eligible for $250 million in new grants. Insurance companies with excessive or unjustified premium exchanges may not be able to participate in the new health insurance Exchanges in 2014. *Grants awarded beginning in 2010.*

Allowing States to Cover More People on Medicaid. States will be able to receive federal matching funds for covering some additional low-income individuals and families under Medicaid for whom federal funds were not previously available. This will make it easier for states that choose to do so to cover more of their residents. *Effective April 1, 2010.*

Increasing Payments for Rural Health Care Providers. Today, 68% of medically underserved communities across the nation are in rural areas. These communities often have trouble attracting and retaining medical professionals. The law provides increased payment to rural health care providers to help them continue to serve their communities. *Effective 2010.*

Strengthening Community Health Centers. The law includes new funding to support the construction of and expand services at community health centers, allowing these centers to serve some 20 million new patients across the country. *Effective 2010.*

2011

IMPROVING QUALITY AND LOWERING COSTS

Offering Prescription Drug Discounts. Seniors who reach the coverage gap will receive a 50% discount when buying Medicare Part D covered brand-name prescription drugs. Over the next ten years, seniors will receive additional savings on brand-name and generic drugs until the coverage gap is closed in 2020. *Effective January 1, 2011.*

Providing Free Preventive Care for Seniors. The law provides certain free preventive services, such as annual wellness visits and personalized prevention plans for seniors on Medicare. *Effective January 1, 2011.*

Improving Health Care Quality and Efficiency. The law establishes a new Center for Medicare & Medicaid Innovation that will begin testing new ways of delivering care to patients. These methods are expected to improve the quality of care, and reduce the rate of growth in health care costs for Medicare, Medicaid, and the Children's Health Insurance Program (CHIP). Additionally, by January 1, 2011, HHS will submit a national strategy for quality improvement in health care, including by these programs. *Effective no later than January 1, 2011.*

Improving Care for Seniors After They Leave the Hospital. The Community Care Transitions Program will help high risk Medicare beneficiaries who are hospitalized avoid unnecessary readmissions by coordinating care and connecting patients to services in their communities. *Effective January 1, 2011.*

Introducing New Innovations to Bring Down Costs. The Independent Payment Advisory Board will begin operations to develop and submit proposals to Congress and the President aimed at extending the life of the Medicare Trust Fund. The Board is expected to focus on ways to target waste in the system, and recommend ways to reduce costs, improve health outcomes for patients, and expand access to high-quality care. *Administrative funding becomes available October 1, 2011.*

INCREASING ACCESS TO AFFORDABLE CARE

Increasing Access to Services at Home and in the Community. The Community First Choice Option allows states to offer home and community based services to disabled individuals through Medicaid rather than institutional care in nursing homes. *Effective beginning October 1, 2011.*

HOLDING INSURANCE COMPANIES ACCOUNTABLE

Bringing Down Health Care Premiums. To ensure premium dollars are spent primarily on health care, the law generally requires that at least 85% of all premium dollars collected by insurance companies for large employer plans are spent on health care services and health care quality improvement. For plans sold to individuals and small employers, at least 80% of the premium must be spent on benefits and quality improvement. If insurance companies do not meet these goals, because their administrative costs or profits are too high, they must provide rebates to consumers. *Effective January 1, 2011.*

Addressing Overpayments to Big Insurance Companies and Strengthening Medicare Advantage. Today, Medicare pays Medicare Advantage insurance companies over $1,000 more per person on average than is spent per person in Traditional Medicare. This results in increased premiums for all Medicare beneficiaries, including the 77% of beneficiaries who are not currently enrolled in a Medicare Advantage plan. The law levels the playing field by gradually eliminating this discrepancy. People enrolled in a Medicare Advantage plan will still receive all guaranteed Medicare benefits, and the law provides bonus payments to Medicare Advantage plans that provide high quality care. *Effective January 1, 2011.*

2012

IMPROVING QUALITY AND LOWERING COSTS

Linking Payment to Quality Outcomes. The law establishes a hospital Value-Based Purchasing program (VBP) in Traditional Medicare. This program offers financial incentives to hospitals to improve the quality of care. Hospital performance is required to be publicly reported, beginning with measures relating to heart attacks, heart failure, pneumonia, surgical care, health-care associated infections, and patients' perception of care. *Effective for payments for discharges occurring on or after October 1, 2012.*

Encouraging Integrated Health Systems. The new law provides incentives for physicians to join together to form "Accountable Care Organizations." These groups allow doctors to better coordinate patient care and improve the quality, help prevent disease and illness and reduce unnecessary hospital admissions. If Accountable Care Organizations provide high quality care and reduce costs to the health care system, they can keep some of the money that they have helped save. *Effective January 1, 2012.*

Reducing Paperwork and Administrative Costs. Health care remains one of the few industries that relies on paper records. The new law will institute a series of changes to standardize billing and requires health plans to begin adopting and implementing rules for the secure, confidential, electronic exchange of health information. Using electronic health records will reduce paperwork and administrative burdens, cut costs, reduce medical errors and most importantly, improve the quality of care. *First regulation effective October 1, 2012.*

Understanding and Fighting Health Disparities. To help understand and reduce persistent health disparities, the law requires any ongoing or new federal health program to collect and report racial, ethnic and language data. The Secretary of Health and Human Services will use this data to help identify and reduce disparities. *Effective March 2012.*

INCREASING ACCESS TO AFFORDABLE CARE

Providing New, Voluntary Options for Long-Term Care Insurance. The law creates a voluntary long-term care insurance program—called CLASS—to provide cash benefits to adults who become disabled. **Note: On October 14, 2011, Secretary Sebelius**

transmitted a report and letter to Congress stating that the Department does not see a viable path forward for CLASS implementation at this time.

2013

IMPROVING QUALITY AND LOWERING COSTS

Improving Preventive Health Coverage. To expand the number of Americans receiving preventive care, the law provides new funding to state Medicaid programs that choose to cover preventive services for patients at little or no cost. *Effective January 1, 2013.*

Expanding Authority to Bundle Payments. The law establishes a national pilot program to encourage hospitals, doctors, and other providers to work together to improve the coordination and quality of patient care. Under payment "bundling," hospitals, doctors, and providers are paid a flat rate for an episode of care rather than the current fragmented system where each service or test or bundles of items or services are billed separately to Medicare. For example, instead of a surgical procedure generating multiple claims from multiple providers, the entire team is compensated with a "bundled" payment that provides incentives to deliver health care services more efficiently while maintaining or improving quality of care. It aligns the incentives of those delivering care, and savings are shared between providers and the Medicare program. *Effective no later than January 1, 2013.*

INCREASING ACCESS TO AFFORDABLE CARE

Increasing Medicaid Payments for Primary Care Doctors. As Medicaid programs and providers prepare to cover more patients in 2014, the Act requires states to pay primary care physicians no less than 100% of Medicare payment rates in 2013 and 2014 for primary care services. The increase is fully funded by the federal government. *Effective January 1, 2013.*

Providing Additional Funding for the Children's Health Insurance Program. Under the law, states will receive two more years of funding to continue coverage for children not eligible for Medicaid. *Effective October 1, 2013.* Learn more about CHIP.

2014

NEW CONSUMER PROTECTIONS

Prohibiting Discrimination Due to Pre-Existing Conditions or Gender. The law implements strong reforms that prohibit insurance companies from refusing to sell coverage or renew policies because of an individual's pre-existing conditions. Also, in the individual and small group market, the law eliminates the ability of insurance companies to charge higher rates due to gender or health status. *Effective January 1, 2014.*

Eliminating Annual Limits on Insurance Coverage. The law prohibits new plans and existing group plans from imposing annual dollar limits on the amount of coverage an individual may receive. *Effective January 1, 2014.*

Ensuring Coverage for Individuals Participating in Clinical Trials. Insurers will be prohibited from dropping or limiting coverage because an individual chooses to participate in a clinical trial. Applies to all clinical trials that treat cancer or other life-threatening diseases. *Effective January 1, 2014.*

IMPROVING QUALITY AND LOWERING COSTS

Making Care More Affordable. Tax credits to make it easier for the middle class to afford insurance will become available for people with income between 100% and 400% of the poverty line who are not eligible for other affordable coverage. (In 2010, 400% of the poverty line comes out to about $43,000 for an individual or $88,000 for a family of four.) The tax credit is advanceable, so it can lower your premium payments each month, rather than making you wait for tax time. It's also refundable, so even moderate-income families can receive the full benefit of the credit. These individuals may also qualify for reduced cost-sharing (copayments, co-insurance, and deductibles). *Effective January 1, 2014.*

Establishing Affordable Insurance Exchanges. Starting in 2014 if your employer doesn't offer insurance, you will be able to buy it directly in an Affordable Insurance Exchange. An Exchange is a new transparent and competitive insurance marketplace where individuals and small businesses can buy affordable and qualified health benefit plans. Exchanges will offer you a choice of health plans that meet certain benefits and cost standards. Starting in 2014, Members of Congress will be getting their health care insurance through Exchanges, and you will be able buy your insurance through Exchanges too. *Effective January 1, 2014.*

Increasing the Small Business Tax Credit. The law implements the second phase of the small business tax credit for qualified small businesses and small non-profit organizations. In this phase, the credit is up to 50% of the employer's contribution to provide health insurance for employees. There is also up to a 35% credit for small non-profit organizations. *Effective January 1, 2014.*

INCREASING ACCESS TO AFFORDABLE CARE

Increasing Access to Medicaid. Americans who earn less than 133% of the poverty level (approximately $14,000 for an individual and $29,000 for a family of four) will be eligible to enroll in Medicaid. States will receive 100% federal funding for the first three years to support this expanded coverage, phasing to 90% federal funding in subsequent years. *Effective January 1, 2014.*

Promoting Individual Responsibility. Under the law, most individuals who can afford it will be required to obtain basic health insurance coverage or pay a fee to help offset the costs of caring for uninsured Americans. If affordable coverage is not available to an individual, he or she will be eligible for an exemption. *Effective January 1, 2014.*

2015

IMPROVING QUALITY AND LOWERING COSTS

Paying Physicians Based on Value Not Volume. A new provision will tie physician payments to the quality of care they provide. Physicians will see their payments modified so that those who provide higher value care will receive higher payments than those who provide lower quality care. *Effective January 1, 2015.*

Source: U.S. Department of Health & Human Services, HealthCare.gov, http://www.healthcare.gov/law/timeline/full.html

State Statistics & Rankings

Covered by Some Type of Health Insurance

All Persons		Under 18 Years		Under 65 Years		65 Years and Over	
State	Percent[1]	State	Percent[1]	State	Percent[1]	State	Percent[1]
Massachusetts	96.3 (0.2)	Massachusetts	98.5 (0.2)	Massachusetts	95.7 (0.2)	New Hampshire	99.9 (0.1)
District of Columbia	93.3 (0.6)	District of Columbia	97.6 (1.0)	District of Columbia	92.6 (0.7)	Maine	99.8 (0.1)
Hawaii	93.3 (0.4)	Hawaii	97.0 (0.7)	Hawaii	92.2 (0.5)	Mississippi	99.8 (0.1)
Vermont	92.8 (0.6)	Vermont	96.9 (1.1)	Vermont	91.4 (0.7)	North Dakota	99.8 (0.1)
Iowa	91.9 (0.3)	New Hampshire	96.2 (0.7)	Minnesota	90.6 (0.3)	West Virginia	99.8 (0.1)
Minnesota	91.8 (0.3)	Michigan	96.0 (0.3)	Iowa	90.5 (0.3)	Iowa	99.7 (0.1)
Delaware	90.9 (0.7)	New York	96.0 (0.2)	Delaware	89.4 (0.8)	Rhode Island	99.7 (0.2)
Wisconsin	90.9 (0.2)	Iowa	95.9 (0.5)	Wisconsin	89.4 (0.3)	Vermont	99.7 (0.2)
Connecticut	90.6 (0.4)	Illinois	95.8 (0.3)	Connecticut	89.1 (0.5)	Wisconsin	99.7 (0.1)
Pennsylvania	90.3 (0.2)	Alabama	95.7 (0.5)	Maryland	88.5 (0.3)	Wyoming	99.7 (0.3)
Maryland	89.8 (0.3)	Connecticut	95.7 (0.5)	Pennsylvania	88.5 (0.2)	Arkansas	99.6 (0.2)
North Dakota	89.6 (0.8)	Maryland	95.6 (0.4)	North Dakota	88.0 (0.9)	District of Columbia	99.6 (0.4)
New Hampshire	89.3 (0.5)	Delaware	95.5 (1.1)	New York	87.7 (0.2)	Kansas	99.6 (0.1)
New York	89.3 (0.2)	Wisconsin	95.3 (0.3)	New Hampshire	87.4 (0.6)	Kentucky	99.6 (0.1)
Michigan	89.0 (0.2)	Ohio	94.7 (0.4)	Michigan	87.2 (0.2)	Massachusetts	99.6 (0.1)
Ohio	89.0 (0.2)	West Virginia	94.7 (0.9)	Ohio	87.1 (0.2)	Montana	99.6 (0.2)
Maine	88.8 (0.5)	Pennsylvania	94.6 (0.3)	Nebraska	87.0 (0.6)	Oregon	99.6 (0.1)
Nebraska	88.7 (0.5)	Rhode Island	94.6 (1.1)	South Dakota	86.9 (0.8)	Alabama	99.5 (0.2)
South Dakota	88.7 (0.7)	Virginia	94.6 (0.4)	Maine	86.5 (0.7)	Indiana	99.5 (0.1)
Rhode Island	88.4 (0.7)	Arkansas	94.5 (0.7)	Rhode Island	86.4 (0.8)	Michigan	99.5 (0.1)
Kansas	87.7 (0.4)	Nebraska	94.5 (0.7)	Virginia	86.0 (0.3)	Minnesota	99.5 (0.2)
Virginia	87.7 (0.3)	Minnesota	94.4 (0.4)	Kansas	85.8 (0.5)	Missouri	99.5 (0.1)
Illinois	87.3 (0.2)	New Jersey	94.4 (0.4)	Illinois	85.5 (0.2)	Ohio	99.5 (0.1)
Missouri	87.0 (0.3)	Louisiana	94.3 (0.4)	New Jersey	84.9 (0.3)	South Dakota	99.5 (0.4)
New Jersey	86.8 (0.2)	Tennessee	94.3 (0.5)	Missouri	84.8 (0.4)	Tennessee	99.5 (0.1)
Wyoming	86.6 (0.9)	Wyoming	94.3 (1.1)	Utah	84.6 (0.5)	North Carolina	99.4 (0.1)
Alabama	86.4 (0.4)	Oregon	94.2 (0.6)	Wyoming	84.6 (1.0)	Pennsylvania	99.4 (0.1)
Tennessee	86.1 (0.3)	Kentucky	94.1 (0.5)	Alabama	84.2 (0.4)	South Carolina	99.4 (0.1)
Indiana	86.0 (0.3)	Maine	94.1 (1.0)	Colorado	84.0 (0.4)	Colorado	99.3 (0.2)
Utah	86.0 (0.5)	Washington	94.1 (0.5)	Indiana	83.9 (0.3)	Nebraska	99.3 (0.3)
Washington	86.0 (0.3)	Kansas	93.9 (0.6)	Tennessee	83.9 (0.3)	Oklahoma	99.3 (0.1)
West Virginia	86.0 (0.5)	North Carolina	93.7 (0.4)	Washington	83.9 (0.4)	Utah	99.2 (0.3)
Colorado	85.9 (0.3)	South Dakota	93.7 (1.1)	Kentucky	83.4 (0.4)	Washington	99.2 (0.2)
Kentucky	85.7 (0.3)	South Carolina	93.3 (0.6)	United States	83.3 (0.1)	Arizona	99.1 (0.2)
United States	85.5 (0.1)	Missouri	93.0 (0.6)	West Virginia	83.2 (0.6)	Connecticut	99.1 (0.2)
Oregon	85.3 (0.4)	United States	92.9 (0.1)	Oregon	82.8 (0.5)	Idaho	99.1 (0.5)
North Carolina	84.4 (0.3)	California	92.6 (0.2)	North Carolina	81.9 (0.3)	Delaware	99.0 (0.4)
South Carolina	84.2 (0.4)	Mississippi	92.4 (0.9)	South Carolina	81.5 (0.5)	Hawaii	99.0 (0.4)
Arkansas	84.0 (0.5)	North Dakota	92.1 (1.2)	Idaho	81.4 (0.9)	Louisiana	99.0 (0.2)
Idaho	83.8 (0.8)	Colorado	91.8 (0.5)	Arkansas	81.2 (0.5)	New York	99.0 (0.1)
Montana	83.5 (0.8)	Indiana	91.8 (0.5)	Louisiana	81.1 (0.4)	United States	99.0 (0.1)
Louisiana	83.4 (0.4)	New Mexico	91.5 (1.0)	California	80.6 (0.2)	Alaska	98.9 (0.5)
Arizona	82.9 (0.4)	Idaho	91.1 (1.0)	Montana	80.5 (0.9)	Virginia	98.9 (0.2)
Mississippi	82.9 (0.5)	Utah	90.5 (0.7)	Mississippi	80.2 (0.6)	Georgia	98.7 (0.2)
California	82.8 (0.2)	Georgia	90.4 (0.5)	Arizona	79.9 (0.4)	Illinois	98.7 (0.2)
Oklahoma	82.3 (0.3)	Oklahoma	90.0 (0.5)	Alaska	79.7 (1.1)	Maryland	98.6 (0.2)
Alaska	81.5 (1.0)	Montana	89.9 (1.4)	Oklahoma	79.6 (0.4)	New Jersey	98.4 (0.2)
New Mexico	81.4 (0.6)	Florida	88.9 (0.4)	Georgia	78.8 (0.3)	New Mexico	98.4 (0.4)
Georgia	81.2 (0.3)	Alaska	88.4 (1.6)	New Mexico	78.4 (0.8)	Florida	98.3 (0.2)
Florida	80.0 (0.2)	Arizona	88.1 (0.7)	Nevada	76.4 (0.7)	California	98.2 (0.1)
Nevada	79.3 (0.6)	Texas	87.4 (0.3)	Florida	75.8 (0.3)	Texas	98.0 (0.2)
Texas	77.9 (0.2)	Nevada	85.1 (1.2)	Texas	75.4 (0.2)	Nevada	97.9 (0.5)

Note: Numbers in thousands; Figures cover 2013; Margin of error appears in parenthesis
Source: U.S. Census Bureau, 2013 American Community Survey, Table HI05. Health Insurance Coverage Status and Type of Coverage by State and Age for All People: 2013

Covered by Private Health Insurance

All Persons		Under 18 Years		Under 65 Years		65 Years and Over	
State	**Percent[1]**	**State**	**Percent[1]**	**State**	**Percent[1]**	**State**	**Percent[1]**
North Dakota	79.1 (1.0)	North Dakota	75.1 (1.9)	North Dakota	79.5 (1.1)	North Dakota	76.5 (1.9)
Minnesota	76.1 (0.4)	Utah	73.7 (0.9)	Hawaii	76.6 (0.8)	Michigan	75.5 (0.5)
Hawaii	75.6 (0.8)	Minnesota	72.6 (0.8)	Minnesota	76.5 (0.5)	Delaware	73.8 (1.9)
Iowa	74.8 (0.5)	Wyoming	71.2 (2.5)	Massachusetts	75.8 (0.4)	Minnesota	73.8 (0.7)
New Hampshire	74.8 (0.8)	Virginia	70.2 (0.8)	New Hampshire	75.3 (0.9)	Maryland	72.7 (0.7)
Massachusetts	74.5 (0.4)	Massachusetts	70.0 (0.9)	Iowa	75.2 (0.5)	Iowa	72.4 (1.0)
Virginia	73.9 (0.4)	Hawaii	69.9 (1.7)	Nebraska	74.5 (0.8)	New Hampshire	72.1 (1.7)
Wyoming	73.9 (1.3)	New Hampshire	69.7 (2.0)	Utah	74.5 (0.7)	Virginia	71.2 (0.7)
Nebraska	73.7 (0.7)	Nebraska	67.5 (1.4)	Wyoming	74.5 (1.3)	Pennsylvania	70.7 (0.4)
Maryland	73.6 (0.5)	Iowa	67.3 (1.0)	Virginia	74.3 (0.5)	Hawaii	70.4 (1.8)
Utah	73.5 (0.6)	New Jersey	66.9 (0.7)	Maryland	73.7 (0.5)	Wyoming	70.2 (2.8)
Kansas	72.2 (0.6)	Maryland	66.7 (0.9)	Kansas	72.6 (0.7)	Kansas	69.7 (1.2)
Pennsylvania	72.2 (0.3)	Connecticut	65.7 (1.2)	South Dakota	72.6 (1.0)	West Virginia	69.1 (1.3)
Wisconsin	71.8 (0.4)	Kansas	65.7 (1.2)	Pennsylvania	72.5 (0.4)	District of Columbia	68.2 (3.0)
South Dakota	71.7 (0.9)	Wisconsin	65.7 (0.8)	Wisconsin	72.5 (0.5)	Nebraska	68.2 (1.3)
Connecticut	70.7 (0.6)	South Dakota	64.5 (1.9)	Connecticut	71.8 (0.7)	Wisconsin	67.6 (0.7)
New Jersey	70.0 (0.3)	Pennsylvania	64.3 (0.7)	New Jersey	71.1 (0.4)	Idaho	67.4 (1.7)
Delaware	69.9 (1.2)	Colorado	63.4 (0.9)	Rhode Island	69.9 (1.2)	Indiana	67.2 (0.9)
Michigan	69.1 (0.3)	Rhode Island	63.2 (2.1)	Colorado	69.8 (0.5)	Washington	67.0 (0.9)
Colorado	68.9 (0.5)	Missouri	62.6 (0.9)	Delaware	69.1 (1.3)	Massachusetts	66.6 (0.7)
Rhode Island	68.9 (1.1)	Ohio	62.6 (0.7)	Missouri	69.1 (0.5)	Vermont	66.4 (1.9)
District of Columbia	68.8 (1.1)	Washington	62.0 (0.8)	Ohio	69.1 (0.4)	Alaska	66.3 (2.7)
Ohio	68.6 (0.4)	Delaware	61.9 (2.5)	District of Columbia	68.9 (1.2)	Oregon	66.2 (1.0)
Washington	68.5 (0.4)	Michigan	61.3 (0.7)	Washington	68.7 (0.5)	South Dakota	66.2 (1.7)
Missouri	68.4 (0.4)	Idaho	60.9 (1.8)	Michigan	68.0 (0.4)	Alabama	65.6 (0.8)
Indiana	67.6 (0.5)	Indiana	60.7 (0.9)	Indiana	67.7 (0.5)	Illinois	65.4 (0.6)
Illinois	66.8 (0.3)	Oregon	60.3 (1.4)	Illinois	67.0 (0.4)	Ohio	65.2 (0.7)
Vermont	66.8 (1.2)	New York	60.2 (0.6)	Vermont	66.8 (1.4)	Maine	65.1 (1.7)
Idaho	66.5 (1.0)	Maine	59.9 (2.0)	Idaho	66.4 (1.2)	Montana	65.1 (1.9)
Oregon	65.7 (0.6)	Nevada	59.5 (1.6)	New York	66.0 (0.3)	Kentucky	64.9 (0.9)
Alaska	65.2 (1.3)	Alaska	59.2 (2.2)	Oregon	65.6 (0.7)	Missouri	64.3 (0.9)
Montana	65.1 (1.0)	Illinois	58.1 (0.6)	United States	65.4 (0.1)	Connecticut	64.2 (1.1)
New York	65.0 (0.3)	United States	58.1 (0.2)	Alaska	65.1 (1.4)	Utah	64.1 (1.4)
United States	65.0 (0.1)	Kentucky	57.0 (1.0)	Montana	65.1 (1.0)	Oklahoma	63.8 (0.8)
Maine	64.9 (0.9)	Montana	56.1 (1.9)	Maine	64.8 (1.0)	North Carolina	63.7 (0.8)
Alabama	64.8 (0.5)	Vermont	56.0 (2.7)	Alabama	64.6 (0.6)	New Jersey	63.3 (0.7)
Kentucky	64.2 (0.6)	Tennessee	55.8 (0.9)	Kentucky	64.1 (0.6)	Rhode Island	63.2 (2.2)
Tennessee	63.8 (0.5)	Alabama	54.8 (1.0)	Tennessee	64.0 (0.5)	South Carolina	63.2 (1.0)
North Carolina	63.3 (0.4)	District of Columbia	54.6 (3.3)	Nevada	63.6 (0.9)	Colorado	63.0 (1.1)
West Virginia	62.8 (0.9)	California	54.1 (0.4)	North Carolina	63.2 (0.4)	Tennessee	62.7 (0.8)
Nevada	62.3 (0.8)	West Virginia	54.0 (1.9)	South Carolina	62.1 (0.7)	United States	62.6 (0.1)
South Carolina	62.3 (0.6)	Arizona	53.9 (0.9)	Georgia	61.7 (0.4)	Georgia	59.8 (0.9)
Georgia	61.5 (0.4)	North Carolina	53.9 (0.8)	West Virginia	61.5 (1.0)	New York	59.2 (0.5)
Oklahoma	61.0 (0.5)	Georgia	53.3 (0.8)	California	60.9 (0.2)	Louisiana	58.4 (1.1)
California	60.0 (0.2)	South Carolina	53.0 (1.1)	Oklahoma	60.6 (0.6)	Arkansas	58.3 (1.2)
Arizona	59.9 (0.4)	Oklahoma	50.8 (1.0)	Arizona	60.2 (0.5)	Arizona	58.2 (0.7)
Louisiana	59.1 (0.6)	Florida	49.9 (0.7)	Louisiana	59.2 (0.7)	Texas	57.1 (0.5)
Arkansas	58.1 (0.7)	Louisiana	49.4 (1.2)	Arkansas	58.1 (0.7)	New Mexico	56.3 (1.6)
Texas	57.9 (0.2)	Texas	49.1 (0.4)	Texas	58.0 (0.3)	Mississippi	55.2 (1.3)
Florida	56.8 (0.3)	Arkansas	45.8 (1.3)	Florida	57.5 (0.3)	Florida	54.0 (0.5)
Mississippi	56.0 (0.7)	Mississippi	44.0 (1.4)	Mississippi	56.1 (0.8)	Nevada	53.9 (1.4)
New Mexico	53.5 (0.8)	New Mexico	42.1 (1.4)	New Mexico	53.0 (0.9)	California	53.4 (0.3)

Note: Numbers in thousands; Figures cover 2013; Margin of error appears in parenthesis
Source: U.S. Census Bureau, 2013 American Community Survey, Table HI05. Health Insurance Coverage Status and Type of Coverage by State and Age for All People: 2013

Covered by Private Health Insurance: Employment Based

All Persons		Under 18 Years		Under 65 Years		65 Years and Over	
State	Percent[1]	State	Percent[1]	State	Percent[1]	State	Percent[1]
Massachusetts	64.6 (0.5)	Minnesota	65.1 (0.9)	Massachusetts	68.5 (0.5)	District of Columbia	54.9 (3.2)
New Hampshire	64.3 (0.8)	Utah	65.0 (1.0)	New Hampshire	68.2 (0.9)	Alaska	51.8 (3.0)
Maryland	63.4 (0.5)	Massachusetts	64.8 (1.0)	Minnesota	67.5 (0.5)	Hawaii	51.0 (1.8)
Utah	62.7 (0.7)	New Hampshire	64.2 (2.0)	North Dakota	66.3 (1.3)	Maryland	50.6 (0.9)
Minnesota	62.3 (0.5)	Wyoming	63.6 (2.6)	Iowa	65.9 (0.6)	Michigan	49.7 (0.6)
Hawaii	61.8 (0.9)	North Dakota	63.0 (2.3)	Wisconsin	65.7 (0.5)	Delaware	47.3 (1.8)
New Jersey	61.8 (0.3)	New Jersey	61.4 (0.7)	Wyoming	65.5 (1.5)	West Virginia	45.8 (1.6)
Wyoming	61.5 (1.4)	Wisconsin	61.3 (0.9)	Utah	65.4 (0.7)	Massachusetts	42.0 (0.8)
North Dakota	61.1 (1.2)	Iowa	60.1 (1.2)	Maryland	65.3 (0.6)	New Hampshire	42.0 (1.8)
Connecticut	61.0 (0.7)	Connecticut	60.0 (1.3)	New Jersey	65.2 (0.4)	Ohio	41.3 (0.6)
Delaware	60.7 (1.3)	Maryland	58.8 (1.0)	Pennsylvania	64.8 (0.3)	New Jersey	41.1 (0.7)
Wisconsin	60.7 (0.4)	Pennsylvania	58.4 (0.7)	Connecticut	64.5 (0.8)	Connecticut	40.8 (1.1)
Iowa	60.2 (0.6)	Nebraska	57.8 (1.4)	Hawaii	63.8 (1.0)	New York	40.4 (0.5)
Pennsylvania	60.1 (0.3)	Ohio	57.8 (0.8)	Delaware	63.2 (1.5)	Virginia	39.8 (0.8)
Ohio	59.7 (0.4)	Virginia	57.0 (0.9)	Nebraska	63.1 (0.8)	Utah	38.0 (1.3)
District of Columbia	59.6 (1.1)	Delaware	56.9 (2.6)	Ohio	62.9 (0.4)	Kentucky	37.2 (0.8)
Michigan	59.4 (0.4)	Michigan	56.6 (0.7)	Virginia	62.1 (0.5)	Alabama	36.8 (0.8)
Virginia	59.1 (0.5)	Rhode Island	56.6 (2.1)	Rhode Island	62.0 (1.1)	Illinois	36.3 (0.6)
Nebraska	57.9 (0.7)	Indiana	55.6 (0.9)	Kansas	61.6 (0.7)	Georgia	35.7 (0.8)
Rhode Island	57.6 (1.0)	Kansas	54.9 (1.4)	Indiana	61.1 (0.5)	Vermont	35.4 (1.8)
Indiana	57.5 (0.5)	Missouri	54.3 (0.9)	Michigan	61.1 (0.4)	Wyoming	35.2 (2.9)
Illinois	57.0 (0.3)	Nevada	53.4 (1.8)	Missouri	60.2 (0.5)	Pennsylvania	35.1 (0.5)
Kansas	56.7 (0.7)	Maine	53.3 (2.2)	District of Columbia	60.1 (1.2)	United States	35.0 (0.1)
New York	56.5 (0.3)	Hawaii	53.2 (2.1)	Illinois	60.1 (0.4)	Washington	34.8 (0.9)
Missouri	56.1 (0.4)	South Dakota	53.1 (2.0)	Vermont	59.8 (1.5)	Indiana	34.7 (0.8)
Alaska	55.9 (1.5)	Illinois	52.9 (0.7)	New York	59.1 (0.3)	New Mexico	34.6 (1.3)
Vermont	55.9 (1.3)	Oregon	52.9 (1.3)	South Dakota	59.1 (1.1)	Louisiana	33.9 (1.0)
Washington	55.5 (0.5)	New York	52.8 (0.5)	Washington	58.8 (0.5)	North Carolina	33.6 (0.7)
West Virginia	54.8 (0.9)	Washington	52.5 (0.9)	Colorado	57.4 (0.6)	South Carolina	33.3 (1.0)
Colorado	54.3 (0.5)	Vermont	51.8 (2.6)	Maine	57.3 (1.1)	Maine	33.1 (1.7)
Kentucky	54.0 (0.5)	Colorado	51.7 (1.0)	United States	57.1 (0.1)	Texas	33.0 (0.4)
United States	54.0 (0.1)	Idaho	51.3 (2.0)	Nevada	56.9 (1.0)	Rhode Island	32.5 (1.9)
Nevada	53.4 (0.9)	United States	50.6 (0.2)	Kentucky	56.8 (0.6)	California	32.4 (0.4)
South Dakota	53.4 (1.0)	Kentucky	50.5 (0.9)	Oregon	56.8 (0.7)	Colorado	32.3 (1.0)
Maine	53.1 (1.0)	West Virginia	50.2 (1.9)	West Virginia	56.7 (1.0)	Missouri	32.2 (0.8)
Oregon	52.8 (0.7)	District of Columbia	48.0 (3.4)	Alaska	56.3 (1.6)	Oklahoma	32.1 (0.8)
Alabama	52.3 (0.5)	Alaska	47.7 (2.5)	Alabama	55.0 (0.6)	Wisconsin	31.3 (0.7)
Idaho	51.4 (1.1)	Tennessee	47.4 (0.9)	Idaho	55.0 (1.2)	Nevada	31.0 (1.1)
Tennessee	51.3 (0.5)	Alabama	46.4 (1.1)	Tennessee	54.8 (0.5)	Oregon	30.4 (1.0)
Georgia	51.0 (0.4)	California	46.4 (0.4)	South Carolina	53.8 (0.6)	Tennessee	30.4 (0.7)
South Carolina	50.7 (0.6)	Arizona	46.2 (0.9)	Montana	53.6 (1.2)	Arizona	29.1 (0.8)
California	49.7 (0.2)	Montana	46.0 (2.2)	Georgia	53.1 (0.4)	Minnesota	28.9 (0.9)
North Carolina	49.6 (0.4)	Georgia	45.4 (0.8)	North Carolina	52.3 (0.4)	Idaho	28.5 (1.7)
Montana	49.2 (1.0)	South Carolina	45.4 (1.0)	California	52.2 (0.2)	Iowa	28.1 (1.0)
Oklahoma	49.1 (0.5)	North Carolina	43.1 (0.8)	Oklahoma	51.8 (0.5)	North Dakota	27.9 (2.3)
Louisiana	49.0 (0.7)	Louisiana	42.9 (1.2)	Arizona	51.5 (0.5)	Florida	27.4 (0.4)
Texas	48.8 (0.3)	Texas	42.5 (0.4)	Louisiana	51.2 (0.8)	Montana	26.5 (1.8)
Arizona	48.1 (0.5)	Oklahoma	42.3 (1.0)	Texas	50.7 (0.3)	Kansas	26.0 (1.2)
Arkansas	46.2 (0.6)	Florida	40.5 (0.7)	Arkansas	49.9 (0.7)	Arkansas	25.3 (1.1)
Mississippi	45.0 (0.6)	Arkansas	39.6 (1.4)	Mississippi	48.3 (0.7)	Nebraska	25.3 (1.3)
Florida	43.7 (0.3)	Mississippi	37.1 (1.3)	Florida	47.4 (0.4)	Mississippi	24.5 (1.1)
New Mexico	43.6 (0.8)	New Mexico	36.9 (1.4)	New Mexico	45.1 (0.9)	South Dakota	19.7 (1.7)

Note: Numbers in thousands; Figures cover 2013; Margin of error appears in parenthesis
Source: U.S. Census Bureau, 2013 American Community Survey, Table HI05. Health Insurance Coverage Status and Type of Coverage by State and Age for All People: 2013

Covered by Private Health Insurance: Direct Purchase

All Persons		Under 18 Years		Under 65 Years		65 Years and Over	
State	Percent[1]	State	Percent[1]	State	Percent[1]	State	Percent[1]
North Dakota	18.9 (0.8)	South Dakota	10.5 (1.0)	South Dakota	13.9 (0.7)	North Dakota	54.6 (2.1)
South Dakota	18.8 (0.7)	North Dakota	10.2 (1.5)	North Dakota	13.2 (0.9)	Minnesota	51.5 (1.0)
Nebraska	16.9 (0.5)	Nebraska	9.2 (0.7)	Nebraska	12.3 (0.5)	Iowa	49.9 (1.1)
Montana	16.7 (0.7)	Montana	9.1 (1.2)	Montana	11.8 (0.7)	South Dakota	48.6 (2.1)
Iowa	16.5 (0.4)	Idaho	8.8 (1.1)	Idaho	11.5 (0.7)	Kansas	47.3 (1.0)
Idaho	15.7 (0.6)	Kansas	8.6 (0.7)	Colorado	11.1 (0.3)	Nebraska	45.9 (1.4)
Minnesota	15.7 (0.3)	Colorado	8.5 (0.6)	Iowa	10.7 (0.4)	Pennsylvania	42.5 (0.5)
Kansas	15.6 (0.3)	New York	8.2 (0.3)	District of Columbia	10.6 (0.8)	Wisconsin	42.5 (0.8)
Oregon	14.5 (0.4)	Utah	8.2 (0.6)	Kansas	10.6 (0.4)	Montana	42.1 (2.3)
Pennsylvania	14.3 (0.2)	Oregon	8.0 (0.7)	Minnesota	10.1 (0.3)	Idaho	41.9 (1.7)
Colorado	13.7 (0.3)	Minnesota	7.9 (0.5)	North Carolina	10.1 (0.2)	Oregon	40.4 (1.2)
North Carolina	13.5 (0.2)	Florida	7.6 (0.3)	Oregon	9.8 (0.4)	Indiana	38.7 (0.8)
Missouri	13.3 (0.3)	Iowa	7.6 (0.6)	Alabama	9.7 (0.4)	Wyoming	37.8 (3.1)
Wisconsin	13.2 (0.2)	North Carolina	7.6 (0.4)	Virginia	9.7 (0.3)	Missouri	36.5 (0.8)
Wyoming	13.1 (0.9)	Alabama	7.3 (0.6)	Utah	9.5 (0.4)	Illinois	35.7 (0.6)
Alabama	13.0 (0.3)	California	7.3 (0.2)	Missouri	9.3 (0.3)	Tennessee	35.1 (0.9)
Virginia	13.0 (0.3)	Missouri	7.3 (0.4)	Wyoming	9.3 (0.9)	Vermont	35.1 (2.2)
Florida	12.8 (0.2)	Washington	7.3 (0.5)	California	9.2 (0.1)	Washington	35.0 (0.9)
Washington	12.7 (0.3)	Virginia	7.2 (0.4)	Florida	9.2 (0.2)	Michigan	34.9 (0.6)
Tennessee	12.6 (0.3)	Arizona	6.8 (0.4)	Washington	9.2 (0.3)	Delaware	34.7 (1.9)
Rhode Island	12.5 (0.6)	Wyoming	6.8 (1.5)	Massachusetts	9.1 (0.3)	Rhode Island	34.7 (2.0)
Massachusetts	12.3 (0.2)	Oklahoma	6.6 (0.5)	Pennsylvania	9.0 (0.2)	Arkansas	34.5 (1.1)
Arizona	12.2 (0.2)	Tennessee	6.6 (0.4)	Tennessee	8.8 (0.3)	North Carolina	34.2 (0.8)
Arkansas	12.2 (0.4)	United States	6.6 (0.1)	Arizona	8.7 (0.2)	Virginia	34.1 (0.7)
Vermont	12.1 (0.6)	District of Columbia	6.5 (1.7)	Maryland	8.7 (0.3)	Maine	33.8 (1.5)
Indiana	11.9 (0.2)	Maryland	6.4 (0.5)	Hawaii	8.6 (0.6)	Kentucky	33.7 (1.1)
Maine	11.9 (0.5)	Pennsylvania	6.4 (0.3)	Rhode Island	8.6 (0.6)	New Hampshire	33.7 (1.7)
Michigan	11.9 (0.2)	New Jersey	6.0 (0.3)	United States	8.6 (0.1)	Oklahoma	33.7 (0.9)
United States	11.9 (0.1)	Mississippi	5.9 (0.7)	Louisiana	8.4 (0.3)	South Carolina	32.6 (1.0)
Oklahoma	11.8 (0.3)	Connecticut	5.8 (0.6)	New York	8.4 (0.2)	Mississippi	32.1 (1.7)
Illinois	11.7 (0.2)	Massachusetts	5.8 (0.4)	Arkansas	8.3 (0.4)	Colorado	32.0 (0.8)
Connecticut	11.6 (0.3)	Rhode Island	5.8 (1.1)	Connecticut	8.3 (0.3)	United States	32.0 (0.1)
District of Columbia	11.6 (0.8)	Kentucky	5.7 (0.5)	Wisconsin	8.3 (0.2)	Alabama	31.9 (0.8)
Utah	11.6 (0.4)	Louisiana	5.7 (0.4)	Oklahoma	8.2 (0.3)	Massachusetts	31.6 (0.7)
Kentucky	11.5 (0.3)	Georgia	5.6 (0.3)	Illinois	8.0 (0.2)	Arizona	31.3 (0.9)
Maryland	11.5 (0.3)	South Carolina	5.6 (0.6)	Georgia	7.9 (0.2)	Ohio	31.1 (0.5)
New Hampshire	11.5 (0.5)	Texas	5.6 (0.2)	Michigan	7.9 (0.2)	Utah	31.0 (1.3)
South Carolina	11.5 (0.3)	Nevada	5.5 (0.6)	Kentucky	7.8 (0.3)	Connecticut	30.7 (1.0)
Hawaii	11.2 (0.6)	Illinois	5.4 (0.2)	Indiana	7.7 (0.2)	Maryland	30.2 (0.8)
Louisiana	11.1 (0.3)	Arkansas	5.2 (0.6)	Mississippi	7.7 (0.3)	New Jersey	29.0 (0.8)
California	11.0 (0.1)	Hawaii	5.2 (0.8)	South Carolina	7.7 (0.3)	Florida	28.6 (0.4)
Mississippi	11.0 (0.4)	Indiana	5.2 (0.4)	Vermont	7.7 (0.6)	Louisiana	28.6 (0.8)
Delaware	10.8 (0.6)	New Hampshire	5.2 (0.9)	New Hampshire	7.6 (0.5)	West Virginia	28.3 (1.3)
New York	10.8 (0.1)	Maine	5.1 (0.7)	Maine	7.3 (0.5)	Texas	26.7 (0.5)
Ohio	10.7 (0.2)	Wisconsin	5.1 (0.4)	Texas	7.3 (0.1)	Georgia	26.6 (0.7)
Georgia	10.2 (0.2)	Michigan	5.0 (0.3)	New Jersey	7.2 (0.2)	New York	25.2 (0.5)
New Jersey	10.2 (0.2)	Ohio	4.8 (0.3)	Ohio	7.2 (0.2)	Hawaii	24.6 (1.6)
Texas	9.5 (0.1)	Alaska	4.6 (1.2)	Nevada	6.9 (0.4)	California	24.0 (0.3)
West Virginia	9.2 (0.4)	Vermont	4.5 (1.0)	New Mexico	6.9 (0.5)	Nevada	22.8 (1.1)
Nevada	9.1 (0.3)	Delaware	4.0 (0.9)	Delaware	6.3 (0.6)	New Mexico	21.8 (1.3)
New Mexico	9.1 (0.4)	West Virginia	3.4 (0.6)	Alaska	5.8 (0.7)	District of Columbia	19.5 (2.3)
Alaska	6.5 (0.7)	New Mexico	3.3 (0.6)	West Virginia	5.3 (0.4)	Alaska	13.1 (2.1)

Note: Numbers in thousands; Figures cover 2013; Margin of error appears in parenthesis
Source: U.S. Census Bureau, 2013 American Community Survey, Table HI05. Health Insurance Coverage Status and Type of Coverage by State and Age for All People: 2013

Covered by Private Health Insurance: TRICARE

All Persons		Under 18 Years		Under 65 Years		65 Years and Over	
State	Percent[1]	State	Percent[1]	State	Percent[1]	State	Percent[1]
Hawaii	9.7 (0.6)	Hawaii	15.8 (1.4)	Hawaii	9.6 (0.6)	Virginia	12.5 (0.5)
Virginia	8.0 (0.2)	Alaska	10.7 (1.5)	Alaska	7.8 (0.7)	Alabama	11.0 (0.6)
Alaska	7.9 (0.6)	Virginia	9.3 (0.4)	Virginia	7.3 (0.2)	Hawaii	10.5 (1.1)
South Carolina	4.7 (0.2)	Colorado	5.2 (0.4)	Colorado	3.9 (0.2)	South Carolina	10.5 (0.6)
Colorado	4.5 (0.2)	North Carolina	4.8 (0.3)	North Dakota	3.8 (0.6)	Alaska	9.5 (2.0)
North Carolina	4.4 (0.1)	North Dakota	4.7 (1.0)	North Carolina	3.7 (0.1)	New Mexico	8.8 (0.8)
Alabama	4.3 (0.2)	Kansas	4.3 (0.5)	South Carolina	3.7 (0.2)	Oklahoma	8.8 (0.6)
Washington	4.3 (0.2)	Washington	4.3 (0.4)	South Dakota	3.6 (0.5)	Washington	8.8 (0.4)
New Mexico	4.2 (0.3)	Georgia	4.0 (0.3)	Georgia	3.5 (0.2)	Colorado	8.7 (0.5)
Georgia	4.1 (0.2)	Wyoming	3.9 (1.3)	Washington	3.5 (0.2)	Delaware	8.7 (1.4)
North Dakota	4.0 (0.5)	Maryland	3.8 (0.3)	Kansas	3.4 (0.3)	Nevada	8.6 (0.7)
South Dakota	4.0 (0.4)	South Carolina	3.8 (0.4)	New Mexico	3.4 (0.3)	Georgia	8.5 (0.5)
Kansas	3.9 (0.2)	South Dakota	3.8 (0.8)	Maryland	3.3 (0.2)	Mississippi	8.5 (0.8)
Oklahoma	3.9 (0.2)	New Mexico	3.4 (0.6)	Alabama	3.2 (0.2)	Arizona	8.4 (0.5)
Maryland	3.8 (0.2)	Oklahoma	3.3 (0.3)	Wyoming	3.2 (0.6)	Arkansas	8.4 (0.7)
Mississippi	3.8 (0.3)	Tennessee	3.2 (0.3)	Mississippi	3.1 (0.3)	Maine	8.4 (0.9)
Florida	3.6 (0.1)	Alabama	3.1 (0.4)	Oklahoma	3.1 (0.2)	North Carolina	8.4 (0.4)
Wyoming	3.6 (0.6)	Montana	3.1 (0.7)	Tennessee	2.9 (0.2)	Texas	7.8 (0.3)
Delaware	3.5 (0.4)	Florida	3.0 (0.2)	Florida	2.7 (0.1)	Tennessee	7.6 (0.6)
Nevada	3.5 (0.2)	Nebraska	3.0 (0.5)	Montana	2.7 (0.4)	Utah	7.6 (0.8)
Tennessee	3.5 (0.2)	Mississippi	2.9 (0.5)	Nebraska	2.7 (0.3)	Idaho	7.5 (0.9)
Maine	3.4 (0.3)	Delaware	2.8 (0.8)	Delaware	2.6 (0.4)	Maryland	7.3 (0.5)
Arkansas	3.3 (0.2)	Maine	2.8 (0.7)	Nevada	2.6 (0.2)	Florida	7.2 (0.3)
Arizona	3.2 (0.1)	Nevada	2.7 (0.5)	Idaho	2.5 (0.3)	New Hampshire	7.0 (0.8)
Idaho	3.2 (0.3)	Kentucky	2.5 (0.3)	Maine	2.4 (0.3)	Kansas	6.5 (0.6)
Montana	3.2 (0.4)	Texas	2.5 (0.2)	Texas	2.4 (0.1)	Nebraska	6.4 (0.7)
Nebraska	3.2 (0.3)	Arizona	2.4 (0.3)	Arizona	2.3 (0.1)	South Dakota	6.4 (1.1)
Texas	3.0 (0.1)	Louisiana	2.4 (0.3)	Arkansas	2.3 (0.3)	Kentucky	6.2 (0.5)
Kentucky	2.7 (0.2)	Missouri	2.4 (0.3)	Kentucky	2.2 (0.2)	Wyoming	6.2 (1.6)
Missouri	2.6 (0.2)	Rhode Island	2.4 (0.7)	Missouri	2.2 (0.2)	Montana	6.0 (1.0)
United States	2.6 (0.1)	United States	2.4 (0.1)	Louisiana	2.1 (0.2)	Vermont	5.9 (1.1)
Louisiana	2.5 (0.2)	Idaho	2.3 (0.6)	United States	2.1 (0.1)	United States	5.8 (0.1)
Utah	2.5 (0.2)	Arkansas	2.2 (0.5)	Utah	1.9 (0.2)	Louisiana	5.7 (0.4)
New Hampshire	2.3 (0.3)	Utah	1.9 (0.4)	Rhode Island	1.6 (0.4)	Oregon	5.7 (0.5)
West Virginia	2.2 (0.2)	District of Columbia	1.7 (0.6)	West Virginia	1.6 (0.2)	North Dakota	5.3 (1.1)
Rhode Island	2.1 (0.4)	California	1.6 (0.1)	New Hampshire	1.4 (0.3)	Missouri	5.2 (0.4)
Vermont	2.0 (0.3)	Connecticut	1.6 (0.4)	California	1.3 (0.1)	Rhode Island	5.0 (0.9)
California	1.8 (0.1)	West Virginia	1.6 (0.4)	District of Columbia	1.3 (0.3)	West Virginia	5.0 (0.7)
Oregon	1.8 (0.1)	New Hampshire	1.3 (0.5)	Vermont	1.3 (0.3)	California	4.7 (0.2)
Iowa	1.6 (0.1)	Iowa	1.2 (0.3)	Connecticut	1.2 (0.2)	Minnesota	3.8 (0.3)
District of Columbia	1.5 (0.3)	Ohio	1.2 (0.2)	Iowa	1.2 (0.1)	Iowa	3.7 (0.4)
Ohio	1.5 (0.1)	Vermont	1.2 (0.6)	Ohio	1.2 (0.1)	Indiana	3.6 (0.3)
Connecticut	1.4 (0.2)	Indiana	1.1 (0.2)	Indiana	1.1 (0.1)	Ohio	3.4 (0.2)
Indiana	1.4 (0.1)	Minnesota	1.0 (0.2)	Oregon	1.1 (0.1)	District of Columbia	3.3 (0.8)
Minnesota	1.4 (0.1)	Illinois	0.9 (0.1)	Minnesota	1.0 (0.1)	Pennsylvania	3.2 (0.2)
Pennsylvania	1.3 (0.1)	Michigan	0.9 (0.1)	Pennsylvania	1.0 (0.1)	Wisconsin	3.2 (0.3)
Michigan	1.2 (0.1)	New Jersey	0.9 (0.1)	Illinois	0.9 (0.1)	Massachusetts	3.1 (0.3)
Wisconsin	1.2 (0.1)	Oregon	0.9 (0.2)	Michigan	0.9 (0.1)	Connecticut	2.8 (0.3)
Illinois	1.1 (0.1)	Pennsylvania	0.9 (0.1)	Wisconsin	0.9 (0.1)	Michigan	2.7 (0.2)
Massachusetts	1.1 (0.1)	New York	0.8 (0.1)	Massachusetts	0.8 (0.1)	Illinois	2.5 (0.2)
New Jersey	1.0 (0.1)	Wisconsin	0.8 (0.1)	New Jersey	0.7 (0.1)	New Jersey	2.3 (0.2)
New York	0.9 (0.1)	Massachusetts	0.7 (0.1)	New York	0.7 (0.1)	New York	1.9 (0.1)

Note: Numbers in thousands; Figures cover 2013; Margin of error appears in parenthesis
Source: U.S. Census Bureau, 2013 American Community Survey, Table HI05. Health Insurance Coverage Status and Type of Coverage by State and Age for All People: 2013

Covered by Government Health Insurance

All Persons		Under 18 Years		Under 65 Years		65 Years and Over	
State	**Percent[1]**	**State**	**Percent[1]**	**State**	**Percent[1]**	**State**	**Percent[1]**
Vermont	39.7 (1.1)	New Mexico	53.7 (1.3)	New Mexico	29.5 (0.7)	Iowa	98.4 (0.3)
New Mexico	39.3 (0.6)	Arkansas	52.5 (1.3)	Vermont	28.7 (1.3)	West Virginia	98.4 (0.3)
Maine	38.8 (0.7)	Mississippi	51.9 (1.3)	District of Columbia	28.2 (1.4)	Arkansas	98.1 (0.4)
West Virginia	38.5 (0.7)	District of Columbia	51.3 (3.0)	Mississippi	28.1 (0.7)	Mississippi	98.0 (0.4)
Arkansas	37.9 (0.4)	Louisiana	48.9 (1.2)	Arkansas	27.2 (0.5)	Wisconsin	98.0 (0.2)
Mississippi	37.7 (0.6)	Vermont	46.3 (2.7)	Maine	26.4 (0.9)	Michigan	97.9 (0.2)
Delaware	35.6 (1.0)	West Virginia	45.0 (1.8)	West Virginia	26.2 (0.8)	Montana	97.9 (0.4)
District of Columbia	35.3 (1.3)	Alabama	44.5 (0.9)	Louisiana	25.3 (0.5)	South Carolina	97.9 (0.3)
New York	35.2 (0.2)	South Carolina	43.7 (1.1)	New York	25.3 (0.3)	Indiana	97.8 (0.2)
Florida	35.0 (0.2)	Oklahoma	43.4 (1.0)	Delaware	24.2 (1.2)	South Dakota	97.8 (0.6)
Alabama	34.8 (0.4)	North Carolina	42.7 (0.8)	Alabama	23.9 (0.4)	Kentucky	97.7 (0.2)
Louisiana	34.5 (0.4)	Tennessee	42.4 (0.9)	Massachusetts	23.7 (0.4)	North Carolina	97.7 (0.2)
Michigan	34.5 (0.3)	Florida	41.6 (0.7)	Tennessee	23.7 (0.4)	Tennessee	97.7 (0.3)
South Carolina	34.5 (0.4)	California	41.5 (0.3)	Michigan	23.5 (0.3)	Oregon	97.6 (0.3)
Arizona	34.4 (0.4)	Illinois	40.9 (0.6)	South Carolina	23.2 (0.5)	Alabama	97.5 (0.3)
Tennessee	34.4 (0.3)	Maine	40.9 (2.0)	Kentucky	23.1 (0.5)	Kansas	97.5 (0.4)
Massachusetts	34.0 (0.4)	Kentucky	40.7 (1.1)	Arizona	23.0 (0.4)	Missouri	97.5 (0.3)
Kentucky	33.7 (0.4)	Texas	40.7 (0.5)	Oklahoma	22.7 (0.4)	Oklahoma	97.5 (0.3)
Oklahoma	33.2 (0.4)	New York	40.6 (0.5)	California	22.2 (0.2)	Maine	97.3 (0.5)
North Carolina	32.7 (0.3)	Georgia	40.0 (0.7)	North Carolina	22.0 (0.3)	Idaho	97.2 (0.7)
Oregon	32.5 (0.5)	Michigan	39.9 (0.7)	Ohio	21.3 (0.4)	North Dakota	97.2 (0.8)
Ohio	32.4 (0.3)	Delaware	38.4 (2.4)	Illinois	21.2 (0.2)	Vermont	97.2 (0.8)
Pennsylvania	32.3 (0.2)	United States	38.3 (0.2)	Florida	21.1 (0.3)	Minnesota	97.1 (0.3)
Montana	31.9 (0.7)	Arizona	37.8 (0.9)	United States	21.1 (0.1)	Nebraska	97.1 (0.5)
Rhode Island	31.8 (0.8)	Montana	37.8 (2.2)	Oregon	20.7 (0.6)	Wyoming	97.1 (1.1)
Wisconsin	31.8 (0.4)	Oregon	37.6 (1.3)	Wisconsin	20.6 (0.4)	Delaware	97.0 (0.6)
United States	31.6 (0.1)	Rhode Island	36.8 (2.2)	Rhode Island	20.4 (1.0)	Ohio	97.0 (0.2)
Hawaii	31.5 (0.6)	Washington	36.4 (0.9)	Georgia	20.1 (0.3)	Pennsylvania	96.9 (0.2)
California	31.2 (0.1)	Ohio	36.2 (0.8)	Connecticut	20.0 (0.6)	Arizona	96.8 (0.3)
Connecticut	31.2 (0.5)	Pennsylvania	35.5 (0.7)	Pennsylvania	20.0 (0.3)	Rhode Island	96.6 (0.7)
Iowa	31.1 (0.4)	Wisconsin	34.6 (0.8)	Texas	20.0 (0.2)	Utah	96.5 (0.6)
Illinois	31.0 (0.2)	Indiana	34.4 (0.9)	Hawaii	19.3 (0.7)	Washington	96.5 (0.3)
Missouri	30.6 (0.3)	South Dakota	34.4 (1.8)	Indiana	19.3 (0.4)	Colorado	96.4 (0.3)
South Dakota	30.3 (0.7)	Iowa	34.2 (1.0)	Iowa	19.2 (0.5)	New Hampshire	96.4 (0.6)
Indiana	29.9 (0.3)	Idaho	34.1 (1.9)	Montana	19.2 (0.8)	United States	96.3 (0.1)
Idaho	29.7 (0.8)	Missouri	33.8 (1.0)	Missouri	19.1 (0.4)	Georgia	96.2 (0.3)
Washington	29.4 (0.3)	Alaska	33.7 (1.9)	South Dakota	19.0 (0.8)	New Mexico	96.0 (0.6)
Georgia	29.1 (0.3)	Connecticut	33.3 (1.2)	Alaska	18.9 (0.9)	Virginia	96.0 (0.3)
Texas	28.3 (0.2)	Massachusetts	33.2 (0.9)	Idaho	18.9 (0.8)	Florida	95.9 (0.2)
Maryland	28.2 (0.3)	Maryland	32.1 (0.9)	Washington	18.9 (0.4)	Louisiana	95.8 (0.4)
Minnesota	28.1 (0.4)	Kansas	31.9 (1.2)	Maryland	18.1 (0.4)	Connecticut	95.7 (0.4)
Kansas	27.7 (0.4)	Colorado	31.5 (0.9)	Colorado	17.3 (0.4)	New York	95.7 (0.2)
New Jersey	27.2 (0.3)	Hawaii	31.1 (1.7)	Minnesota	17.3 (0.4)	Illinois	95.6 (0.3)
New Hampshire	27.0 (0.7)	Nebraska	30.3 (1.4)	Kansas	16.6 (0.5)	Hawaii	95.4 (0.6)
Colorado	26.9 (0.4)	New Jersey	30.0 (0.6)	New Jersey	16.0 (0.3)	Massachusetts	95.2 (0.3)
Nebraska	26.8 (0.4)	New Hampshire	29.7 (2.3)	Nevada	15.7 (0.7)	Texas	95.1 (0.2)
Nevada	26.4 (0.6)	Nevada	28.5 (1.7)	Nebraska	15.6 (0.5)	New Jersey	94.8 (0.3)
Alaska	25.8 (0.8)	Wyoming	27.8 (2.8)	New Hampshire	14.9 (0.8)	California	94.5 (0.2)
Virginia	25.6 (0.3)	Virginia	27.1 (0.7)	Virginia	14.7 (0.3)	Maryland	94.4 (0.4)
Wyoming	25.2 (0.9)	Minnesota	25.9 (0.9)	Wyoming	14.3 (1.1)	Nevada	94.2 (0.6)
North Dakota	23.8 (0.6)	North Dakota	21.7 (1.8)	Utah	12.9 (0.5)	Alaska	94.1 (1.6)
Utah	21.0 (0.4)	Utah	20.0 (0.9)	North Dakota	12.2 (0.7)	District of Columbia	92.0 (1.3)

Note: Numbers in thousands; Figures cover 2013; Margin of error appears in parenthesis
Source: U.S. Census Bureau, 2013 American Community Survey, Table HI05. Health Insurance Coverage Status and Type of Coverage by State and Age for All People: 2013

Covered by Government Health Insurance: Medicaid

All Persons		Under 18 Years		Under 65 Years		65 Years and Over	
State	**Percent[1]**	**State**	**Percent[1]**	**State**	**Percent[1]**	**State**	**Percent[1]**
District of Columbia	26.3 (1.2)	New Mexico	52.6 (1.3)	District of Columbia	26.6 (1.4)	District of Columbia	23.6 (2.6)
New Mexico	24.6 (0.6)	Arkansas	52.0 (1.4)	Vermont	26.5 (1.3)	Mississippi	20.1 (1.0)
Vermont	24.4 (1.1)	Mississippi	51.4 (1.3)	New Mexico	26.1 (0.7)	California	19.4 (0.3)
Mississippi	24.0 (0.5)	District of Columbia	50.9 (3.1)	Mississippi	24.6 (0.6)	New York	18.7 (0.4)
New York	22.8 (0.2)	Louisiana	48.5 (1.2)	Maine	23.5 (0.9)	Massachusetts	18.0 (0.7)
Maine	22.5 (0.7)	Vermont	46.0 (2.7)	New York	23.4 (0.3)	Maine	17.5 (1.3)
Louisiana	21.8 (0.4)	West Virginia	44.5 (1.9)	Arkansas	22.8 (0.5)	Louisiana	17.4 (0.7)
Massachusetts	21.7 (0.4)	Alabama	44.0 (0.9)	Louisiana	22.5 (0.5)	New Mexico	15.8 (0.9)
Arkansas	21.6 (0.4)	South Carolina	43.2 (1.1)	Massachusetts	22.3 (0.4)	Texas	15.3 (0.4)
California	20.3 (0.1)	Oklahoma	42.5 (1.0)	Delaware	21.5 (1.2)	Georgia	15.0 (0.6)
Delaware	19.8 (1.0)	North Carolina	42.4 (0.8)	West Virginia	21.2 (0.8)	Alabama	14.9 (0.7)
Michigan	19.6 (0.3)	Tennessee	42.0 (0.9)	Michigan	21.0 (0.3)	Arkansas	14.6 (0.7)
West Virginia	19.6 (0.6)	Florida	41.1 (0.7)	Arizona	20.4 (0.4)	Rhode Island	14.5 (1.6)
Tennessee	19.4 (0.3)	California	40.9 (0.3)	California	20.4 (0.2)	Alaska	14.0 (1.8)
Alabama	19.2 (0.4)	Maine	40.7 (2.0)	Tennessee	20.4 (0.4)	Kentucky	14.0 (0.6)
Arizona	19.0 (0.4)	Illinois	40.5 (0.7)	Alabama	19.9 (0.4)	Florida	13.8 (0.3)
South Carolina	18.6 (0.4)	Kentucky	40.4 (1.1)	South Carolina	19.6 (0.5)	United States	13.8 (0.1)
Kentucky	18.3 (0.4)	Texas	40.3 (0.5)	Illinois	19.2 (0.3)	Vermont	13.8 (1.4)
Illinois	18.1 (0.2)	New York	40.2 (0.5)	Kentucky	19.0 (0.4)	Tennessee	13.7 (0.6)
North Carolina	17.9 (0.3)	Michigan	39.7 (0.7)	North Carolina	18.8 (0.3)	Hawaii	13.2 (1.1)
United States	17.9 (0.1)	Georgia	39.4 (0.8)	Oklahoma	18.8 (0.4)	South Carolina	13.0 (0.7)
Rhode Island	17.8 (0.8)	United States	37.9 (0.2)	Ohio	18.6 (0.3)	Wisconsin	13.0 (0.5)
Oklahoma	17.7 (0.4)	Delaware	37.8 (2.4)	United States	18.5 (0.1)	North Carolina	12.8 (0.5)
Wisconsin	17.6 (0.4)	Arizona	37.6 (0.9)	Wisconsin	18.4 (0.4)	Connecticut	12.7 (0.7)
Florida	17.4 (0.2)	Montana	37.2 (2.1)	Rhode Island	18.3 (1.0)	Oregon	12.6 (0.7)
Texas	17.4 (0.2)	Oregon	37.2 (1.3)	Florida	18.2 (0.3)	New Jersey	12.5 (0.5)
Connecticut	17.3 (0.5)	Rhode Island	36.8 (2.2)	Connecticut	18.1 (0.6)	Nevada	12.4 (0.8)
Ohio	17.3 (0.3)	Washington	36.1 (0.9)	Oregon	17.8 (0.5)	Michigan	12.0 (0.4)
Georgia	17.0 (0.3)	Ohio	35.9 (0.8)	Pennsylvania	17.6 (0.3)	Washington	11.8 (0.6)
Oregon	17.0 (0.5)	Pennsylvania	35.3 (0.7)	Texas	17.6 (0.2)	Arizona	11.7 (0.5)
Pennsylvania	16.6 (0.2)	South Dakota	34.1 (1.8)	Georgia	17.3 (0.3)	Maryland	11.6 (0.6)
Hawaii	16.4 (0.7)	Wisconsin	34.1 (0.8)	Hawaii	17.1 (0.8)	Iowa	11.5 (0.5)
Iowa	16.3 (0.4)	Indiana	34.0 (0.8)	Iowa	17.1 (0.5)	North Dakota	11.5 (1.4)
Alaska	15.8 (0.8)	Iowa	34.0 (1.0)	Indiana	16.5 (0.4)	Pennsylvania	11.5 (0.3)
Indiana	15.7 (0.3)	Alaska	33.6 (2.0)	Washington	16.3 (0.3)	West Virginia	11.5 (1.0)
Washington	15.7 (0.3)	Missouri	33.5 (1.0)	Alaska	16.0 (0.8)	Illinois	11.1 (0.3)
Maryland	15.3 (0.3)	Idaho	33.2 (2.0)	Idaho	15.9 (0.9)	Nebraska	11.1 (0.8)
Idaho	15.2 (0.8)	Connecticut	33.1 (1.2)	Maryland	15.9 (0.4)	South Dakota	11.1 (1.3)
South Dakota	15.1 (0.7)	Massachusetts	33.0 (0.9)	Montana	15.9 (0.8)	Colorado	10.9 (0.5)
Missouri	14.8 (0.3)	Maryland	31.8 (0.9)	South Dakota	15.8 (0.8)	Oklahoma	10.9 (0.6)
Montana	14.8 (0.6)	Kansas	31.6 (1.1)	Missouri	15.7 (0.4)	Delaware	10.6 (1.2)
Colorado	14.5 (0.4)	Hawaii	31.0 (1.7)	Minnesota	15.3 (0.4)	Kansas	10.6 (0.7)
Minnesota	14.5 (0.4)	Colorado	30.9 (0.9)	Colorado	15.0 (0.4)	Idaho	10.3 (1.3)
New Jersey	14.1 (0.3)	Nebraska	29.9 (1.4)	New Jersey	14.3 (0.3)	Ohio	10.3 (0.4)
Kansas	13.7 (0.4)	New Jersey	29.8 (0.6)	Kansas	14.2 (0.4)	Indiana	10.2 (0.5)
Nebraska	13.0 (0.5)	New Hampshire	29.6 (2.3)	Nebraska	13.3 (0.5)	Utah	10.1 (0.7)
Nevada	12.7 (0.6)	Nevada	28.1 (1.7)	Nevada	12.8 (0.6)	Wyoming	10.0 (1.7)
New Hampshire	11.3 (0.6)	Wyoming	27.4 (2.7)	New Hampshire	12.0 (0.7)	Minnesota	9.8 (0.5)
Utah	11.2 (0.4)	Virginia	26.2 (0.8)	Virginia	11.4 (0.3)	Missouri	9.6 (0.5)
Virginia	11.1 (0.3)	Minnesota	25.7 (0.9)	Utah	11.3 (0.4)	Virginia	9.6 (0.4)
Wyoming	11.0 (1.0)	North Dakota	21.5 (1.8)	Wyoming	11.1 (1.0)	Montana	9.4 (0.9)
North Dakota	10.2 (0.7)	Utah	19.9 (0.9)	North Dakota	10.0 (0.7)	New Hampshire	7.0 (0.9)

Note: Numbers in thousands; Figures cover 2013; Margin of error appears in parenthesis
Source: U.S. Census Bureau, 2013 American Community Survey, Table HI05. Health Insurance Coverage Status and Type of Coverage by State and Age for All People: 2013

Covered by Medicaid and Private Health Insurance

All Persons		Under 18 Years		Under 65 Years		65 Years and Over	
State	Percent[1]	State	Percent[1]	State	Percent[1]	State	Percent[1]
District of Columbia	4.5 (0.6)	District of Columbia	8.1 (2.2)	District of Columbia	3.8 (0.7)	District of Columbia	9.7 (1.6)
Maine	4.0 (0.4)	Maine	6.6 (1.1)	Maine	3.4 (0.4)	Maine	7.2 (0.9)
Massachusetts	3.6 (0.1)	Iowa	5.5 (0.6)	Massachusetts	3.0 (0.2)	Massachusetts	6.9 (0.4)
Iowa	3.4 (0.2)	Rhode Island	5.4 (1.2)	Vermont	3.0 (0.4)	Alabama	6.8 (0.5)
Michigan	3.4 (0.1)	Vermont	5.3 (1.0)	Michigan	2.9 (0.1)	North Dakota	6.6 (1.2)
Vermont	3.4 (0.4)	Michigan	5.2 (0.3)	Rhode Island	2.9 (0.4)	Iowa	6.5 (0.4)
Rhode Island	3.3 (0.4)	Pennsylvania	5.2 (0.3)	Iowa	2.8 (0.2)	Louisiana	6.5 (0.5)
Delaware	3.2 (0.3)	South Dakota	5.1 (0.8)	Delaware	2.7 (0.3)	Wisconsin	6.4 (0.3)
Pennsylvania	3.2 (0.1)	Wisconsin	4.9 (0.3)	New York	2.7 (0.1)	Michigan	6.3 (0.3)
South Dakota	3.2 (0.3)	New York	4.7 (0.2)	Pennsylvania	2.7 (0.1)	South Dakota	6.2 (1.0)
Wisconsin	3.2 (0.1)	Wyoming	4.7 (1.4)	South Dakota	2.7 (0.4)	Kentucky	6.1 (0.5)
Alabama	3.1 (0.2)	Massachusetts	4.6 (0.4)	Wisconsin	2.7 (0.1)	Mississippi	6.1 (0.6)
Mississippi	3.0 (0.2)	North Dakota	4.6 (0.9)	New Mexico	2.6 (0.3)	Nebraska	6.1 (0.6)
New Mexico	3.0 (0.3)	Delaware	4.5 (0.9)	Alabama	2.5 (0.2)	Oregon	6.1 (0.4)
New York	3.0 (0.1)	Alaska	4.4 (1.0)	Mississippi	2.5 (0.2)	Pennsylvania	6.1 (0.2)
North Dakota	3.0 (0.4)	Washington	4.2 (0.3)	Hawaii	2.4 (0.3)	Delaware	6.0 (0.8)
Louisiana	2.9 (0.2)	West Virginia	4.2 (0.8)	Idaho	2.4 (0.3)	Maryland	5.9 (0.3)
Oregon	2.9 (0.2)	New Mexico	4.1 (0.7)	North Dakota	2.4 (0.4)	Tennessee	5.8 (0.4)
Arkansas	2.8 (0.2)	Hawaii	4.0 (0.7)	Arkansas	2.3 (0.2)	Connecticut	5.7 (0.6)
Hawaii	2.8 (0.3)	Louisiana	4.0 (0.5)	Louisiana	2.3 (0.2)	Georgia	5.6 (0.3)
Tennessee	2.8 (0.1)	Minnesota	4.0 (0.4)	Oregon	2.3 (0.2)	Kansas	5.5 (0.5)
Idaho	2.7 (0.3)	Ohio	4.0 (0.3)	Tennessee	2.3 (0.2)	South Carolina	5.4 (0.5)
Kentucky	2.7 (0.2)	Oklahoma	4.0 (0.4)	Washington	2.3 (0.1)	Washington	5.4 (0.4)
Washington	2.7 (0.1)	Idaho	3.9 (0.8)	Alaska	2.2 (0.5)	Arkansas	5.3 (0.4)
West Virginia	2.7 (0.2)	Tennessee	3.8 (0.4)	Montana	2.2 (0.3)	New Mexico	5.3 (0.7)
Kansas	2.6 (0.2)	Montana	3.7 (0.7)	West Virginia	2.2 (0.2)	Rhode Island	5.3 (0.8)
Maryland	2.6 (0.1)	Oregon	3.7 (0.5)	Wyoming	2.2 (0.5)	Utah	5.2 (0.6)
South Carolina	2.6 (0.1)	Arkansas	3.6 (0.5)	Arizona	2.1 (0.2)	Vermont	5.2 (1.0)
Wyoming	2.6 (0.5)	Kansas	3.6 (0.4)	Kansas	2.1 (0.2)	Wyoming	5.2 (1.1)
Arizona	2.5 (0.1)	Alabama	3.5 (0.4)	Kentucky	2.1 (0.2)	North Carolina	5.1 (0.3)
Minnesota	2.5 (0.1)	Arizona	3.5 (0.3)	Maryland	2.1 (0.1)	United States	5.1 (0.1)
Nebraska	2.5 (0.2)	Kentucky	3.5 (0.5)	Minnesota	2.1 (0.1)	Minnesota	5.0 (0.3)
Ohio	2.5 (0.1)	Mississippi	3.5 (0.5)	Ohio	2.1 (0.1)	Colorado	4.9 (0.4)
United States	2.5 (0.1)	United States	3.5 (0.1)	South Carolina	2.1 (0.1)	Indiana	4.9 (0.3)
Connecticut	2.4 (0.2)	Missouri	3.4 (0.4)	United States	2.1 (0.1)	New Jersey	4.9 (0.3)
Montana	2.4 (0.3)	Connecticut	3.3 (0.4)	Utah	2.1 (0.2)	New York	4.9 (0.2)
Oklahoma	2.4 (0.1)	Indiana	3.3 (0.3)	Nebraska	2.0 (0.2)	West Virginia	4.9 (0.6)
Utah	2.4 (0.2)	Nebraska	3.3 (0.5)	Oklahoma	2.0 (0.2)	Hawaii	4.8 (0.6)
Alaska	2.3 (0.4)	South Carolina	3.3 (0.3)	Colorado	1.9 (0.1)	Ohio	4.7 (0.2)
Colorado	2.3 (0.1)	Maryland	3.2 (0.4)	California	1.8 (0.1)	Texas	4.7 (0.2)
North Carolina	2.3 (0.1)	New Hampshire	3.2 (0.8)	Connecticut	1.8 (0.2)	Virginia	4.7 (0.3)
Georgia	2.2 (0.1)	Utah	3.2 (0.4)	Georgia	1.8 (0.1)	Arizona	4.6 (0.3)
Indiana	2.2 (0.1)	Colorado	3.1 (0.3)	Illinois	1.8 (0.1)	Idaho	4.6 (0.8)
California	2.1 (0.1)	Illinois	3.1 (0.2)	Indiana	1.8 (0.1)	Nevada	4.6 (0.5)
Florida	2.1 (0.1)	California	2.9 (0.1)	Missouri	1.8 (0.1)	Illinois	4.5 (0.3)
Illinois	2.1 (0.1)	Nevada	2.9 (0.4)	North Carolina	1.8 (0.1)	Oklahoma	4.4 (0.4)
Missouri	2.1 (0.1)	North Carolina	2.9 (0.3)	Florida	1.6 (0.1)	California	4.3 (0.2)
Nevada	2.0 (0.2)	Georgia	2.8 (0.2)	Nevada	1.6 (0.2)	Florida	4.2 (0.2)
New Jersey	2.0 (0.1)	Florida	2.4 (0.2)	New Jersey	1.5 (0.1)	Missouri	4.0 (0.3)
Texas	1.9 (0.1)	New Jersey	2.4 (0.2)	Texas	1.5 (0.1)	Montana	3.8 (0.7)
New Hampshire	1.7 (0.2)	Texas	2.4 (0.1)	New Hampshire	1.4 (0.3)	Alaska	3.6 (0.9)
Virginia	1.7 (0.1)	Virginia	2.3 (0.2)	Virginia	1.3 (0.1)	New Hampshire	3.4 (0.6)

Note: Numbers in thousands; Figures cover 2013; Margin of error appears in parenthesis
Source: U.S. Census Bureau, 2013 American Community Survey, Table HI05. Health Insurance Coverage Status and Type of Coverage by State and Age for All People: 2013

Covered by Government Health Insurance: Medicare

All Persons		Under 18 Years		Under 65 Years		65 Years and Over	
State	Percent[1]	State	Percent[1]	State	Percent[1]	State	Percent[1]
West Virginia	21.3 (0.3)	New Mexico	1.4 (0.4)	West Virginia	5.6 (0.3)	Iowa	98.3 (0.3)
Maine	20.5 (0.3)	Alabama	1.1 (0.2)	Arkansas	5.1 (0.2)	West Virginia	98.1 (0.4)
Florida	20.4 (0.1)	Delaware	1.0 (0.6)	Alabama	5.0 (0.2)	Arkansas	97.9 (0.4)
Arkansas	19.1 (0.2)	Oklahoma	1.0 (0.2)	Mississippi	4.7 (0.3)	Mississippi	97.9 (0.4)
Vermont	19.0 (0.4)	Virginia	0.9 (0.2)	Kentucky	4.6 (0.2)	Montana	97.9 (0.4)
Alabama	18.6 (0.2)	California	0.8 (0.1)	Maine	4.4 (0.3)	Wisconsin	97.9 (0.2)
Delaware	18.4 (0.4)	Georgia	0.8 (0.2)	Vermont	4.1 (0.4)	Michigan	97.8 (0.2)
Montana	18.1 (0.2)	Mississippi	0.8 (0.2)	South Carolina	3.9 (0.2)	Indiana	97.7 (0.2)
Pennsylvania	18.1 (0.1)	Arkansas	0.7 (0.2)	Tennessee	3.9 (0.2)	North Carolina	97.7 (0.2)
South Carolina	18.1 (0.2)	Colorado	0.7 (0.2)	Louisiana	3.8 (0.2)	South Carolina	97.7 (0.3)
Kentucky	17.9 (0.2)	District of Columbia	0.7 (0.4)	New Mexico	3.8 (0.2)	South Dakota	97.7 (0.7)
Michigan	17.6 (0.1)	Louisiana	0.7 (0.1)	Delaware	3.7 (0.4)	Kentucky	97.6 (0.3)
Mississippi	17.5 (0.2)	Maryland	0.7 (0.2)	Missouri	3.7 (0.1)	Tennessee	97.6 (0.3)
Missouri	17.4 (0.1)	New York	0.7 (0.2)	Oklahoma	3.7 (0.2)	Alabama	97.4 (0.3)
Oregon	17.4 (0.2)	South Carolina	0.7 (0.2)	Michigan	3.6 (0.1)	Kansas	97.4 (0.4)
Tennessee	17.4 (0.1)	Wisconsin	0.7 (0.1)	North Carolina	3.5 (0.1)	Missouri	97.4 (0.3)
New Mexico	17.3 (0.2)	Wyoming	0.7 (0.5)	Rhode Island	3.4 (0.3)	Oregon	97.4 (0.3)
Rhode Island	17.3 (0.3)	Connecticut	0.6 (0.2)	Florida	3.2 (0.1)	Oklahoma	97.2 (0.3)
Arizona	17.0 (0.1)	Florida	0.6 (0.1)	Indiana	3.2 (0.1)	Vermont	97.2 (0.8)
New Hampshire	17.0 (0.3)	Illinois	0.6 (0.1)	New Hampshire	3.1 (0.3)	Maine	97.1 (0.5)
Hawaii	16.9 (0.2)	Indiana	0.6 (0.1)	Pennsylvania	3.1 (0.1)	North Dakota	97.1 (0.8)
Iowa	16.9 (0.1)	Kentucky	0.6 (0.1)	Ohio	3.0 (0.1)	Wyoming	97.1 (1.1)
Ohio	16.9 (0.1)	Ohio	0.6 (0.1)	Oregon	3.0 (0.2)	Delaware	97.0 (0.6)
North Carolina	16.8 (0.1)	Tennessee	0.6 (0.2)	Georgia	2.9 (0.1)	Idaho	97.0 (0.8)
Oklahoma	16.8 (0.1)	Texas	0.6 (0.1)	United States	2.9 (0.1)	Minnesota	96.9 (0.3)
Wisconsin	16.6 (0.1)	United States	0.6 (0.1)	Virginia	2.9 (0.1)	Nebraska	96.9 (0.5)
South Dakota	16.3 (0.3)	Vermont	0.6 (0.3)	Montana	2.8 (0.3)	Ohio	96.9 (0.2)
Connecticut	16.2 (0.2)	West Virginia	0.6 (0.2)	New York	2.8 (0.1)	Pennsylvania	96.8 (0.2)
Indiana	16.1 (0.1)	Arizona	0.5 (0.1)	Wisconsin	2.8 (0.1)	Arizona	96.5 (0.3)
Massachusetts	15.9 (0.1)	Iowa	0.5 (0.2)	Idaho	2.7 (0.2)	Rhode Island	96.4 (0.7)
New York	15.9 (0.1)	Maine	0.5 (0.2)	South Dakota	2.7 (0.3)	Utah	96.4 (0.6)
United States	15.9 (0.1)	Massachusetts	0.5 (0.1)	District of Columbia	2.6 (0.3)	Washington	96.4 (0.3)
Idaho	15.7 (0.2)	Montana	0.5 (0.3)	Iowa	2.6 (0.1)	Colorado	96.3 (0.3)
Louisiana	15.7 (0.2)	Nebraska	0.5 (0.3)	Kansas	2.6 (0.2)	New Hampshire	96.2 (0.6)
Kansas	15.6 (0.2)	New Jersey	0.5 (0.1)	Washington	2.6 (0.1)	United States	96.2 (0.1)
New Jersey	15.4 (0.1)	North Carolina	0.5 (0.1)	Arizona	2.5 (0.1)	Georgia	96.1 (0.3)
Virginia	15.3 (0.1)	Washington	0.5 (0.1)	Connecticut	2.5 (0.2)	New Mexico	95.9 (0.6)
Washington	15.3 (0.1)	Alaska	0.4 (0.3)	Massachusetts	2.5 (0.1)	Florida	95.8 (0.2)
Nebraska	15.2 (0.2)	Idaho	0.4 (0.2)	Nevada	2.5 (0.2)	Virginia	95.8 (0.3)
Minnesota	14.9 (0.1)	Kansas	0.4 (0.1)	Illinois	2.4 (0.1)	New York	95.6 (0.2)
Nevada	14.9 (0.2)	Michigan	0.4 (0.1)	New Jersey	2.4 (0.1)	Connecticut	95.5 (0.4)
North Dakota	14.9 (0.3)	Missouri	0.4 (0.1)	Maryland	2.3 (0.1)	Louisiana	95.5 (0.5)
Illinois	14.7 (0.1)	Nevada	0.4 (0.2)	Texas	2.3 (0.1)	Illinois	95.4 (0.3)
Wyoming	14.6 (0.3)	North Dakota	0.4 (0.3)	California	2.2 (0.1)	Hawaii	95.2 (0.7)
Maryland	14.4 (0.1)	Oregon	0.4 (0.2)	Colorado	2.2 (0.1)	Massachusetts	95.1 (0.3)
Georgia	14.0 (0.1)	Pennsylvania	0.4 (0.1)	Nebraska	2.2 (0.2)	Texas	94.9 (0.2)
California	13.6 (0.1)	South Dakota	0.4 (0.2)	Minnesota	2.1 (0.1)	New Jersey	94.7 (0.3)
Colorado	13.6 (0.1)	Minnesota	0.3 (0.1)	Wyoming	2.1 (0.3)	California	94.3 (0.2)
District of Columbia	12.6 (0.3)	Rhode Island	0.3 (0.3)	Hawaii	2.0 (0.2)	Maryland	94.3 (0.4)
Texas	12.6 (0.1)	Hawaii	0.2 (0.1)	North Dakota	1.9 (0.3)	Nevada	94.0 (0.6)
Utah	10.9 (0.1)	New Hampshire	0.2 (0.2)	Utah	1.7 (0.1)	Alaska	93.3 (1.8)
Alaska	9.9 (0.3)	Utah	0.2 (0.1)	Alaska	1.6 (0.3)	District of Columbia	91.5 (1.4)

Note: Numbers in thousands; Figures cover 2013; Margin of error appears in parenthesis
Source: U.S. Census Bureau, 2013 American Community Survey, Table HI05. Health Insurance Coverage Status and Type of Coverage by State and Age for All People: 2013

Covered by Medicare and Private Health Insurance

All Persons		Under 18 Years		Under 65 Years		65 Years and Over	
State	Percent[1]	State	Percent[1]	State	Percent[1]	State	Percent[1]
West Virginia	13.0 (0.3)	Virginia	0.4 (0.1)	West Virginia	1.8 (0.2)	Michigan	73.9 (0.5)
Delaware	12.3 (0.4)	Montana	0.3 (0.2)	Alabama	1.5 (0.1)	North Dakota	73.8 (2.0)
Michigan	12.0 (0.1)	Delaware	0.2 (0.2)	Kentucky	1.3 (0.1)	Delaware	71.9 (1.9)
Pennsylvania	11.8 (0.1)	District of Columbia	0.2 (0.1)	Arkansas	1.2 (0.1)	Minnesota	71.3 (0.7)
Maine	11.6 (0.3)	Massachusetts	0.2 (0.1)	Delaware	1.2 (0.2)	Iowa	71.1 (1.0)
Hawaii	11.3 (0.3)	Oklahoma	0.2 (0.1)	Michigan	1.2 (0.1)	New Hampshire	68.5 (1.8)
Iowa	11.3 (0.2)	South Carolina	0.2 (0.1)	Mississippi	1.2 (0.1)	Maryland	68.4 (0.8)
New Hampshire	11.0 (0.3)	South Dakota	0.2 (0.2)	South Carolina	1.2 (0.1)	Virginia	68.2 (0.7)
Vermont	11.0 (0.4)	Vermont	0.2 (0.1)	Missouri	1.1 (0.1)	Pennsylvania	68.1 (0.4)
Montana	10.9 (0.3)	Alabama	0.1 (0.1)	North Carolina	1.0 (0.1)	Wyoming	67.6 (2.8)
Alabama	10.7 (0.2)	Alaska	0.1 (0.2)	Pennsylvania	1.0 (0.1)	Kansas	67.5 (1.1)
North Dakota	10.6 (0.3)	Arizona	0.1 (0.1)	Rhode Island	1.0 (0.2)	West Virginia	67.5 (1.4)
Oregon	10.6 (0.2)	Arkansas	0.1 (0.1)	Tennessee	1.0 (0.1)	Hawaii	66.6 (1.9)
South Carolina	10.3 (0.2)	California	0.1 (0.1)	Virginia	1.0 (0.1)	Nebraska	65.8 (1.3)
Wisconsin	10.3 (0.1)	Colorado	0.1 (0.1)	Idaho	0.9 (0.1)	Wisconsin	65.8 (0.7)
Florida	10.2 (0.1)	Connecticut	0.1 (0.1)	Indiana	0.9 (0.1)	Idaho	65.4 (1.8)
Minnesota	10.2 (0.1)	Florida	0.1 (0.1)	Louisiana	0.9 (0.1)	Indiana	65.4 (0.9)
Kentucky	10.1 (0.2)	Georgia	0.1 (0.1)	Maine	0.9 (0.1)	South Dakota	64.4 (1.8)
Missouri	10.1 (0.1)	Hawaii	0.1 (0.1)	Montana	0.9 (0.2)	Washington	64.3 (0.9)
Ohio	10.0 (0.1)	Indiana	0.1 (0.1)	New Hampshire	0.9 (0.2)	Oregon	64.2 (1.1)
Virginia	10.0 (0.1)	Iowa	0.1 (0.1)	Oklahoma	0.9 (0.1)	Vermont	63.9 (2.1)
Kansas	9.9 (0.2)	Louisiana	0.1 (0.1)	Oregon	0.9 (0.1)	Alabama	63.6 (0.8)
South Dakota	9.9 (0.3)	Maine	0.1 (0.1)	Vermont	0.9 (0.2)	Montana	63.4 (2.0)
Rhode Island	9.8 (0.3)	Maryland	0.1 (0.1)	Wyoming	0.9 (0.2)	Kentucky	63.0 (0.9)
Idaho	9.7 (0.3)	Michigan	0.1 (0.1)	Georgia	0.8 (0.1)	Ohio	62.7 (0.6)
Wyoming	9.7 (0.4)	Minnesota	0.1 (0.1)	Iowa	0.8 (0.1)	Maine	62.4 (1.7)
Arkansas	9.6 (0.2)	Mississippi	0.1 (0.1)	Kansas	0.8 (0.1)	Illinois	62.3 (0.6)
Indiana	9.6 (0.1)	Missouri	0.1 (0.1)	Massachusetts	0.8 (0.1)	Missouri	62.3 (0.8)
Maryland	9.6 (0.1)	New Hampshire	0.1 (0.1)	New Mexico	0.8 (0.1)	Massachusetts	62.1 (0.8)
Massachusetts	9.6 (0.1)	New Jersey	0.1 (0.1)	New York	0.8 (0.1)	North Carolina	61.9 (0.8)
Nebraska	9.6 (0.2)	New Mexico	0.1 (0.1)	Ohio	0.8 (0.1)	Oklahoma	61.9 (0.8)
North Carolina	9.6 (0.1)	New York	0.1 (0.1)	South Dakota	0.8 (0.1)	South Carolina	61.5 (1.0)
Tennessee	9.6 (0.1)	North Carolina	0.1 (0.1)	United States	0.8 (0.1)	Utah	61.3 (1.4)
Connecticut	9.5 (0.2)	North Dakota	0.1 (0.1)	Washington	0.8 (0.1)	Tennessee	60.9 (0.8)
Oklahoma	9.5 (0.1)	Ohio	0.1 (0.1)	Wisconsin	0.8 (0.1)	Alaska	60.7 (3.0)
Washington	9.4 (0.1)	Pennsylvania	0.1 (0.1)	Arizona	0.7 (0.1)	Connecticut	60.7 (1.1)
Arizona	9.2 (0.1)	Tennessee	0.1 (0.1)	Colorado	0.7 (0.1)	District of Columbia	60.3 (2.8)
New Jersey	9.1 (0.1)	Texas	0.1 (0.1)	Connecticut	0.7 (0.1)	Rhode Island	60.1 (2.0)
United States	9.0 (0.1)	United States	0.1 (0.1)	Florida	0.7 (0.1)	Colorado	60.0 (1.2)
Illinois	8.8 (0.1)	Washington	0.1 (0.1)	Hawaii	0.7 (0.1)	United States	59.8 (0.1)
New Mexico	8.6 (0.3)	West Virginia	0.1 (0.1)	Maryland	0.7 (0.1)	New Jersey	59.5 (0.7)
New York	8.5 (0.1)	Wisconsin	0.1 (0.1)	Minnesota	0.7 (0.1)	Georgia	57.3 (0.9)
Mississippi	8.3 (0.2)	Wyoming	0.1 (0.1)	New Jersey	0.7 (0.1)	Arkansas	56.8 (1.2)
Colorado	7.9 (0.1)	Idaho	0.0 (0.1)	North Dakota	0.7 (0.2)	New York	55.9 (0.5)
Louisiana	7.9 (0.1)	Illinois	0.0 (0.1)	District of Columbia	0.6 (0.1)	Arizona	55.8 (0.7)
Georgia	7.5 (0.1)	Kansas	0.0 (0.1)	Illinois	0.6 (0.1)	Louisiana	55.0 (1.0)
Nevada	7.4 (0.2)	Kentucky	0.0 (0.1)	Nebraska	0.6 (0.1)	Texas	54.1 (0.5)
District of Columbia	7.3 (0.3)	Nebraska	0.0 (0.1)	Nevada	0.6 (0.1)	New Mexico	53.8 (1.6)
California	6.6 (0.1)	Nevada	0.0 (0.1)	Texas	0.6 (0.1)	Mississippi	53.4 (1.4)
Texas	6.5 (0.1)	Oregon	0.0 (0.1)	California	0.5 (0.1)	Florida	51.5 (0.5)
Utah	6.4 (0.1)	Rhode Island	0.0 (0.1)	Utah	0.5 (0.1)	Nevada	50.1 (1.4)
Alaska	5.9 (0.3)	Utah	0.0 (0.1)	Alaska	0.4 (0.1)	California	49.6 (0.4)

Note: Numbers in thousands; Figures cover 2013; Margin of error appears in parenthesis
Source: U.S. Census Bureau, 2013 American Community Survey, Table HI05. Health Insurance Coverage Status and Type of Coverage by State and Age for All People: 2013

Covered by Medicaid and Medicare

All Persons		Under 18 Years		Under 65 Years		65 Years and Over	
State	Percent[1]	State	Percent[1]	State	Percent[1]	State	Percent[1]
Maine	5.4 *(0.3)*	Alabama	0.8 *(0.2)*	Maine	2.9 *(0.2)*	District of Columbia	23.6 *(2.6)*
Mississippi	4.8 *(0.2)*	Delaware	0.5 *(0.4)*	Vermont	2.6 *(0.3)*	Mississippi	20.1 *(1.0)*
Vermont	4.4 *(0.4)*	New Mexico	0.5 *(0.2)*	Mississippi	2.3 *(0.2)*	California	19.4 *(0.3)*
District of Columbia	4.3 *(0.4)*	Connecticut	0.4 *(0.2)*	Alabama	2.2 *(0.1)*	New York	18.7 *(0.4)*
Alabama	4.0 *(0.2)*	Louisiana	0.4 *(0.1)*	Arkansas	2.2 *(0.2)*	Massachusetts	18.0 *(0.7)*
Arkansas	4.0 *(0.2)*	Maryland	0.4 *(0.2)*	West Virginia	2.2 *(0.2)*	Maine	17.5 *(1.3)*
Louisiana	4.0 *(0.1)*	Mississippi	0.4 *(0.1)*	Louisiana	2.0 *(0.1)*	Louisiana	17.4 *(0.7)*
Massachusetts	3.9 *(0.1)*	Arizona	0.3 *(0.1)*	Rhode Island	1.9 *(0.3)*	New Mexico	15.8 *(0.9)*
New Mexico	3.9 *(0.2)*	Arkansas	0.3 *(0.1)*	District of Columbia	1.8 *(0.3)*	Texas	15.3 *(0.4)*
New York	3.8 *(0.1)*	California	0.3 *(0.1)*	Kentucky	1.8 *(0.1)*	Georgia	15.0 *(0.6)*
Rhode Island	3.8 *(0.3)*	Colorado	0.3 *(0.1)*	Michigan	1.8 *(0.1)*	Alabama	14.9 *(0.7)*
West Virginia	3.8 *(0.3)*	District of Columbia	0.3 *(0.3)*	New Mexico	1.8 *(0.2)*	Arkansas	14.6 *(0.7)*
Florida	3.7 *(0.1)*	Florida	0.3 *(0.1)*	Delaware	1.7 *(0.3)*	Rhode Island	14.5 *(1.6)*
Kentucky	3.6 *(0.1)*	Georgia	0.3 *(0.1)*	Tennessee	1.7 *(0.1)*	Alaska	14.0 *(1.8)*
Tennessee	3.4 *(0.1)*	Illinois	0.3 *(0.1)*	Massachusetts	1.6 *(0.1)*	Kentucky	14.0 *(0.6)*
California	3.3 *(0.1)*	Iowa	0.3 *(0.1)*	South Carolina	1.6 *(0.1)*	Florida	13.8 *(0.3)*
Michigan	3.3 *(0.1)*	Kentucky	0.3 *(0.1)*	Wisconsin	1.6 *(0.1)*	United States	13.8 *(0.1)*
South Carolina	3.3 *(0.2)*	Maine	0.3 *(0.2)*	Iowa	1.5 *(0.1)*	Vermont	13.8 *(1.4)*
Wisconsin	3.2 *(0.1)*	Massachusetts	0.3 *(0.1)*	Missouri	1.5 *(0.1)*	Tennessee	13.7 *(0.6)*
Delaware	3.1 *(0.3)*	Michigan	0.3 *(0.1)*	North Carolina	1.5 *(0.1)*	Hawaii	13.2 *(1.1)*
North Carolina	3.1 *(0.1)*	New York	0.3 *(0.1)*	Pennsylvania	1.5 *(0.1)*	South Carolina	13.0 *(0.7)*
Oregon	3.1 *(0.1)*	North Dakota	0.3 *(0.3)*	Florida	1.4 *(0.1)*	Wisconsin	13.0 *(0.5)*
Pennsylvania	3.1 *(0.1)*	Ohio	0.3 *(0.1)*	Indiana	1.4 *(0.1)*	North Carolina	12.8 *(0.5)*
United States	3.1 *(0.1)*	Oklahoma	0.3 *(0.1)*	New York	1.4 *(0.1)*	Connecticut	12.7 *(0.7)*
Iowa	3.0 *(0.1)*	Rhode Island	0.3 *(0.3)*	Georgia	1.3 *(0.1)*	Oregon	12.6 *(0.7)*
Connecticut	2.9 *(0.1)*	South Carolina	0.3 *(0.1)*	Idaho	1.3 *(0.2)*	New Jersey	12.5 *(0.5)*
Georgia	2.9 *(0.1)*	Tennessee	0.3 *(0.1)*	Oklahoma	1.3 *(0.1)*	Nevada	12.4 *(0.8)*
Arizona	2.8 *(0.1)*	United States	0.3 *(0.1)*	Oregon	1.3 *(0.1)*	Michigan	12.0 *(0.4)*
Hawaii	2.8 *(0.2)*	Vermont	0.3 *(0.2)*	South Dakota	1.3 *(0.2)*	Washington	11.8 *(0.6)*
Missouri	2.7 *(0.1)*	Wisconsin	0.3 *(0.1)*	United States	1.3 *(0.1)*	Arizona	11.7 *(0.5)*
New Jersey	2.7 *(0.1)*	Wyoming	0.3 *(0.3)*	Connecticut	1.2 *(0.1)*	Maryland	11.6 *(0.6)*
Oklahoma	2.7 *(0.1)*	Alaska	0.2 *(0.2)*	Kansas	1.2 *(0.1)*	Iowa	11.5 *(0.5)*
South Dakota	2.7 *(0.3)*	Hawaii	0.2 *(0.1)*	Montana	1.2 *(0.2)*	North Dakota	11.5 *(1.4)*
Washington	2.7 *(0.1)*	Indiana	0.2 *(0.1)*	New Hampshire	1.2 *(0.2)*	Pennsylvania	11.5 *(0.3)*
Idaho	2.6 *(0.2)*	Kansas	0.2 *(0.1)*	Ohio	1.2 *(0.1)*	West Virginia	11.5 *(1.0)*
Indiana	2.6 *(0.1)*	Minnesota	0.2 *(0.1)*	Washington	1.2 *(0.1)*	Illinois	11.1 *(0.3)*
Nevada	2.6 *(0.2)*	Missouri	0.2 *(0.1)*	Arizona	1.1 *(0.1)*	Nebraska	11.1 *(0.8)*
Ohio	2.6 *(0.1)*	New Jersey	0.2 *(0.1)*	California	1.1 *(0.1)*	South Dakota	11.1 *(1.3)*
Texas	2.6 *(0.1)*	North Carolina	0.2 *(0.1)*	Illinois	1.1 *(0.1)*	Colorado	10.9 *(0.5)*
Kansas	2.5 *(0.1)*	Oregon	0.2 *(0.1)*	Texas	1.1 *(0.1)*	Oklahoma	10.9 *(0.6)*
Montana	2.5 *(0.2)*	Pennsylvania	0.2 *(0.1)*	Colorado	1.0 *(0.1)*	Delaware	10.6 *(1.2)*
Illinois	2.4 *(0.1)*	South Dakota	0.2 *(0.1)*	Maryland	1.0 *(0.1)*	Kansas	10.6 *(0.7)*
Maryland	2.4 *(0.1)*	Texas	0.2 *(0.1)*	Minnesota	1.0 *(0.1)*	Idaho	10.3 *(1.3)*
Nebraska	2.4 *(0.1)*	Virginia	0.2 *(0.1)*	Nebraska	1.0 *(0.1)*	Ohio	10.3 *(0.4)*
North Dakota	2.4 *(0.3)*	Washington	0.2 *(0.1)*	Nevada	1.0 *(0.1)*	Indiana	10.2 *(0.5)*
Colorado	2.2 *(0.1)*	West Virginia	0.2 *(0.1)*	New Jersey	1.0 *(0.1)*	Utah	10.1 *(0.7)*
Minnesota	2.2 *(0.1)*	Idaho	0.1 *(0.1)*	North Dakota	1.0 *(0.2)*	Wyoming	10.0 *(1.7)*
Alaska	2.1 *(0.3)*	Nebraska	0.1 *(0.1)*	Alaska	0.9 *(0.2)*	Minnesota	9.8 *(0.5)*
New Hampshire	2.1 *(0.2)*	Nevada	0.1 *(0.1)*	Virginia	0.9 *(0.1)*	Missouri	9.6 *(0.5)*
Virginia	2.1 *(0.1)*	New Hampshire	0.1 *(0.1)*	Hawaii	0.8 *(0.2)*	Virginia	9.6 *(0.4)*
Wyoming	2.0 *(0.3)*	Utah	0.1 *(0.1)*	Wyoming	0.8 *(0.2)*	Montana	9.4 *(0.9)*
Utah	1.7 *(0.1)*	Montana	0.0 *(0.1)*	Utah	0.7 *(0.1)*	New Hampshire	7.0 *(0.9)*

Note: Numbers in thousands; Figures cover 2013; Margin of error appears in parenthesis
Source: U.S. Census Bureau, 2013 American Community Survey, Table HI05. Health Insurance Coverage Status and Type of Coverage by State and Age for All People: 2013

Covered by Government Health Insurance: VA Care

All Persons		Under 18 Years		Under 65 Years		65 Years and Over	
State	Percent[1]	State	Percent[1]	State	Percent[1]	State	Percent[1]
Montana	3.8 (0.3)	Idaho	0.6 (0.5)	Alaska	2.5 (0.3)	Montana	13.0 (0.9)
South Dakota	3.6 (0.3)	Virginia	0.4 (0.1)	Montana	2.1 (0.2)	South Dakota	12.7 (1.1)
West Virginia	3.6 (0.2)	Oklahoma	0.3 (0.1)	South Dakota	2.1 (0.3)	Alaska	12.2 (2.0)
Alaska	3.4 (0.3)	Alabama	0.2 (0.1)	Wyoming	2.1 (0.3)	Nebraska	11.9 (0.8)
Arkansas	3.4 (0.1)	Arizona	0.2 (0.1)	West Virginia	2.0 (0.2)	Wyoming	11.7 (1.5)
Maine	3.4 (0.2)	Arkansas	0.2 (0.1)	Arkansas	1.9 (0.1)	Arkansas	11.6 (0.6)
Wyoming	3.4 (0.3)	Colorado	0.2 (0.1)	Oklahoma	1.9 (0.1)	West Virginia	11.6 (0.9)
Oklahoma	3.3 (0.1)	Minnesota	0.2 (0.1)	South Carolina	1.9 (0.1)	Oklahoma	11.5 (0.5)
Idaho	3.1 (0.2)	Mississippi	0.2 (0.1)	Idaho	1.8 (0.3)	North Dakota	11.3 (1.0)
New Mexico	3.1 (0.2)	Missouri	0.2 (0.1)	Maine	1.8 (0.2)	Maine	11.2 (0.7)
Nevada	3.0 (0.2)	Montana	0.2 (0.1)	Nevada	1.8 (0.2)	Idaho	10.8 (0.9)
South Carolina	3.0 (0.1)	New Mexico	0.2 (0.2)	New Mexico	1.8 (0.2)	Iowa	10.8 (0.6)
Oregon	2.9 (0.1)	North Dakota	0.2 (0.1)	Alabama	1.6 (0.1)	Minnesota	10.8 (0.4)
Florida	2.8 (0.1)	South Carolina	0.2 (0.1)	Kentucky	1.6 (0.1)	Nevada	10.7 (0.6)
Kentucky	2.8 (0.1)	Vermont	0.2 (0.2)	Mississippi	1.6 (0.1)	New Mexico	10.6 (0.8)
Missouri	2.8 (0.1)	West Virginia	0.2 (0.1)	Missouri	1.6 (0.1)	Kentucky	10.2 (0.6)
Nebraska	2.8 (0.2)	Alaska	0.1 (0.1)	North Carolina	1.6 (0.1)	Missouri	10.0 (0.5)
Arizona	2.7 (0.1)	California	0.1 (0.1)	Oregon	1.6 (0.1)	Oregon	9.8 (0.5)
Iowa	2.7 (0.1)	Delaware	0.1 (0.1)	Virginia	1.6 (0.1)	New Hampshire	9.5 (0.8)
North Dakota	2.7 (0.3)	Florida	0.1 (0.1)	Washington	1.6 (0.1)	South Carolina	9.5 (0.4)
Alabama	2.6 (0.1)	Georgia	0.1 (0.1)	Arizona	1.5 (0.1)	Kansas	9.3 (0.5)
Mississippi	2.6 (0.1)	Hawaii	0.1 (0.1)	Colorado	1.4 (0.1)	Mississippi	9.2 (0.6)
North Carolina	2.6 (0.1)	Illinois	0.1 (0.1)	Florida	1.4 (0.1)	Vermont	9.2 (0.8)
Minnesota	2.5 (0.1)	Indiana	0.1 (0.1)	Georgia	1.4 (0.1)	Indiana	9.1 (0.4)
Washington	2.5 (0.1)	Kansas	0.1 (0.1)	North Dakota	1.4 (0.2)	North Carolina	9.1 (0.3)
Kansas	2.4 (0.1)	Kentucky	0.1 (0.1)	Tennessee	1.4 (0.1)	Wisconsin	9.1 (0.4)
New Hampshire	2.4 (0.2)	Louisiana	0.1 (0.1)	Hawaii	1.3 (0.2)	Arizona	9.0 (0.5)
Tennessee	2.4 (0.1)	Maine	0.1 (0.1)	Iowa	1.3 (0.1)	Florida	9.0 (0.2)
Wisconsin	2.4 (0.1)	Maryland	0.1 (0.1)	Kansas	1.3 (0.1)	Alabama	8.6 (0.4)
Indiana	2.3 (0.1)	Massachusetts	0.1 (0.1)	Louisiana	1.3 (0.1)	Texas	8.6 (0.3)
Vermont	2.3 (0.2)	Michigan	0.1 (0.1)	Nebraska	1.3 (0.1)	Rhode Island	8.5 (1.0)
Virginia	2.3 (0.1)	Nevada	0.1 (0.1)	Texas	1.3 (0.1)	Tennessee	8.3 (0.4)
Colorado	2.2 (0.1)	New Jersey	0.1 (0.1)	Indiana	1.2 (0.1)	Louisiana	8.2 (0.4)
Georgia	2.2 (0.1)	New York	0.1 (0.1)	Maryland	1.2 (0.1)	Washington	8.2 (0.4)
Hawaii	2.2 (0.2)	North Carolina	0.1 (0.1)	Minnesota	1.2 (0.1)	United States	8.1 (0.1)
Louisiana	2.2 (0.1)	Ohio	0.1 (0.1)	New Hampshire	1.2 (0.2)	Georgia	7.9 (0.3)
Ohio	2.2 (0.1)	Oregon	0.1 (0.1)	Ohio	1.2 (0.1)	Ohio	7.9 (0.3)
United States	2.2 (0.1)	South Dakota	0.1 (0.1)	United States	1.2 (0.1)	Utah	7.8 (0.6)
Pennsylvania	2.1 (0.1)	Tennessee	0.1 (0.1)	Wisconsin	1.2 (0.1)	Colorado	7.6 (0.5)
Texas	2.1 (0.1)	Texas	0.1 (0.1)	Michigan	1.1 (0.1)	Pennsylvania	7.6 (0.2)
Maryland	1.9 (0.1)	United States	0.1 (0.1)	District of Columbia	1.0 (0.2)	Illinois	7.1 (0.3)
Michigan	1.9 (0.1)	Washington	0.1 (0.1)	Pennsylvania	1.0 (0.1)	Connecticut	7.0 (0.5)
Rhode Island	1.9 (0.2)	Wisconsin	0.1 (0.1)	Vermont	1.0 (0.2)	Hawaii	6.9 (0.8)
Connecticut	1.7 (0.1)	Wyoming	0.1 (0.1)	Delaware	0.9 (0.2)	Michigan	6.9 (0.2)
Delaware	1.7 (0.2)	Connecticut	0.0 (0.1)	California	0.8 (0.1)	Virginia	6.7 (0.3)
Illinois	1.6 (0.1)	District of Columbia	0.0 (0.1)	Connecticut	0.8 (0.1)	Maryland	6.4 (0.3)
California	1.5 (0.1)	Iowa	0.0 (0.1)	Illinois	0.8 (0.1)	Massachusetts	6.3 (0.3)
District of Columbia	1.5 (0.2)	Nebraska	0.0 (0.1)	Rhode Island	0.8 (0.2)	Delaware	6.2 (0.8)
Utah	1.5 (0.1)	New Hampshire	0.0 (0.1)	Utah	0.8 (0.1)	California	6.0 (0.1)
Massachusetts	1.4 (0.1)	Pennsylvania	0.0 (0.1)	New York	0.7 (0.1)	District of Columbia	5.8 (1.1)
New York	1.4 (0.1)	Rhode Island	0.0 (0.1)	Massachusetts	0.6 (0.1)	New York	5.8 (0.2)
New Jersey	1.1 (0.1)	Utah	0.0 (0.1)	New Jersey	0.4 (0.1)	New Jersey	5.0 (0.3)

Note: Numbers in thousands; Figures cover 2013; Margin of error appears in parenthesis
Source: U.S. Census Bureau, 2013 American Community Survey, Table HI05. Health Insurance Coverage Status and Type of Coverage by State and Age for All People: 2013

Not Covered by Health Insurance at any Time During the Year

All Persons		Under 18 Years		Under 65 Years		65 Years and Over	
State	Percent[1]	State	Percent[1]	State	Percent[1]	State	Percent[1]
Texas	22.1 (0.2)	Nevada	14.9 (1.2)	Texas	24.6 (0.2)	Nevada	2.1 (0.5)
Nevada	20.7 (0.6)	Texas	12.6 (0.3)	Florida	24.2 (0.3)	Texas	2.0 (0.2)
Florida	20.0 (0.2)	Arizona	11.9 (0.7)	Nevada	23.6 (0.7)	California	1.8 (0.1)
Georgia	18.8 (0.3)	Alaska	11.6 (1.6)	New Mexico	21.6 (0.8)	Florida	1.7 (0.2)
New Mexico	18.6 (0.6)	Florida	11.1 (0.4)	Georgia	21.2 (0.3)	New Jersey	1.6 (0.2)
Alaska	18.5 (1.0)	Montana	10.1 (1.4)	Oklahoma	20.4 (0.4)	New Mexico	1.6 (0.4)
Oklahoma	17.7 (0.3)	Oklahoma	10.0 (0.5)	Alaska	20.3 (1.1)	Maryland	1.4 (0.2)
California	17.2 (0.2)	Georgia	9.6 (0.5)	Arizona	20.1 (0.4)	Georgia	1.3 (0.2)
Arizona	17.1 (0.4)	Utah	9.5 (0.7)	Mississippi	19.8 (0.6)	Illinois	1.3 (0.2)
Mississippi	17.1 (0.5)	Idaho	8.9 (1.0)	Montana	19.5 (0.9)	Alaska	1.1 (0.5)
Louisiana	16.6 (0.4)	New Mexico	8.5 (1.0)	California	19.4 (0.2)	Virginia	1.1 (0.2)
Montana	16.5 (0.8)	Colorado	8.2 (0.5)	Louisiana	18.9 (0.4)	Delaware	1.0 (0.4)
Idaho	16.2 (0.8)	Indiana	8.2 (0.5)	Arkansas	18.8 (0.5)	Hawaii	1.0 (0.4)
Arkansas	16.0 (0.5)	North Dakota	7.9 (1.2)	Idaho	18.6 (0.9)	Louisiana	1.0 (0.2)
South Carolina	15.8 (0.4)	Mississippi	7.6 (0.9)	South Carolina	18.5 (0.5)	New York	1.0 (0.1)
North Carolina	15.6 (0.3)	California	7.4 (0.2)	North Carolina	18.1 (0.3)	United States	1.0 (0.1)
Oregon	14.7 (0.4)	United States	7.1 (0.1)	Oregon	17.2 (0.5)	Arizona	0.9 (0.2)
United States	14.5 (0.1)	Missouri	7.0 (0.6)	West Virginia	16.8 (0.6)	Connecticut	0.9 (0.2)
Kentucky	14.3 (0.3)	South Carolina	6.7 (0.6)	United States	16.7 (0.1)	Idaho	0.9 (0.5)
Colorado	14.1 (0.3)	North Carolina	6.3 (0.4)	Kentucky	16.6 (0.4)	Utah	0.8 (0.3)
Indiana	14.0 (0.3)	South Dakota	6.3 (1.1)	Indiana	16.1 (0.3)	Washington	0.8 (0.2)
Utah	14.0 (0.5)	Kansas	6.1 (0.6)	Tennessee	16.1 (0.3)	Colorado	0.7 (0.2)
Washington	14.0 (0.3)	Kentucky	5.9 (0.5)	Washington	16.1 (0.4)	Nebraska	0.7 (0.3)
West Virginia	14.0 (0.5)	Maine	5.9 (1.0)	Colorado	16.0 (0.4)	Oklahoma	0.7 (0.1)
Tennessee	13.9 (0.3)	Washington	5.9 (0.5)	Alabama	15.8 (0.4)	North Carolina	0.6 (0.1)
Alabama	13.6 (0.4)	Oregon	5.8 (0.6)	Utah	15.4 (0.5)	Pennsylvania	0.6 (0.1)
Wyoming	13.4 (0.9)	Louisiana	5.7 (0.4)	Wyoming	15.4 (1.0)	South Carolina	0.6 (0.1)
New Jersey	13.2 (0.2)	Tennessee	5.7 (0.5)	Missouri	15.2 (0.4)	Alabama	0.5 (0.2)
Missouri	13.0 (0.3)	Wyoming	5.7 (1.1)	New Jersey	15.1 (0.3)	Indiana	0.5 (0.1)
Illinois	12.7 (0.2)	Minnesota	5.6 (0.4)	Illinois	14.5 (0.2)	Michigan	0.5 (0.1)
Kansas	12.3 (0.4)	New Jersey	5.6 (0.4)	Kansas	14.2 (0.5)	Minnesota	0.5 (0.2)
Virginia	12.3 (0.3)	Arkansas	5.5 (0.7)	Virginia	14.0 (0.3)	Missouri	0.5 (0.1)
Rhode Island	11.6 (0.7)	Nebraska	5.5 (0.7)	Rhode Island	13.6 (0.8)	Ohio	0.5 (0.1)
Nebraska	11.3 (0.5)	Pennsylvania	5.4 (0.3)	Maine	13.5 (0.7)	South Dakota	0.5 (0.4)
South Dakota	11.3 (0.7)	Rhode Island	5.4 (1.1)	South Dakota	13.1 (0.8)	Tennessee	0.5 (0.1)
Maine	11.2 (0.5)	Virginia	5.4 (0.4)	Nebraska	13.0 (0.6)	Arkansas	0.4 (0.2)
Michigan	11.0 (0.2)	Ohio	5.3 (0.4)	Ohio	12.9 (0.2)	District of Columbia	0.4 (0.4)
Ohio	11.0 (0.2)	West Virginia	5.3 (0.9)	Michigan	12.8 (0.2)	Kansas	0.4 (0.1)
New Hampshire	10.7 (0.5)	Wisconsin	4.7 (0.3)	New Hampshire	12.6 (0.6)	Kentucky	0.4 (0.1)
New York	10.7 (0.2)	Delaware	4.5 (1.1)	New York	12.3 (0.2)	Massachusetts	0.4 (0.1)
North Dakota	10.4 (0.8)	Maryland	4.4 (0.4)	North Dakota	12.0 (0.9)	Montana	0.4 (0.2)
Maryland	10.2 (0.3)	Alabama	4.3 (0.5)	Maryland	11.5 (0.3)	Oregon	0.4 (0.1)
Pennsylvania	9.7 (0.2)	Connecticut	4.3 (0.5)	Pennsylvania	11.5 (0.2)	Iowa	0.3 (0.1)
Connecticut	9.4 (0.4)	Illinois	4.2 (0.3)	Connecticut	10.9 (0.5)	Rhode Island	0.3 (0.2)
Delaware	9.1 (0.7)	Iowa	4.1 (0.5)	Delaware	10.6 (0.8)	Vermont	0.3 (0.2)
Wisconsin	9.1 (0.2)	Michigan	4.0 (0.3)	Wisconsin	10.6 (0.3)	Wisconsin	0.3 (0.1)
Minnesota	8.2 (0.3)	New York	4.0 (0.2)	Iowa	9.5 (0.3)	Wyoming	0.3 (0.3)
Iowa	8.1 (0.3)	New Hampshire	3.8 (0.7)	Minnesota	9.4 (0.3)	Maine	0.2 (0.1)
Vermont	7.2 (0.6)	Vermont	3.1 (1.1)	Vermont	8.6 (0.7)	Mississippi	0.2 (0.1)
District of Columbia	6.7 (0.6)	Hawaii	3.0 (0.7)	Hawaii	7.8 (0.5)	North Dakota	0.2 (0.1)
Hawaii	6.7 (0.4)	District of Columbia	2.4 (1.0)	District of Columbia	7.4 (0.7)	West Virginia	0.2 (0.1)
Massachusetts	3.7 (0.2)	Massachusetts	1.5 (0.2)	Massachusetts	4.3 (0.2)	New Hampshire	0.1 (0.1)

Note: Numbers in thousands; Figures cover 2013; Margin of error appears in parenthesis
Source: U.S. Census Bureau, 2013 American Community Survey, Table HI05. Health Insurance Coverage Status and Type of Coverage by State and Age for All People: 2013

Managed Care Organizations Ranked by Total Enrollment

State	Total Enrollment	Organization	Plan Type
Alabama	70,000,000	UnitedHealthCare of Alabama	HMO/PPO
Alabama	8,000,000	United Concordia: Dental Corporation of Alabama	Dental
Alabama	4,800,000	CompBenefits: Alabama	Multiple
Alabama	3,200,000	Blue Cross & Blue Shield of Alabama	HMO
Alabama	3,200,000	Blue Cross Preferred Care	PPO
Alabama	480,000	Behavioral Health Systems	PPO
Alabama	80,000	VIVA Health	HMO
Alabama	66,000	North Alabama Managed Care Inc	PPO
Alabama	47,000	Assurant Employee Benefits: Alabama	Multiple
Alabama	45,000	Health Choice of Alabama	PPO
Alabama	30,000	Cigna-HealthSpring of Alabama	Medicare
Alabama	8,147	Great-West Healthcare Alabama	HMO/PPO
Alaska	75,000,000	UnitedHealthCare of Alaska	HMO/PPO
Alaska	11,596,230	Aetna Health of Alaska	PPO
Alaska	1,700,000	Premera Blue Cross Blue Shield of Alaska	PPO
Alaska	800,000	Moda Health Alaska	Multiple
Alaska	8,097	Humana Health Insurance of Alaska	HMO/PPO
Alaska	1,003	CCN: Alaska	PPO
Arizona	75,000,000	UnitedHealthCare of Arizona	HMO/PPO
Arizona	60,000,000	Preferred Therapy Providers	PPO
Arizona	55,000,000	VSP: Vision Service Plan of Arizona	Vision
Arizona	54,000,000	Delta Dental of Arizona	Dental
Arizona	8,000,000	United Concordia: Arizona	Dental
Arizona	7,000,000	Outlook Vision Service	Vision
Arizona	2,700,000	Desert Canyon Community Care	Medicare
Arizona	2,000,000	Avesis: Corporate Headquarters	PPO
Arizona	1,300,000	CoreSource: Arizona	Multiple
Arizona	1,000,000	Blue Cross & Blue Shield of Arizona	HMO/PPO
Arizona	300,000	Mercy Care Plan/Mercy Care Advantage	Medicare
Arizona	175,000	Arizona Foundation for Medical Care	Multiple
Arizona	127,564	Humana Health Insurance of Arizona	HMO/PPO
Arizona	120,000	Employers Dental Services	Dental
Arizona	119,000	Health Net of Arizona	HMO
Arizona	115,000	Health Choice Arizona	HMO
Arizona	109,089	Aetna Health of Arizona	HMO
Arizona	103,561	CIGNA HealthCare of Arizona	HMO/PPO
Arizona	98,500	Action Healthcare Management Services	PPO
Arizona	80,000	Magellan Health Services Arizona	PPO
Arizona	55,000	SecureCare Dental	Dental
Arizona	50,715	Maricopa Integrated Health System/Maricopa Health Plan	HMO
Arizona	37,459	Great-West Healthcare Arizona	HMO/PPO
Arizona	7,000	Pima Health System	HMO
Arizona	3,000	Phoenix Health Plans	Multiple
Arkansas	75,000,000	CIGNA HealthCare of Arkansas	HMO
Arkansas	75,000,000	UnitedHealthCare of Arkansas	HMO/PPO
Arkansas	54,000,000	Delta Dental of Arkansas	Dental
Arkansas	11,596,230	Aetna Health of Arkansas	PPO
Arkansas	1,100,000	CoreSource: Arkansas	Multiple
Arkansas	475,000	HealthSCOPE Benefits	Other
Arkansas	400,000	Arkansas Blue Cross and Blue Shield	Multiple

State	Total Enrollment	Organization	Plan Type
Arkansas	200,000	Arkansas Managed Care Organization	PPO
Arkansas	73,000	Mercy Health Plans: Arkansas	HMO
Arkansas	50,000	American Denticare	HMO
Arkansas	36,000	QualChoice/QCA Health Plan	HMO/PPO
Arkansas	7,000	Arkansas Community Care	Medicare
California	100,000,000	ChiroSource Inc	Multiple
California	94,000,000	American Specialty Health	HMO
California	75,000,000	UnitedHealthCare of Northern California	HMO/PPO
California	75,000,000	UnitedHealthCare of Southern California	HMO/PPO
California	55,000,000	VSP: Vision Service Plan	Vision
California	55,000,000	VSP: Vision Service Plan of California	Vision
California	43,000,000	United Behavioral Health	Other
California	26,000,000	Delta Dental of California	Dental
California	16,000,000	Beech Street Corporation: Corporate Office	PPO
California	12,225,000	Beech Street Corporation: Northeast Region	PPO
California	12,225,000	Beech Street Corporation: Western Region	HMO
California	10,000,000	Managed Health Network	PPO
California	10,000,000	CIGNA HealthCare of Northern California	HMO
California	10,000,000	CIGNA HealthCare of Southern California	HMO
California	8,569,000	Kaiser Permanente Health Plan: Corporate Office	HMO
California	8,000,000	United Concordia: California	Dental
California	6,700,000	Health Net Medicare Plan	Medicare
California	6,600,000	Dental Benefit Providers: California	Dental
California	6,000,000	Health Net: Corporate Headquarters	HMO
California	3,500,000	Blue Shield of California	HMO/PPO
California	3,284,000	Kaiser Permanente Health Plan of Southern California	HMO
California	3,223,235	Kaiser Permanente Health Plan of Northern California	HMO
California	3,000,000	eHealthInsurance Services Inc. Corporate Office	HMO/PPO
California	2,900,000	Interplan Health Group	PPO
California	2,000,000	Superior Vision Services, Inc.	Vision
California	1,915,829	PacifiCare Health Systems	HMO
California	1,800,000	March Vision Care	Vision
California	1,800,000	SafeGuard Health Enterprises: Corporate Office	Dental
California	1,400,000	Molina Healthcare: Corporate Office	HMO
California	1,283,000	PacifiCare of California	HMO
California	1,100,000	Orange County Foundation for Medical Care	PPO
California	1,100,000	Physical Therapy Provider Network	Multiple
California	1,000,000	California Foundation for Medical Care	PPO
California	950,000	Bright Now! Dental	Dental
California	857,252	L.A. Care Health Plan	HMO
California	700,000	Los Angeles County Department of Health Services	HMO
California	650,000	Pacific Dental Benefits	Dental
California	575,000	Inland Empire Health Plan	HMO
California	540,000	Health Net Dental	Dental
California	427,039	Aetna Health of California	HMO
California	413,795	CalOptima	HMO
California	390,000	Dental Alternatives Insurance Services	Dental
California	338,000	Pacific Health Alliance	PPO
California	315,440	Western Dental Services	Dental
California	300,000	Pacific Foundation for Medical Care	Multiple
California	291,000	Care 1st Health Plan: California	HMO
California	250,000	Lakeside Community Healthcare Network	HMO
California	234,072	CIGNA HealthCare of California	HMO
California	210,000	Central California Alliance for Health	HMO
California	204,077	Great-West Healthcare California	HMO/PPO

State	Total Enrollment	Organization	Plan Type
California	200,473	Golden West Dental & Vision Plan	Multiple
California	200,000	Community Health Plan of Los Angeles County	HMO
California	150,000	Landmark Healthplan of California	HMO/PPO
California	146,000	Community Health Group	HMO
California	140,462	PacifiCare Dental and Vision Administrators	Multiple
California	140,000	Alameda Alliance for Health	HMO
California	128,272	SCAN Health Plan	HMO
California	125,000	Premier Access Insurance/Access Dental	PPO
California	123,880	Access Dental Services	Dental
California	121,794	Santa Clara Family Health Foundations Inc	HMO
California	109,000	Health Plan of San Joaquin	HMO
California	100,000	Contra Costa Health Plan	HMO
California	97,000	Kern Family Health Care	HMO
California	93,000	Partnership HealthPlan of California	Medicare
California	92,000	Western Health Advantage	HMO
California	90,000	BEST Life and Health Insurance Co.	PPO
California	90,000	Dental Health Services of California	Dental
California	87,740	Health Plan of San Mateo	HMO
California	60,000	Foundation for Medical Care for Kern & Santa Barbara County	PPO
California	55,000	Arta Medicare Health Plan	Medicare
California	55,000	San Francisco Health Plan	HMO
California	49,000	Sharp Health Plan	HMO
California	47,000	Assurant Employee Benefits: California	Multiple
California	41,266	Coastal Healthcare Administrators	PPO
California	34,000	Foundation for Medical Care for Mendocino and Lake Counties	PPO
California	17,000	Primecare Dental Plan	Dental
California	14,600	Inter Valley Health Plan	Multiple
California	13,582	Chinese Community Health Plan	HMO
California	8,000	Easy Choice Health Plan	Medicare
California	3,000	Central Health Medicare Plan	Medicare
California	1,000	On Lok Lifeways	HMO
Colorado	75,000,000	UnitedHealthCare of Colorado	HMO/PPO
Colorado	57,000,000	VSP: Vision Service Plan of Colorado	Vision
Colorado	54,000,000	Delta Dental of Colorado	Dental
Colorado	14,000,000	Anthem Blue Cross & Blue Shield of Nevada	HMO/PPO
Colorado	8,000,000	United Concordia: Colorado	Dental
Colorado	3,000,000	eHealthInsurance Services Inc.	HMO/PPO
Colorado	2,000,000	Great-West/One Health Plan	HMO/PPO
Colorado	880,475	Anthem Blue Cross & Blue Shield of Colorado	HMO/PPO
Colorado	535,000	Kaiser Permanente Health Plan of Colorado	HMO
Colorado	328,000	PacifiCare of Colorado	HMO
Colorado	270,000	CNA Insurance Companies: Colorado	PPO
Colorado	207,180	Rocky Mountain Health Plans	HMO/PPO
Colorado	160,000	Colorado Health Partnerships	HMO
Colorado	126,000	HMO Colorado	HMO
Colorado	113,229	Humana Health Insurance of Colorado Springs	HMO/PPO
Colorado	60,000	Boulder Valley Individual Practice Association	PPO
Colorado	56,000	Beta Health Plan	Multiple
Colorado	47,000	Assurant Employee Benefits: Colorado	Multiple
Colorado	36,611	CIGNA HealthCare of Colorado	HMO
Colorado	36,423	Aetna Health of Colorado	HMO
Colorado	15,000	Denver Health Medical Plan Inc	HMO
Colorado	5,000	Colorado Choice Health Plans	HMO
Connecticut	75,000,000	UnitedHealthCare of Connecticut	HMO/PPO

State	Total Enrollment	Organization	Plan Type
Connecticut	18,602,000	Aetna Health, Inc. Corporate Headquarters	HMO
Connecticut	1,600,000	Oxford Health Plans: Corporate Headquarters	HMO/PPO
Connecticut	1,535,753	Anthem Blue Cross & Blue Shield Connecticut	HMO/PPO
Connecticut	1,500,000	Delta Dental of New Jersey & Connecticut	Dental
Connecticut	1,300,000	Health Plan of New York: Connecticut	HMO/PPO
Connecticut	240,000	ConnectiCare	HMO/PPO
Connecticut	29,506	CIGNA HealthCare of Connecticut	HMO
Delaware	75,000,000	UnitedHealthCare of Maryland	HMO/PPO
Delaware	54,000,000	Delta Dental of the Mid-Atlantic	Dental
Delaware	400,000	Highmark Blue Cross & Blue Shield Delaware	HMO/PPO
Delaware	265,000	AmeriHealth HMO	HMO/PPO
Delaware	180,000	Mid Atlantic Medical Services: Delaware	HMO/PPO
Delaware	101,900	Mid Atlantic Psychiatric Services (MAMSI)	Multiple
Delaware	100,000	Coventry Health Care of Delaware	HMO/PPO
Delaware	27,179	Aetna Health of Delaware	HMO
Delaware	2,718	Great-West Healthcare Delaware	HMO/PPO
Delaware	984	CIGNA HealthCare of Delaware	HMO
District of Columbia	75,000,000	UnitedHealthCare of the District of Columbia	HMO/PPO
District of Columbia	54,000,000	Delta Dental of the Mid-Atlantic	Dental
District of Columbia	3,400,000	CareFirst Blue Cross Blue Shield	HMO/PPO
District of Columbia	211,156	Aetna Health District of Columbia	HMO
District of Columbia	180,000	Mid Atlantic Medical Services: DC	HMO/PPO
District of Columbia	109,186	CIGNA HealthCare of the Mid-Atlantic	HMO/PPO
District of Columbia	100,000	DC Chartered Health Plan	HMO
District of Columbia	90,000	Quality Plan Administrators	HMO/PPO
Florida	75,000,000	UnitedHealthCare of Florida	HMO/PPO
Florida	75,000,000	UnitedHealthCare of South Florida	HMO/PPO
Florida	57,000,000	VSP: Vision Service Plan of Florida	Vision
Florida	54,000,000	Delta Dental of Florida	Dental
Florida	8,000,000	United Concordia: Florida	Dental
Florida	4,500,000	CompBenefits: Florida	Multiple
Florida	4,000,000	Florida Blue: Jacksonville	HMO/PPO
Florida	2,600,000	WellCare Health Plans	Medicare
Florida	1,900,000	Amerigroup Florida	HMO
Florida	1,800,000	Molina Healthcare: Florida	HMO
Florida	1,800,000	SafeGuard Health Enterprises: Florida	Dental
Florida	900,000	CompCare: Comprehensive Behavioral Care	Multiple
Florida	521,696	Aetna Health of Florida	HMO
Florida	400,000	Dimension Health PPO	PPO
Florida	350,000	AvMed Health Plan: Orlando	HMO
Florida	350,000	AvMed Health Plan: Tampa Bay	HMO
Florida	350,000	AvMed Health Plan: Corporate Office	HMO
Florida	350,000	AvMed Health Plan: Gainesville	HMO
Florida	350,000	AvMed Health Plan: Fort Lauderdale	HMO
Florida	350,000	AvMed Health Plan: Jacksonville	HMO
Florida	320,000	First Medical Health Plan of Florida	Medicare
Florida	310,000	Coventry Health Care of Florida	HMO/PPO
Florida	194,944	CIGNA HealthCare of Florida	HMO
Florida	125,000	Capital Health Plan	HMO
Florida	125,000	Humana Health Insurance of Tampa - Pinellas	HMO/PPO
Florida	125,000	Humana Health Insurance of Jacksonville	HMO/PPO
Florida	108,000	Neighborhood Health Partnership	HMO
Florida	105,000	JMH Health Plan	HMO

State	Total Enrollment	Organization	Plan Type
Florida	81,822	Great-West Healthcare Florida	HMO/PPO
Florida	69,000	Coventry Health Care of Southern Florida	Multiple
Florida	67,440	Florida Health Care Plan	HMO
Florida	67,000	CarePlus Health Plans, Inc	HMO
Florida	63,700	Health First Health Plans	HMO
Florida	56,000	Humana Health Insurance of Orlando	HMO/PPO
Florida	54,000	Citrus Health Care	Medicare
Florida	54,000	Florida Blue: Pensacola	HMO/PPO
Florida	52,000	Preferred Medical Plan	HMO
Florida	47,000	Assurant Employee Benefits: Florida	Multiple
Florida	45,000	Preferred Care Partners	Multiple
Florida	35,000	Healthchoice Orlando	PPO
Florida	27,000	Leon Medical Centers Health Plan	HMO
Florida	12,000	Medica HealthCare Plans, Inc	Medicare
Florida	10,000	Total Health Choice	HMO
Florida	6,000	Risk Placement Services, Inc.	PPO
Georgia	75,000,000	UnitedHealthCare of Georgia	HMO/PPO
Georgia	59,000,000	Delta Dental of Alabama	Dental
Georgia	57,000,000	VSP: Vision Service Plan of Georgia	Vision
Georgia	54,000,000	Delta Dental of Georgia	Dental
Georgia	54,000,000	Delta Dental of Nevada	Dental
Georgia	8,000,000	United Concordia: Georgia	Dental
Georgia	4,800,000	CompBenefits Corporation	Multiple
Georgia	3,300,000	Blue Cross & Blue Shield of Georgia	HMO
Georgia	2,000,000	Avesis: Arizona	PPO
Georgia	1,900,000	Amerigroup Georgia	HMO
Georgia	1,000,000	National Better Living Association	PPO
Georgia	270,000	CNA Insurance Companies: Georgia	PPO
Georgia	238,000	Kaiser Foundation Health Plan of Georgia	HMO
Georgia	150,000	Coventry Health Care of GA	HMO/PPO
Georgia	116,375	Aetna Health of Georgia	HMO
Georgia	73,000	Humana Health Insurance of Georgia	HMO/PPO
Georgia	68,000	Secure Health PPO Newtork	PPO
Georgia	49,984	Great-West Healthcare Georgia	HMO/PPO
Georgia	47,000	Assurant Employee Benefits: Georgia	Multiple
Georgia	42,000	Northeast Georgia Health Partners	PPO
Georgia	25,769	CIGNA HealthCare of Georgia	HMO
Georgia	23,241	Athens Area Health Plan Select	HMO
Georgia	15,000	Alliant Health Plans	HMO/PPO
Hawaii	75,000,000	UnitedHealthCare of Hawaii	HMO/PPO
Hawaii	57,000,000	VSP: Vision Service Plan of Hawaii	Vision
Hawaii	11,596,230	Aetna Health of Hawaii	PPO
Hawaii	229,186	Kaiser Permanente Health Plan of Hawaii	HMO
Hawaii	80,000	AlohaCare	HMO
Hawaii	42,000	Hawaii Medical Assurance Association	PPO
Hawaii	36,505	University Health Alliance	PPO
Hawaii	2,407	CIGNA HealthCare of Hawaii	HMO
Hawaii	368	Great-West Healthcare Hawaii	HMO/PPO
Idaho	75,000,000	UnitedHealthCare of Idaho	HMO/PPO
Idaho	54,000,000	Delta Dental of Idaho	Dental
Idaho	11,596,230	Aetna Health of Idaho	PPO
Idaho	2,200,000	Regence BlueShield of Idaho	Multiple
Idaho	563,000	Blue Cross of Idaho Health Service, Inc.	HMO/PPO

State	Total Enrollment	Organization	Plan Type
Idaho	456,719	IHC: Intermountain Healthcare Health Plan	HMO
Idaho	402,000	SelectHealth	HMO
Idaho	280,000	PacificSource Health Plans: Idaho	HMO/PPO
Idaho	27,000	CIGNA HealthCare of Idaho	PPO
Idaho	14,000	Primary Health Plan	Multiple
Illinois	75,000,000	UnitedHealthCare of Illinois	HMO/PPO
Illinois	57,000,000	VSP: Vision Service Plan of Illinois	Vision
Illinois	54,000,000	Delta Dental of Illinois	Dental
Illinois	13,000,000	Health Care Service Corporation	HMO/PPO
Illinois	7,000,000	Blue Cross & Blue Shield of Illinois	HMO/PPO
Illinois	6,200,000	Dental Network of America	Dental
Illinois	4,500,000	CompBenefits: Illinois	Multiple
Illinois	2,000,000	First Health	PPO
Illinois	1,500,000	OSF Healthcare	HMO
Illinois	1,100,000	CoreSource: Corporate Headquarters	Multiple
Illinois	763,175	Humana Health Insurance of Illinois	HMO/PPO
Illinois	750,000	HealthSmart Preferred Care	PPO
Illinois	475,000	Trustmark Companies	PPO
Illinois	335,000	Health Alliance Medical Plans	HMO/PPO
Illinois	316,000	Preferred Network Access	PPO
Illinois	300,000	First Commonwealth	HMO
Illinois	270,000	CNA Insurance Companies: Illinois	PPO
Illinois	255,494	Health Alliance Medicare	Medicare
Illinois	145,000	Unicare: Illinois	HMO/PPO
Illinois	115,313	Great-West Healthcare Illinois	HMO/PPO
Illinois	100,000	Coventry Health Care of Illinois	HMO
Illinois	64,973	OSF HealthPlans	PPO
Illinois	47,000	Assurant Employee Benefits: Illinois	Multiple
Illinois	45,014	Aetna Health of Illinois	HMO
Illinois	45,000	Medical Associates Health Plan	HMO
Illinois	18,588	CIGNA HealthCare of Illinois	HMO
Indiana	75,000,000	UnitedHealthCare of Indiana	HMO/PPO
Indiana	57,000,000	VSP: Vision Service Plan of Indiana	Vision
Indiana	54,000,000	Delta Dental of Michigan, Ohio and Indiana	Dental
Indiana	36,500,000	Magellan Health Services Indiana	PPO
Indiana	35,000,000	WellPoint: Corporate Office	HMO
Indiana	28,000,000	Anthem Dental Services	Dental
Indiana	2,000,000	Avesis: Indiana	PPO
Indiana	1,600,818	Anthem Blue Cross & Blue Shield of Indiana	HMO
Indiana	900,000	Anthem Blue Cross & Blue Shield of Indiana	HMO/PPO
Indiana	664,318	Encore Health Network	PPO
Indiana	500,000	Meritain Health: Indiana	PPO
Indiana	360,561	Sagamore Health Network	PPO
Indiana	200,000	Health Resources, Inc.	Dental
Indiana	140,000	Deaconess Health Plans	PPO
Indiana	102,506	Humana Health Insurance of Indiana	HMO/PPO
Indiana	90,000	Parkview Total Health	PPO
Indiana	86,000	Advantage Health Solutions	HMO
Indiana	45,014	Aetna Health of Indiana	HMO
Indiana	43,620	Great-West Healthcare Indiana	HMO/PPO
Indiana	43,000	Physicians Health Plan of Northern Indiana	HMO
Indiana	40,000	Cardinal Health Alliance	HMO
Indiana	38,515	Welborn Health Plans	HMO
Indiana	15,153	American Health Network of Indiana	PPO

State	Total Enrollment	Organization	Plan Type
Indiana	10,231	Southeastern Indiana Health Organization	HMO
Indiana	9,678	CIGNA HealthCare of Indiana	HMO
Indiana	8,000	Arnett Health Plans	HMO
Iowa	75,000,000	UnitedHealthCare of Iowa	HMO/PPO
Iowa	54,000,000	Delta Dental of Iowa	Dental
Iowa	11,596,230	Aetna Health of Iowa	PPO
Iowa	7,000,000	Humana Health Insurance of Iowa	HMO/PPO
Iowa	2,000,000	Avesis: Iowa	PPO
Iowa	250,000	Wellmark Blue Cross Blue Shield	HMO
Iowa	50,000	Sanford Health Plan	HMO
Iowa	47,000	Coventry Health Care of Iowa	HMO/PPO
Iowa	45,000	Medical Associates Health Plan: West	HMO
Iowa	34,284	CIGNA HealthCare of Iowa	HMO
Iowa	10,082	Great-West Healthcare Iowa	HMO/PPO
Kansas	75,000,000	UnitedHealthCare of Kansas	HMO/PPO
Kansas	57,000,000	VSP: Vision Service Plan of Kansas	Vision
Kansas	54,000,000	Delta Dental of Kansas	Dental
Kansas	11,596,230	Aetna Health of Kansas	PPO
Kansas	5,000,000	PCC Preferred Chiropractic Care	PPO
Kansas	1,100,000	CoreSource: Kansas (FMH CoreSource)	Multiple
Kansas	898,111	Blue Cross & Blue Shield of Kansas	HMO
Kansas	400,000	Preferred Mental Health Management	Multiple
Kansas	152,000	ProviDRs Care Network	PPO
Kansas	145,000	Unicare: Kansas	HMO/PPO
Kansas	135,000	Advance Insurance Company of Kansas	Multiple
Kansas	100,000	Preferred Vision Care	Vision
Kansas	95,000	Health Partners of Kansas	PPO
Kansas	84,841	Humana Health Insurance of Kansas	HMO/PPO
Kansas	83,151	Preferred Plus of Kansas	HMO
Kansas	73,000	Coventry Health Care of Kansas	HMO/PPO
Kansas	73,000	Mercy Health Plans: Kansas	HMO
Kansas	47,000	Assurant Employee Benefits: Kansas	Multiple
Kansas	33,153	Preferred Health Systems Insurance Company	PPO
Kansas	21,580	Great-West Healthcare Kansas	HMO/PPO
Kansas	9,848	CIGNA HealthCare of Kansas	HMO
Kentucky	75,000,000	CIGNA HealthCare of Kentucky	HMO
Kentucky	75,000,000	UnitedHealthCare of Kentucky	HMO/PPO
Kentucky	54,000,000	Delta Dental of Kentucky	Dental
Kentucky	11,596,230	Aetna Health of Kentucky	PPO
Kentucky	4,000,000	Humana Medicare Plan	Medicare
Kentucky	894,531	Anthem Blue Cross & Blue Shield of Kentucky	HMO
Kentucky	500,000	Meritain Health: Kentucky	PPO
Kentucky	190,000	CHA Health	HMO
Kentucky	170,000	Passport Health Plan	HMO
Kentucky	136,472	Bluegrass Family Health	HMO/PPO
Kentucky	110,000	Preferred Health Plan Inc	PPO
Louisiana	75,000,000	CIGNA HealthCare of Louisiana	HMO
Louisiana	75,000,000	UnitedHealthCare of Louisiana	HMO/PPO
Louisiana	54,000,000	Delta Dental of Georgia	Dental
Louisiana	11,596,230	Aetna Health of Louisiana	PPO
Louisiana	1,172,000	Blue Cross & Blue Shield of Louisiana	HMO/PPO
Louisiana	500,000	Meritain Health: Louisiana	PPO

State	Total Enrollment	Organization	Plan Type
Louisiana	142,000	Humana Health Insurance of Louisiana	HMO/PPO
Louisiana	137,000	Calais Health	Multiple
Louisiana	42,000	Peoples Health	Medicare
Louisiana	41,000	Peoples Health	HMO
Louisiana	30,000	Coventry Health Care of Louisiana	HMO
Louisiana	30,000	DINA Dental Plans	Dental
Louisiana	30,000	Health Plus of Louisiana	HMO
Louisiana	14,000	Vantage Medicare Advantage	Medicare
Louisiana	14,000	Vantage Health Plan	HMO
Maine	75,000,000	UnitedHealthCare of Maine	HMO/PPO
Maine	1,100,000	Harvard Pilgrim Health Care: Maine	Multiple
Maine	545,610	Anthem Blue Cross & Blue Shield of Maine	HMO/PPO
Maine	85,000	Martin's Point HealthCare	Multiple
Maine	22,417	Aetna Health of Maine	HMO
Maine	8,184	Great-West Healthcare Maine	HMO/PPO
Maine	6,343	CIGNA HealthCare of Maine	HMO
Maryland	75,000,000	UnitedHealthCare of the Mid-Atlantic	HMO/PPO
Maryland	54,000,000	Delta Dental of the Mid-Atlantic	Dental
Maryland	36,500,000	Magellan Health Services: Corporate Headquarters	Multiple
Maryland	17,000,000	Spectera	Multiple
Maryland	8,000,000	United Concordia: Maryland	Dental
Maryland	6,600,000	Dental Benefit Providers	Dental
Maryland	5,000,000	Coventry Health Care: Corporate Headquarters	HMO/PPO
Maryland	3,000,000	Block Vision	Vision
Maryland	3,000,000	Catalyst Health Solutions Inc	HMO
Maryland	2,000,000	Avesis: Maryland	PPO
Maryland	1,900,000	Amerigroup Maryland	HMO
Maryland	1,100,000	CoreSource: Maryland	Multiple
Maryland	970,000	OneNet PPO	PPO
Maryland	471,360	Kaiser Permanente Health Plan of the Mid-Atlantic States	HMO
Maryland	360,000	Cigna Health-Spring	Medicare
Maryland	211,156	Aetna Health of Maryland	HMO
Maryland	185,000	Priority Partners Health Plans	HMO
Maryland	180,000	Mid Atlantic Medical Services: Corporate Office	HMO/PPO
Maryland	151,000	Optimum Choice	HMO
Maryland	141,000	American Postal Workers Union (APWU) Health Plan	HMO/PPO
Maryland	109,186	CIGNA HealthCare of the Mid-Atlantic	HMO/PPO
Maryland	10,000	Denta-Chek of Maryland	Multiple
Maryland	8,000	Graphic Arts Benefit Corporation	HMO/PPO
Massachusetts	70,000,000	UnitedHealthCare of Massachusetts	HMO/PPO
Massachusetts	55,000,000	VSP: Vision Service Plan of Massachusetts	Vision
Massachusetts	14,000,000	Dentaquest	Dental
Massachusetts	3,000,000	Blue Cross & Blue Shield of Massachusetts	HMO
Massachusetts	2,000,000	Avesis: Massachusetts	PPO
Massachusetts	2,000,000	Great-West Healthcare of Massachusetts	HMO/PPO
Massachusetts	1,200,000	Health Plan of New York: Massachusetts	HMO/PPO
Massachusetts	1,079,674	Harvard Pilgrim Health Care	Multiple
Massachusetts	737,411	Tufts Health Plan	HMO/PPO
Massachusetts	240,890	Boston Medical Center Healthnet Plan	HMO
Massachusetts	240,000	ConnectiCare of Massachusetts	HMO/PPO
Massachusetts	186,000	Neighborhood Health Plan	HMO
Massachusetts	178,000	Fallon Community Health Plan	HMO/PPO
Massachusetts	106,000	Health New England	HMO

State	Total Enrollment	Organization	Plan Type
Massachusetts	80,000	Unicare: Massachusetts	HMO/PPO
Massachusetts	47,000	Assurant Employee Benefits: Massachusetts	Multiple
Massachusetts	12,000	Health Plans, Inc.	Other
Massachusetts	11,121	Aetna Health of Massachusetts	HMO
Massachusetts	10,315	CIGNA HealthCare of Massachusetts	PPO
Massachusetts	6,443	Harvard University Group Health Plan	HMO
Michigan	75,000,000	UnitedHealthCare of Michigan	HMO/PPO
Michigan	55,000,000	VSP: Vision Service Plan of Michigan	Vision
Michigan	54,000,000	Delta Dental: Corporate Headquarters	Dental
Michigan	11,596,230	Aetna Health of Michigan	PPO
Michigan	8,000,000	United Concordia: Michigan	Dental
Michigan	4,500,000	DenteMax	Dental
Michigan	4,300,000	Blue Cross Blue Shield of Michigan	PPO
Michigan	2,500,000	Cofinity	PPO
Michigan	1,700,000	Unicare: Michigan	HMO
Michigan	1,400,000	Molina Healthcare: Michigan	HMO
Michigan	1,100,000	CoreSource: Michigan (NGS CoreSource)	Multiple
Michigan	620,000	Blue Care Network of Michigan: Corporate Headquarters	HMO
Michigan	620,000	Blue Care Network: Ann Arbor	HMO
Michigan	620,000	Blue Care Network: Flint	HMO
Michigan	620,000	Blue Care Network: Great Lakes, Muskegon Heights	HMO
Michigan	596,220	Priority Health: Corporate Headquarters	HMO
Michigan	500,000	Health Alliance Plan	HMO/PPO
Michigan	500,000	Meritain Health: Michigan	PPO
Michigan	390,000	SVS Vision	Vision
Michigan	383,000	Health Alliance Medicare	Medicare
Michigan	290,000	Health Plan of Michigan	HMO
Michigan	220,000	M-Care	PPO
Michigan	215,000	Great Lakes Health Plan	HMO
Michigan	200,000	HealthPlus of Michigan: Flint	HMO
Michigan	200,000	HealthPlus of Michigan: Saginaw	HMO
Michigan	187,000	Paramount Care of Michigan	HMO/PPO
Michigan	185,000	American Community Mutual Insurance Company	PPO
Michigan	130,000	Golden Dental Plans	Dental
Michigan	112,011	Humana Health Insurance of Michigan	HMO/PPO
Michigan	90,000	Total Health Care	HMO
Michigan	68,942	Physicians Health Plan of Mid-Michigan	HMO
Michigan	50,000	OmniCare: A Coventry Health Care Plan	HMO
Michigan	50,000	CareSource: Michigan	HMO
Michigan	47,000	Assurant Employee Benefits: Michigan	Multiple
Michigan	35,992	Great-West Healthcare Michigan	HMO/PPO
Michigan	25,278	Upper Peninsula Health Plan	HMO
Michigan	17,000	ConnectCare	PPO
Michigan	14,000	HealthPlus Senior Medicare Plan	Medicare
Michigan	8,000	Grand Valley Health Plan	HMO
Minnesota	75,000,000	UnitedHealthCare of Minnesota	HMO/PPO
Minnesota	75,000,000	UnitedHealthCare of Wisconsin: Central	HMO/PPO
Minnesota	70,000,000	UnitedHealthCare of Pennsylvania	HMO/PPO
Minnesota	60,000,000	OptumHealth Care Solutions: Physical Health	Multiple
Minnesota	55,000,000	Security Life Insurance Company of America	Multiple
Minnesota	55,000,000	VSP: Vision Service Plan of Minnesota	Vision
Minnesota	54,000,000	Delta Dental of Minnesota	Dental
Minnesota	11,596,230	Aetna Health of Minnesota	PPO
Minnesota	2,700,000	Blue Cross & Blue Shield of Minnesota	HMO

State	Total Enrollment	Organization	Plan Type
Minnesota	2,000,000	Avesis: Minnesota	PPO
Minnesota	1,600,000	Medica: Corporate Office	PPO
Minnesota	1,250,000	HealthPartners	HMO
Minnesota	500,000	Meritain Health: Minnesota	PPO
Minnesota	250,000	Araz Group	PPO
Minnesota	200,000	UCare Minnesota	HMO/PPO
Minnesota	97,800	PreferredOne	HMO/PPO
Minnesota	80,000	Patient Choice	PPO
Minnesota	75,000	UCare Medicare Plan	Medicare
Minnesota	64,977	CIGNA HealthCare of Minnesota	HMO
Minnesota	47,000	Assurant Employee Benefits: Minnesota	Multiple
Minnesota	21,000	Metropolitan Health Plan	HMO
Minnesota	18,556	Great-West Healthcare Minnesota	HMO/PPO
Minnesota	3,971	Evercare Health Plans	Medicare
Mississippi	75,000,000	CIGNA HealthCare of Mississippi	HMO
Mississippi	75,000,000	UnitedHealthCare of Mississippi	HMO/PPO
Mississippi	54,000,000	Delta Dental Insurance Company	Dental
Mississippi	11,596,230	Aetna Health of Mississippi	PPO
Mississippi	155,070	Health Link PPO	PPO
Mississippi	78,600	Humana Health Insurance of Mississippi	HMO/PPO
Missouri	75,000,000	UnitedHealthCare of Missouri	HMO/PPO
Missouri	54,000,000	Delta Dental of Missouri	Dental
Missouri	1,700,000	Dental Health Alliance	Dental
Missouri	1,450,000	Centene Corporation	HMO
Missouri	1,400,000	Molina Healthcare: Missouri	HMO
Missouri	1,159,875	BlueChoice	HMO
Missouri	1,100,000	Anthem Blue Cross & Blue Shield of Missouri	PPO
Missouri	1,000,000	Blue Cross & Blue Shield of Kansas City	PPO
Missouri	1,000,000	HealthLink HMO	HMO
Missouri	942,000	American Health Care Alliance	PPO
Missouri	900,000	GEHA-Government Employees Hospital Association	Multiple
Missouri	500,000	Meritain Health: Missouri	PPO
Missouri	330,000	GHP Coventry Health Plan	HMO/PPO
Missouri	238,976	Preferred Care Blue	PPO
Missouri	185,375	Healthcare USA of Missouri	HMO
Missouri	119,600	Mid America Health	HMO/PPO
Missouri	73,000	Mercy Health Plans: Corporate Office	HMO
Missouri	67,308	Great-West Healthcare Missouri	HMO/PPO
Missouri	49,976	Children's Mercy Pediatric Care Network	HMO
Missouri	47,000	Assurant Employee Benefits: Corporate Headquarters	Multiple
Missouri	10,885	Aetna Health of Missouri	HMO
Missouri	8,049	CIGNA HealthCare of St. Louis	HMO
Missouri	7,000	Community Health Improvement Solutions	HMO
Missouri	5,000	Cox Healthplans	HMO/PPO
Montana	75,000,000	UnitedHealthCare of Montana	HMO/PPO
Montana	54,000,000	Delta Dental of Montana	Dental
Montana	11,596,230	Aetna Health of Montana	PPO
Montana	236,000	Blue Cross & Blue Shield of Montana	HMO
Montana	80,000	Health InfoNet	PPO
Montana	43,000	New West Health Services	HMO/PPO
Montana	43,000	New West Medicare Plan	Medicare
Montana	7,642	CIGNA HealthCare of Montana	HMO
Montana	4,970	Great-West Healthcare Montana	HMO/PPO

State	Total Enrollment	Organization	Plan Type
Nebraska	75,000,000	UnitedHealthCare of Nebraska	HMO/PPO
Nebraska	54,000,000	Delta Dental of Nebraska	Dental
Nebraska	11,596,230	Aetna Health of Nebraska	PPO
Nebraska	2,543,705	Ameritas Group	Dental
Nebraska	717,000	Blue Cross & Blue Shield of Nebraska	PPO
Nebraska	615,000	Midlands Choice	PPO
Nebraska	54,418	Mutual of Omaha Health Plans	HMO/PPO
Nebraska	54,000	Coventry Health Care of Nebraska	HMO/PPO
Nebraska	18,322	CIGNA HealthCare of Nebraska	PPO
Nevada	600,000	Behavioral Healthcare Options, Inc.	HMO/PPO
Nevada	580,000	UnitedHealthcare Nevada	HMO/PPO
Nevada	418,000	Health Plan of Nevada	HMO/PPO
Nevada	150,000	Nevada Preferred Healthcare Providers	HMO/PPO
Nevada	150,000	Nevada Preferred Healthcare Providers	PPO
Nevada	109,089	Aetna Health of Nevada	HMO
Nevada	85,000	Amerigroup Nevada	HMO
Nevada	32,000	Hometown Health Plan	Multiple
Nevada	26,000	PacifiCare of Nevada	HMO
Nevada	15,000	Saint Mary's Health Plans	HMO
Nevada	3,000	NevadaCare	HMO
New Hampshire	75,000,000	UnitedHealthCare of New Hampshire	HMO/PPO
New Hampshire	11,596,230	Aetna Health of New Hampshire	PPO
New Hampshire	1,100,000	Harvard Pilgrim Health Care of New England	Multiple
New Hampshire	750,000	MVP Health Care: New Hampshire	HMO/PPO
New Hampshire	745,000	Delta Dental of New Hampshire	Dental
New Hampshire	560,000	Anthem Blue Cross & Blue Shield of New Hampshire	HMO
New Hampshire	23,559	CIGNA HealthCare of New Hampshire	HMO
New Jersey	75,000,000	UnitedHealthCare of New Jersey	HMO/PPO
New Jersey	55,000,000	VSP: Vision Service Plan of New Jersey	Vision
New Jersey	54,000,000	Delta Dental of New Jersey & Connecticut	Dental
New Jersey	5,183,333	Aetna Health of New Jersey	HMO
New Jersey	3,600,000	Horizon Blue Cross & Blue Shield of New Jersey	HMO/PPO
New Jersey	3,600,000	Horizon Healthcare of New Jersey	HMO/PPO
New Jersey	1,900,000	Amerigroup New Jersey	HMO
New Jersey	975,000	CHN PPO	PPO
New Jersey	750,000	QualCare	HMO/PPO
New Jersey	500,000	HealthFirst New Jersey Medicare Plan	Medicare
New Jersey	467,000	Horizon NJ Health	PPO
New Jersey	332,840	Oxford Health Plans: New Jersey	HMO
New Jersey	300,000	Block Vision of New Jersey	Vision
New Jersey	265,000	AmeriHealth HMO	HMO/PPO
New Jersey	200,871	AmeriChoice by UnitedHealthCare	HMO
New Jersey	150,000	Atlanticare Health Plans	HMO/PPO
New Jersey	68,935	CIGNA HealthCare of New Jersey	HMO
New Jersey	47,000	Assurant Employee Benefits: New Jersey	Multiple
New Jersey	21,000	Rayant Insurance Company	Dental
New Jersey	12,317	WellChoice	HMO
New Mexico	75,000,000	UnitedHealthCare of New Mexico	HMO/PPO
New Mexico	54,000,000	Delta Dental of New Mexico	Dental
New Mexico	11,596,230	Aetna Health of New Mexico	PPO
New Mexico	8,000,000	United Concordia: New Mexico	Dental

State	Total Enrollment	Organization	Plan Type
New Mexico	1,900,000	Amerigroup New Mexico	HMO
New Mexico	1,400,000	Molina Healthcare: New Mexico	HMO
New Mexico	400,000	Presbyterian Health Plan	HMO
New Mexico	367,000	Blue Cross & Blue Shield of New Mexico	HMO/PPO
New Mexico	200,000	Lovelace Medicare Health Plan	HMO/PPO
New Mexico	163,000	Lovelace Health Plan	HMO
New Mexico	10,816	Great-West Healthcare New Mexico	HMO/PPO
New York	75,000,000	UnitedHealthCare of New York	HMO/PPO
New York	55,000,000	Davis Vision	Vision
New York	54,000,000	Delta Dental of the Mid-Atlantic	Dental
New York	19,000,000	MultiPlan, Inc.	PPO
New York	8,000,000	United Concordia: New York	Dental
New York	4,450,116	Coalition America's National Preferred Provider Network	PPO
New York	2,000,000	Healthplex	Dental
New York	2,000,000	Universal American Medicare Plans	Medicare
New York	1,900,000	Amerigroup New York	HMO
New York	1,850,000	National Medical Health Card	Multiple
New York	1,700,000	Excellus Blue Cross Blue Shield: Central New York	HMO
New York	1,700,000	Excellus Blue Cross Blue Shield: Rochester Region	HMO
New York	1,700,000	Excellus Blue Cross Blue Shield: Utica Region	HMO
New York	1,700,000	Univera Healthcare	HMO
New York	1,601,000	GHI	HMO/PPO
New York	1,500,000	Oxford Health Plans: New York	HMO
New York	1,326,000	MagnaCare	PPO
New York	1,200,000	Health Plan of New York	HMO/PPO
New York	750,000	MVP Health Care: Buffalo Region	HMO/PPO
New York	750,000	MVP Health Care: Central New York	HMO/PPO
New York	750,000	MVP Health Care: Corporate Office	HMO/PPO
New York	750,000	MVP Health Care: Mid-State Region	HMO/PPO
New York	750,000	MVP Health Care: Western New York	HMO/PPO
New York	625,000	Fidelis Care	Multiple
New York	555,405	Blue Cross & Blue Shield of Western New York	HMO/PPO
New York	553,000	HealthNow New York - Emblem Health	HMO
New York	500,000	Meritain Health: Corporate Headquarters	PPO
New York	400,000	CDPHP Medicare Plan	Medicare
New York	365,000	Independent Health	HMO
New York	350,000	CDPHP: Capital District Physicians' Health Plan	HMO/PPO
New York	332,128	MetroPlus Health Plan	HMO
New York	240,000	ConnectiCare of New York	HMO/PPO
New York	205,677	Guardian Life Insurance Company of America	HMO/PPO
New York	200,000	Vytra Health Plans	HMO/PPO
New York	193,498	BlueShield of Northeastern New York	HMO/PPO
New York	171,028	Empire Blue Cross & Blue Shield	HMO/PPO
New York	154,162	Aetna Health of New York	PPO
New York	134,837	Affinity Health Plan	HMO
New York	107,387	AmeriChoice by UnitedHealthCare	HMO
New York	81,000	Humana Health Insurance of New York	HMO/PPO
New York	80,000	NOVA Healthcare Administrators	Other
New York	53,000	GHI Medicare Plan	Medicare
New York	52,000	Island Group Administration, Inc.	Multiple
New York	40,319	CIGNA HealthCare of New York	HMO
New York	30,000	Easy Choice Health Plan	HMO
New York	28,785	Great-West Healthcare New York	HMO/PPO
New York	19,000	Quality Health Plans of New York	Medicare
New York	19,000	Quality Health Plans	Medicare

State	Total Enrollment	Organization	Plan Type
New York	16,000	Elderplan	Medicare
New York	11,000	Touchstone Health HMO	Medicare
New York	9,000	Perfect Health Insurance Company	PPO
North Carolina	75,000,000	UnitedHealthCare of North Carolina	HMO/PPO
North Carolina	54,000,000	Delta Dental of North Carolina	Dental
North Carolina	8,000,000	United Concordia: North Carolina	Dental
North Carolina	5,000,000	Catalyst RX	PPO
North Carolina	3,718,355	Blue Cross & Blue Shield of North Carolina	HMO/PPO
North Carolina	1,100,000	CoreSource: North Carolina	Multiple
North Carolina	1,000,000	OptiCare Managed Vision	Vision
North Carolina	670,000	MedCost	PPO
North Carolina	494,200	Humana Health Insurance of North Carolina	HMO/PPO
North Carolina	180,000	Mid Atlantic Medical Services: North Carolina	HMO/PPO
North Carolina	160,000	WellPath: A Coventry Health Care Plan	HMO
North Carolina	56,422	Great-West Healthcare North Carolina	HMO/PPO
North Carolina	47,000	Assurant Employee Benefits: North Carolina	Multiple
North Carolina	40,000	Crescent Health Solutions	PPO
North Carolina	29,583	CIGNA HealthCare of North Carolina	HMO
North Carolina	18,960	Aetna Health of the Carolinas	HMO
North Carolina	13,000	FirstCarolinaCare	HMO
North Dakota	75,000,000	UnitedHealthCare of North Dakota	HMO/PPO
North Dakota	54,000,000	Delta Dental of North Dakota	Dental
North Dakota	11,596,230	Aetna Health of North Dakota	PPO
North Dakota	1,600,000	Medica: North Dakota	HMO
North Dakota	434,000	Noridian Insurance Services	PPO
North Dakota	1,000	Heart of America Health Plan	HMO
North Dakota	884	Great-West Healthcare North Dakota	HMO/PPO
Ohio	159,000,000	EyeMed Vision Care	Vision
Ohio	75,000,000	UnitedHealthCare of Ohio: Columbus	HMO/PPO
Ohio	75,000,000	UnitedHealthCare of Ohio: Dayton & Cincinnati	HMO/PPO
Ohio	55,000,000	VSP: Vision Service Plan of Ohio	Vision
Ohio	54,000,000	Delta Dental of Michigan, Ohio and Indiana	Dental
Ohio	3,000,000	Anthem Blue Cross & Blue Shield of Ohio	PPO
Ohio	1,900,000	Amerigroup Ohio	HMO
Ohio	1,400,000	Molina Healthcare: Ohio	HMO
Ohio	1,107,000	Medical Mutual of Ohio	HMO/PPO
Ohio	1,100,000	CoreSource: Ohio	Multiple
Ohio	1,000,000	Interplan Health Group	PPO
Ohio	840,000	CareSource	HMO
Ohio	500,000	Aultcare Corporation	HMO/PPO
Ohio	500,000	Meritain Health: Ohio	PPO
Ohio	380,000	The Health Plan of the Ohio Valley/Mountaineer Region	HMO/PPO
Ohio	370,000	Ohio Health Choice	PPO
Ohio	269,392	The Dental Care Plus Group	Dental
Ohio	187,000	Paramount Elite Medicare Plan	Medicare
Ohio	187,000	Paramount Health Care	HMO/PPO
Ohio	159,375	Aetna Health of Ohio	HMO
Ohio	155,000	SummaCare Health Plan	HMO/PPO
Ohio	110,000	Kaiser Permanente Health Plan Ohio	HMO
Ohio	108,000	HealthSpan	PPO
Ohio	103,000	Unison Health Plan of Ohio	HMO
Ohio	100,000	Humana Health Insurance of Ohio	HMO/PPO
Ohio	100,000	OhioHealth Group	PPO

State	Total Enrollment	Organization	Plan Type
Ohio	52,000	Ohio State University Health Plan Inc.	Multiple
Ohio	47,000	Assurant Employee Benefits: Ohio	Multiple
Ohio	28,125	Mount Carmel Health Plan Inc (MediGold)	Medicare
Ohio	26,000	SummaCare Medicare Advantage Plan	Medicare
Oklahoma	75,000,000	CIGNA HealthCare of Oklahoma	HMO/PPO
Oklahoma	70,000,000	UnitedHealthCare of Oklahoma	HMO/PPO
Oklahoma	54,000,000	Delta Dental of Oklahoma	Dental
Oklahoma	22,000,000	Aetna Health of Oklahoma	HMO
Oklahoma	600,000	Blue Cross & Blue Shield of Oklahoma	HMO/PPO
Oklahoma	522,248	BlueLincs HMO	HMO
Oklahoma	250,000	CommunityCare Managed Healthcare Plans of Oklahoma	HMO/PPO
Oklahoma	73,000	Mercy Health Plans: Oklahoma	HMO
Oklahoma	47,000	Assurant Employee Benefits: Oklahoma	Multiple
Oklahoma	43,000	PacifiCare of Oklahoma	HMO
Oklahoma	18,335	Great-West Healthcare Oklahoma	HMO/PPO
Oregon	75,000,000	UnitedHealthCare of Oregon	HMO/PPO
Oregon	55,000,000	VSP: Vision Service Plan of Oregon	Vision
Oregon	11,596,230	Aetna Health of Oregon	PPO
Oregon	8,000,000	United Concordia: Oregon	Dental
Oregon	2,500,000	Regence Blue Cross & Blue Shield of Oregon	PPO
Oregon	1,500,000	Lifewise Health Plan of Oregon	PPO
Oregon	1,500,000	ODS Health Plan	Multiple
Oregon	471,000	Kaiser Permanente Health Plan of the Northwest	HMO
Oregon	350,000	Providence Health Plans	HMO/PPO
Oregon	280,000	PacificSource Health Plans: Corporate Headquarters	HMO/PPO
Oregon	131,096	CareOregon Health Plan	Medicare
Oregon	129,120	Managed HealthCare Northwest	PPO
Oregon	126,000	CIGNA HealthCare of Oregon	PPO
Oregon	123,000	Health Net Health Plan of Oregon	HMO/PPO
Oregon	47,000	Assurant Employee Benefits: Oregon	Multiple
Oregon	39,334	Great-West Healthcare Oregon	HMO/PPO
Oregon	35,000	Clear One Health Plans	Multiple
Oregon	30,000	Samaritan Health Plan	Multiple
Oregon	29,000	PacifiCare of Oregon	HMO
Oregon	2,000	FamilyCare Health Medicare Plan	Medicare
Pennsylvania	54,000,000	Delta Dental of the Mid-Atlantic	Dental
Pennsylvania	22,000,000	Value Behavioral Health of Pennsylvania	PPO
Pennsylvania	11,000,000	CIGNA: Corporate Headquarters	HMO
Pennsylvania	6,000,000	United Concordia	Dental
Pennsylvania	4,900,000	Highmark Blue Cross & Blue Shield	HMO/PPO
Pennsylvania	3,400,000	Keystone Health Plan East	HMO/PPO
Pennsylvania	3,300,000	Independence Blue Cross	HMO/PPO
Pennsylvania	3,100,000	American WholeHealth Network	PPO
Pennsylvania	3,000,000	Devon Health Services	PPO
Pennsylvania	1,100,000	CoreSource: Pennsylvania	Multiple
Pennsylvania	700,000	InterGroup Services Corporation	PPO
Pennsylvania	600,000	Highmark Blue Shield	PPO
Pennsylvania	550,000	Blue Cross of Northeastern Pennsylvania	HMO/PPO
Pennsylvania	500,000	HealthAmerica	Multiple
Pennsylvania	500,000	HealthAmerica Pennsylvania	Multiple
Pennsylvania	409,265	Aetna Health of Pennsylvania	HMO
Pennsylvania	360,000	Bravo Health: Pennsylvania	Medicare
Pennsylvania	290,000	Geisinger Health Plan	HMO/PPO

State	Total Enrollment	Organization	Plan Type
Pennsylvania	244,000	Gateway Health Plan	HMO
Pennsylvania	186,425	Preferred Care	PPO
Pennsylvania	180,000	Mid Atlantic Medical Services: Pennsylvania	HMO/PPO
Pennsylvania	174,309	Valley Preferred	Multiple
Pennsylvania	170,000	Health Partners Medicare Plan	Medicare
Pennsylvania	160,000	Unison Health Plan of Pennsylvania	Multiple
Pennsylvania	143,488	CIGNA HealthCare of Pennsylvania	HMO
Pennsylvania	121,000	Capital Blue Cross	HMO/PPO
Pennsylvania	115,400	First Priority Health	HMO
Pennsylvania	101,000	UPMC Health Plan	Multiple
Pennsylvania	93,000	Keystone Health Plan Central	HMO
Pennsylvania	80,316	Preferred Health Care	PPO
Pennsylvania	71,000	Americhoice of Pennsylvania	Multiple
Pennsylvania	60,353	Berkshire Health Partners	PPO
Pennsylvania	60,000	American Health Care Group	HMO/PPO
Pennsylvania	56,000	South Central Preferred	PPO
Pennsylvania	50,000	Blue Ridge Health Network	PPO
Pennsylvania	47,000	Assurant Employee Benefits: Pennsylvania	Multiple
Pennsylvania	45,000	Susquehanna Health Care	PPO
Pennsylvania	33,000	Prime Source Health Network	PPO
Pennsylvania	26,411	Great-West Healthcare Pennsylvania	HMO/PPO
Pennsylvania	20,000	Preferred Healthcare System	PPO
Pennsylvania	18,500	Penn Highlands Health Plan	PPO
Pennsylvania	15,700	SelectCare Access Corporation	PPO
Pennsylvania	12,700	Central Susquehanna Healthcare Providers	PPO
Pennsylvania	2,375	Val-U-Health	PPO
Puerto Rico	75,000,000	CIGNA HealthCare of Puerto Rico	PPO
Puerto Rico	75,000,000	UnitedHealthCare of Puerto Rico	HMO/PPO
Puerto Rico	370,000	Humana Health Insurance of Puerto Rico	HMO/PPO
Puerto Rico	300,000	Medical Card System (MCS)	Multiple
Puerto Rico	180,000	First Medical Health Plan	Multiple
Puerto Rico	126,000	MMM Healthcare	Multiple
Puerto Rico	100,000	Triple-S Salud Blue Cross Blue Shield of Puerto Rico	Multiple
Puerto Rico	53,000	PMC Medicare Choice	Medicare
Rhode Island	70,000,000	CVS CareMark	Other
Rhode Island	70,000,000	UnitedHealthCare of Rhode Island	HMO/PPO
Rhode Island	59,500,000	Delta Dental of Rhode Island	Dental
Rhode Island	11,596,230	Aetna Health of Rhode Island	PPO
Rhode Island	1,018,589	Tufts Health Plan: Rhode Island	HMO/PPO
Rhode Island	600,000	Blue Cross & Blue Shield of Rhode Island	HMO
Rhode Island	90,000	Neighborhood Health Plan of Rhode Island	HMO
South Carolina	75,000,000	CIGNA HealthCare of South Carolina	HMO
South Carolina	70,000,000	UnitedHealthCare of South Carolina	HMO/PPO
South Carolina	55,000,000	VSP: Vision Service Plan of South Carolina	Vision
South Carolina	1,400,000	Delta Dental of South Carolina	Dental
South Carolina	950,000	Blue Cross & Blue Shield of South Carolina	HMO/PPO
South Carolina	234,000	Select Health of South Carolina	HMO
South Carolina	205,000	BlueChoice Health Plan of South Carolina	Multiple
South Carolina	144,000	Medical Mutual Services	PPO
South Carolina	123,000	Carolina Care Plan	HMO
South Carolina	47,000	Assurant Employee Benefits: South Carolina	Multiple
South Carolina	30,000	InStil Health	Medicare
South Carolina	19,468	Kanawha Healthcare Solutions	PPO

State	Total Enrollment	Organization	Plan Type
South Carolina	18,960	Aetna Health of the Carolinas	HMO
South Carolina	16,852	Great-West Healthcare South Carolina	HMO/PPO
South Dakota	75,000,000	UnitedHealthCare of South Dakota	HMO/PPO
South Dakota	60,000,000	Delta Dental of South Dakota	Dental
South Dakota	11,596,230	Aetna Health of South Dakota	PPO
South Dakota	3,000,000	eHealthInsurance Services Inc.	HMO/PPO
South Dakota	1,800,000	Wellmark Blue Cross & Blue Shield of South Dakota	PPO
South Dakota	1,600,000	Medica: South Dakota	HMO
South Dakota	118,600	DakotaCare	HMO
South Dakota	87,000	First Choice of the Midwest	PPO
South Dakota	63,000	Avera Health Plans	HMO
South Dakota	8,135	CIGNA HealthCare of South Dakota	PPO
South Dakota	1,685	Great-West Healthcare South Dakota	HMO/PPO
Tennessee	75,000,000	CIGNA HealthCare of Tennessee	HMO
Tennessee	70,000,000	UnitedHealthCare of Tennessee	HMO/PPO
Tennessee	3,000,000	Blue Cross & Blue Shield of Tennessee	HMO/PPO
Tennessee	2,700,000	Amerigroup Tennessee	HMO
Tennessee	1,200,000	Delta Dental of Tennessee	Dental
Tennessee	551,309	John Deere Health	HMO/PPO
Tennessee	518,000	Health Choice LLC	PPO
Tennessee	423,244	Baptist Health Services Group	Other
Tennessee	345,000	HealthSpring: Corporate Offices	Medicare
Tennessee	200,000	Initial Group	PPO
Tennessee	172,000	Humana Health Insurance of Tennessee	HMO/PPO
Tennessee	80,000	Signature Health Alliance	PPO
Tennessee	75,000	Windsor Medicare Extra	Medicare
Tennessee	73,000	Cariten Healthcare	Multiple
Tennessee	50,919	Cariten Preferred	PPO
Tennessee	48,477	HealthPartners	PPO
Tennessee	47,000	Assurant Employee Benefits: Tennessee	Multiple
Tennessee	24,054	Aetna Health of Tennessee	HMO
Texas	75,000,000	CIGNA HealthCare of North Texas	HMO/PPO
Texas	75,000,000	CIGNA HealthCare of South Texas	HMO
Texas	70,000,000	UnitedHealthCare of Texas	HMO/PPO
Texas	59,000,000	Delta Dental of Texas	Dental
Texas	55,000,000	VSP: Vision Service Plan of Texas	Vision
Texas	22,000,000	Aetna Health of Texas	HMO
Texas	8,000,000	United Concordia: Texas	Dental
Texas	5,427,579	USA Managed Care Organization	PPO
Texas	4,000,000	Blue Cross & Blue Shield of Texas: Houston	HMO/PPO
Texas	3,800,000	HMO Blue Texas	HMO
Texas	3,645,891	Blue Cross & Blue Shield of Texas	HMO/PPO
Texas	3,500,000	Galaxy Health Network	PPO
Texas	2,000,000	Avesis: Texas	PPO
Texas	2,000,000	MHNet Behavioral Health	Multiple
Texas	1,900,000	Amerigroup Texas	HMO
Texas	1,800,000	Molina Healthcare: Texas	HMO
Texas	1,800,000	SafeGuard Health Enterprises: Texas	Dental
Texas	1,080,000	HAS-Premier Providers	PPO
Texas	1,080,000	Texas True Choice	PPO
Texas	1,000,000	HealthSpring of Texas	Medicare
Texas	470,623	HealthSmart Preferred Care	PPO
Texas	360,000	Bravo Health: Texas	Medicare

State	Total Enrollment	Organization	Plan Type
Texas	300,000	WellPoint NextRx	Multiple
Texas	230,000	Texas Community Care	Medicare
Texas	203,856	Great-West Healthcare Texas	HMO/PPO
Texas	200,000	Scott & White Health Plan	HMO
Texas	172,000	Humana Health Insurance of Corpus Christi	HMO/PPO
Texas	172,000	Humana Health Insurance of San Antonio	HMO/PPO
Texas	170,000	Parkland Community Health Plan	HMO
Texas	146,000	PacifiCare of Texas	HMO
Texas	130,000	First Care Health Plans	Multiple
Texas	120,000	Horizon Health Corporation	PPO
Texas	110,000	Community First Health Plans	HMO/PPO
Texas	107,539	Healthcare Partners of East Texas	PPO
Texas	80,000	Alliance Regional Health Network	PPO
Texas	73,000	Mercy Health Plans: Texas	HMO
Texas	65,300	Brazos Valley Health Network	PPO
Texas	47,000	Assurant Employee Benefits: Texas	Multiple
Texas	42,000	TexanPlus Medicare Advantage HMO	Medicare
Texas	38,000	Unicare: Texas	HMO/PPO
Texas	30,000	Concentra: Corporate Office	HMO/PPO
Texas	22,000	Valley Baptist Health Plan	HMO
Texas	15,000	Seton Health Plan	HMO
Texas	1,000	UTMB HealthCare Systems	HMO
Texas	1,000	Legacy Health Plan	HMO
Utah	75,000,000	UnitedHealthCare of Utah	HMO/PPO
Utah	54,000,000	Delta Dental of Utah	Dental
Utah	11,596,230	Aetna Health of Utah	PPO
Utah	1,400,000	Molina Healthcare: Utah	HMO
Utah	500,000	Meritain Health: Utah	PPO
Utah	402,000	SelectHealth	HMO
Utah	320,000	Regence Blue Cross & Blue Shield of Utah	PPO
Utah	177,854	Public Employees Health Program	PPO
Utah	150,000	Opticare of Utah	Vision
Utah	148,000	Altius Health Plans	Multiple
Utah	86,000	University Health Plans	HMO/PPO
Utah	47,724	CIGNA HealthCare of Utah	HMO/PPO
Utah	6,000	Educators Mutual	HMO/PPO
Vermont	75,000,000	UnitedHealthCare of Vermont	HMO/PPO
Vermont	54,000,000	Delta Dental of Vermont	Dental
Vermont	11,596,230	Aetna Health of Vermont	PPO
Vermont	750,000	MVP Health Care: Vermont	HMO/PPO
Vermont	180,000	Blue Cross & Blue Shield of Vermont	PPO
Virginia	75,000,000	UnitedHealthCare of Virginia	HMO/PPO
Virginia	56,000,000	Delta Dental of Virginia	Dental
Virginia	24,000,000	Dominion Dental Services	Dental
Virginia	8,000,000	United Concordia: Virginia	Dental
Virginia	3,400,000	CareFirst Blue Cross & Blue Shield of Virginia	HMO/PPO
Virginia	2,800,000	Anthem Blue Cross & Blue Shield of Virginia	HMO
Virginia	1,900,000	Amerigroup Corporation	HMO
Virginia	430,000	Optima Health Plan	HMO/PPO
Virginia	324,600	CIGNA HealthCare of Virginia	HMO
Virginia	211,156	Aetna Health of Virginia	HMO
Virginia	200,000	Coventry Health Care Virginia	HMO/PPO
Virginia	180,000	Mid Atlantic Medical Services: Virginia	HMO/PPO

State	Total Enrollment	Organization	Plan Type
Virginia	143,725	Virginia Premier Health Plan	HMO
Virginia	105,200	Trigon Health Care	HMO
Virginia	100,000	National Capital PPO	PPO
Virginia	88,366	Virginia Health Network	PPO
Virginia	53,000	Peninsula Health Care	HMO/PPO
Virginia	30,000	Piedmont Community Health Plan	PPO
Washington	75,000,000	UnitedHealthCare of Washington	HMO/PPO
Washington	55,000,000	VSP: Vision Service Plan of Washington	Vision
Washington	54,000,000	Delta Dental of Washington	Dental
Washington	11,596,230	Aetna Health of Washington	PPO
Washington	8,000,000	United Concordia: Washington	Dental
Washington	2,200,000	Regence Blue Shield	PPO
Washington	1,500,000	Lifewise Health Plan of Washington	PPO
Washington	1,500,000	Premera Blue Cross	PPO
Washington	1,400,000	Molina Healthcare: Washington	HMO
Washington	600,000	Group Health Cooperative	Multiple
Washington	270,000	Community Health Plan of Washington	Multiple
Washington	240,000	PacifiCare Benefit Administrators	PPO
Washington	120,000	CIGNA HealthCare of Washington	PPO
Washington	47,000	Assurant Employee Benefits: Washington	Multiple
Washington	45,000	PacifiCare of Washington	HMO
Washington	17,000	Puget Sound Health Partners	Medicare
West Virginia	75,000,000	UnitedHealthCare of West Virginia	HMO/PPO
West Virginia	54,000,000	Delta Dental of the Mid-Atlantic	Dental
West Virginia	11,596,230	Aetna Health of West Virginia	PPO
West Virginia	400,000	Mountain State Blue Cross Blue Shield	PPO
West Virginia	180,000	Mid Atlantic Medical Services: West Virginia	HMO/PPO
West Virginia	100,000	Coventry Health Care of West Virginia	HMO/PPO
West Virginia	80,000	Unicare: West Virginia	HMO/PPO
West Virginia	65,000	SelectNet Plus, Inc.	PPO
West Virginia	35,316	CIGNA HealthCare of West Virginia	PPO
West Virginia	11,745	Great-West Healthcare West Virginia	HMO/PPO
Wisconsin	75,000,000	UnitedHealthCare of Wisconsin: Central	HMO/PPO
Wisconsin	54,000,000	Delta Dental of Wisconsin	Dental
Wisconsin	11,596,230	Aetna Health of Wisconsin	PPO
Wisconsin	5,000,000	Vision Insurance Plan of America	Vision
Wisconsin	820,000	HealthEOS	PPO
Wisconsin	247,881	Dean Health Plan	Multiple
Wisconsin	200,000	Care Plus Dental Plans	Dental
Wisconsin	187,000	Security Health Plan of Wisconsin	Multiple
Wisconsin	175,000	Wisconsin Physician's Service	PPO
Wisconsin	150,000	ChiroCare of Wisconsin	PPO
Wisconsin	130,000	Managed Health Services	HMO
Wisconsin	119,712	Prevea Health Network	PPO
Wisconsin	118,000	Network Health Plan of Wisconsin	HMO/PPO
Wisconsin	112,000	Physicians Plus Insurance Corporation	HMO/PPO
Wisconsin	95,000	Group Health Cooperative of Eau Claire	HMO
Wisconsin	90,000	Gundersen Lutheran Health Plan	HMO
Wisconsin	90,000	Unity Health Insurance	Multiple
Wisconsin	72,853	CIGNA HealthCare of Wisconsin	PPO
Wisconsin	61,000	Group Health Cooperative of South Central Wisconsin	HMO
Wisconsin	49,000	Humana Health Insurance of Wisconsin	HMO/PPO
Wisconsin	47,000	Assurant Employee Benefits: Wisconsin	Multiple

State	Total Enrollment	Organization	Plan Type
Wisconsin	40,000	MercyCare Health Plans	HMO
Wisconsin	34,000	Health Tradition	HMO
Wisconsin	28,619	Great-West Healthcare Wisconsin	HMO/PPO
Wisconsin	24,000	ABRI Health Plan, Inc.	Multiple
Wisconsin	5,000	Trilogy Health Insurance	PPO
Wyoming	75,000,000	UnitedHealthCare of Wyoming	HMO/PPO
Wyoming	54,000,000	Delta Dental of Wyoming	Dental
Wyoming	11,596,230	Aetna Health of Wyoming	PPO
Wyoming	100,000	Blue Cross & Blue Shield of Wyoming	PPO
Wyoming	11,234	CIGNA HealthCare of Wyoming	PPO
Wyoming	11,000	WINhealth Partners	Multiple

Managed Care Organizations Ranked by State Enrollment

State	State Enrollment	Organization	Plan Type
Alabama	2,842,000	Blue Cross Preferred Care	PPO
Alabama	2,100,000	Blue Cross & Blue Shield of Alabama	HMO
Alabama	831,000	Beech Street Corporation: Alabama	PPO
Alabama	107,210	UnitedHealthCare of Alabama	HMO/PPO
Alabama	80,000	VIVA Health	HMO
Alabama	45,000	Health Choice of Alabama	PPO
Alabama	17,844	Cigna-HealthSpring of Alabama	Medicare
Alabama	6,662	Great-West Healthcare Alabama	HMO/PPO
Alaska	100,000	Premera Blue Cross Blue Shield of Alaska	PPO
Alaska	6,000	Beech Street: Alaska	PPO
Arizona	1,270,000	UnitedHealthCare of Arizona	HMO/PPO
Arizona	1,000,000	Blue Cross & Blue Shield of Arizona	HMO/PPO
Arizona	435,000	Delta Dental of Arizona	Dental
Arizona	300,000	Mercy Care Plan/Mercy Care Advantage	Medicare
Arizona	120,000	Employers Dental Services	Dental
Arizona	103,561	CIGNA HealthCare of Arizona	HMO/PPO
Arizona	100,000	Phoenix Health Plan	HMO
Arizona	80,000	Magellan Health Services Arizona	PPO
Arizona	60,500	Health Net of Arizona	HMO
Arizona	39,997	Maricopa Integrated Health System/Maricopa Health Plan	HMO
Arizona	26,120	Humana Health Insurance of Arizona	HMO/PPO
Arizona	7,000	Pima Health System	HMO
Arizona	5,048	Great-West Healthcare Arizona	HMO/PPO
Arkansas	1,000,000	Delta Dental of Arkansas	Dental
Arkansas	400,000	Arkansas Blue Cross and Blue Shield	Multiple
Arkansas	200,000	Arkansas Managed Care Organization	PPO
Arkansas	92,995	UnitedHealthCare of Arkansas	HMO/PPO
Arkansas	84,176	QualChoice/QCA Health Plan	HMO/PPO
California	6,700,000	Health Net Medicare Plan	Medicare
California	6,400,000	Kaiser Permanente Health Plan: Corporate Office	HMO
California	3,500,000	Blue Shield of California	HMO/PPO
California	3,284,540	Kaiser Permanente Health Plan of Southern California	HMO
California	3,223,235	Kaiser Permanente Health Plan of Northern California	HMO
California	2,300,000	UnitedHealthCare of Northern California	HMO/PPO
California	2,300,000	UnitedHealthCare of Southern California	HMO/PPO
California	1,700,000	Interplan Health Group	PPO
California	1,345,473	PacifiCare Health Systems	HMO
California	836,724	L.A. Care Health Plan	HMO
California	773,000	Beech Street Corporation: Northeast Region	PPO
California	653,000	Beech Street Corporation: Corporate Office	PPO
California	653,000	Beech Street Corporation: Western Region	HMO
California	575,000	Inland Empire Health Plan	HMO
California	450,000	CIGNA HealthCare of Northern California	HMO
California	450,000	CIGNA HealthCare of Southern California	HMO
California	427,039	Aetna Health of California	HMO
California	402,000	CalOptima	HMO
California	250,000	Lakeside Community Healthcare Network	HMO
California	234,072	CIGNA HealthCare of California	HMO
California	200,000	Community Health Plan of Los Angeles County	HMO

State	State Enrollment	Organization	Plan Type
California	197,000	Pacific Health Alliance	PPO
California	190,000	Central California Alliance for Health	HMO
California	146,000	Community Health Group	HMO
California	121,794	Santa Clara Family Health Foundations Inc	HMO
California	110,000	Alameda Alliance for Health	HMO
California	109,000	Health Plan of San Joaquin	HMO
California	100,000	Contra Costa Health Plan	HMO
California	92,000	Western Health Advantage	HMO
California	90,074	Kern Family Health Care	HMO
California	87,740	Health Plan of San Mateo	HMO
California	57,459	Great-West Healthcare California	HMO/PPO
California	55,000	Arta Medicare Health Plan	Medicare
California	55,000	San Francisco Health Plan	HMO
California	49,000	Sharp Health Plan	HMO
California	34,000	Foundation for Medical Care for Mendocino and Lake Counties	PPO
California	12,283	SCAN Health Plan	HMO
California	8,000	Easy Choice Health Plan	Medicare
California	6,336	Chinese Community Health Plan	HMO
California	942	On Lok Lifeways	HMO
Colorado	1,000,000	Delta Dental of Colorado	Dental
Colorado	735,900	UnitedHealthCare of Colorado	HMO/PPO
Colorado	535,000	Kaiser Permanente Health Plan of Colorado	HMO
Colorado	462,000	CIGNA HealthCare of Colorado	HMO
Colorado	207,180	Rocky Mountain Health Plans	HMO/PPO
Colorado	160,000	Colorado Health Partnerships	HMO
Colorado	154,503	Anthem Blue Cross & Blue Shield of Nevada	HMO/PPO
Colorado	115,262	Great-West/One Health Plan	HMO/PPO
Colorado	113,229	Humana Health Insurance of Colorado Springs	HMO/PPO
Colorado	60,270	Anthem Blue Cross & Blue Shield of Colorado	HMO/PPO
Colorado	36,423	Aetna Health of Colorado	HMO
Colorado	15,000	Denver Health Medical Plan Inc	HMO
Connecticut	391,301	Anthem Blue Cross & Blue Shield Connecticut	HMO/PPO
Connecticut	160,000	ConnectiCare	HMO/PPO
Connecticut	70,139	Oxford Health Plans: Corporate Headquarters	HMO/PPO
Connecticut	61,677	Aetna Health, Inc. Corporate Headquarters	HMO
Connecticut	29,506	CIGNA HealthCare of Connecticut	HMO
Delaware	1,500,000	UnitedHealthCare of Maryland	HMO/PPO
Delaware	321,000	Highmark Blue Cross & Blue Shield Delaware	HMO/PPO
Delaware	27,179	Aetna Health of Delaware	HMO
Delaware	2,508	Great-West Healthcare Delaware	HMO/PPO
Delaware	984	CIGNA HealthCare of Delaware	HMO
District of Columbia	550,000	CareFirst Blue Cross Blue Shield	HMO/PPO
District of Columbia	176,000	UnitedHealthCare of the District of Columbia	HMO/PPO
District of Columbia	100,000	DC Chartered Health Plan	HMO
District of Columbia	90,000	Quality Plan Administrators	HMO/PPO
Florida	2,200,000	WellCare Health Plans	Medicare
Florida	1,373,917	Florida Blue: Jacksonville	HMO/PPO
Florida	870,159	UnitedHealthCare of Florida	HMO/PPO
Florida	521,696	Aetna Health of Florida	HMO
Florida	400,000	Dimension Health PPO	PPO
Florida	350,000	AvMed Health Plan: Orlando	HMO

State	State Enrollment	Organization	Plan Type
Florida	350,000	AvMed Health Plan: Tampa Bay	HMO
Florida	350,000	AvMed Health Plan: Corporate Office	HMO
Florida	350,000	AvMed Health Plan: Fort Lauderdale	HMO
Florida	350,000	AvMed Health Plan: Gainesville	HMO
Florida	350,000	AvMed Health Plan: Jacksonville	HMO
Florida	320,000	First Medical Health Plan of Florida	Medicare
Florida	295,000	UnitedHealthCare of South Florida	HMO/PPO
Florida	237,000	Amerigroup Florida	HMO
Florida	194,944	CIGNA HealthCare of Florida	HMO
Florida	191,000	Universal Health Care Group	Medicare
Florida	141,178	Neighborhood Health Partnership	HMO
Florida	125,000	Capital Health Plan	HMO
Florida	105,000	JMH Health Plan	HMO
Florida	69,000	Molina Healthcare: Florida	HMO
Florida	67,000	CarePlus Health Plans, Inc	HMO
Florida	63,700	Health First Health Plans	HMO
Florida	54,000	Citrus Health Care	Medicare
Florida	39,776	Preferred Medical Plan	HMO
Florida	39,511	Florida Health Care Plan	HMO
Florida	35,000	Healthchoice Orlando	PPO
Florida	15,347	Total Health Choice	HMO
Florida	1,771	Great-West Healthcare Florida	HMO/PPO
Georgia	1,051,334	UnitedHealthCare of Georgia	HMO/PPO
Georgia	500,733	Blue Cross & Blue Shield of Georgia	HMO
Georgia	287,000	Amerigroup Georgia	HMO
Georgia	238,000	Kaiser Foundation Health Plan of Georgia	HMO
Georgia	183,000	Coventry Health Care of GA	HMO/PPO
Georgia	116,375	Aetna Health of Georgia	HMO
Georgia	82,000	Humana Health Insurance of Georgia	HMO/PPO
Georgia	68,000	Secure Health PPO Newtork	PPO
Georgia	42,000	Northeast Georgia Health Partners	PPO
Georgia	25,769	CIGNA HealthCare of Georgia	HMO
Georgia	23,241	Athens Area Health Plan Select	HMO
Georgia	15,000	Alliant Health Plans	HMO/PPO
Georgia	1,545	Great-West Healthcare Georgia	HMO/PPO
Hawaii	692,000	Hawaii Medical Services Association	PPO
Hawaii	229,186	Kaiser Permanente Health Plan of Hawaii	HMO
Hawaii	42,000	Hawaii Medical Assurance Association	PPO
Hawaii	3,902	UnitedHealthCare of Hawaii	HMO/PPO
Hawaii	1,602	CIGNA HealthCare of Hawaii	HMO
Hawaii	213	Great-West Healthcare Hawaii	HMO/PPO
Idaho	2,200,000	Regence BlueShield of Idaho	Multiple
Idaho	563,000	Blue Cross of Idaho Health Service, Inc.	HMO/PPO
Idaho	296,175	IHC: Intermountain Healthcare Health Plan	HMO
Idaho	40,618	UnitedHealthCare of Idaho	HMO/PPO
Illinois	13,000,000	Health Care Service Corporation	HMO/PPO
Illinois	7,000,000	Blue Cross & Blue Shield of Illinois	HMO/PPO
Illinois	2,000,000	Delta Dental of Illinois	Dental
Illinois	763,175	Humana Health Insurance of Illinois	HMO/PPO
Illinois	646,192	UnitedHealthCare of Illinois	HMO/PPO
Illinois	585,000	First Health	PPO
Illinois	316,000	Preferred Network Access	PPO

State	State Enrollment	Organization	Plan Type
Illinois	100,000	Coventry Health Care of Illinois	HMO
Illinois	45,014	Aetna Health of Illinois	HMO
Illinois	37,792	Medical Associates Health Plan	HMO
Illinois	18,588	CIGNA HealthCare of Illinois	HMO
Illinois	9,662	Great-West Healthcare Illinois	HMO/PPO
Illinois	2,732	OSF HealthPlans	PPO
Indiana	450,000	Meritain Health: Indiana	PPO
Indiana	244,441	UnitedHealthCare of Indiana	HMO/PPO
Indiana	132,000	Deaconess Health Plans	PPO
Indiana	61,064	Advantage Health Solutions	HMO
Indiana	48,000	Physicians Health Plan of Northern Indiana	HMO
Indiana	45,086	Arnett Health Plans	HMO
Indiana	40,136	Anthem Blue Cross & Blue Shield of Indiana	HMO
Indiana	10,231	Southeastern Indiana Health Organization	HMO
Indiana	9,678	CIGNA HealthCare of Indiana	HMO
Indiana	900	Humana Health Insurance of Indiana	HMO/PPO
Indiana	718	Great-West Healthcare Indiana	HMO/PPO
Iowa	250,000	Wellmark Blue Cross Blue Shield	HMO
Iowa	74,000	Delta Dental of Iowa	Dental
Iowa	41,644	Coventry Health Care of Iowa	HMO/PPO
Iowa	28,259	CIGNA HealthCare of Iowa	HMO
Iowa	14,412	Medical Associates Health Plan: West	HMO
Iowa	8,337	Great-West Healthcare Iowa	HMO/PPO
Kansas	1,000,000	Preferred Vision Care	Vision
Kansas	880,000	Delta Dental of Kansas	Dental
Kansas	680,466	Blue Cross & Blue Shield of Kansas	HMO
Kansas	132,716	Coventry Health Care of Kansas	HMO/PPO
Kansas	95,000	Health Partners of Kansas	PPO
Kansas	82,778	Preferred Plus of Kansas	HMO
Kansas	40,800	Humana Health Insurance of Kansas	HMO/PPO
Kansas	31,453	Preferred Health Systems Insurance Company	PPO
Kansas	17,258	Great-West Healthcare Kansas	HMO/PPO
Kentucky	570,000	Delta Dental of Kentucky	Dental
Kentucky	450,000	Meritain Health: Kentucky	PPO
Kentucky	170,000	Passport Health Plan	HMO
Kentucky	135,106	UnitedHealthCare of Kentucky	HMO/PPO
Kentucky	110,000	Preferred Health Plan Inc	PPO
Kentucky	67,948	CHA Health	HMO
Kentucky	65,428	Bluegrass Family Health	HMO/PPO
Kentucky	63,698	Anthem Blue Cross & Blue Shield of Kentucky	HMO
Louisiana	1,172,000	Blue Cross & Blue Shield of Louisiana	HMO/PPO
Louisiana	450,000	Meritain Health: Louisiana	PPO
Louisiana	272,972	UnitedHealthCare of Louisiana	HMO/PPO
Louisiana	155,722	Humana Health Insurance of Louisiana	HMO/PPO
Louisiana	71,716	Coventry Health Care of Louisiana	HMO
Louisiana	50,000	Peoples Health	Medicare
Louisiana	30,000	Health Plus of Louisiana	HMO
Louisiana	14,000	Vantage Health Plan	HMO
Louisiana	4,707	Peoples Health	HMO
Maine	85,917	Anthem Blue Cross & Blue Shield of Maine	HMO/PPO

State	State Enrollment	Organization	Plan Type
Maine	67,000	Harvard Pilgrim Health Care: Maine	Multiple
Maine	22,417	Aetna Health of Maine	HMO
Maine	8,078	Great-West Healthcare Maine	HMO/PPO
Maine	6,343	CIGNA HealthCare of Maine	HMO
Maryland	471,360	Kaiser Permanente Health Plan of the Mid-Atlantic States	HMO
Maryland	185,000	Priority Partners Health Plans	HMO
Maryland	176,000	UnitedHealthCare of the Mid-Atlantic	HMO/PPO
Massachusetts	3,000,000	Blue Cross & Blue Shield of Massachusetts	HMO
Massachusetts	240,890	Boston Medical Center Healthnet Plan	HMO
Massachusetts	135,581	Fallon Community Health Plan	HMO/PPO
Massachusetts	106,000	Health New England	HMO
Massachusetts	65,000	Harvard Pilgrim Health Care	Multiple
Massachusetts	25,804	Neighborhood Health Plan	HMO
Massachusetts	19,053	Great-West Healthcare of Massachusetts	HMO/PPO
Massachusetts	11,121	Aetna Health of Massachusetts	HMO
Massachusetts	10,315	CIGNA HealthCare of Massachusetts	PPO
Massachusetts	9,000	ConnectiCare of Massachusetts	HMO/PPO
Michigan	4,300,000	Blue Cross Blue Shield of Michigan	PPO
Michigan	620,000	Blue Care Network of Michigan: Corporate Headquarters	HMO
Michigan	620,000	Blue Care Network: Ann Arbor	HMO
Michigan	620,000	Blue Care Network: Flint	HMO
Michigan	620,000	Blue Care Network: Great Lakes, Muskegon Heights	HMO
Michigan	500,000	Health Alliance Plan	HMO/PPO
Michigan	450,000	Meritain Health: Michigan	PPO
Michigan	250,863	Health Plan of Michigan	HMO
Michigan	215,000	Great Lakes Health Plan	HMO
Michigan	207,319	UnitedHealthCare of Michigan	HMO/PPO
Michigan	200,000	HealthPlus of Michigan: Flint	HMO
Michigan	200,000	HealthPlus of Michigan: Saginaw	HMO
Michigan	146,000	Priority Health	HMO/PPO
Michigan	102,752	Care Choices	HMO
Michigan	90,000	Total Health Care	HMO
Michigan	68,942	Physicians Health Plan of Mid-Michigan	HMO
Michigan	50,000	OmniCare: A Coventry Health Care Plan	HMO
Michigan	50,000	CareSource: Michigan	HMO
Michigan	47,400	Humana Health Insurance of Michigan	HMO/PPO
Michigan	36,000	ConnectCare	PPO
Michigan	31,314	Great-West Healthcare Michigan	HMO/PPO
Michigan	26,599	Grand Valley Health Plan	HMO
Michigan	25,278	Upper Peninsula Health Plan	HMO
Michigan	20,000	Dencap Dental Plans	Dental
Michigan	14,000	HealthPlus Senior Medicare Plan	Medicare
Michigan	3,944	M-Care	PPO
Minnesota	3,500,000	Delta Dental of Minnesota	Dental
Minnesota	2,700,000	Blue Cross & Blue Shield of Minnesota	HMO
Minnesota	450,000	Meritain Health: Minnesota	PPO
Minnesota	392,782	UnitedHealthCare of Wisconsin: Central	HMO/PPO
Minnesota	349,070	HealthPartners	HMO
Minnesota	283,106	UnitedHealthCare of Pennsylvania	HMO/PPO
Minnesota	216,150	PreferredOne	HMO/PPO
Minnesota	160,000	Araz Group	PPO
Minnesota	53,490	CIGNA HealthCare of Minnesota	HMO

State	State Enrollment	Organization	Plan Type
Minnesota	17,322	Great-West Healthcare Minnesota	HMO/PPO
Minnesota	3,971	Evercare Health Plans	Medicare
Mississippi	53,490	CIGNA HealthCare of Mississippi	HMO
Mississippi	2,900	Humana Health Insurance of Mississippi	HMO/PPO
Missouri	1,400,000	Delta Dental of Missouri	Dental
Missouri	1,000,000	Blue Cross & Blue Shield of Kansas City	PPO
Missouri	900,000	Anthem Blue Cross & Blue Shield of Missouri	PPO
Missouri	860,000	American Health Care Alliance	PPO
Missouri	450,000	Meritain Health: Missouri	PPO
Missouri	395,996	HealthLink HMO	HMO
Missouri	330,000	GHP Coventry Health Plan	HMO/PPO
Missouri	185,375	Healthcare USA of Missouri	HMO
Missouri	68,070	BlueChoice	HMO
Missouri	60,000	UnitedHealthCare of Missouri	HMO/PPO
Missouri	49,976	Children's Mercy Pediatric Care Network	HMO
Missouri	47,367	Great-West Healthcare Missouri	HMO/PPO
Missouri	26,000	Med-Pay	Other
Missouri	25,335	Community Health Improvement Solutions	HMO
Missouri	10,885	Aetna Health of Missouri	HMO
Missouri	8,049	CIGNA HealthCare of St. Louis	HMO
Missouri	1,964	Cox Healthplans	HMO/PPO
Montana	236,000	Blue Cross & Blue Shield of Montana	HMO
Montana	56,000	Health InfoNet	PPO
Montana	43,000	New West Health Services	HMO/PPO
Montana	43,000	New West Medicare Plan	Medicare
Montana	17,853	UnitedHealthCare of Montana	HMO/PPO
Montana	5,008	CIGNA HealthCare of Montana	HMO
Montana	3,405	Great-West Healthcare Montana	HMO/PPO
Nebraska	818,531	Ameritas Group	Dental
Nebraska	717,000	Blue Cross & Blue Shield of Nebraska	PPO
Nebraska	602,578	Mutual of Omaha DentaBenefits	Dental
Nebraska	63,000	Coventry Health Care of Nebraska	HMO/PPO
Nebraska	44,000	UnitedHealthCare of Nebraska	HMO/PPO
Nebraska	28,978	Mutual of Omaha Health Plans	HMO/PPO
Nebraska	15,405	CIGNA HealthCare of Nebraska	PPO
Nevada	600,000	Behavioral Healthcare Options, Inc.	HMO/PPO
Nevada	150,000	Nevada Preferred Healthcare Providers	HMO/PPO
Nevada	150,000	Nevada Preferred Healthcare Providers	PPO
Nevada	107,963	UnitedHealthcare Nevada	HMO/PPO
Nevada	28,591	PacifiCare of Nevada	HMO
Nevada	25,576	Health Plan of Nevada	HMO/PPO
Nevada	19,642	NevadaCare	HMO
Nevada	10,000	Hometown Health Plan	Multiple
New Hampshire	700,000	Delta Dental of New Hampshire	Dental
New Hampshire	400,000	Anthem Blue Cross & Blue Shield of New Hampshire	HMO
New Hampshire	139,000	Harvard Pilgrim Health Care of New England	Multiple
New Hampshire	23,559	CIGNA HealthCare of New Hampshire	HMO
New Jersey	3,600,000	Horizon Blue Cross & Blue Shield of New Jersey	HMO/PPO
New Jersey	3,000,000	Horizon Healthcare of New Jersey	HMO/PPO

State	State Enrollment	Organization	Plan Type
New Jersey	750,000	QualCare	HMO/PPO
New Jersey	518,333	Aetna Health of New Jersey	HMO
New Jersey	500,000	HealthFirst New Jersey Medicare Plan	Medicare
New Jersey	467,000	Horizon NJ Health	PPO
New Jersey	431,833	UnitedHealthCare of New Jersey	HMO/PPO
New Jersey	200,000	National Health Plan Corporation	PPO
New Jersey	199,018	AmeriChoice by UnitedHealthCare	HMO
New Jersey	150,000	Atlanticare Health Plans	HMO/PPO
New Jersey	115,000	Family Choice Health Alliance	PPO
New Jersey	105,000	Amerigroup New Jersey	HMO
New Jersey	77,761	AmeriHealth HMO	HMO/PPO
New Jersey	68,935	CIGNA HealthCare of New Jersey	HMO
New Jersey	59,800	Oxford Health Plans: New Jersey	HMO
New Jersey	30,000	Managed Healthcare Systems of New Jersey	HMO
New Jersey	12,317	WellChoice	HMO
New Mexico	400,000	Presbyterian Health Plan	HMO
New Mexico	367,000	Blue Cross & Blue Shield of New Mexico	HMO/PPO
New Mexico	200,000	Delta Dental of New Mexico	Dental
New Mexico	120,937	UnitedHealthCare of New Mexico	HMO/PPO
New Mexico	83,000	Molina Healthcare: New Mexico	HMO
New Mexico	68,674	Lovelace Health Plan	HMO
New Mexico	7,417	Great-West Healthcare New Mexico	HMO/PPO
New York	2,475,666	GHI	HMO/PPO
New York	1,700,000	Excellus Blue Cross Blue Shield: Central New York	HMO
New York	1,700,000	Excellus Blue Cross Blue Shield: Rochester Region	HMO
New York	1,700,000	Excellus Blue Cross Blue Shield: Utica Region	HMO
New York	1,700,000	Univera Healthcare	HMO
New York	928,200	MagnaCare	PPO
New York	625,000	Fidelis Care	Multiple
New York	553,000	HealthNow New York - Emblem Health	HMO
New York	450,000	Meritain Health: Corporate Headquarters	PPO
New York	365,000	Independent Health	HMO
New York	350,000	CDPHP: Capital District Physicians' Health Plan	HMO/PPO
New York	332,128	MetroPlus Health Plan	HMO
New York	295,841	Dentcare Delivery Systems	Dental
New York	222,000	UnitedHealthCare of New York	HMO/PPO
New York	197,194	Blue Cross & Blue Shield of Western New York	HMO/PPO
New York	154,162	Aetna Health of New York	PPO
New York	134,837	Affinity Health Plan	HMO
New York	100,000	NOVA Healthcare Administrators	Other
New York	76,753	Coalition America's National Preferred Provider Network	PPO
New York	76,213	Vytra Health Plans	HMO/PPO
New York	72,563	BlueShield of Northeastern New York	HMO/PPO
New York	40,319	CIGNA HealthCare of New York	HMO
New York	30,000	Easy Choice Health Plan	HMO
New York	24,502	Great-West Healthcare New York	HMO/PPO
New York	15,000	Elderplan	Medicare
New York	3,000	Perfect Health Insurance Company	PPO
North Carolina	3,718,355	Blue Cross & Blue Shield of North Carolina	HMO/PPO
North Carolina	822,170	Preferred Care Select	PPO
North Carolina	670,000	MedCost	PPO
North Carolina	357,768	UnitedHealthCare of North Carolina	HMO/PPO
North Carolina	325,000	Catalyst RX	PPO

State	State Enrollment	Organization	Plan Type
North Carolina	160,000	WellPath: A Coventry Health Care Plan	HMO
North Carolina	53,379	Great-West Healthcare North Carolina	HMO/PPO
North Carolina	40,000	Crescent Health Solutions	PPO
North Carolina	29,583	CIGNA HealthCare of North Carolina	HMO
North Carolina	17,400	Humana Health Insurance of North Carolina	HMO/PPO
North Carolina	13,000	FirstCarolinaCare	HMO
North Dakota	2,049	Heart of America Health Plan	HMO
North Dakota	503	Great-West Healthcare North Dakota	HMO/PPO
Ohio	3,000,000	Anthem Blue Cross & Blue Shield of Ohio	PPO
Ohio	952,000	Delta Dental of Michigan, Ohio and Indiana	Dental
Ohio	501,086	CareSource	HMO
Ohio	450,000	Meritain Health: Ohio	PPO
Ohio	404,052	Humana Health Insurance of Ohio	HMO/PPO
Ohio	380,000	The Health Plan of the Ohio Valley/Mountaineer Region	HMO/PPO
Ohio	370,000	Ohio Health Choice	PPO
Ohio	300,000	Emerald Health PPO	PPO
Ohio	159,375	Aetna Health of Ohio	HMO
Ohio	155,000	SummaCare Health Plan	HMO/PPO
Ohio	135,000	Superior Dental Care	Dental
Ohio	134,949	Kaiser Permanente Health Plan Ohio	HMO
Ohio	100,000	OhioHealth Group	PPO
Ohio	82,000	UnitedHealthCare of Ohio: Columbus	HMO/PPO
Ohio	82,000	UnitedHealthCare of Ohio: Dayton & Cincinnati	HMO/PPO
Ohio	81,760	HealthSpan	PPO
Ohio	73,724	SummaCare Medicare Advantage Plan	Medicare
Ohio	55,000	HMO Health Ohio	HMO
Ohio	52,000	Ohio State University Health Plan Inc.	Multiple
Ohio	28,125	Mount Carmel Health Plan Inc (MediGold)	Medicare
Ohio	5,151	Aultcare Corporation	HMO/PPO
Oklahoma	700,000	Delta Dental of Oklahoma	Dental
Oklahoma	600,000	Blue Cross & Blue Shield of Oklahoma	HMO/PPO
Oklahoma	250,000	CommunityCare Managed Healthcare Plans of Oklahoma	HMO/PPO
Oklahoma	177,243	UnitedHealthCare of Oklahoma	HMO/PPO
Oklahoma	78,785	PacifiCare of Oklahoma	HMO
Oklahoma	31,363	Aetna Health of Oklahoma	HMO
Oklahoma	22,300	CIGNA HealthCare of Oklahoma	HMO/PPO
Oklahoma	16,882	Great-West Healthcare Oklahoma	HMO/PPO
Oklahoma	15,248	BlueLincs HMO	HMO
Oregon	1,500,000	ODS Health Plan	Multiple
Oregon	800,000	Regence Blue Cross & Blue Shield of Oregon	PPO
Oregon	471,000	Kaiser Permanente Health Plan of the Northwest	HMO
Oregon	350,000	Providence Health Plans	HMO/PPO
Oregon	231,125	UnitedHealthCare of Oregon	HMO/PPO
Oregon	131,096	CareOregon Health Plan	Medicare
Oregon	129,120	Managed HealthCare Northwest	PPO
Oregon	82,000	Lifewise Health Plan of Oregon	PPO
Oregon	49,455	PacifiCare of Oregon	HMO
Oregon	35,000	Clear One Health Plans	Multiple
Oregon	30,000	Samaritan Health Plan	Multiple
Oregon	17,100	Health Net Health Plan of Oregon	HMO/PPO
Oregon	3,487	Great-West Healthcare Oregon	HMO/PPO

State	State Enrollment	Organization	Plan Type
Pennsylvania	4,900,000	Highmark Blue Cross & Blue Shield	HMO/PPO
Pennsylvania	3,300,000	Independence Blue Cross	HMO/PPO
Pennsylvania	3,000,000	Devon Health Services	PPO
Pennsylvania	2,600,000	Keystone Health Plan East	HMO/PPO
Pennsylvania	550,000	Blue Cross of Northeastern Pennsylvania	HMO/PPO
Pennsylvania	409,265	Aetna Health of Pennsylvania	HMO
Pennsylvania	395,000	HealthAmerica	Multiple
Pennsylvania	395,000	HealthAmerica Pennsylvania	Multiple
Pennsylvania	375,300	Highmark Blue Shield	PPO
Pennsylvania	244,000	Gateway Health Plan	HMO
Pennsylvania	209,211	UPMC Health Plan	Multiple
Pennsylvania	174,209	Valley Preferred	Multiple
Pennsylvania	170,000	Health Partners Medicare Plan	Medicare
Pennsylvania	146,000	Preferred Care	PPO
Pennsylvania	116,465	Capital Blue Cross	HMO/PPO
Pennsylvania	110,736	Americhoice of Pennsylvania	Multiple
Pennsylvania	60,353	Berkshire Health Partners	PPO
Pennsylvania	56,000	South Central Preferred	PPO
Pennsylvania	50,000	Blue Ridge Health Network	PPO
Pennsylvania	45,000	Susquehanna Health Care	PPO
Pennsylvania	33,000	Prime Source Health Network	PPO
Pennsylvania	21,997	Great-West Healthcare Pennsylvania	HMO/PPO
Pennsylvania	18,500	Penn Highlands Health Plan	PPO
Pennsylvania	12,700	Central Susquehanna Healthcare Providers	PPO
Pennsylvania	11,969	CIGNA: Corporate Headquarters	HMO
Pennsylvania	13	CIGNA HealthCare of Pennsylvania	HMO
Puerto Rico	180,000	First Medical Health Plan	Multiple
Puerto Rico	100,000	Triple-S Salud Blue Cross Blue Shield of Puerto Rico	Multiple
Rhode Island	587,000	Delta Dental of Rhode Island	Dental
Rhode Island	92,000	UnitedHealthCare of Rhode Island	HMO/PPO
Rhode Island	90,000	Neighborhood Health Plan of Rhode Island	HMO
South Carolina	950,000	Blue Cross & Blue Shield of South Carolina	HMO/PPO
South Carolina	234,000	Select Health of South Carolina	HMO
South Carolina	205,000	BlueChoice Health Plan of South Carolina	Multiple
South Carolina	148,404	UnitedHealthCare of South Carolina	HMO/PPO
South Carolina	123,000	Carolina Care Plan	HMO
South Carolina	19,468	Kanawha Healthcare Solutions	PPO
South Carolina	15,452	Great-West Healthcare South Carolina	HMO/PPO
South Carolina	14,341	CIGNA HealthCare of South Carolina	HMO
South Dakota	300,000	Wellmark Blue Cross & Blue Shield of South Dakota	PPO
South Dakota	245,000	Americas PPO	PPO
South Dakota	204,000	Delta Dental of South Dakota	Dental
South Dakota	63,000	Avera Health Plans	HMO
South Dakota	25,000	First Choice of the Midwest	PPO
South Dakota	24,310	DakotaCare	HMO
South Dakota	6,570	CIGNA HealthCare of South Dakota	PPO
South Dakota	1,430	Great-West Healthcare South Dakota	HMO/PPO
Tennessee	3,000,000	Blue Cross & Blue Shield of Tennessee	HMO/PPO
Tennessee	518,000	Health Choice LLC	PPO
Tennessee	379,224	Signature Health Alliance	PPO
Tennessee	270,665	UnitedHealthCare of Tennessee	HMO/PPO

State	State Enrollment	Organization	Plan Type
Tennessee	251,418	John Deere Health	HMO/PPO
Tennessee	229,356	CIGNA HealthCare of Tennessee	HMO
Tennessee	106,364	Initial Group	PPO
Tennessee	50,919	Cariten Preferred	PPO
Tennessee	48,477	HealthPartners	PPO
Tennessee	35,800	Humana Health Insurance of Tennessee	HMO/PPO
Tennessee	24,054	Aetna Health of Tennessee	HMO
Tennessee	17,844	HealthSpring: Corporate Offices	Medicare
Tennessee	14,477	Cariten Healthcare	Multiple
Texas	4,000,000	Block Vision of Texas	Vision
Texas	3,200,000	Galaxy Health Network	PPO
Texas	2,720,162	Blue Cross & Blue Shield of Texas: Houston	HMO/PPO
Texas	1,862,466	UnitedHealthCare of Texas	HMO/PPO
Texas	1,118,582	USA Managed Care Organization	PPO
Texas	1,080,000	HAS-Premier Providers	PPO
Texas	1,080,000	Texas True Choice	PPO
Texas	394,011	HealthSmart Preferred Care	PPO
Texas	310,853	Blue Cross & Blue Shield of Texas	HMO/PPO
Texas	294,566	Aetna Health of Texas	HMO
Texas	275,000	Interplan Health Group	PPO
Texas	200,000	Scott & White Health Plan	HMO
Texas	177,539	Healthcare Partners of East Texas	PPO
Texas	130,000	First Care Health Plans	Multiple
Texas	111,877	CIGNA HealthCare of North Texas	HMO/PPO
Texas	111,877	CIGNA HealthCare of South Texas	HMO
Texas	110,000	Community First Health Plans	HMO/PPO
Texas	79,500	Alliance Regional Health Network	PPO
Texas	78,139	Brazos Valley Health Network	PPO
Texas	65,000	Medical Care Referral Group	PPO
Texas	47,755	PacifiCare of Texas	HMO
Texas	12,334	Great-West Healthcare Texas	HMO/PPO
Texas	12,004	Valley Baptist Health Plan	HMO
Texas	1,500	Dental Source: Dental Health Care Plans	Dental
Utah	450,000	Meritain Health: Utah	PPO
Utah	231,824	Regence Blue Cross & Blue Shield of Utah	PPO
Utah	177,854	Public Employees Health Program	PPO
Utah	150,000	Opticare of Utah	Vision
Utah	109,709	UnitedHealthCare of Utah	HMO/PPO
Utah	84,000	Altius Health Plans	Multiple
Utah	65,000	Educators Mutual	HMO/PPO
Utah	50,000	University Health Plans	HMO/PPO
Utah	4,198	CIGNA HealthCare of Utah	HMO/PPO
Vermont	54,023	Blue Cross & Blue Shield of Vermont	PPO
Virginia	2,800,000	Anthem Blue Cross & Blue Shield of Virginia	HMO
Virginia	490,000	Dominion Dental Services	Dental
Virginia	430,000	Optima Health Plan	HMO/PPO
Virginia	200,000	Coventry Health Care Virginia	HMO/PPO
Virginia	169,621	Virginia Premier Health Plan	HMO
Virginia	88,366	Virginia Health Network	PPO
Virginia	55,017	Peninsula Health Care	HMO/PPO
Virginia	44,458	National Capital PPO	PPO
Virginia	30,000	Piedmont Community Health Plan	PPO

State	State Enrollment	Organization	Plan Type
Virginia	28,460	CIGNA HealthCare of Virginia	HMO
Washington	2,000,000	Delta Dental of Washington	Dental
Washington	1,500,000	Premera Blue Cross	PPO
Washington	624,000	UnitedHealthCare of Washington	HMO/PPO
Washington	270,000	Community Health Plan of Washington	Multiple
Washington	263,795	Molina Healthcare: Washington	HMO
Washington	87,000	Lifewise Health Plan of Washington	PPO
Washington	52,186	PacifiCare of Washington	HMO
Washington	49,135	CIGNA HealthCare of Washington	PPO
Washington	40,000	Asuris Northwest Health	Multiple
Washington	21,633	Regence Blue Shield	PPO
Washington	17,000	Puget Sound Health Partners	Medicare
Washington	7,550	PacifiCare Benefit Administrators	PPO
West Virginia	400,000	Mountain State Blue Cross Blue Shield	PPO
West Virginia	100,000	Coventry Health Care of West Virginia	HMO/PPO
West Virginia	50,000	SelectNet Plus, Inc.	PPO
West Virginia	27,783	CIGNA HealthCare of West Virginia	PPO
West Virginia	10,417	Great-West Healthcare West Virginia	HMO/PPO
Wisconsin	700,000	HealthEOS	PPO
Wisconsin	392,782	UnitedHealthCare of Wisconsin: Central	HMO/PPO
Wisconsin	223,000	Wisconsin Physician's Service	PPO
Wisconsin	187,000	Security Health Plan of Wisconsin	Multiple
Wisconsin	164,700	Managed Health Services	HMO
Wisconsin	112,000	Physicians Plus Insurance Corporation	HMO/PPO
Wisconsin	95,000	Group Health Cooperative of Eau Claire	HMO
Wisconsin	90,000	Gundersen Lutheran Health Plan	HMO
Wisconsin	75,000	Unity Health Insurance	Multiple
Wisconsin	67,812	Network Health Plan of Wisconsin	HMO/PPO
Wisconsin	53,255	CIGNA HealthCare of Wisconsin	PPO
Wisconsin	48,202	Group Health Cooperative of South Central Wisconsin	HMO
Wisconsin	40,000	Health Tradition	HMO
Wisconsin	40,000	MercyCare Health Plans	HMO
Wisconsin	22,450	Great-West Healthcare Wisconsin	HMO/PPO
Wisconsin	15,706	Prevea Health Network	PPO
Wyoming	100,000	Blue Cross & Blue Shield of Wyoming	PPO
Wyoming	21,919	UnitedHealthCare of Wyoming	HMO/PPO
Wyoming	9,864	WINhealth Partners	Multiple
Wyoming	3,334	CIGNA HealthCare of Wyoming	PPO

HMO/PPO Profiles

Health Insurance Coverage Status and Type of Coverage by Age

Category	All Persons		Under 18 years		Under 65 years		65 years and over	
	Number	%	Number	%	Number	%	Number	%
Total population	4,755	-	1,108	-	4,053	-	702	-
Covered by some type of health insurance	4,110 *(17)*	86.4 *(0.4)*	1,060 *(6)*	95.7 *(0.5)*	3,412 *(17)*	84.2 *(0.4)*	698 *(3)*	99.5 *(0.2)*
Covered by private health insurance	3,080 *(25)*	64.8 *(0.5)*	607 *(11)*	54.8 *(1.0)*	2,619 *(24)*	64.6 *(0.6)*	460 *(6)*	65.6 *(0.8)*
Employment based	2,489 *(25)*	52.3 *(0.5)*	514 *(12)*	46.4 *(1.1)*	2,231 *(24)*	55.0 *(0.6)*	258 *(6)*	36.8 *(0.8)*
Direct purchase	619 *(16)*	13.0 *(0.3)*	81 *(7)*	7.3 *(0.6)*	395 *(16)*	9.7 *(0.4)*	224 *(6)*	31.9 *(0.8)*
Covered by TRICARE	206 *(10)*	4.3 *(0.2)*	34 *(4)*	3.1 *(0.4)*	129 *(8)*	3.2 *(0.2)*	77 *(5)*	11.0 *(0.6)*
Covered by government health insurance	1,655 *(18)*	34.8 *(0.4)*	493 *(11)*	44.5 *(0.9)*	970 *(18)*	23.9 *(0.4)*	685 *(3)*	97.5 *(0.3)*
Covered by Medicaid	912 *(18)*	19.2 *(0.4)*	487 *(11)*	44.0 *(0.9)*	807 *(17)*	19.9 *(0.4)*	105 *(5)*	14.9 *(0.7)*
Also by private insurance	149 *(8)*	3.1 *(0.2)*	39 *(4)*	3.5 *(0.4)*	102 *(7)*	2.5 *(0.2)*	47 *(3)*	6.8 *(0.5)*
Covered by Medicare	886 *(8)*	18.6 *(0.2)*	13 *(3)*	1.1 *(0.2)*	202 *(7)*	5.0 *(0.2)*	684 *(3)*	97.4 *(0.3)*
Also by private insurance	509 *(7)*	10.7 *(0.2)*	1 *(1)*	0.1 *(0.1)*	63 *(4)*	1.5 *(0.1)*	446 *(6)*	63.6 *(0.8)*
Also by Medicaid	192 *(7)*	4.0 *(0.2)*	9 *(2)*	0.8 *(0.2)*	88 *(5)*	2.2 *(0.1)*	105 *(5)*	14.9 *(0.7)*
Covered by VA Care	125 *(6)*	2.6 *(0.1)*	2 *(2)*	0.2 *(0.1)*	64 *(5)*	1.6 *(0.1)*	61 *(3)*	8.6 *(0.4)*
Not covered at any time during the year	645 *(17)*	13.6 *(0.4)*	48 *(6)*	4.3 *(0.5)*	642 *(17)*	15.8 *(0.4)*	4 *(1)*	0.5 *(0.2)*

Note: Numbers in thousands; Figures cover 2013; Margin of error appears in parenthesis; A "Z" indicates that the value either represents or rounds to zero.
Source: U.S. Census Bureau, 2013 American Community Survey, Table HI05. Health Insurance Coverage Status and Type of Coverage by State and Age for All People: 2013

Alabama

2 Aetna Health of Alabama

151 Farmington Avenue
Hartford, CT 06156
Toll-Free: 800-872-3862
Phone: 860-273-0123
www.aetna.com
Partnered with: eHealthInsurance Services Inc.
For Profit Organization: Yes

Healthplan and Services Defined
PLAN TYPE: HMO
Plan Specialty: EPO
Benefits Offered: Dental, Disease Management, Long-Term Care,
    Prescription, Wellness, Life, LTD, STD

Type of Coverage
Commercial, Individual

Type of Payment Plans Offered
POS, FFS

Geographic Areas Served
Statewide

Key Personnel
Chairman/CEO/President. Mark T Bertolini
EVP/General Counsel . . . . William J Casazza
EVP/CFO . . . . Shawn M Guertin

3 Assurant Employee Benefits: Alabama

2700 Corporate Drive
Suite 150
Birmingham, AL 35242
Phone: 202-909-5700
www.assurantemployeebenefits.com
Subsidiary of: Assurant, Inc
For Profit Organization: Yes
Number of Primary Care Physicians: 112,000
Total Enrollment: 47,000

Healthplan and Services Defined
PLAN TYPE: Multiple
Plan Specialty: Dental, Vision, Long & Short-Term Disability
Benefits Offered: Dental, Vision, Wellness, AD&D, Life, LTD, STD,
    Long & Short-Term Disability

Type of Coverage
Commercial, Indemnity, Individual Dental Plans

Geographic Areas Served
Statewide

Subscriber Information
Average Monthly Fee Per Subscriber
    (Employee + Employer Contribution):
        Employee Only (Self): Varies by plan

Accreditation Certification
NCQA

Key Personnel
President/CEO. . . . . John S Roberts
Sr. Vice President, Sales. J. Marc Warrington
Senior Vice President - S . . . . J. Marc Warrington

4 Beech Street Corporation: Alabama

3460 Preston Ridge Road
Suite 300
Alpharetta, GA 30005
Toll-Free: 800-877-1444
Phone: 770-346-0520
Fax: 770-346-0506
www.beechstreet.com

Subsidiary of: Viant
Acquired by: MultiPlan
For Profit Organization: Yes
Year Founded: 1983
Number of Affiliated Hospitals: 76
Number of Primary Care Physicians: 2,963
Number of Referral/Specialty Physicians: 4,678
State Enrollment: 831,000

Healthplan and Services Defined
PLAN TYPE: PPO
Model Type: Network
Benefits Offered: Behavioral Health, Chiropractic, Disease
    Management, Home Care, Inpatient SNF, Long-Term Care,
    Physical Therapy, Podiatry, Transplant, Wellness, Worker's
    Compensation

Type of Coverage
Commercial, Individual, Medicaid

Geographic Areas Served
Southeastern states

Accreditation Certification
TJC, URAC, NCQA

Key Personnel
Chairman of the Board . . . . William A Fickling, Jr
President/CEO . . . . William Hale
Sr VP Legal, Regulatory . . . . Norman Werthwein
Executive VP . . . . Rick Markus
Sr VP/CFO. . . . . Jon Bird
Sr VP Operations Support . . . . Greg DeVille

5 Behavioral Health Systems

Two Metroplex Drive
Suite 500
Birmingham, AL 35209
Toll-Free: 800-245-1150
Phone: 205-879-1150
Fax: 205-879-1178
info@behavioralhealthsystems.com
www.bhs-inc.com
For Profit Organization: Yes
Physician Owned Organization: No
Federally Qualified: No
Number of Affiliated Hospitals: 617
Number of Primary Care Physicians: 11,000
Total Enrollment: 480,000

Healthplan and Services Defined
PLAN TYPE: PPO
Benefits Offered: Behavioral Health, Psychiatric, Worker's
    Compensation, EAP, Drug Testing

Type of Coverage
Commercial

Geographic Areas Served
Nationwide

Network Qualifications
Minimum Years of Practice: 5
Pre-Admission Certification: Yes

Peer Review Type
Utilization Review: Yes
Case Management: Yes

Publishes and Distributes Report Card: Yes

Accreditation Certification
AAAHC, TJC, URAC, CARF
Utilization Review, Pre-Admission Certification, Quality Assurance
    Program

Key Personnel
Founder, Chairman & CEO . . . . Deborah L Stephens
Executive Vice President. . . . . Pat Friedley

Executive Vice President . . . . .Kyle Strange
EVP/CFO. . . . . .Mark Gordon
Medical Director. . . . . .William M. Patterson, MD
Vice President, Business . . . . .Judi Braswell
VP, Public & Corporate Re. . . . . Shannon Goff Flanagan
   205-443-5483

Specialty Managed Care Partners
State of Alabama, Drummond Co, MTD Products
Enters into Contracts with Regional Business Coalitions: Yes
Employers Coalition on Healthcare Options (ECHO), Louisiana
   Business Group on Health (LBGH), Louisiana Health Care
   Alliance (LHCA)

6   Blue Cross & Blue Shield of Alabama

450 Riverchase Parkway East
Birmingham, AL 35244
Toll-Free: 888-267-2955
www.bcbsal.com
Year Founded: 1936
Total Enrollment: 3,200,000
State Enrollment: 2,100,000

Healthplan and Services Defined
  PLAN TYPE: HMO
  Model Type: IPA

Type of Coverage
  Commercial, Individual, Supplemental Medicare

Geographic Areas Served
  Alabama

Accreditation Certification
  URAC

Key Personnel
  President/CEO . . . . .Terry D Kellogg
  Media Contact. . . . . .Koko Mackin
     205-220-2713

7   Blue Cross Preferred Care

450 Riverchase Parkway East
Birmingham, AL 35244
Toll-Free: 800-213-7930
www.bcbsal.com
Non-Profit Organization: Yes
Year Founded: 1936
Number of Affiliated Hospitals: 130
Number of Primary Care Physicians: 9,000
Total Enrollment: 3,200,000
State Enrollment: 2,842,000

Healthplan and Services Defined
  PLAN TYPE: PPO
  Model Type: Network
  Plan Specialty: Behavioral Health, Chiropractic, Dental, Disease
    Management, Lab, Radiology, UR
  Benefits Offered: Behavioral Health, Chiropractic, Dental, Disease
    Management, Home Care, Inpatient SNF, Long-Term Care,
    Physical Therapy, Podiatry, Prescription, Psychiatric, Transplant,
    Vision, Wellness, AD&D, Life, LTD, STD, Hospital,
    Miscellaneous

Type of Coverage
  Commercial, Individual, Medicare, Supplemental Medicare

Type of Payment Plans Offered
  DFFS

Publishes and Distributes Report Card: Yes

Accreditation Certification
  URAC

Key Personnel
  President/CEO . . . . .Terry D Kellogg

8   Cigna-HealthSpring of Alabama

2 Chase Corporate Drive
Suite 300
Birmingham, AL 35244
Toll-Free: 800-668-3813
LetUsHelpYou@healthspring.com
www.cignahealthspring.com
Subsidiary of: The Oath of Alabama
For Profit Organization: Yes
Year Founded: 2000
Number of Affiliated Hospitals: 50
Total Enrollment: 30,000
State Enrollment: 17,844

Healthplan and Services Defined
  PLAN TYPE: Medicare
  Model Type: Network
  Plan Specialty: Disease Management, Lab, MSO, Vision, Radiology,
    UR, Group Medical
  Benefits Offered: Behavioral Health, Chiropractic, Disease
    Management, Home Care, Inpatient SNF, Long-Term Care,
    Physical Therapy, Podiatry, Prescription, Psychiatric, Transplant,
    Wellness

Type of Coverage
  Commercial, Individual, Medicare

Type of Payment Plans Offered
  DFFS

Geographic Areas Served
  Autauga, Baldwin, Bibb, Blount, Bullock, Butler, Calhoun, Cherokee,
  Chilton, Clarke, Clay, Cleburn, Colbert, Conecuh, Coosa, Cullman,
  Dallas, DeKalb, Elmore, Escambia, Etowah, Fayette, Franklin, Green,
  Hale, Jefferson, Lamar, Lauderdale, Lawrence, Lowndes, Macon,
  Madison, Marion, Marshall, Mobile, Monroe, Montgomery, Morgan,
  Perry, Pickens, Randolph, Saint Clair, Shelby, Talladega, Tucaloosa,
  Walker, Washington, Wilcox, Winston counties

Accreditation Certification
  NCQA
  TJC Accreditation

Key Personnel
  President. . . . . .Bob Dawson
  CFO . . . . .David Beauchaine
  Financial Analysis Senior . . . . .Brent Sander
     215-761-5417

Specialty Managed Care Partners
  MHNet, Express Script

Employer References
  Hertz, USX, Public Education Employees Health Plan

9   CompBenefits: Alabama

2204 Lakeshore Drive
Suite 100
Birmingham, AL 35209
Toll-Free: 800-942-0605
Phone: 205-879-7374
Fax: 205-879-5307
www.compbenefits.com
Subsidiary of: Humana Healthcare of Birmingham
Year Founded: 1978
Owned by an Integrated Delivery Network (IDN): Yes
Total Enrollment: 4,800,000

Healthplan and Services Defined
  PLAN TYPE: Multiple
  Model Type: Network, HMO, PPO, POS, TPA
  Plan Specialty: ASO, Dental, Vision
  Benefits Offered: Dental, Vision

Type of Coverage
  Commercial, Individual, Indemnity

Type of Payment Plans Offered
DFFS, Capitated, FFS

Geographic Areas Served
Alabama, Arkansas, Illinois, Indiana, Georgia, Florida, Mississippi, Missouri, Kentucky, Kansas, North Carolina, South Carolina, West Virginia, Texas, Tennessee, Ohio, Louisiana

Publishes and Distributes Report Card: Yes

Key Personnel
Chairman/CEO . . . . Michael McCallister
President . . . . Bruce Broussard
COO . . . . James Murray
SVP/CFO . . . . James Bloen

Specialty Managed Care Partners
Enters into Contracts with Regional Business Coalitions: Yes

10 eHealthInsurance Services Inc.

11919 Foundation Place
Gold River, CA 95670
Toll-Free: 800-977-8860
info@ehealthinsurance.com
www.e.healthinsurance.com
Year Founded: 1997

Healthplan and Services Defined
PLAN TYPE: HMO/PPO
Benefits Offered: Dental, Life, STD

Type of Coverage
Commercial, Individual, Medicare

Key Personnel
Chairman & CEO . . . . Gary L. Lauer
EVP/Business & Corp. Dev. . . . . Bruce Telkamp
EVP/Chief Technology . . . . Dr. Sheldon X. Wang
SVP & CFO . . . . Stuart M. Huizinga
Pres. of eHealth Gov. Sys . . . . Samuel C. Gibbs
SVP of Sales & Operations . . . . Robert S. Hurley
Director Public Relations . . . . Nate Purpura
650-210-3115

11 Great-West Healthcare Alabama

2 Securities Center
3500 Piedmont Road, Suite
Atlanta, GA 30305
Toll-Free: 866-494-2111
Phone: 404-443-8800
eliginquiries@cigna.com
www.cignaforhealth.com
Subsidiary of: CIGNA HealthCare
Acquired by: CIGNA
For Profit Organization: Yes
Total Enrollment: 8,147
State Enrollment: 6,662

Healthplan and Services Defined
PLAN TYPE: HMO/PPO
Benefits Offered: Disease Management, Prescription, Wellness

Type of Coverage
Commercial

Type of Payment Plans Offered
POS, FFS

Geographic Areas Served
Alabama

Accreditation Certification
URAC

Specialty Managed Care Partners
Caremark Rx

12 Health Choice of Alabama

Ridge Park Place
1130 22nd Street South; Suite 1000
Birmingham, AL 35205
Toll-Free: 866-508-4800
Phone: 205-715-4801
Fax: 205-715-4802
www.healthchoiceofalabama.com
Mailing Address: PO Box 830605, Birmingham, AL 35283
Subsidiary of: Alabama Premier Network (APN)
Non-Profit Organization: Yes
Year Founded: 1984
Number of Affiliated Hospitals: 90
Number of Primary Care Physicians: 4,600
Number of Referral/Specialty Physicians: 2,681
Total Enrollment: 45,000
State Enrollment: 45,000

Healthplan and Services Defined
PLAN TYPE: PPO
Model Type: Group, Network
Plan Specialty: Chiropractic
Benefits Offered: Chiropractic

Type of Coverage
Commercial

Type of Payment Plans Offered
POS, DFFS, FFS

Geographic Areas Served
Statewide

Specialty Managed Care Partners
Aetna, Superien, MNHO

13 Humana Health Insurance of Huntsville

600 Boulevard Street
Suite 104
Huntsville, AL 35802
Toll-Free: 800-942-0605
Phone: 256-705-3551
Fax: 205-876-8791
www.humana.com
Secondary Address: 2100 Southbridge Parkway, Suite 650, Birmingham, AL 35209
For Profit Organization: Yes

Healthplan and Services Defined
PLAN TYPE: HMO/PPO

Type of Coverage
Commercial, Individual

Accreditation Certification
URAC, NCQA, CORE

Key Personnel
President & CEO . . . . Bruce D. Broussard
Executive Vice President . . . . James E. Murray
Senior Vice President . . . . Jody Bilney
Senior Vice President . . . . Roy A. Beveridge, MD
Senior Vice President . . . . Brian LeClaire
Senior Vice President - P . . . . Heidi S. Margulis

14 North Alabama Managed Care Inc

PO Box 18788
Huntsville, AL 35804
beth.couch@compone.org
www.namci.com
Non-Profit Organization: Yes
Year Founded: 1991
Number of Affiliated Hospitals: 31
Number of Primary Care Physicians: 498

Number of Referral/Specialty Physicians: 1,014
Total Enrollment: 66,000

Healthplan and Services Defined
PLAN TYPE: PPO
Model Type: Network
Plan Specialty: Group Health
Benefits Offered: PPO Network

Type of Coverage
Commercial, Individual

Type of Payment Plans Offered
Combination FFS & DFFS

Geographic Areas Served
Alabama counties: Madison, Morgan, Marshall, Jackson, Colbert, Limestone, Lauderdale, and Franklin. Also Lincoln county, Tennessee, Tishomingo, MS

Subscriber Information
Average Subscriber Co-Payment:
Primary Care Physician: Varies by plan
Nursing Home: Varies

Network Qualifications
Pre-Admission Certification: Yes

Key Personnel
Executive Director . . . . Sheree Clark
256-532-2755
sherreh@namci.com
Operations Manager . . . . Brenda Willoughby
256-532-2754
brenda.willoughby@namci.com
Credentialing Claims Spec . . . . Nichelle Russell
256-532-2759
Marketing Manager. . . . . Dana Sellers
256-532-2770
danas@namci.com
Sales/Marketing . . . . Beth Couch
beth.couch@compone.org

Specialty Managed Care Partners
Enters into Contracts with Regional Business Coalitions: Yes
ECHO

Employer References
Huntsville HospitalSunshine Homes

---

15 **United Concordia: Dental Corporation of Alabama**
400 Vestavia Parkway
Suite 205
Birmingham, AL 35216
Toll-Free: 800-972-4191
Phone: 205-824-1235
Fax: 717-433-9871
ucproducer@ucci.com
www.ucci.com
For Profit Organization: Yes
Year Founded: 1971
Number of Primary Care Physicians: 111,000
Total Enrollment: 8,000,000

Healthplan and Services Defined
PLAN TYPE: Dental
Plan Specialty: Dental
Benefits Offered: Dental

Type of Coverage
Commercial, Individual

Geographic Areas Served
Military personnel and their families, nationwide

Accreditation Certification
URAC, NCQA

Key Personnel
Chief Dental Officer. . . . . James Bramson
SVP/Business Operations . . . . Dow Briggs, MD
Account Representataive . . . . David Belrose

---

16 **UnitedHealthCare of Alabama**
33 Inverness Center Parkway
Suite 350
Birmingham, AL 35242
Toll-Free: 800-345-1520
www.uhc.com
Subsidiary of: UnitedHealth Group
For Profit Organization: Yes
Year Founded: 1991
Number of Affiliated Hospitals: 5,622
Number of Primary Care Physicians: 720,301
Total Enrollment: 70,000,000
State Enrollment: 107,210

Healthplan and Services Defined
PLAN TYPE: HMO/PPO
Plan Specialty: Dental, Vision
Benefits Offered: Dental, Long-Term Care, Vision, Life

Type of Coverage
Medicare, Medicaid

Geographic Areas Served
Statewide

Accreditation Certification
NCQA

Key Personnel
President/CEO . . . . Glen Golemi
Chairman . . . . Richard Burke, Sr
CFO . . . . Frank Ulibarri
Media Contact. . . . . Roger Rollman
roger_f_rollman@uhc.com

---

17 **VIVA Health**
417 20th Street North
Suite 1100
Birmingham, AL 35205
Toll-Free: 800-633-1542
Phone: 205-918-2067
vivamemberhelp@uabmc.edu
www.vivahealth.com
Mailing Address: PO Box 55209, Birmingham, AL 35255
Subsidiary of: Triton Health Systems or UAB Health Systems
Total Enrollment: 80,000
State Enrollment: 80,000

Healthplan and Services Defined
PLAN TYPE: HMO
Other Type: Medicare
Plan Specialty: Medicare
Benefits Offered: Medicare

Type of Coverage
Medicare, Supplemental Medicare

Geographic Areas Served
Alabama

Key Personnel
CEO . . . . Brad Rollow
COO. . . . . Card Feagin
VP of Provider Services . . . . Terry Knight
CFO. . . . . Letitia Watkins
VP, Corporate Development . . . . Libba Yates
VP, Information Systems . . . . Doug Cannon
VP, Provider Relations . . . . Terry Knight

Health Insurance Coverage Status and Type of Coverage by Age

Category	All Persons		Under 18 years		Under 65 years		65 years and over	
	Number	%	Number	%	Number	%	Number	%
Total population	712	-	188	-	648	-	65	-
Covered by some type of health insurance	580 (7)	81.5 (1.0)	166 (3)	88.4 (1.6)	516 (7)	79.7 (1.1)	64 (1)	98.9 (0.5)
Covered by private health insurance	464 (9)	65.2 (1.3)	111 (4)	59.2 (2.2)	422 (9)	65.1 (1.4)	43 (2)	66.3 (2.7)
Employment based	398 (11)	55.9 (1.5)	90 (5)	47.7 (2.5)	365 (11)	56.3 (1.6)	33 (2)	51.8 (3.0)
Direct purchase	46 (5)	6.5 (0.7)	9 (2)	4.6 (1.2)	38 (4)	5.8 (0.7)	8 (1)	13.1 (2.1)
Covered by TRICARE	57 (4)	7.9 (0.6)	20 (3)	10.7 (1.5)	50 (4)	7.8 (0.7)	6 (1)	9.5 (2.0)
Covered by government health insurance	183 (6)	25.8 (0.8)	63 (4)	33.7 (1.9)	123 (6)	18.9 (0.9)	61 (1)	94.1 (1.6)
Covered by Medicaid	112 (6)	15.8 (0.8)	63 (4)	33.6 (2.0)	103 (5)	16.0 (0.8)	9 (1)	14.0 (1.8)
Also by private insurance	16 (3)	2.3 (0.4)	8 (2)	4.4 (1.0)	14 (3)	2.2 (0.5)	2 (1)	3.6 (0.9)
Covered by Medicare	71 (2)	9.9 (0.3)	1 (Z)	0.4 (0.3)	10 (2)	1.6 (0.3)	60 (1)	93.3 (1.8)
Also by private insurance	42 (2)	5.9 (0.3)	Z (Z)	0.1 (0.2)	3 (1)	0.4 (0.1)	39 (2)	60.7 (3.0)
Also by Medicaid	15 (2)	2.1 (0.3)	Z (Z)	0.2 (0.2)	6 (1)	0.9 (0.2)	9 (1)	14.0 (1.8)
Covered by VA Care	24 (2)	3.4 (0.3)	Z (Z)	0.1 (0.1)	17 (2)	2.5 (0.3)	8 (1)	12.2 (2.0)
Not covered at any time during the year	132 (7)	18.5 (1.0)	22 (3)	11.6 (1.6)	131 (7)	20.3 (1.1)	1 (Z)	1.1 (0.5)

Note: Numbers in thousands; Figures cover 2013; Margin of error appears in parenthesis; A "Z" indicates that the value either represents or rounds to zero.
Source: U.S. Census Bureau, 2013 American Community Survey, Table HI05. Health Insurance Coverage Status and Type of Coverage by State and Age for All People: 2013

Alaska

18 Aetna Health of Alaska

151 Farmington Avenue
Hartford, CT 06156
Toll-Free: 800-872-3862
Phone: 860-273-0123
www.aetna.com
For Profit Organization: Yes
Total Enrollment: 11,596,230

Healthplan and Services Defined
  PLAN TYPE: PPO
  Other Type: POS
  Plan Specialty: EPO
  Benefits Offered: Dental, Disease Management, Long-Term Care,
    Prescription, Wellness, Life, LTD, STD

Type of Coverage
  Commercial, Individual

Type of Payment Plans Offered
  POS, FFS

Geographic Areas Served
  Statewide

Subscriber Information
  Average Monthly Fee Per Subscriber
    (Employee + Employer Contribution):
      Employee Only (Self): Varies
      Employee & 2 Family Members: Varies
  Average Annual Deductible Per Subscriber:
      Employee Only (Self): Varies
      Employee & 2 Family Members: Varies
  Average Subscriber Co-Payment:
      Primary Care Physician: Varies
      Prescription Drugs: Varies

Key Personnel
  Chairman/CEO/President....................Mark T Bertolini
  EVP/General Counsel.....................William J Casazza
  EVP/CFO...............................Shawn M Guertin

19 Beech Street: Alaska

25500 Commercentre Drive
Lake Forest, CA 92630
Toll-Free: 800-877-1444
Phone: 949-672-1000
Fax: 949-672-1111
www.beechstreet.com
Subsidiary of: Viant
Acquired by: MultiPlan
For Profit Organization: Yes
Year Founded: 1951
Number of Affiliated Hospitals: 6
Number of Primary Care Physicians: 12
Number of Referral/Specialty Physicians: 68
State Enrollment: 6,000

Healthplan and Services Defined
  PLAN TYPE: PPO
  Benefits Offered: Behavioral Health, Chiropractic, Home Care,
    Inpatient SNF, Long-Term Care, Podiatry, Psychiatric, Transplant,
    Worker's Compensation

Type of Coverage
  Commercial, Individual, Supplemental Medicare

Geographic Areas Served
  AK (Aleutians East, Aleutians West, Anchorage, Central, Lake &
    Peninsula, Matanustka-Susitn, Northwestern, Prince Wales
    Ketchikan, Southcentral, Southeastern)

Accreditation Certification
  URAC, NCQA

Key Personnel
  President......................................William Hale
  Chairman of the Board....................William Fickling, Jr
  Sr VP Legal, Regulatory....................Norman Werthwein
  Executive VP...............................Rick Markus
  Sr VP/CFO..................................Jon Bird
  Sr VP Operations Support.....................Greg DeVille

20 CCN: Alaska

615 East 82nd Avenue
Anchorage, AK 99518
alaskaccn@gmail.com
www.alaskaccn.com
Subsidiary of: First Health: A Coventry Health Care Company
Acquired by: First Health/Coventry
For Profit Organization: Yes
Year Founded: 1984
Number of Affiliated Hospitals: 4
Number of Primary Care Physicians: 11
Number of Referral/Specialty Physicians: 19
Total Enrollment: 1,003

Healthplan and Services Defined
  PLAN TYPE: PPO
  Model Type: Network
  Benefits Offered: Chiropractic, Dental, Home Care, Inpatient SNF,
    Long-Term Care, Physical Therapy, Podiatry, Prescription,
    Psychiatric, Transplant, Worker's Compensation

Type of Coverage
  Commercial

Accreditation Certification
  URAC

Key Personnel
  CEO...Dale Wolf
  Senior VP...................................Marty Sholder

21 CIGNA HealthCare of Alaska

3900 East Mexico Avenue
Suite 1100
Denver, CO 80210
Toll-Free: 800-832-3211
Phone: 303-782-1500
Fax: 303-691-3197
www.cigna.com
For Profit Organization: Yes
Number of Affiliated Hospitals: 200

Healthplan and Services Defined
  PLAN TYPE: HMO
  Plan Specialty: Behavioral Health, Dental, Vision
  Benefits Offered: Behavioral Health, Dental, Disease Management,
    Prescription, Transplant, Vision, Wellness, Life

Type of Coverage
  Commercial

Type of Payment Plans Offered
  POS, FFS

Geographic Areas Served
  Montana

Key Personnel
  Director At Cigna..........................Sallie Vanasdale
  VP Provider Relations.........................William Cetti
  VP Client Relations..........................Gregg Prussing

22   eHealthInsurance Services Inc.

11919 Foundation Place
Gold River, CA 95670
Toll-Free: 800-644-3491
webmaster@healthinsurance.com
www.e.healthinsurance.com
Year Founded: 1997

Healthplan and Services Defined
  PLAN TYPE: HMO/PPO
  Benefits Offered: Dental, Life, STD

Type of Coverage
  Commercial, Individual, Medicare

Geographic Areas Served
  All 50 states in the USA and District of Columbia

Key Personnel
  Chairman & CEO . . . . Gary L. Lauer
  EVP/Business & Corp. Dev. Bruce Telkamp
  EVP/Chief Technology . . . . Dr. Sheldon X. Wang
  SVP & CFO . . . . Stuart M. Huizinga
  Pres. of eHealth Gov. Sys . . . . Samuel C. Gibbs
  SVP of Sales & Operations . . . . Robert S. Hurley
  Director Public Relations. . . . . Nate Purpura
    650-210-3115

23   Humana Health Insurance of Alaska

1498 SE Tech Center Place
Suite 300
Vancouver, WA 98683
Toll-Free: 800-781-4203
Phone: 360-253-7523
Fax: 360-253-7524
www.humana.com
For Profit Organization: Yes
Year Founded: 1961
Federally Qualified: Yes
Total Enrollment: 8,097

Healthplan and Services Defined
  PLAN TYPE: HMO/PPO
  Model Type: IPA
  Benefits Offered: Behavioral Health, Chiropractic, Dental,
    Prescription, Psychiatric, Transplant, Vision, Worker's
    Compensation

Type of Coverage
  Commercial, Individual

Geographic Areas Served
  Nationwide

Accreditation Certification
  TJC, URAC, NCQA, CORE

Key Personnel
  President/CEO . . . . Michael McCallister

24   Liberty Health Plan Anchorage

2700 Gambell Street
Suite 405
Anchorage, AK 99503-2835
Toll-Free: 866-893-1541
Phone: 907-561-2030
Fax: 800-254-5728
customerservice.center@libertynorthwest.com
www.libertynorthwest.com
For Profit Organization: Yes
Year Founded: 1983

Healthplan and Services Defined
  PLAN TYPE: PPO
  Model Type: Group

Plan Specialty: Worker's Compensation, Property & Casualty
Benefits Offered: Prescription, Property & Casualty

Type of Payment Plans Offered
  POS, DFFS, FFS, Combination FFS & DFFS

Geographic Areas Served
  Statewide

Network Qualifications
  Pre-Admission Certification: Yes

Peer Review Type
  Case Management: Yes

Publishes and Distributes Report Card: No

Key Personnel
  Manager. . . . . Lori Forlande
  Manager . . . . Nancie Linley
  Senior PR Consultant . . . . Chris Goetcheus

Specialty Managed Care Partners
  Enters into Contracts with Regional Business Coalitions: No

25   Moda Health Alaska

510 L Street
Suite 270
Anchorage, AK 99501-6303
Toll-Free: 888-277-7820
medical@modahealth.com
www.modahealth.com
Secondary Address: 601 S.W. Second Avenue, Portland, OR 97240
Year Founded: 1955
Total Enrollment: 800,000

Healthplan and Services Defined
  PLAN TYPE: Multiple
  Other Type: PPO, POS, Dental
  Plan Specialty: Dental
  Benefits Offered: Chiropractic, Dental, Disease Management, Home
    Care, Inpatient SNF, Physical Therapy, Podiatry, Prescription,
    Psychiatric, Vision, Wellness

Type of Coverage
  Commercial, Individual, Medicare

Subscriber Information
  Average Monthly Fee Per Subscriber
    (Employee + Employer Contribution):
      Employee Only (Self): Varies
      Medicare: Varies
  Average Annual Deductible Per Subscriber:
      Employee Only (Self): Varies
      Medicare: Varies
  Average Subscriber Co-Payment:
      Primary Care Physician: Varies
      Non-Network Physician: Varies
      Prescription Drugs: Varies
      Hospital ER: Varies
      Home Health Care: Varies
      Home Health Care Max. Days/Visits Covered: Varies
      Nursing Home: Varies
      Nursing Home Max. Days/Visits Covered: Varies

Accreditation Certification
  URAC

Key Personnel
  Chief Executive Officer. . . . . Robert Gootee
  President . . . . William Johnson, MD, MBA
  Executive Vice President . . . . Steve Wynee
  Senior Vice President. . . . . Robin Richardson
  Senior Vice President . . . . Bill Ten Pas, DMD
  Senior Vice President . . . . Tracie Murphy
  Senior Vice President. . . . . Dave Evans
  Senior Vice President . . . . Kraig Anderson
  Senior Vice President. . . . . Jay Lamb

VP, Marketing . . . . Jonathan Nicholas
    503-219-3673
    jonathan.nicholas@modahealth.com

26 Premera Blue Cross Blue Shield of Alaska

2550 Denali Street
Suite 1404
Anchorage, AK 99503
Toll-Free: 800-508-4722
www.premera.com
For Profit Organization: Yes
Year Founded: 1952
Number of Affiliated Hospitals: 20
Total Enrollment: 1,700,000
State Enrollment: 100,000

Healthplan and Services Defined
  PLAN TYPE: PPO
  Other Type: EPO
  Plan Specialty: Dental
  Benefits Offered: Dental, Long-Term Care, Vision, Life

Type of Coverage
  Supplemental Medicare

Accreditation Certification
  AAAHC, URAC, TJC

Key Personnel
  President/CEO . . . . H.R. Brereton Barlow
  President, Alaska . . . . Jim Grazko
  Director, Sales . . . . Lynn Rust Henderson

27 UnitedHealthCare of Alaska

7632 SW Durham Road
Tigard, OR 97224
Toll-Free: 866-432-5992
www.uhc.com
Subsidiary of: UnitedHealth Group
For Profit Organization: Yes
Total Enrollment: 75,000,000

Healthplan and Services Defined
  PLAN TYPE: HMO/PPO

Geographic Areas Served
  Statewide

Key Personnel
  Chief Executive Officer . . . . David Hansen
  Marketing . . . . Lya Selby
  Medical Director . . . . Roger Muller, MD
  Media Contact . . . . Will Shanley
    will.shanley@uhc.com

Health Insurance Coverage Status and Type of Coverage by Age

Category	All Persons		Under 18 years		Under 65 years		65 years and over	
	Number	%	Number	%	Number	%	Number	%
Total population	6,521	-	1,614	-	5,514	-	1,007	-
Covered by some type of health insurance	5,403 *(24)*	82.9 *(0.4)*	1,422 *(11)*	88.1 *(0.7)*	4,405 *(24)*	79.9 *(0.4)*	998 *(2)*	99.1 *(0.2)*
Covered by private health insurance	3,904 *(29)*	59.9 *(0.4)*	869 *(14)*	53.9 *(0.9)*	3,318 *(28)*	60.2 *(0.5)*	586 *(8)*	58.2 *(0.7)*
Employment based	3,135 *(29)*	48.1 *(0.5)*	746 *(15)*	46.2 *(0.9)*	2,842 *(28)*	51.5 *(0.5)*	293 *(8)*	29.1 *(0.8)*
Direct purchase	796 *(15)*	12.2 *(0.2)*	110 *(7)*	6.8 *(0.4)*	480 *(13)*	8.7 *(0.2)*	316 *(9)*	31.3 *(0.9)*
Covered by TRICARE	209 *(9)*	3.2 *(0.1)*	39 *(4)*	2.4 *(0.3)*	125 *(8)*	2.3 *(0.1)*	84 *(5)*	8.4 *(0.5)*
Covered by government health insurance	2,242 *(24)*	34.4 *(0.4)*	611 *(14)*	37.8 *(0.9)*	1,267 *(24)*	23.0 *(0.4)*	974 *(3)*	96.8 *(0.3)*
Covered by Medicaid	1,242 *(25)*	19.0 *(0.4)*	606 *(14)*	37.6 *(0.9)*	1,124 *(24)*	20.4 *(0.4)*	118 *(5)*	11.7 *(0.5)*
Also by private insurance	162 *(10)*	2.5 *(0.1)*	56 *(5)*	3.5 *(0.3)*	117 *(9)*	2.1 *(0.2)*	46 *(3)*	4.6 *(0.3)*
Covered by Medicare	1,111 *(8)*	17.0 *(0.1)*	7 *(2)*	0.5 *(0.1)*	139 *(7)*	2.5 *(0.1)*	972 *(4)*	96.5 *(0.3)*
Also by private insurance	599 *(8)*	9.2 *(0.1)*	1 *(1)*	0.1 *(0.1)*	37 *(4)*	0.7 *(0.1)*	562 *(8)*	55.8 *(0.7)*
Also by Medicaid	181 *(7)*	2.8 *(0.1)*	6 *(1)*	0.3 *(0.1)*	63 *(5)*	1.1 *(0.1)*	118 *(5)*	11.7 *(0.5)*
Covered by VA Care	174 *(8)*	2.7 *(0.1)*	3 *(2)*	0.2 *(0.1)*	83 *(6)*	1.5 *(0.1)*	91 *(5)*	9.0 *(0.5)*
Not covered at any time during the year	1,118 *(24)*	17.1 *(0.4)*	192 *(11)*	11.9 *(0.7)*	1,109 *(25)*	20.1 *(0.4)*	9 *(2)*	0.9 *(0.2)*

Note: Numbers in thousands; Figures cover 2013; Margin of error appears in parenthesis; A "Z" indicates that the value either represents or rounds to zero.
Source: U.S. Census Bureau, 2013 American Community Survey, Table HI05. Health Insurance Coverage Status and Type of Coverage by State and Age for All People: 2013

Arizona

28 Action Healthcare Management Services

6245 N 24th Parkway
Suite 112
Phoenix, AZ 85016
Toll-Free: 800-433-6915
Phone: 602-265-0681
Fax: 602-265-0202
jeanr@actionhealthcare.com
www.actionhealthcare.com
For Profit Organization: Yes
Year Founded: 1987
Physician Owned Organization: No
Federally Qualified: No
Total Enrollment: 98,500

Healthplan and Services Defined
  PLAN TYPE: PPO
  Model Type: Medical Mgmt Company
  Plan Specialty: Disease Management
  Benefits Offered: Behavioral Health, Disease Management, Home
    Care, Inpatient SNF, Long-Term Care, Podiatry, Psychiatric,
    Transplant, Wellness, Worker's Compensation

Type of Coverage
  Commercial, Self-Funded Healthcare Benefits

Geographic Areas Served
  Nationwide

Network Qualifications
  Pre-Admission Certification: No

Peer Review Type
  Utilization Review: Yes

Publishes and Distributes Report Card: No

Accreditation Certification
  TJC

Key Personnel
  President/CEO . . . . .Jean Rice
  Medical Director . . . . .Joel V Brill, MD
  Clinical Operations Mgr. . . . . Mary Kim Brown, RN-BC

Specialty Managed Care Partners
  Enters into Contracts with Regional Business Coalitions: No

29 Aetna Health of Arizona

2625 Shadelands Drive
Suite 240
Walnut Creek, CA 94598
Toll-Free: 866-582-9629
Fax: 602-427-2176
www.aetna.com
For Profit Organization: Yes
Year Founded: 1988
Number of Affiliated Hospitals: 44
Number of Primary Care Physicians: 1,554
Number of Referral/Specialty Physicians: 4,374
Total Enrollment: 109,089

Healthplan and Services Defined
  PLAN TYPE: HMO
  Other Type: POS
  Benefits Offered: Dental, Disease Management, Long-Term Care,
    Prescription, Wellness, LTD, STD
  Offers Demand Management Patient Information Service: Yes

Type of Coverage
  Commercial, Individual

Type of Payment Plans Offered
  POS, Capitated, Combination FFS & DFFS

Geographic Areas Served
  Statewide

Network Qualifications
  Minimum Years of Practice: 2
  Pre-Admission Certification: Yes

Peer Review Type
  Utilization Review: Yes

Publishes and Distributes Report Card: Yes

Accreditation Certification
  NCQA

Specialty Managed Care Partners
  Behavioral Health, Prescription, Dental, Vision

30 Arizona Foundation for Medical Care

326 East Coronado Road
Phoenix, AZ 85004
Toll-Free: 800-624-4277
Phone: 602-252-4042
Fax: 602-254-3086
marketing@azfmc.com
www.azfmc.com
Subsidiary of: Ancillary Benefit Systems
Non-Profit Organization: Yes
Year Founded: 1969
Number of Affiliated Hospitals: 78
Number of Primary Care Physicians: 14,000
Total Enrollment: 175,000

Healthplan and Services Defined
  PLAN TYPE: Multiple
  Other Type: HMO, PPO, POS, EPO
  Model Type: Group, Network
  Plan Specialty: Chiropractic, Disease Management, EPO, Worker's
    Compensation, PPO, POS, Medical Management, Case
    Management, Utilization Management, Wellness Services, 24/7
    Nurse Line
  Benefits Offered: Disease Management, Wellness, Maternity
    Management
  Offers Demand Management Patient Information Service: Yes
  DMPI Services Offered: 24-Hour Nurse Care Line

Type of Coverage
  Commercial, Individual, Indemnity

Type of Payment Plans Offered
  POS

Geographic Areas Served
  Arizona (Statewide)

Network Qualifications
  Pre-Admission Certification: Yes

Peer Review Type
  Utilization Review: Yes
  Case Management: Yes

Accreditation Certification
  TJC, URAC, NCQA

Key Personnel
  Executive VP . . . . .Roger Stinton
  President. . . . . .Stanley A. Gering, MD
  Administration/Finance . . . . .Sandra D Flowers
  Chief Medical Officer. . . . . Terry Murphy
  Dir, Network Management . . . . .Coleen Hamilton
  Manager. . . . . .Kay Banda, 74
  Mgr, Bus Implementation . . . . .Ashley Rogers
  Director/Claims. . . . . .Theresa Murphy
  Medical Management and Pr . . . . Kerry Kovaleski
  Information Services . . . . .Tracy Mitchell

31   Arizona Physicians IPA

3141 North Third Avenue
Phoenix, AZ 85013
Phone: 602-651-6127
www.myapipa.com
Subsidiary of: AmeriChoice, A UnitedHealth Group Company
For Profit Organization: Yes

Healthplan and Services Defined
  PLAN TYPE: HMO

Type of Coverage
  Medicare, Supplemental Medicare, Medicaid

Geographic Areas Served
  Apache, Cochise, Coconino, Graham, Greenlee, La Paz, Maricopa, Mohave, Navajo, Pima, Santa Cruz, Yavapai, Yuma

Key Personnel
Principal . . . . .Donna Payne
Media Contact. . . . . .Jeff Smith
  952-931-5685
  jeff.smith@uhc.com

32   Avesis: Corporate Headquarters

3030 N Central Avenue
Suite 300
Phoenix, AZ 85012
Toll-Free: 800-522-0258
www.avesis.com
Year Founded: 1978
Number of Primary Care Physicians: 18,000
Total Enrollment: 2,000,000

Healthplan and Services Defined
  PLAN TYPE: PPO
  Other Type: Vision, Dental
  Model Type: Network
  Plan Specialty: Dental, Vision, Hearing
  Benefits Offered: Dental, Vision

Type of Coverage
  Commercial

Type of Payment Plans Offered
  POS, Capitated, Combination FFS & DFFS

Geographic Areas Served
  Nationwide and Puerto Rico

Publishes and Distributes Report Card: Yes

Accreditation Certification
  AAAHC, NCQA
  TJC Accreditation

Key Personnel
Vice Chairman . . . . .William Cohen
CEO . . . . .Alan Cohen
Chief Operations Officer. . . . . .Linda Chirichella
CFO. . . . . .Joel Alperstein
Chief Marketing Officer . . . . .Michael Reamer
Chief Information Officer. .Laura Gill
Government Sales. . . . . .Josh Cohn
  410-581-8700
  jcohn@avesis.com

33   Banner MediSun Medicare Plan

13632 N 99th Avenue
Sun City, AZ 85351
Toll-Free: 800-446-8331
Phone: 623-974-7430
www.bannerhealth.com

Healthplan and Services Defined
  PLAN TYPE: Medicare

Type of Coverage
  Medicare, Supplemental Medicare

Geographic Areas Served
  Maricopa County

Key Personnel
President/CEO . . . . .Peter S. Fine
EVP, CAO. . . . . .Ron Bunnell
EVP/CMO. . . . . .John Hensing

34   Blue Cross & Blue Shield of Arizona

2444 West Las Palmaritas Drive
Phoenix, AZ 85021
Phone: 602-864-4100
www.azblue.com
Mailing Address: PO Box 13466, Phoenix, AZ 85002-3466
Non-Profit Organization: Yes
Year Founded: 1939
Number of Affiliated Hospitals: 65
Number of Primary Care Physicians: 1,611
Total Enrollment: 1,000,000
State Enrollment: 1,000,000

Healthplan and Services Defined
  PLAN TYPE: HMO/PPO
  Model Type: Network
  Benefits Offered: Behavioral Health, Chiropractic, Dental, Prescription, Wellness

Type of Coverage
  Commercial, Individual, Indemnity, Supplemental Medicare

Geographic Areas Served
  Statewide

Accreditation Certification
  URAC
  TJC Accreditation, Medicare Approved, Utilization Review, Pre-Admission Certification, State Licensure, Quality Assurance Program

Key Personnel
President/CEO. . . . . .Richard L Boals
EVP, External Operations. . . . . .Sandra Lee Gibson
EVP, Internal Operations . . . . .Susan Navran
Sr VP Claims Services . . . . .H Jody Chandler
SVP & CFO. . . . . .Karen Abraham
SVP, General Counsel . . . . .Deanna Salazar
  602-864-5870
SVP, Business Development. . . . . .Tony M Astorga
SVP, Marketing . . . . .Richard M Hannon
SVP/Chief Medical Officer . . . . .Vishu J Jhaveri, MD
SVP/Chief Finance Officer . . . . .Karen Abraham
SVP, Chief Info Officer .Elizabeth A Messina

35   Care 1st Health Plan: Arizona

2355 East Camelback Road
Suite 300
Phoenix, AZ 85016
Toll-Free: 866-560-4042
Phone: 602-778-1800
Fax: 602778-1863
www.care1st.com
For Profit Organization: Yes
Year Founded: 1994

Healthplan and Services Defined
  PLAN TYPE: HMO
  Benefits Offered: Disease Management, Wellness

Type of Coverage
  Supplemental Medicare, Medicaid

Geographic Areas Served
  Maricopa County

Accreditation Certification
 NCQA

Key Personnel
 Chief Admin Officer. . . . . Scott Cummings
 Chief Operating Officer . . . . Susan Cordier
 Chief Financial Officer . . . . Deena Sigel
 Director, Claims. . . . . Steffanie Costal
 Dir, Pharmacy. . . . . Nirali Soni, RPh, CDE
 Dir, Sales & Marketing. . . . . Anna Maria Maldonado
 Dir, Quality Management . . . . Pat Seabert, RN
 Health Plan Services . . . . Kathy Thurman
 Dir, Member Services. . . . . Mike Ferguson
 Dir, Information Tech. . . . . Jim Solinsky
 Dir, Provider Network . . . . Jessica Sedita-Igneri

36 CIGNA HealthCare of Arizona

900 Cottage Grove Road
Bloomfield, AZ 06002
Toll-Free: 800-997-1654
www.cigna.com
Secondary Address: Two Liberty Place, 1601 Chestnut Street,
 Philadephia, PA 19102, 480-922-6508
For Profit Organization: Yes
Year Founded: 1972
Number of Primary Care Physicians: 1,150
Number of Referral/Specialty Physicians: 3,180
Total Enrollment: 103,561
State Enrollment: 103,561

Healthplan and Services Defined
 PLAN TYPE: HMO/PPO
 Other Type: POS
 Model Type: IPA, Network
 Benefits Offered: Behavioral Health, Chiropractic, Complementary
 Medicine, Disease Management, Home Care, Inpatient SNF,
 Long-Term Care, Physical Therapy, Podiatry, Prescription,
 Psychiatric, Transplant, Vision, Wellness

Type of Coverage
 Commercial, Individual, Medicare

Type of Payment Plans Offered
 POS

Accreditation Certification
 NCQA

Key Personnel
 President/CEO. . . . . David Cordani
 EVP,GCMO. . . . . Lisa Bacus
 EVP, GCIO. . . . . Mark Boxer
 Network Manager. . . . . Wendy Woske
 Pharmacy Compliance Offc. . . . . David Hu
 Marketing Manager . . . . Jay Headley
 Chief Medical Officer . . . . Alan Muney, MD, MHA
 VP, Sales. . . . . Frank Benedetto

37 CoreSource: Arizona

7830 E Broadway Blvd
Tucson, AZ 85710
Toll-Free: 800-888-7202
Phone: 520-290-4600
www.coresource.com
Subsidiary of: Trustmark
Year Founded: 1980
Total Enrollment: 1,300,000

Healthplan and Services Defined
 PLAN TYPE: Multiple
 Other Type: TPA
 Model Type: Network
 Plan Specialty: Claims Administration, TPA

Benefits Offered: Behavioral Health, Home Care, Prescription,
 Transplant

Type of Coverage
 Commercial

Geographic Areas Served
 Nationwide

Accreditation Certification
 URAC, NCQA
 Utilization Review, Pre-Admission Certification

Key Personnel
 Regional President . . . . Dave Parrish
 VP, Claims Operations. . . . . Pam Corso

38 Delta Dental of Arizona

5656 West Talavi Blvd
Glendale, AZ 85306
Toll-Free: 800-352-6132
Phone: 602-938-3131
Fax: 602-588-3636
customerservice@deltadentalaz.com
www.deltadentalaz.com
Mailing Address: PO Box 43000, Phoenix, AZ 85080-3000
Subsidiary of: Canyon Insurance Services
Non-Profit Organization: Yes
Year Founded: 1972
Number of Primary Care Physicians: 2,700
Total Enrollment: 54,000,000
State Enrollment: 435,000

Healthplan and Services Defined
 PLAN TYPE: Dental
 Other Type: Dental PPO
 Model Type: Network
 Plan Specialty: Dental, Vision
 Benefits Offered: Dental, Vision

Type of Coverage
 Commercial, Indemnity

Type of Payment Plans Offered
 FFS

Geographic Areas Served
 Statewide

Accreditation Certification
 NCQA

Key Personnel
 President/CEO. . . . . Allan Allford
 VP, CFO. . . . . Mark Anderson
 Communications Mgr . . . . Tiffany Di Gracinto, DDS
 VP/Sales . . . . David Hurley
 Dir. Legal Affairs. . . . . Anne Bishop
 VP, Sales . . . . David Hurley
 Media Contact . . . . Shannon Keller
 602-346-2575
 shannonk@barclaycomm.com

39 Desert Canyon Community Care

3767 Karicio Lane
Suite D
Prescott, AZ 86303
Toll-Free: 800-887-6177
Phone: 928-777-9226
Fax: 928-777-9243
www.wellcare.com
Subsidiary of: Arcadian Health Plans
Total Enrollment: 2,700,000

Healthplan and Services Defined
 PLAN TYPE: Medicare

Type of Coverage
  Medicare

Accreditation Certification
  NCQA

Key Personnel
  Chief Executive Officer . . . . Alec Cunningham
  Chief Sales Officer . . . . Garrison Rios
  Senior Vice President and . . . . Lawrence D. Anderson

40 eHealthInsurance Services Inc.
11919 Foundation Place
Gold River, CA 95670
Toll-Free: 800-644-3491
webmaster@healthinsurance.com
www.e.healthinsurance.com
Year Founded: 1997

Healthplan and Services Defined
  PLAN TYPE: HMO/PPO
  Benefits Offered: Dental, Life, STD

Type of Coverage
  Commercial, Individual, Medicare

Geographic Areas Served
  All 50 states in the USA and District of Columbia

Key Personnel
  Chairman & CEO . . . . Gary L. Lauer
  EVP/Business & Corp. Dev. Bruce Telkamp
  EVP/Chief Technology . . . . Dr. Sheldon X. Wang
  SVP & CFO . . . . Stuart M. Huizinga
  Pres. of eHealth Gov. Sys . . . . Samuel C. Gibbs
  SVP of Sales & Operations . . . . Robert S. Hurley
  Director Public Relations . . . . Nate Purpura
    650-210-3115

41 Employers Dental Services
2355 E Camelback Road
Suite 601
Phoenix, AZ 85016
Toll-Free: 800-722-9772
Phone: 602-248-8912
edscs@mydentalplan.net
www.mydentalplan.net
Mailing Address: PO Box 36600, Tucson, AZ 85740
Year Founded: 1974
Owned by an Integrated Delivery Network (IDN): Yes
Number of Primary Care Physicians: 1,340
Total Enrollment: 120,000
State Enrollment: 120,000

Healthplan and Services Defined
  PLAN TYPE: Dental
  Model Type: Group, Individual
  Plan Specialty: Dental
  Benefits Offered: Dental, Prepaid

Type of Coverage
  DHMO

Geographic Areas Served
  Arizona Statewide

Peer Review Type
  Utilization Review: Yes
  Case Management: Yes

Accreditation Certification
  Utilization Review, Quality Assurance Program

Specialty Managed Care Partners
  Enters into Contracts with Regional Business Coalitions: Yes

42 Fortified Provider Network
8712 East Via De Commercio
Suite 2
Scottsdale, AZ 85258
Toll-Free: 866-955-4376
Phone: 480-607-0222
Fax: 480-223-6373
fpn@fortifiedprovider.com
www.fortifiedprovider.com
Year Founded: 1997

Healthplan and Services Defined
  PLAN TYPE: PPO

Key Personnel
  President . . . . Michael Reagan
  Marketing Manager . . . . Rebecca Chesley
  VP Contracting . . . . Michael Olson

43 Great-West Healthcare Arizona
6909 East Greenway Parkway
Suite 180
Scottsdale, AZ 85254
Toll-Free: 800-274-4950
Phone: 480-922-6508
eliginquiries@cigna.com
www.cigna.com/betterhealth
Subsidiary of: CIGNA HealthCare
Acquired by: CIGNA
For Profit Organization: Yes
Total Enrollment: 37,459
State Enrollment: 5,048

Healthplan and Services Defined
  PLAN TYPE: HMO/PPO
  Benefits Offered: Disease Management, Prescription, Wellness

Type of Coverage
  Commercial

Type of Payment Plans Offered
  POS, FFS

Geographic Areas Served
  Arizona

Accreditation Certification
  URAC

Specialty Managed Care Partners
  Caremark Rx

44 Health Choice Arizona
410 N 44th Street
Suite 900
Phoenix, AZ 85008
Toll-Free: 800-322-8670
Phone: 480-968-6866
comments@healthchoiceaz.com
www.healthchoiceaz.com
Subsidiary of: IASIS Healthcare
For Profit Organization: Yes
Year Founded: 1990
Number of Affiliated Hospitals: 16
Number of Primary Care Physicians: 400
Total Enrollment: 115,000

Healthplan and Services Defined
  PLAN TYPE: HMO
  Model Type: IPA
  Plan Specialty: Services to AHCCCS members
  Benefits Offered: Behavioral Health, Dental, Disease Management,
    Prescription, Wellness, Care Coordination, Maternal Child Health

Type of Coverage
Medicaid, Managed Medicaid

Geographic Areas Served
Apache, Coconino, Gila, Maricopa, Mohave, Navajo, Pima, Pinal counties

Network Qualifications
Pre-Admission Certification: Yes

Peer Review Type
Utilization Review: Yes
Second Surgical Opinion: Yes
Case Management: Yes

Accreditation Certification
TJC Accreditation, Utilization Review

Key Personnel
President/CEO...............................Carolyn Rose
Claims...................................Adrian Brown
Member Services............................Suzan Irmer
Info Tech Manager ....Mike Uchrin
Information Systems.......................Jesse Perlmutter

---

45   Health Net of Arizona

1230 West Washington Street
Suite 401
Tempe, AZ 85281
Toll-Free: 866-458-1047
Phone: 602-286-9194
Fax: 602-286-9244
www.healthnet.com
Subsidiary of: Health Net
For Profit Organization: Yes
Year Founded: 1981
Number of Affiliated Hospitals: 52
Number of Primary Care Physicians: 1,200
Number of Referral/Specialty Physicians: 3,800
Total Enrollment: 119,000
State Enrollment: 60,500

Healthplan and Services Defined
PLAN TYPE: HMO
Model Type: Network
Plan Specialty: Behavioral Health, Chiropractic, Disease Management, Lab, MSO, PBM, Vision, Radiology, UR
Benefits Offered: Behavioral Health, Chiropractic, Complementary Medicine, Dental, Disease Management, Home Care, Inpatient SNF, Physical Therapy, Podiatry, Prescription, Psychiatric, Transplant, Vision, Wellness, AD&D, Life, Alternative Medicine

Type of Coverage
Commercial, Individual, Indemnity, Medicare

Type of Payment Plans Offered
POS, DFFS, Combination FFS & DFFS

Geographic Areas Served
Apache, Cochise, Coconino, Gila, Graham, Greenlee, La Paz, Maricipa, Mohave, Navajo, Pima, Pinal, Santa Cruz, Yuma counties

Subscriber Information
Average Monthly Fee Per Subscriber
(Employee + Employer Contribution):
Employee Only (Self): Varies
Employee & 1 Family Member: Varies
Employee & 2 Family Members: Varies
Medicare: Varies
Average Annual Deductible Per Subscriber:
Employee Only (Self): Varies
Employee & 1 Family Member: Varies
Employee & 2 Family Members: Varies
Medicare: Varies

Network Qualifications
Minimum Years of Practice: 3
Pre-Admission Certification: Yes

Peer Review Type
Utilization Review: Yes
Second Surgical Opinion: Yes
Case Management: Yes

Accreditation Certification
NCQA
Medicare Approved, Utilization Review, Pre-Admission Certification, State Licensure, Quality Assurance Program

Key Personnel
President ....Brett A Morris
CFO ....Alec Mahmood
Regional CFO ....Lorry Bottrill
Chief Medical Officer ....Richard Jacobs, MD
VP Provider Services.........................Carolyn Pace
Mgr, Public Relations.........................Lori Rieger
602-794-1415
lori.rieger@healthnet.com

Specialty Managed Care Partners
Preferred Home Care, Infusion Care Systems, Catalina Behavioral Health Services, Sonoma Quest Laboratory, Health South, Southwest Footcare

Employer References
FEHB, IBM

---

46   Humana Health Insurance of Arizona

2231 East Camelback Road
Suite 400
Phoenix, AZ 85016
Toll-Free: 800-889-0301
Phone: 602-760-1700
www.humana.com
Secondary Address: 5120 E Williams Circle, Suite 200, Tucson, AZ 85711, 520-571-6548
For Profit Organization: Yes
Year Founded: 1984
Number of Affiliated Hospitals: 33
Number of Primary Care Physicians: 500
Total Enrollment: 127,564
State Enrollment: 26,120

Healthplan and Services Defined
PLAN TYPE: HMO/PPO
Model Type: IPA
Benefits Offered: Dental, Disease Management, Prescription, Transplant, Vision, Wellness, Life, LTD, STD

Type of Coverage
Commercial, Individual

Type of Payment Plans Offered
POS, Combination FFS & DFFS

Geographic Areas Served
Apache, Cochise, Coconino, Gila, Graham, Greenlee, La Paz, Maricipa, Mohave, Navajo, Pima, Pinal, Santa Cruz, Yavapai, Yuma counties

Subscriber Information
Average Monthly Fee Per Subscriber
(Employee + Employer Contribution):
Employee Only (Self): Varies
Employee & 1 Family Member: Varies
Employee & 2 Family Members: Varies
Medicare: Varies
Average Subscriber Co-Payment:
Prescription Drugs: Varies

Network Qualifications
Pre-Admission Certification: Yes

Peer Review Type
Utilization Review: Yes
Second Surgical Opinion: Yes
Case Management: Yes

Publishes and Distributes Report Card: Yes

Accreditation Certification
URAC, NCQA, CORE
TJC Accreditation

Key Personnel
President/CEO . . . . Bruce D. Broussard
EVP, COO . . . . James E. Murray
SVP, CFO, Treasurer . . . . James H. Bloem, FSA MAAA
SVP, General Counsel . . . . Christopher M. Todoroff
SVP, CDO . . . . Paul B. Kusserow
SVP, CHRO . . . . Tim Huval
Sr VP Marketing Officer . . . . Steven Moya
Sr VP Government Relation . . . . Heidi Margulis
SVP, CMO . . . . Roy A. Beveridge, MD
VP/Controller . . . . Steven McCulley
SVP, CIO . . . . Brian LeClaire
SVP, Public Affairs . . . . Heidi S. Margulis

Specialty Managed Care Partners
Enters into Contracts with Regional Business Coalitions: Yes

47   Magellan Health Services Arizona

4129 E Van Buren Street
Suite 250
Phoenix, AZ 85008
Toll-Free: 800-564-5465
www.magellanofaz.com
For Profit Organization: Yes
Total Enrollment: 80,000
State Enrollment: 80,000

Healthplan and Services Defined
PLAN TYPE: PPO

Type of Coverage
Medicaid, Title XXI/KidsCare

Accreditation Certification
URAC, NCQA

Key Personnel
CEO . . . . Richard Clarke, PhD
Deputy CEO . . . . Shawn Thiele
Chief Medical Officer . . . . Shareh Ghani, MD
Chief Financial Officer . . . . Alex Nunez
Chief Comm Relations Offc . . . . Nolberto Machiche

48   Maricopa Integrated Health System/Maricopa Health Plan

2601 East Roosevelt Street
Phoenix, AZ 85008
Phone: 602-344-5011
Fax: 602-344-5190
www.mihs.org
Subsidiary of: University of Arizona Health Network
Non-Profit Organization: Yes
Year Founded: 1981
Number of Affiliated Hospitals: 10
Number of Primary Care Physicians: 124
Number of Referral/Specialty Physicians: 317
Total Enrollment: 50,715
State Enrollment: 39,997

Healthplan and Services Defined
PLAN TYPE: HMO
Model Type: Network
Plan Specialty: Lab, Radiology
Benefits Offered: Dental, Physical Therapy, Prescription, Wellness

Type of Coverage
Individual, Medicare, Medicaid

Type of Payment Plans Offered
Capitated, FFS

Geographic Areas Served
Maricopa County

Network Qualifications
Pre-Admission Certification: Yes

Peer Review Type
Utilization Review: Yes
Second Surgical Opinion: No
Case Management: Yes

Publishes and Distributes Report Card: Yes

Accreditation Certification
TJC Accreditation, Medicare Approved, Utilization Review,
Pre-Admission Certification, State Licensure, Quality Assurance
Program

Key Personnel
President/CEO . . . . Steve Purves

Specialty Managed Care Partners
Enters into Contracts with Regional Business Coalitions: Yes

49   Mercy Care Plan/Mercy Care Advantage

4350 East Cotton Center Boulevard
Building D
Phoenix, AZ 85040
Toll-Free: 800-624-3879
Phone: 602-263-3000
www.mercycareplan.com
Subsidiary of: Southwest Catholic Health Network
Non-Profit Organization: Yes
Year Founded: 1985
Total Enrollment: 300,000
State Enrollment: 300,000

Healthplan and Services Defined
PLAN TYPE: Medicare
Model Type: Group
Benefits Offered: Disease Management, Prescription, Wellness

Type of Coverage
Medicare, Medicaid

Geographic Areas Served
Cochise, Gila, Graham, Greenlee, La Paz, Maricopa, Pima, Pinal,
Santa Cruz, Yavapai, Yuma counties

50   Outlook Vision Service

1550 E McKellips Road
Suite 112
Mesa, AZ 85203
Toll-Free: 800-342-7188
Phone: 480-461-9001
Fax: 480-461-9021
customerservice@outlookvision.com
www.outlookvision.com
Year Founded: 1990
Federally Qualified: Yes
Total Enrollment: 7,000,000

Healthplan and Services Defined
PLAN TYPE: Vision
Plan Specialty: Vision
Benefits Offered: Prescription, Vision, Hearing

Type of Coverage
Commercial, Individual

Geographic Areas Served
Nationwide

Key Personnel
Owner/President . . . . Ron Johnson
Dir Provider Services . . . . Joan Vander Pluym

51   PacifiCare of Arizona

6245 E Broadway
Tucson, AZ 85711
Toll-Free: 800-624-8822
Phone: 602-244-8200
Fax: 602-681-7680
www.uhcwest.com
Acquired by: United Healthcare
For Profit Organization: Yes

Healthplan and Services Defined
   PLAN TYPE: HMO/PPO

Type of Coverage
   Commercial, Individual, Indemnity, Medicare

Key Personnel
   President......................................Ace Hodgin
   Manager Facilities ....Julie Carter

52   Phoenix Health Plan

7878 North 16th Street
Suite 105
Phoenix, AZ 85020
Toll-Free: 800-747-7997
Phone: 602-824-3700
www.phoenixhealthplan.com
Non-Profit Organization: Yes
Year Founded: 1982
Number of Affiliated Hospitals: 27
Number of Primary Care Physicians: 300
State Enrollment: 100,000

Healthplan and Services Defined
   PLAN TYPE: HMO
   Model Type: IPA
   Benefits Offered: Behavioral Health, Dental, Disease Management,
      Prescription, Wellness
   Offers Demand Management Patient Information Service: Yes
   DMPI Services Offered: 24 Hour Nurse Hotline

Type of Coverage
   Medicaid

Type of Payment Plans Offered
   POS, Combination FFS & DFFS

Geographic Areas Served
   Apache, Coconino, Gila, Maricopa, Mohave, Najavo, Pima, Pinal,
   Yavapai counties

Publishes and Distributes Report Card: Yes

Accreditation Certification
   NCQA
   TJC Accreditation, Medicare Approved, Utilization Review,
      Pre-Admission Certification, State Licensure, Quality Assurance
      Program

Key Personnel
   President/CEO ....Nancy Novick
   Marketing.....................................Mark Sands
   Medical Affairs ....Nancy Hirst
   Information Systems ....James Mathew
   Provider Services............................Mark Jokisch

Specialty Managed Care Partners
   Enters into Contracts with Regional Business Coalitions: Yes

53   Phoenix Health Plans

7878 North 16th Street
Suite 105
Phoenix, AZ 85020
Toll-Free: 888-864-1114
Phone: 602-824-3900
www.abrazoadvantage.com

Mailing Address: PO Box 81200, Phoenix, AZ 85069
Total Enrollment: 3,000

Healthplan and Services Defined
   PLAN TYPE: Multiple
   Benefits Offered: Chiropractic, Home Care, Inpatient SNF, Physical
      Therapy, Podiatry, Prescription, Vision, Wellness, Mental Health,
      Hospice

Type of Coverage
   Supplemental Medicare

Geographic Areas Served
   Arizona

Accreditation Certification
   TJC, URAC, NCQA

Key Personnel
   CEO ....Jeff Egbert
   CFO ....Brian Steines

54   Pima Health System

3950 S Country Club Road
Suite 350
Tucson, AZ 85714
Toll-Free: 866-518-6843
Phone: 520-243-8060
Fax: 866-472-4568
www.pimahealthsystem.org
Mailing Address: PO Box 7777, Phoenix, AZ 85011-777
Non-Profit Organization: Yes
Year Founded: 1982
Number of Affiliated Hospitals: 1
Number of Primary Care Physicians: 350
Total Enrollment: 7,000
State Enrollment: 7,000

Healthplan and Services Defined
   PLAN TYPE: HMO
   Model Type: Group
   Benefits Offered: Disease Management, Long-Term Care,
      Prescription, Wellness, Home Support Programs

Type of Coverage
   Medicaid

Type of Payment Plans Offered
   Capitated, FFS

Geographic Areas Served
   Pima, Santa Cruz counties

Subscriber Information
   Average Subscriber Co-Payment:
      Nursing Home Max. Days/Visits Covered: Fully covered

Publishes and Distributes Report Card: Yes

Accreditation Certification
   TJC Accreditation, Medicare Approved, Utilization Review,
      Pre-Admission Certification, State Licensure, Quality Assurance
      Program

Key Personnel
   President/CEO ....Karen Fields
   CFO...Donna Terry
   Materials Management......................Mona Berkowitz
   Medical Affairs ....Fred Miller, Md
   Member Services ....Virginia Rountree

55   Preferred Therapy Providers

23460 North 19th Avenue
Suite 250
Phoenix, AZ 85027
Toll-Free: 800-664-5240
Phone: 623-869-9101
contact@preferredtherapy.com

www.preferredtherapy.com
For Profit Organization: Yes
Year Founded: 1992
Physician Owned Organization: No
Federally Qualified: No
Number of Referral/Specialty Physicians: 3,000
Total Enrollment: 60,000,000

Healthplan and Services Defined
  PLAN TYPE: PPO
  Model Type: Network
  Plan Specialty: Physical, Occupational, Speech Therapies
  Benefits Offered: Physical Therapy, Ocupational Therapy, Speech Therapy
  Offers Demand Management Patient Information Service: No

Type of Coverage
  Commercial

Geographic Areas Served
  35 states

Network Qualifications
  Pre-Admission Certification: No

Publishes and Distributes Report Card: No

Accreditation Certification
  NCQA, AAPPO

Specialty Managed Care Partners
  Enters into Contracts with Regional Business Coalitions: No

---

56   SecureCare Dental
777 East Missouri Avenue
Suite 121
Phoenix, AZ 85014
Toll-Free: 888-429-0914
Phone: 602-241-0914
Fax: 602-285-0121
customer@securedental.com
www.securecaredental.com
Mailing Address: PO Box 29697, Phoenix, AZ 85038-9697
Year Founded: 1987
Number of Primary Care Physicians: 1,850
Total Enrollment: 55,000

Healthplan and Services Defined
  PLAN TYPE: Dental
  Other Type: Dental PPO
  Model Type: Network
  Plan Specialty: Dental
  Benefits Offered: Dental

Type of Coverage
  Commercial, Group

Type of Payment Plans Offered
  FFS, Combination FFS & DFFS

Geographic Areas Served
  Arizona and Nevada

Key Personnel
  President/CEO..............................David Popejoy
  Principal ....Thomas Abrams
  Marketing Director ....Mike Popejoy

---

57   Total Dental Administrators
2111 E Highland Avenue
Suite 250
Phoenix, AZ 85016-4735
Toll-Free: 888-422-1995
Phone: 602-266-1995
Fax: 602-266-1948
www.tdadental.com

Secondary Address: 6985 Union Park Center, Suite 675, Cottonwood Heights, UT 84047, 800-880-3536
Healthplan and Services Defined
  PLAN TYPE: Dental

Key Personnel
  President....................................Jane Morrison
  Provider Relations Mgr ....Meg Pipken
  VP, Technology ....Chad Cranston
  VP Sales/Marketing..........................Paulette Gafney
  Mgr Of Info Systems ....Chris Parrott
  Dental Director.............................Donald Peterson

---

58   United Concordia: Arizona
2198 E Camelback Road
Suite 260
Phoenix, AZ 85016
Toll-Free: 800-972-4191
Phone: 602-667-2201
ucproducer@ucci.com
www.ucci.com
For Profit Organization: Yes
Year Founded: 1971
Number of Primary Care Physicians: 111,000
Total Enrollment: 8,000,000

Healthplan and Services Defined
  PLAN TYPE: Dental
  Plan Specialty: Dental
  Benefits Offered: Dental

Type of Coverage
  Commercial, Individual

Geographic Areas Served
  Military personnel and their families, nationwide

---

59   UnitedHealthCare of Arizona
1 E Eashington Street
Suite 1700
Phoenix, AZ 85016
Toll-Free: 800-985-2356
www.uhc.com
Secondary Address: 6245 E Broadway, #600, Tucson, AZ 85711, 866-374-6057
Subsidiary of: UnitedHealth Group
For Profit Organization: Yes
Total Enrollment: 75,000,000
State Enrollment: 1,270,000

Healthplan and Services Defined
  PLAN TYPE: HMO/PPO

Geographic Areas Served
  Statewide

Key Personnel
  Chief Executive Officer ....Benton Davis
  Marketing.................................Janet Bollman
  Senior Medical Director.............. Robert Beauchamp, MD
  Media Contact ....Will Shanley
    will.shanley@uhc.com

---

60   University Family Care Health Plan

, AZ
Toll-Free: 800-582-8686
Phone: 520-874-5290
www.ufcaz.com
Subsidiary of: University Physicians Health Plans
Non-Profit Organization: Yes

Healthplan and Services Defined
  PLAN TYPE: HMO

Geographic Areas Served
  Maricopa County

---

61 ## VSP: Vision Service Plan of Arizona
2111 E Highland Avenue
Suite B160
Phoenix, AZ 85016-4757
Toll-Free: 800-877-7195
Phone: 602-956-1820
webmaster@vsp.com
www.vsp.com
Year Founded: 1955
Number of Primary Care Physicians: 26,000
Total Enrollment: 55,000,000

Healthplan and Services Defined
  PLAN TYPE: Vision
  Plan Specialty: Vision
  Benefits Offered: Vision

Type of Payment Plans Offered
  Capitated

Geographic Areas Served
  Statewide

Network Qualifications
  Pre-Admission Certification: Yes

Peer Review Type
  Utilization Review: Yes

Accreditation Certification
  Utilization Review, Quality Assurance Program

Health Insurance Coverage Status and Type of Coverage by Age

Category	All Persons		Under 18 years		Under 65 years		65 years and over	
	Number	%	Number	%	Number	%	Number	%
Total population	2,907	-	709	-	2,469	-	438	-
Covered by some type of health insurance	2,442 *(13)*	84.0 *(0.5)*	670 *(6)*	94.5 *(0.7)*	2,006 *(14)*	81.2 *(0.5)*	436 *(2)*	99.6 *(0.2)*
Covered by private health insurance	1,689 *(19)*	58.1 *(0.7)*	325 *(9)*	45.8 *(1.3)*	1,433 *(18)*	58.1 *(0.7)*	256 *(5)*	58.3 *(1.2)*
Employment based	1,343 *(18)*	46.2 *(0.6)*	281 *(10)*	39.6 *(1.4)*	1,232 *(17)*	49.9 *(0.7)*	111 *(5)*	25.3 *(1.1)*
Direct purchase	356 *(12)*	12.2 *(0.4)*	37 *(4)*	5.2 *(0.6)*	205 *(10)*	8.3 *(0.4)*	151 *(5)*	34.5 *(1.1)*
Covered by TRICARE	95 *(7)*	3.3 *(0.2)*	16 *(4)*	2.2 *(0.5)*	58 *(7)*	2.3 *(0.3)*	37 *(3)*	8.4 *(0.7)*
Covered by government health insurance	1,101 *(12)*	37.9 *(0.4)*	372 *(10)*	52.5 *(1.3)*	671 *(12)*	27.2 *(0.5)*	430 *(3)*	98.1 *(0.4)*
Covered by Medicaid	627 *(13)*	21.6 *(0.4)*	369 *(10)*	52.0 *(1.4)*	562 *(12)*	22.8 *(0.5)*	64 *(3)*	14.6 *(0.7)*
Also by private insurance	81 *(5)*	2.8 *(0.2)*	26 *(3)*	3.6 *(0.5)*	58 *(5)*	2.3 *(0.2)*	23 *(2)*	5.3 *(0.4)*
Covered by Medicare	555 *(7)*	19.1 *(0.2)*	5 *(2)*	0.7 *(0.2)*	126 *(5)*	5.1 *(0.2)*	429 *(3)*	97.9 *(0.4)*
Also by private insurance	279 *(6)*	9.6 *(0.2)*	Z *(Z)*	0.1 *(0.1)*	30 *(2)*	1.2 *(0.1)*	249 *(5)*	56.8 *(1.2)*
Also by Medicaid	118 *(5)*	4.0 *(0.2)*	2 *(1)*	0.3 *(0.1)*	53 *(4)*	2.2 *(0.2)*	64 *(3)*	14.6 *(0.7)*
Covered by VA Care	99 *(4)*	3.4 *(0.1)*	1 *(1)*	0.2 *(0.1)*	48 *(3)*	1.9 *(0.1)*	51 *(2)*	11.6 *(0.6)*
Not covered at any time during the year	465 *(14)*	16.0 *(0.5)*	39 *(5)*	5.5 *(0.7)*	463 *(14)*	18.8 *(0.5)*	2 *(1)*	0.4 *(0.2)*

Note: Numbers in thousands; Figures cover 2013; Margin of error appears in parenthesis; A "Z" indicates that the value either represents or rounds to zero.
Source: U.S. Census Bureau, 2013 American Community Survey, Table HI05. Health Insurance Coverage Status and Type of Coverage by State and Age for All People: 2013

Arkansas

62 Aetna Health of Arkansas

151 Farmington Avenue
Hartford, CT 06156
Toll-Free: 800-872-3862
Phone: 860-273-0123
www.aetna.com
Partnered with: eHealthInsurance Services Inc.
For Profit Organization: Yes
Total Enrollment: 11,596,230

Healthplan and Services Defined
PLAN TYPE: PPO
Other Type: POS
Plan Specialty: EPO
Benefits Offered: Dental, Disease Management, Long-Term Care,
Prescription, Wellness, Life, LTD, STD

Type of Coverage
Commercial, Individual

Type of Payment Plans Offered
POS, FFS

Geographic Areas Served
Statewide

Key Personnel
Chairman/CEO/President. Mark T Bertolini
EVP/General Counsel . . . . William J Casazza
EVP/CFO . . . . Shawn M Guertin

63 American Denticare

1525 Merrill Drive
Little Rock, AR 72211
Toll-Free: 877-537-6453
marketing@aiba.com
www.americandenticare.com
For Profit Organization: Yes
Year Founded: 1985
Number of Primary Care Physicians: 70
Number of Referral/Specialty Physicians: 25
Total Enrollment: 50,000

Healthplan and Services Defined
PLAN TYPE: HMO
Model Type: IPA
Plan Specialty: Dental
Benefits Offered: Dental
Offers Demand Management Patient Information Service: Yes

Type of Coverage
Commercial, Individual

Type of Payment Plans Offered
POS, Capitated

Geographic Areas Served
Arkansas, Chicot, Columbia, Craighead, Crawford, Crittenden,
Cross, Desha, Faulkner, Garland, Hot Springs, Jackson, Jefferson,
Lincoln, Lonoke, Miller, Mississippi, Poinsette, Pope, Pulaski,
Saline, Sebastian, St. Francis, Union, Washington, White counties

Network Qualifications
Pre-Admission Certification: Yes

Peer Review Type
Second Surgical Opinion: Yes
Case Management: Yes

Publishes and Distributes Report Card: Yes

Accreditation Certification
URAC
Quality Assurance Program

Key Personnel
President . . . . J Matt Lile III, RHU

64 Arkansas Blue Cross and Blue Shield

320 West Capitol
Suite 900
Little Rock, AR 72201
Toll-Free: 800-238-8379
Phone: 501-379-4600
Fax: 501-379-4659
www.arkansasbluecross.com
Mailing Address: PO Box 2181, Little Rock, AR 72203-2181
Subsidiary of: BlueAdvantage Administrators of Arkansas, Blue & You
Foundat
Total Enrollment: 400,000
State Enrollment: 400,000

Healthplan and Services Defined
PLAN TYPE: Multiple
Other Type: HMO, Medicare
Benefits Offered: Chiropractic, Dental, Home Care, Inpatient SNF,
Physical Therapy, Podiatry, Prescription, Vision, Worker's
Compensation, Life, Mental Health, Substance Abuse, Emergency

Type of Coverage
Commercial, Individual, Medicare, Supplemental Medicare
Catastrophic Illness Benefit: Varies per case

Geographic Areas Served
Arkansas

Subscriber Information
Average Subscriber Co-Payment:
Hospital ER: $250.00
Home Health Care: Varies
Nursing Home: Varies

Accreditation Certification
TJC, URAC, NCQA

Key Personnel
EVP/Chief of Strategy. . . . . Carl Kellogg, PhD
President & CEO . . . . P. Mark White
Executive VP & COO. . . . . Mike Brown
EVP, Internal Operations . . . . David Bridges
VP, Human Resources . . . . Richard Cooper
Vice President. . . . . Steve Abell
Senior Vice President. . . . . Jim Bailey
Chief Medical Officer/SVP. . . . . Robert Griffin, MD, MD
SVP, Statewide Business . . . . Ron DeBerry
SVP, Private Programs. . . . . Joseph Smith
SVP, Government Relations . . . . Lee Douglass
Media Contact. . . . . Max Heuer
501-378-2131
mxheuer@arkbluecross.com
VP, Communications. . . . . Karen Raley

65 Arkansas Community Care

10025 West Markham Street
Suite 220
Little Rock, AR 72205-2178
Toll-Free: 800-705-0766
Phone: 501-223-9889
lhenry@arcadianhealth.com
www.arkansascommunitycare.com
Subsidiary of: Arcadian Health Plans
Year Founded: 1998
Physician Owned Organization: Yes
Total Enrollment: 7,000

Healthplan and Services Defined
PLAN TYPE: Medicare
Plan Specialty: Dental, Vision
Benefits Offered: Dental, Prescription, Vision

Type of Coverage
Medicare, Supplemental Medicare

Geographic Areas Served
Benton, Carroll, Lonoke, Madison, Pulaski, Saline, Washington, and White counties

Key Personnel
President .... John Austin, MD
Executive Director............................ Ray Blaylock
Vice President .... Nancy Freeman

66 Arkansas Managed Care Organization

10 Corporate Hill Drive
Suite 200
Little Rock, AR 72205
Toll-Free: 800-278-8470
Phone: 501-225-8470
Fax: 501-225-7954
info@amcoppo.com
www.amcoppo.com
Non-Profit Organization: Yes
Year Founded: 1993
Owned by an Integrated Delivery Network (IDN): Yes
Number of Affiliated Hospitals: 100
Number of Primary Care Physicians: 1,000
Number of Referral/Specialty Physicians: 5,000
Total Enrollment: 200,000
State Enrollment: 200,000

Healthplan and Services Defined
PLAN TYPE: PPO
Model Type: Network
Plan Specialty: ASO, Behavioral Health, Chiropractic, Lab, PBM, Vision, Radiology, Burns, Cardiovascular Care, Neonatal Intensive Care, Neurological & Physical Rehabilitation, Organ Transplants
Benefits Offered: Behavioral Health, Chiropractic, Home Care, Long-Term Care, Physical Therapy, Podiatry, Transplant, Vision

Type of Coverage
Commercial, Individual

Accreditation Certification
NCQA
TJC Accreditation, Medicare Approved, State Licensure

Key Personnel
Associate Executive Dir......................... Jo Anna Gist
Director, Customer Serv......................... Pamela Loux
Credentialing Coordinator .... Sandra Sowell

Specialty Managed Care Partners
Enters into Contracts with Regional Business Coalitions: Yes

67 CIGNA HealthCare of Arkansas

3400 Players Club Parkway
Suite 140
Memphis, TN 38125
Toll-Free: 866-438-2446
Phone: 901-748-4100
Fax: 901-748-4104
www.cigna.com
For Profit Organization: Yes
Year Founded: 1985
Number of Affiliated Hospitals: 31
Number of Primary Care Physicians: 300
Number of Referral/Specialty Physicians: 1,668
Total Enrollment: 75,000,000

Healthplan and Services Defined
PLAN TYPE: HMO
Model Type: IPA
Benefits Offered: Behavioral Health, Disease Management, Home Care, Physical Therapy, Prescription, Psychiatric, Transplant, Vision, Wellness
Offers Demand Management Patient Information Service: Yes

DMPI Services Offered: Language Links Service, 24 hour Health Information Line, Health Information Library, Automated ReferralLine

Type of Coverage
Commercial
Catastrophic Illness Benefit: Varies per case

Type of Payment Plans Offered
POS

Geographic Areas Served
Cannon, Cheatham, Coffee, Davidson, DeKalb, Dickson, Franlin, Hickney, Maury, Montgomery, Overton, Robertson, Rutherford, Smith, Sumner, Warren, Williamson and Wilson counties, Tennessee

Subscriber Information
Average Subscriber Co-Payment:
Primary Care Physician: $10.00
Non-Network Physician: $10.00
Prescription Drugs: $10.00
Hospital ER: $500.00

Publishes and Distributes Report Card: Yes

Accreditation Certification
URAC, NCQA
TJC Accreditation, Medicare Approved

Key Personnel
President/CEO............................... David Mathis
CFO .... Stuart Wright
Network Contracting......................... David Mathis
In House Formulary .... Tim Moore
Medical Affairs......................... Frederick Buckwold
Member Services .... Chuck Utterbeck

Average Claim Compensation
Physician's Fees Charged: 82%
Hospital's Fees Charged: 56%

Specialty Managed Care Partners
Enters into Contracts with Regional Business Coalitions: Yes

68 CoreSource: Arkansas

1811 Rahling Road
Suite 100
Little Rock, AR 72223
Toll-Free: 888-604-9397
Phone: 501-221-9905
www.coresource.com
Subsidiary of: Trustmark
Year Founded: 1980
Total Enrollment: 1,100,000

Healthplan and Services Defined
PLAN TYPE: Multiple
Other Type: TPA
Model Type: Network
Plan Specialty: Claims Administration, TPA
Benefits Offered: Behavioral Health, Home Care, Prescription, Transplant

Type of Coverage
Commercial

Geographic Areas Served
Nationwide

Accreditation Certification
Utilization Review, Pre-Admission Certification

Key Personnel
President .... Nancy Eckrich
Vice President .... Rob Corrigan
Chief Financial Officer .... Clare Smith

69   Delta Dental of Arkansas

, AR
Toll-Free: 800-462-5410
Phone: 501-835-3400
Fax: 877-992-1854
eob@ddpar.com
www.deltadentalar.com
Non-Profit Organization: Yes
Year Founded: 1982
Total Enrollment: 54,000,000
State Enrollment: 1,000,000

Healthplan and Services Defined
  PLAN TYPE: Dental
  Other Type: Dental\Vision PPO
  Model Type: Network
  Plan Specialty: Dental, Vision
  Benefits Offered: Dental, Vision

Type of Coverage
  Commercial

Type of Payment Plans Offered
  DFFS

Geographic Areas Served
  Statewide

Subscriber Information
  Average Monthly Fee Per Subscriber
    (Employee + Employer Contribution):
      Employee Only (Self): $17
      Employee & 2 Family Members: $50
  Average Annual Deductible Per Subscriber:
      Employee Only (Self): $150
      Employee & 2 Family Members: $50
  Average Subscriber Co-Payment:
      Primary Care Physician: 80%
      Non-Network Physician: 50%

Network Qualifications
  Pre-Admission Certification: Yes

Publishes and Distributes Report Card: Yes

Key Personnel
  President/CEO . . . . Eddie Choate
  Chairman . . . . Ron Ownbey
  Vice Chairman . . . . Robert Gladden
  Media Contact . . . . Melissa Masingill
    501-992-1666
    mmasingill@ddpar.com

70   eHealthInsurance Services Inc.

11919 Foundation Place
Gold River, CA 95670
Toll-Free: 800-644-3491
webmaster@healthinsurance.com
www.e.healthinsurance.com
Year Founded: 1997

Healthplan and Services Defined
  PLAN TYPE: HMO/PPO
  Benefits Offered: Dental, Life, STD

Type of Coverage
  Commercial, Individual, Medicare

Geographic Areas Served
  All 50 states in the USA and District of Columbia

Key Personnel
  Chairman & CEO . . . . Gary L. Lauer
  EVP/Business & Corp. Dev. . . . . Bruce Telkamp
  EVP/Chief Technology . . . . Dr. Sheldon X. Wang
  SVP & CFO . . . . Stuart M. Huizinga
  Pres. of eHealth Gov. Sys . . . . Samuel C. Gibbs

SVP of Sales & Operations . . . . Robert S. Hurley
Director Public Relations . . . . Nate Purpura
  650-210-3115

71   HealthSCOPE Benefits

27 Corporate Hill Drive
Little Rock, AR 72205
Toll-Free: 800-972-3025
Phone: 501-218-7578
Fax: 501-218-7799
www.healthscopebenefits.com
Mailing Address: PO Box 1224, Little Rock, AR 72203
For Profit Organization: Yes
Year Founded: 1985
Total Enrollment: 475,000

Healthplan and Services Defined
  PLAN TYPE: Other
  Model Type: IPA, Group, Network, PHO
  Plan Specialty: ASO, Behavioral Health, Chiropractic, Dental,
    Disease Management, EPO, Lab, PBM, Vision, Radiology, UR,
    COBRA, HIPAA, FSA, Retiree
  Benefits Offered: Behavioral Health, Chiropractic, Complementary
    Medicine, Dental, Disease Management, Home Care, Inpatient
    SNF, Physical Therapy, Podiatry, Prescription, Psychiatric,
    Transplant, Vision, Wellness, STD

Type of Coverage
  Medicare, Catastrophic
  Catastrophic Illness Benefit: Maximum $1M

Type of Payment Plans Offered
  POS, DFFS, FFS, Combination FFS & DFFS

Geographic Areas Served
  Nationwide

Network Qualifications
  Minimum Years of Practice: 3
  Pre-Admission Certification: Yes

Peer Review Type
  Utilization Review: Yes
  Second Surgical Opinion: Yes
  Case Management: Yes

Accreditation Certification
  TJC, URAC
  Utilization Review, State Licensure

Key Personnel
  Chief Executive Officer . . . . Joe Edwards
  President . . . . Mary Catherine Person
  VP, Claims Administration . . . . Cathleen Armstrong
  SVP, Legal & Compliance . . . . Brett Edwards
  VP, IT . . . . Ross Johnston
  VP, Sales . . . . Scott Barnes
  SVP, Network Services . . . . Mike Castleberry
  Director, Operations . . . . Mel Cox
  VP, Business Systems . . . . Ed Grooms
  VP, Sales . . . . Wesley Jones

Specialty Managed Care Partners
  American Health Holdings, PHCS, Advance PCS, Caremark, CCN
  Enters into Contracts with Regional Business Coalitions: Yes
  Alaska Business Coalition

Employer References
  American Greetings, Alcoa, MedCath, Whirlpool

72   Humana Health Insurance of Little Rock

650 S Shackleford
Suite 125
Little Rock, AR 72211
Toll-Free: 800-941-4951
Fax: 501-223-2094
www.humana.com
For Profit Organization: Yes

Healthplan and Services Defined
PLAN TYPE: HMO/PPO
Plan Specialty: Vision
Benefits Offered: Dental, Prescription

Type of Coverage
Commercial, Individual, Medicare, Medicaid

Accreditation Certification
URAC, NCQA, CORE

73   Mercy Health Plans: Arkansas

521 President Clinton Ave
Suite 700
Little Rock, AR 72201
Toll-Free: 866-647-1551
Phone: 501-372-0065
Fax: 501-372-0211
www.mercyhealthplans.com
Non-Profit Organization: Yes
Total Enrollment: 73,000

Healthplan and Services Defined
PLAN TYPE: HMO

Type of Coverage
Commercial, Individual

74   Novasys Health

PO Box 25230
Little Rock, AR 72221
Toll-Free: 800-294-3557
Phone: 501-954-6100
Fax: 877-658-0306
customerservice@novasyshealth.com
www.novasyshealth.com

Healthplan and Services Defined
PLAN TYPE: PPO

Key Personnel
President . . . . .John Glassford
Executive Director/Claims . . . . .Michael Boone
CEO . . . . .John Ryan
VP of IT . . . . .Scott Shell

75   QualChoice/QCA Health Plan

12615 Chenal Parkway
Suite 300
Little Rock, AR 72211
Toll-Free: 800-235-7111
Phone: 501-228-7111
christy.garrett@qualchoice.com
www.qualchoice.com
Secondary Address: 4100 Corporate Center Drive, Suite 102,
    Springdale, AR 72762, 479-442-0700
Year Founded: 1994
Number of Affiliated Hospitals: 80
Number of Primary Care Physicians: 3,200
Total Enrollment: 36,000
State Enrollment: 84,176

Healthplan and Services Defined
PLAN TYPE: HMO/PPO
Other Type: POS
Benefits Offered: Behavioral Health, Dental, Prescription, Worker's
    Compensation, Life

Type of Coverage
Commercial, Individual, Indemnity

Geographic Areas Served
Statewide

Key Personnel
President . . . . .Francis Browning
VP, COO, CIO . . . . .M Haley Wilson
Chief Financial Officer . . . . .Randall A Crow
VP, Compliance . . . . .Jim Couch
Dir, Network Services. . . . . .Rose Anne Cato
VP, Underwriting . . . . .Jon Foose
VP, Operations . . . . .Joni S Daniels
VP, Pharmacy . . . . .Barry Fielder, PharmD
VP, Sales & Marketing . . . . .BJ Himes
Dir, Actuarial Services . . . . .Graham Sutherlin
VP, Medical Affairs . . . . .Richard Armstrong, MD
VP, Quality & Care Mgmt . . . . .Cindy Reese Furgerson, RN
VP/Information Svcs. . . . . .Jeff Brinsfield, Jr
Director/Provider Svcs . . . . .Mark Johnson
VP Sales/Marketing. . . . . .Roy Lamm

Specialty Managed Care Partners
Express Scripts

76   UnitedHealthCare

PO Box 29675
Hot Springs, AR 71903-9802
Toll-Free: 877-596-3258
www.uhcmedicaresolutions.com
Subsidiary of: UnitedHealthCare
For Profit Organization: Yes

Healthplan and Services Defined
PLAN TYPE: Medicare
Model Type: Network
Benefits Offered: Prescription

Type of Coverage
Medicare, Supplemental Medicare

Publishes and Distributes Report Card: Yes

Key Personnel
Chairman/CEO Health Sys. . . . . .Howard Phanstiel
CFO . . . . .Greg Scott
President/CEO Health Plan .Brad Bowlus
Exec VP/Specialty Plans . . . . .Jacqueline Kosecoff
Exec VP/Enterprise Svce. . . . . .Sharon Garrett
Exec VP/General Counsel . . . . .Joseph Konowiecki
Exec VP/Secure Horizons . . . . .Kathy Feeny
Exec VP/Major Accounts . . . . .James Frey
Exec VP/Chief Med Officer. .Sam Ho
Pres/CEO Behavioral Healt. . . . . .Jerome V Vaccaro, MD
Sr VP/Human Resources . . . . .Carol Black

Specialty Managed Care Partners
Enters into Contracts with Regional Business Coalitions: Yes

77   UnitedHealthCare of Arkansas

1401 Capital Avenue
Suite 375
Little Rock, AR 72201
Toll-Free: 800-678-3176
www.uhc.com
Subsidiary of: UnitedHealth Group
For Profit Organization: Yes
Year Founded: 1991
Total Enrollment: 75,000,000

State Enrollment: 92,995

Healthplan and Services Defined
  PLAN TYPE: HMO/PPO
  Model Type: IPA
  Benefits Offered: Dental, Disease Management, Prescription, Vision,
    Wellness, LTD, STD

Type of Coverage
  Commercial, Individual, Indemnity, Medicare

Type of Payment Plans Offered
  POS, FFS

Geographic Areas Served
  Statewide

Network Qualifications
  Pre-Admission Certification: Yes

Peer Review Type
  Utilization Review: Yes

Publishes and Distributes Report Card: Yes

Accreditation Certification
  URAC, NCQA
  TJC Accreditation, Medicare Approved, Utilization Review,
    Pre-Admission Certification, State Licensure, Quality Assurance
    Program

Key Personnel
  CEO . . . . Ken Hoverman
  Marketing . . . . David Johnson
  Sales. . . . . David Johnson

Specialty Managed Care Partners
  Enters into Contracts with Regional Business Coalitions: Yes

Health Insurance Coverage Status and Type of Coverage by Age

Category	All Persons		Under 18 years		Under 65 years		65 years and over	
	Number	%	Number	%	Number	%	Number	%
Total population	37,832	-	9,158	-	33,134	-	4,697	-
Covered by some type of health insurance	31,331 *(58)*	82.8 *(0.2)*	8,485 *(18)*	92.6 *(0.2)*	26,718 *(57)*	80.6 *(0.2)*	4,614 *(6)*	98.2 *(0.1)*
Covered by private health insurance	22,694 *(71)*	60.0 *(0.2)*	4,954 *(32)*	54.1 *(0.4)*	20,185 *(68)*	60.9 *(0.2)*	2,509 *(16)*	53.4 *(0.3)*
Employment based	18,809 *(76)*	49.7 *(0.2)*	4,248 *(34)*	46.4 *(0.4)*	17,287 *(72)*	52.2 *(0.2)*	1,522 *(16)*	32.4 *(0.4)*
Direct purchase	4,175 *(35)*	11.0 *(0.1)*	668 *(16)*	7.3 *(0.2)*	3,049 *(34)*	9.2 *(0.1)*	1,126 *(15)*	24.0 *(0.3)*
Covered by TRICARE	662 *(21)*	1.8 *(0.1)*	142 *(10)*	1.6 *(0.1)*	443 *(19)*	1.3 *(0.1)*	220 *(7)*	4.7 *(0.2)*
Covered by government health insurance	11,802 *(54)*	31.2 *(0.1)*	3,803 *(31)*	41.5 *(0.3)*	7,362 *(53)*	22.2 *(0.2)*	4,440 *(10)*	94.5 *(0.2)*
Covered by Medicaid	7,678 *(54)*	20.3 *(0.1)*	3,747 *(32)*	40.9 *(0.3)*	6,767 *(52)*	20.4 *(0.2)*	911 *(14)*	19.4 *(0.3)*
Also by private insurance	786 *(20)*	2.1 *(0.1)*	263 *(10)*	2.9 *(0.1)*	585 *(17)*	1.8 *(0.1)*	200 *(7)*	4.3 *(0.2)*
Covered by Medicare	5,150 *(20)*	13.6 *(0.1)*	74 *(7)*	0.8 *(0.1)*	719 *(17)*	2.2 *(0.1)*	4,432 *(10)*	94.3 *(0.2)*
Also by private insurance	2,491 *(18)*	6.6 *(0.1)*	8 *(2)*	0.1 *(0.1)*	160 *(6)*	0.5 *(0.1)*	2,331 *(17)*	49.6 *(0.4)*
Also by Medicaid	1,267 *(18)*	3.3 *(0.1)*	25 *(4)*	0.3 *(0.1)*	355 *(11)*	1.1 *(0.1)*	911 *(14)*	19.4 *(0.3)*
Covered by VA Care	560 *(11)*	1.5 *(0.1)*	9 *(3)*	0.1 *(0.1)*	280 *(9)*	0.8 *(0.1)*	280 *(7)*	6.0 *(0.1)*
Not covered at any time during the year	6,500 *(57)*	17.2 *(0.2)*	673 *(18)*	7.4 *(0.2)*	6,417 *(56)*	19.4 *(0.2)*	83 *(6)*	1.8 *(0.1)*

Note: Numbers in thousands; Figures cover 2013; Margin of error appears in parenthesis; A "Z" indicates that the value either represents or rounds to zero.
Source: U.S. Census Bureau, 2013 American Community Survey, Table HI05. Health Insurance Coverage Status and Type of Coverage by State and Age for All People: 2013

California

78 Access Dental Services

2693 Florin Road
Sacramento, CA 95822
Phone: 916-424-5500
Fax: 916-424-7634
104m@accessdental.com
www.accessdental.com
Secondary Address: 5200 Stockton Boulevard, Suite 110, Sacramento, CA 95820, 916-455-6600
For Profit Organization: Yes
Year Founded: 1989
Number of Primary Care Physicians: 2,000
Total Enrollment: 123,880

Healthplan and Services Defined
PLAN TYPE: Dental
Model Type: Staff
Plan Specialty: Dental
Benefits Offered: Dental

Type of Coverage
Commercial, Individual, Medicare, Supplemental Medicare, Medicaid

Geographic Areas Served
Statewide

Key Personnel
Office Manager . . . . Shilo Cortes

79 Aetna Health of California

2625 Shadelands Drive
Suite 1100, MSF915
Walnut Creek, CA 94598
Toll-Free: 866-582-9629
www.aetna.com
For Profit Organization: Yes
Total Enrollment: 427,039
State Enrollment: 427,039

Healthplan and Services Defined
PLAN TYPE: HMO
Plan Specialty: EPO
Benefits Offered: Dental, Disease Management, Long-Term Care, Prescription, Wellness, Life, LTD, STD

Type of Coverage
Commercial, Individual

Type of Payment Plans Offered
POS, FFS

Geographic Areas Served
Statewide

Key Personnel
Chairman/CEO . . . . Mark Bertollini
General Counsel . . . . William Casazza
EVP/Government Svcs . . . . Kristi Matus
EVP/Operations . . . . Meg McCarthy

80 Alameda Alliance for Health

1240 South Loop Road
Alameda, CA 94502
Phone: 510-747-4500
www.alamedaalliance.org
Secondary Address: 3075 Adeline Street, Suite 160, Berkeley, CA 94703, 510-747-6100
Non-Profit Organization: Yes
Year Founded: 1996
Federally Qualified: Yes
Number of Affiliated Hospitals: 15

Number of Primary Care Physicians: 1,700
Total Enrollment: 140,000
State Enrollment: 110,000

Healthplan and Services Defined
PLAN TYPE: HMO
Model Type: Network
Plan Specialty: Dental
Benefits Offered: Dental, Prescription, Vision, Medi-Cal, Healthy Families, Alliance Group Care, Alliance CompleteCare

Type of Coverage
Individual, Government Sponsored Programs

Type of Payment Plans Offered
POS

Geographic Areas Served
California

Peer Review Type
Second Surgical Opinion: Yes

Accreditation Certification
State Licensure

81 American Specialty Health

10221 Wateridge Circle
San Diego, CA 92121
Toll-Free: 800-848-3555
Fax: 619-237-3859
www.ashcompanies.com
For Profit Organization: Yes
Year Founded: 1987
Total Enrollment: 94,000,000

Healthplan and Services Defined
PLAN TYPE: HMO
Model Type: Network
Plan Specialty: Chiropractic
Benefits Offered: Chiropractic, Complementary Medicine, Acupuncture

Type of Coverage
Commercial, Supplemental Medicare

Type of Payment Plans Offered
POS, Capitated

Geographic Areas Served
Nationwide - ASH Network, California - ASH Plans

Network Qualifications
Pre-Admission Certification: Yes

Peer Review Type
Utilization Review: Yes
Case Management: Yes

Accreditation Certification
URAC

Specialty Managed Care Partners
Enters into Contracts with Regional Business Coalitions: Yes

82 Arcadian Health Plans

500 12th Street
Suite 350
Oakland, CA 94607
Phone: 510-832-0311
Fax: 510-832-0170
www.arcadianhealth.com
Subsidiary of: Humana Healthcare
For Profit Organization: Yes

Healthplan and Services Defined
PLAN TYPE: HMO/PPO

Key Personnel
President/CEO . . . . Bruce D. Broussard

EVP, COO . . . . James E. Murray
SVP, CFO & Treasurer . . . . James H. Bloem
SVP, General Counsel . . . . Christopher M. Todoroff
SVP, CHRO . . . . Tim Huval
SVP, Human Capital . . . . Heidi Sullivan
Executive Manager . . . . Terrence Cullen
SVP, Chief Sales & Mktg . . . . Garrison Rios
SVP, CMO . . . . Roy A. Beveridge, MD
SVP, CIO . . . . Brian LeClaire
SVP, Public Affairs . . . . Heidi S. Margulis

---

83 Arta Medicare Health Plan

1640 E Hill Street
Signal Hill, CA 90755
Toll-Free: 800-735-2929
Phone: 888-327-2730
www.mdcarehealthplan.com
Mailing Address: PO Box 92919, Long Beach, CA 90809
Year Founded: 1995
Number of Affiliated Hospitals: 15
Number of Primary Care Physicians: 800
Total Enrollment: 55,000
State Enrollment: 55,000

Healthplan and Services Defined
 PLAN TYPE: Medicare
 Other Type: HMO

Type of Coverage
 Individual, Medicare, Supplemental Medicare

Key Personnel
 President . . . . Baruch Fogel
 Chief Medical Officer . . . . Robert Sorrentine

---

84 Assurant Employee Benefits: California

2323 Grand Boulevard
Kansas City, CA 64108
Phone: 816-474-2345
www.assurantemployeebenefits.com
Subsidiary of: Assurant, Inc
For Profit Organization: Yes
Number of Primary Care Physicians: 112,000
Total Enrollment: 47,000

Healthplan and Services Defined
 PLAN TYPE: Multiple
 Plan Specialty: Dental, Vision, Long & Short-Term Disability
 Benefits Offered: Dental, Vision, Wellness, AD&D, Life, LTD, STD

Type of Coverage
 Commercial, Indemnity, Individual Dental Plans

Geographic Areas Served
 Statewide

Subscriber Information
 Average Monthly Fee Per Subscriber
 (Employee + Employer Contribution):
  Employee Only (Self): Varies by plan

Key Personnel
 President/CEO . . . . John S. Roberts
 SVP,CFO . . . . Miles B. Yakre
 SVP, General Counsel . . . . Kenneth D. Bowen
 SVP, Marketing . . . . Joseph A. Sevcik
 SVP, Human Resources & De . . . . Rosemary Polk
 SVP, CIO . . . . Karla J. Schacht
 SVP, Sales . . . . J. Marc Warrington
 PR Specialist . . . . Megan Hutchison
  816-556-7815
  megan.hutchinson@assurant.com

---

85 Basic Chiropractic Health Plan

2027 Grand Canal Blvd
Suite 21
Stockton, CA 95207
Toll-Free: 866-224-7462
Phone: 209-476-1435
www.chpc.com
Year Founded: 1999

Healthplan and Services Defined
 PLAN TYPE: PPO
 Plan Specialty: Chiropractic
 Benefits Offered: Chiropractic

Key Personnel
 President . . . . Don Smallie, DC
  dsmallie@bchpinc.com
 CEO/COO . . . . David Moscovic
  david@bchpinc.com
 Accounting Manager . . . . Venus Giacomotti
  venus@bchpinc.com
 Member Services . . . . Kimberly Randolph
  kimberly@bchpinc.com
 Provider Relations . . . . Kimberly Randolph
  kimberly@bchpinc.com

---

86 Beech Street Corporation: Corporate Office

25500 Commercentre Drive
Lake Forest, CA 92630-8855
Toll-Free: 800-877-1444
Phone: 949-672-1000
Fax: 949-672-1111
viantinquiries@multiplan.com
www.beechstreet.com
Subsidiary of: Viant
Acquired by: MultiPlan
For Profit Organization: Yes
Year Founded: 1951
Owned by an Integrated Delivery Network (IDN): Yes
Number of Affiliated Hospitals: 3,800
Number of Primary Care Physicians: 400,000
Total Enrollment: 16,000,000
State Enrollment: 653,000

Healthplan and Services Defined
 PLAN TYPE: PPO
 Model Type: Network
 Plan Specialty: Behavioral Health, Chiropractic, Disease
  Management, Lab, Radiology, Worker's Compensation, UR
 Benefits Offered: Behavioral Health, Chiropractic, Disease
  Management, Home Care, Inpatient SNF, Long-Term Care,
  Physical Therapy, Podiatry, Psychiatric, Transplant, Wellness,
  Worker's Compensation

Type of Payment Plans Offered
 Capitated, FFS

Network Qualifications
 Pre-Admission Certification: Yes

Peer Review Type
 Utilization Review: Yes
 Second Surgical Opinion: Yes
 Case Management: Yes

Accreditation Certification
 URAC, NCQA

Key Personnel
 CEO . . . . Deborah Gage
 President, Viant . . . . Tom Bartlett
 EVP, Finance & CFO . . . . David Redmund
 General Counsel . . . . Bryan Adel
 EVP, Network Development . . . . Keith Vangeison
 EVP, Chief Info Officer . . . . Meridith Herdes

SVP, Information Tech ....Santosh Dave
SVP, Sales & Marketing ....Terry Harris
Media Contact.................................Cliff Greifer
  630-649-5345
  cliff.greifer@viant.com

Specialty Managed Care Partners
Enters into Contracts with Regional Business Coalitions: Yes

---

87 Beech Street Corporation: Northeast Region

25500 Commercentre Drive
Lake Forest, CA 92630
Toll-Free: 866-875-0030
Phone: 212-944-7600
Fax: 212-944-7655
www.beechstreet.com
Subsidiary of: Viant
Acquired by: MultiPlan
For Profit Organization: Yes
Total Enrollment: 12,225,000
State Enrollment: 773,000

Healthplan and Services Defined
  PLAN TYPE: PPO
  Benefits Offered: Disease Management, Wellness

Accreditation Certification
  NCQA

Key Personnel
President and CEO ....Bill Hale

---

88 Beech Street Corporation: Western Region

PO Box 5061
Lake Forest, CA 92609-5061
Phone: 949-639-3800
Fax: 949-639-3880
Subsidiary of: Viant
Acquired by: MultiPlan
Total Enrollment: 12,225,000
State Enrollment: 653,000

Healthplan and Services Defined
  PLAN TYPE: HMO
  Benefits Offered: Disease Management, Home Care, Inpatient SNF,
    Long-Term Care, Prescription, Psychiatric, Wellness

---

89 BEST Life and Health Insurance Co.

17701 Mitchell North
Irvine, CA 92614-6028
Toll-Free: 800-433-0088
Fax: 208-893-5040
cs@bestlife.com
www.bestlife.com
Mailing Address: PO Box 890, Meridian, ID 83680-0890
For Profit Organization: Yes
Year Founded: 1970
Number of Affiliated Hospitals: 5,005
Number of Primary Care Physicians: 772,292
Total Enrollment: 90,000

Healthplan and Services Defined
  PLAN TYPE: PPO
  Model Type: PPO/Indemnity
  Benefits Offered: Dental, Disease Management, Vision, Wellness,
    Life, STD

Type of Coverage
  Commercial

Geographic Areas Served
  AK, AL, AR, AZ, CA, CO, DC, FL, GA, HI, ID, IL, IN, KS, KY, LA,
  MD, MI, MS, MO, MT, NC, ND, NE, NM, NV, OH, OK, OR, PA, SC,
  SD, TN, TX, UT, VA, WA, WY

Network Qualifications
  Pre-Admission Certification: Yes

Peer Review Type
  Case Management: Yes

Accreditation Certification
  URAC, NCQA
  Quality Assurance Program

Key Personnel
President ....Donald Lawerence

---

90 Blue Shield of California

50 Beale Street
San Francisco, CA 94105-1808
Toll-Free: 800-393-6130
Phone: 415-229-5000
www.blueshieldca.com
Mailing Address: P.O. Box 272540, Chico, CA 95927-2540
Subsidiary of: California Physicians' Service, Inc
Non-Profit Organization: Yes
Year Founded: 1939
Number of Affiliated Hospitals: 354
Number of Primary Care Physicians: 67,000
Total Enrollment: 3,500,000
State Enrollment: 3,500,000

Healthplan and Services Defined
  PLAN TYPE: HMO/PPO
  Benefits Offered: Home Care, Prescription

Type of Coverage
  Supplemental Medicare

Geographic Areas Served
  California

Accreditation Certification
  NCQA

Key Personnel
President/CEO...............................Paul Markovich
EVP, Health Care Quality ....Juan Davila
SVP/CIO..................................Michael Mathias
SVP/CFO..................................Michael Murray
SVP, Customer Quality ....Rob Geyer
SVP/Chief HR Officer.......................Mary O'Hara
SVP, Enterprise Sales.........................Jeff Hermosillo
SVP/Chief Health Officer ....Marcus Thygeson, MD
EVP, Markets ....Janet Widmann
SVP/General Counsel......................Seth A. Jacobs, Esq.
SVP, Consumer Markets ....Ken Wood

---

91 Brand New Day HMO

5455 Garden Grove Boulevard
Suite 500
Westminster, CA 92683
Toll-Free: 866-255-4795
Fax: 657-400-1212
www.hmocalif.com

Healthplan and Services Defined
  PLAN TYPE: HMO
  Plan Specialty: Behavioral Health
  Benefits Offered: Behavioral Health, Dental, Disease Management,
    Prescription, Psychiatric, Vision, Wellness

Type of Coverage
  Individual, Medicare, Medicaid

92 Bright Now! Dental

3358 South Bristol Street
Santa Ana, CA 92704
Toll-Free: 844-400-7645
Phone: 714-361-2141
www.brightnow.com
Secondary Address: 1601 West 17th Street, Suite G, Santa Ana, CA
92706, 714-567-9255
Year Founded: 1998
Number of Primary Care Physicians: 300
Number of Referral/Specialty Physicians: 416
Total Enrollment: 950,000

Healthplan and Services Defined
PLAN TYPE: Dental
Model Type: Staff, Network
Plan Specialty: Dental
Benefits Offered: Dental

Type of Payment Plans Offered
Capitated

Geographic Areas Served
Nationwide

Subscriber Information
Average Monthly Fee Per Subscriber
(Employee + Employer Contribution):
Employee Only (Self): $40.00
Employee & 1 Family Member: $75.00
Employee & 2 Family Members: $110.00

Network Qualifications
Pre-Admission Certification: Yes

Key Personnel
President/CEO.................................Steven Bilt
sbilt@brightnow.com
CFO ....Bradley Schmidt
CIO ....George Suda
Human Resource Mgr.........................Beth Goldstein
VP Dental Affairs ....Charles Stirewalt, DDS
cstirewalt@brightnow.com
Medical Affairs ....Charles Stirewalt, DMD
Member Services ....Lanchi Hua

Specialty Managed Care Partners
Enters into Contracts with Regional Business Coalitions: No

93 California Dental Network

23291 Mill Creek Drive
Suite 100
Laguna Hills, CA 92653
Toll-Free: 877-433-6825
Fax: 949-830-1655
www.caldental.net

Healthplan and Services Defined
PLAN TYPE: Dental
Plan Specialty: Dental
Benefits Offered: Dental

Type of Coverage
Individual

Key Personnel
Chairman......................................James Lindsey
President ....Steven Casey

94 California Foundation for Medical Care

3993 Jurupa Avenue
Riverside, CA 92506
Phone: 951-686-9049
RFP@CFMCNet.org
www.cfmcnet.org

Non-Profit Organization: Yes
Year Founded: 1983
Number of Affiliated Hospitals: 300
Number of Primary Care Physicians: 34,000
Number of Referral/Specialty Physicians: 5,500
Total Enrollment: 1,000,000

Healthplan and Services Defined
PLAN TYPE: PPO
Other Type: EPO and Workers Comp
Plan Specialty: Behavioral Health, Lab, Worker's Compensation, UR
Benefits Offered: Worker's Compensation, EPO

Geographic Areas Served
California

Key Personnel
President.................................Steve Beargeon
559-734-1321
steve@tkfmc.org
CEO ....Dolores L Green
951-686-9094
dgreen@rcmanet.org
Dir Of Administration ....Ester M Sanchez
951-686-9049
esanchez@rfasi.com
Network Coordinator ....Bianca Scarborough
951-686-9049
bscraborough@rfasi.com

95 CalOptima

505 City Parkway West
Orange, CA 92868
Toll-Free: 888-587-8088
Phone: 714-246-8500
www.caloptima.org
For Profit Organization: Yes
Year Founded: 1995
Owned by an Integrated Delivery Network (IDN): Yes
Number of Primary Care Physicians: 3,500
Total Enrollment: 413,795
State Enrollment: 402,000

Healthplan and Services Defined
PLAN TYPE: HMO
Model Type: Group
Plan Specialty: ASO, Behavioral Health, Chiropractic, Dental,
Disease Management, EPO, Lab, MSO, PBM, Vision, Radiology,
Worker's Compensation
Benefits Offered: Prescription

Type of Coverage
Individual, Supplemental Medicare, Medicaid, Medi-Cal

Geographic Areas Served
Orange County

Key Personnel
Chief Executive Officer ....Michael Schrader
Chief Counsel.................................Gary Crockett
Chief Medical Officer....................Richard Helmer, MD
Chief Operating Officer ....Bill Jones
Chief Information Officer ....Len Rosignoli
Chief of Strategy.............................Michael Ruane
Chief Network Officer ....Javier Sanchez
Chief Financial Officer.........................Chet C. Uma
Executive Director, Ops......................Ladan Khamseh

96   Care 1st Health Plan: California
601 Potrero Grande Drive
Monterey Park, CA 91755
Toll-Free: 800-847-1222
Phone: 323-889-6638
Fax: 323-889-6255
www.care1st.com
Secondary Address: 3131 Camino del Rio North, Suite 350, San
    Diego, CA 92108, 619-528-4800
For Profit Organization: Yes
Year Founded: 1995
Number of Affiliated Hospitals: 69
Number of Primary Care Physicians: 3,000
Total Enrollment: 291,000

Healthplan and Services Defined
    PLAN TYPE: HMO
    Benefits Offered: Disease Management, Wellness

Type of Coverage
    Supplemental Medicare, Medicaid

Geographic Areas Served
    Southern California & Arizona

Accreditation Certification
    NCQA

Key Personnel
    CEO .... Anna Tran
    Chief Financial Officer .... Janet Jan
    Chief Medical Info Office .... Darryl Leong
    VP, Legal & Regulator Ser .... Alan Bloom
    VP, Compliance .... Brooks Jones
    VP, Medical Services .... Josie Wong, RN
    VP, Pharmacy & Medicare .... Michael Lasconia
    Dir, Legal & Regulatory S .... Gamini Gunawardane, PhD
    Assoc VP, Quality Improve .... David Wedemeyer
    Chief Medical Officer .... Jorge Weingarten, Md
    Medi-Cal Operations .... Tracie Howell
    Information Technology .... Michael Rowan
    VP, Business Development .... Walter Gray
    Dir, Medicare Sales .... Ed Gorner

97   CareMore Health Plan
12900 Park Plaza Drive
Suite 150, MS-6150
Cerritos, CA 90703
Toll-Free: 800-499-2793
Fax: 562-741-4406
www.caremore.com

Healthplan and Services Defined
    PLAN TYPE: Medicare

Type of Coverage
    Medicare

Geographic Areas Served
    Arizona, California, Nevada

Key Personnel
    Chief Executive Officer .... Leeba Lessin
    President .... Jason Barker
    Chief Operations Officer .... Vish Sankaran
    Chief Financial Officer .... Michael Plumb
    Chief, Clinical Services .... Balu Gadhe
    Chief Development Officer .... Robert Lonardo
    VP/Chief Info Officer .... Jamie Myers
    Chief Nurse Practitioner .... Peggy Salazar, RN, MSN

**98   CenCal Health: The Regional Health
Authority**
4050 Calle Real
Santa Barbara, CA 93110
Toll-Free: 800-421-2560
Phone: 805-685-9525
webmaster@cencalhealth.org
www.cencalhealth.org
Non-Profit Organization: Yes

Healthplan and Services Defined
    PLAN TYPE: HMO
    Benefits Offered: Complementary Medicine, Disease Management,
        Prescription, Wellness

Type of Coverage
    Individual, Medicare, Medicaid, Medi-Cal, Healthly Families

Geographic Areas Served
    Santa Barbara and San Luis Obispo counties

Key Personnel
    Chief Executive Officer .... Bob Freeman, MBA
    CFO/Treasurer .... David Ambrose
        dambrose@cencalhealth.org
    Chief Operation Officer .... Paul Jaconette, MD, MBA
    Claims Operations Directo .... Lulu Van Alvensleben
    Chief Medical Officer .... Lowell Gordon
    Member Services Director .... Donna Slimak
    Information Technology .... Dave Seibel
    Provider Services Directo .... Marina Gordon

99   Central California Alliance for Health
1600 Green Hills Road
Suite 101
Scotts Valley, CA 95066-4981
Toll-Free: 800-700-3874
Phone: 831-430-5500
www.ccah-alliance.org
Secondary Address: 339 Pajaro Street, Suite E, Salinas, CA
    93901-3400, 831-755-6000
Non-Profit Organization: Yes
Year Founded: 1996
Physician Owned Organization: No
Federally Qualified: No
Number of Primary Care Physicians: 1,590
Total Enrollment: 210,000
State Enrollment: 190,000

Healthplan and Services Defined
    PLAN TYPE: HMO
    Model Type: County Org Health System
    Benefits Offered: Medi-Cal, Healthy Families, Healthy Kids, Alliance
        Care Access for Infants and Mothers, Alliance Care IHSS
    Offers Demand Management Patient Information Service: No

Geographic Areas Served
    Santa Cruz, Monterey and Merced counties

Network Qualifications
    Pre-Admission Certification: No

Publishes and Distributes Report Card: No

Key Personnel
    Executive Director .... Alan McCay
    Chief Financial Officer .... Patti McFarland
    Chief Operating Officer .... Rachael Nava
    Provider Services Dir. .... Stephanie Sonnenshine
    Finance Director .... Frank Souza
    Utilization Management .... Christine Gerbo, RN
    Human Resources Director .... Scott Fortner
    Pharmacy Director .... Richard Johnson, PharmD
    Quality Improvement Dir .... Barbara Flynn, RN
    Reg Dir, Monterey County .... Lilia Chagolla

Medical Director . . . . Richard Helmer, MD
Assoc Medical Director . . . . David Altman, MD
Information Tech Director . . . . Bob Chernis
Govt Relations Director . . . . Danita Carlson
Reg Dir, Merced County. . . . . Jennifer Mockus, RN
Business Devlopment Mgr . . . . Traci Webb
   831-430-5500
   press@ccah-alliance.org
Member Services Director . . . . Jan Wolf

Specialty Managed Care Partners
Enters into Contracts with Regional Business Coalitions: No

---

100 Central Health Medicare Plan
1540 Bridgegate Drive
Diamond Bar, CA 91765
Toll-Free: 866-314-2427
Phone: 626-388-2300
Fax: 626-388-2329
compliance@centralhealthplan.com
www.centralhealthplan.com
Subsidiary of: Central Health Plan of California, Inc
Year Founded: 2004
Total Enrollment: 3,000

Healthplan and Services Defined
   PLAN TYPE: Medicare
   Other Type: HMO
   Benefits Offered: Chiropractic, Dental, Home Care, Inpatient SNF,
      Podiatry, Vision, Wellness

Type of Coverage
   Medicare, Supplemental Medicare

Geographic Areas Served
   Los Angeles, San Bernardino, Orange counties

Subscriber Information
   Average Monthly Fee Per Subscriber
      (Employee + Employer Contribution):
         Employee Only (Self): $89.00
   Average Subscriber Co-Payment:
         Primary Care Physician: $5.00/10.00
         Prescription Drugs: Varies
         Hospital ER: $50.00
         Home Health Care: Varies
         Nursing Home: Varies

---

101 Chinese Community Health Plan
445 Grant Avenue
Suite 700
San Francisco, CA 94108
Toll-Free: 888-775-7888
Phone: 415-955-8800
Fax: 415-955-8818
www.cchphmo.com
Secondary Address: 827 Pacific Ave, San Francisco, CA 94133
For Profit Organization: Yes
Year Founded: 1986
Owned by an Integrated Delivery Network (IDN): Yes
Number of Affiliated Hospitals: 5
Number of Primary Care Physicians: 160
Number of Referral/Specialty Physicians: 144
Total Enrollment: 13,582
State Enrollment: 6,336

Healthplan and Services Defined
   PLAN TYPE: HMO
   Model Type: IPA
   Benefits Offered: Prescription, Acupuncture Services, Worldwide
      Emergency

Type of Coverage
   Medicare

Geographic Areas Served
   San Francisco, Northern San Mateo

Subscriber Information
   Average Monthly Fee Per Subscriber
      (Employee + Employer Contribution):
         Employee Only (Self): $218.00
         Employee & 1 Family Member: $419.00
         Employee & 2 Family Members: $384.53
   Average Subscriber Co-Payment:
         Primary Care Physician: $10.00
         Non-Network Physician: Not covered
         Prescription Drugs: $6.00
         Hospital ER: $25.00
         Home Health Care Max. Days/Visits Covered: None except
            mental
         Nursing Home Max. Days/Visits Covered: 10 days

Network Qualifications
   Pre-Admission Certification: Yes

Peer Review Type
   Utilization Review: Yes
   Second Surgical Opinion: Yes
   Case Management: Yes

Accreditation Certification
   TJC Accreditation, Medicare Approved, Utilization Review,
      Pre-Admission Certification, State Licensure, Quality Assurance
      Program

Key Personnel
   CEO/Executive Director . . . . Richard Loosn
   CFO . . . . Steve Tsang
   Executive Director. . . . . Tom Tsang
   Claims Manager . . . . Amy Lee
   Dir, Business Development . . . . Deena Louie
   Manager, Sales . . . . Yolanda Lee
   Dir, Clinical Services . . . . Dana Samples
   Chief Medical Officer . . . . Edward Chow, MD
   Member Services Manager. . . . . Irene Louie
   IT Manager . . . . JC Tucker
   Provider Services Manager. . . . . Heather Brandenburg

Specialty Managed Care Partners
   Enters into Contracts with Regional Business Coalitions: No

---

102 Chiropractic Health Plan of California
5356 Clayton Road #201
Concord, CA 94521
Toll-Free: 800-995-2442
Phone: 925-844-3100
Fax: 925-844-3124
info@chpc.com
www.chpc.com
Mailing Address: PO Box 190, Clayton, CA 94517
For Profit Organization: Yes
Year Founded: 1986
Number of Primary Care Physicians: 795

Healthplan and Services Defined
   PLAN TYPE: PPO
   Model Type: Network
   Plan Specialty: ASO, Chiropractic, EPO, Worker's Compensation, UR
   Benefits Offered: Chiropractic, Worker's Compensation, Group
      Health

Type of Coverage
   Commercial

Type of Payment Plans Offered
   POS, DFFS, FFS, Combination FFS & DFFS

Geographic Areas Served
   California, Nevada, Texas

Network Qualifications
   Pre-Admission Certification: Yes

Peer Review Type
Utilization Review: Yes

Key Personnel
CEO . . . . Ronald Cataldo
CFO . . . . Amy Tsui
Claims . . . . Gloria Spahn
Medical Affairs . . . . Ronald Cataldo, DC
Provider Services . . . . Ronald Cataldo, DC

Specialty Managed Care Partners
Enters into Contracts with Regional Business Coalitions: Yes

---

103   ChiroSource Inc

5356 Clayton Road
Suite 201
Concord, CA 94521
Toll-Free: 800-680-9997
Phone: 925-672-5333
Fax: 925-844-3124
info@chirosource.com
www.chirosource.com
Mailing Address: PO Box 130, Clayton, CA 94517
Subsidiary of: Discover Health, A Product of ChiroSource, Inc.
For Profit Organization: Yes
Year Founded: 1993
Number of Primary Care Physicians: 2,133
Total Enrollment: 100,000,000

Healthplan and Services Defined
PLAN TYPE: Multiple
Model Type: Network
Plan Specialty: Chiropractic, Physical Medicine, Accupuncture, Massage
Benefits Offered: Worker's Compensation, Health-Group & Individual, Medicare Advantage, IME Networks

Type of Coverage
PPO, EPO, POS, MPN, HCN, IME

Type of Payment Plans Offered
FFS

Geographic Areas Served
National

Network Qualifications
Pre-Admission Certification: Yes

Peer Review Type
Utilization Review: Yes

Publishes and Distributes Report Card: No

Key Personnel
President/CEO . . . . Christopher DeRosa, DC
CFO . . . . Jean Francois Beaule
Executive Director . . . . Debbie Turner
Claims . . . . Glorie Spahn
Chief Medical Officer . . . . James K Wang

Specialty Managed Care Partners
Enters into Contracts with Regional Business Coalitions: Yes

---

104   CIGNA HealthCare of California

400 North Brand Blvd
Suite 400
Glendale, CA 91203
Toll-Free: 866-621-8270
Phone: 818-500-6262
www.cigna.com
For Profit Organization: Yes
Total Enrollment: 234,072
State Enrollment: 234,072

Healthplan and Services Defined
PLAN TYPE: HMO

Other Type: POS
Type of Coverage
Commercial

---

105   CIGNA HealthCare of Northern California

1 Front Street
7th Floor
San Francisco, CA 94111
Toll-Free: 888-802-4462
Phone: 415-374-2500
Fax: 860-298-2443
www.cigna.com
Secondary Address: Great-West Healthcare, now part of CIGNA, 1340 Treat Blvd, Suite 599, Walnut Creek, CA 94597, 925-938-7788
For Profit Organization: Yes
Year Founded: 1929
Number of Affiliated Hospitals: 100
Number of Primary Care Physicians: 52,300
Number of Referral/Specialty Physicians: 20,766
Total Enrollment: 10,000,000
State Enrollment: 450,000

Healthplan and Services Defined
PLAN TYPE: HMO
Model Type: Network
Plan Specialty: ASO, HMO, POS, PPO, CDHP, Fully Insured Funding, Minimum Premium Funding
Benefits Offered: Chiropractic, Dental, Disease Management, Home Care, Physical Therapy, Podiatry, Psychiatric, Transplant, Vision, Wellness, Behavioral Health, Pharmacy, Radiology

Type of Coverage
Commercial, Individual, Indemnity
Catastrophic Illness Benefit: Covered

Type of Payment Plans Offered
DFFS, Capitated, FFS, Combination FFS & DFFS

Geographic Areas Served
Northern and Southern California, Nationwide

Subscriber Information
Average Monthly Fee Per Subscriber
(Employee + Employer Contribution):
Employee Only (Self): $140
Employee & 1 Family Member: $280
Employee & 2 Family Members: $420
Average Subscriber Co-Payment:
Primary Care Physician: $10.00
Prescription Drugs: $7.00/14.00
Hospital ER: $50.00

Network Qualifications
Pre-Admission Certification: Yes

Peer Review Type
Utilization Review: Yes
Case Management: Yes

Publishes and Distributes Report Card: Yes

Accreditation Certification
NCQA
TJC Accreditation, Medicare Approved, Utilization Review, Pre-Admission Certification, State Licensure, Quality Assurance Program

Key Personnel
President/CEO . . . . David Cordani
CFO . . . . Ralph Nicolletti
Claims . . . . Doug Stewart
Chief Communications Ofc . . . . Maggie Fitzpatrick
EVP/Global CIO . . . . Mark Boxer
Member Services . . . . Doug Stewart
Provider Services . . . . Ben Katz
Sales . . . . Kirby Hutson
VP Sales . . . . Peter Welch

Specialty Managed Care Partners
CIGNA Dental, CIGNA Vision, CIGNA Voluntary, CIGNA Behavioral

Employer References
Intel, Cisco, Safeway

106   CIGNA HealthCare of Southern California

26 Executive Park
Suite 200
Irvine, CA 92614
Phone: 949-255-1400
Fax: 949-255-1483
www.cigna.com
Secondary Address: 400 North Brand Blvd, Suite 400, Glendale, CA 91203, 818-500-6262
Subsidiary of: CIGNA
For Profit Organization: Yes
Year Founded: 1929
Owned by an Integrated Delivery Network (IDN): Yes
Number of Affiliated Hospitals: 234
Number of Primary Care Physicians: 52,300
Number of Referral/Specialty Physicians: 20,766
Total Enrollment: 10,000,000
State Enrollment: 450,000

Healthplan and Services Defined
PLAN TYPE: HMO
Model Type: Network
Plan Specialty: ASO, HMO, POS, PPO, CDHP, Fully Insured Funding, Minimum Premium Funding
Benefits Offered: Behavioral Health, Chiropractic, Dental, Disease Management, Home Care, Physical Therapy, Podiatry, Psychiatric, Transplant, Vision, Wellness, Pharmacy, Radiology

Type of Coverage
Commercial, Individual, Indemnity
Catastrophic Illness Benefit: Varies per case

Type of Payment Plans Offered
DFFS, Capitated, FFS, Combination FFS & DFFS

Geographic Areas Served
Northern and Southern California, Nationwide

Network Qualifications
Pre-Admission Certification: Yes

Peer Review Type
Utilization Review: Yes
Case Management: Yes

Publishes and Distributes Report Card: Yes

Accreditation Certification
NCQA

Key Personnel
President/CEO . . . . David Cordani
CFO . . . . Ralph Nicolletti
Claims . . . . Doug Stewart
Communications Officer . . . . Maggie Fitzpatrick
EVP/Global CIO . . . . Mark Boxer
Member Services. . . . . Doug Stewart
Provider Services . . . . Randy Mathews

Specialty Managed Care Partners
CIGNA Behavioral, CIGNA Dental, CIGNA Vision, CIGNA Voluntary

Employer References
Disney, Los Angeles School District, County of Orange

107   Citizens Choice Healthplan

17315 Studebaker Road
Suite #200
Cerritos, CA 90703
Toll-Free: 866-646-2247
Phone: 323-728-7232
Fax: 323-728-8494
info@mycchp.com
www.citizenschoicehealth.com
Year Founded: 2005

Healthplan and Services Defined
PLAN TYPE: HMO

Type of Coverage
Supplemental Medicare

Geographic Areas Served
California

Key Personnel
Media Contact . . . . Mayra Merrick
323-728-7232

108   Coastal Healthcare Administrators

928 East Blanco Road
Suite 235
Salinas, CA 93901
Toll-Free: 800-564-7475
Phone: 831-754-3800
Fax: 831-754-3830
info@coastalmgmt.com
www.coastalmgmt.com
Mailing Address: PO Box 80308, Salinas, CA 93912
For Profit Organization: Yes
Year Founded: 1961
Number of Affiliated Hospitals: 21
Number of Primary Care Physicians: 2,594
Number of Referral/Specialty Physicians: 3,241
Total Enrollment: 41,266

Healthplan and Services Defined
PLAN TYPE: PPO
Model Type: PPO Network
Benefits Offered: Prescription, PPO Network

Type of Coverage
Commercial
Catastrophic Illness Benefit: Unlimited

Type of Payment Plans Offered
FFS

Geographic Areas Served
Monterey, San Benito, San Luis Obispo, Santa Clara and Santa Cruz counties

Subscriber Information
Average Subscriber Co-Payment:
Primary Care Physician: $20.00
Prescription Drugs: $10.00
Home Health Care Max. Days/Visits Covered: 120 days
Nursing Home Max. Days/Visits Covered: 60 days

Peer Review Type
Utilization Review: No
Second Surgical Opinion: Yes
Case Management: No

Accreditation Certification
NCQA

Key Personnel
President/CEO. . . . . Deborah (Debi) Hardwick
831-754-3800
dhardwick@coastalmgmt.com

Accounting Manager..........................Peggy Kalekos
  831-754-3800
Office Manager................................Shari Griffin
Claims Supervisor ....Maria Rodriguez
Dir Network Management......................Betty Yancey
  831-754-3800
  byancey@coastalmgmt.com

Average Claim Compensation
Physician's Fees Charged: 70%
Hospital's Fees Charged: 85%

109 Community Health Group

, CA
Toll-Free: 800-840-0089
Phone: 619-422-0422
Fax: 619-422-5930
info@chgsd.com
www.chgsd.com
Non-Profit Organization: Yes
Year Founded: 1982
Number of Affiliated Hospitals: 28
Number of Primary Care Physicians: 488
Number of Referral/Specialty Physicians: 1,820
Total Enrollment: 146,000
State Enrollment: 146,000

Healthplan and Services Defined
  PLAN TYPE: HMO
  Model Type: Network
  Plan Specialty: Behavioral Health, Disease Management, Lab,
    Vision, Radiology, UR
  Benefits Offered: Behavioral Health, Disease Management, Home
    Care, Inpatient SNF, Physical Therapy, Podiatry, Prescription,
    Psychiatric, Transplant, Wellness
  Offers Demand Management Patient Information Service: Yes

Type of Coverage
  Medi-Cal, Healthy Families, SNP
  Catastrophic Illness Benefit: None

Type of Payment Plans Offered
  Capitated, FFS

Geographic Areas Served
  San Diego and Riverside counties

Network Qualifications
  Pre-Admission Certification: Yes

Peer Review Type
  Utilization Review: Yes
  Second Surgical Opinion: Yes
  Case Management: Yes

Publishes and Distributes Report Card: Yes

Accreditation Certification
  NCQA
  Utilization Review, Pre-Admission Certification, State Licensure,
    Quality Assurance Program

Key Personnel
  CEO ....Norma Diaz

Specialty Managed Care Partners
  Enters into Contracts with Regional Business Coalitions: No

110 Community Health Plan of Los Angeles County

1000 South Fremont Ave
Bldg A-9 East, 2nd Floor, Unit 4
Alhambra, CA 91803-8859
Toll-Free: 800-353-7988
Phone: 855-830-9222
Fax: 626-299-7258
chpwebmaster@dhs.lacounty.gov
http://chp.dhs.lacounty.gov
Non-Profit Organization: Yes
Total Enrollment: 200,000
State Enrollment: 200,000

Healthplan and Services Defined
  PLAN TYPE: HMO
  Offers Demand Management Patient Information Service: Yes
  DMPI Services Offered: 24-hour Nurse Line

Type of Coverage
  Individual, Medicare, Medicaid

Key Personnel
  Director ....Mitchel H. Katz
  Chief Information Officer ....Kevin Lynch

111 CONCERN: Employee Assistance Program

1503 Grant Road
Suite 120
Mountain View, CA 94040
Toll-Free: 800-344-4222
info@concern-eap.com
www.concern-eap.com

Healthplan and Services Defined
  PLAN TYPE: Other
  Other Type: EAP

Type of Coverage
  Commercial, EAP

Key Personnel
  Chief Executive Officer ....Cecile Currier
  Chief Technology Officer ....Jim Carroll
  Chief Financial Officer ....Michael Rigeor
  Dir/Business Development....................Paulette Hannah
  Marketing Manager........................Ann McCammond

112 Contra Costa Health Plan

50 Douglas Drive
Martinez, CA 94553
Toll-Free: 877-661-6230
Phone: 925-313-6000
Fax: 925-313-6047
3chp@hsd.cccounty.us
www.cchealth.org
Non-Profit Organization: Yes
Year Founded: 1973
Federally Qualified: Yes
Number of Affiliated Hospitals: 7
Number of Primary Care Physicians: 150
Number of Referral/Specialty Physicians: 210
Total Enrollment: 100,000
State Enrollment: 100,000

Healthplan and Services Defined
  PLAN TYPE: HMO
  Model Type: Staff, Network
  Benefits Offered: Disease Management, Wellness

Geographic Areas Served
  Contra Costa County

Subscriber Information
　Average Monthly Fee Per Subscriber
　　(Employee + Employer Contribution):
　　　Employee Only (Self): $389.00
　　　Employee & 1 Family Member: $985.00
　　　Employee & 2 Family Members: $1530.00
　Average Annual Deductible Per Subscriber:
　　　Employee Only (Self): $0.00
　　　Employee & 1 Family Member: $0.00
　　　Employee & 2 Family Members: $0.00
　Average Subscriber Co-Payment:
　　　Primary Care Physician: $15.00
　　　Non-Network Physician: $15.00
　　　Prescription Drugs: $15/30
　　　Hospital ER: $35.00
　　　Nursing Home: $100.00
　　　Nursing Home Max. Days/Visits Covered: 100.00/200.00 max

Network Qualifications
　Pre-Admission Certification: No

Peer Review Type
　Utilization Review: Yes
　Second Surgical Opinion: Yes
　Case Management: Yes

Publishes and Distributes Report Card: Yes

Accreditation Certification
　URAC Accredition
　TJC Accreditation, Medicare Approved, Utilization Review, State
　　Licensure, Quality Assurance Program

Key Personnel
　CEO . . . . Patricia Tanquary, MPH, PhD
　CFO/COO . . . . Patrick Godley
　　925-957-5405
　CIO/Health Officer . . . . David J Runt, MD
　Manager Claims . . . . Cindy Shelby
　　925-957-5185
　In-House Formulary . . . . Curt Le
　　925-957-7260
　Marketing/Sales Manger . . . . Wendy Mailer
　　800-211-8040
　Communications Officer . . . . Kate Fowlie
　　925-313-6268
　　kate.fowlie@hsd.ccounty.us

Specialty Managed Care Partners
　Enters into Contracts with Regional Business Coalitions: Yes

---

113　CorVel Corporation

2010 Main Street
Suite 600
Irvine, CA 92614
Toll-Free: 888-726-7835
Phone: 949-851-1473
Fax: 949-851-1469
marketing@corvel.com
www.corvel.com
For Profit Organization: Yes
Year Founded: 1988

Healthplan and Services Defined
　PLAN TYPE: PPO
　Benefits Offered: Disease Management, Wellness, Worker's
　　Compensation

Type of Coverage
　Commercial, Indemnity

Geographic Areas Served
　Nationwide

Accreditation Certification
　URAC

Key Personnel
　Chairman/CEO . . . . Gordon Clemons
　Chief Information Officer . . . . Donald C. McFarlane
　Director, Legal Services . . . . Sharon O'Connor
　Chief Financial Officer . . . . Scott McCloud
　Secretary . . . . Richard Schweppe
　SVP, Sales/Account Mgmt. Diane J. Blaha

114　Delta Dental of California

12898 Towne Center Drive
Cerritos, CA 90703-8546
Toll-Free: 800-422-4234
Phone: 562-403-4040
Fax: 562-924-3172
scasales@delta.org
www.deltadentalca.org
Mailing Address: PO Box 997330, Sacramento, CA 95899-7330
Non-Profit Organization: Yes
Year Founded: 1955
Number of Primary Care Physicians: 2,476
Number of Referral/Specialty Physicians: 924
Total Enrollment: 26,000,000

Healthplan and Services Defined
　PLAN TYPE: Dental
　Other Type: Dental PPO
　Model Type: Network
　Plan Specialty: Dental
　Benefits Offered: Dental

Type of Coverage
　Commercial, Dental Benefits

Type of Payment Plans Offered
　DFFS, Capitated, FFS

Geographic Areas Served
　Statewide

Subscriber Information
　Average Monthly Fee Per Subscriber
　　(Employee + Employer Contribution):
　　　Employee Only (Self): Varies
　　　Employee & 1 Family Member: Varies
　　　Employee & 2 Family Members: Varies
　　　Medicare: Varies
　Average Annual Deductible Per Subscriber:
　　　Employee Only (Self): Varies
　Average Subscriber Co-Payment:
　　　Primary Care Physician: Varies
　　　Non-Network Physician: Varies

Network Qualifications
　Pre-Admission Certification: No

Peer Review Type
　Utilization Review: Yes
　Second Surgical Opinion: Yes
　Case Management: Yes

Publishes and Distributes Report Card: Yes

Key Personnel
　President/CEO . . . . Gary Radine
　　415-972-8300
　Director Product Mtkg/Dev . . . . Lynette Crosby
　　415-972-8300
　Information Systems . . . . Martin Whelan
　　415-972-8300
　VP Sales . . . . John Crooms, Jr.
　　415-972-8300
　VP, Public & Govt Affairs . . . . Jeff Album
　　415-972-8418
　Dir/Media & Public Affair . . . . Elizabeth Risberg
　　415-972-8423

Specialty Managed Care Partners
PMI Dental Health Plan
Enters into Contracts with Regional Business Coalitions: Yes

115   Dental Alternatives Insurance Services

, CA
Toll-Free: 800-445-8119
info@gotodais.com
www.gotodais.com
For Profit Organization: Yes
Year Founded: 1979
Total Enrollment: 390,000

Healthplan and Services Defined
PLAN TYPE: Dental
Model Type: IPA
Plan Specialty: Dental
Benefits Offered: Dental
Offers Demand Management Patient Information Service: Yes

Network Qualifications
Pre-Admission Certification: Yes

Peer Review Type
Utilization Review: Yes
Second Surgical Opinion: Yes
Case Management: Yes

Publishes and Distributes Report Card: Yes

Accreditation Certification
NCQA

Key Personnel
President . . . . .Maribeth Tennison

Specialty Managed Care Partners
Enters into Contracts with Regional Business Coalitions: Yes

116   Dental Benefit Providers: California

425 Market Street
12th Floor
San Francisco, CA 94105
Toll-Free: 800-445-9090
Phone: 415-778-3800
Fax: 415-778-3833
www.dbp.com
Secondary Address: 6220 Old Dobbin Lane, Columbia, MD 21045
For Profit Organization: Yes
Year Founded: 1984
Number of Primary Care Physicians: 125,000
Total Enrollment: 6,600,000

Healthplan and Services Defined
PLAN TYPE: Dental
Model Type: IPA
Plan Specialty: ASO, Dental, EPO, DHMO, PPO, CSO, Preventive,
Claims Repricing and Network Access
Benefits Offered: Dental

Type of Coverage
Indemnity, Medicare, Medicaid

Type of Payment Plans Offered
POS, DFFS, Capitated, FFS

Geographic Areas Served
48 states including District of Columbia, Puerto Rico and Virgin
Islands

Accreditation Certification
NCQA

Key Personnel
CEO. . . . . .Diane Souza
President. . . . . .Paul Hebert

Vice President . . . . .Scott Murphy
760-452-6552
smurphy@dbp.com

117   Dental Health Services of California

3833 Atlantic Avenue
Long Beach, CA 90807
Toll-Free: 800-637-6453
www.dentalhealthservices.com
For Profit Organization: Yes
Year Founded: 1974
Physician Owned Organization: Yes
Federally Qualified: Yes
Number of Primary Care Physicians: 1,000
Number of Referral/Specialty Physicians: 400
Total Enrollment: 90,000

Healthplan and Services Defined
PLAN TYPE: Dental
Model Type: Network
Plan Specialty: Dental
Benefits Offered: Dental

Type of Coverage
Commercial, Individual
Catastrophic Illness Benefit: None

Type of Payment Plans Offered
DFFS

Geographic Areas Served
California and Washington

Subscriber Information
Average Monthly Fee Per Subscriber
(Employee + Employer Contribution):
Employee Only (Self): Varies
Employee & 1 Family Member: Varies
Employee & 2 Family Members: Varies

Network Qualifications
Pre-Admission Certification: Yes

Peer Review Type
Second Surgical Opinion: Yes
Case Management: Yes

Publishes and Distributes Report Card: Yes

Accreditation Certification
Dhm
TJC Accreditation, Utilization Review, State Licensure, Quality
Assurance Program

Key Personnel
Pres/Employee Benfits Mgr . . . . .Godfrey Pernell

Specialty Managed Care Partners
United Association, 7up
Enters into Contracts with Regional Business Coalitions: No

118   Dentistat

1688 Dell Avenue
Suite 210
Campbell, CA 95008
Toll-Free: 800-336-8250
Phone: 408-376-0336
Fax: 408-376-0736
info@dentistat.com
www.dentistat.com
For Profit Organization: Yes
Year Founded: 1968
Number of Primary Care Physicians: 80,000

Healthplan and Services Defined
PLAN TYPE: Dental
Model Type: Network
Plan Specialty: Dental

Benefits Offered: Dental

Type of Payment Plans Offered
DFFS, Capitated, FFS, Combination FFS & DFFS

Geographic Areas Served
Nationwide

Accreditation Certification
NCQA
Utilization Review, Quality Assurance Program

Key Personnel
President . . . . Bret Guenther
Chief Information Officer . . . . Sondra Zambino

Specialty Managed Care Partners
Enters into Contracts with Regional Business Coalitions: Yes

---

119   Easy Choice Health Plan

180 E Ocean Blvd
Suite 700
Long Beach, CA 90802
Toll-Free: 866-999-3945
Phone: 562-343-9710
Fax: 877-999-3945
info@easychoicehp.com
www.easychoicehealthplan.com
Mailing Address: PO Box 22653, Long Beach, CA 90801
Total Enrollment: 8,000
State Enrollment: 8,000

Healthplan and Services Defined
PLAN TYPE: Medicare
Benefits Offered: Dental, Disease Management, Prescription, Vision, Wellness

Type of Coverage
Medicare

Geographic Areas Served
Los Angeles & Orange County

Key Personnel
President . . . . Eric E Spencer, MBA
COO & CFO . . . . Frank Vo
Medical Director . . . . Alexis Martin, MD
Chief Info Officer . . . . Koh Kedsri

---

120   eHealthInsurance Services Inc.

11919 Foundation Place
Gold River, CA 95670
Toll-Free: 800-644-3491
webmaster@healthinsurance.com
www.e.healthinsurance.com

Healthplan and Services Defined
PLAN TYPE: HMO/PPO

Key Personnel
Chairman & CEO . . . . Gary L. Lauer
EVP/Business & Corp. Dev. Bruce Telkamp
EVP/Chief Technology . . . . Dr. Sheldon X. Wang
SVP & CFO . . . . Stuart M. Huizinga
Pres. of eHealth Gov. Sys . . . . Samuel C. Gibbs
SVP of Sales & Operations . . . . Robert S. Hurley
Director Public Relations . . . . Nate Purpura
650-210-3115

---

121   eHealthInsurance Services Inc.

11919 Foundation Place
Gold River, CA 95670
Toll-Free: 800-644-3491
webmaster@healthinsurance.com
www.e.healthinsurance.com
Year Founded: 1997

Healthplan and Services Defined
PLAN TYPE: HMO/PPO
Benefits Offered: Dental, Life, STD

Type of Coverage
Commercial, Individual, Medicare

Geographic Areas Served
All 50 states in the USA and District of Columbia

Key Personnel
Chairman & CEO . . . . Gary L. Lauer
EVP/Business & Corp. Dev. Bruce Telkamp
EVP/Chief Technology . . . . Dr. Sheldon X. Wang
SVP & CFO . . . . Stuart M. Huizinga
Pres. of eHealth Gov. Sys . . . . Samuel C. Gibbs
SVP of Sales & Operations . . . . Robert S. Hurley
Director Public Relations . . . . Nate Purpura
650-210-3115

---

122   eHealthInsurance Services Inc. Corporate Office

440 East Middlefield Road
Mountain View, CA 94043
Toll-Free: 877-456-7180
headquarters@ehealth.com
www.ehealthinsurance.com
Year Founded: 1997
Total Enrollment: 3,000,000

Healthplan and Services Defined
PLAN TYPE: HMO/PPO
Benefits Offered: Dental, Life, STD

Type of Coverage
Commercial, Individual, Medicare

Geographic Areas Served
All 50 states in the USA and District of Columbia

Key Personnel
Chairman & CEO . . . . Gary L. Lauer
EVP/Business & Corp. Dev. Bruce Telkamp
EVP/Chief Technology . . . . Dr. Sheldon X. Wang
SVP & CFO . . . . Stuart M. Huizinga
Pres. of eHealth Gov. Sys . . . . Samuel C. Gibbs
SVP of Sales & Operations . . . . Robert S. Hurley
Director Public Relations . . . . Nate Purpura
650-210-3115

---

123   Foundation for Medical Care for Kern & Santa Barbara County

5701 Truxtun Avenue
Suite 100
Bakersfield, CA 93309
Phone: 661-327-7581
Fax: 661-327-5129
ctemple@kernfmc.com
www.kernfmc.com
Non-Profit Organization: Yes
Year Founded: 1983
Physician Owned Organization: Yes
Number of Affiliated Hospitals: 400
Number of Primary Care Physicians: 30,000
Number of Referral/Specialty Physicians: 7,000
Total Enrollment: 60,000

Healthplan and Services Defined
PLAN TYPE: PPO
Model Type: IPA, Group, Network
Benefits Offered: Prescription
Offers Demand Management Patient Information Service: Yes

Type of Payment Plans Offered
POS, DFFS, FFS, Combination FFS & DFFS

Geographic Areas Served
Kern, Santa Barbara, Mono and Inyo counties

Network Qualifications
Pre-Admission Certification: Yes

Peer Review Type
Utilization Review: Yes
Second Surgical Opinion: Yes
Case Management: Yes

Accreditation Certification
TJC Accreditation, Medicare Approved, Utilization Review,
Pre-Admission Certification, State Licensure

Key Personnel
CEO.......................................Carolyn J Temple
ctemple@kernfmc.com
COO...Lori Howell
lhowell@kernfmc.com
Dir, Admin & Finance ....Elizabeth Maynard
lizmaynard@kernfmc.com
Chief Marketing Officer ....George Stephenson, II
gstephenson@kernfmc.com
Executive Assistant ....Lisa Garzelli
lgarzelli@kernfmc.com
Manager, Customer Service ....Ellen Wright
ewright@kernfmc.com
Provider Relations ....D'Ln Brown
dbrown@kernfmc.com
Mgr, Provider Relations ....Jeanne Simpson
jsimpson@kernfmc.com
Sales & Mktg Supervisor ....Keith Salyards
ksalyards@kernfmc.com
Exec Admin Supervisor ....Lisa Garzelli
lgarzelli@kernfmc.com

Specialty Managed Care Partners
Enters into Contracts with Regional Business Coalitions: No

---

124 Foundation for Medical Care for Mendocino and Lake Counties

620 S Dora Street
Suite 201
Ukiah, CA 95482
Phone: 707-462-7607
Fax: 707-462-1206
mendolake_counties@sbcglobal.net
www.mendolake-physicians.com
Subsidiary of: California Foundation for Medical Care
Non-Profit Organization: Yes
Year Founded: 1962
Number of Affiliated Hospitals: 5
Number of Primary Care Physicians: 350
Number of Referral/Specialty Physicians: 5,500
Total Enrollment: 34,000
State Enrollment: 34,000

Healthplan and Services Defined
PLAN TYPE: PPO
Model Type: PPO
Benefits Offered: Prescription
Offers Demand Management Patient Information Service: Yes

Geographic Areas Served
Lake & Mendocino counties

Network Qualifications
Pre-Admission Certification: Yes

Peer Review Type
Utilization Review: Yes
Second Surgical Opinion: No
Case Management: No

Accreditation Certification
TJC Accreditation, Utilization Review, Pre-Admission Certification,
State Licensure, Quality Assurance Program

Key Personnel
Executive Director ....Kathy King
CEO ....Gene Draper
Controller ....Shawn Lowry
Medical Affairs ....Mark Apfel, MD

---

125 GEMCare Health Plan

4550 California Avenue
Suite 100
Bakersfield, CA 93309
Toll-Free: 877-697-2464
Phone: 661-716-8800
info@gemcarehealthplan.com
www.gemcarehealthplan.com

Healthplan and Services Defined
PLAN TYPE: Medicare

Type of Coverage
Medicare, Supplemental Medicare

Geographic Areas Served
Kern County

Key Personnel
President/CEO.............................Michael R Myers
Chief Medical Officer.....................Dr Ramen Neufeld
Director/Health Svcs...........................Janice Jones
Dir/Operations...........................Jennifer Del Villar

---

126 Golden West Dental & Vision Plan

888 West Ventura Blvd
Carmarillo, CA 93010
Toll-Free: 877-494-9202
Fax: 805-499-0842
agent.support@wellpoint.com
www.goldenwestdental.com
Subsidiary of: WellPoint
For Profit Organization: Yes
Year Founded: 1974
Number of Primary Care Physicians: 2,011
Number of Referral/Specialty Physicians: 733
Total Enrollment: 200,473

Healthplan and Services Defined
PLAN TYPE: Multiple
Model Type: IPA, Network
Plan Specialty: Dental, Vision
Benefits Offered: Dental, Vision
Offers Demand Management Patient Information Service: Yes

Type of Payment Plans Offered
Capitated, Combination FFS & DFFS

Geographic Areas Served
Statewide

Subscriber Information
Average Monthly Fee Per Subscriber
(Employee + Employer Contribution):
Employee Only (Self): Varies
Employee & 1 Family Member: Varies
Employee & 2 Family Members: Varies
Medicare: Varies

Peer Review Type
Second Surgical Opinion: Yes

Publishes and Distributes Report Card: Yes

Key Personnel
CFO ....Steve Sheehan
CIO..Shenoy Manju
Marketing ....Chris McConathy

Dental Director . . . . Karen Feldman

Average Claim Compensation
Physician's Fees Charged: 80%

Specialty Managed Care Partners
Enters into Contracts with Regional Business Coalitions: Yes

---

127   Great-West Healthcare California

2355 Main Street
Suite 240
Irvine, CA 92614
Toll-Free: 866-494-2111
Phone: 949-225-2500
eliginquiries@cigna.com
www.cignaforhealth.com
Subsidiary of: CIGNA HealthCare
Acquired by: CIGNA
For Profit Organization: Yes
Total Enrollment: 204,077
State Enrollment: 57,459

Healthplan and Services Defined
  PLAN TYPE: HMO/PPO
  Benefits Offered: Disease Management, Prescription, Wellness

Type of Coverage
Commercial

Type of Payment Plans Offered
POS, FFS

Geographic Areas Served
California

Accreditation Certification
URAC

Specialty Managed Care Partners
Caremark Rx

---

128   Health Net Dental

21281 Burbank Blvd
Woodland Hills, CA 91367
Toll-Free: 800-865-6288
Phone: 818-676-5000
Fax: 818-676-5382
www.healthnet.com
Mailing Address: PO Box 30930, Laguna Hills, CA 92654-0930
For Profit Organization: Yes
Year Founded: 1972
Number of Primary Care Physicians: 2,700
Total Enrollment: 540,000

Healthplan and Services Defined
  PLAN TYPE: Dental
  Plan Specialty: Dental
  Benefits Offered: Dental

Key Personnel
Presdient/CEO . . . . Jay M Gellert
Mgr, Public Relations . . . . Brad Kieffer
  818-676-6833
  brad.kieffer@healthnet.com

---

129   Health Net Medicare Plan

21281 Burbank Blvd
Woodland Hills, CA 91367
Toll-Free: 800-291-6911
Phone: 818-676-5000
Fax: 818-676-5382
www.healthnet.com/portal/medicare/home.do
Mailing Address: PO Box 10198, Van Nuys, CA 91410-0198
Year Founded: 1978
Total Enrollment: 6,700,000

State Enrollment: 6,700,000

Healthplan and Services Defined
  PLAN TYPE: Medicare
  Benefits Offered: Chiropractic, Dental, Disease Management, Home
    Care, Inpatient SNF, Physical Therapy, Podiatry, Prescription,
    Psychiatric, Vision, Wellness

Type of Coverage
Individual, Medicare

Geographic Areas Served
Available in multiple states

Subscriber Information
Average Monthly Fee Per Subscriber
  (Employee + Employer Contribution):
    Employee Only (Self): Varies
    Medicare: Varies
Average Annual Deductible Per Subscriber:
    Employee Only (Self): Varies
    Medicare: Varies
Average Subscriber Co-Payment:
    Primary Care Physician: Varies
    Non-Network Physician: Varies
    Prescription Drugs: Varies
    Hospital ER: Varies
    Home Health Care: Varies
    Home Health Care Max. Days/Visits Covered: Varies
    Nursing Home: Varies
    Nursing Home Max. Days/Visits Covered: Varies

Key Personnel
President/CEO . . . . Jay M Gellert
SVP/Speciality Services . . . . Gerald V Coil
Regional Health Plans . . . . Stephen D Lynch
SVP/Organization Mgmt. . . . . Karin D Mayhew
SVP/Communications . . . . David W Olson
EVP/CFO. . . . . Anthony S Piszel
Compliance Officer. . . . . Ann Williams
Pharmaceutical Division . . . . John P Sivori
SVP/General Counsel . . . . B Curtis Westen, Esq
President/Government Svcs . . . . James E Woys
Dir, Communications . . . . Amy Sheyer
  818-676-8304
  amy.l.sheyer@healthnet.org

---

130   Health Net: Corporate Headquarters

21281 Burbank Blvd
Woodland Hills, CA 91367
Toll-Free: 800-291-6911
Phone: 818-676-5000
Fax: 818676-5382
www.healthnet.com
Mailing Address: PO Box 9103, Van Nuys, CA 91409-9103
For Profit Organization: Yes
Year Founded: 1979
Number of Affiliated Hospitals: 419
Number of Primary Care Physicians: 1,207
Total Enrollment: 6,000,000

Healthplan and Services Defined
  PLAN TYPE: HMO
  Model Type: IPA, Group
  Benefits Offered: Disease Management, Prescription, Wellness
  Offers Demand Management Patient Information Service: Yes

Type of Coverage
Catastrophic Illness Benefit: Covered

Type of Payment Plans Offered
POS, DFFS, FFS

Geographic Areas Served
Alameda, Amador, Butte, Calaveras, Colusa, Contra Costa, El
Dorado, Fresno, Glenn, Humboldt, Kern, Kings, Lake, Lassen, Los
Angeles, Madera, Marin, Mariposa, Mendocino, Merced, Napa,

Nevada, Orange, Placer, Plumas, Riverside, Sacramento, San Bernardino, San Diego, San Francisco, San Joaquin, San Luis Obispo, San Mateo, Santa Barbara, Santa Clara, Santa Cruz, Shasta, Sierra, Solano, Sonoma, Stanislaus, Sutter, Tehama, Trinity, Tulare, Tuolumne, Ventura, Yolo & Yuba

Subscriber Information
Average Monthly Fee Per Subscriber
    (Employee + Employer Contribution):
        Employee Only (Self): $139.08
        Employee & 1 Family Member: $305.98/236.44
        Employee & 2 Family Members: $403.34
        Medicare: $0-52.00
Average Subscriber Co-Payment:
        Primary Care Physician: $10.00
        Non-Network Physician: Not covered
        Prescription Drugs: $6.00
        Hospital ER: $35.00
        Home Health Care Max. Days/Visits Covered: Unlimited
        Nursing Home Max. Days/Visits Covered: 100 days

Network Qualifications
Pre-Admission Certification: Yes

Peer Review Type
Utilization Review: Yes
Second Surgical Opinion: Yes
Case Management: Yes

Publishes and Distributes Report Card: Yes

Accreditation Certification
NCQA
TJC Accreditation, Medicare Approved, Utilization Review,
    Pre-Admission Certification, State Licensure, Quality Assurance
    Program

Key Personnel
President/Ceo . . . . Jay M Gellert
SVP, General Counsel . . . . Angelee F Bouchard, Esq
EVP, Chief Financial Offc . . . . Joseph C Capezza, CPA
SVP, Chief Regulatory Ofc . . . . Patricia T Clarey
Chief Govt Prog Officer . . . . Scott R Kelly
SVP, Org. Effectiveness . . . . Karin D Mayhew
VP, Treasurer. . . . . Jonathan Rollins, CFA
Health Care Svcs Officer. . . . . John P Sivori
VP, Ext Communications . . . . Margita Thompson
    818-676-7912
    margita.thompson@healthnet.com
President, Govt Programs . . . . Steven D Tough
Chief Operating Officer. . . . . James E Woys
Mgr, Public Relations . . . . Brad Kieffer
    818-676-6833
    brad.kieffer@healthnet.com
Corporate Communications . . . . Lori Hillman
    818-676-8684
    lori.a.hillman@healthnet.com

Specialty Managed Care Partners
Enters into Contracts with Regional Business Coalitions: Yes

---

131   Health Plan of San Joaquin
7751 South Manthey Road
French Camp, CA 95231
Toll-Free: 888-936-7526
Phone: 209-942-6300
Fax: 209-942-6305
www.hpsj.com
Mailing Address: PO Box 30490, Stockton, CA 95213-0490
Non-Profit Organization: Yes
Year Founded: 1996
Number of Primary Care Physicians: 180
Number of Referral/Specialty Physicians: 1,400
Total Enrollment: 109,000
State Enrollment: 109,000

Healthplan and Services Defined
PLAN TYPE: HMO
Benefits Offered: Inpatient SNF, Podiatry, Vision, Wellness
Offers Demand Management Patient Information Service: Yes
DMPI Services Offered: 24 Hour Nurse Advice Hotline

Type of Coverage
Commercial, Medicaid

Geographic Areas Served
San Joaquin county

Key Personnel
CEO . . . . John Hackworth, PhD
    209-461-2211
    jhackworth@hpsj.com
CFO . . . . Paul Antigua
    209-461-2268
    pantigua@hpsj.com
COO. . . . . Kathryn Kutz
Marketing Director . . . . David Hurst
    209-461-2241
    dhurst@hpsj.com
Medical Director. . . . . Dale Bishop, MD
    209-461-2281
    dbishop@hpsj.com
Dir, Marketing . . . . David Hurst
    209-491-2241
    dhurst@hpsj.com

---

132   Health Plan of San Mateo
701 Gateway Boulevard
Suite 400
South San Francisco, CA 94080
Toll-Free: 800-750-4776
Phone: 650-616-0050
Fax: 650-616-0060
info@hpsm.org
www.hpsm.org
Non-Profit Organization: Yes
Year Founded: 1987
Number of Affiliated Hospitals: 12
Number of Primary Care Physicians: 197
Total Enrollment: 87,740
State Enrollment: 87,740

Healthplan and Services Defined
PLAN TYPE: HMO
Model Type: IPA
Benefits Offered: Disease Management, Prescription, Wellness

Type of Coverage
Medi-Cal, Healthy Families

Type of Payment Plans Offered
Capitated, FFS

Geographic Areas Served
San Mateo county

Key Personnel
Chief Executive Officer . . . . Maya Altman
Finance & Administrative . . . . Ron Robinson
MIS Director . . . . Eben Yong
Dir, Systems Improvement. . . . . Chris Baughman
Medical Director . . . . Fiona Donald
Dir/Provider Network Deve . . . . Ed Ortiz
Dir, Compliance & Regulat . . . . Ellen Dunn-Malhotra
Member Services & Outreac. . . . . Carolyn Thon
Human Resources Director. . . . . Cindy Lem

133   Humana Health Insurance of Fresno

1676 N California Blvd
Suite 600
Walnut Creek, CA 94596
Toll-Free: 888-486-0257
Phone: 925-934-0284
Fax: 925-934-1347
www.humana.com
For Profit Organization: Yes

Healthplan and Services Defined
    PLAN TYPE: HMO/PPO

Type of Coverage
    Commercial, Individual

Accreditation Certification
    URAC, NCQA, CORE

Key Personnel
    Chairman/CEO . . . . Michael McCallister
    President . . . . Bruce Broussard
    COO . . . . James Murray
    SVP/CFO . . . . James Bloem

134   Humana Health Insurance of Southern California

5421 Avenida Encinas
Suite N
Carlsbad, CA 92008
Toll-Free: 800-795-2403
Phone: 760-918-0152
Fax: 760-918-0654
www.humana.com
For Profit Organization: Yes

Healthplan and Services Defined
    PLAN TYPE: HMO
    Model Type: POS

Type of Coverage
    Commercial, Individual

Accreditation Certification
    URAC, NCQA, CORE

Key Personnel
    Chairman/CEO . . . . Michael McCallister
    President . . . . Bruce Broussard
    COO . . . . James Murray
    SVP/CFO . . . . James Bloem

135   Inland Empire Health Plan

10801 Sixth Street
Suite 120
Rancho Cucamonga, CA 91730
Phone: 909-890-2000
Fax: 909-890-2003
memberservices@iehp.org
www.iehp.org
Mailing Address: P.O. Box 19026, San Bernardino, CA 92423
Non-Profit Organization: Yes
Year Founded: 1996
Number of Affiliated Hospitals: 27
Number of Primary Care Physicians: 1,700
Total Enrollment: 575,000
State Enrollment: 575,000

Healthplan and Services Defined
    PLAN TYPE: HMO
    Model Type: Staff, IPA
    Benefits Offered: Inpatient SNF, Physical Therapy, Prescription,
        Transplant, Vision, Wellness

Type of Coverage
    Commercial, Medicaid

Geographic Areas Served
    San Bernardino and Riverside counties

Accreditation Certification
    NCQA

Key Personnel
    CEO . . . . Bradley P Gilbert, MD
    Chief Operations Officer . . . . Rohan C. Reid
    Chief Financial Officer . . . . Chet C. Uma
    Chief Network Officer . . . . Kurt Hubler
    Chief Info Officer . . . . Michael Deering
    Chief Marketing Officer . . . . Susan Arcidiacono
    Chief Medical Officer . . . . William Henning, MD
    Marketing Director . . . . Thomas Pham
        909-890-2176
        pham-t@iehp.org

136   Inter Valley Health Plan

300 S Park Avenue
PO Box 6002
Pomona, CA 91769-6002
Toll-Free: 800-251-8191
info@ivhp.com
www.ivhp.com
Non-Profit Organization: Yes
Year Founded: 1979
Owned by an Integrated Delivery Network (IDN): No
Federally Qualified: Yes
Number of Affiliated Hospitals: 24
Number of Primary Care Physicians: 1,161
Number of Referral/Specialty Physicians: 4,791
Total Enrollment: 14,600

Healthplan and Services Defined
    PLAN TYPE: Multiple
    Model Type: Network
    Benefits Offered: Behavioral Health, Home Care, Inpatient SNF,
        Physical Therapy, Prescription, Psychiatric, Transplant, Wellness

Type of Coverage
    Medicare
    Catastrophic Illness Benefit: Unlimited

Type of Payment Plans Offered
    Capitated

Geographic Areas Served
    Southern California counties including Los Angeles, Riverside, San
    Bernardino

Subscriber Information
    Average Subscriber Co-Payment:
        Primary Care Physician: $7/15/30/55
        Hospital ER: $50.00
        Nursing Home: $40/day,day 2/thru100
        Nursing Home Max. Days/Visits Covered: 100

Network Qualifications
    Pre-Admission Certification: No

Peer Review Type
    Utilization Review: Yes
    Second Surgical Opinion: Yes
    Case Management: Yes

Accreditation Certification
    URAC, PBGH, CCHRI
    TJC Accreditation, Medicare Approved, Utilization Review, State
        Licensure, Quality Assurance Program

Key Personnel
    President and CEO . . . . Ron Bolding
    CFO . . . . Donald D McCain
    Chief Medical Officer . . . . Kenneth E. Smith, MD, MBA
    VP/Health Services . . . . Susan Tenorio

VP, Sales/Marketing . . . . Cyndie O'Brien

Average Claim Compensation
Physician's Fees Charged: 75%
Hospital's Fees Charged: 55%

Specialty Managed Care Partners
Vision Service Plan

137   Interplan Health Group

2575 Grand Canal Boulevard
Suite 100
Stockton, CA 95207
Toll-Free: 800-444-4036
Phone: 209-473-0811
Fax: 209-473-0863
info@interplanhealth.com
www.interplanhealth.com
Subsidiary of: A HealthSmart Network
Acquired by: HealthSmart
For Profit Organization: Yes
Year Founded: 1984
Number of Affiliated Hospitals: 380
Number of Primary Care Physicians: 58,170
Number of Referral/Specialty Physicians: 13,157
Total Enrollment: 2,900,000
State Enrollment: 1,700,000

Healthplan and Services Defined
PLAN TYPE: PPO
Model Type: Network
Plan Specialty: Behavioral Health, Chiropractic, Disease
Management, Lab, PBM, Vision, Radiology, Worker's
Compensation

Type of Coverage
Commercial, Individual

Geographic Areas Served
Arizona, California, Florida, Illinois, Indiana, Iowa, Kentucky,
Michigan, Nebraska, Nevada, North Dakota, Ohio, South Dakota,
Tenessee, Texas, Washington, West Virginia, Wisconsin

Peer Review Type
Utilization Review: Yes
Case Management: Yes

Publishes and Distributes Report Card: No

Key Personnel
President-PPO Division . . . . Peter Osenar
800-683-6830
CEO . . . . Ted Parker
806-473-3075
CFO. . . . . Lisa Cobb
806-473-3075
SVP Provider Networks . . . . Reagan Bruce
806-473-3075
Dental. . . . . Cornelia Outten
800-683-6830
Chief Sales, Mktg Officer . . . . Michael Schotz
800-444-4036
Medical Director . . . . John Sizer, MD
Client Services . . . . Kathy Polenske
800-444-4036
President-Cost Contain. . . . . Maureen Starr
860-678-7877
Executive Vice President . . . . Bill Dembereckyj
806-473-3075

Specialty Managed Care Partners
Enters into Contracts with Regional Business Coalitions: Yes

138   Kaiser Permanente Health Plan of Northern California

1950 Franklin Street
Oakland, CA 94612-2911
Phone: 510-987-1000
Fax: 510-271-6493
marc.t.brown@kp.org
www.kaiserpermanente.org
Non-Profit Organization: Yes
Year Founded: 1945
Number of Affiliated Hospitals: 35
Number of Primary Care Physicians: 15,129
Total Enrollment: 3,223,235
State Enrollment: 3,223,235

Healthplan and Services Defined
PLAN TYPE: HMO
Model Type: Group, Network
Benefits Offered: Disease Management, Home Care, Inpatient SNF,
Long-Term Care, Physical Therapy, Podiatry, Prescription,
Psychiatric, Transplant, Vision, Wellness

Type of Payment Plans Offered
POS, Combination FFS & DFFS

Geographic Areas Served
Alameda, Amador, Contra Costa, El Dorado, Francisco, San Joaquin,
San Mateo, Santa Clara, Solano, Sonoma, Sutter, Tulcare, Yolo &
Yuba counties

Subscriber Information
Average Monthly Fee Per Subscriber
(Employee + Employer Contribution):
Employee Only (Self): Varies by plan
Average Subscriber Co-Payment:
Home Health Care: $5.00
Home Health Care Max. Days/Visits Covered: Unlimited
Nursing Home Max. Days/Visits Covered: 100 days

Network Qualifications
Pre-Admission Certification: Yes

Publishes and Distributes Report Card: Yes

Accreditation Certification
TJC Accreditation, Medicare Approved, Utilization Review,
Pre-Admission Certification, State Licensure, Quality Assurance
Program

Key Personnel
CEO/Chairman. . . . . George C Halvorson
President/COO. . . . . Bernard Tyson
Sr VP/Community Benefit . . . . Raymond J Baxter, PhD
SVP, Corp Development. . . . . Chris Grant
SVP, Chief Diversity Offc . . . . Ronald Knox
Consultant . . . . Louise L Liang, MD
Exec VP/Health Plan Ops . . . . Bernard J Tyson
Exec Dir, Clinical Care . . . . Scott Young, MD
EVP/Health Plan Operation . . . . Arthur M Southam, MD
SVP, Communications . . . . Diane Gage Lofgren
SVP, General Counsel. . . . . Steven Zatkin
SVP, Human Resources . . . . Church Columbus
SVP, Chief Info Officer . . . . Phil Fasano
SVP, Quality Care . . . . Jed Weissberg, MD
CEO, Northern Calif Reg. . . . . Robert M Pearl, MD
Media Contact. . . . . Marc Brown
510-987-4672
marc.t.brown@kp.org
Pres, Northern Calif Reg . . . . Gregory A Adams

Specialty Managed Care Partners
Enters into Contracts with Regional Business Coalitions: Yes

139　Kaiser Permanente Health Plan of Southern California

393 E Walnut Street
2nd Floor
Pasadena, CA 91188
Toll-Free: 800-464-4000
Phone: 626-405-3665
Fax: 626-405-5186
kpsc.isb@kp.org
www.kaiserpermanente.org
Non-Profit Organization: Yes
Year Founded: 1945
Physician Owned Organization: Yes
Federally Qualified: Yes
Number of Affiliated Hospitals: 32
Number of Primary Care Physicians: 13,729
Total Enrollment: 3,284,000
State Enrollment: 3,284,540

Healthplan and Services Defined
PLAN TYPE: HMO
Model Type: Group
Plan Specialty: Behavioral Health, Chiropractic, Dental, Disease
Management, Lab, PBM, Vision, Radiology, Worker's
Compensation, UR, All Types of Medical Services
Benefits Offered: Behavioral Health, Chiropractic, Complementary
Medicine, Dental, Disease Management, Home Care, Inpatient
SNF, Long-Term Care, Physical Therapy, Podiatry, Prescription,
Psychiatric, Transplant, Vision, Wellness, Worker's Compensation,
AD&D, Life
Offers Demand Management Patient Information Service: Yes

Type of Coverage
Commercial, Individual, Indemnity, Medicare, Supplemental
Medicare, Catastrophic
Catastrophic Illness Benefit: Unlimited

Type of Payment Plans Offered
POS

Geographic Areas Served
East Bay, Fresno, Golden Gate, North East Bay, South Bay,
Sanislaus, Coachella Valley, Inland Empire, Metropolitan Los
Angeles/West Los Angeles, Orange, San Diego, Tri-Central and
Western Ventura counties

Subscriber Information
Average Monthly Fee Per Subscriber
(Employee + Employer Contribution):
Employee Only (Self): Varies by plan
Average Subscriber Co-Payment:
Home Health Care Max. Days/Visits Covered: Unlimited
Nursing Home Max. Days/Visits Covered: 100 days

Network Qualifications
Pre-Admission Certification: Yes

Peer Review Type
Utilization Review: Yes
Second Surgical Opinion: No
Case Management: Yes

Publishes and Distributes Report Card: Yes

Accreditation Certification
NCQA
TJC Accreditation, Medicare Approved, Utilization Review, State
Licensure, Quality Assurance Program

Key Personnel
CEO/Chairman . . . . George C Halvorson
President/COO . . . . Bernard Tyson
Sr VP/Community Benefit . . . . Raymond J Baxter, PhD
Managing Director . . . . Chris Grant
SVP, Chief Diversity Offc . . . . Ronald Knox
Consultant . . . . Louise L Liang, MD
Exec VP/Health Plan Ops . . . . Bernard J Tyson

Exec Dir, Clinical Care . . . . Scott Young, MD
EVP/Health Plan Operation . . . . Arthur M Southam, MD
SVP, Communications . . . . Diane Gage Lofgren
SVP, General Counsel . . . . Steven Zatkin
SVP, Human Resources . . . . Chuck Columbus
SVP, Chief Info Officer . . . . Phil Fasano
SVP, Quality Care . . . . Jed Weissberg, MD
Exec Med Dir, South Calif . . . . Jeffery A Weisz, MD
Media Contact . . . . Jim Anderson
626-405-5157
jim.h.anderson@kp.org
Pres, Southern Calif Reg . . . . Benjamin K Chu, MPH

Specialty Managed Care Partners
Enters into Contracts with Regional Business Coalitions: Yes

140　Kaiser Permanente Health Plan: Corporate Office

One Kaiser Plaza
Oakland, CA 94612-3610
Phone: 510-271-5800
Fax: 510-267-7524
newscenter@kp.org
www.kaiserpermanente.org
Non-Profit Organization: Yes
Year Founded: 1945
Number of Affiliated Hospitals: 35
Number of Primary Care Physicians: 15,129
Total Enrollment: 8,569,000
State Enrollment: 6,400,000

Healthplan and Services Defined
PLAN TYPE: HMO
Model Type: Group
Benefits Offered: Disease Management, Home Care, Inpatient SNF,
Long-Term Care, Physical Therapy, Podiatry, Prescription,
Psychiatric, Transplant, Vision, Wellness
Offers Demand Management Patient Information Service: Yes

Type of Coverage
Catastrophic Illness Benefit: Covered

Type of Payment Plans Offered
POS

Geographic Areas Served
The 12 Kaiser Permanente Regions cover service areas in 16 states
and the District of Columbia: portions of California, Colorado,
Connecticut, Washington, DC, Georgia, Hawaii, Idaho, Kansas,
Maryland, Massachusetts, Missouri, New York, North Carolina, Ohio,
Oregon, South Carolina, Texas, Virginia, Vermont & Washington

Network Qualifications
Pre-Admission Certification: Yes

Peer Review Type
Utilization Review: Yes
Second Surgical Opinion: Yes
Case Management: Yes

Publishes and Distributes Report Card: Yes

Accreditation Certification
NCQA
TJC Accreditation, Medicare Approved, Utilization Review,
Pre-Admission Certification, State Licensure, Quality Assurance
Program

Key Personnel
CEO/Chairman . . . . George C Halvorson
President/COO VP . . . . Bernard Tyson
Sr VP/Community Benefit . . . . Raymond J Baxter, PhD
SVP, Corp Development . . . . Chris Grant
SVP, Chief Diversity Offc . . . . Ronald Knox
Consultant . . . . Louise L Liang, MD
Exec VP/Health Plan Ops . . . . Bernard J Tyson
Exec Dir, Clinical Care . . . . Scott Young, MD

EVP/Health Plan Operation . . . . Arthur M Southam, MD
SVP, Communications . . . . Diane Gage Lofgren
SVP, General Counsel. . . . . Steven Zatkin
SVP, Human Resources . . . . Church Columbus
SVP, Chief Info Officer . . . . Phil Fasano
SVP, Quality Care . . . . Jed Weissberg, MD
Media Contact. . . . . Danielle Cass
    510-267-5354
    newscenter@kp.org

Specialty Managed Care Partners
Enters into Contracts with Regional Business Coalitions: No

---

141 Kaiser Permanente Medicare Plan

1950 Franklin Street
Oakland, CA 94612
Toll-Free: 877-220-3956
Phone: 510-987-1000
http://medicare.kaiserpermanente.org

Healthplan and Services Defined
  PLAN TYPE: Medicare
  Benefits Offered: Chiropractic, Dental, Disease Management, Home
    Care, Inpatient SNF, Physical Therapy, Podiatry, Prescription,
    Psychiatric, Vision, Wellness

Type of Coverage
  Individual, Medicare

Geographic Areas Served
  Available within multiple states

Subscriber Information
  Average Monthly Fee Per Subscriber
    (Employee + Employer Contribution):
      Employee Only (Self): Varies
      Medicare: Varies
  Average Annual Deductible Per Subscriber:
    Employee Only (Self): Varies
    Medicare: Varies
  Average Subscriber Co-Payment:
    Primary Care Physician: Varies
    Non-Network Physician: Varies
    Prescription Drugs: Varies
    Hospital ER: Varies
    Home Health Care: Varies
    Home Health Care Max. Days/Visits Covered: Varies
    Nursing Home: Varies
    Nursing Home Max. Days/Visits Covered: Varies

Key Personnel
CEO/Chairman. . . . . George C Halvorson
President/COO. . . . . Bernard Tyson
Sr VP/Community Benefit . . . . Raymond J Baxter, PhD
SVP, Corp Development. . . . . Chris Grant
SVP, Chief Diversity Offc . . . . Ronald Knox
Consultant . . . . Louise L Liang, MD
Exec VP/Health Plan Ops . . . . Bernard J Tyson
Exec Dir, Clinical Care . . . . Scott Young, MD
EVP/Health Plan Operation . . . . Arthur M Southam, MD
SVP, Communications . . . . Diane Gage Lofgren
SVP, General Counsel. . . . . Steven Zatkin
SVP, Human Resources . . . . Church Columbus
SVP, Chief Info Officer . . . . Phil Fasano
SVP, Quality Care . . . . Jed Weissberg, MD

---

142 Kern Family Health Care

9700 Stockdale Highway
Bakersfield, CA 93311
Toll-Free: 800-391-2000
Phone: 661-664-5000
louiei@khs-net.com
www.kernfamilyhealthcare.com

Subsidiary of: Kern Health Systems
Non-Profit Organization: Yes
Year Founded: 1996
Number of Affiliated Hospitals: 9
Number of Primary Care Physicians: 213
Number of Referral/Specialty Physicians: 400
Total Enrollment: 97,000
State Enrollment: 90,074

Healthplan and Services Defined
  PLAN TYPE: HMO
  Model Type: Network
  Benefits Offered: Disease Management, Wellness
  Offers Demand Management Patient Information Service: Yes
  DMPI Services Offered: 24 Hour Nurse Advice Hotline

Type of Coverage
  Individual, Medicaid

Key Personnel
Chief Executive Officer. . . . . Douglas A. Hayward, RN
Chief Financial Officer . . . . Keith Quinlinvan
Chief Operations Officer. Becky Davenport
Chief Compliance Officer . . . . Clayton Carlos, MPA
Manager/Public Affairs . . . . Louis Iturriria
    661-664-5120
    louiei@khs-net.com
Associate Medical Dir . . . . G. Remmington Brooks, MD
Health Services Officer. . . . . Bob Woodard
Manager, Marketing . . . . Louis Iturriria
    661-664-5120
    louiei@khs-net.com

---

143 L.A. Care Health Plan

1055 W 7th Street
10th Floor
Los Angeles, CA 90017
Toll-Free: 888-452-2273
Phone: 213-694-1250
Fax: 213-694-1246
webmaster@lacare.org
www.lacare.org
Non-Profit Organization: Yes
Year Founded: 1994
Number of Affiliated Hospitals: 83
Number of Primary Care Physicians: 3,555
Number of Referral/Specialty Physicians: 6,286
Total Enrollment: 857,252
State Enrollment: 836,724

Healthplan and Services Defined
  PLAN TYPE: HMO
  Model Type: Staff
  Benefits Offered: Dental, Vision, Comprehensive Health Coverage,
    Medical

Type of Coverage
  Medicaid, Healthy Families, L.A. Care's Healt

Geographic Areas Served
  Los Angeles County

Key Personnel
Chief Executive Officer . . . . Howard A Kahn
Chief Operations Officer . . . . John Wallace
Chief Financial Officer . . . . Tim Reilly
Chief Of Strategy, Regula . . . . Jonathan Freedman
Chief HR . . . . Barbara Cook
CIO . . . . Gene Fernandez
General Counsel . . . . Augustavia J. Haydel
Chief Medical Officer . . . . Gertrude Carter, MD
Chief Of Human & Communit . . . . Barbara Cook
Public Relations Spec. . . . . Marissa Jiminez
    213-694-1250
    mjiminez@lacare.org

144   Lakeside Community Healthcare Network

8510 Balboa Boulevard
Northridge, CA 91325
Phone: 866-654-3471
info@lakesidecommunityhealthcare.com
www.lakesidecommunityhealthcare.com
For Profit Organization: Yes
Year Founded: 1997
Number of Primary Care Physicians: 300
Number of Referral/Specialty Physicians: 1,500
Total Enrollment: 250,000
State Enrollment: 250,000

Healthplan and Services Defined
 PLAN TYPE: HMO
 Model Type: IPA

Key Personnel
 President/CEO . . . . Francesco Federico, MD
 EVP, Corporate Dev . . . . Keith S Richman, MD
 COO . . . . Joan Rose, MPH
 CFO . . . . Kermit Newman
 SVP, Medical Operations . . . . Jeffrey Hay
 Medical Director . . . . Ziad Dabuni, MD
 Chief Medical Officer . . . . Bernard Siegel, MD
 Media Contact . . . . Pamela Pollock
  pam.pollock@lakesidecommunityhealthcare.

145   Landmark Healthplan of California

1610 Arden Way
Suite 280
Sacramento, CA 95815
Toll-Free: 800-638-4557
Fax: 800-599-8350
info@LMhealthcare.com
www.landmarkhealthcare.com
For Profit Organization: Yes
Year Founded: 1985
Number of Referral/Specialty Physicians: 4,500
Total Enrollment: 150,000

Healthplan and Services Defined
 PLAN TYPE: HMO/PPO
 Model Type: IPA, Network
 Plan Specialty: Chiropractic, Acupuncture
 Benefits Offered: Chiropractic, Acupuncture

Type of Payment Plans Offered
 Combination FFS & DFFS

Geographic Areas Served
 California

Network Qualifications
 Pre-Admission Certification: Yes

Peer Review Type
 Utilization Review: Yes
 Case Management: Yes

Key Personnel
 Chief Executive Officer . . . . John J. Arlotta, Jr
 President . . . . Douglas K. Tardio
 VP Operations . . . . Debra Tull
 EVP, Sales & Marketing . . . . Michael Joslin
 Chief Medical Officer . . . . A. Bartley Bryt, DC
 VP/Clinical & Quality Adm . . . . Debbie Enigl
 Sales Account Manager . . . . Michelle Kulton
  800-638-4557
  mkulton@lmhealthcare.com

146   Liberty Dental Plan

340 Commerce
Suite 100
Irvine, CA 92602
Toll-Free: 888-703-6999
www.libertydentalplan.com
Mailing Address: PO Box 26110, Santa Ana, CA 92799-9547
For Profit Organization: Yes

Healthplan and Services Defined
 PLAN TYPE: Dental
 Other Type: Dental HMO
 Plan Specialty: Dental
 Benefits Offered: Dental

Type of Coverage
 Commercial

Key Personnel
 CEO, President . . . . Amir Neshat, DDS
 Executive Vice President . . . . John Carvelli
 Chief Financial Officer . . . . Maja Kapic
 VP, Liberty Nevada . . . . Randy Brecher
 VP, Business Development . . . . Bill Henderson
 Chief Financial Officer . . . . Maja Kapic
 Dental Director . . . . Richard Hague, DMD, MPA
 VP, Client Services . . . . Marsha Hazlewood
 Dental Dir, Utiliz Mgmt . . . . Brian Benjamin, DDS
 Dir, Administrative Svcs . . . . Rob Linfield
 Gen Mgr, Nevada Operation . . . . Terry Allen

147   Los Angeles County Department of Health Services

313 North Figueroa Street
Los Angeles, CA 90012
www.ladhs.org
Subsidiary of: Los Angeles County Department of Health Services
Non-Profit Organization: Yes
Year Founded: 1983
Federally Qualified: Yes
Number of Affiliated Hospitals: 12
Number of Primary Care Physicians: 800
Total Enrollment: 700,000

Healthplan and Services Defined
 PLAN TYPE: HMO
 Model Type: Staff
 Benefits Offered: Prescription

Type of Coverage
 Catastrophic Illness Benefit: Unlimited

Geographic Areas Served
 Los Angeles County

Subscriber Information
 Average Monthly Fee Per Subscriber
  (Employee + Employer Contribution):
   Employee Only (Self): $143.05
   Employee & 1 Family Member: $286.15
   Employee & 2 Family Members: $332.01
 Average Subscriber Co-Payment:
   Primary Care Physician: $5.00
   Prescription Drugs: $4.00
   Home Health Care Max. Days/Visits Covered: Unlimited
   Nursing Home Max. Days/Visits Covered: 60 days

Network Qualifications
 Pre-Admission Certification: Yes

Peer Review Type
 Utilization Review: Yes
 Second Surgical Opinion: Yes
 Case Management: Yes

Accreditation Certification
TJC Accreditation, Medicare Approved, Utilization Review, State Licensure, Quality Assurance Program

Key Personnel
Director..................................Michael Katz, PhD
Interim Admin Deputy ....Gregory Polk, MPA
Planning & Prog Oversight ....Cheri Todoroff, MPH
Deputy Dir/Planning..........................Cheri Todoroff
Chief Network Officer ....Carol Meyer
CFO......................................Allan Wecker
Interim Chief Medical Off...............Gail V Anderson Jr, MD
Chief Nursing Officer ....Vivian C Branchick, RN
Director, Ambulatory Care ....Gretchen McGinley
Chief Information Officer.....................Kevin Lynch, MS

148 Managed Health Network

2370 Kerner Blvd
San Rafael, CA 94901
Toll-Free: 800-327-2133
www.mhn.com
Subsidiary of: Health Net Inc
For Profit Organization: Yes
Year Founded: 1974
Number of Affiliated Hospitals: 1,400
Number of Primary Care Physicians: 51,000
Total Enrollment: 10,000,000

Healthplan and Services Defined
PLAN TYPE: PPO
Model Type: IPA, Group
Plan Specialty: Behavioral Health, Disease Management
Benefits Offered: Behavioral Health, Disease Management, Prescription, Substance Abuse

Type of Coverage
Commercial, TRICARE, EAP

Type of Payment Plans Offered
POS, FFS

Geographic Areas Served
Nationwide

Network Qualifications
Pre-Admission Certification: Yes

Peer Review Type
Case Management: Yes

Publishes and Distributes Report Card: Yes

Accreditation Certification
URAC, NCQA

Key Personnel
President/CEO ....Jeffrey Barstow
Executive Director ....Brian Oleary
President ....Steven Sell
COO....................................Juanell Hefner
CIO.....................................Rick Simmons
Chief Medical Officer ....Ian A Schaffer
Chief Sales Officer..........................Gidget Peddie
Media Contact............................Gina Clemente
  415-460-8054
  gina.clemente@mhn.com
Media Contact ....Margita Thompson
  818-676-7912
  margita.thompson@healthnet.com

Specialty Managed Care Partners
Enters into Contracts with Regional Business Coalitions: Yes

149 March Vision Care

6701 Center Drive West
Suite 790
Los Angeles, CA 90045
Toll-Free: 888-493-4070
marchinfo@marchvisioncare.com
www.marchvisioncare.com
For Profit Organization: Yes
Total Enrollment: 1,800,000

Healthplan and Services Defined
PLAN TYPE: Vision
Plan Specialty: Vision
Benefits Offered: Vision

Type of Coverage
Commercial

Geographic Areas Served
Nationwide

Key Personnel
Founder & CEO.....................Glenville A March, Jr, MD
Founder & CEO.........................Cabrini T March, MD

150 MD Care Healthplan

1640 E Hill Street
Signal Hill, CA 90755
Toll-Free: 888-285-9676
Phone: 562-344-3400
Fax: 866-237-3578
www.mdcareadvantage.com
Subsidiary of: Humana Healthcare

Healthplan and Services Defined
PLAN TYPE: Medicare

Type of Coverage
Medicare

Key Personnel
President ....Long Dang

151 Medfocus Radiology Network

2811 Wilshire Boulevard
Suite 900
Santa Monica, CA 90403
Toll-Free: 800-398-8999
Fax: 800-950-4700
webmaster@medfocus.net
www.medfocuslogin.net
Year Founded: 1988
Number of Primary Care Physicians: 3,400

Healthplan and Services Defined
PLAN TYPE: PPO
Model Type: Network
Plan Specialty: UR

Geographic Areas Served
42 States, including District of Columbia and Puerto Rico

Peer Review Type
Utilization Review: Yes
Second Surgical Opinion: Yes

Accreditation Certification
NCQA

Key Personnel
Medical Director ....Stephen Meisel, MD

152 Mida Dental Plan

PO Box 10194
Van Nuys, CA 91410
Toll-Free: 800-876-6432
Phone: 818-710-9400
Fax: 818-704-9817
Acquired by: United Concordia

Healthplan and Services Defined
 PLAN TYPE: Dental
 Plan Specialty: Dental
 Benefits Offered: Dental

Type of Payment Plans Offered
 POS, FFS

Publishes and Distributes Report Card: Yes

Key Personnel
 Dental Director............................Paul Manos, DDS
  paul.manos@ucci.com
 Medical Affairs ....Don Gross
 Provider Relations Coordinator.................Carrie Ahluwalia
  carrie.ahluwalia@ucci.com

153 Molina Healthcare: Corporate Office

200 Oceangate
Suite 100
Long Beach, CA 90802
Toll-Free: 888-562-5442
Phone: 562-435-3666
Fax: 562-499-0790
www.molinahealthcare.com
Secondary Address: 2277 Fair Oaks Blvd, Suite 195, Sacramento, CA
 95825
For Profit Organization: Yes
Year Founded: 1980
Physician Owned Organization: Yes
Number of Affiliated Hospitals: 84
Number of Primary Care Physicians: 2,167
Number of Referral/Specialty Physicians: 6,184
Total Enrollment: 1,400,000

Healthplan and Services Defined
 PLAN TYPE: HMO
 Model Type: Network
 Benefits Offered: Chiropractic, Dental, Home Care, Inpatient SNF,
  Long-Term Care, Podiatry, Vision

Type of Coverage
 Commercial, Medicare, Supplemental Medicare, Medicaid

Geographic Areas Served
 Los Angeles, Riverside, San Bernardino, Sacramento, Yolo and San
 Diego counties

Accreditation Certification
 URAC, NCQA

Key Personnel
 President/CEO..........................J Mario Molina, MD
 Chief Financial Officer.....................John C Molina, JD
 Chief Operations Officer ....Terry T Bayer, JD
 Chief Accounting Officer ....Joseph W. White
 SVP, Secretary & General ....Jeff D. Barlow
 VP Medical Affairs ....Richard A Helmer, MD
 Chief Information Officer.........................Rick Hopper
 VP Finance....................................Harvey A Fein
 VP, Investor Relations & ....Juan Jose Orellano
 Chief Medical Officer ....James W Howatt, MD

154 Omni IPA/Medcore Medical Group

2609 E Hammer Lane
Stockton, CA 95210
Toll-Free: 877-963-2673
Phone: 209-320-2600
Fax: 209-320-2644
webmaster@medcoreipa.com
www.medcoreipa.com
Year Founded: 1985
Number of Primary Care Physicians: 400

Healthplan and Services Defined
 PLAN TYPE: Other
 Other Type: IPA

Geographic Areas Served
 San Joaquin County

Key Personnel
 CEO.......................................Kirit Patel, Md
 COO.....................................Sheila Stephens
 CIO...Jack Duguc
 Marketing......................................Arlene Lind

155 On Lok Lifeways

1333 Bush Street
San Francisco, CA 94109
Phone: 415-292-8888
Fax: 415-292-8745
info@onlok.org
www.onlok.org
Non-Profit Organization: Yes
Year Founded: 1971
Number of Affiliated Hospitals: 7
Number of Primary Care Physicians: 10
Number of Referral/Specialty Physicians: 100
Total Enrollment: 1,000
State Enrollment: 942

Healthplan and Services Defined
 PLAN TYPE: HMO
 Model Type: Staff
 Benefits Offered: Home Care, Long-Term Care, Physical Therapy,
  Prescription, Vision, Wellness

Type of Coverage
 Medicaid
 Catastrophic Illness Benefit: Covered

Geographic Areas Served
 San Francisco, Fremont, Newark, Union City and Santa Clara County

Subscriber Information
 Average Monthly Fee Per Subscriber
  (Employee + Employer Contribution):
   Employee & 1 Family Member: None if medicare/med
   Medicare: $2100.00
 Average Subscriber Co-Payment:
   Home Health Care Max. Days/Visits Covered: Unlimited
   Nursing Home Max. Days/Visits Covered: Unlimited

Accreditation Certification
 TJC Accreditation, Medicare Approved, Utilization Review,
  Pre-Admission Certification, State Licensure, Quality Assurance
  Program

Key Personnel
 Chief Executive Officer ....Robert E Edmondson
 Chief Financial Officer..........................Sue Wong
 Chief Admin Officer.............................Kelvin Quan
 Dir, Policy & Govt Rel.....................Eileen Kunz, MPH
 Chief Operating Officer........................Grace Li, MHA
 Chief Medical Officer ....Jay Luxenberg

156   Orange County Foundation for Medical Care

17322 Murphy Avenue
Irvine, CA 92614-5920
Toll-Free: 800-345-8643
info@ocfmc.com
www.ocfmc.com
Non-Profit Organization: Yes
Year Founded: 1959
Number of Affiliated Hospitals: 283
Number of Primary Care Physicians: 6,000
Total Enrollment: 1,100,000

Healthplan and Services Defined
  PLAN TYPE: PPO
  Other Type: EPO
  Model Type: Network
  Plan Specialty: Medical
  Benefits Offered: Claims Management/Utilization Management, Case
    Management/Claims Repricing/Customer Service/Provider
    Services/Cobra
  Offers Demand Management Patient Information Service: Yes

Type of Payment Plans Offered
  DFFS

Geographic Areas Served
  Orange County, Los Angeles County and Statewide

Subscriber Information
  Average Monthly Fee Per Subscriber
    (Employee + Employer Contribution):
      Employee Only (Self): $5.00
      Employee & 1 Family Member: $5.00
      Employee & 2 Family Members: $5.00
  Average Annual Deductible Per Subscriber:
      Employee Only (Self): $500.00
      Employee & 1 Family Member: $500.00
      Employee & 2 Family Members: $250.00
  Average Subscriber Co-Payment:
      Primary Care Physician: $10.00
      Non-Network Physician: $35.00
      Hospital ER: $50.00

Network Qualifications
  Pre-Admission Certification: Yes

Peer Review Type
  Utilization Review: Yes
  Second Surgical Opinion: Yes
  Case Management: Yes

Accreditation Certification
  URAC
  TJC Accreditation, Medicare Approved, Utilization Review, State
    Licensure, Quality Assurance Program

Key Personnel
  President . . . . .Dawn Bruner
  Vice President. . . . . .Jay Ross Zubrin, MD
  Treasurer/Secretary . . . . .Kerri Shiller
  Medical Director. . . . . .Mark Krugman

157   Pacific Dental Benefits

1390 Willow Pass Road
Suite 800
Concord, CA 94520-5240
Toll-Free: 800-999-3367
Phone: 925-363-6000
Fax: 925-363-6099
vbrembt@pdbi.com
www.pdbi.com
Acquired by: UnitedHealthcare Dental
For Profit Organization: Yes

Year Founded: 1973
Number of Primary Care Physicians: 3,600
Number of Referral/Specialty Physicians: 1,700
Total Enrollment: 650,000

Healthplan and Services Defined
  PLAN TYPE: Dental
  Model Type: IPA, Group
  Plan Specialty: Dental
  Benefits Offered: Dental, Vision

Type of Payment Plans Offered
  POS, Capitated, Combination FFS & DFFS

Geographic Areas Served
  California, Nevada, Texas, Illinois, District of Columbia, Virginia,
  Georgia, North Carolina and South Carolina

Subscriber Information
  Average Monthly Fee Per Subscriber
    (Employee + Employer Contribution):
      Employee Only (Self): $15-19
      Employee & 1 Family Member: $22-26
      Employee & 2 Family Members: $32-36

Network Qualifications
  Pre-Admission Certification: Yes

Peer Review Type
  Utilization Review: Yes

Publishes and Distributes Report Card: No

Accreditation Certification
  Medicare Approved, Utilization Review, State Licensure

Key Personnel
  CEO. . . . . .John Gaebel
    jgaebel@pdbi.com
  VP Administration/CFO . . . . .Randy Brecher
  Director Operations . . . . .Nilesh Patel
  Executive VP Claims. . . . . .Martin Brennan
    mbrennan@pdbi.com
  Controller . . . . .Burt Weinstein
  Dental Services Director . . . . .Gary Dougan
  Chief Marketing Officer. . . . . .James Fuhrman
  VP Health Services . . . . .Dan Maher
    dmaher@pdbi.com

Specialty Managed Care Partners
  Enters into Contracts with Regional Business Coalitions: No

158   Pacific Foundation for Medical Care

3510 Unocal Place
Suite 108
Santa Rosa, CA 95403
Toll-Free: 800-548-7677
Phone: 707-525-4281
Fax: 707-525-4311
kpass@rhs.org
www.pfmc.org
Non-Profit Organization: Yes
Year Founded: 1957
Number of Affiliated Hospitals: 75
Number of Primary Care Physicians: 3,000
Number of Referral/Specialty Physicians: 4,430
Total Enrollment: 300,000

Healthplan and Services Defined
  PLAN TYPE: Multiple
  Model Type: Network
  Plan Specialty: EPO, PPO, LOCO

Geographic Areas Served
  Sonoma, Alameda, Contra Costa, El Dorado, Imperial, Napa, Nevada,
  Placer, Sacramento, San Diego, Solano, Marin and Yolo counties.
  Butte, Colusa, Glenn, Lassen, Modoc, Pluma, Shasta, Sierra,
  Siskiquou, Sutter counties

Network Qualifications
Pre-Admission Certification: Yes

Peer Review Type
Utilization Review: Yes
Second Surgical Opinion: Yes
Case Management: Yes

Publishes and Distributes Report Card: No

Key Personnel
Chief Executive Officer ....John Nacol
    707-525-4370
    jnacol@rhs.org
Medical Director ....William Pitt
Claims.......................................Sandy Sylvers
Network Contracting...........................Kathy Pass
Medical Review Services ....Nancy Manchee
    619-401-6843
    nmanchee@rhs.org
Marketing Manager............................Kathy Pass
Medical Affairs ....William Pitt, MD
Member Services...............................Kathy Pass
    707-525-4281
    kpass@rhs.org
Provider Services.............................Kathy Pass
    707-525-4281
    kpass@rhs.org

Specialty Managed Care Partners
Enters into Contracts with Regional Business Coalitions: No

---

159   Pacific Health Alliance
1525 Rollins Road
Suite B
Burlingame, CA 94010
Toll-Free: 800-533-4742
Fax: 650-375-5820
pha@pacifichealthalliance.com
www.pacifichealthalliance.com
For Profit Organization: Yes
Year Founded: 1986
Number of Affiliated Hospitals: 400
Number of Primary Care Physicians: 50,000
Number of Referral/Specialty Physicians: 1,500
Total Enrollment: 338,000
State Enrollment: 197,000

Healthplan and Services Defined
    PLAN TYPE: PPO
    Model Type: Group
    Plan Specialty: Behavioral Health, Chiropractic, EPO, Lab, Worker's
        Compensation, UR
    Benefits Offered: Behavioral Health, Chiropractic, Dental, Home
        Care, Inpatient SNF, Long-Term Care, Physical Therapy, Podiatry,
        Psychiatric, Transplant, Vision, Worker's Compensation

Type of Coverage
Commercial, Individual, Indemnity

Type of Payment Plans Offered
DFFS, FFS

Geographic Areas Served
California, Nevada

Network Qualifications
Pre-Admission Certification: Yes

Peer Review Type
Utilization Review: Yes
Second Surgical Opinion: Yes
Case Management: Yes

Publishes and Distributes Report Card: No

Accreditation Certification
TJC Accreditation, Medicare Approved, Utilization Review,
    Pre-Admission Certification, State Licensure, Quality Assurance
    Program

Average Claim Compensation
Physician's Fees Charged: 70%
Hospital's Fees Charged: 75%

Specialty Managed Care Partners
Daughters of Charity, Saint Rose Hospital, San Monterry
Enters into Contracts with Regional Business Coalitions: No

---

160   Pacific IPA
9700 Flair Drive
El Monte, CA 91731
Toll-Free: 888-888-7472
Phone: 626-652-3526
Fax: 626-401-1670
admin@pacificipa.com
http://pacificipa.net
Year Founded: 1986
Number of Primary Care Physicians: 800

Healthplan and Services Defined
    PLAN TYPE: Other
    Other Type: IPA
    Model Type: IPA
    Benefits Offered: Disease Management, Wellness

---

161   PacifiCare Dental and Vision Administrators
3110 West Lake Center Dr
Santa Ana, CA 92704-6921
Toll-Free: 800-228-3384
Phone: 661-631-8613
Fax: 714-513-6486
www.myuhdental.com
Mailing Address: PO Box 30968, Salt Lake City, UT 84130-0968
Subsidiary of: UnitedHealthCare
For Profit Organization: Yes
Year Founded: 1973
Number of Primary Care Physicians: 8,986
Number of Referral/Specialty Physicians: 2,705
Total Enrollment: 140,462

Healthplan and Services Defined
    PLAN TYPE: Multiple
    Model Type: IPA
    Plan Specialty: Dental, Vision
    Benefits Offered: Dental, Vision

Type of Coverage
Commercial, Individual, Indemnity, Medicare

Type of Payment Plans Offered
POS, Capitated, FFS

Geographic Areas Served
Arizona, California, Colorado, Nevada, Oklahoma, Oregon, Texas and
    Washington

Network Qualifications
Pre-Admission Certification: Yes

Peer Review Type
Utilization Review: Yes

Key Personnel
President/CEO ....Kelly McCrann
VP/General Manager.....................Claire L Hannan, CPA
CFO ....Christopher D Boles
Managing Director ....Moody Kyal
VP Information Services.....................Kerry Matsumoto
VP Sales/Marketing ....John W Whalley

162 PacifiCare Health Systems

5995 Plaza Drive
Cypress, CA 90630
Toll-Free: 800-411-0191
Phone: 714-952-1121
Fax: 714-236-5803
www.pacificare.com
Mailing Address: PO Box 6006, Cypress, CA 90630-0006
Subsidiary of: UnitedHealthCare
For Profit Organization: Yes
Year Founded: 1978
Number of Affiliated Hospitals: 305
Number of Primary Care Physicians: 1,050
Number of Referral/Specialty Physicians: 1,791
Total Enrollment: 1,915,829
State Enrollment: 1,345,473

Healthplan and Services Defined
  PLAN TYPE: HMO
  Model Type: Network
  Benefits Offered: Disease Management, Prescription, Wellness

Type of Coverage
  Commercial, Individual, Indemnity, Medicare

Geographic Areas Served
  California, Texas, Oklahoma, Oregon & Washington

Peer Review Type
  Second Surgical Opinion: Yes

Publishes and Distributes Report Card: Yes

Accreditation Certification
  TJC Accreditation, Medicare Approved, Utilization Review,
  Pre-Admission Certification, State Licensure, Quality Assurance
  Program

Key Personnel
  Chairman/CEO . . . . Howard Phanstiel
  Exec VP/CFO. . . . . Gregory W Scott
  Vice President . . . . Edward Cymerys
  Facilities Managaer. . . . . Pam Palumbo
  Chief Medical Officer . . . . Sam Ho
  Director Member Services. . . . . Judu Bernauer
  Chief Information Officer. . . . . Mike Connelly
  Provider Services . . . . Carol Ackerman

Specialty Managed Care Partners
  Enters into Contracts with Regional Business Coalitions: Yes

163 PacifiCare of California

5995 Plaza Drive
Cypress, CA 90630
Toll-Free: 800-624-8822
Phone: 909-274-3045
www.pacificare.com
Mailing Address: PO Box 6006, Cypress, CA 90963
Subsidiary of: UnitedHealthCare
For Profit Organization: Yes
Year Founded: 1978
Number of Affiliated Hospitals: 304
Number of Primary Care Physicians: 8,271
Number of Referral/Specialty Physicians: 1,466
Total Enrollment: 1,283,000

Healthplan and Services Defined
  PLAN TYPE: HMO
  Model Type: Network
  Benefits Offered: Behavioral Health, Dental, Prescription, Vision,
  Life

Type of Coverage
  Commercial, Individual, Indemnity, Medicare

Type of Payment Plans Offered
  POS, DFFS, Capitated, FFS, Combination FFS & DFFS

Geographic Areas Served
  Licensed in areas comprising 90% of California's population

Subscriber Information
  Average Monthly Fee Per Subscriber
    (Employee + Employer Contribution):
      Employee Only (Self): $139.68
      Employee & 1 Family Member: $312.69
      Employee & 2 Family Members: $428.93
      Medicare: $19.80
  Average Subscriber Co-Payment:
      Primary Care Physician: $5.00
      Prescription Drugs: $5.00
      Hospital ER: $35.00
      Home Health Care: $5.00
      Home Health Care Max. Days/Visits Covered: As necessary

Network Qualifications
  Pre-Admission Certification: Yes

Peer Review Type
  Utilization Review: Yes
  Case Management: Yes

Publishes and Distributes Report Card: Yes

Accreditation Certification
  NCQA
  TJC Accreditation, Medicare Approved, Utilization Review,
  Pre-Admission Certification, State Licensure, Quality Assurance
  Program

Key Personnel
  President . . . . James Frey
  james.frey@phs.com

164 Partnership HealthPlan of California

4665 Business Center Drive
Fairfield, CA 94534-1675
Toll-Free: 800-863-4144
Phone: 707-863-4100
Fax: 707-863-4117
www.partnershiphp.org
Non-Profit Organization: Yes
Year Founded: 1994
Total Enrollment: 93,000

Healthplan and Services Defined
  PLAN TYPE: Medicare
  Other Type: Medicare HMO
  Benefits Offered: Chiropractic, Inpatient SNF, Long-Term Care,
  Vision

Type of Coverage
  Individual, Medicare, Medicaid

Geographic Areas Served
  Miami-Dade, Broward and Palm Beach counties

Accreditation Certification
  NCQA

165 Physical Therapy Provider Network

26635 W Agoura Road
Suite 250
Calabasas, CA 91302
Toll-Free: 800-766-7876
info@ptpn.com
www.ptpn.com
For Profit Organization: Yes
Year Founded: 1985
Physician Owned Organization: No
Federally Qualified: No
Number of Referral/Specialty Physicians: 1,200
Total Enrollment: 1,100,000

Healthplan and Services Defined
  PLAN TYPE: Multiple
  Model Type: Network
  Benefits Offered: Physical Therapy, Occupational Therapy, Hand
    Therapy, Pediatric Therapy and Speech/Language Therapy
  Offers Demand Management Patient Information Service: No

Geographic Areas Served
  Arizona, California, Colorado, Florida, Georgia, Louisiana,
  Massachusetts, Maryland, Maine, Michigan, Missouri, Mississippi,
  New Hampshire, New Jersey, New York, Ohio, Oklahoma,
  Pennsylvania, Rhode Island, Tennessee, Texas, Vermont, West
  Virginia

Network Qualifications
  Pre-Admission Certification: Yes

Peer Review Type
  Utilization Review: Yes
  Case Management: Yes

Publishes and Distributes Report Card: No

Accreditation Certification
  State Licensure

Key Personnel
  President..........................Michael Weinper, PT/DPT
  Vice President............................Nancy Rothenberg
  Direction, QA...........................Mitchel Kaye, PT

Specialty Managed Care Partners
  Enters into Contracts with Regional Business Coalitions: No

---

166 Preferred Utilization Management Inc
5356 Clayton Road
Suite 201
Concord, CA 94521
Phone: 925-844-3100
Fax: 925-844-3124
www.suptullog.com
Mailing Address: PO Box 190, Clayton, CA 94517
For Profit Organization: Yes
Year Founded: 1982

Healthplan and Services Defined
  PLAN TYPE: Other
  Other Type: VRO
  Model Type: URO
  Plan Specialty: Chiropractic
  Benefits Offered: Concurrent Review and Retro-Review, prospective
    review

Type of Coverage
  Health & Workers Comp, Pers Injury

Geographic Areas Served
  Nationwide

Peer Review Type
  Utilization Review: Yes

Key Personnel
  President/CEO...........................Ronald Cataldo, Sr
  CFO..Jeanette Cataldo

Specialty Managed Care Partners
  ChiroSource Inc, Chiropractic Health Plan of California Inc, Basic
    Chiropractic Health Plan Inc, Preferred Therapy Provider of
    America
  Enters into Contracts with Regional Business Coalitions: Yes

---

167 Premier Access Insurance/Access Dental
P.O. Box 659010
Sacramento, CA 95826-9010
Toll-Free: 888-634-6074
Phone: 916-920-2500
Fax: 916-563-9000
info@premierlife.com
www.premierppo.com
For Profit Organization: Yes
Year Founded: 1998
Number of Primary Care Physicians: 1,000
Total Enrollment: 125,000

Healthplan and Services Defined
  PLAN TYPE: PPO
  Model Type: Network
  Plan Specialty: Dental
  Benefits Offered: Dental

Type of Payment Plans Offered
  FFS

Geographic Areas Served
  California and outside of California

Accreditation Certification
  TJC Accreditation, Medicare Approved, Utilization Review,
    Pre-Admission Certification, State Licensure, Quality Assurance
    Program

Key Personnel
  President/CEO.......................Reza Abbaszadeh, DDS
  CFO......................................Katherine Smith
  SVP, Strategic Plan Ops.........................Robin Muck
  Chief Marketing Officer........................Richard Fulton

---

168 Primecare Dental Plan
10700 Civic Center Drive
Suite 100-A
Rancho Cucamonga, CA 91730
Toll-Free: 800-937-3400
contact@primecaredental.net
www.primecaredental.net
Subsidiary of: Jaimini Health Inc. Companies, Healthdent of California
For Profit Organization: Yes
Year Founded: 1983
Physician Owned Organization: Yes
Number of Referral/Specialty Physicians: 3,700
Total Enrollment: 17,000

Healthplan and Services Defined
  PLAN TYPE: Dental
  Model Type: Staff
  Plan Specialty: Dental
  Benefits Offered: Dental
  Offers Demand Management Patient Information Service: Yes

Type of Coverage
  Commercial, Individual

Type of Payment Plans Offered
  DFFS, Capitated

Geographic Areas Served
  Alameda, Butte, Colusa, Contra Costa, El Dorado, Fresno, Glenn,
  Kern, Kings, Los Angeles, Madera, Mariposa, Merced Monterey,
  Napa, Nevada, Orange, Placer, Riverside, Sacramento, San Benito,
  San Bernardino, San Diego, San Francisco, San Joaquin, San Luis
  Opispo, San Mateo, Santa Barbara, Santa Clara, Santa Cruz, Shasta,
  Siskiyou, Solano, Sonoma, Stanislaus, Sutter, Tehama, Tuolumne,
  Tulare, Ventura, Yolo, and Yuba counties

Subscriber Information
  Average Monthly Fee Per Subscriber
    (Employee + Employer Contribution):
      Employee Only (Self): $9.50

Employee & 1 Family Member: $12.00
Employee & 2 Family Members: $14.00

Network Qualifications
Pre-Admission Certification: Yes

Peer Review Type
Utilization Review: Yes

Publishes and Distributes Report Card: No

Accreditation Certification
URAC, NCQA
Utilization Review

Key Personnel
President and CEO . . . . .Mohender Narula
CFO . . . . .Mahesh Manchandia
COO . . . . .Carolyn Brodt

Specialty Managed Care Partners
Enters into Contracts with Regional Business Coalitions: No

---

169   PTPN

26635 W Agoura Road
Suite 250
Calabasas, CA 91302
Toll-Free: 800-766-7876
info@ptpn.com
www.ptpn.com
Year Founded: 1985
Number of Primary Care Physicians: 1,200

Healthplan and Services Defined
  PLAN TYPE: PPO
  Other Type: Rehab Network
  Model Type: Network
  Plan Specialty: Outpatient Rehabilitation (Physical, Occupational and
    Speech Therapy)
  Benefits Offered: Physical Therapy, Worker's Compensation,
    Occupational Therapy, Speech Therapy, Physical Therapy, Hand
    Therapy, Speech/Language Therapy and Pediatric Therapy.

Type of Payment Plans Offered
DFFS

Geographic Areas Served
Nationwide

Network Qualifications
Minimum Years of Practice: 3

Peer Review Type
Utilization Review: Yes

Accreditation Certification
NCQA

Key Personnel
President. . . . . .Michael Weinper, PT, DPT
Vice President . . . . .Nancy Rothenberg
Quality Assurance. . . . . .Michael Kaye
Media Contact. . . . . .Ruben Marroquin
  818-737-0207
  rmarroquin@ptpn.com

---

170   SafeGuard Health Enterprises: Corporate Office

95 Enterprise
Suite 100
Aliso Viejo, CA 92656
Toll-Free: 800-880-1800
Phone: 949-425-4300
Fax: 949-425-4586
www.safeguard.net
Subsidiary of: MetLife
For Profit Organization: Yes
Year Founded: 1974

Number of Primary Care Physicians: 2,073
Number of Referral/Specialty Physicians: 2,030
Total Enrollment: 1,800,000

Healthplan and Services Defined
  PLAN TYPE: Dental
  Other Type: Dental HMO
  Model Type: IPA
  Plan Specialty: ASO, Dental, Vision
  Benefits Offered: Dental, Vision

Type of Coverage
Individual, Indemnity, Medicaid

Type of Payment Plans Offered
DFFS, Capitated

Geographic Areas Served
California, Texas, Florida

Subscriber Information
Average Annual Deductible Per Subscriber:
  Employee Only (Self): $50.00
  Employee & 1 Family Member: $100.00
  Employee & 2 Family Members: $150.00

Network Qualifications
Pre-Admission Certification: Yes

Peer Review Type
Utilization Review: Yes

Publishes and Distributes Report Card: No

Key Personnel
Chairman/CEO . . . . .James E Buncher
  949-425-4500
President/COO . . . . .Stephen J Baker
SVP/CFO . . . . .Dennis L Gates
VP/CIO . . . . .Michael J Lauffenburger
SVP/General Counsel . . . . .Ronald I Brendzel
Dir/Human Resources . . . . .William Wolff
VP . . . . .Robin Muck

Specialty Managed Care Partners
Enters into Contracts with Regional Business Coalitions: Yes

Employer References
State of California, Boeing, County of Los Angeles, Farmers
  Insurance, Automobile Club

---

171   San Francisco Health Plan

201 Third Street
7th Floor
San Francisco, CA 94103
Phone: 415-547-7818
Fax: 415-547-7826
memberservices@sfhp.org
www.sfhp.org
Non-Profit Organization: Yes
Year Founded: 1994
Number of Affiliated Hospitals: 6
Number of Primary Care Physicians: 2,300
Total Enrollment: 55,000
State Enrollment: 55,000

Healthplan and Services Defined
  PLAN TYPE: HMO
  Benefits Offered: Disease Management, Wellness

Type of Coverage
Medicare, Medicaid, Medi-Cal, Healthy Families, Healthy

Geographic Areas Served
San Francisco

Key Personnel
Chief Executive Officer. . . . . .John F Grgurina, Jr
Chief Financial Officer. . . . . .John Gregoire
Chief Operating Officer . . . . .Deena Louie
Chief Information Officer .Sunny Cooper

Compliance Officer . . . . Nina Maruyama
Medical Director . . . . Kelly Pfeifer, MD
General Counsel . . . . Richard Rubinstein
Human Res Consultant . . . . Kate Gormley
Dir, Marketing & Comm . . . . Bob Menezes
Dir, Clinical Services . . . . Alison Lum, PharmD
Dir, Clinical Informatics . . . . Kimberley Higgins-Mays
Dir, Finance . . . . Skip Bishop
Dir, Technology Services . . . . Cecil Newton
Dir, Business Services . . . . Van Wong
Dir, Qual & Performance . . . . Tammy Fisher
Media Contact . . . . Bob Memezes
  bmenezes@sfhp.org

172 Santa Clara Family Health Foundations Inc

210 East Hacienda Avenue
Campbell, CA 95008-6617
Toll-Free: 800-260-2055
Phone: 408-376-2000
mainoffice@scfhp.com
www.scfhp.com
Secondary Address: 1153 King Road, San Jose, CA 95122,
  877-688-7234
Non-Profit Organization: Yes
Year Founded: 1997
Number of Affiliated Hospitals: 8
Number of Primary Care Physicians: 890
Number of Referral/Specialty Physicians: 2,309
Total Enrollment: 121,794
State Enrollment: 121,794

Healthplan and Services Defined
  PLAN TYPE: HMO
  Benefits Offered: Behavioral Health, Disease Management,
    Prescription, Wellness
  Offers Demand Management Patient Information Service: Yes
  DMPI Services Offered: 24 hour nurse advice line

Type of Coverage
  Commercial, Medicaid, Medicare Advantage SNP, Medi-Cal, H

Geographic Areas Served
  Santa Clara County

Subscriber Information
  Average Monthly Fee Per Subscriber
    (Employee + Employer Contribution):
      Employee & 2 Family Members: $18 max per family

Key Personnel
  President/CEO . . . . Ronald Cohn
  Executive Director . . . . Craig Walsh
  CFO . . . . Michael Weatherford
  CMO . . . . R Dennis Collins, MD
  General Counsel . . . . Sheila Maloney
  Provider Relations . . . . Lisa Kraymer
  Marketing . . . . Janie Tyre
  Member Relations . . . . Pat McClelland
  Pharmacy Director . . . . Angeli Garg
  Public Relations . . . . Elisabeth Handler

Specialty Managed Care Partners
  Medimpact

173 SCAN Health Plan

3800 Kilroy Airport Way
Suite 100
Long Beach, CA 90806
Toll-Free: 800-559-3500
www.scanhealthplan.com
Non-Profit Organization: Yes
Year Founded: 1977
Number of Affiliated Hospitals: 151

Number of Primary Care Physicians: 6,560
Number of Referral/Specialty Physicians: 17,186
Total Enrollment: 128,272
State Enrollment: 12,283

Healthplan and Services Defined
  PLAN TYPE: HMO
  Plan Specialty: Medicare

Type of Coverage
  Medicare

Geographic Areas Served
  California & Arizona

Subscriber Information
  Average Annual Deductible Per Subscriber:
    Medicare: $0
  Average Subscriber Co-Payment:
    Primary Care Physician: $0-$5
    Hospital ER: $50
    Home Health Care: $0
    Nursing Home: $0
    Nursing Home Max. Days/Visits Covered: 100

Key Personnel
  CEO . . . . Christopher Wing
  CFO . . . . Randy Stone
  Chief Risk Officer . . . . Nancy J. Monk
  Chief Operating Officer . . . . Bill Roth
  SVP/GM, All Markets . . . . Cathy Batteer
  SVP Public & Gov. Affairs . . . . Peter Begans
  SVP, Healthcare Services . . . . Eve Gelb
  SVP, Healthcare Info. . . . . Moon Leung, PhD
  SVP, National Sales . . . . Gil Miller
  VP/GM, Northern Cal. . . . . Karen Sugano
  SVP/GM, Southern Cal. . . . . Sherry L Stanislaw
  Corporate Medical Dir. Romilla Batra
  Corporate Medical Dir. Raymond Chan

174 Sharp Health Plan

8520 Tech Way
Suite 200
San Diego, CA 92123
Toll-Free: 800-359-2002
Phone: 858-499-8300
www.sharphealthplan.com
Subsidiary of: Sharp HealthCare
Non-Profit Organization: Yes
Total Enrollment: 49,000
State Enrollment: 49,000

Healthplan and Services Defined
  PLAN TYPE: HMO

Geographic Areas Served
  San Diego and Southern Riverside counties

Key Personnel
  CEO & President . . . . Melissa Hayden Cook
  Vice President/CFO . . . . Rita Datko
  Vice President/COO . . . . Leslie Pels-Beck
  Vice President/CBDO . . . . Michael Byrd
  VP, Chief Medical Officer . . . . Dr Lori Stone, MD

175 Stanislaus Foundation for Medical Care

2339 St Pauls Way
Modesto, CA 95355
Phone: 209-527-1704
www.stanislausmedicalsociety.com
Mailing Address: PO Box 576007, Modesto, CA 95357-6007
Non-Profit Organization: Yes
Year Founded: 1957
Number of Affiliated Hospitals: 400
Number of Primary Care Physicians: 27,000

Number of Referral/Specialty Physicians: 5,000

Healthplan and Services Defined
  PLAN TYPE: PPO
  Model Type: Network
  Benefits Offered: Prescription
  Offers Demand Management Patient Information Service: Yes

Geographic Areas Served
  Stanislaus, Tuolumne counties

Network Qualifications
  Pre-Admission Certification: Yes

Publishes and Distributes Report Card: No

Key Personnel
  President . . . . .Steve Benak, MD
  President-Elect. . . . . .Peter Broderick, MD
  Director . . . . .Delaine Fortson, MD
  Nurse Case Manager . . . . .Jannell Cipponeri, MD

Specialty Managed Care Partners
  Enters into Contracts with Regional Business Coalitions: No

176   Superior Vision Services, Inc.

11101 White Rock Road
Rancho Cordova, CA 95670
Toll-Free: 800-507-3800
contactus@supervision.com
www.superiorvision.com
For Profit Organization: Yes
Year Founded: 1993
Number of Primary Care Physicians: 46,000
Total Enrollment: 2,000,000

Healthplan and Services Defined
  PLAN TYPE: Vision
  Model Type: Group
  Plan Specialty: Vision, Vision Benefits, Exams, Glasses, Contact
    Lenses
  Benefits Offered: Vision, Managed Vision Care

Type of Coverage
  Commercial, Indemnity, Medicaid, Catastrophic

Geographic Areas Served
  Nationwide

Subscriber Information
  Average Monthly Fee Per Subscriber
    (Employee + Employer Contribution):
      Employee Only (Self): Varies
      Employee & 1 Family Member: Varies
      Employee & 2 Family Members: Varies
      Medicare: Varies

Accreditation Certification
  AAPI, NCQA

Key Personnel
  Chief Executive Officer. . . . . .Kirk Rothrock
  Chief Information Officer . . . . .Greg Pontius
  Chief Financial Officer. .Brian Silverberg
  SVP, Operations . . . . .Kimberly Hess
  VP, Provider Relations . . . . .Zon Dunn
  VP, Marketing . . . . .Carol Misso
  VP, Corporate Development. . . . . .Josh Silverman
  VP, Sales . . . . .Thomas Luchetta

177   UDC Dental Care of California

6310 Greenwich Drive
Suite 210
San Diego, CA 92122
Toll-Free: 800-821-1294
Phone: 858-812-8230
Fax: 858-678-0692
www.udcdentalcalifornia.com

For Profit Organization: Yes

Healthplan and Services Defined
  PLAN TYPE: Dental
  Other Type: Prepaid Dental Plan
  Plan Specialty: Dental
  Benefits Offered: Dental

Type of Coverage
  Commercial

178   United Behavioral Health

425 Market Street
27th Floor
San Francisco, CA 94105
Toll-Free: 800-888-2998
Phone: 415-547-5000
www.unitedbehavioralhealth.com
Subsidiary of: UnitedHealth Group
Year Founded: 1997
Number of Affiliated Hospitals: 3,500
Number of Primary Care Physicians: 85,000
Total Enrollment: 43,000,000

Healthplan and Services Defined
  PLAN TYPE: Other
  Other Type: EAP
  Model Type: Network
  Plan Specialty: Behavioral Health
  Benefits Offered: Behavioral Health, Prescription, Psychiatric
  Offers Demand Management Patient Information Service: Yes

Type of Payment Plans Offered
  POS

Geographic Areas Served
  Nationwide

Peer Review Type
  Case Management: Yes

Publishes and Distributes Report Card: Yes

Accreditation Certification
  TJC, URAC, NCQA

Key Personnel
  CEO . . . . .Gregory A Bayer, PhD
  CFO . . . . .Randall Odzer
  VP, Human Capital . . . . .Pamela Russo
  VP . . . . .Joe Guinn
  Chief Strategy Officer. . . . . .David Whitehouse, MD
  Chief Medical Officer . . . . .Rhonda Robinson-Beale, MD
  Human Capital Partner . . . . .Pamela Russo
  Chief Marketing Officer . . . . .Rick Bates
  Media Relations. . . . . .Brad Lotterman
    714-445-0453

Specialty Managed Care Partners
  Enters into Contracts with Regional Business Coalitions: Yes

179   United Concordia: California

21700 Oxnard Street
Suite 500
Woodland Hills, CA 91367
Toll-Free: 800-345-3837
Phone: 810-823-7835
ucproducer@ucci.com
www.secure.ucci.com
Secondary Address: 4370 La Jolla Village Drive, Suite 429, San Diego,
  CA 92122, 858-646-3041
For Profit Organization: Yes
Year Founded: 1971
Number of Primary Care Physicians: 111,000
Total Enrollment: 8,000,000

Healthplan and Services Defined
  PLAN TYPE: Dental
  Plan Specialty: Dental
  Benefits Offered: Dental

Type of Coverage
  Commercial, Individual

Geographic Areas Served
  Military personnel and their families, nationwide

---

180 UnitedHealthCare of Northern California
8880 Cal Center Drive
Suite 300
Sacramento, CA 95826
Toll-Free: 866-288-4993
www.uhc.com
Subsidiary of: UnitedHealth Group
For Profit Organization: Yes
Year Founded: 1986
Total Enrollment: 75,000,000
State Enrollment: 2,300,000

Healthplan and Services Defined
  PLAN TYPE: HMO/PPO
  Model Type: Network
  Benefits Offered: Disease Management, Prescription, Wellness
  Offers Demand Management Patient Information Service: Yes

Type of Coverage
  Catastrophic Illness Benefit: Covered

Type of Payment Plans Offered
  DFFS, Capitated

Geographic Areas Served
  Statewide

Subscriber Information
  Average Monthly Fee Per Subscriber
    (Employee + Employer Contribution):
      Employee Only (Self): $120.00
      Employee & 1 Family Member: $240.00
      Employee & 2 Family Members: $375.00
  Average Annual Deductible Per Subscriber:
      Employee & 2 Family Members: Varies
  Average Subscriber Co-Payment:
      Primary Care Physician: $5.00-10.00
      Prescription Drugs: $5.00/10.00/25.00
      Hospital ER: $50.00
      Nursing Home Max. Days/Visits Covered: 120 per year

Publishes and Distributes Report Card: Yes

Accreditation Certification
  NCQA
  TJC Accreditation, Utilization Review, State Licensure

Key Personnel
  President/CEO . . . . Dan Rosenthal
  Chief Financial Officer . . . . Peter Horn
  Marketing . . . . Devon Waggoner
  CMO/West Region . . . . Sandra Nichols, MD
  Media Contact . . . . Will Shanley
    will.shanley@uhc.com

Specialty Managed Care Partners
  Enters into Contracts with Regional Business Coalitions: Yes

---

181 UnitedHealthCare of Southern California
5701 Katella Ave
Cypress, CA 90630
Toll-Free: 800-357-0978
Phone: 877-511-3039
www.uhc.com
Secondary Address: 505 N Brand Blvd, Suite 1200, Glendale, CA
  91203

Subsidiary of: UnitedHealth Group
For Profit Organization: Yes
Year Founded: 1987
Total Enrollment: 75,000,000
State Enrollment: 2,300,000

Healthplan and Services Defined
  PLAN TYPE: HMO/PPO
  Model Type: IPA
  Benefits Offered: Disease Management, Prescription, Wellness
  Offers Demand Management Patient Information Service: Yes

Type of Coverage
  Catastrophic Illness Benefit: Unlimited

Type of Payment Plans Offered
  POS

Geographic Areas Served
  Statewide

Subscriber Information
  Average Monthly Fee Per Subscriber
    (Employee + Employer Contribution):
      Employee Only (Self): $120.00
      Employee & 1 Family Member: $240.00
      Employee & 2 Family Members: $370.00
  Average Subscriber Co-Payment:
      Primary Care Physician: $10.00
      Prescription Drugs: $5.00
      Hospital ER: $50.00

Network Qualifications
  Pre-Admission Certification: Yes

Peer Review Type
  Utilization Review: Yes
  Second Surgical Opinion: Yes
  Case Management: Yes

Publishes and Distributes Report Card: Yes

Accreditation Certification
  NCQA
  TJC Accreditation, Medicare Approved, Utilization Review,
    Pre-Admission Certification, State Licensure, Quality Assurance
    Program

Key Personnel
  Chief Executive Officer . . . . David Anderson
  Chief Financial Officer. . . . . Alex Uhm
  Marketing . . . . Devon Waggoner
  Chief Medical Officer . . . . Sandra Nichols, MD
  Media Contact. . . . . Matt Yi
    will.shanley@uhc.com

Specialty Managed Care Partners
  Enters into Contracts with Regional Business Coalitions: Yes

---

182 Ventura County Health Care Plan
2220 East Gonzales Road
Suite 210 B
Oxnard, CA 93036
Phone: 805-981-5050
Fax: 805-981-5051
vchcp.memberservices@ventura.org
www.vchealthcareplan.org
Non-Profit Organization: Yes
Year Founded: 1993

Healthplan and Services Defined
  PLAN TYPE: HMO
  Benefits Offered: Disease Management, Prescription, Wellness

Geographic Areas Served
  Ventura County

183 Vision Plan of America
3255 Wilshire Boulevard
Suite 1610
Los Angeles, CA 90010
Toll-Free: 800-400-4872
Fax: 213-384-0084
info@visionplanofamerica.com
www.visionplanofamerica.com
Subsidiary of: The Camden Insurance Agency
For Profit Organization: Yes
Year Founded: 1986
Number of Primary Care Physicians: 700
Number of Referral/Specialty Physicians: 165

Healthplan and Services Defined
  PLAN TYPE: Vision
  Model Type: IPA
  Plan Specialty: Vision
  Benefits Offered: Vision

Type of Coverage
  Commercial, Individual

Type of Payment Plans Offered
  POS, Capitated

Geographic Areas Served
  Statewide

Peer Review Type
  Case Management: Yes

Key Personnel
  President and CEO . . . . Stuart Needleman, OD
  CFO . . . . Phillip Needleman
  Manager . . . . Milori Lopez Duarte
  Optometric Director . . . . Adolphus Lages, OD
  Provider Relations . . . . Mayra Castillo

184 VSP: Vision Service Plan
3333 Quality Drive
Rancho Cordova, CA 95670
Toll-Free: 800-852-7600
Phone: 916-851-5000
Fax: 916-851-4858
webmaster@vsp.com
www.vsp.com
Secondary Address: 3400 Morse Crossing, Columbus, OH 43219
Year Founded: 1955
Number of Primary Care Physicians: 26,000
Total Enrollment: 55,000,000

Healthplan and Services Defined
  PLAN TYPE: Vision
  Plan Specialty: Vision
  Benefits Offered: Vision

Type of Payment Plans Offered
  Capitated

Geographic Areas Served
  Nationwide

Network Qualifications
  Pre-Admission Certification: Yes

Peer Review Type
  Utilization Review: Yes

Accreditation Certification
  Utilization Review, Quality Assurance Program

Key Personnel
  President/CEO . . . . Rob Lynch
  CEO, Marchon Eyewear . . . . Al Berg
  President, Vision Care . . . . Gary Brooks
  Pres/Opthalmic Operations . . . . Donald Oakley
  Pres/Practice Solutions . . . . Jim McGrann

Chairman . . . . Tim Jankowski
CFO . . . . Donald Ball, Jr
VSP, Public Relations . . . . Pat McNeil
  patrmc@vps.com

185 VSP: Vision Service Plan of California
1 Market Plaza
Suite 2625
San Francisco, CA 94105-1101
Phone: 415-957-0977
Fax: 415-546-9755
webmaster@vsp.com
www.vsp.com
Year Founded: 1955
Number of Primary Care Physicians: 28,000
Total Enrollment: 55,000,000

Healthplan and Services Defined
  PLAN TYPE: Vision
  Plan Specialty: Vision
  Benefits Offered: Vision

Type of Payment Plans Offered
  Capitated

Geographic Areas Served
  Statewide

Network Qualifications
  Pre-Admission Certification: Yes

Peer Review Type
  Utilization Review: Yes

Accreditation Certification
  Utilization Review, Quality Assurance Program

Key Personnel
  Regional Vice President . . . . Janet Findlay
  Regional Manager . . . . Daniel Morgan
  Marketing Manager . . . . Phyllis Moore

186 Western Dental Services
530 South Main Street
Orange, CA 92868
Toll-Free: 800-4579-3783
www.westerndental.com
For Profit Organization: Yes
Year Founded: 1903
Number of Primary Care Physicians: 1,700
Number of Referral/Specialty Physicians: 1,400
Total Enrollment: 315,440

Healthplan and Services Defined
  PLAN TYPE: Dental
  Other Type: Dental HMO
  Model Type: Staff, IPA
  Plan Specialty: Dental
  Benefits Offered: Dental

Type of Coverage
  Indemnity

Type of Payment Plans Offered
  POS, Combination FFS & DFFS

Geographic Areas Served
  California and Arizona

Subscriber Information
  Average Monthly Fee Per Subscriber
    (Employee + Employer Contribution):
      Employee Only (Self): $10.28
      Employee & 1 Family Member: $19.48
      Employee & 2 Family Members: $25.62

Network Qualifications
  Pre-Admission Certification: Yes

Peer Review Type
    Utilization Review: Yes
    Second Surgical Opinion: Yes
    Case Management: Yes

Publishes and Distributes Report Card: No

Accreditation Certification
    Utilization Review

Key Personnel
Chief Executive Officer . . . . Simon Castellanos
Chief Dental Officer. . . . . Louis Amendola
SVP, Operations . . . . Roderick Place
SVP/General Counsel . . . . Jeffrey Miller
Chief Marketing Officer . . . . Joshua Marder
VP, Real Estate . . . . Andrew Eddy
Chief Information Officer . . . . Michael Warter

Average Claim Compensation
    Physician's Fees Charged: 80%

Specialty Managed Care Partners
    Enters into Contracts with Regional Business Coalitions: No

187   Western Health Advantage

2349 Gateway Oaks Drive
Suite 100
Sacramento, CA 95833
Phone: 916-563-2250
hr@westernhealth.com
www.westernhealth.com
Non-Profit Organization: Yes
Year Founded: 1996
Total Enrollment: 92,000
State Enrollment: 92,000

Healthplan and Services Defined
    PLAN TYPE: HMO

Geographic Areas Served
    Sacramento, Yolo, Solano, western El Dorado, western Placer
    counties

Key Personnel
President & CEO . . . . Garry Maisel
Chief Financial Officer . . . . Rita Ruecker
Chief Legal Officer . . . . Rebecca Downing
Chief Sales Officer . . . . Bill Figenshu
Chief Marketing/Branding . . . . Rick Heron
Chief, Client Services . . . . Glenn Hamburg
Chief Medical Officer . . . . Don Hufford, MD
Chief Financial Officer . . . . Rita Ruecker
Chief Sales Officer . . . . Bill Figenshu

Health Insurance Coverage Status and Type of Coverage by Age

Category	All Persons		Under 18 years		Under 65 years		65 years and over	
	Number	%	Number	%	Number	%	Number	%
Total population	5,173	-	1,239	-	4,544	-	629	-
Covered by some type of health insurance	4,444 *(18)*	85.9 *(0.3)*	1,137 *(6)*	91.8 *(0.5)*	3,819 *(18)*	84.0 *(0.4)*	625 *(2)*	99.3 *(0.2)*
Covered by private health insurance	3,567 *(24)*	68.9 *(0.5)*	786 *(11)*	63.4 *(0.9)*	3,170 *(24)*	69.8 *(0.5)*	396 *(7)*	63.0 *(1.1)*
Employment based	2,811 *(27)*	54.3 *(0.5)*	641 *(13)*	51.7 *(1.0)*	2,608 *(27)*	57.4 *(0.6)*	203 *(6)*	32.3 *(1.0)*
Direct purchase	707 *(18)*	13.7 *(0.3)*	106 *(7)*	8.5 *(0.6)*	506 *(16)*	11.1 *(0.3)*	201 *(5)*	32.0 *(0.8)*
Covered by TRICARE	231 *(10)*	4.5 *(0.2)*	65 *(5)*	5.2 *(0.4)*	176 *(10)*	3.9 *(0.2)*	55 *(3)*	8.7 *(0.5)*
Covered by government health insurance	1,394 *(19)*	26.9 *(0.4)*	390 *(12)*	31.5 *(0.9)*	788 *(19)*	17.3 *(0.4)*	606 *(3)*	96.4 *(0.3)*
Covered by Medicaid	749 *(19)*	14.5 *(0.4)*	384 *(11)*	30.9 *(0.9)*	681 *(18)*	15.0 *(0.4)*	68 *(3)*	10.9 *(0.5)*
Also by private insurance	117 *(7)*	2.3 *(0.1)*	38 *(4)*	3.1 *(0.3)*	87 *(6)*	1.9 *(0.1)*	31 *(2)*	4.9 *(0.4)*
Covered by Medicare	706 *(6)*	13.6 *(0.1)*	8 *(2)*	0.7 *(0.2)*	100 *(5)*	2.2 *(0.1)*	606 *(3)*	96.3 *(0.3)*
Also by private insurance	409 *(8)*	7.9 *(0.1)*	1 *(Z)*	0.1 *(0.1)*	32 *(3)*	0.7 *(0.1)*	377 *(7)*	60.0 *(1.2)*
Also by Medicaid	112 *(5)*	2.2 *(0.1)*	3 *(2)*	0.3 *(0.1)*	43 *(3)*	1.0 *(0.1)*	68 *(3)*	10.9 *(0.5)*
Covered by VA Care	113 *(6)*	2.2 *(0.1)*	2 *(1)*	0.2 *(0.1)*	65 *(5)*	1.4 *(0.1)*	48 *(3)*	7.6 *(0.5)*
Not covered at any time during the year	729 *(18)*	14.1 *(0.3)*	102 *(6)*	8.2 *(0.5)*	725 *(18)*	16.0 *(0.4)*	4 *(1)*	0.7 *(0.2)*

Note: Numbers in thousands; Figures cover 2013; Margin of error appears in parenthesis; A "Z" indicates that the value either represents or rounds to zero.
Source: U.S. Census Bureau, 2013 American Community Survey, Table HI05. Health Insurance Coverage Status and Type of Coverage by State and Age for All People: 2013

Colorado

188 Aetna Health of Colorado
1 South Wacker Drive
Mail Stop F643
Chicago, IL 60606
Toll-Free: 877-751-9310
www.aetna.com
Partnered with: eHealthInsurance Services Inc.
For Profit Organization: Yes
Year Founded: 1987
Number of Affiliated Hospitals: 19
Number of Primary Care Physicians: 2,292
Total Enrollment: 36,423
State Enrollment: 36,423

Healthplan and Services Defined
PLAN TYPE: HMO
Other Type: POS
Model Type: Network
Plan Specialty: Behavioral Health, Dental, Vision
Benefits Offered: Behavioral Health, Dental, Disease Management,
    Home Care, Physical Therapy, Podiatry, Prescription, Vision,
    Worker's Compensation, Life

Type of Coverage
Commercial, Individual

Type of Payment Plans Offered
POS, Capitated, FFS, Combination FFS & DFFS

Geographic Areas Served
Statewide

Peer Review Type
Case Management: Yes

Publishes and Distributes Report Card: Yes

Accreditation Certification
TJC Accreditation, Medicare Approved, Utilization Review,
    Pre-Admission Certification, State Licensure, Quality Assurance
    Program

Key Personnel
CEO .... Ronald A Williams
President................................. Mark T Bertolini
CFO................................... Joseph Rubretsky
General Counsel .... William Carsazza
Chief Medical Officer...................... Lonny ReismanD

Specialty Managed Care Partners
Enters into Contracts with Regional Business Coalitions: Yes

189 American Dental Group
PO Box 25517
Colorado Springs, CO 80917
Toll-Free: 800-633-3010
Phone: 719-633-3000
www.americandentalgroup.org
For Profit Organization: Yes
Year Founded: 1991
Physician Owned Organization: Yes
Number of Primary Care Physicians: 54,000
Number of Referral/Specialty Physicians: 73

Healthplan and Services Defined
PLAN TYPE: Dental
Model Type: Group
Plan Specialty: Dental
Benefits Offered: Dental, Vision

Type of Coverage
Commercial, Individual

Type of Payment Plans Offered
DFFS, FFS, Combination FFS & DFFS

Geographic Areas Served
Allen Park, Ann Arbor, Bloomfield Hills, Brighton, Canton, Clinton
Twp, Dearborn, Dearborn Hts, Detroit, Eastpointe, Farmington Hills,
Flint, Grand Blanc, Gross Pointe, Lansing, Livonia, Monroe, Novi,
Oak Park, Pontiac, Rochester Hills, Rochester, Roseville, Southfield,
Shelby Twp, Southgate, Sterling Hts, Troy, Walled Lakes, Warren,
Waterford, Wayne, W Bloomfield. Also, Toledo, OH; Richmond, VA
and Atlanta, Douglasville, Kennesaw, Lawrenceville, Marietta, GA

Subscriber Information
Average Monthly Fee Per Subscriber
    (Employee + Employer Contribution):
        Employee Only (Self): $9.95/month
        Employee & 1 Family Member: $16.95/mont
Average Annual Deductible Per Subscriber:
    Employee Only (Self): $0
    Employee & 1 Family Member: $0
    Employee & 2 Family Members: $0
    Medicare: $0

Key Personnel
President/CEO.................................. T McGinty
Owner .... Don Whaley

190 Anthem Blue Cross & Blue Shield of Colorado
700 Broadway
Denver, CO 80273
Toll-Free: 866-293-2892
Phone: 303-831-2131
Fax: 303-831-2631
www.anthem.com
Secondary Address: 555 Middlecreek Parkway, Colorado Springs, CO
    80921, 719-488-7400
For Profit Organization: Yes
Year Founded: 1978
Total Enrollment: 880,475
State Enrollment: 60,270

Healthplan and Services Defined
PLAN TYPE: HMO/PPO
Plan Specialty: Dental, Vision
Benefits Offered: Dental, Disease Management, Prescription, Vision,
    Wellness, Life

Type of Coverage
Commercial, Individual, Medicare

Type of Payment Plans Offered
POS, FFS

Geographic Areas Served
Colorado

Key Personnel
CEO.. Larry Glasscock
President/GM .... Mike Ramseier
CFO.. Michael Smith
CMO .... Dr Elizabeth Kraft
General Counsel............................... Dave Harris
Media Contact .... Joyzelle Davis
    303-831-2005
    joyzelle.davis@anthem.com

191 Anthem Blue Cross & Blue Shield of Nevada
P.O. Box 5747
Denver, CO 80217
Toll-Free: 877-811-3106
www.anthem.com
For Profit Organization: Yes
Year Founded: 1995
Number of Affiliated Hospitals: 27
Number of Primary Care Physicians: 3,474
Number of Referral/Specialty Physicians: 2,518

Total Enrollment: 14,000,000
State Enrollment: 154,503

Healthplan and Services Defined
  PLAN TYPE: HMO/PPO
  Model Type: IPA
  Benefits Offered: Behavioral Health, Chiropractic, Complementary
    Medicine, Dental, Disease Management, Home Care, Inpatient
    SNF, Long-Term Care, Physical Therapy, Podiatry, Prescription,
    Psychiatric, Transplant, Vision, Wellness, AD&D, Life, LTD, STD

Type of Coverage
  Commercial, Individual, Indemnity, Medicare, Supplemental
  Medicare, Medicaid, Catastrophic

Geographic Areas Served
  Statewide

Network Qualifications
  Pre-Admission Certification: Yes

Peer Review Type
  Utilization Review: Yes
  Second Surgical Opinion: Yes
  Case Management: Yes

Accreditation Certification
  Medicare Approved, Utilization Review, Pre-Admission
    Certification, State Licensure, Quality Assurance Program

---

192   Assurant Employee Benefits: Colorado

2323 Grand Boulevard
Kansas City, CO 64108
Phone: 816-474-2345
Fax: 303-796-2769
Denver.rfp@assurant.com
www.assurantemployeebenefits.com
Subsidiary of: Assurant, Inc
For Profit Organization: Yes
Number of Primary Care Physicians: 112,000
Total Enrollment: 47,000

Healthplan and Services Defined
  PLAN TYPE: Multiple
  Plan Specialty: Dental, Vision, Long & Short-Term Disability
  Benefits Offered: Dental, Vision, Wellness, AD&D, Life, LTD, STD

Type of Coverage
  Commercial, Indemnity, Individual Dental Plans

Geographic Areas Served
  Statewide

Subscriber Information
  Average Monthly Fee Per Subscriber
    (Employee + Employer Contribution):
      Employee Only (Self): Varies by plan

Key Personnel
  President/CEO . . . . John S. Roberts
  SVP & General Counsel . . . . Kenneth D. Brown
  SVP/CFO. . . . . Miles B. Yakre
  PR Specialist. . . . . Megan Hutchison
    816-556-7815
    megan.hutchison@assurant.com

---

193   Behavioral Healthcare

155 Inverness Drive West
Suite 201
Englewood, CO 80112
Phone: 720-490-4400
Fax: 720-490-4395
www.bhicares.org
Non-Profit Organization: Yes

Healthplan and Services Defined
  PLAN TYPE: Other
  Model Type: Network

Plan Specialty: Behavioral Health
Benefits Offered: Behavioral Health

Type of Coverage
  Medicaid

Geographic Areas Served
  Arapahoe, Adams, Douglas counties & City of Aurora

Key Personnel
  Chief Executive Officer . . . . Roger Gunter
  Chief Financial Officer . . . . Rian Nowitzki
  Director, Quality Imprv. . . . . Samantha Kommana
  Chief Medical Officer. . . . . Kimberly Nordstrom, MD, JD
  Director, Member Affairs . . . . Scott Utash
  Director, Technology Svcs . . . . Jeff George

---

194   Beta Health Plan

9725 E Hampden Avenue
Suite 400
Denver, CO 80231
Toll-Free: 800-807-0706
Phone: 303-744-3007
Fax: 303-744-2890
www.betadental.com
Subsidiary of: Beta Health Association Inc
For Profit Organization: Yes
Year Founded: 1990
Physician Owned Organization: Yes
Number of Primary Care Physicians: 480
Number of Referral/Specialty Physicians: 120
Total Enrollment: 56,000

Healthplan and Services Defined
  PLAN TYPE: Multiple
  Model Type: Discount FFS Network
  Plan Specialty: Dental, Vision
  Benefits Offered: Dental, Vision

Type of Coverage
  Commercial, Individual, Indemnity
  Catastrophic Illness Benefit: Unlimited

Geographic Areas Served
  Statewide

Subscriber Information
  Average Monthly Fee Per Subscriber
    (Employee + Employer Contribution):
      Employee Only (Self): $11.00
      Employee & 1 Family Member: $21.75
      Employee & 2 Family Members: $31.75

Network Qualifications
  Pre-Admission Certification: No

Publishes and Distributes Report Card: Yes

Accreditation Certification
  State Dental Board

Key Personnel
  President. . . . . Rod Henningsen
  Senior Account Executive . . . . Linda Krueger
  VP . . . . Gail Burk

Specialty Managed Care Partners
  Enters into Contracts with Regional Business Coalitions: Yes

---

195   Boulder Valley Individual Practice Association

6676 Gunpark Drive
Suite B
Boulder, CO 80301
Phone: 303-530-3405
Fax: 303-530-2441
www.bvipa.com

Non-Profit Organization: Yes
Year Founded: 1978
Physician Owned Organization: Yes
Number of Affiliated Hospitals: 3
Number of Primary Care Physicians: 110
Number of Referral/Specialty Physicians: 190
Total Enrollment: 60,000

Healthplan and Services Defined
PLAN TYPE: PPO
  Model Type: IPA
  Offers Demand Management Patient Information Service: Yes

Type of Payment Plans Offered
  POS

Geographic Areas Served
  Boulder, Lafayette, Longmont & Louisville

Network Qualifications
  Pre-Admission Certification: Yes

Peer Review Type
  Utilization Review: Yes
  Second Surgical Opinion: Yes
  Case Management: Yes

Publishes and Distributes Report Card: No

Accreditation Certification
  TJC Accreditation, Utilization Review, State Licensure

Key Personnel
  President.................................Susan Roach, MD
  Vice President...........................Drigan Weider, CPA
  Treasurer.................................Jeffrey Perkins
  Medical Director.........................Laird Cagan, MD
    lcagan@bvipa.com

Specialty Managed Care Partners
  Enters into Contracts with Regional Business Coalitions: No

196 CIGNA HealthCare of Colorado
3900 E Mexico Avenue
Suite 1100
Denver, CO 80210
Toll-Free: 800-245-2471
Phone: 303-782-1500
Fax: 303-691-3197
www.cigna.com
Secondary Address: Great-West Healthcare, now part of CIGNA, 5445 DTC Parkway, Suite 400, Greenwood Village, CO 80111, 303-323-0000
For Profit Organization: Yes
Year Founded: 1986
Number of Affiliated Hospitals: 80
Number of Primary Care Physicians: 500
Total Enrollment: 36,611
State Enrollment: 462,000

Healthplan and Services Defined
PLAN TYPE: HMO
  Other Type: POS
  Model Type: IPA, Network
  Plan Specialty: Behavioral Health, Dental, Vision
  Benefits Offered: Behavioral Health, Dental, Disease Management, Prescription, Vision, Wellness, Life, LTD, STD
  Offers Demand Management Patient Information Service: Yes

Type of Coverage
  Commercial, Individual
  Catastrophic Illness Benefit: Covered

Type of Payment Plans Offered
  POS, Combination FFS & DFFS

Geographic Areas Served
  Adams, Arapahoe, Boulder, Denver, Douglas, El Paso, Elbert, Jefferson, Larimer, Pueblo, Teller and Weld counties

Subscriber Information
  Average Monthly Fee Per Subscriber
    (Employee + Employer Contribution):
      Employee Only (Self): $128.00
      Medicare: $396.00
  Average Subscriber Co-Payment:
      Primary Care Physician: $10.00
      Prescription Drugs: $5.00
      Hospital ER: $50.00

Network Qualifications
  Pre-Admission Certification: Yes

Peer Review Type
  Utilization Review: Yes
  Second Surgical Opinion: Yes
  Case Management: Yes

Publishes and Distributes Report Card: Yes

Accreditation Certification
  NCQA
  TJC Accreditation, Medicare Approved, Utilization Review, Pre-Admission Certification, State Licensure, Quality Assurance Program

Key Personnel
  President/CEO............................David Cordani
  Director At Cigna.......................Sallie Vanasdale
  VP Provider Relations...................William Cetti
  VP Client Relations.....................Gregg Prussing

Specialty Managed Care Partners
  Enters into Contracts with Regional Business Coalitions: Yes

197 CNA Insurance Companies: Colorado
10375 Park Meadows Drive
Suite 300
Littleton, CO 80124
Phone: 303-858-4100
Fax: 303-858-4427
cna_help@cna.com
www.cna.com
Year Founded: 1986
Number of Affiliated Hospitals: 57
Number of Primary Care Physicians: 3,400
Total Enrollment: 270,000

Healthplan and Services Defined
PLAN TYPE: PPO

Geographic Areas Served
  Metro Denver area

Key Personnel
  Chairman/CEO............................Thomas F Motamed
  President/COO...........................Bob Lindemann
  EVP, Chief Actuary......................Larry A Haefner
  EVP, Worldwide P&C Claim................George R Fay
  SVP/Dep. General Counsel................Michael P Warnick
  EVP/CFO................................D Craig Mense
  EVP, Chief Admin Officer...............Thomas Pontarelli
  President, COO CNA Spec................Peter W Wilson
  President, Field Oper..................Tim Szerlong
  SVP, CNA Select Risk...................John Angerami
  SVP, Human Resources...................Debbie Nutley
  Western Zone Officer...................Steve Stonehouse
  Central Zone Officer...................Greg Vezzosi
  Northern Zone Officer..................Steve Wachtel
  Media Contact..........................Sarah Pang

198   Colorado Access

10065 E Harvard Avenue
Suite 600
Denver, CO 80231
Toll-Free: 877-441-6032
Phone: 303-751-2657
customer.service@coaccess.com
www.coaccess.com
Non-Profit Organization: Yes
Year Founded: 1994

Healthplan and Services Defined
   PLAN TYPE: HMO

Type of Coverage
   Medicare, Medicaid

Key Personnel
   President/CEO/CMO . . . . .Marshall Thomas, MD
   Chief Financial Officer . . . . .Philip J Reed
   SVP/Chief Operating Offic. . . . . .Marie Steckbeck, MBA
   SVP, Clinical Operations. . . . . .Mike L McKitterick, RN
   VP, Admin Services & Corp .Rene Gallegos
   SVP, Public Policy & Perf. . . . . .Gretchen Flanders McGinnis, MSPH
   SVP, Behavioral Health . . . . .Alexis Giese, MD
   Chief Information Officer . . . . .Bobby Sherrill
   Media Relations . . . . .Ballard Pritchett
      mediarelations@coaccess.com

199   Colorado Choice Health Plans

700 Main Street
Suite 100
Alamosa, CO 81101
Toll-Free: 800-475-8466
Phone: 718-589-3696
Fax: 719-589-4901
www.slvhmo.com; coloradochoicehp.com
Non-Profit Organization: Yes
Year Founded: 1972
Total Enrollment: 5,000

Healthplan and Services Defined
   PLAN TYPE: HMO
   Benefits Offered: Dental, Disease Management, Prescription, Vision,
      Wellness, Life

Type of Coverage
   Commercial, Individual, Medicare

Geographic Areas Served
   Southern Colorado, San Luis Valley, Arkansas Valley, Durango,
   Pueblo, Colorado Springs, Denver

Key Personnel
   CEO . . . . .Cynthia Palmer
   VP Innovation & Dev. .Jerry Howell, PHD
   Director Sales/Marketing . . . . .Paul Roberts
   Director of Finance. . . . . .Sue Gray

200   Colorado Health Partnerships

7150 Campus Drive
Suite 300
Colorado Springs, CO 80920
Toll-Free: 800-804-5008
Fax: 719-538-1433
coproviderrelations@valueoptions.com
www.coloradohealthpartnerships.com
Non-Profit Organization: Yes
Year Founded: 1995
Number of Affiliated Hospitals: 8
Total Enrollment: 160,000
State Enrollment: 160,000

Healthplan and Services Defined
   PLAN TYPE: HMO
   Plan Specialty: Behavioral Health
   Benefits Offered: Behavioral Health

Type of Coverage
   Medicaid

Geographic Areas Served
   Alamosa, Archuleta, Baca, Bent, Chaffee, Conejos, Costilla, Crowley,
   Custer, Delta, Dolores, Eagle, El Paso, Fremont, Garfield, Grand,
   Gunnison, Hinsdale, Huerfano, Jackson, Kiowa, Lake, La Plata, Las
   Animas, Mesa, Mineral, Moffat, Montezuma, Montrose, Otero, Ouray,
   Park, Pitkin, Pueblo, Prowers, Rio Blanco, Rio Grande, Routt,
   Saguache, San Juan, San Miguel, Summit, Teller counties

201   Delta Dental of Colorado

4582 South Ulster Street
Suite 800
Denver, CO 80237
Toll-Free: 800-610-0201
customer_service@ddpco.com
www.deltadentalco.com
Non-Profit Organization: Yes
Year Founded: 1958
Total Enrollment: 54,000,000
State Enrollment: 1,000,000

Healthplan and Services Defined
   PLAN TYPE: Dental
   Other Type: Dental PPO
   Model Type: Network
   Plan Specialty: Dental
   Benefits Offered: Dental

Type of Coverage
   Commercial, Individual

Type of Payment Plans Offered
   DFFS

Geographic Areas Served
   Statewide

Subscriber Information
   Average Monthly Fee Per Subscriber
      (Employee + Employer Contribution):
         Employee Only (Self): $14.25
         Employee & 2 Family Members: $36.25
   Average Annual Deductible Per Subscriber:
         Employee Only (Self): $50
         Employee & 2 Family Members: $102
   Average Subscriber Co-Payment:
         Primary Care Physician: 80%
         Non-Network Physician: 50%

Network Qualifications
   Pre-Admission Certification: Yes

Publishes and Distributes Report Card: Yes

Key Personnel
   President & CEO . . . . .Kathryn Paul
   VP & COO . . . . .Linda Arneson, JD
   VP/CFO. . . . . .David Beal
   General Counsel & VP Admi . . . . .Barbara Springer
   VP, Sales & Marketing. . . . . .Jean Lawhead

202   Denver Health Medical Plan Inc

777 Bannock Street
MC600
Denver, CO 80204
Toll-Free: 800-700-8140
Phone: 303-602-2100
Fax: 303-436-5131
DHMPinfo@dhha.org

www.denverhealthmedicalplan.com
For Profit Organization: Yes
Year Founded: 1997
Number of Primary Care Physicians: 5,000
Total Enrollment: 15,000
State Enrollment: 15,000

Healthplan and Services Defined
  PLAN TYPE: HMO
  Benefits Offered: Chiropractic, Home Care, Inpatient SNF, Physical
    Therapy, Podiatry, Psychiatric, Transplant, Vision, Wellness

Type of Coverage
  Commercial, Medicare, Medicare Advantage, CHP+

Key Personnel
  CEO/Executive Director . . . . Leann Donovan
  Medical Director . . . . David Brody, MD

203 eHealthInsurance Services Inc.
11919 Foundation Place
Gold River, CA 95670
Toll-Free: 800-644-3491
webmaster@healthinsurance.com
www.ehealthinsurance.com
Year Founded: 1997
Total Enrollment: 3,000,000

Healthplan and Services Defined
  PLAN TYPE: HMO/PPO
  Benefits Offered: Dental, Prescription, Vision, Life, STD, pet, travel

Type of Coverage
  Commercial, Individual, Medicare

Type of Payment Plans Offered
  POS

Geographic Areas Served
  All 50 states in the USA and District of Columbia

Key Personnel
  Chairman & CEO . . . . Gary L. Lauer
  President/COO . . . . Bill Shaughnessy
  SVP, Engineering . . . . Dr. Jiang Wu
  SVP & CFO . . . . Stuart M. Huizinga
  SVP, Carrier Relations . . . . Robert S. Hurley
  SVP, Product Management . . . . Tom Tsao
  VP Communications . . . . Brian Mast
  SVP of Sales. . . . . Samuel C. Gibbs, III
  Director Public Relations. . . . . Nate Purpura
    650-210-3115
    nate.purpura@ehealth.com

204 Great-West/One Health Plan
8515 E Orchard Road
Greenwood Village, CO 80111
Toll-Free: 800-537-2033
Phone: 303-737-3000
greatwestcomments@gwl.com
www.greatwest.com
Mailing Address: PO Box 1700, Denver, CO 80201
Subsidiary of: Great-West Lifeco Inc
Acquired by: CIGNA
For Profit Organization: Yes
Year Founded: 1996
Owned by an Integrated Delivery Network (IDN): Yes
Number of Affiliated Hospitals: 3,700
Number of Primary Care Physicians: 400,000
Number of Referral/Specialty Physicians: 3,276
Total Enrollment: 2,000,000
State Enrollment: 115,262

Healthplan and Services Defined
  PLAN TYPE: HMO/PPO

Model Type: Network
Plan Specialty: ASO, Behavioral Health, Chiropractic, Disease
  Management, Lab, Radiology
Benefits Offered: Behavioral Health, Chiropractic, Complementary
  Medicine, Disease Management, Physical Therapy, Prescription,
  AD&D, Life
Offers Demand Management Patient Information Service: Yes

Type of Coverage
  Commercial

Type of Payment Plans Offered
  Combination FFS & DFFS

Geographic Areas Served
  We offer managed care in all fifty states

Network Qualifications
  Pre-Admission Certification: Yes

Peer Review Type
  Utilization Review: Yes
  Case Management: Yes

Publishes and Distributes Report Card: Yes

Accreditation Certification
  URAC

Key Personnel
  President/CEO. . . . . Mitchell T.G. Graye
  EVP/Chief Investment Offi. . . . . S. Mark Corbett
  SVP/Chief Marketing Offic. . . . . Joseph S. Greene
  In House Formulary . . . . David Burton
  Materials Management . . . . Jim Hicks
  Medical Affairs. . . . . John Tudor, MD
  Member Services. . . . . Martha Spoor
  Provider Services. . . . . Josh Nelson
  Sales . . . . Robert Immitt

Specialty Managed Care Partners
  ESI
  Enters into Contracts with Regional Business Coalitions: No

205 HMO Colorado
700 Broadway
9th Floor
Denver, CO 80203
Toll-Free: 800-654-9338
Phone: 303-831-2131
Fax: 303-831-2011
www.anthem.com
Subsidiary of: Anthem Blue Cross/Blue Shield
For Profit Organization: Yes
Year Founded: 1979
Owned by an Integrated Delivery Network (IDN): Yes
Number of Affiliated Hospitals: 66
Number of Primary Care Physicians: 1,941
Number of Referral/Specialty Physicians: 5,454
Total Enrollment: 126,000

Healthplan and Services Defined
  PLAN TYPE: HMO
  Model Type: IPA
  Benefits Offered: Behavioral Health, Chiropractic, Complementary
    Medicine, Dental, Disease Management, Home Care, Inpatient
    SNF, Long-Term Care, Physical Therapy, Podiatry, Prescription,
    Psychiatric, Transplant, Vision, Wellness, AD&D, Life, LTD, STD

Type of Coverage
  Commercial, Individual, Indemnity, Medicare, Supplemental
    Medicare, Medicaid, Catastrophic
  Catastrophic Illness Benefit: Maximum $1M

Type of Payment Plans Offered
  POS, FFS, Combination FFS & DFFS

Geographic Areas Served
Statewide outside of Adams, Arapahoe, Bloomfield, Denver, Douglas and Jefferson counties

Network Qualifications
Pre-Admission Certification: Yes

Peer Review Type
Utilization Review: Yes
Second Surgical Opinion: Yes
Case Management: Yes

Publishes and Distributes Report Card: No

Accreditation Certification
NCQA
TJC Accreditation, Medicare Approved, Utilization Review, Pre-Admission Certification, State Licensure, Quality Assurance Program

Key Personnel
Vice President . . . . Blair Christianson
Senior Vice President . . . . Beverly Sloan

Specialty Managed Care Partners
Enters into Contracts with Regional Business Coalitions: No

Employer References
Proprietary

---

206   Humana Health Insurance of Colorado Springs

8033 N Academy Blvd.
Colorado Springs, CO 80920
Toll-Free: 800-871-6270
Phone: 719-598-1317
Fax: 719-531-7089
www.humana.com
Secondary Address: 7400 E Orchard Road, Suite 1000 N, Greenwood Village, CO 80111, 303-773-0300
For Profit Organization: Yes
Year Founded: 1987
Number of Affiliated Hospitals: 72
Number of Primary Care Physicians: 2,811
Number of Referral/Specialty Physicians: 3,653
Total Enrollment: 113,229
State Enrollment: 113,229

Healthplan and Services Defined
PLAN TYPE: HMO/PPO
Plan Specialty: ASO, Dental, Vision, Fully Insured
Benefits Offered: Dental, Disease Management, Transplant, Vision, Personal Nurse, Case Management, On-Site Hospital Review, Utilization Management, Transplant Management, Humana First

Type of Coverage
Commercial, Individual, Group, Medicare

Geographic Areas Served
Colorado

Accreditation Certification
URAC, NCQA

Key Personnel
Regional Leader . . . . Leslie Andrews
Market Medical Officer . . . . Richard W Jones
VP . . . . Katherine Trease
Director Small Group Sale . . . . Robb Scheele
Media Relations . . . . Ross McLerran
210-617-1771

---

207   Kaiser Permanente Health Plan of Colorado

10350 E Dakota Avenue
Denver, CO 80247
Toll-Free: 888-681-7878
Phone: 303-338-3700
Fax: 303-338-3797
www.kaiserpermanente.org
Subsidiary of: Kaiser Permanente
Non-Profit Organization: Yes
Year Founded: 1969
Physician Owned Organization: Yes
Federally Qualified: Yes
Number of Affiliated Hospitals: 26
Number of Primary Care Physicians: 844
Total Enrollment: 535,000
State Enrollment: 535,000

Healthplan and Services Defined
PLAN TYPE: HMO
Model Type: Staff
Plan Specialty: Behavioral Health, Chiropractic, Dental, Disease Management, Vision, Radiology, UR
Benefits Offered: Behavioral Health, Chiropractic, Dental, Disease Management, Home Care, Inpatient SNF, Long-Term Care, Physical Therapy, Podiatry, Prescription, Psychiatric, Transplant, Vision, Wellness
Offers Demand Management Patient Information Service: Yes

Type of Coverage
Major Medical Plan
Catastrophic Illness Benefit: Unlimited

Geographic Areas Served
Southern Colorado, Denver, Boulder, Longmont metropolitan area and Colorado Springs

Publishes and Distributes Report Card: Yes

Accreditation Certification
NCQA

Key Personnel
Regional President . . . . Donna Lynne, DrPH
VP, Govt Relations . . . . Jandel Allen-Davis, MD
Assoc. Med Dir, Quality . . . . Michael D Chase, MD
Assoc. Med Dir, Network . . . . Elizabeth Kincannon, MD
VP, Health Plan Admin . . . . Anne McDow
VP, Operations . . . . Ginny McLain
VP, Finance . . . . Rick Newsome
VP, Business Operations . . . . Nancy Wollen
Med Dir, Clinical Process . . . . Bill Marsh, MD
Exec Medical Director . . . . William Wright, MD
Med Dir, Human Resources . . . . Rudy Kadota, MD
VP, Human Resources . . . . Robin Sadler
Med Dir, Primary Care . . . . Scott Smith
VP, Sales & Marketing . . . . Keith J Evans
Mgr, Integrated Communic. . . . . Art Luebke
303-344-7619
arthur.j.luebke@kp.org
Media Contact . . . . Amy D Whited
303-344-7518
amy.l.whited@kp.org

Specialty Managed Care Partners
Dental, Prescription, Vision, Good Samaritan, Saint Joseph
Enters into Contracts with Regional Business Coalitions: Yes

---

208   PacifiCare of Colorado

6455 S Yosemite Street
Greenwood Village, CO 80111
Phone: 303-714-3427
www.pacificare.com
Mailing Address: PO Box 4306, Englewood, CO 80155
Subsidiary of: UnitedHealthCare

For Profit Organization: Yes
Year Founded: 1974
Number of Affiliated Hospitals: 43
Number of Primary Care Physicians: 1,100
Number of Referral/Specialty Physicians: 2,400
Total Enrollment: 328,000

Healthplan and Services Defined
PLAN TYPE: HMO
Model Type: Network
Benefits Offered: Prescription

Type of Coverage
Commercial, Individual, Indemnity, Medicare
Catastrophic Illness Benefit: Covered

Type of Payment Plans Offered
DFFS, Capitated, FFS, Combination FFS & DFFS

Geographic Areas Served
Adams, Arapahoe, Boulder, Broomfield, Clear Creek, Denver, Douglas, Elbert, El Paso, Fremont, Gilpin, Jefferson, Larimer, Lincoln, Logan, Morgan, Park, Teller, Washington and Weld counties

Subscriber Information
Average Monthly Fee Per Subscriber
(Employee + Employer Contribution):
Employee Only (Self): $148.11
Employee & 2 Family Members: $473.96
Average Subscriber Co-Payment:
Primary Care Physician: $10.00
Non-Network Physician: 30%
Prescription Drugs: $10.00
Hospital ER: $50.00
Home Health Care: $0
Nursing Home: $0
Nursing Home Max. Days/Visits Covered: 120/yr.

Network Qualifications
Pre-Admission Certification: Yes

Peer Review Type
Utilization Review: Yes
Case Management: Yes

Accreditation Certification
NCQA
TJC Accreditation, Medicare Approved, Utilization Review, Pre-Admission Certification, State Licensure, Quality Assurance Program

Key Personnel
Chairman/CEO . . . . Howard Phanstiel
Executive VP/CFO. . . . . Greg Scott
VP/Chief Medical Officer . . . . Sam Ho

Average Claim Compensation
Physician's Fees Charged: 1%
Hospital's Fees Charged: 1%

Specialty Managed Care Partners
Enters into Contracts with Regional Business Coalitions: Yes

209 Pueblo Health Care
400 West 16th Street
Pueblo, CO 81003
Phone: 719-584-4806
Fax: 719-584-4038
www.pueblohealthcare.com
Number of Primary Care Physicians: 265

Healthplan and Services Defined
PLAN TYPE: PPO
Model Type: Network

Key Personnel
Executive Director . . . . Ann Bellah
719-584-4371
ann_bellah@parkviewmc.com

Provider Relations . . . . Sandra Proud
719-584-4642
sandra_proud@parkviewmc.com

210 Rocky Mountain Health Plans
2775 Crossroads Boulevard
Grand Junction, CO 81506-8712
Toll-Free: 800-843-0719
Phone: 970-244-7760
customer_service@rmph.org
www.rmhp.org
Mailing Address: PO Box 10600, Grand Junction, CO 81502-5600
Subsidiary of: Rocky Mountain Health Maintenance Organization
Non-Profit Organization: Yes
Year Founded: 1974
Owned by an Integrated Delivery Network (IDN): Yes
Number of Affiliated Hospitals: 107
Number of Primary Care Physicians: 2,425
Number of Referral/Specialty Physicians: 6,866
Total Enrollment: 207,180
State Enrollment: 207,180

Healthplan and Services Defined
PLAN TYPE: HMO/PPO
Other Type: HSA
Model Type: Mixed
Benefits Offered: Disease Management, Home Care, Prescription, Wellness

Type of Coverage
Commercial, Individual, Medicare, Supplemental Medicare, Medicaid
Catastrophic Illness Benefit: Unlimited

Type of Payment Plans Offered
FFS

Geographic Areas Served
Plans are available throughout Colorado

Subscriber Information
Average Subscriber Co-Payment:
Primary Care Physician: $20.00
Home Health Care Max. Days/Visits Covered: Unlimited

Network Qualifications
Minimum Years of Practice: 3
Pre-Admission Certification: Yes

Peer Review Type
Utilization Review: Yes
Second Surgical Opinion: Yes
Case Management: Yes

Publishes and Distributes Report Card: Yes

Accreditation Certification
NCQA
Medicare Approved, Utilization Review, Pre-Admission Certification, State Licensure, Quality Assurance Program

Key Personnel
President/CEO . . . . Steven ErkenBrack
COO. . . . . Laurel Walters
CFO. . . . . Pat Duncan
VP, Human Resources. . . . . Jan Rohr
Pres/CEO CNIC Health Sol. . . . . Jim Swayze
VP, Legal & Govt Affairs . . . . Mike Huotari
Chief Marketing Officer . . . . Neil Waldron
Chief Medical Officer . . . . Kevin R Fitzgerald, MD

Specialty Managed Care Partners
Delta Dental, Landmark Chiropractic, Vision Service Plan, Life Strategies

211   United Concordia: Colorado

999 18th Street
Suite 3023
Denver, CO 80202
Phone: 303-357-2388
Fax: 303-357-2389
ucproducer@ucci.com
www.secure.ucci.com
For Profit Organization: Yes
Year Founded: 1971
Number of Primary Care Physicians: 111,000
Total Enrollment: 8,000,000

Healthplan and Services Defined
  PLAN TYPE: Dental
  Plan Specialty: Dental
  Benefits Offered: Dental

Type of Coverage
  Commercial, Individual

Geographic Areas Served
  Military personnel and their families, nationwide

212   UnitedHealthCare of Colorado

6465 S Greenwood Plaza Boulevard
Suite 300
Centennial, CO 80111
Toll-Free: 866-574-6088
www.uhc.com
Subsidiary of: UnitedHealth Group
For Profit Organization: Yes
Year Founded: 1986
Number of Affiliated Hospitals: 47
Number of Primary Care Physicians: 1,600
Number of Referral/Specialty Physicians: 3,500
Total Enrollment: 75,000,000
State Enrollment: 735,900

Healthplan and Services Defined
  PLAN TYPE: HMO/PPO
  Model Type: Mixed Model
  Plan Specialty: MSO
  Benefits Offered: Behavioral Health, Chiropractic, Complementary
    Medicine, Dental, Disease Management, Home Care, Inpatient
    SNF, Long-Term Care, Physical Therapy, Podiatry, Prescription,
    Psychiatric, Transplant, Vision, Wellness, AD&D, Life

Type of Coverage
  Commercial, Individual, Medicaid, Commercial Group

Type of Payment Plans Offered
  DFFS, FFS, Combination FFS & DFFS

Geographic Areas Served
  HMO: Front Range Colorado; PPO/POS statewide

Subscriber Information
  Average Monthly Fee Per Subscriber
    (Employee + Employer Contribution):
      Employee Only (Self): Varies
  Average Subscriber Co-Payment:
    Primary Care Physician: $10
    Prescription Drugs: $10/15/30
    Hospital ER: $50

Network Qualifications
  Pre-Admission Certification: Yes

Peer Review Type
  Case Management: Yes

Publishes and Distributes Report Card: Yes

Accreditation Certification
  URAC, NCQA
  State Licensure, Quality Assurance Program

Key Personnel
  CEO . . . . .Beth Sorberg
  Marketing . . . . .Janet Bollman
  VP Small Business Sales . . . . .Chad Zechiel
  VP Key Account Sales . . . . .Cory Foreman
  Regional Media Contact . . . . .Kristen Hellmer
    602-255-8466
    kristen_hellmer@uhc.com

Average Claim Compensation
  Physician's Fees Charged: 70%
  Hospital's Fees Charged: 55%

Specialty Managed Care Partners
  United Behavioral Health
  Enters into Contracts with Regional Business Coalitions: No

213   VSP: Vision Service Plan of Colorado

1050 17th Street
Suite 1430
Denver, CO 80265-1501
Phone: 303-892-7663
webmaster@vsp.com
www.vsp.com
Year Founded: 1955
Number of Primary Care Physicians: 28,000
Total Enrollment: 57,000,000

Healthplan and Services Defined
  PLAN TYPE: Vision
  Plan Specialty: Vision
  Benefits Offered: Vision

Type of Payment Plans Offered
  Capitated

Geographic Areas Served
  Statewide

Network Qualifications
  Pre-Admission Certification: Yes

Peer Review Type
  Utilization Review: Yes

Accreditation Certification
  Utilization Review, Quality Assurance Program

Key Personnel
  Manager . . . . .Paula Palmer

Health Insurance Coverage Status and Type of Coverage by Age

Category	All Persons		Under 18 years		Under 65 years		65 years and over	
	Number	%	Number	%	Number	%	Number	%
Total population	3,541	-	784	-	3,020	-	522	-
Covered by some type of health insurance	3,209 *(14)*	90.6 *(0.4)*	751 *(4)*	95.7 *(0.5)*	2,692 *(14)*	89.1 *(0.5)*	517 *(2)*	99.1 *(0.2)*
Covered by private health insurance	2,504 *(23)*	70.7 *(0.6)*	515 *(10)*	65.7 *(1.2)*	2,169 *(21)*	71.8 *(0.7)*	335 *(6)*	64.2 *(1.1)*
Employment based	2,161 *(24)*	61.0 *(0.7)*	470 *(11)*	60.0 *(1.3)*	1,948 *(23)*	64.5 *(0.8)*	213 *(6)*	40.8 *(1.1)*
Direct purchase	410 *(12)*	11.6 *(0.3)*	45 *(4)*	5.8 *(0.6)*	250 *(10)*	8.3 *(0.3)*	160 *(5)*	30.7 *(1.0)*
Covered by TRICARE	51 *(6)*	1.4 *(0.2)*	12 *(3)*	1.6 *(0.4)*	36 *(6)*	1.2 *(0.2)*	15 *(2)*	2.8 *(0.3)*
Covered by government health insurance	1,103 *(18)*	31.2 *(0.5)*	261 *(9)*	33.3 *(1.2)*	604 *(17)*	20.0 *(0.6)*	499 *(2)*	95.7 *(0.4)*
Covered by Medicaid	611 *(18)*	17.3 *(0.5)*	260 *(9)*	33.1 *(1.2)*	545 *(17)*	18.1 *(0.6)*	66 *(4)*	12.7 *(0.7)*
Also by private insurance	84 *(6)*	2.4 *(0.2)*	26 *(4)*	3.3 *(0.4)*	54 *(5)*	1.8 *(0.2)*	30 *(3)*	5.7 *(0.6)*
Covered by Medicare	574 *(6)*	16.2 *(0.2)*	4 *(2)*	0.6 *(0.2)*	76 *(6)*	2.5 *(0.2)*	498 *(2)*	95.5 *(0.4)*
Also by private insurance	338 *(7)*	9.5 *(0.2)*	Z *(Z)*	0.1 *(0.1)*	21 *(3)*	0.7 *(0.1)*	317 *(6)*	60.7 *(1.1)*
Also by Medicaid	101 *(5)*	2.9 *(0.1)*	3 *(2)*	0.4 *(0.2)*	35 *(4)*	1.2 *(0.1)*	66 *(4)*	12.7 *(0.7)*
Covered by VA Care	60 *(4)*	1.7 *(0.1)*	Z *(Z)*	0.0 *(0.1)*	23 *(3)*	0.8 *(0.1)*	37 *(2)*	7.0 *(0.5)*
Not covered at any time during the year	333 *(14)*	9.4 *(0.4)*	34 *(4)*	4.3 *(0.5)*	328 *(14)*	10.9 *(0.5)*	5 *(1)*	0.9 *(0.2)*

Note: Numbers in thousands; Figures cover 2013; Margin of error appears in parenthesis; A "Z" indicates that the value either represents or rounds to zero.
Source: U.S. Census Bureau, 2013 American Community Survey, Table HI05. Health Insurance Coverage Status and Type of Coverage by State and Age for All People: 2013

Connecticut

214 Aetna Health, Inc. Corporate Headquarters

151 Farmington Avenue
Hartford, CT 06156
Toll-Free: 800-872-3862
Phone: 860-273-0123
www.aetna.com
For Profit Organization: Yes
Year Founded: 1853
Number of Affiliated Hospitals: 5,200
Number of Primary Care Physicians: 546,000
Number of Referral/Specialty Physicians: 981,000
Total Enrollment: 18,602,000
State Enrollment: 61,677

Healthplan and Services Defined
  PLAN TYPE: HMO
  Other Type: POS
  Plan Specialty: Dental, Lab, PBM, Vision, Radiology
  Benefits Offered: Behavioral Health, Dental, Disease Management,
    Long-Term Care, Physical Therapy, Podiatry, Prescription,
    Psychiatric, Vision, Life

Type of Coverage
  Commercial, Individual

Type of Payment Plans Offered
  FFS

Geographic Areas Served
  Nationwide

Key Personnel
  Chairman/CEO/President.....................Mark T Bertolini
  EVP/General Counsel ....William J Casazza
  EVP/CFO ....Shawn M Guertin

215 Aetna Health, Inc. Medicare Plan

Aetna Golden Medicare Plan
151 Farmington Avenue
Hartford, CT 06156
Toll-Free: 866-582-9629
Phone: 860-273-0123
www.aetnamedicare.com

Healthplan and Services Defined
  PLAN TYPE: Medicare
  Benefits Offered: Chiropractic, Dental, Disease Management, Home
    Care, Inpatient SNF, Physical Therapy, Podiatry, Prescription,
    Psychiatric, Vision, Wellness

Type of Coverage
  Individual, Medicare

Geographic Areas Served
  Available in multiple states

Subscriber Information
  Average Monthly Fee Per Subscriber
    (Employee + Employer Contribution):
      Employee Only (Self): Varies
      Medicare: Varies
  Average Annual Deductible Per Subscriber:
      Employee Only (Self): Varies
      Medicare: Varies
  Average Subscriber Co-Payment:
      Primary Care Physician: Varies
      Non-Network Physician: Varies
      Prescription Drugs: Varies
      Hospital ER: Varies
      Home Health Care: Varies
      Home Health Care Max. Days/Visits Covered: Varies

Key Personnel
  CEO ....Ronald A Williams

President...............................Mark T Bertolini
SVP, General Counsel ....William J Casazza
EVP, CFO ....Joseph M Zubretsky
Head, M&A Integration ....Kay Mooney
SVP, Marketing...........................Robert E Mead
Chief Medical Officer ....Lonny Reisman, MD
SVP, Human Resources.....................Elease E Wright
SVP, CIO...............................Meg McCarthy

216 AmeriChoice by UnitedHealthcare

400 Capital Blvd
Rocky Hill, CT 06067
www.americhoice.com
Subsidiary of: UnitedHealth Group

Healthplan and Services Defined
  PLAN TYPE: HMO

Key Personnel
  Media Contact...........................Alice Ferreira
    203-459-7775
    aferreira@uhc.com

217 Anthem Blue Cross & Blue Shield Connecticut

370 Bassett Road
Building Three, Fourth Floor
North Haven, CT 06473
Toll-Free: 800-545-0948
Phone: 203-239-4911
www.anthem.com
Subsidiary of: Wellpoint
For Profit Organization: Yes
Total Enrollment: 1,535,753
State Enrollment: 391,301

Healthplan and Services Defined
  PLAN TYPE: HMO/PPO
  Benefits Offered: Behavioral Health, Chiropractic, Complementary
    Medicine, Disease Management, Home Care, Inpatient SNF,
    Physical Therapy, Podiatry, Prescription, Psychiatric, Transplant,
    Vision, Wellness

Type of Coverage
  Commercial, Individual, Supplemental Medicare, Medicaid

Type of Payment Plans Offered
  POS, FFS

Geographic Areas Served
  Connecticut

Network Qualifications
  Pre-Admission Certification: Yes

Peer Review Type
  Utilization Review: Yes

Publishes and Distributes Report Card: Yes

Accreditation Certification
  NCQA

Key Personnel
  CEO...................................Larry Glasscock
  President ....Marjorie Dorr
  COO ....Claudia Lindsey
  CFO ....Guy W Marszalek
  CMO ....Dr Eleanor Seiler
  General Counsel ....Alfred Jarvis
  Provider Relations..........................DiJuana Lewis
  Marketing.................................Dave Fusco
  Member Relations ....Rita Marcinkus
  Pharmacy Director ....Glen Smyth
  Public Relations ....Deborah New

Media Contact . . . . Sarah Yeager
203-234-5402
sarah.yeager@anthem.com

Average Claim Compensation
Physician's Fees Charged: 40%
Hospital's Fees Charged: 33%

Specialty Managed Care Partners
Psychiatric Management, Quest Diagnostics
Enters into Contracts with Regional Business Coalitions: Yes

---

218 Charter Oak Health Plan

25 Sigourney Street
Hartford, CT 06106-5033
Toll-Free: 877-772-8625
dss.healthcare@ct.gov
www.charteroakhealthplan.com
Subsidiary of: Community Health Network of Connecticut
Year Founded: 2008

Healthplan and Services Defined
PLAN TYPE: HMO
Benefits Offered: Behavioral Health, Disease Management,
Prescription, Wellness

Type of Coverage
Individual
Catastrophic Illness Benefit: Maximum $1M

Subscriber Information
Average Monthly Fee Per Subscriber
(Employee + Employer Contribution):
Employee Only (Self): $446
Average Annual Deductible Per Subscriber:
Employee Only (Self): Varies
Average Subscriber Co-Payment:
Primary Care Physician: $25
Non-Network Physician: $35
Prescription Drugs: $10
Hospital ER: $100

---

219 CIGNA HealthCare of Connecticut

900 Cottage Grove Road
C8NAS
Hartford, CT 06002
Toll-Free: 866-438-2446
Phone: 860-226-2300
Fax: 860-226-2333
www.cigna.com
Secondary Address: 612 Wheelers Farm Rd, Milford, CT 06461,
203-874-1122
For Profit Organization: Yes
Year Founded: 1986
Number of Affiliated Hospitals: 100
Number of Primary Care Physicians: 11,300
Number of Referral/Specialty Physicians: 4,500
Total Enrollment: 29,506
State Enrollment: 29,506

Healthplan and Services Defined
PLAN TYPE: HMO
Model Type: IPA
Benefits Offered: Dental, Disease Management, Prescription,
Transplant, Wellness, Life

Type of Coverage
Commercial, Individual
Catastrophic Illness Benefit: Varies per case

Type of Payment Plans Offered
FFS

Geographic Areas Served
Fairfield, Hartford, Litchfield, Middlesex, New Haven, New London,
Tolland, Windham counties

Subscriber Information
Average Annual Deductible Per Subscriber:
Employee Only (Self): $0
Employee & 1 Family Member: $0
Employee & 2 Family Members: $0
Medicare: $0
Average Subscriber Co-Payment:
Primary Care Physician: $5.00-15.00
Prescription Drugs: $10.00
Hospital ER: $50.00
Home Health Care Max. Days/Visits Covered: Varies

Publishes and Distributes Report Card: Yes

Accreditation Certification
NCQA
TJC Accreditation

Key Personnel
President . . . . David Cordani
CEO . . . . H Edward Hanway
CFO . . . . Michael W Bell
EVP/General Counsel. . . . . Nicole Jones
Chief Medical Officer . . . . Alan Muney, MD, MHA

---

220 ConnectiCare

175 Scott Swamp Road
PO Box 4050
Farmington, CT 06034-4050
Toll-Free: 800-251-7722
Phone: 860-674-5757
Fax: 860-674-2011
info@connecticare.com
www.connecticare.com
Mailing Address: PO Box 416191, Boston, MA 02241-6191
For Profit Organization: Yes
Year Founded: 1981
Owned by an Integrated Delivery Network (IDN): Yes
Number of Affiliated Hospitals: 126
Number of Primary Care Physicians: 5,580
Number of Referral/Specialty Physicians: 11,800
Total Enrollment: 240,000
State Enrollment: 160,000

Healthplan and Services Defined
PLAN TYPE: HMO/PPO
Other Type: POS
Model Type: IPA, HMO, POS
Plan Specialty: Disease Management, Vision, UR
Benefits Offered: Behavioral Health, Chiropractic, Complementary
Medicine, Dental, Disease Management, Home Care, Inpatient
SNF, Physical Therapy, Podiatry, Prescription, Psychiatric,
Transplant, Vision, Wellness, Medical

Type of Coverage
Commercial, Individual, Medicare, Medicare Advantage
Catastrophic Illness Benefit: Unlimited

Type of Payment Plans Offered
Capitated, FFS

Geographic Areas Served
All of Connecticut; Hampshire, Hampden, Franklin and Berkshire
counties in Massachusetts; five boroughs of NYC

Subscriber Information
Average Monthly Fee Per Subscriber
(Employee + Employer Contribution):
Employee Only (Self): Proprietary
Employee & 1 Family Member: Proprietary
Employee & 2 Family Members: Proprietary
Medicare: Proprietary

Average Subscriber Co-Payment:
  Non-Network Physician: $10.00
  Prescription Drugs: $10.00
  Hospital ER: $25.00
  Nursing Home Max. Days/Visits Covered: 90

Network Qualifications
Pre-Admission Certification: Yes

Peer Review Type
Utilization Review: Yes
Second Surgical Opinion: Yes
Case Management: Yes

Publishes and Distributes Report Card: Yes

Accreditation Certification
TJC, NCQA
Utilization Review, Pre-Admission Certification, State Licensure, Quality Assurance Program

Key Personnel
President/CEO............................Michael Wise
VP Network Operations....................Kathleen Madden
Credentialing Manager........................Joyce Vagts
Pharmacy Serv Director....................Jeff Casberg, RPh
Marketing Director..........................Ezio Sabatino
VP/CIO.......................................Mark Verre
Media Contact...........................Stephen Jewett
  860-674-7068
  publicrelations@connecticare.com

Average Claim Compensation
Physician's Fees Charged: 100%
Hospital's Fees Charged: 100%

Specialty Managed Care Partners
United Behavioral Health, Express Scripts
Enters into Contracts with Regional Business Coalitions: No

Employer References
Federal Government, Hartford Insurance Company, United Technologies, State of Connecticut

221 Delta Dental of New Jersey & Connecticut
1639 Route 10
PO Box 222
Parsippany, NJ 07054
Toll-Free: 800-452-9310
Phone: 973-285-4000
Fax: 973-285-4141
marketing@deltadentalnj.com
www.deltadentalnj.com
Non-Profit Organization: Yes
Year Founded: 1969
Total Enrollment: 1,500,000

Healthplan and Services Defined
  PLAN TYPE: Dental
  Other Type: Dental HMO/PPO/POS
  Model Type: Staff
  Plan Specialty: Dental
  Benefits Offered: Dental

Type of Coverage
Commercial

Type of Payment Plans Offered
POS, DFFS, Capitated, FFS, Combination FFS & DFFS

Geographic Areas Served
New Jersey and Connecticut

Key Personnel
President/CEO............................Walter VanBrunt
SVP/CFO....................................James Suleski
SVP, Operations...........................Bruce Silverman
VP/Claims & Cust Service.....................Lori Acker
VP/Dental Director......................Scott Navarro, DDS

VP, Marketing..............................Steven Fleischer
Dir/Media & Public Affair...................Elizabeth Risberg
  415-972-8423

222 Health Plan of New York: Connecticut
55 Water Street
New York, NY 10041
Toll-Free: 800-447-8255
Phone: 646-447-5000
Fax: 646-447-3011
www.hipusa.com
Subsidiary of: An Emblem Health Company
Year Founded: 1947
Number of Affiliated Hospitals: 160
Total Enrollment: 1,300,000

Healthplan and Services Defined
  PLAN TYPE: HMO/PPO
  Other Type: POS, EPO, ASO
  Benefits Offered: Chiropractic, Dental, Disease Management, Home Care, Inpatient SNF, Physical Therapy, Podiatry, Prescription, Psychiatric, Vision, Wellness

Type of Coverage
Individual, Medicare

Geographic Areas Served
New York, Connecticut, Massachusetts

Subscriber Information
Average Monthly Fee Per Subscriber
  (Employee + Employer Contribution):
    Employee Only (Self): Varies
    Medicare: Varies
Average Annual Deductible Per Subscriber:
    Employee Only (Self): Varies
    Medicare: Varies
Average Subscriber Co-Payment:
    Primary Care Physician: Varies
    Non-Network Physician: Varies
    Prescription Drugs: Varies
    Hospital ER: Varies
    Home Health Care: Varies
    Home Health Care Max. Days/Visits Covered: Varies
    Nursing Home: Varies
    Nursing Home Max. Days/Visits Covered: Varies

Accreditation Certification
URAC, NCQA

223 Humana Health Insurance of Connecticut
One International Boulevard
Suite 904
Mahwah, NJ 07495
Toll-Free: 800-967-2370
Fax: 201-934-1369
www.humana.com
For Profit Organization: Yes

Healthplan and Services Defined
  PLAN TYPE: HMO/PPO

Type of Coverage
Commercial, Individual

Accreditation Certification
URAC, NCQA, CORE

224   Oxford Health Plans: Corporate Headquarters
48 Monroe Turnpike
Trumbull, CT 06611
Toll-Free: 800-444-6222
Phone: 203-459-6000
Fax: 203-459-6464
groupservices@oxfordhealth.com
www.oxfordhealth.com
Subsidiary of: UnitedHealthCare
For Profit Organization: Yes
Year Founded: 1984
Owned by an Integrated Delivery Network (IDN): Yes
Number of Affiliated Hospitals: 219
Number of Primary Care Physicians: 17,000
Total Enrollment: 1,600,000
State Enrollment: 70,139

Healthplan and Services Defined
 PLAN TYPE: HMO/PPO
 Model Type: IPA, Network, POS
 Benefits Offered: Behavioral Health, Chiropractic, Complementary
  Medicine, Dental, Disease Management, Home Care, Inpatient
  SNF, Podiatry, Prescription, Psychiatric, Transplant, Vision,
  Wellness
 Offers Demand Management Patient Information Service: Yes

Type of Coverage
 Commercial, Individual, Indemnity, Medicare, Catastrophic
 Catastrophic Illness Benefit: Varies per case

Type of Payment Plans Offered
 FFS

Geographic Areas Served
 Connecticut: Fairfield, New Haven, Litchfield, Hartford, Middlesex,
 New London, Tolland & Windham counties; New Jersey: Essex,
 Hudson, Middlesex, Monmouth, Morris, Ocean, Passaic & Somerset
 counties; New York: Bronx, Dutchess, Kings, Nassau, New York,
 Putnam, Queens, Richmond, Rockland, Suffolk, & Westchester
 counties

Subscriber Information
 Average Monthly Fee Per Subscriber
  (Employee + Employer Contribution):
   Employee Only (Self): Varies
   Employee & 1 Family Member: Varies
   Employee & 2 Family Members: Varies
   Medicare: Varies
 Average Annual Deductible Per Subscriber:
   Employee Only (Self): Varies
   Employee & 1 Family Member: Varies
   Employee & 2 Family Members: Varies
   Medicare: Varies

Network Qualifications
 Pre-Admission Certification: Yes

Peer Review Type
 Utilization Review: Yes
 Second Surgical Opinion: Yes
 Case Management: Yes

Publishes and Distributes Report Card: Yes

Accreditation Certification
 NCQA
 TJC Accreditation, Medicare Approved, Utilization Review,
  Pre-Admission Certification, State Licensure, Quality Assurance
  Program

Key Personnel
 EVP/CFO...................................Kurt Thompson

Specialty Managed Care Partners
 Enters into Contracts with Regional Business Coalitions: Yes

225   UnitedHealthCare of Connecticut
185 Asylum Street
Hartford, CT 06103
Toll-Free: 877-832-7734
Phone: 860-702-5000
www.uhc.com
Subsidiary of: UnitedHealth Group
For Profit Organization: Yes
Year Founded: 1991
Total Enrollment: 75,000,000

Healthplan and Services Defined
 PLAN TYPE: HMO/PPO

Key Personnel
 Media Contact ....Ben Goldstein
  240-683-5372
  benjamin_j_goldstein@uhc.com

Health Insurance Coverage Status and Type of Coverage by Age

Category	All Persons		Under 18 years		Under 65 years		65 years and over	
	Number	%	Number	%	Number	%	Number	%
Total population	912	-	203	-	768	-	143	-
Covered by some type of health insurance	828 (6)	90.9 (0.7)	194 (2)	95.5 (1.1)	687 (6)	89.4 (0.8)	142 (1)	99.0 (0.4)
Covered by private health insurance	637 (11)	69.9 (1.2)	126 (5)	61.9 (2.5)	531 (10)	69.1 (1.3)	106 (3)	73.8 (1.9)
Employment based	554 (12)	60.7 (1.3)	116 (5)	56.9 (2.6)	486 (11)	63.2 (1.5)	68 (3)	47.3 (1.8)
Direct purchase	98 (6)	10.8 (0.6)	8 (2)	4.0 (0.9)	48 (5)	6.3 (0.6)	50 (3)	34.7 (1.9)
Covered by TRICARE	32 (4)	3.5 (0.4)	6 (2)	2.8 (0.8)	20 (3)	2.6 (0.4)	12 (2)	8.7 (1.4)
Covered by government health insurance	325 (9)	35.6 (1.0)	78 (5)	38.4 (2.4)	186 (9)	24.2 (1.2)	139 (1)	97.0 (0.6)
Covered by Medicaid	180 (9)	19.8 (1.0)	77 (5)	37.8 (2.4)	165 (9)	21.5 (1.2)	15 (2)	10.6 (1.2)
Also by private insurance	29 (3)	3.2 (0.3)	9 (2)	4.5 (0.9)	21 (3)	2.7 (0.3)	9 (1)	6.0 (0.8)
Covered by Medicare	167 (3)	18.4 (0.4)	2 (1)	1.0 (0.6)	29 (3)	3.7 (0.4)	139 (1)	97.0 (0.6)
Also by private insurance	112 (3)	12.3 (0.4)	Z (Z)	0.2 (0.2)	9 (1)	1.2 (0.2)	103 (3)	71.9 (1.9)
Also by Medicaid	28 (3)	3.1 (0.3)	1 (1)	0.5 (0.4)	13 (2)	1.7 (0.3)	15 (2)	10.6 (1.2)
Covered by VA Care	16 (2)	1.7 (0.2)	Z (Z)	0.1 (0.1)	7 (1)	0.9 (0.2)	9 (1)	6.2 (0.8)
Not covered at any time during the year	83 (6)	9.1 (0.7)	9 (2)	4.5 (1.1)	82 (6)	10.6 (0.8)	1 (1)	1.0 (0.4)

Note: Numbers in thousands; Figures cover 2013; Margin of error appears in parenthesis; A "Z" indicates that the value either represents or rounds to zero.
Source: U.S. Census Bureau, 2013 American Community Survey, Table HI05. Health Insurance Coverage Status and Type of Coverage by State and Age for All People: 2013

Delaware

226 Aetna Health of Delaware

151 Farmington Avenue
Hartford, CT 06156
Toll-Free: 800-872-3862
Phone: 860-273-0123
www.aetna.com
For Profit Organization: Yes
Total Enrollment: 27,179
State Enrollment: 27,179

Healthplan and Services Defined
PLAN TYPE: HMO
Other Type: POS
Plan Specialty: EPO
Benefits Offered: Dental, Disease Management, Long-Term Care,
  Prescription, Wellness, Life, LTD, STD

Type of Coverage
Commercial, Individual

Type of Payment Plans Offered
POS, FFS

Geographic Areas Served
Statewide

Key Personnel
Chairman/CEO/President.....................Mark T Bertolini
EVP/General Counsel ....William J Casazza
EVP/CFO ....Shawn M Guertin

227 AmeriHealth HMO

Mellon Bank Center
919 Market Street, Suite 1200
Wilmington, DE 19801
Toll-Free: 800-444-6282
Phone: 302-777-6400
Fax: 302-777-6444
www.amerihealth.com
Secondary Address: 1901 Market Street, Philadelphia, PA 19103-1480
Year Founded: 1995
Number of Affiliated Hospitals: 250
Number of Primary Care Physicians: 35,000
Total Enrollment: 265,000

Healthplan and Services Defined
PLAN TYPE: HMO/PPO
Model Type: IPA
Plan Specialty: Health Insurance
Benefits Offered: Dental, Disease Management, Prescription, Vision,
  Wellness, HMO, POS, PPO, HSA

Type of Coverage
Commercial

Geographic Areas Served
Delaware, New Jersey, Pennsylvania

Subscriber Information
Average Subscriber Co-Payment:
  Primary Care Physician: $10.00

Network Qualifications
Pre-Admission Certification: Yes

Peer Review Type
Utilization Review: Yes
Second Surgical Opinion: Yes
Case Management: Yes

Publishes and Distributes Report Card: No

Accreditation Certification
NCQA

TJC Accreditation, Medicare Approved, Utilization Review,
  Pre-Admission Certification, State Licensure, Quality Assurance
  Program

Key Personnel
President........................G. Fred DiBona
CFO............................John Foos
VP/General Manager ....Jay Moorehead
Marketing..............................Robin Colantuono

228 CIGNA HealthCare of Delaware

1777 Sentry Park West
Gwynedd Hall, Suite 100
Bluebell, PA 19422
Toll-Free: 800-441-7150
Phone: 215-283-3300
www.cigna.com
For Profit Organization: Yes
Federally Qualified: Yes
Total Enrollment: 984
State Enrollment: 984

Healthplan and Services Defined
PLAN TYPE: HMO
Other Type: POS
Model Type: IPA, Group, Network
Benefits Offered: Disease Management, Prescription, Transplant,
  Wellness

Type of Coverage
Commercial

Publishes and Distributes Report Card: Yes

Accreditation Certification
NCQA
TJC Accreditation, Medicare Approved, Utilization Review,
  Pre-Admission Certification, State Licensure, Quality Assurance
  Program

Key Personnel
AVP National Contracting ....Diane Exline Van De Beek
General Manager ....Vincent Sobocinski
Care Senior Associate ....Lorraine Gray

229 Coventry Health Care of Delaware

750 Prides Crossing
Suite 200
Newark, DE 19713
Toll-Free: 800-833-7423
DECustomerService@cvty.com
http://chcdelaware.coventryhealthcare.com
Subsidiary of: Coventry Health Care Inc.
For Profit Organization: Yes
Year Founded: 1986
Number of Affiliated Hospitals: 120
Number of Primary Care Physicians: 24,000
Total Enrollment: 100,000

Healthplan and Services Defined
PLAN TYPE: HMO/PPO
Other Type: POS
Model Type: Group, Individual
Benefits Offered: Behavioral Health, Worker's Compensation

Type of Coverage
Medicare, Medicaid

Geographic Areas Served
Delaware, Maryland, southern Pennsylvania, southern New Jersey

Accreditation Certification
URAC

Key Personnel
Chief Executive Officer....................Allen F Wise
Chief Operating Officer......................Michael D Bahr

EVP/CFO. . . . . .Randy Giles

230   Delta Dental of the Mid-Atlantic

One Delta Drive
Mechanicsburg, PA 17055-6999
Toll-Free: 800-932-0783
Fax: 717-766-8719
www.deltadentalins.com
Non-Profit Organization: Yes
Total Enrollment: 54,000,000

Healthplan and Services Defined
 PLAN TYPE: Dental
 Other Type: Dental PPO

Type of Coverage
 Commercial

Geographic Areas Served
 Delaware, District of Columbia, New York, Pennsylvania, Maryland,
 West Virginia

Key Personnel
 President/CEO. . . . . .Gary D Radine
 VP, Public & Govt Affairs . . . . .Jeff Album
  415-972-8418
 Dir/Media & Public Affair .Elizabeth Risberg
  415-972-8423

231   eHealthInsurance Services Inc.

11919 Foundation Place
Gold River, CA 95670
Toll-Free: 800-644-3491
webmaster@healthinsurance.com
www.e.healthinsurance.com
Year Founded: 1997

Healthplan and Services Defined
 PLAN TYPE: HMO/PPO
 Benefits Offered: Dental, Life, STD

Type of Coverage
 Commercial, Individual, Medicare

Geographic Areas Served
 All 50 states in the USA and District of Columbia

Key Personnel
 Chairman & CEO. . . . . .Gary L. Lauer
 EVP/Business & Corp. Dev. .Bruce Telkamp
 EVP/Chief Technology. . . . . .Dr. Sheldon X. Wang
 SVP & CFO . . . . .Stuart M. Huizinga
 Pres. of eHealth Gov. Sys . . . . .Samuel C. Gibbs
 SVP of Sales & Operations . . . . .Robert S. Hurley
 Director Public Relations. . . . . .Nate Purpura
  650-210-3115

232   Great-West Healthcare Delaware

1777 Sentry Park West, Suite 100
Gwynedd Hall
Bluebell, PA 19422
Toll-Free: 866-494-2111
Phone: 215-283-3300
eliginquiries@cigna.com
www.cignaforhealth.com
Subsidiary of: CIGNA HealthCare
Acquired by: CIGNA
For Profit Organization: Yes
Total Enrollment: 2,718
State Enrollment: 2,508

Healthplan and Services Defined
 PLAN TYPE: HMO/PPO
 Benefits Offered: Disease Management, Prescription, Wellness

Type of Coverage
 Commercial

Type of Payment Plans Offered
 POS, FFS

Geographic Areas Served
 Delaware

Accreditation Certification
 URAC

Key Personnel
 Senior VP, Healthcare Ops. . . . . .Donna Goldin
 Chief Medical Officer . . . . .Terry Fouts, MD
 Vice President, Sales . . . . .Marc Neely

Specialty Managed Care Partners
 Caremark Rx

233   Highmark Blue Cross & Blue Shield Delaware

P.O. Box 1991
Wilmington, DE 19899-1991
Toll-Free: 800-633-2563
info@highmarkbcbsde.com
www.highmarkbcbsde.com
Non-Profit Organization: Yes
Year Founded: 1935
Number of Affiliated Hospitals: 11
Number of Primary Care Physicians: 762
Number of Referral/Specialty Physicians: 826
Total Enrollment: 400,000
State Enrollment: 321,000

Healthplan and Services Defined
 PLAN TYPE: HMO/PPO
 Other Type: POS
 Model Type: IPA, Network
 Benefits Offered: Dental, Disease Management, Prescription, Vision,
 Wellness

Type of Coverage
 Commercial, Individual, Medicare, Supplemental Medicare

Type of Payment Plans Offered
 Combination FFS & DFFS

Geographic Areas Served
 Statewide

Key Personnel
 President/CEO . . . . .William Winkenwerder, Jr
 Director, Enterprise Apps. .Sally Retzko
  sretzko@bcbsde.com
 Community Relations . . . . .Melissa Lukach
 VP Operations . . . . .George English
  302-421-3290
  genglish@bcbsde.com
 Media Contact. . . . . .Michael Weinstein
  412-544-7903
  michael.weinstein@highmark.com

234   Humana Health Insurance of Delaware

325 Sentry Parkway
Suite 200
Blue Bell, PA 19422
www.humana.com
For Profit Organization: Yes

Healthplan and Services Defined
 PLAN TYPE: HMO/PPO

Type of Coverage
 Commercial, Individual

Accreditation Certification
 URAC, NCQA, CORE

Key Personnel
Media Contact. . . . . .Nancy A Hanewinckel
941-585-4763
nhanewinckel1@humana.com

---

235   Mid Atlantic Medical Services: Delaware
2 West Rolling Crossroads
Suite 11
Baltimore, MD 21228
Toll-Free: 800-782-1966
Phone: 410-869-7400
Fax: 410-869-7583
masales99@uhc.com
www.mamsiunitedhealthcare.com
Subsidiary of: United Healthcare/United Health Group
Year Founded: 1986
Number of Affiliated Hospitals: 342
Number of Primary Care Physicians: 3,276
Total Enrollment: 180,000

Healthplan and Services Defined
   PLAN TYPE: HMO/PPO
   Model Type: IPA, Network
   Benefits Offered: Dental, Disease Management, Prescription, Vision,
      Wellness, Life, LTD, STD

Type of Payment Plans Offered
   Combination FFS & DFFS

Geographic Areas Served
   Delaware, Maryland, North Carolina, Pennsylvania, Virginia,
   Washington DC, West Virginia

Network Qualifications
   Pre-Admission Certification: Yes

Peer Review Type
   Utilization Review: Yes
   Second Surgical Opinion: Yes
   Case Management: Yes

Publishes and Distributes Report Card: No

Accreditation Certification
   TJC, NCQA

Key Personnel
   CFO. . . . . .Robert E Foss
   EVP/CIO. . . . . .R Larry Mauzy

Specialty Managed Care Partners
   Enters into Contracts with Regional Business Coalitions: Yes

---

236   Mid Atlantic Psychiatric Services (MAMSI)
910 S Chapel Street
Suite 102
Newark, DE 19713
Phone: 302-224-1400
Fax: 302-224-1402
www.midatlanticbh.com
Subsidiary of: United Healthcare/United Health Group
Acquired by: UnitedHealthcare/A UnitedHealth Group
For Profit Organization: Yes
Number of Affiliated Hospitals: 340
Number of Primary Care Physicians: 3,276
Total Enrollment: 101,900

Healthplan and Services Defined
   PLAN TYPE: Multiple
   Model Type: Network
   Benefits Offered: Disease Management, Prescription, Wellness

Type of Payment Plans Offered
   FFS

Geographic Areas Served
   Maryland, Virginia, West Virginia, North Carolina, Pennsylvania,
   Delaware & Washington DC

Network Qualifications
   Minimum Years of Practice: 2
   Pre-Admission Certification: Yes

Peer Review Type
   Utilization Review: No
   Second Surgical Opinion: No
   Case Management: No

Publishes and Distributes Report Card: No

Accreditation Certification
   TJC Accreditation, Medicare Approved, Utilization Review,
      Pre-Admission Certification, State Licensure, Quality Assurance
      Program

Key Personnel
   President/CEO . . . . .Thomas P Barbera
   SEVP/CFO . . . . .Robert E Foss
   EVP/CIO. . . . . .R Larry Mauzy

Specialty Managed Care Partners
   Enters into Contracts with Regional Business Coalitions: No

---

237   UnitedHealthcare Community Plan
3844 Kennett Pike
Powder Mill Square, Suite 210
Greenville, DE 19807
Phone: 302-429-7800
Fax: 866-915-0309
www.uhccommunityplan.com
Subsidiary of: AmeriChoice, A UnitedHealth Group Company

Healthplan and Services Defined
   PLAN TYPE: HMO

Type of Coverage
   Supplemental Medicare

Key Personnel
   Executive Director. . . . . .Allison Davenport
   Marketing Director. . . . . .Dorinda Borer

---

238   UnitedHealthCare of Maryland
6095 Marshalee Drive
Suite 200
Elkridge, MD 21075
Toll-Free: 800-307-7820
www.uhc.com
Subsidiary of: UnitedHealth Group
Non-Profit Organization: Yes
Year Founded: 1976
Number of Affiliated Hospitals: 215
Number of Primary Care Physicians: 2,559
Number of Referral/Specialty Physicians: 8,300
Total Enrollment: 75,000,000
State Enrollment: 1,500,000

Healthplan and Services Defined
   PLAN TYPE: HMO/PPO
   Model Type: Network
   Benefits Offered: Disease Management, Prescription, Wellness
   Offers Demand Management Patient Information Service: Yes

Geographic Areas Served
   Statewide; MD, VA, DC

Subscriber Information
   Average Monthly Fee Per Subscriber
      (Employee + Employer Contribution):
         Employee Only (Self): $104.00-135.00
         Employee & 1 Family Member: $143.00-184.00
         Employee & 2 Family Members: $331.00-440.00
         Medicare: $112.00-156.00

Average Annual Deductible Per Subscriber:
    Employee Only (Self): $100.00-250.00
    Employee & 1 Family Member: $500.00-1500.00
    Employee & 2 Family Members: $200.00-500.00
    Medicare: $0
Average Subscriber Co-Payment:
    Primary Care Physician: $5.00/10.00
    Non-Network Physician: Deductible
    Prescription Drugs: $5.00/10.00
    Hospital ER: $25.00/50.00
    Home Health Care: $5.00/10.00

Network Qualifications
Pre-Admission Certification: Yes

Peer Review Type
Utilization Review: Yes
Second Surgical Opinion: Yes
Case Management: Yes

Publishes and Distributes Report Card: Yes

Accreditation Certification
TJC Accreditation, Medicare Approved, Utilization Review,
    Pre-Admission Certification, State Licensure, Quality Assurance
    Program

Key Personnel
Region CEO . . . . Jim Cronin

Specialty Managed Care Partners
Enters into Contracts with Regional Business Coalitions: Yes

Health Insurance Coverage Status and Type of Coverage by Age

Category	All Persons		Under 18 years		Under 65 years		65 years and over	
	Number	%	Number	%	Number	%	Number	%
Total population	636	-	111	-	564	-	71	-
Covered by some type of health insurance	594 (4)	93.3 (0.6)	109 (1)	97.6 (1.0)	522 (4)	92.6 (0.7)	71 (1)	99.6 (0.4)
Covered by private health insurance	438 (7)	68.8 (1.1)	61 (4)	54.6 (3.3)	389 (7)	68.9 (1.2)	49 (2)	68.2 (3.0)
Employment based	379 (7)	59.6 (1.1)	53 (4)	48.0 (3.4)	339 (7)	60.1 (1.2)	39 (2)	54.9 (3.2)
Direct purchase	74 (5)	11.6 (0.8)	7 (2)	6.5 (1.7)	60 (5)	10.6 (0.8)	14 (2)	19.5 (2.3)
Covered by TRICARE	10 (2)	1.5 (0.3)	2 (1)	1.7 (0.6)	7 (1)	1.3 (0.3)	2 (1)	3.3 (0.8)
Covered by government health insurance	225 (8)	35.3 (1.3)	57 (3)	51.3 (3.0)	159 (8)	28.2 (1.4)	66 (1)	92.0 (1.3)
Covered by Medicaid	167 (8)	26.3 (1.2)	57 (3)	50.9 (3.1)	150 (8)	26.6 (1.4)	17 (2)	23.6 (2.6)
Also by private insurance	29 (4)	4.5 (0.6)	9 (2)	8.1 (2.2)	22 (4)	3.8 (0.7)	7 (1)	9.7 (1.6)
Covered by Medicare	80 (2)	12.6 (0.3)	1 (Z)	0.7 (0.4)	15 (2)	2.6 (0.3)	65 (1)	91.5 (1.4)
Also by private insurance	46 (2)	7.3 (0.3)	Z (Z)	0.2 (0.1)	3 (1)	0.6 (0.1)	43 (2)	60.3 (2.8)
Also by Medicaid	27 (3)	4.3 (0.4)	Z (Z)	0.3 (0.3)	10 (2)	1.8 (0.3)	17 (2)	23.6 (2.6)
Covered by VA Care	10 (1)	1.5 (0.2)	Z (Z)	0.0 (0.1)	6 (1)	1.0 (0.2)	4 (1)	5.8 (1.1)
Not covered at any time during the year	42 (4)	6.7 (0.6)	3 (1)	2.4 (1.0)	42 (4)	7.4 (0.7)	Z (Z)	0.4 (0.4)

Note: Numbers in thousands; Figures cover 2013; Margin of error appears in parenthesis; A "Z" indicates that the value either represents or rounds to zero.
Source: U.S. Census Bureau, 2013 American Community Survey, Table HI05. Health Insurance Coverage Status and Type of Coverage by State and Age for All People: 2013

District of Columbia

239　Aetna Health District of Columbia
151 Farmintgon Avenue
Hartford, CT 06156
Toll-Free: 800-872-3862
Phone: 860-273-0123
www.aetna.com
For Profit Organization: Yes
Year Founded: 1986
Number of Affiliated Hospitals: 64
Number of Primary Care Physicians: 1,898
Total Enrollment: 211,156

Healthplan and Services Defined
　PLAN TYPE: HMO
　Benefits Offered: Disease Management, Wellness

Geographic Areas Served
　Statewide

Accreditation Certification
　TJC Accreditation, Medicare Approved, Utilization Review,
　　Pre-Admission Certification, State Licensure, Quality Assurance
　　Program

Key Personnel
　Chairman/CEO/President. . . . . Mark T Bertolini
　EVP/General Counsel . . . . William J Casazza
　EVP/CFO . . . . Shawn M Guertin

240　CareFirst Blue Cross Blue Shield
840 First Street NE
Union Center Plaza
Washington, DC 20065
Toll-Free: 866-520-6099
Phone: 202-479-8000
mediarelations@carefirst.com
www.carefirst.com
Subsidiary of: CareFirst Of Maryland Inc.
Non-Profit Organization: Yes
Year Founded: 1984
Number of Affiliated Hospitals: 165
Number of Primary Care Physicians: 4,500
Total Enrollment: 3,400,000
State Enrollment: 550,000

Healthplan and Services Defined
　PLAN TYPE: HMO/PPO
　Model Type: Network
　Benefits Offered: Prescription

Type of Coverage
　Commercial, Individual, Medicare
　Catastrophic Illness Benefit: Unlimited

Geographic Areas Served
　Areas of Fairfax and Prince William counties, Maryland, District of
　Columbia, Arlington county, town of Vienna and the cities of
　Alexandria and Fairfax

Accreditation Certification
　NCQA
　TJC Accreditation, Medicare Approved, Utilization Review,
　　Pre-Admission Certification, State Licensure, Quality Assurance
　　Program

Key Personnel
　Chairman/CEO . . . . Chester Burrell
　EVP/CFO . . . . G. Mark Chaney
　EVP/General Counsel. . . . . John A Picciotto, Esq
　EVP/Chief Marketing Offcr. . . . . Gregory A Devou
　SVP, Community Affairs . . . . Maria Tildon

Specialty Managed Care Partners
　Enters into Contracts with Regional Business Coalitions: Yes

241　CIGNA HealthCare of the Mid-Atlantic
9700 Patuxent Woods Drive
Columbia, MD 20146
Toll-Free: 866-438-2446
Phone: 410-837-4005
Fax: 800-657-3073
www.cigna.com
For Profit Organization: Yes
Year Founded: 1984
Physician Owned Organization: No
Number of Affiliated Hospitals: 54
Number of Primary Care Physicians: 2,032
Number of Referral/Specialty Physicians: 5,028
Total Enrollment: 109,186

Healthplan and Services Defined
　PLAN TYPE: HMO/PPO
　Model Type: IPA
　Benefits Offered: Disease Management, Prescription, Transplant,
　　Wellness
　Offers Demand Management Patient Information Service: Yes

Type of Coverage
　Commercial

Type of Payment Plans Offered
　Combination FFS & DFFS

Geographic Areas Served
　District of Columbia, Maryland, Virginia

Network Qualifications
　Pre-Admission Certification: Yes

Peer Review Type
　Utilization Review: Yes
　Second Surgical Opinion: Yes
　Case Management: Yes

Publishes and Distributes Report Card: Yes

Accreditation Certification
　NCQA

Specialty Managed Care Partners
　CIGNA Dental, CIGNA Behavioral Health
　Enters into Contracts with Regional Business Coalitions: No

242　DC Chartered Health Plan
1025 15th Street NW
Washington, DC 20005-4205
Toll-Free: 800-408-7511
Phone: 202-408-4720
Fax: 202-408-4730
member-services@chartered-health.com
www.chartered-health.com
Subsidiary of: AmeriHealth Family Of Companies
For Profit Organization: Yes
Year Founded: 1987
Total Enrollment: 100,000
State Enrollment: 100,000

Healthplan and Services Defined
　PLAN TYPE: HMO
　Model Type: IPA
　Benefits Offered: Prescription

Type of Coverage
　Medicaid

Geographic Areas Served
　District of Columbia

Publishes and Distributes Report Card: Yes

Accreditation Certification
　NCQA

Key Personnel
　President/CEO. . . . . Maynard G McAlpin

EVP, Strategic Health . . . . Karen M Dale, RN, MSN
SVP, General Counsel . . . . Francis S Smith
SVP, Health Plan Services . . . . Keith Maccannon
Chief Medical Officer . . . . Lavdena Adams, MD
Chief Information Officer . . . . Parminder Sethi

Specialty Managed Care Partners
Enters into Contracts with Regional Business Coalitions: Yes

243　Delta Dental of the Mid-Atlantic

One Delta Drive
Mechanicsburg, PA 17055-6999
Toll-Free: 800-932-0783
Fax: 717-766-8719
www.deltadentalins.com
Non-Profit Organization: Yes
Total Enrollment: 54,000,000

Healthplan and Services Defined
PLAN TYPE: Dental
Other Type: Dental PPO

Type of Coverage
Commercial

Geographic Areas Served
Statewide

Key Personnel
President/CEO . . . . Gary D Radine
VP, Public & Govt Affairs . . . . Jeff Album
415-972-8418
Dir/Media & Public Affair . . . . Elizabeth Risberg
415-972-8423

244　eHealthInsurance Services Inc.

11919 Foundation Place
Gold River, CA 95670
Toll-Free: 800-644-3491
webmaster@healthinsurance.com
www.e.healthinsurance.com
Year Founded: 1997

Healthplan and Services Defined
PLAN TYPE: HMO/PPO
Benefits Offered: Dental, Life, STD

Type of Coverage
Commercial, Individual, Medicare

Geographic Areas Served
All 50 states in the USA and District of Columbia

Key Personnel
Chairman & CEO . . . . Gary L. Lauer
EVP/Business & Corp. Dev. . . . . Bruce Telkamp
EVP/Chief Technology . . . . Dr. Sheldon X. Wang
SVP & CFO . . . . Stuart M. Huizinga
Pres. of eHealth Gov. Sys . . . . Samuel C. Gibbs
SVP of Sales & Operations . . . . Robert S. Hurley
Director Public Relations . . . . Nate Purpura
650-210-3115

245　Humana Health Insurance of D.C.

1 International Blvd
Suite 400
Mahwah, NJ 07495
Toll-Free: 800-967-2370
Phone: 201-512-8818
www.humana.com
For Profit Organization: Yes

Healthplan and Services Defined
PLAN TYPE: HMO/PPO

Type of Coverage
Commercial, Individual

Accreditation Certification
URAC, NCQA, CORE

246　Mid Atlantic Medical Services: DC

4 Taft Court
Rockville, MD 20850-5310
Toll-Free: 800-884-5188
Phone: 301-762-8205
Fax: 301-545-5380
masales99@uhc.com
www.mamsiunitedhealthcare.com
Subsidiary of: United Healthcare/United Health Group
Year Founded: 1986
Number of Affiliated Hospitals: 342
Number of Primary Care Physicians: 3,276
Total Enrollment: 180,000

Healthplan and Services Defined
PLAN TYPE: HMO/PPO
Model Type: IPA, Network
Benefits Offered: Disease Management, Prescription, Wellness

Type of Payment Plans Offered
Combination FFS & DFFS

Geographic Areas Served
Delaware, Maryland, North Carolina, Pennsylvania, Virginia,
Washington DC, West Virginia

Network Qualifications
Pre-Admission Certification: Yes

Peer Review Type
Utilization Review: Yes
Second Surgical Opinion: Yes
Case Management: Yes

Publishes and Distributes Report Card: No

Accreditation Certification
TJC, NCQA

Specialty Managed Care Partners
Enters into Contracts with Regional Business Coalitions: Yes

247　Quality Plan Administrators

7824 Eastern Avenue NW
Suite 100
Washington, DC 20012
Toll-Free: 800-900-4112
Phone: 202-722-2744
Fax: 202-291-5703
qpa2000@aol.com
www.qualityplanadmin.com
For Profit Organization: Yes
Year Founded: 1986
Number of Primary Care Physicians: 175
Total Enrollment: 90,000
State Enrollment: 90,000

Healthplan and Services Defined
PLAN TYPE: HMO/PPO
Other Type: Dental/Vision
Plan Specialty: Dental, Vision
Benefits Offered: Dental, Vision

Key Personnel
President/CEO . . . . Milton Bernard, DDS
CFO . . . . Alphonzo L Davidson, DDS
Manager . . . . Barry Scott
Credentialing . . . . Grace Coward
Dental Manager . . . . Martha McClary
Materials Management . . . . Desi Bernard
Member Services . . . . Nasia Eudell

Information Systems . . . . Wilfred Welsh

Employer References

DC Chartered Health Plan, Healthright, Vision Plan for DC
Government, Health Services for Children with Special Needs, DC
Healthcare Alliance, DC Healthy Smiles (Medicaid)

248 UnitedHealthcare Community Plan Capital Area

PO Box 29675
Hot Springs, DC 71903-9802
Toll-Free: 800-905-8671
www.unisonhealthplan.com
Subsidiary of: AmeriChoice, A UnitedHealth Group Company

Healthplan and Services Defined
PLAN TYPE: HMO

Key Personnel
Executive Director. . . . . Karen Johnson
Media Contact. . . . . Jeff Smith
952-931-5685
jeff.smith@uhc.com

249 UnitedHealthCare of the District of Columbia

4416 East West Highway
Suite 310
Bethesda, MD 20814
www.uhc.com
Secondary Address: 4 Taft Court, Rockville, MD 20814,
877-842-3210
Subsidiary of: UnitedHealth Group
Non-Profit Organization: Yes
Year Founded: 1976
Number of Affiliated Hospitals: 215
Number of Primary Care Physicians: 2,559
Number of Referral/Specialty Physicians: 8,300
Total Enrollment: 75,000,000
State Enrollment: 176,000

Healthplan and Services Defined
PLAN TYPE: HMO/PPO
Model Type: Network
Benefits Offered: Disease Management, Prescription, Wellness
Offers Demand Management Patient Information Service: Yes

Geographic Areas Served
Statewide

Subscriber Information
Average Monthly Fee Per Subscriber
(Employee + Employer Contribution):
Employee Only (Self): $104.00-135.00
Employee & 1 Family Member: $143.00-184.00
Employee & 2 Family Members: $331.00-440.00
Medicare: $112.00-156.00
Average Annual Deductible Per Subscriber:
Employee Only (Self): $100.00-250.00
Employee & 1 Family Member: $500.00-1500.00
Employee & 2 Family Members: $200.00-500.00
Medicare: $0
Average Subscriber Co-Payment:
Primary Care Physician: $5.00/10.00
Non-Network Physician: Deductible
Prescription Drugs: $5.00/10.00
Hospital ER: $25.00/50.00
Home Health Care: $5.00/10.00

Network Qualifications
Pre-Admission Certification: Yes

Peer Review Type
Utilization Review: Yes

Second Surgical Opinion: Yes
Case Management: Yes

Publishes and Distributes Report Card: Yes

Accreditation Certification
TJC Accreditation, Medicare Approved, Utilization Review,
Pre-Admission Certification, State Licensure, Quality Assurance
Program

Key Personnel
Region CEO . . . . Jim Cronin

Specialty Managed Care Partners
Enters into Contracts with Regional Business Coalitions: Yes

Health Insurance Coverage Status and Type of Coverage by Age

Category	All Persons		Under 18 years		Under 65 years		65 years and over	
	Number	%	Number	%	Number	%	Number	%
Total population	19,245	-	4,020	-	15,667	-	3,578	-
Covered by some type of health insurance	15,392 (44)	80.0 (0.2)	3,575 (17)	88.9 (0.4)	11,873 (43)	75.8 (0.3)	3,519 (7)	98.3 (0.2)
Covered by private health insurance	10,935 (55)	56.8 (0.3)	2,004 (27)	49.9 (0.7)	9,002 (53)	57.5 (0.3)	1,933 (18)	54.0 (0.5)
Employment based	8,414 (58)	43.7 (0.3)	1,628 (28)	40.5 (0.7)	7,433 (56)	47.4 (0.4)	981 (15)	27.4 (0.4)
Direct purchase	2,473 (35)	12.8 (0.2)	305 (13)	7.6 (0.3)	1,449 (31)	9.2 (0.2)	1,024 (14)	28.6 (0.4)
Covered by TRICARE	688 (21)	3.6 (0.1)	120 (9)	3.0 (0.2)	430 (19)	2.7 (0.1)	258 (9)	7.2 (0.3)
Covered by government health insurance	6,733 (46)	35.0 (0.2)	1,671 (30)	41.6 (0.7)	3,302 (46)	21.1 (0.3)	3,431 (9)	95.9 (0.2)
Covered by Medicaid	3,344 (48)	17.4 (0.2)	1,651 (30)	41.1 (0.7)	2,849 (47)	18.2 (0.3)	495 (11)	13.8 (0.3)
Also by private insurance	395 (13)	2.1 (0.1)	97 (7)	2.4 (0.2)	246 (11)	1.6 (0.1)	150 (6)	4.2 (0.2)
Covered by Medicare	3,923 (17)	20.4 (0.1)	26 (4)	0.6 (0.1)	495 (15)	3.2 (0.1)	3,428 (9)	95.8 (0.2)
Also by private insurance	1,957 (18)	10.2 (0.1)	2 (1)	0.1 (0.1)	114 (5)	0.7 (0.1)	1,844 (17)	51.5 (0.5)
Also by Medicaid	718 (19)	3.7 (0.1)	10 (3)	0.3 (0.1)	223 (11)	1.4 (0.1)	495 (11)	13.8 (0.3)
Covered by VA Care	547 (13)	2.8 (0.1)	5 (2)	0.1 (0.1)	226 (9)	1.4 (0.1)	321 (8)	9.0 (0.2)
Not covered at any time during the year	3,853 (43)	20.0 (0.2)	445 (17)	11.1 (0.4)	3,794 (42)	24.2 (0.3)	59 (5)	1.7 (0.2)

Note: Numbers in thousands; Figures cover 2013; Margin of error appears in parenthesis; A "Z" indicates that the value either represents or rounds to zero.
Source: U.S. Census Bureau, 2013 American Community Survey, Table HI05. Health Insurance Coverage Status and Type of Coverage by State and Age for All People: 2013

Florida

250 Aetna Health of Florida

11675 Great Oaks Way
Alpharetta, GA 30022
Toll-Free: 866-582-9629
www.aetna.com
For Profit Organization: Yes
Total Enrollment: 521,696
State Enrollment: 521,696

Healthplan and Services Defined
PLAN TYPE: HMO
Other Type: POS
Plan Specialty: EPO
Benefits Offered: Dental, Disease Management, Long-Term Care,
Prescription, Wellness, Life, LTD, STD

Type of Coverage
Commercial, Individual

Type of Payment Plans Offered
POS, FFS

Geographic Areas Served
Statewide

251 American Pioneer Life Insurance Co

1001 Heathrow Park Lane
Suite 5001
Lake Mary, FL 32741
Toll-Free: 877-504-3918
Phone: 407-628-1776
www.universalamericaninsuranceplans.com
Secondary Address: 1289 Airport Blvd, Suite 310, Pensacola, FL
32504
Subsidiary of: Universal American
For Profit Organization: Yes
Year Founded: 1961

Healthplan and Services Defined
PLAN TYPE: Medicare
Benefits Offered: Life

Type of Coverage
Medicare, Supplemental Medicare

Key Personnel
Chairman/CEO . . . . Richard A Barasch
President & CEO . . . . Gary W Bryant, CPA
President, Medicare Advtg . . . . Theodore M Carpenter, Jr
VP, Marketing . . . . Harry Jenkins
EVP, CFO . . . . Robert A Waegelein
VP, Marketing & Staff Op . . . . Mark E Yeager
SVP, Project Management . . . . Dana Adams
VP, Marketing Support . . . . Nancy Walko
VP, Financial Reporting . . . . William H Cushman
VP, Underwriting . . . . James Kalmer
SVP, Finance & Treasurer . . . . John Squarok, CPA
VP, Product Filing . . . . Michelle Doherty
SVP, Corporate Dvlpmnt . . . . Gary M Jacobs
VP, Market Conduct . . . . John T Mackin, Jr
SVP, Operations . . . . Roslind Nelles

252 Amerigroup Florida

4200 W Cypress Street
Suite 900
Tampa, FL 33607
Toll-Free: 800-600-4441
Phone: 813-830-6900
Fax: 813-314-2050
www.amerigroupcorp.com

Secondary Address: 621 NW 53rd Street, Suite 175, Boca Raton, FL
33487
Subsidiary of: Amerigroup Corporation
For Profit Organization: Yes
Year Founded: 1998
Owned by an Integrated Delivery Network (IDN): Yes
Number of Affiliated Hospitals: 30
Number of Primary Care Physicians: 1,000
Total Enrollment: 1,900,000
State Enrollment: 237,000

Healthplan and Services Defined
PLAN TYPE: HMO
Model Type: Network
Plan Specialty: ASO, Behavioral Health, Chiropractic, Dental,
Disease Management, EPO, Lab, MSO, PBM, Vision, Radiology,
Medicaid
Benefits Offered: Behavioral Health, Chiropractic, Complementary
Medicine, Dental, Disease Management, Home Care, Inpatient
SNF, Long-Term Care, Physical Therapy, Podiatry, Prescription,
Psychiatric, Transplant, Vision, Wellness, AD&D, Medicaid
Offers Demand Management Patient Information Service: Yes

Type of Coverage
Individual, Medicare, Medicaid, Healthy Kids

Geographic Areas Served
35 counties in the Tampa, Orlando and Miami-Fort Lauderdale areas

Publishes and Distributes Report Card: Yes

Key Personnel
CEO . . . . Don Gilmore
813-830-6900
Marketing President . . . . David Rodriguez
Chief Medical Officer . . . . John Knispel

Specialty Managed Care Partners
Enters into Contracts with Regional Business Coalitions: Yes

253 Assurant Employee Benefits: Florida

5401 W Kennedy Blvd
Suite 760
Tampa, FL 33609-2428
Toll-Free: 800-277-2300
Phone: 850-886-2300
Fax: 813-289-8315
claims.dental@assurant.com
www.assurantemployeebenefits.com
Subsidiary of: Assurant, Inc
For Profit Organization: Yes
Number of Primary Care Physicians: 112,000
Total Enrollment: 47,000

Healthplan and Services Defined
PLAN TYPE: Multiple
Plan Specialty: Dental, Vision, Long & Short-Term Disability
Benefits Offered: Dental, Vision, Wellness, AD&D, Life, LTD, STD

Type of Coverage
Commercial, Indemnity, Individual Dental Plans

Geographic Areas Served
Statewide

Subscriber Information
Average Monthly Fee Per Subscriber
(Employee + Employer Contribution):
Employee Only (Self): Varies by plan

Key Personnel
President/CEO . . . . Robert B Pollock
PR Specialist . . . . Megan Hutchison
816-556-7815
megan.hutchison@assurant.com

254 AvMed Health Plan: Corporate Office

9400 S Dadeland Boulevard
Corporate Headquarters
Miami, FL 33156
Toll-Free: 800-477-8768
Phone: 305-671-5437
Fax: 305-671-4764
rxcoaching@avmed.com
www.avmed.org
Subsidiary of: SanteFe Healthcare, Inc.
Non-Profit Organization: Yes
Year Founded: 1973
Number of Affiliated Hospitals: 126
Number of Primary Care Physicians: 2,061
Number of Referral/Specialty Physicians: 7,629
Total Enrollment: 350,000
State Enrollment: 350,000

Healthplan and Services Defined
PLAN TYPE: HMO
Model Type: IPA
Benefits Offered: Disease Management, Prescription, Wellness

Type of Payment Plans Offered
POS

Geographic Areas Served
Dade county

Subscriber Information
Average Annual Deductible Per Subscriber:
Employee Only (Self): $0
Employee & 1 Family Member: $0
Employee & 2 Family Members: $0
Medicare: $0

Network Qualifications
Pre-Admission Certification: Yes

Peer Review Type
Utilization Review: Yes
Second Surgical Opinion: Yes
Case Management: Yes

Publishes and Distributes Report Card: Yes

Accreditation Certification
NCQA
TJC Accreditation, Medicare Approved, Utilization Review,
Pre-Admission Certification, State Licensure, Quality Assurance
Program

Key Personnel
CEO/President . . . . Michael P Gallagher
SVP/General Counsel . . . . Steven M Ziegler
VP, CFO . . . . Randall L Stuart
SVP, Operations . . . . Susan Knapp Pinnas
SVP, Sales & Marketing . . . . James M Repp
SVP, Chief Medical Offc . . . . Ann O Wehr, MD
SVP, Member Services. . . . . Kay Ayers
Director, Communications. . . . . Conchita Ruiz-Topinka
305-671-7306
conchita.ruiz@avmed.org

Specialty Managed Care Partners
Enters into Contracts with Regional Business Coalitions: No

255 AvMed Health Plan: Fort Lauderdale

13450 W Sunrise Boulevard
Suite 370
Fort Lauderdale, FL 33323
Toll-Free: 800-368-9189
Phone: 954-462-2520
www.avmed.org
Non-Profit Organization: Yes
Year Founded: 1973

Federally Qualified: Yes
Number of Affiliated Hospitals: 22
Number of Primary Care Physicians: 328
Number of Referral/Specialty Physicians: 564
Total Enrollment: 350,000
State Enrollment: 350,000

Healthplan and Services Defined
PLAN TYPE: HMO
Model Type: IPA
Benefits Offered: Disease Management, Prescription, Wellness

Geographic Areas Served
Broward county

Subscriber Information
Average Monthly Fee Per Subscriber
(Employee + Employer Contribution):
Employee Only (Self): $145.00
Employee & 1 Family Member: $320.00
Employee & 2 Family Members: $410.00
Medicare: $0
Average Subscriber Co-Payment:
Primary Care Physician: $5.00/10.00/15.00
Prescription Drugs: $5.00/7.00/12.00
Hospital ER: $30.00/50.00

Accreditation Certification
TJC, NCQA

Key Personnel
CEO/President . . . . Michael P Gallagher
SVP/General Counsel . . . . Steven M Ziegler
VP, CFO . . . . Randall L Stuart
SVP, Operations . . . . Susan Knapp Pinnas
SVP, Sales & Marketing . . . . James M Repp
SVP, Chief Medical Offc . . . . Ann O Wehr, MD
SVP, Member Services. . . . . Kay Ayers
Director, Communications. . . . . Conchita Ruiz-Topinka
305-671-7306
conchita.ruiz@avmed.org

256 AvMed Health Plan: Gainesville

4300 NW 89th Boulevard
Gainesville, FL 32606
Toll-Free: 800-346-0231
Phone: 352-372-8400
www.avmed.org
Non-Profit Organization: Yes
Year Founded: 1986
Number of Affiliated Hospitals: 11
Number of Primary Care Physicians: 219
Number of Referral/Specialty Physicians: 596
Total Enrollment: 350,000
State Enrollment: 350,000

Healthplan and Services Defined
PLAN TYPE: HMO
Model Type: IPA
Benefits Offered: Disease Management, Prescription, Wellness
Offers Demand Management Patient Information Service: Yes

Type of Coverage
Catastrophic Illness Benefit: Unlimited

Type of Payment Plans Offered
POS, DFFS, Combination FFS & DFFS

Geographic Areas Served
Alachua, Bradford, Citrus, Columbia, Dixie, Gilchrist, Hamilton,
Levy, Marion, Suwannee and Union counties

Subscriber Information
Average Monthly Fee Per Subscriber
(Employee + Employer Contribution):
Employee Only (Self): $110.00-135.00
Employee & 1 Family Member: $385.00-460.00

Employee & 2 Family Members: $220.00-260.00
Average Annual Deductible Per Subscriber:
Employee Only (Self): $0
Employee & 1 Family Member: $0
Employee & 2 Family Members: $0
Medicare: $0
Average Subscriber Co-Payment:
Primary Care Physician: $5.00-15.00
Prescription Drugs: $7.00/12.00
Hospital ER: $30.00/50.00
Home Health Care: $0
Nursing Home: $0
Nursing Home Max. Days/Visits Covered: 20

Network Qualifications
Minimum Years of Practice: 5
Pre-Admission Certification: Yes

Peer Review Type
Utilization Review: Yes
Second Surgical Opinion: Yes
Case Management: Yes

Publishes and Distributes Report Card: Yes

Accreditation Certification
NCQA
TJC Accreditation, Medicare Approved, Utilization Review,
Pre-Admission Certification, State Licensure, Quality Assurance
Program

Key Personnel
CEO/President . . . . Michael P Gallagher
SVP/General Counsel . . . . Steven M Ziegler
VP, CFO . . . . Randall L Stuart
SVP, Operations . . . . Susan Knapp Pinnas
SVP, Sales & Marketing . . . . James M Repp
SVP, Chief Medical Offc . . . . Ann O Wehr, MD
SVP, Member Services. . . . . Kay Ayers
Director, Communications. . . . . Conchita Ruiz-Topinka
305-671-7306
conchita.ruiz@avmed.org

Average Claim Compensation
Physician's Fees Charged: 85%
Hospital's Fees Charged: 70%

Specialty Managed Care Partners
Enters into Contracts with Regional Business Coalitions: No

257   AvMed Health Plan: Jacksonville

1300 Riverplace Boulevard
Suite 640
Jacksonville, FL 32207
Toll-Free: 800-227-4184
Phone: 904-858-1300
Fax: 904-858-1355
www.avmed.org
Non-Profit Organization: Yes
Year Founded: 1969
Federally Qualified: Yes
Number of Affiliated Hospitals: 12
Number of Primary Care Physicians: 267
Total Enrollment: 350,000
State Enrollment: 350,000

Healthplan and Services Defined
PLAN TYPE: HMO
Model Type: IPA
Benefits Offered: Disease Management, Prescription, Wellness

Type of Coverage
Commercial, Individual, Supplemental Medicare

Geographic Areas Served
Baker, Clay, Duval, Nassau, & St. Johns counties

Subscriber Information
Average Subscriber Co-Payment:
Primary Care Physician: $10.00
Non-Network Physician: Not covered
Prescription Drugs: $7.00
Hospital ER: $50.00

Peer Review Type
Second Surgical Opinion: Yes
Case Management: Yes

Publishes and Distributes Report Card: Yes

Accreditation Certification
NCQA

Key Personnel
President/CEO . . . . Michael P Gallagher
Dir, Communications. . . . . Conchita Ruiz-Topinka
305-671-7306
conchita.ruiz@avmed.org

258   AvMed Health Plan: Orlando

541 S Orlando Ave
Maitland, FL 32571
Toll-Free: 800-227-4848
Phone: 407-539-0007
www.avmed.org
Non-Profit Organization: Yes
Year Founded: 1988
Number of Primary Care Physicians: 1,400
Number of Referral/Specialty Physicians: 775
Total Enrollment: 350,000
State Enrollment: 350,000

Healthplan and Services Defined
PLAN TYPE: HMO
Model Type: IPA
Plan Specialty: ASO, Behavioral Health, Chiropractic, Disease
Management, EPO, Lab, Vision, Radiology, UR
Benefits Offered: Disease Management, Prescription, Wellness
Offers Demand Management Patient Information Service: Yes

Type of Coverage
Commercial

Type of Payment Plans Offered
FFS, Combination FFS & DFFS

Geographic Areas Served
Orange, Osceola and Seminole counties

Subscriber Information
Average Subscriber Co-Payment:
Primary Care Physician: $5.00/10.00/15.00
Prescription Drugs: $5.00/7.00/12.00
Hospital ER: $30.00/50.00

Network Qualifications
Pre-Admission Certification: Yes

Peer Review Type
Second Surgical Opinion: Yes

Publishes and Distributes Report Card: Yes

Accreditation Certification
TJC, NCQA
Utilization Review, Quality Assurance Program

Key Personnel
CEO/President . . . . Michael P Gallagher
SVP/General Counsel . . . . Steven M Ziegler
VP, CFO . . . . Randall L Stuart
SVP, Operations . . . . Susan Knapp Pinnas
SVP, Sales & Marketing . . . . James M Repp
SVP, Chief Medical Offc . . . . Ann O Wehr, MD
SVP, Member Services. . . . . Kay Ayers

Director, Communications. . . . . Conchita Ruiz-Topinka
305-671-7306
conchita.ruiz@avmed.org

Specialty Managed Care Partners
Enters into Contracts with Regional Business Coalitions: Yes

259 AvMed Health Plan: Tampa Bay
1511 North WestShore Blvd
Suite 450
Tampa, FL 33607
Phone: 813-281-5650
www.avmed.org
Non-Profit Organization: Yes
Year Founded: 1969
Federally Qualified: Yes
Number of Affiliated Hospitals: 14
Number of Primary Care Physicians: 240
Number of Referral/Specialty Physicians: 550
Total Enrollment: 350,000
State Enrollment: 350,000

Healthplan and Services Defined
　PLAN TYPE: HMO
　Model Type: IPA
　Benefits Offered: Disease Management, Prescription, Wellness
　Offers Demand Management Patient Information Service: Yes

Geographic Areas Served
　Hernando, Hillsborough, Lee, Pasco, Pinellas, Polk and Sarasota
　counties

Subscriber Information
　Average Monthly Fee Per Subscriber
　　(Employee + Employer Contribution):
　　　Employee Only (Self): Varies
　　　Employee & 1 Family Member: Varies
　　　Employee & 2 Family Members: Varies
　Average Annual Deductible Per Subscriber:
　　　Employee Only (Self): Varies
　　　Employee & 1 Family Member: Varies
　　　Employee & 2 Family Members: Varies
　Average Subscriber Co-Payment:
　　　Primary Care Physician: Varies
　　　Non-Network Physician: Varies
　　　Prescription Drugs: Varies
　　　Hospital ER: Varies

Network Qualifications
　Pre-Admission Certification: Yes

Peer Review Type
　Utilization Review: Yes
　Second Surgical Opinion: Yes

Publishes and Distributes Report Card: Yes

Accreditation Certification
　AAAHC, TJC, NCQA

Key Personnel
　CEO/President . . . . Michael P Gallagher
　SVP/General Counsel . . . . Steven M Ziegler
　VP, CFO . . . . Randall L Stuart
　SVP, Operations . . . . Susan Knapp Pinnas
　SVP, Sales & Marketing . . . . James M Repp
　SVP, Chief Medical Offc . . . . Ann O Wehr, MD
　SVP, Member Services . . . . Kay Ayers
　Director, Communications. . . . . Conchita Ruiz-Topinka
　305-671-7306
　conchita.ruiz@avmed.org

Specialty Managed Care Partners
Enters into Contracts with Regional Business Coalitions: Yes

260 AvMed Medicare Preferred
9400 South Dadeland Boulevard
Miami, FL 33156
Toll-Free: 800-782-8633
Phone: 305-671-5437
www.avmed.org
Non-Profit Organization: Yes
Year Founded: 1969
Federally Qualified: Yes

Healthplan and Services Defined
　PLAN TYPE: Medicare

Type of Coverage
　Medicare, Supplemental Medicare

Key Personnel
　President & CEO . . . . Michael P. Gallagher
　SVP, Member Services . . . . Kay Ayers
　SVP, Underwriting . . . . Brad Bentley
　SVP, Sales & Marketing . . . . James M. Repp
　SVP/CFO . . . . Randall L. Stuart
　SVP/Chief Medical Officer . . . . Ann O. Wehr, MD, FACP
　SVP/General Counsel. . . . . Steven M. Ziegler
　SVP/Chief Info Officer. . . . . Tony Tardugno

261 Capital Health Plan
2140 Centerville Place
Tallahassee, FL 32308
Toll-Free: 800-390-1434
Phone: 850-383-3400
Fax: 850-383-1031
memberservices@chp.com
www.capitalhealth.com
Mailing Address: PO Box 15349, Tallahaseee, FL 32317-5349
Subsidiary of: Blue Cross Blue Shield of Florida
Non-Profit Organization: Yes
Year Founded: 1982
Owned by an Integrated Delivery Network (IDN): Yes
Number of Affiliated Hospitals: 4
Number of Primary Care Physicians: 150
Number of Referral/Specialty Physicians: 400
Total Enrollment: 125,000
State Enrollment: 125,000

Healthplan and Services Defined
　PLAN TYPE: HMO
　Model Type: Staff, Mixed Model
　Plan Specialty: Chiropractic, Lab, Vision, Radiology, UR
　Benefits Offered: Behavioral Health, Chiropractic, Disease
　　Management, Home Care, Inpatient SNF, Physical Therapy,
　　Podiatry, Prescription, Psychiatric, Transplant, Vision, Wellness

Type of Coverage
　Commercial, Medicare, Supplemental Medicare, Catastrophic
　Catastrophic Illness Benefit: Unlimited

Geographic Areas Served
　Calhoun, Liberty, Franklin, Leon, Gadsden, Jefferson and Wakulla
　counties

Subscriber Information
　Average Annual Deductible Per Subscriber:
　　　Employee Only (Self): $0
　　　Employee & 1 Family Member: $0
　　　Employee & 2 Family Members: $0
　　　Medicare: $0
　Average Subscriber Co-Payment:
　　　Primary Care Physician: $15.00
　　　Prescription Drugs: $7.00
　　　Hospital ER: $50.00
　　　Nursing Home Max. Days/Visits Covered: 60

Peer Review Type
　Second Surgical Opinion: Yes

Publishes and Distributes Report Card: Yes

Accreditation Certification
NCQA

Key Personnel
President/CEO ....John Hogan
CFO/COO ....Kearney Pool
Principal...................................Summer Knight
Director of Claims.............................Amy Adams
Network Development...........................Eric Smith
Chief Marketing Officer.........................Sue Conte
Chief Medical Officer ....Nancy Van Vessem, MD
Chief Information Officer ....Eric Smith

Specialty Managed Care Partners
Enters into Contracts with Regional Business Coalitions: Yes

262 CarePlus Health Plans, Inc
11430 NW 20th Street
Suite 300
Doral, FL 33172
Toll-Free: 855-605-6171
Phone: 800-794-5907
CPHP_memberservices@careplus-hp.com
www.care-plus-health-plans.com
Year Founded: 2003
Total Enrollment: 67,000
State Enrollment: 67,000

Healthplan and Services Defined
PLAN TYPE: HMO
Plan Specialty: Dental, Vision
Benefits Offered: Dental, Prescription, Vision, Transportation in
some areas

Type of Coverage
Medicare, Supplemental Medicare

Geographic Areas Served
Miami-Dade, Broward, Palm Beach, Hillsborough, Pinellas, Pasco,
Polk, Seminole, Sumter, Orange, Osceola, Brevard, Okeechobee and
Saint Lucie counties. 2010 expansion to Indian River, Martin, Lake,
Marion, Charlotte, Lee and Sarasota

Accreditation Certification
AAAHC

263 CIGNA HealthCare of Florida
255 Primera Blvd
Suite 264
Lake Mary, FL 32746
Toll-Free: 866-621-8270
Phone: 407-833-3100
www.cigna.com
Secondary Address: 1571 Sawgrass Corporate Parkway, Suite 140,
Sunrise, FL 33323, 954-514-6600
For Profit Organization: Yes
Year Founded: 1981
Number of Affiliated Hospitals: 230
Number of Primary Care Physicians: 32,300
Number of Referral/Specialty Physicians: 797
Total Enrollment: 194,944
State Enrollment: 194,944

Healthplan and Services Defined
PLAN TYPE: HMO
Other Type: POS
Model Type: Network
Benefits Offered: Dental, Disease Management, Prescription,
Transplant, Vision, Wellness, Life, LTD, STD

Type of Coverage
Commercial

Type of Payment Plans Offered
POS, DFFS, FFS, Combination FFS & DFFS

Geographic Areas Served
Tampa

Network Qualifications
Minimum Years of Practice: 3

Peer Review Type
Second Surgical Opinion: Yes
Case Management: Yes

Publishes and Distributes Report Card: Yes

Accreditation Certification
NCQA
TJC Accreditation, Medicare Approved, Utilization Review,
Pre-Admission Certification, State Licensure, Quality Assurance
Program

Key Personnel
Chief Medical Officer ....William Alexander, MD

264 Citrus Health Care
5420 Bay Center Drive
Suite 250
Tampa, FL 33609
Toll-Free: 877-624-8787
Phone: 813-490-8900
Fax: 813-490-8909
www.uhcmedicaresolutions.com
Mailing Address: PO Box 690670, San Antonio, TX 78269-0670
Subsidiary of: Physicians Health Choice/WellMed Medical
Management
For Profit Organization: Yes
Year Founded: 2003
Physician Owned Organization: Yes
Total Enrollment: 54,000
State Enrollment: 54,000

Healthplan and Services Defined
PLAN TYPE: Medicare
Other Type: HMO
Benefits Offered: Disease Management, Wellness

Type of Coverage
Commercial, Medicare, Medicaid, Long Term Care

Geographic Areas Served
Florida

Key Personnel
President ....Dan J Comrie
VP, Marketing & Dev...........................Jeff White
Chief Medical Officer ....Robert S Grossman, MD
VP, Customer Service.......................Donna L Debner
Compliance Officer ....Laura Ketterman
VP, Sales ....Tamara Schumacher-Konick

265 CompBenefits: Florida
5775 Blue Lagoon Drive
Suite 400
Miami, FL 33126-1333
Toll-Free: 800-223-6447
Phone: 305-262-1333
Fax: 305-269-2118
www.compbenefits.com
Secondary Address: 1511 North Westshore Blvd, Suite 1000, Tampa,
FL 33607
Subsidiary of: Humana
Year Founded: 1978
Owned by an Integrated Delivery Network (IDN): Yes
Total Enrollment: 4,500,000

Healthplan and Services Defined
  PLAN TYPE: Multiple
  Model Type: Network, HMO, PPO, POS, TPA
  Plan Specialty: ASO, Dental, Vision
  Benefits Offered: Dental, Vision

Type of Coverage
  Commercial, Individual, Indemnity

Type of Payment Plans Offered
  DFFS, Capitated, FFS

Geographic Areas Served
  Alabama, Arkansas, Illinois, Indiana, Georgia, Florida, Mississippi, Missouri, Kentucky, Kansas, North Carolina, South Carolina, West Virginia, Texas, Tennessee, Ohio, Louisiana

Publishes and Distributes Report Card: Yes

Specialty Managed Care Partners
  Enters into Contracts with Regional Business Coalitions: Yes

---

266 CompCare: Comprehensive Behavioral Care

3405 W Dr Martin Luther King Jr Blvd
Suite 101
Tampa, FL 33607
Toll-Free: 800-435-5348
Phone: 813-288-4808
Fax: 813-288-4844
info@compcare.com
www.compcare.com
For Profit Organization: Yes
Year Founded: 1969
Total Enrollment: 900,000

Healthplan and Services Defined
  PLAN TYPE: Multiple
  Model Type: Network
  Plan Specialty: ASO, Behavioral Health, Disease Management, PBM
  Benefits Offered: Behavioral Health
  Offers Demand Management Patient Information Service: Yes

Type of Coverage
  Commercial, Medicare, Medicaid

Type of Payment Plans Offered
  POS, DFFS, Capitated, FFS, Combination FFS & DFFS

Geographic Areas Served
  Nationwide and Puerto Rico

Peer Review Type
  Utilization Review: Yes
  Second Surgical Opinion: Yes

Publishes and Distributes Report Card: Yes

Accreditation Certification
  TJC, NCQA

Key Personnel
  Chairman & CEO . . . . Clark A. Marcus
  Chief Financial Officer . . . . Robert J. Landis
  SVP, Operations . . . . Susan Norris, PhD
  Acting CFO . . . . Robert J Landis
  Medical Director . . . . Jayendra Choksi
  Medical Director . . . . Jayendra Choksi, MD
  Corporate Communications . . . . Darnell Albarado
    813-367-4519
    dalbarado@compcare.com

---

267 Coventry Health Care of Florida

1340 Concord Terrace
Sunrise, FL 33323
Toll-Free: 866-847-8235
Phone: 954-858-3000
Fax: 954-846-0331
www.chcflorida.com

Secondary Address: 3611 Queen Palm Drive, Suite 200, Tampa, FL 33619, 866-576-1094
For Profit Organization: Yes
Number of Affiliated Hospitals: 16
Number of Primary Care Physicians: 1,500
Total Enrollment: 310,000

Healthplan and Services Defined
  PLAN TYPE: HMO/PPO
  Other Type: Other Health Plans
  Benefits Offered: Disease Management, Prescription, Wellness

Type of Coverage
  Commercial, Individual, Medicare, Medicaid

Type of Payment Plans Offered
  POS

Geographic Areas Served
  Hernando, Pasco, Pinellas, Hillsborough, St. Lucie, Martin, Palm Beach, Broward, Miami-Dade counties

Accreditation Certification
  URAC

Key Personnel
  CEO . . . . Allen F Wise
  COO . . . . Michael D Bahr
  EVP/CFO . . . . Randy Giles
  CMO . . . . Mark Bloom, MD
  General Counsel . . . . Thomas C Zielinski
  Provider Relations . . . . Duell Wise
  Marketing . . . . Peter Joseph
  Member Relations . . . . Frank Appel
  Pharmacy Director . . . . Hal Goldman
  Public Relations . . . . Pam Gadinsky

---

268 Coventry Health Care of Southern Florida

1340 Concord Terrace
Sunrise, FL 33323
Toll-Free: 866-847-8235
http://chcflorida.coventryhealthcare.com
Number of Primary Care Physicians: 5,000
Total Enrollment: 69,000

Healthplan and Services Defined
  PLAN TYPE: Multiple

Type of Coverage
  Supplemental Medicare

Geographic Areas Served
  Miami-Dade, Broward, Palm Beach, Martin and St. Lucie counties and 21 counties in North Floridda from Ocala to Pensacola

---

269 Delta Dental of Florida

258 Southhall Lane
Suite 350
Maitland, FL 32751
Toll-Free: 800-662-9034
Phone: 407-660-9034
Fax: 407-660-2899
flsales@delta.org
www.deltadentalins.com
Secondary Address: 5200 Blue Lagoon Drive, Suite 110, Miami, FL 33126
Non-Profit Organization: Yes
Total Enrollment: 54,000,000

Healthplan and Services Defined
  PLAN TYPE: Dental
  Other Type: Dental PPO

Type of Coverage
  Commercial

Geographic Areas Served
Statewide

Key Personnel
President/CEO..............................Gary D Radine
VP, Public & Govt Affairs ....Jeff Album
415-972-8418
Dir/Media & Public Affair ....Elizabeth Risberg
415-972-8423

270 Dimension Health PPO
5881 NW 151st Street
Suite 201
Miami Lakes, FL 33014
Toll-Free: 800-483-4992
Phone: 305-823-7664
Fax: 305-818-8814
info@dimensionhealth.com
www.dimensionhealth.com
Year Founded: 1985
Number of Affiliated Hospitals: 34
Number of Primary Care Physicians: 6,000
Number of Referral/Specialty Physicians: 3,660
Total Enrollment: 400,000
State Enrollment: 400,000

Healthplan and Services Defined
PLAN TYPE: PPO
Model Type: Network, PPO
Benefits Offered: Disease Management, Wellness, Worker's
Compensation

Type of Coverage
Commercial

Type of Payment Plans Offered
POS, DFFS, Capitated, FFS, Combination FFS & DFFS

Geographic Areas Served
Monroe, Dade, Broward and Palm Beach counties

Network Qualifications
Pre-Admission Certification: Yes

Peer Review Type
Utilization Review: Yes
Second Surgical Opinion: Yes
Case Management: Yes

Publishes and Distributes Report Card: No

Key Personnel
President/CEO ....Charles A. Lindgren
clindgren@dimensionhealth.com
Sr. Executive Assistant t ....Rosemary Osorio
rosorio@dimensionhealth.com
VP, Network Development.......................Creta Diehs
Chief Medical Officer.......................Ray Mummery
Chief Medical Director....................Ray Mummery, MD
rmummery@dimensionhealth.com
VP, Network Development.......................Creta Diehs
cdiehs@dimensionhealth.com

Average Claim Compensation
Physician's Fees Charged: 110%

Specialty Managed Care Partners
Enters into Contracts with Regional Business Coalitions: No

271 eHealthInsurance Services Inc.
11919 Foundation Place
Gold River, CA 95670
Toll-Free: 800-644-3491
webmaster@healthinsurance.com
www.e.healthinsurance.com
Year Founded: 1997

Healthplan and Services Defined
PLAN TYPE: HMO/PPO
Benefits Offered: Dental, Life, STD

Type of Coverage
Commercial, Individual, Medicare

Geographic Areas Served
All 50 states in the USA and District of Columbia

Key Personnel
Chairman & CEO............................Gary L. Lauer
EVP/Business & Corp. Dev.....................Bruce Telkamp
EVP/Chief Technology..................Dr. Sheldon X. Wang
SVP & CFO ....Stuart M. Huizinga
Pres. of eHealth Gov. Sys ....Samuel C. Gibbs
SVP of Sales & Operations ....Robert S. Hurley
Director Public Relations......................Nate Purpura
650-210-3115

272 First Medical Health Plan of Florida
9455 SW 39th Street
Miami, FL 33165-4017
Toll-Free: 888-364-7535
Phone: 305-269-7995
www.firstmedicalflorida.com
For Profit Organization: Yes
Year Founded: 1977
Number of Primary Care Physicians: 5,000
Total Enrollment: 320,000
State Enrollment: 320,000

Healthplan and Services Defined
PLAN TYPE: Medicare
Benefits Offered: Behavioral Health, Prescription, Wellness

Type of Coverage
Medicare, Supplemental Medicare

Geographic Areas Served
Southern Florida and Puerto Rico

Key Personnel
President ....Patricia Serrano

273 Florida Blue: Jacksonville
4800 Deerwood Campus Parkway
Jacksonville, FL 32246
Toll-Free: 800-477-3736
Phone: 904-791-6111
Fax: 904-905-6638
corporatecommunications@bcbsfl.com
www.floridablue.com; www.bcbsfl.com
Mailing Address: PO Box 1798, Jacksonville, FL 32231-0014
Non-Profit Organization: Yes
Year Founded: 1985
Owned by an Integrated Delivery Network (IDN): Yes
Number of Affiliated Hospitals: 211
Number of Primary Care Physicians: 8,977
Number of Referral/Specialty Physicians: 18,451
Total Enrollment: 4,000,000
State Enrollment: 1,373,917

Healthplan and Services Defined
PLAN TYPE: HMO/PPO
Benefits Offered: Behavioral Health, Chiropractic, Complementary
Medicine, Disease Management, Home Care, Inpatient SNF,
Physical Therapy, Podiatry, Prescription, Psychiatric, Transplant,
Wellness
Offers Demand Management Patient Information Service: Yes
DMPI Services Offered: Nurse Line 24x7x365, Health Coaching,
Support for Chronic Conditions, Health Risk Assessments, Web
Tools & Resources

Type of Coverage
Commercial, Individual, Indemnity, Medicare

Type of Payment Plans Offered
FFS

Geographic Areas Served
State of Florida

Subscriber Information
Average Subscriber Co-Payment:
Primary Care Physician: Varies
Non-Network Physician: Varies
Prescription Drugs: Varies
Hospital ER: Varies
Home Health Care: Varies
Nursing Home: Varies

Network Qualifications
Pre-Admission Certification: Yes

Peer Review Type
Utilization Review: Yes

Publishes and Distributes Report Card: No

Accreditation Certification
Utilization Review

Key Personnel
CEO/Chairman ....Patrick J Geraghty
Senior Director CEO Offc. ....Camille Harrison
EVP/CFO ....R Chris Doerr
VP Pharmacy Programs ....Lowell Sterler
SVP, Corporate Affairs ....Charles Joseph
Chief Medical Officer ....Jonathan B Gavras, MD
EVP, Business ....Steve Booma
SVP, Sales & Marketing........................Jon Urbanek
SVP, Consumer Markets........................Craig Thomas
SVP, Enterprise Comm. ....Sharon Wamble-King

Specialty Managed Care Partners
Prime Therapeutics, LLC-PBM and Mental Health Network
(MHnet), Health Dialog, Accordant and Quest Diagnostics
Enters into Contracts with Regional Business Coalitions: Yes

Employer References
State of Florida, Gevity HR (formerly Staff Leasing), Publix,
Lincare, Miami Dade County

---

274 Florida Blue: Pensacola
2190 Airport Boulevard
Suite 3000
Pensacola, FL 32504-8907
Toll-Free: 800-477-3736
Phone: 904-791-6111
Fax: 904-905-6638
corporatecommunications@bcbsfl.com
www.floridablue.com; www.bcbsfl.com
Mailing Address: PO Box 1798, Jacksonville, FL 32231-0014
Subsidiary of: Blue Cross Blue Shield
For Profit Organization: Yes
Year Founded: 1985
Number of Affiliated Hospitals: 7
Number of Primary Care Physicians: 240
Number of Referral/Specialty Physicians: 350
Total Enrollment: 54,000

Healthplan and Services Defined
PLAN TYPE: HMO/PPO
Model Type: IPA
Plan Specialty: Worker's Compensation
Benefits Offered: Dental, Disease Management, Prescription,
Wellness, Worker's Compensation, AD&D, Life

Type of Coverage
Commercial, Individual, Medicare, Supplemental Medicare
Catastrophic Illness Benefit: Unlimited

Type of Payment Plans Offered
POS, DFFS, Capitated, FFS, Combination FFS & DFFS

Geographic Areas Served
Escambia, Okaloosa, Walton and Santa Rosa counties

Subscriber Information
Average Subscriber Co-Payment:
Primary Care Physician: $10.00
Non-Network Physician: $10.00
Prescription Drugs: $7.00/14.00
Hospital ER: $50.00
Home Health Care Max. Days/Visits Covered: Unlimited

Network Qualifications
Pre-Admission Certification: Yes

Peer Review Type
Utilization Review: Yes
Second Surgical Opinion: Yes
Case Management: Yes

Publishes and Distributes Report Card: Yes

Accreditation Certification
NCQA
TJC Accreditation, Medicare Approved, Utilization Review,
Pre-Admission Certification, State Licensure, Quality Assurance
Program

Key Personnel
CEO/Chairman ....Patrick J Geraghty
Senior Director CEO Offc. ....Camille Harrison
EVP/CFO ....R Chris Doerr
VP Pharmacy Programs ....Lowell Sterler
SVP, Corporate Affairs ....Charles Joseph
Chief Medical Officer ....Jonathan B Gavras, MD
EVP, Business ....Steve Booma
SVP, Sales & Marketing........................Jon Urbanek
SVP, Consumer Markets........................Craig Thomas
SVP, Enterprise Comm. ....Sharon Wamble-King

---

275 Florida Health Care Plan
1340 Ridgewood Avenue
Holly Hill, FL 32117
Toll-Free: 800-352-9824
Phone: 386-676-7100
Fax: 386-676-7119
www.fhcp.com
Mailing Address: PO Box 9910, Daytona Beach, FL 32120
Subsidiary of: Blue Cross Blue Shield
Non-Profit Organization: Yes
Year Founded: 1974
Owned by an Integrated Delivery Network (IDN): Yes
Federally Qualified: Yes
Number of Affiliated Hospitals: 10
Number of Primary Care Physicians: 71
Number of Referral/Specialty Physicians: 241
Total Enrollment: 67,440
State Enrollment: 39,511

Healthplan and Services Defined
PLAN TYPE: HMO
Model Type: Mixed
Benefits Offered: Behavioral Health, Chiropractic, Dental, Disease
Management, Home Care, Inpatient SNF, Podiatry, Prescription,
Psychiatric, Transplant, Vision, Wellness
Offers Demand Management Patient Information Service: Yes
DMPI Services Offered: Asthma Disease Management, Complex Case
Management, Diabetes Health Management, Depression Healing
Management, Congestive Heart Failure

Type of Coverage
Commercial, Individual, Medicare, Supplemental Medicare, Healthy
Kids
Catastrophic Illness Benefit: Varies per case

Geographic Areas Served
Volusia and Flagler counties, Florida

Subscriber Information
Average Annual Deductible Per Subscriber:
Employee Only (Self): $0
Employee & 1 Family Member: $0
Employee & 2 Family Members: $0
Medicare: $0

Peer Review Type
Utilization Review: Yes
Second Surgical Opinion: Yes
Case Management: Yes

Publishes and Distributes Report Card: Yes

Accreditation Certification
TJC

Key Personnel
President/CEO . . . . Dr Wendy Myers
386-676-7100
CFO . . . . David Schandel
386-676-7100
Chief Marketing Officer . . . . Mikelle Streicher, RN, PhD
Pharmacy Administrator. Gary Klein, RPh
386-676-7100
Adm. Membership/Retention . . . . Pamela C Mims
386-676-7110
Materials Management . . . . Tom Beall
Chief Medical Officer. . . . . Joseph Zuckerman, MD
Member Service Manager. . . . . Mickey Linse-weiss
386-676-7100
CIO . . . . James W Bare
386-238-3200
Administrator of Contact . . . . Sherri Hutchinson
386-676-7100
Sales. . . . . Pamela C Mims
386-676-7100

Specialty Managed Care Partners
Enters into Contracts with Regional Business Coalitions: Yes

Employer References
State of Florida, Volusia County School District, City of Daytona Beach, Florida, Publix Super-Markets, Walgreen Company

276 Freedom Health, Inc
PO Box 151137
Tampa, FL 33684
Toll-Free: 800-401-2740
Phone: 800-955-8771
Fax: 813-506-6150
contact@freedomhealth.com
www.freedomhealth.com
Mailing Address: PO Box 151257, Tampa, FL 33684-9850
Physician Owned Organization: Yes

Healthplan and Services Defined
PLAN TYPE: Medicare
Benefits Offered: Dental, Prescription, Vision, Hearing, and Preventative health care services

Type of Coverage
Supplemental Medicare, Medicaid

Geographic Areas Served
Broward, Hillsborough, Pasco, Sumter, Dade, Lake, Pinellas, Hernando, Marion and Orange counties

Accreditation Certification
NCQA

277 Great-West Healthcare Florida
2701 N Rocky Point
Suite 800
Tampa, FL 33607-5954
Toll-Free: 800-663-8081
Phone: 813-207-0216
eliginquiries@cigna.com
www.cignaforhealth.com
Secondary Address: 1572 Sawgrass Corporate Parkway, Suite 140, Sunrise, FL 33323
Subsidiary of: CIGNA HealthCare
Acquired by: CIGNA
For Profit Organization: Yes
Total Enrollment: 81,822
State Enrollment: 1,771

Healthplan and Services Defined
PLAN TYPE: HMO/PPO
Benefits Offered: Disease Management, Prescription, Wellness

Type of Coverage
Commercial

Type of Payment Plans Offered
POS, FFS

Geographic Areas Served
Florida

Accreditation Certification
URAC

Specialty Managed Care Partners
Caremark Rx

278 Health First Health Plans
6450 US Highway 1
Rockledge, FL 32955
Toll-Free: 800-716-7737
Phone: 321-434-5665
Fax: 321-434-4362
hfhpinfo@health-first.org
www.health-first.org/health_plans
Subsidiary of: Health First
Non-Profit Organization: Yes
Year Founded: 1995
Number of Affiliated Hospitals: 5
Number of Primary Care Physicians: 228
Number of Referral/Specialty Physicians: 537
Total Enrollment: 63,700
State Enrollment: 63,700

Healthplan and Services Defined
PLAN TYPE: HMO
Other Type: POS
Model Type: IPA, Network
Plan Specialty: Fully Insured HMO
Benefits Offered: Behavioral Health, Chiropractic, Disease Management, Home Care, Inpatient SNF, Long-Term Care, Physical Therapy, Podiatry, Prescription, Psychiatric, Transplant, Vision, Wellness

Type of Coverage
Commercial, Medicare
Catastrophic Illness Benefit: Covered

Type of Payment Plans Offered
FFS

Geographic Areas Served
All of Brevard County, the town of Sebastian in Indian River County

Subscriber Information
Average Subscriber Co-Payment:
Primary Care Physician: $15.00
Prescription Drugs: $2.00/7/15/35/70
Hospital ER: $75

Home Health Care: $0
Nursing Home: $0
Nursing Home Max. Days/Visits Covered: 60 days

Peer Review Type
Utilization Review: Yes
Second Surgical Opinion: Yes
Case Management: Yes

Accreditation Certification
NCQA

Key Personnel
President/CEO.............................Margaret Haney
VP/Finance ....Joseph Felkner, CPA
VP, Human Resources ....Robert Suttles
Chief Nursing Officer ....Ed Hannah, RN
Chief Medical Officer ....Scott Gettings, MD
Chief Information Officer ....Lori DeLone

Average Claim Compensation
Physician's Fees Charged: 110%

Specialty Managed Care Partners
SXC, Ameripharm

Employer References
Boeing/McDonnell Douglas Corp., ITT, Computer Science
Raytheon, Intersil Corp.

---

279 Health First Medicare Plans

6450 US Highway 1
Rockledge, FL 32955
Toll-Free: 800-716-7737
Phone: 321-434-5665
Fax: 321-434-4362
www.health-first.org/health_plans/medicare
Subsidiary of: Health First
Year Founded: 1997

Healthplan and Services Defined
PLAN TYPE: Medicare

Type of Coverage
Medicare, MA and MA-PD

Geographic Areas Served
Brevard county, zip codes of 32957, 32958, 32978 and in the city of
Sebastian in Indian River county

Key Personnel
Chairman ....Nicholas E Pellegrino
Vice Chairman ....Larry F Garrison

---

280 Healthchoice Orlando

102 W Pineloch Avenue
Suite 23
Orlando, FL 32806
Toll-Free: 800-635-4345
Phone: 407-481-7100
Fax: 407-481-7190
hcweb@orlandohealth.com
www.healthchoiceorlando.org
Subsidiary of: Orlando Health
For Profit Organization: Yes
Year Founded: 1984
Number of Affiliated Hospitals: 16
Number of Primary Care Physicians: 2,000
Number of Referral/Specialty Physicians: 2,221
Total Enrollment: 35,000
State Enrollment: 35,000

Healthplan and Services Defined
PLAN TYPE: PPO
Model Type: IPA
Plan Specialty: Worker's Compensation, UR
Benefits Offered: Disease Management

Offers Demand Management Patient Information Service: Yes

Type of Coverage
Commercial
Catastrophic Illness Benefit: Varies per case

Type of Payment Plans Offered
FFS

Geographic Areas Served
PPO: Brevard, Orange, Osceola, Seminole and Lake counties; EPO:
Orange, Osceola, Seminole, and Lake counties

Network Qualifications
Pre-Admission Certification: Yes

Peer Review Type
Utilization Review: Yes
Second Surgical Opinion: Yes
Case Management: Yes

Publishes and Distributes Report Card: Yes

Accreditation Certification
AAAHC
TJC Accreditation, Medicare Approved, Utilization Review,
Pre-Admission Certification, State Licensure, Quality Assurance
Program

Key Personnel
COO......................................Christy Pearson
Medical Director.......................Michael Howell, MD
Marketing/Sales.......................Stephanie Scarbrough

Specialty Managed Care Partners
Enters into Contracts with Regional Business Coalitions: Yes

---

281 HealthSun Health Plans

3250 Mary Street
Suite 400
Coconut Grove, FL 33133
Toll-Free: 877-207-4900
Phone: 305-234-9292
Fax: 305-234-9275
info@healthsun.com
www.health-sun.com

Healthplan and Services Defined
PLAN TYPE: Medicare
Other Type: HMO

Type of Coverage
Medicare

Geographic Areas Served
Miami-Dade and Broward counties

---

282 Humana Health Insurance of Jacksonville

76 S Laura Street
10th Floor
Jacksonville, FL 32202
Toll-Free: 800-639-1133
Phone: 904-376-1234
Fax: 904-376-1270
www.humana.com
For Profit Organization: Yes
Year Founded: 1985
Owned by an Integrated Delivery Network (IDN): Yes
Number of Affiliated Hospitals: 13
Number of Primary Care Physicians: 3,200
Total Enrollment: 125,000

Healthplan and Services Defined
PLAN TYPE: HMO/PPO
Model Type: IPA
Plan Specialty: ASO, Behavioral Health, Chiropractic, Dental,
Disease Management, EPO, Lab, Vision, Radiology, Worker's
Compensation

Benefits Offered: Behavioral Health, Chiropractic, Complementary
   Medicine, Dental, Disease Management, Home Care, Inpatient
   SNF, Physical Therapy, Podiatry, Prescription, Psychiatric,
   Transplant, Vision, Worker's Compensation
Offers Demand Management Patient Information Service: Yes

Type of Coverage
   Commercial, Individual, Indemnity, Medicare, Catastrophic
   Catastrophic Illness Benefit: Maximum $1M

Geographic Areas Served
   Statewide

Peer Review Type
   Utilization Review: Yes
   Second Surgical Opinion: Yes

Accreditation Certification
   TJC, URAC, NCQA, CORE

Key Personnel
   President/CEO . . . . .Alan Guzzino
   CFO . . . . .Michael Lynch
   Florida Employer Grp Pres. . . . . .Dan Fenik
   East Region CEO . . . . .Paul Kraemer
   Marketing . . . . .Monica Colquette
   Medical Affairs. . . . . .Robert Blalock, MD
   Sales . . . . .Laura Taravaglia
   Media Relations Manager .Mitch Lubitz
      813-287-6180
      mlubitz@humana.com

Specialty Managed Care Partners
   University of Florida

---

283   Humana Health Insurance of Orlando
385 Douglas Avenue
Suite 1050
Alamonte Springs, FL 32714
Toll-Free: 800-797-2273
Phone: 407-772-3140
Fax: 407-862-0355
www.humana.com
For Profit Organization: Yes
Year Founded: 1962
Number of Affiliated Hospitals: 12
Number of Primary Care Physicians: 250
Total Enrollment: 56,000

Healthplan and Services Defined
   PLAN TYPE: HMO/PPO
   Model Type: IPA
   Benefits Offered: Disease Management, Prescription, Wellness

Type of Coverage
   Commercial, Individual

Type of Payment Plans Offered
   POS

Geographic Areas Served
   Alachua, Lake, Marion, Orange, Osceola & Seminole counties

Subscriber Information
   Average Annual Deductible Per Subscriber:
      Employee Only (Self): $0
      Medicare: $0
   Average Subscriber Co-Payment:
      Primary Care Physician: $10.00
      Prescription Drugs: $7.00
      Hospital ER: $25.00

Network Qualifications
   Pre-Admission Certification: Yes

Peer Review Type
   Utilization Review: Yes
   Second Surgical Opinion: Yes
   Case Management: Yes

Publishes and Distributes Report Card: Yes
Accreditation Certification
   URAC, NCQA, CORE
   TJC Accreditation, Medicare Approved, Utilization Review,
      Pre-Admission Certification, State Licensure, Quality Assurance
      Program
Key Personnel
   President/CEO . . . . .Nancy Smith
   CFO . . . . .Brenda Radhe
   In House Formulary . . . . .Mauro Florentine
   Marketing . . . . .Michelle McPhail
   Materials Management . . . . .Kathy Basher
   Medical Affairs . . . . .Mark Reinecke, MD
   Provider Services . . . . .Julie Brown
Specialty Managed Care Partners
   Enters into Contracts with Regional Business Coalitions: Yes

---

**284   Humana Health Insurance of Tampa -
Pinellas**
1530 N. McMullen Booth Road
Suite D2
Clearwater, FL 33759
Toll-Free: 800-421-2491
Phone: 727-793-2100
Fax: 239-225-7315
www.humana.com
For Profit Organization: Yes
Year Founded: 1984
Number of Affiliated Hospitals: 29
Number of Primary Care Physicians: 600
Total Enrollment: 125,000

Healthplan and Services Defined
   PLAN TYPE: HMO/PPO
   Model Type: Staff, IPA, Network
   Benefits Offered: Disease Management, Prescription, Wellness

Type of Coverage
   Commercial, Individual
   Catastrophic Illness Benefit: Varies per case

Type of Payment Plans Offered
   DFFS, Capitated

Geographic Areas Served
   Citrus, DeSoto, Hardee, Highlands, Hillsborough, Hernando,
   Manatee, Pasco, Pinellas, Polk, Sarasota counties

Subscriber Information
   Average Monthly Fee Per Subscriber
      (Employee + Employer Contribution):
         Employee Only (Self): Varies
         Employee & 1 Family Member: Varies
         Employee & 2 Family Members: Varies
         Medicare: Varies
   Average Annual Deductible Per Subscriber:
         Employee Only (Self): Varies
         Employee & 1 Family Member: Varies
         Employee & 2 Family Members: Varies
         Medicare: Varies
   Average Subscriber Co-Payment:
         Primary Care Physician: Varies
         Non-Network Physician: Varies
         Prescription Drugs: Varies
         Hospital ER: Varies
         Home Health Care: Varies
         Home Health Care Max. Days/Visits Covered: Varies
         Nursing Home: Varies
         Nursing Home Max. Days/Visits Covered: Varies

Publishes and Distributes Report Card: Yes

Accreditation Certification
   AAAHC, URAC, NCQA

TJC Accreditation, State Licensure

Key Personnel
Chairman of The Board/CEO . . . . Michael B McCallister
COO . . . . James E Murray
SVP/CFO/Treasurer . . . . James H Bloem
In House Formulary . . . . Richard Nissenbaum, RPh
Media Relations Manager . . . . Mitch Lubitz
    813-287-6180
    mlubitz@humana.com

Specialty Managed Care Partners
Enters into Contracts with Regional Business Coalitions: Yes

285   JMH Health Plan

1801 NW 9th Avenue
Suite 100
Miami, FL 33136
Toll-Free: 877-547-2279
inquiries@jmhhp.com
www.jmhhp.com
Subsidiary of: Jackson Health System
Non-Profit Organization: Yes
Year Founded: 1985
Number of Affiliated Hospitals: 32
Number of Primary Care Physicians: 3,000
Total Enrollment: 105,000
State Enrollment: 105,000

Healthplan and Services Defined
  PLAN TYPE: HMO
  Model Type: Staff, Group
  Benefits Offered: Prescription

Type of Coverage
  Catastrophic Illness Benefit: Covered

Type of Payment Plans Offered
  POS, DFFS, Capitated

Geographic Areas Served
  South FL: Miami-Dade county

Subscriber Information
  Average Subscriber Co-Payment:
    Primary Care Physician: $10.00
    Prescription Drugs: $5.00
    Hospital ER: $25.00
    Home Health Care: $0
    Home Health Care Max. Days/Visits Covered: 60 days
    Nursing Home: $0
    Nursing Home Max. Days/Visits Covered: 90 days

Network Qualifications
  Pre-Admission Certification: No

Peer Review Type
  Utilization Review: Yes
  Second Surgical Opinion: Yes
  Case Management: Yes

Accreditation Certification
  AAAHC
  TJC Accreditation

Average Claim Compensation
  Physician's Fees Charged: 30%
  Hospital's Fees Charged: 19%

286   Leon Medical Centers Health Plan

11401 SW 40th Street
Suite 400
Miami, FL 33165
Toll-Free: 866-393-5366
Phone: 305-229-7461
membersupport@lmchealthplans.com
www.lmchealthplans.com

Subsidiary of: HealthSpring
For Profit Organization: Yes
Year Founded: 1996
Number of Affiliated Hospitals: 5
Number of Primary Care Physicians: 1,200
Total Enrollment: 27,000

Healthplan and Services Defined
  PLAN TYPE: HMO

Type of Coverage
  Supplemental Medicare, Medicare Advantage

Geographic Areas Served
  Miami-Dade County

Key Personnel
Director, Finance . . . . Mercy Kirkpatrick
Vice President, IT . . . . Jennifer Puglisi
Medical Director . . . . Alina Campos, MD
Human Resources Manager . . . . Carolina Garcia Castillo
Chief Operating Officer . . . . Henry Hernandez
President/CEO . . . . Albert Maury
Vice President, Claims . . . . Luis Fernandez

287   Medica HealthCare Plans, Inc

4000 Ponce de Leon Blvd
Suite 650
Coral Gables, FL 33146
Toll-Free: 800-407-9069
Phone: 305-460-0600
Fax: 305-460-0613
membersvc@medicaplans.com
www.medicaplans.com
Total Enrollment: 12,000

Healthplan and Services Defined
  PLAN TYPE: Medicare
  Benefits Offered: Disease Management, Wellness

Type of Coverage
  Medicare, Supplemental Medicare

Geographic Areas Served
  Miami-Dade & Broward counties

288   Molina Healthcare: Florida

8300 NW 33rd Street
Doral, FL 33122
Toll-Free: 866-472-4585
www.molinahealthcare.com
For Profit Organization: Yes
Year Founded: 1980
Physician Owned Organization: Yes
Number of Affiliated Hospitals: 84
Number of Primary Care Physicians: 2,167
Number of Referral/Specialty Physicians: 6,184
Total Enrollment: 1,800,000
State Enrollment: 69,000

Healthplan and Services Defined
  PLAN TYPE: HMO
  Model Type: Network
  Benefits Offered: Chiropractic, Dental, Home Care, Inpatient SNF,
    Long-Term Care, Podiatry, Vision

Type of Coverage
  Commercial, Medicare, Supplemental Medicare, Medicaid

Accreditation Certification
  URAC, NCQA

Key Personnel
President . . . . David Pollack

289 Neighborhood Health Partnership

7600 Corporate Center Drive
Miami, FL 33126
Toll-Free: 877-972-8845
Phone: 305-715-2500
www.neighborhood-health.com
Subsidiary of: UnitedHealthcare
For Profit Organization: Yes
Year Founded: 1993
Number of Affiliated Hospitals: 29
Number of Primary Care Physicians: 1,282
Total Enrollment: 108,000
State Enrollment: 141,178

Healthplan and Services Defined
PLAN TYPE: HMO
Other Type: POS

Type of Coverage
Commercial, Medicare

Type of Payment Plans Offered
Capitated

Geographic Areas Served
Miami-Dade, Broward and Palm Beach counties

Peer Review Type
Utilization Review: Yes

Publishes and Distributes Report Card: Yes

Accreditation Certification
NCQA

Key Personnel
President & CEO..........................Daniel Rosenthal
Chief Financial Officer........................Ramon Coto
VP, Provider Relations....................Maritza Borrajero

290 Optimum HealthCare, Inc

5403 North Church Ave
Tampa, FL 33614
Toll-Free: 866-245-5360
Fax: 813-506-6150
www.youroptimumhealthcare.com
Secondary Address: 8373 Northcliffe Blvd, Springhill, FL 34606

Healthplan and Services Defined
PLAN TYPE: Medicare

Geographic Areas Served
Brevard, Broward, Charlotte, Citrus, Clay, Collier, Dade, De Soto, Duval, Escambia, Hernando, Hillsborough, Indian River, Lake, Lee, Manatee, Marion, Martin, Orange, Osceola, Palm Beach, Pasco, Pinellas, Polk, Sarasota, Seminole, St. Lucie, Sumter and Volusia counties

Accreditation Certification
NCQA

291 Physicians United Plan

9102 SouthPark Circle
Suite 500
Orlando, FL 32819
Toll-Free: 888-827-5787
www.pupcorp.com
Secondary Address: 1372 6th St NW, Winter Haven, FL 33881,
863-293-6354
Year Founded: 2005

Healthplan and Services Defined
PLAN TYPE: Multiple
Other Type: HMO, Medicare
Benefits Offered: Dental, Prescription, Vision

Type of Coverage
Supplemental Medicare

Geographic Areas Served
Brevard, Broward, Palm Beach, Hillsborough, Pasco, Pinellas, Miami-Dade, Lake, Marion, Orange, Osceola, Polk, Seminole and Sumter counties

Accreditation Certification
URAC

Key Personnel
Chief Executive Officer......................James Kollefrath
President.................................Sandeep Bajaj
Chief Financial Officer......................Aaron S Henry
Compliance Officer............................Paul Christy
Dir, Enrollment.............................Ryan Horbal
Human Resources Manager.....................Jennifer Blue
VP, Sales & Operations.........................Shawn Holt
Media Contact..............................Ana Handshuh
407-619-3016
ahandshuh@pupcorp.com

292 Preferred Care Partners

9100 South Dadeland Boulevard
Miami, FL 33156
Toll-Free: 866-231-7201
Fax: 888-659-0618
memberservices@mypreferredcare.com
www.mypreferredcare.com
Mailing Address: PO Box 56-5748, Miami, FL 33256
Number of Affiliated Hospitals: 27
Number of Primary Care Physicians: 1,500
Total Enrollment: 45,000

Healthplan and Services Defined
PLAN TYPE: Multiple
Benefits Offered: Dental, Prescription, Vision, Hearing, Transportation, Fitness Programs

Type of Coverage
Supplemental Medicare

Geographic Areas Served
Miami-Dade, Broward, Marion, Lake & Sumter counties

Accreditation Certification
URAC

Key Personnel
President..................................Justo Luis Pozo
CEO..................................Joseph L Caruncho
SVP, COO...............................Roger Rodriguez
SVP/Chief Compliance Offc..............Annette C Onorati, Esq
Chairman, CMO..............Orlando Lopez-Fernandez, Jr, MD

293 Preferred Medical Plan

4950 SW 8th Street
Coral Gables, FL 33134
Toll-Free: 800-767-5551
Phone: 305-447-8373
Fax: 305-648-0420
info@pmphmo.com
www.pmphmo.com
For Profit Organization: Yes
Year Founded: 1972
Number of Affiliated Hospitals: 30
Number of Primary Care Physicians: 600
Total Enrollment: 52,000
State Enrollment: 39,776

Healthplan and Services Defined
PLAN TYPE: HMO
Model Type: Staff, Group
Benefits Offered: Disease Management, Prescription, Wellness

Type of Coverage
Individual, Family

Geographic Areas Served
Miami-Dade, Broward counties

Accreditation Certification
AAAHC

Key Personnel
President/CEO ....Tamara Meyerson
CFO ....Albert Arca
COO ....Nancy Garcia
Marketing ....Estella Ginoris
Dir, Patient Relations ....Rosie Lopez-Casiro
Chief Information Officer ....Paul Bell

---

294 Risk Placement Services, Inc.
3030 North Rocky Point Drive West
Suite 161
Tampa, FL 33607
Toll-Free: 866-595-8413
Phone: 813-288-8522
Fax: 719-528-8323
www.avalonhealthcare.com
For Profit Organization: Yes
Total Enrollment: 6,000

Healthplan and Services Defined
PLAN TYPE: PPO
Benefits Offered: Dental, Prescription, Vision

Type of Coverage
Commercial, Individual

---

295 SafeGuard Health Enterprises: Florida
8207 SW 124th Street
Pinecrest, CA 33156
Toll-Free: 800-880-1800
Phone: 305-252-9304
Fax: 305-252-9306
office@floridasafeguard.com
www.safeguard.net
Subsidiary of: MetLife
For Profit Organization: Yes
Year Founded: 1974
Number of Primary Care Physicians: 2,073
Number of Referral/Specialty Physicians: 2,030
Total Enrollment: 1,800,000

Healthplan and Services Defined
PLAN TYPE: Dental
Other Type: Dental HMO
Model Type: IPA
Plan Specialty: ASO, Dental, Vision
Benefits Offered: Dental, Vision

Type of Coverage
Individual, Indemnity, Medicaid

Type of Payment Plans Offered
DFFS, Capitated

Geographic Areas Served
California, Texas, Florida

Subscriber Information
Average Annual Deductible Per Subscriber:
Employee Only (Self): $50.00
Employee & 1 Family Member: $100.00
Employee & 2 Family Members: $150.00

Network Qualifications
Pre-Admission Certification: Yes

Peer Review Type
Utilization Review: Yes

Publishes and Distributes Report Card: No
Key Personnel
Chairman/CEO ....Steven A Kandarian
EVP/CFO ....John Hele
VP/CIO ....Michael J Lauffenburger
SVP/General Counsel.......................Nicholas Latrenta
Dir/Human Resources ....Frans Hijkoop
Director ....Jack R Anderson

Specialty Managed Care Partners
Enters into Contracts with Regional Business Coalitions: Yes
Employer References
State of California, Gulfstream Aerospace, AFGE, Boward County,
City of San Antonio

---

296 Total Health Choice
PO Box 830010
Miami, FL 33283-0010
Toll-Free: 800-887-6888
Phone: 305-408-5700
Fax: 305-408-5858
info@thc-online.com
www.fl.thconline.us
Subsidiary of: Total Health Care, Inc. of Michigan
Non-Profit Organization: Yes
Year Founded: 1997
Owned by an Integrated Delivery Network (IDN): Yes
Number of Affiliated Hospitals: 28
Number of Primary Care Physicians: 600
Number of Referral/Specialty Physicians: 1,200
Total Enrollment: 10,000
State Enrollment: 15,347

Healthplan and Services Defined
PLAN TYPE: HMO
Model Type: Group
Plan Specialty: Disease Management, Worker's Compensation,
Prescription
Benefits Offered: Behavioral Health, Chiropractic, Disease
Management, Physical Therapy, Podiatry, Prescription, Wellness,
Worker's Compensation, Life, LTD

Type of Coverage
Commercial, Individual, Supplemental Medicare, Medicaid,
Catastrophic
Catastrophic Illness Benefit: Varies per case

Type of Payment Plans Offered
POS, DFFS, FFS

Geographic Areas Served
Broward, Miami-Dade counties

Subscriber Information
Average Subscriber Co-Payment:
Primary Care Physician: $5.00
Prescription Drugs: $5.00

Network Qualifications
Pre-Admission Certification: Yes

Peer Review Type
Utilization Review: No
Second Surgical Opinion: Yes
Case Management: Yes

Publishes and Distributes Report Card: Yes

Accreditation Certification
AAAHC
Medicare Approved, State Licensure, Quality Assurance Program

Key Personnel
Owner....................................Kenneth Rimmer
CEO.......................................Michael Ross
CFO ....Gerry Hammond
Marketing ....Carlos Martinez

Medical Affairs . . . . Robyn Arrington, MD
Provider Services . . . . Sergie Covas

Specialty Managed Care Partners
Enters into Contracts with Regional Business Coalitions: Yes

297 United Concordia: Florida

1408 N Westshore Blvd
Suite 512
Tampa, FL 33607
Toll-Free: 800-972-4191
Phone: 813-287-1823
Fax: 813-287-1819
ucproducer@ucci.com
www.secure.ucci.com
For Profit Organization: Yes
Year Founded: 1971
Number of Primary Care Physicians: 111,000
Total Enrollment: 8,000,000

Healthplan and Services Defined
PLAN TYPE: Dental
Plan Specialty: Dental
Benefits Offered: Dental

Type of Coverage
Commercial, Individual

Geographic Areas Served
Military personnel and their families, nationwide

298 UnitedHealthCare of Florida

10151 Deerwood Park
Bldg 100, Suite 420
Jacksonville, FL 32256
Toll-Free: 800-250-6178
www.uhc.com
Secondary Address: 495 North Keller Road, Maitland, FL 32751,
800-899-6500
Subsidiary of: UnitedHealth Group
For Profit Organization: Yes
Owned by an Integrated Delivery Network (IDN): Yes
Total Enrollment: 75,000,000
State Enrollment: 870,159

Healthplan and Services Defined
PLAN TYPE: HMO/PPO
Model Type: Group
Plan Specialty: Full Service
Benefits Offered: Behavioral Health, Chiropractic, Dental, Disease
Management, Home Care, Inpatient SNF, Physical Therapy,
Podiatry, Prescription, Psychiatric, Transplant, Vision, Wellness,
AD&D, Life, LTD, STD

Type of Coverage
Commercial

Geographic Areas Served
Central/North Florida

Subscriber Information
Average Monthly Fee Per Subscriber
(Employee + Employer Contribution):
Employee Only (Self): Varies

Peer Review Type
Case Management: Yes

Accreditation Certification
TJC, NCQA

Key Personnel
President/CEO . . . . Matthew Davies
Media Contact . . . . Liz Calzadilla-Fiallo
elizabeth.calzadilla-fiallo@uhc.com

Specialty Managed Care Partners
Own Network
Enters into Contracts with Regional Business Coalitions: Yes

299 UnitedHealthCare of South Florida

13621 NW 12th Street
Sunrise, FL 33323
Toll-Free: 800-825-8792
www.uhc.com
Secondary Address: 9009 Corporate Lake Drive, Suite 200, Tampa, FL
33634, 800-595-0440
Subsidiary of: UnitedHealth Group
For Profit Organization: Yes
Year Founded: 1970
Number of Affiliated Hospitals: 58
Number of Primary Care Physicians: 2,500
Number of Referral/Specialty Physicians: 4,500
Total Enrollment: 75,000,000
State Enrollment: 295,000

Healthplan and Services Defined
PLAN TYPE: HMO/PPO
Model Type: Network
Plan Specialty: ASO, Behavioral Health, Chiropractic, Dental,
Disease Management
Benefits Offered: Behavioral Health, Chiropractic, Complementary
Medicine, Dental, Disease Management, Physical Therapy,
Podiatry, Prescription, Psychiatric, Vision, Wellness, AD&D, Life,
LTD, STD
Offers Demand Management Patient Information Service: Yes

Type of Coverage
Commercial
Catastrophic Illness Benefit: Varies per case

Type of Payment Plans Offered
POS, DFFS, Capitated, FFS, Combination FFS & DFFS

Geographic Areas Served
Palm Beach, Broward & Dade counties

Subscriber Information
Average Subscriber Co-Payment:
Primary Care Physician: $5.00-15.00
Non-Network Physician: Varies
Prescription Drugs: $5.00-10.00
Hospital ER: $100.00

Network Qualifications
Pre-Admission Certification: Yes

Peer Review Type
Utilization Review: Yes
Second Surgical Opinion: Yes
Case Management: Yes

Publishes and Distributes Report Card: Yes

Accreditation Certification
AAAHC, URAC, NCQA
TJC Accreditation, Medicare Approved, Utilization Review,
Pre-Admission Certification, State Licensure, Quality Assurance
Program

Key Personnel
CEO . . . . Dan Rosenthal
CFO . . . . Jon Schwarz
Network Contracting . . . . Jonathan Gavras, MD
Marketing . . . . Lawrence J Kissner
Medical Affairs . . . . Jonathan Gavras, MD
Sales . . . . Albert Fernandez
Media Contact . . . . Liz Calzadilla-Fiallo
elizabeth.calzadilla-fiallo@uhc.com

Specialty Managed Care Partners
Enters into Contracts with Regional Business Coalitions: No

300 Universal Health Care Group

100 Central Ave
Suite 200
St Petersburg, FL 33701
Toll-Free: 866-690-4842
www.univhc.com
Secondary Address: 2713 Forest Road, Spring Hill, FL 34606
Year Founded: 2002
State Enrollment: 191,000

Healthplan and Services Defined
PLAN TYPE: Medicare

Type of Coverage
Individual, Medicare, Supplemental Medicare, Medicaid

Key Personnel
Chairman & CEO . . . . A.K. Desai, MD, MPH
Chief Operating Officer . . . . Michael P Holohan
CAO/General Counsel . . . . Sandip Patel
Interim CFO . . . . Deepak Desai
SVP, Sales & Marketing . . . . Jeff Ludy

301 VSP: Vision Service Plan of Florida

3001 N Rocky Point Drive East
Suite 200
Tampa, FL 33607-5806
Fax: 813-281-4605
webmaster@vsp.com
www.vsp.com
Non-Profit Organization: Yes
Year Founded: 1955
Number of Primary Care Physicians: 28,000
Total Enrollment: 57,000,000

Healthplan and Services Defined
PLAN TYPE: Vision
Plan Specialty: Vision
Benefits Offered: Vision

Type of Payment Plans Offered
Capitated

Geographic Areas Served
Statewide

Network Qualifications
Pre-Admission Certification: Yes

Peer Review Type
Utilization Review: Yes

Accreditation Certification
Utilization Review, Quality Assurance Program

Key Personnel
VSP Global President/CEO . . . . Rob Lynch

302 WellCare Health Plans

PO Box 31372
Tampa, FL 33631-3372
Toll-Free: 866-530-9491
Phone: 813-290-6200
Fax: 813-262-2802
www.wellcare.com
For Profit Organization: Yes
Year Founded: 1985
Number of Affiliated Hospitals: 83
Number of Primary Care Physicians: 2,091
Total Enrollment: 2,600,000
State Enrollment: 2,200,000

Healthplan and Services Defined
PLAN TYPE: Medicare
Model Type: IPA
Benefits Offered: Disease Management, Prescription, Wellness

Type of Coverage
Medicare, Medicaid
Catastrophic Illness Benefit: Unlimited

Type of Payment Plans Offered
POS, Combination FFS & DFFS

Geographic Areas Served
Connecticut, Florida, Georgia, Hawaii, Illinois, Indiana, Missouri,
New Jersey, New York, Ohio, Texas

Subscriber Information
Average Subscriber Co-Payment:
Primary Care Physician: $10.00
Prescription Drugs: $8.00
Hospital ER: $35.00
Home Health Care: $10.00
Home Health Care Max. Days/Visits Covered: Unlimited
Nursing Home Max. Days/Visits Covered: 120 days

Network Qualifications
Pre-Admission Certification: Yes

Peer Review Type
Utilization Review: Yes
Second Surgical Opinion: Yes
Case Management: Yes

Publishes and Distributes Report Card: Yes

Accreditation Certification
NCQA
TJC Accreditation, Medicare Approved, Utilization Review,
Pre-Admission Certification, State Licensure, Quality Assurance
Program

Key Personnel
Chief Executive Officer . . . . Alec Cunningham
SVP/Chief Human Resources . . . . Lawrence D. Anderson
SVP/Chief Financial Offic . . . . Thomas L. Tran
SVP/Chief Compliance Offi . . . . Blaire W. Todt
SVP/General Counsel & Sec . . . . Lisa G. Iglesias
President, North Division . . . . Marc S Russo
SVP/Chief Medical Officer . . . . Steven Goldberg

Health Insurance Coverage Status and Type of Coverage by Age

Category	All Persons		Under 18 years		Under 65 years		65 years and over	
	Number	%	Number	%	Number	%	Number	%
Total population	9,801	-	2,487	-	8,639	-	1,162	-
Covered by some type of health insurance	7,955 *(29)*	81.2 *(0.3)*	2,249 *(12)*	90.4 *(0.5)*	6,808 *(29)*	78.8 *(0.3)*	1,146 *(5)*	98.7 *(0.2)*
Covered by private health insurance	6,029 *(40)*	61.5 *(0.4)*	1,326 *(20)*	53.3 *(0.8)*	5,334 *(39)*	61.7 *(0.4)*	695 *(10)*	59.8 *(0.9)*
Employment based	4,998 *(39)*	51.0 *(0.4)*	1,129 *(20)*	45.4 *(0.8)*	4,583 *(39)*	53.1 *(0.4)*	415 *(9)*	35.7 *(0.8)*
Direct purchase	995 *(22)*	10.2 *(0.2)*	140 *(8)*	5.6 *(0.3)*	686 *(20)*	7.9 *(0.2)*	309 *(8)*	26.6 *(0.7)*
Covered by TRICARE	399 *(16)*	4.1 *(0.2)*	99 *(7)*	4.0 *(0.3)*	301 *(16)*	3.5 *(0.2)*	98 *(6)*	8.5 *(0.5)*
Covered by government health insurance	2,856 *(28)*	29.1 *(0.3)*	996 *(19)*	40.0 *(0.7)*	1,738 *(27)*	20.1 *(0.3)*	1,118 *(5)*	96.2 *(0.3)*
Covered by Medicaid	1,671 *(25)*	17.0 *(0.3)*	980 *(19)*	39.4 *(0.8)*	1,496 *(26)*	17.3 *(0.3)*	174 *(7)*	15.0 *(0.6)*
Also by private insurance	219 *(11)*	2.2 *(0.1)*	71 *(6)*	2.8 *(0.2)*	154 *(10)*	1.8 *(0.1)*	65 *(4)*	5.6 *(0.3)*
Covered by Medicare	1,370 *(12)*	14.0 *(0.1)*	21 *(4)*	0.8 *(0.2)*	253 *(11)*	2.9 *(0.1)*	1,117 *(5)*	96.1 *(0.3)*
Also by private insurance	735 *(12)*	7.5 *(0.1)*	3 *(1)*	0.1 *(0.1)*	69 *(4)*	0.8 *(0.1)*	666 *(10)*	57.3 *(0.9)*
Also by Medicaid	285 *(9)*	2.9 *(0.1)*	8 *(2)*	0.3 *(0.1)*	111 *(6)*	1.3 *(0.1)*	174 *(7)*	15.0 *(0.6)*
Covered by VA Care	213 *(8)*	2.2 *(0.1)*	3 *(2)*	0.1 *(0.1)*	121 *(7)*	1.4 *(0.1)*	92 *(4)*	7.9 *(0.3)*
Not covered at any time during the year	1,846 *(30)*	18.8 *(0.3)*	238 *(12)*	9.6 *(0.5)*	1,831 *(29)*	21.2 *(0.3)*	16 *(3)*	1.3 *(0.2)*

Note: Numbers in thousands; Figures cover 2013; Margin of error appears in parenthesis; A "Z" indicates that the value either represents or rounds to zero.
Source: U.S. Census Bureau, 2013 American Community Survey, Table HI05. Health Insurance Coverage Status and Type of Coverage by State and Age for All People: 2013

Georgia

303 Aetna Health of Georgia

11675 Great Oaks Way
Atlanta, GA 30022
Toll-Free: 866-582-9629
Phone: 770-346-4300
Fax: 770-346-4490
www.aetna.com
For Profit Organization: Yes
Year Founded: 1986
Number of Affiliated Hospitals: 28
Number of Primary Care Physicians: 469
Number of Referral/Specialty Physicians: 1,200
Total Enrollment: 116,375
State Enrollment: 116,375

Healthplan and Services Defined
PLAN TYPE: HMO
Model Type: IPA
Benefits Offered: Disease Management, Prescription, Wellness

Type of Coverage
Catastrophic Illness Benefit: Unlimited

Type of Payment Plans Offered
DFFS, Capitated

Geographic Areas Served
Statewide

Subscriber Information
Average Annual Deductible Per Subscriber:
Employee Only (Self): $0
Employee & 2 Family Members: $0
Average Subscriber Co-Payment:
Primary Care Physician: $10.00
Non-Network Physician: Not covered
Prescription Drugs: $5.00
Hospital ER: $35.00
Home Health Care: $0
Home Health Care Max. Days/Visits Covered: Unlimited
Nursing Home: $0
Nursing Home Max. Days/Visits Covered: 100/yr.

Network Qualifications
Pre-Admission Certification: Yes

Peer Review Type
Second Surgical Opinion: Yes
Case Management: Yes

Accreditation Certification
NCQA
TJC Accreditation, Pre-Admission Certification

Key Personnel
Chmn/President/CEO . . . . Mark T Bertolini

Specialty Managed Care Partners
Enters into Contracts with Regional Business Coalitions: No

304 Alere Health

51 Sawyer Road
Suite 200
Waltham, GA 02453-3448
Toll-Free: 800-456-4060
Phone: 781-647-3900
salesinquiry@alere.com
www.alere.com
Secondary Address: 10615 Professional Circle, Reno, NV 89521
For Profit Organization: Yes
Year Founded: 2008
Number of Primary Care Physicians: 1,200

Healthplan and Services Defined
PLAN TYPE: PPO

Key Personnel
President/CEO . . . . Ron Zwanziger
President, Free & Clear . . . . Tim Kilgallon
President, Health Improv. . . . . Michael L Cotton
President, Women's Health . . . . Gregg E Raybuck
EVP, Technology Solutions . . . . Douglas Albro
EVP, General Counsel . . . . Craig Apolinsky
EVP, Performance . . . . Julie Griffin
SVP, Enterprise Marketing . . . . Scott McClintock
Chief Innovation Officer . . . . Gordon K Norman, MD/MBA
Media Contact. . . . . Jan McClure
770-559-1016
janm@mccluremedia.com

305 Alliant Health Plans

600 TownPark Lane NW
Suite LL-1000
Kennesaw, GA 30144
Toll-Free: 877-668-1015
Phone: 800-811-4793
Fax: 770-499-9876
information@alliantplans.com
www.alliantplans.com
Non-Profit Organization: Yes
Year Founded: 1998
Physician Owned Organization: Yes
Number of Affiliated Hospitals: 9,999
Number of Primary Care Physicians: 500,000
Total Enrollment: 15,000
State Enrollment: 15,000

Healthplan and Services Defined
PLAN TYPE: HMO/PPO
Model Type: PSHCC

Type of Coverage
Commercial, Individual

Key Personnel
CEO . . . . Judy Pair
CFO . . . . Sara Carpenter
COO . . . . Al Ertel
VP/Sales & Marketing . . . . Mark Mixer

306 Amerigroup Georgia

303 Perimeter Center North
Suite 400
Atlanta, GA 30346
Toll-Free: 888-423-6765
Phone: 757-490-6900
www.realsolutions.com
Secondary Address: 621 Northwest Frontage Road, Suite 100, Augusta, GA 30907
For Profit Organization: Yes
Year Founded: 2006
Total Enrollment: 1,900,000
State Enrollment: 287,000

Healthplan and Services Defined
PLAN TYPE: HMO
Benefits Offered: Prescription

Type of Coverage
Medicaid, PeachCare, Planning for Healthy Bab

Accreditation Certification
NCQA

Key Personnel
Chief Compliance Officer . . . . Georgia Dodds Foley
VP, External Comms. . . . . Maureen C McDonnell

307   Assurant Employee Benefits: Georgia

780 Johnson Ferry Road NE
Atlanta, GA 30342-1434
benefits@assurant.com
www.assurantemployeebenefits.com
Subsidiary of: Assurant, Inc
For Profit Organization: Yes
Number of Primary Care Physicians: 112,000
Total Enrollment: 47,000

Healthplan and Services Defined
  PLAN TYPE: Multiple
  Plan Specialty: Dental, Vision, Long & Short-Term Disability
  Benefits Offered: Dental, Vision, Wellness, AD&D, Life, LTD, STD

Type of Coverage
  Commercial, Indemnity, Individual Dental Plans

Geographic Areas Served
  Statewide

Subscriber Information
  Average Monthly Fee Per Subscriber
    (Employee + Employer Contribution):
      Employee Only (Self): Varies by plan

Key Personnel
  Partner .... Pace Schuchmann
  VP, Sales & Marketing........................... Mike Geren
  PR Specialist.............................. Megan Hutchison
    816-556-7815
    megan.hutchison@assurant.com

308   Athens Area Health Plan Select

295 West Clayton Street
Athens, GA 30601
Toll-Free: 800-293-6260
Phone: 706-549-0549
Fax: 706-549-8004
memberservices@aahps.com
www.aahps.com
Subsidiary of: Athens Regional Health Services
Non-Profit Organization: Yes
Year Founded: 1997
Number of Affiliated Hospitals: 1
Number of Primary Care Physicians: 1,000
Total Enrollment: 23,241
State Enrollment: 23,241

Healthplan and Services Defined
  PLAN TYPE: HMO
  Other Type: POS
  Benefits Offered: Disease Management, Prescription, Wellness,
    Durable Medical Equipment
  Offers Demand Management Patient Information Service: Yes
  DMPI Services Offered: 24 hour nurse line

Type of Coverage
  Commercial, Self-Insured

Geographic Areas Served
  27 counties in northeast Georgia

Accreditation Certification
  URAC

Key Personnel
  Medical Director .... Thomas Wells, MD
  Chief Medical Officer .... Geoffrey Cole, MD
    gcole@aahps.com

309   Avesis: Arizona

3030 N Central Ave
Suite 300
Phoenix, AZ 85012
Toll-Free: 800-522-0258
Fax: 602-240-9100
www.avesis.com
Year Founded: 1978
Number of Primary Care Physicians: 18,000
Total Enrollment: 2,000,000

Healthplan and Services Defined
  PLAN TYPE: PPO
  Model Type: Network
  Plan Specialty: Dental, Vision, Hearing
  Benefits Offered: Dental, Vision

Type of Coverage
  Commercial

Type of Payment Plans Offered
  POS, Capitated, Combination FFS & DFFS

Geographic Areas Served
  Nationwide and Puerto Rico

Publishes and Distributes Report Card: Yes

Accreditation Certification
  AAAHC
  TJC Accreditation

Key Personnel
  Chief Executive Officer........................... Alan Cohn
  Chief Financial Officer .... Joel Alperstein
  Chief Operation Officer .... Linda Chirichella
  Chief Marketing Officer..................... Michael Reamer
  Chief Information Officer......................... Laura Gill

310   Blue Cross & Blue Shield of Georgia

3350 Peachtree Road NE
Atlanta, GA 30326
Phone: 404-842-8000
www.bcbsga.com
Secondary Address: 2357 Warm Springs Road, Columbus, GA 31909
For Profit Organization: Yes
Year Founded: 1937
Number of Affiliated Hospitals: 196
Number of Primary Care Physicians: 19,000
Total Enrollment: 3,300,000
State Enrollment: 500,733

Healthplan and Services Defined
  PLAN TYPE: HMO
  Model Type: Network
  Plan Specialty: ASO, Behavioral Health, Chiropractic, Dental,
    Disease Management, EPO, Lab, MSO, PBM, Vision, Radiology,
    Worker's Compensation, UR
  Benefits Offered: Behavioral Health, Chiropractic, Complementary
    Medicine, Dental, Disease Management, Home Care, Inpatient
    SNF, Physical Therapy, Podiatry, Prescription, Psychiatric,
    Transplant, Vision, Wellness, AD&D, Life
  Offers Demand Management Patient Information Service: Yes

Type of Coverage
  Commercial, Individual, Indemnity, Medicare, Supplemental
    Medicare

Type of Payment Plans Offered
  POS, DFFS, Capitated, FFS

Geographic Areas Served
  Statewide

Network Qualifications
  Pre-Admission Certification: Yes

Peer Review Type
  Utilization Review: Yes

Case Management: Yes

Publishes and Distributes Report Card: Yes

Accreditation Certification
AAAHC, URAC, NCQA
TJC Accreditation, Medicare Approved, Utilization Review,
Pre-Admission Certification, State Licensure, Quality Assurance
Program

Average Claim Compensation
Physician's Fees Charged: 1%
Hospital's Fees Charged: 1%

Specialty Managed Care Partners
Wellpoint Dental Services, Greater Georgia Life, Wellpoint
Pharmacy Management, Wellpoint Behavioral Health
Enters into Contracts with Regional Business Coalitions: Yes

311 CIGNA HealthCare of Georgia

3500 Piedmont Road NE
Suite 200
Atlanta, GA 30305
Toll-Free: 800-526-5481
Phone: 404-443-8800
Fax: 404-443-8932
www.cigna.com
Mailing Address: PO Box 740022, Atlanta, GA 30374
Subsidiary of: CIGNA Corporation
For Profit Organization: Yes
Year Founded: 1981
Owned by an Integrated Delivery Network (IDN): Yes
Number of Primary Care Physicians: 16,000
Number of Referral/Specialty Physicians: 7,683
Total Enrollment: 25,769
State Enrollment: 25,769

Healthplan and Services Defined
PLAN TYPE: HMO
Other Type: POS
Model Type: IPA
Plan Specialty: ASO, Behavioral Health, Chiropractic, Dental,
Disease Management, EPO, Lab, MSO, PBM, Vision, Radiology,
UR
Benefits Offered: Behavioral Health, Chiropractic, Dental, Disease
Management, Home Care, Inpatient SNF, Physical Therapy,
Podiatry, Prescription, Psychiatric, Transplant, Vision, Wellness,
Life

Type of Coverage
Commercial

Type of Payment Plans Offered
FFS, Combination FFS & DFFS

Geographic Areas Served
Atlanta & Metro Area

Subscriber Information
Average Annual Deductible Per Subscriber:
Employee Only (Self): $0
Employee & 1 Family Member: $0
Employee & 2 Family Members: $0
Average Subscriber Co-Payment:
Primary Care Physician: $15.00
Non-Network Physician: Varies
Prescription Drugs: $10.00
Hospital ER: $50.00
Home Health Care: $0

Network Qualifications
Pre-Admission Certification: Yes

Peer Review Type
Utilization Review: Yes
Second Surgical Opinion: Yes
Case Management: Yes

Publishes and Distributes Report Card: Yes

Accreditation Certification
NCQA
TJC Accreditation, Utilization Review, Pre-Admission Certification,
State Licensure, Quality Assurance Program

Key Personnel
President/General Manager . . . . .Scott Evelyn
Network Contracting. . . . . .Vernice Gailey
Credentialing . . . . .Rita Rakestraw
In House Formulary. .Marybeth Luptowski
Marketing. . . . . .Stephen Joiner
Chief Medical Officer . . . . .Mary Caufield, MD
Provider Services . . . . .Karen Little

Specialty Managed Care Partners
Enters into Contracts with Regional Business Coalitions: No

312 CNA Insurance Companies: Georgia

2435 Commerce Avenue
Building 2200 Satellite Place
Duluth, GA 30096
Toll-Free: 800-282-7084
Phone: 678-473-3700
Fax: 866-512-2301
cna_help@cna.com
www.cna.com
Year Founded: 1897
Number of Affiliated Hospitals: 57
Number of Primary Care Physicians: 3,400
Total Enrollment: 270,000

Healthplan and Services Defined
PLAN TYPE: PPO
Model Type: Network
Plan Specialty: Worker's Compensation
Benefits Offered: Prescription

Type of Coverage
Catastrophic Illness Benefit: Varies per case

Type of Payment Plans Offered
POS, DFFS, Capitated, FFS, Combination FFS & DFFS

Geographic Areas Served
Nationwide

Network Qualifications
Pre-Admission Certification: Yes

Peer Review Type
Utilization Review: Yes
Second Surgical Opinion: Yes
Case Management: Yes

Accreditation Certification
TJC Accreditation, Medicare Approved, Utilization Review,
Pre-Admission Certification, State Licensure, Quality Assurance
Program

Key Personnel
Chairman/CEO . . . . .Thomas F Motamed
President/COO . . . . .Bob Lindemann
EVP, Chief Actuary. . . . . .Larry A Haefner
EVP, Worldwide P&C Claim .George R Fay
EVP, General Counsel. .Johnathan D Kantor
EVP/CFO . . . . .D Craig Mense
EVP, Chief Admin Officer. . . . . .Thomas Pontarelli
President, COO CNA Spec . . . . .Peter W Wilson
President, Field Oper . . . . .Tim Szerlong
SVP, CNA Select Risk . . . . .John Angerami
SVP, Business Insurance .Michael W Covne
Mid-Atlantic Zone Officer. . . . . .George Agven
Western Zone Officer . . . . .Steve Stonehouse
Central Zone Officer . . . . .Greg Vezzosi
Northern Zone Officer . . . . .Steve Wachtel

Media Contact . . . . Katrina W Parker
312-822-5167

Specialty Managed Care Partners
Enters into Contracts with Regional Business Coalitions: No

---

313   CompBenefits Corporation

100 Mansell Court East
Suite 400
Roswell, GA 30076-4859
Toll-Free: 800-633-1262
Fax: 770-998-6871
www.compbenefits.com
Subsidiary of: Humana
Year Founded: 1978
Owned by an Integrated Delivery Network (IDN): Yes
Total Enrollment: 4,800,000

Healthplan and Services Defined
PLAN TYPE: Multiple
Model Type: Network, HMO, PPO, POS, TPA
Plan Specialty: ASO, Dental, Vision
Benefits Offered: Dental, Vision

Type of Coverage
Commercial, Individual, Indemnity

Type of Payment Plans Offered
DFFS, Capitated, FFS

Geographic Areas Served
Alabama, Arkansas, Illinois, Indiana, Georgia, Florida, Mississippi, Missouri, Kentucky, Kansas, North Carolina, South Carolina, West Virginia, Texas, Tennessee, Ohio, Louisiana

Publishes and Distributes Report Card: Yes

Key Personnel
President/CEO . . . . Gerald L Ganoni
Exec VP/CFO . . . . George Dunaway
Dir, Vice Chairman . . . . Stanley Shapiro
Director . . . . Larry Fisher
Sr VP Marketing . . . . Judith Herron

Specialty Managed Care Partners
Enters into Contracts with Regional Business Coalitions: Yes

Employer References
Royal Caribbean Cruise Line, Tupperware

---

314   Coventry Health Care of GA

1100 Circle 75 Parkway
Suite 1400
Atlanta, GA 30339
Toll-Free: 800-470-2004
Phone: 678-202-2100
http://chcgeorgia.coventryhealthcare.com
Secondary Address: 7402 Hodgson Memorial Drive, 1st Floor, Suite 105, Savannah, GA 31406, 866-875-7284
Subsidiary of: Coventry Health Care Inc.
For Profit Organization: Yes
Year Founded: 1994
Number of Affiliated Hospitals: 86
Number of Primary Care Physicians: 17,000
Total Enrollment: 150,000
State Enrollment: 183,000

Healthplan and Services Defined
PLAN TYPE: HMO/PPO
Other Type: POS
Model Type: Group, Individual, Medicare Adv
Benefits Offered: Disease Management, Prescription, Wellness

Geographic Areas Served
71 counties in Georgia

Publishes and Distributes Report Card: Yes

Accreditation Certification
AAAHC, URAC

Key Personnel
CEO . . . . Thomas Davis
CFO . . . . Paul Farrell
COO . . . . Angela Meoli
Director . . . . Mark Norato
VP Sales/Marketing . . . . Cory Scott

Specialty Managed Care Partners
Enters into Contracts with Regional Business Coalitions: Yes

---

315   Delta Dental of Alabama

P.O. Box 1809
Alpharetta, GA 30023-1809
Toll-Free: 800-521-2651
www.deltadentalins.com
Non-Profit Organization: Yes
Total Enrollment: 59,000,000

Healthplan and Services Defined
PLAN TYPE: Dental
Other Type: Dental PPO
Plan Specialty: Dental
Benefits Offered: Dental

Type of Coverage
Commercial

Geographic Areas Served
Statewide

Key Personnel
Director Sales . . . . Frazier Sherrill
VP, Public & Govt Affairs . . . . Chris Pyle
630-574-6850

---

316   Delta Dental of Georgia

1130 Sanctuary Parkway
Suite 600
Alpharetta, GA 30004
Toll-Free: 888-858-5252
Phone: 770-645-8700
Fax: 770-641-5234
4gasales@delta.org
www.deltadentalins.com
Non-Profit Organization: Yes
Number of Primary Care Physicians: 198,000
Total Enrollment: 54,000,000

Healthplan and Services Defined
PLAN TYPE: Dental
Other Type: Dental PPO
Plan Specialty: Dental
Benefits Offered: Dental

Type of Coverage
Commercial

Type of Payment Plans Offered
POS, DFFS, FFS

Geographic Areas Served
Statewide

Key Personnel
President/CEO . . . . Gary D Radine
Director, Sales . . . . Frazier Sherrill
770-641-5196
VP, Public & Govt Affairs . . . . Jeff Album
415-972-8418
Dir/Media & Public Affair . . . . Elizabeth Risberg
415-972-8423

317 Delta Dental of Nevada

P.O. Box 1803
Alpharetta, GA 30023-1809
Toll-Free: 800-521-2651
www.deltadentalins.com
Non-Profit Organization: Yes
Total Enrollment: 54,000,000

Healthplan and Services Defined
  PLAN TYPE: Dental
  Other Type: Dental PPO

Type of Coverage
  Commercial

Geographic Areas Served
  Statewide

Key Personnel
  VP, Public & Govt Affairs . . . . .Jeff Album
    415-972-8418
  Dir/Media & Public Affair . . . . .Elizabeth Risberg
    415-972-8423

318 eHealthInsurance Services Inc.

11919 Foundation Place
Gold River, CA 95670
Toll-Free: 800-644-3491
webmaster@healthinsurance.com
www.e.healthinsurance.com
Year Founded: 1997

Healthplan and Services Defined
  PLAN TYPE: HMO/PPO
  Benefits Offered: Dental, Life, STD

Type of Coverage
  Commercial, Individual, Medicare

Geographic Areas Served
  All 50 states in the USA and District of Columbia

Key Personnel
  Chairman & CEO . . . . .Gary L. Lauer
  EVP/Business & Corp. Dev. .Bruce Telkamp
  EVP/Chief Technology .Dr. Sheldon X. Wang
  SVP & CFO . . . . .Stuart M. Huizinga
  Pres. of eHealth Gov. Sys . . . . .Samuel C. Gibbs
  SVP of Sales & Operations . . . . .Robert S. Hurley
  Director Public Relations. . . . . .Nate Purpura
    650-210-3115

319 Great-West Healthcare Georgia

245 Perimeter Center Parkway
Tenth Floor
Atlanta, GA 30346
Toll-Free: 866-225-0736
Phone: 770-290-7000
eliginquiries@cigna.com
www.cignaforhealth.com
Subsidiary of: CIGNA HealthCare
Acquired by: CIGNA
For Profit Organization: Yes
Total Enrollment: 49,984
State Enrollment: 1,545

Healthplan and Services Defined
  PLAN TYPE: HMO/PPO
  Benefits Offered: Disease Management, Prescription, Wellness

Type of Coverage
  Commercial

Type of Payment Plans Offered
  POS, FFS

Geographic Areas Served
  Georgia

Accreditation Certification
  URAC

Specialty Managed Care Partners
  Caremark Rx

320 Humana Health Insurance of Georgia

1200 Ashwood Parkway
Sutie 180
Atlanta, GA 30328
Toll-Free: 800-986-9527
Phone: 770-508-2388
Fax: 770-391-1423
www.humana.com
For Profit Organization: Yes
Year Founded: 1961
Number of Affiliated Hospitals: 144
Number of Primary Care Physicians: 3,464
Number of Referral/Specialty Physicians: 6,452
Total Enrollment: 73,000
State Enrollment: 82,000

Healthplan and Services Defined
  PLAN TYPE: HMO/PPO
  Model Type: Network
  Benefits Offered: Behavioral Health, Chiropractic, Dental, Disease
    Management, Prescription, Psychiatric, Transplant, Wellness,
    Worker's Compensation

Type of Coverage
  Commercial, Individual, Medicare, Supplemental Medicare

Geographic Areas Served
  Statewide

Accreditation Certification
  URAC, NCQA, CORE

Key Personnel
  Chairman. . . . . .David A Jones, Jr
  Executive Director . . . . .Dan Feruck
  Media Relations Manager. . . . . .Nancy A Hanewinckel
    941-585-4763
    nhanewinckel1@humana.com

321 Kaiser Foundation Health Plan of Georgia

9 Piedmont Center
3495 Piedmont Road NE
Atlanta, GA 30300-1736
Toll-Free: 800-232-4404
Phone: 404-233-3700
www.kaiserpermanente.org
Non-Profit Organization: Yes
Year Founded: 1985
Number of Affiliated Hospitals: 29
Number of Primary Care Physicians: 15,129
Total Enrollment: 238,000
State Enrollment: 238,000

Healthplan and Services Defined
  PLAN TYPE: HMO
  Model Type: Group
  Benefits Offered: Disease Management, Prescription, Wellness
  Offers Demand Management Patient Information Service: Yes

Geographic Areas Served
  28 counties in the Metro-Atlanta Area

Subscriber Information
  Average Subscriber Co-Payment:
    Primary Care Physician: $10.00
    Prescription Drugs: $10.00
    Hospital ER: $50.00

Home Health Care: $10.00
Nursing Home Max. Days/Visits Covered: 100/yr.

Publishes and Distributes Report Card: Yes

Accreditation Certification
NCQA
TJC Accreditation, Medicare Approved, Utilization Review,
Pre-Admission Certification, State Licensure, Quality Assurance
Program

Key Personnel
Exec Medical Director . . . . Rob Schreiner, MD
Media Contact . . . . Bill Auer
404-869-5952
billy.auer@kp.org

322 National Better Living Association

6470 East Johns Crossing
Suite 170
Duluth, GA 30097
Toll-Free: 888-774-0848
Phone: 770-448-4677
Fax: 888-774-0456
www.nblaplans.com
Year Founded: 1995
Number of Affiliated Hospitals: 5,500
Total Enrollment: 1,000,000

Healthplan and Services Defined
PLAN TYPE: PPO
Model Type: Network
Plan Specialty: Chiropractic, Dental, Lab, PBM, Vision, Radiology,
Act Med
Benefits Offered: Chiropractic, Complementary Medicine, Dental,
Home Care, Long-Term Care, Physical Therapy, Prescription,
Vision, Wellness, AD&D, LTD, Indemnity

Type of Coverage
Commercial, Individual, Indemnity, Medicare, Catastrophic,
Discount Programs
Catastrophic Illness Benefit: Maximum $2M

Type of Payment Plans Offered
DFFS

Geographic Areas Served
Nationwide

Subscriber Information
Average Monthly Fee Per Subscriber
(Employee + Employer Contribution):
Employee Only (Self): $150.00
Employee & 1 Family Member: $250.00
Employee & 2 Family Members: $350.00
Average Annual Deductible Per Subscriber:
Employee Only (Self): $0
Employee & 1 Family Member: $0
Employee & 2 Family Members: $6

Network Qualifications
Minimum Years of Practice: 3
Pre-Admission Certification: Yes

Publishes and Distributes Report Card: No

Accreditation Certification
NCQA, Internally Performed
Pre-Admission Certification, State Licensure, Quality Assurance
Program

Key Personnel
President . . . . George E Spalding, Jr, CPA
800-669-8682
gspalding@corpsavershealthcare.com
CEO . . . . Dan Siewert, III
800-669-8682
dsiewert@corpsavershealthcare.com

COO . . . . Timothy Siewert
800-669-8682
tsiewert@corpsavershealthcare.com
VP Provider Relations . . . . Susan Spalding

Specialty Managed Care Partners
Guardian Life Insurance Co, Coalition America
Enters into Contracts with Regional Business Coalitions: Yes

Employer References
Aegon Financial Services, Memberworks, Ses, Goodhealth Services
LLC, Global Care

323 Northeast Georgia Health Partners

451 EE Butler Parkway
Suite 5
Gainesville, FL 30501
Phone: 770-219-6600
Fax: 770-219-6609
steven.mcneilly@nghs.com
www.healthpartnersnetwork.com
Subsidiary of: Northeast Georgia Health System
Non-Profit Organization: Yes
Number of Affiliated Hospitals: 8
Number of Primary Care Physicians: 500
Number of Referral/Specialty Physicians: 35
Total Enrollment: 42,000
State Enrollment: 42,000

Healthplan and Services Defined
PLAN TYPE: PPO
Benefits Offered: Behavioral Health, Home Care, Prescription,
Psychiatric, Wellness

Type of Coverage
Commercial

Geographic Areas Served
Banks, Barrow, Dawson, Forsyth, Gwinnet, Habersham, Hall,
Jackson, Lumplin, Rabun, Stephens, Towns, Union and White
counties

Accreditation Certification
NCQA

Key Personnel
Sales/Marketing Director . . . . Steven McNeilly
678-897-6601
steven.mcneilly@nghs.com
QI Specialist . . . . Janet Lathem
janet.lathem@nghs.com
Credentialing Coordinator . . . . Pam Short
pam.short@nghs.com
Provider Relations Rep . . . . Melissa D Corral
melissa.corral@nghs.com

324 Secure Health PPO Newtork

577 Mulberry Street
Suite 1000
Macon, GA 31201
Toll-Free: 800-648-7563
Phone: 478-314-2400
sales@shpg.com
www.shpg.com
Mailing Address: PO Box 4088, Macon, GA 31028
For Profit Organization: Yes
Year Founded: 1992
Physician Owned Organization: Yes
Number of Affiliated Hospitals: 16
Number of Primary Care Physicians: 950
Total Enrollment: 68,000
State Enrollment: 68,000

Healthplan and Services Defined
  PLAN TYPE: PPO
  Other Type: TPA
  Benefits Offered: Disease Management, Prescription, Wellness, EAP

Type of Coverage
  Commercial

Geographic Areas Served
  Georgia

Peer Review Type
  Utilization Review: Yes
  Case Management: Yes

Accreditation Certification
  URAC

Key Personnel
  President/CEO . . . . .Robbin Morton
  Dir, Sales & Marketing . . . . .Lisa Gilbert
    478-314-2426

325 Southeast Community Care

3920 Arkwright Road, Suite 370
Macon, GA 31210
Toll-Free: 888-701-2678
Phone: 478-474-2678
Fax: 484-477-9958
www.southeastcommunitycare.com
Subsidiary of: Humana

Healthplan and Services Defined
  PLAN TYPE: Medicare
  Benefits Offered: Prescription

Type of Coverage
  Medicare, Medicare Advantage

326 United Concordia: Georgia

Three Northwinds Center
2500 Northwinds Parkway, Suite 360
Alpharetta, GA 30009
Toll-Free: 800-972-4191
Phone: 678-893-8654
Fax: 678-297-9920
ucproducer@ucci.com
www.secure.ucci.com
For Profit Organization: Yes
Year Founded: 1971
Number of Primary Care Physicians: 111,000
Total Enrollment: 8,000,000

Healthplan and Services Defined
  PLAN TYPE: Dental
  Plan Specialty: Dental
  Benefits Offered: Dental

Type of Coverage
  Commercial, Individual

Geographic Areas Served
  Military personnel and their families, nationwide

Key Personnel
  Sales . . . . .Brent Shelly
    brent-shelly@ucci.com

327 UnitedHealthCare of Georgia

3720 Davinci Court, Suite 300
Norcross, GA 30092
Phone: 770-300-3501
georgiaprteam@uhc.com
www.uhc.com
Subsidiary of: UnitedHealth Group

For Profit Organization: Yes
Year Founded: 1980
Number of Affiliated Hospitals: 47
Number of Primary Care Physicians: 2,200
Number of Referral/Specialty Physicians: 4,000
Total Enrollment: 75,000,000
State Enrollment: 1,051,334

Healthplan and Services Defined
  PLAN TYPE: HMO/PPO
  Model Type: Network
  Benefits Offered: Disease Management, Physical Therapy,
    Prescription, Wellness
  Offers Demand Management Patient Information Service: Yes

Type of Coverage
  Catastrophic Illness Benefit: Unlimited

Type of Payment Plans Offered
  POS, FFS

Geographic Areas Served
  Statewide

Network Qualifications
  Pre-Admission Certification: Yes

Peer Review Type
  Utilization Review: Yes
  Case Management: Yes

Publishes and Distributes Report Card: Yes

Accreditation Certification
  NCQA
  TJC Accreditation, Medicare Approved, Utilization Review,
    Pre-Admission Certification, State Licensure, Quality Assurance
    Program

Key Personnel
  Regional CEO . . . . .Daniel Laurence Ohman
  CEO . . . . .Rick Elliott
  Media Contact. . . . . .Tracey Lempner
    770-300-3573
    tracey.lempner@uhc.com

Specialty Managed Care Partners
  Enters into Contracts with Regional Business Coalitions: Yes

328 VSP: Vision Service Plan of Georgia

3091 Governors Lake Drive, #240
Norcross, GA 30071-1143
Phone: 770-447-6128
Fax: 770-263-6008
webmaster@vsp.com
www.vsp.com
Year Founded: 1955
Number of Primary Care Physicians: 28,000
Total Enrollment: 57,000,000

Healthplan and Services Defined
  PLAN TYPE: Vision
  Plan Specialty: Vision
  Benefits Offered: Vision

Type of Payment Plans Offered
  Capitated

Geographic Areas Served
  Statewide

Network Qualifications
  Pre-Admission Certification: Yes

Peer Review Type
  Utilization Review: Yes

Accreditation Certification
  Utilization Review, Quality Assurance Program

Key Personnel
  Manager . . . . .Cheryl Rains

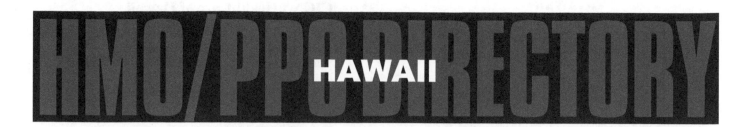

Health Insurance Coverage Status and Type of Coverage by Age

Category	All Persons		Under 18 years		Under 65 years		65 years and over	
	Number	%	Number	%	Number	%	Number	%
Total population	1,345	-	307	-	1,129	-	216	-
Covered by some type of health insurance	1,254 (6)	93.3 (0.4)	298 (2)	97.0 (0.7)	1,041 (6)	92.2 (0.5)	214 (1)	99.0 (0.4)
Covered by private health insurance	1,017 (11)	75.6 (0.8)	215 (5)	69.9 (1.7)	865 (10)	76.6 (0.8)	152 (4)	70.4 (1.8)
Employment based	831 (12)	61.8 (0.9)	163 (6)	53.2 (2.1)	721 (12)	63.8 (1.0)	110 (4)	51.0 (1.8)
Direct purchase	150 (8)	11.2 (0.6)	16 (3)	5.2 (0.8)	97 (7)	8.6 (0.6)	53 (3)	24.6 (1.6)
Covered by TRICARE	131 (8)	9.7 (0.6)	49 (4)	15.8 (1.4)	108 (7)	9.6 (0.6)	23 (2)	10.5 (1.1)
Covered by government health insurance	424 (9)	31.5 (0.6)	95 (5)	31.1 (1.7)	218 (8)	19.3 (0.7)	206 (2)	95.4 (0.6)
Covered by Medicaid	221 (9)	16.4 (0.7)	95 (5)	31.0 (1.7)	193 (8)	17.1 (0.8)	29 (2)	13.2 (1.1)
Also by private insurance	38 (4)	2.8 (0.3)	12 (2)	4.0 (0.7)	27 (4)	2.4 (0.3)	10 (1)	4.8 (0.6)
Covered by Medicare	228 (3)	16.9 (0.2)	1 (Z)	0.2 (0.1)	23 (2)	2.0 (0.2)	205 (2)	95.2 (0.7)
Also by private insurance	152 (5)	11.3 (0.3)	Z (Z)	0.1 (0.1)	8 (1)	0.7 (0.1)	144 (4)	66.6 (1.9)
Also by Medicaid	38 (3)	2.8 (0.2)	1 (Z)	0.2 (0.1)	9 (2)	0.8 (0.2)	29 (2)	13.2 (1.1)
Covered by VA Care	30 (3)	2.2 (0.2)	Z (Z)	0.1 (0.1)	15 (2)	1.3 (0.2)	15 (2)	6.9 (0.8)
Not covered at any time during the year	91 (6)	6.7 (0.4)	9 (2)	3.0 (0.7)	89 (5)	7.8 (0.5)	2 (1)	1.0 (0.4)

Note: Numbers in thousands; Figures cover 2013; Margin of error appears in parenthesis; A "Z" indicates that the value either represents or rounds to zero.
Source: U.S. Census Bureau, 2013 American Community Survey, Table HI05. Health Insurance Coverage Status and Type of Coverage by State and Age for All People: 2013

Hawaii

329　Aetna Health of Hawaii

151 Farmington Avenue
Hartford, CT 06156
Toll-Free: 800-872-3862
Phone: 860-273-0123
www.aetna.com
Partnered with: eHealthInsurance Services Inc.
For Profit Organization: Yes
Total Enrollment: 11,596,230

Healthplan and Services Defined
　PLAN TYPE: PPO
　Other Type: POS
　Plan Specialty: EPO
　Benefits Offered: Dental, Disease Management, Long-Term Care,
　　Prescription, Wellness, Life, LTD, STD

Type of Coverage
　Commercial, Individual

Type of Payment Plans Offered
　POS, FFS

Geographic Areas Served
　Statewide

Key Personnel
　Chairman/President/CEO . . . . Mark T Bertolini
　EVP/General Counsel . . . . William J Casazza
　EVP/CFO . . . . Shawn M Guertin

330　AlohaCare

1357 Kapiolani Boulevard
Suite 1250
Honolulu, HI 96814
Toll-Free: 800-830-7222
Phone: 808-973-1650
Fax: 808-973-0726
info@alohacare.org
www.alohacare.org
Non-Profit Organization: Yes
Year Founded: 1994
Number of Primary Care Physicians: 3,000
Total Enrollment: 80,000

Healthplan and Services Defined
　PLAN TYPE: HMO

Type of Coverage
　Medicare, Supplemental Medicare

Geographic Areas Served
　Oahu & Big Island

Peer Review Type
　Case Management: Yes

Publishes and Distributes Report Card: Yes

Key Personnel
　CEO . . . . John McComas
　VP, Governance. . . . . David Bess
　Provider Relations . . . . Machille Pedro
　Business Development . . . . Nolan Namba
　Medical Director . . . . Sharon Tisza, MD
　Senior Dir, Cmty Rltns . . . . Daryl Huff
　　808-973-1569
　　druff@alohacare.org

331　CIGNA HealthCare of Hawaii

1 Front Street
7th Floor
San Francisco, CA 94111
Toll-Free: 888-802-4462
Fax: 860-298-2443
www.cigna.com
For Profit Organization: Yes
Total Enrollment: 2,407
State Enrollment: 1,602

Healthplan and Services Defined
　PLAN TYPE: HMO
　Benefits Offered: Disease Management, Prescription, Transplant,
　　Wellness

Type of Coverage
　Commercial

Type of Payment Plans Offered
　POS, FFS

Geographic Areas Served
　Hawaii

332　eHealthInsurance Services Inc.

11919 Foundation Place
Gold River, CA 95670
Toll-Free: 800-644-3491
webmaster@healthinsurance.com
www.e.healthinsurance.com
Year Founded: 1997

Healthplan and Services Defined
　PLAN TYPE: HMO/PPO
　Benefits Offered: Dental, Life, STD

Type of Coverage
　Commercial, Individual, Medicare

Geographic Areas Served
　All 50 states in the USA and District of Columbia

Key Personnel
　Chairman & CEO . . . . Gary L. Lauer
　EVP/Business & Corp. Dev. . . . . Bruce Telkamp
　EVP/Chief Technology . . . . Dr. Sheldon X. Wang
　SVP & CFO . . . . Stuart M. Huizinga
　Pres. of eHealth Gov. Sys . . . . Samuel C. Gibbs
　SVP of Sales & Operations . . . . Robert S. Hurley
　Director Public Relations. Nate Purpura
　　650-210-3115

333　Great-West Healthcare Hawaii

1999 Harrison Street
Suite 1000
Oakland, CA 94612
Phone: 510-273-8400
eliginquiries@cigna.com
www.cignaforhealth.com
Subsidiary of: CIGNA HealthCare
Acquired by: CIGNA
For Profit Organization: Yes
Total Enrollment: 368
State Enrollment: 213

Healthplan and Services Defined
　PLAN TYPE: HMO/PPO
　Benefits Offered: Disease Management, Prescription, Wellness

Type of Coverage
　Commercial

Geographic Areas Served
　Hawaii

Accreditation Certification
   URAC

Specialty Managed Care Partners
   Caremark Rx

---

334   Hawaii Medical Assurance Association

737 Bishop Street
Suite 1200
Honolulu, HI 96813
Toll-Free: 800-621-6998
Phone: 808-591-0088
Fax: 808-591-0463
www.hmaa.com
For Profit Organization: Yes
Year Founded: 1989
Number of Primary Care Physicians: 1,874
Total Enrollment: 42,000
State Enrollment: 42,000

Healthplan and Services Defined
   PLAN TYPE: PPO
   Benefits Offered: Dental, Prescription, Vision, Wellness, AD&D,
   Life

Type of Coverage
   Commercial

Accreditation Certification
   URAC

Key Personnel
   Chairman/President/CEO . . . . John Henry Felix

---

335   Hawaii Medical Services Association

818 Keeaumoku Street
Honolulu, HI 96814
Phone: 808-948-6111
Fax: 808-948-5567
www.hmsa.com
Mailing Address: PO Box 860HI 96808-0860
Subsidiary of: Blue Cross/Blue Shield
Non-Profit Organization: Yes
Year Founded: 1938
State Enrollment: 692,000

Healthplan and Services Defined
   PLAN TYPE: PPO
   Benefits Offered: Quest

Accreditation Certification
   URAC, NCQA

Key Personnel
   CEO . . . . Robert P Hiam
   President/COO . . . . Michael A Gold
   Exec VP/CFO/Treasurer . . . . Steve Van Ribbink
   Executive Vice President . . . . Gwen S Miyasato
   Senior Vice President . . . . Michael Cheng
   Senior Vice President . . . . Timothy E Johns
   SVP/CIO . . . . Michel Danon
   Media Relations . . . . Robyn Kuroaka
   808-948-6826
   robyn_kuraoka@hmsa.com

---

336   Humana Health Insurance of Hawaii

Seven Waterfront Plaza
500 Ala Moana Blvd., Suite 400
Honolulu, HI 96813
Phone: 808-396-9213
Fax: 808-543-2085
www.humana.com
For Profit Organization: Yes

Healthplan and Services Defined
   PLAN TYPE: HMO/PPO

Type of Coverage
   Commercial, Individual

Accreditation Certification
   URAC, NCQA, CORE

Key Personnel
   Media Relations Manager . . . . Marina Renneke, APR
   480-515-6435
   mrenneke@humana.com

---

337   Kaiser Permanente Health Plan of Hawaii

711 Kapiolani Boulevard
Tower Suite 400
Honolulu, HI 96813
Toll-Free: 800-805-2739
www.kaiserpermanente.org
Non-Profit Organization: Yes
Year Founded: 1958
Number of Affiliated Hospitals: 35
Number of Primary Care Physicians: 15,129
Total Enrollment: 229,186
State Enrollment: 229,186

Healthplan and Services Defined
   PLAN TYPE: HMO
   Model Type: Group
   Benefits Offered: Chiropractic, Complementary Medicine, Disease
   Management, Prescription, Vision, Wellness, Worker's
   Compensation
   Offers Demand Management Patient Information Service: Yes

Type of Coverage
   Commercial, Individual, Medicare, Medicaid
   Catastrophic Illness Benefit: Unlimited

Type of Payment Plans Offered
   POS, Capitated, FFS

Geographic Areas Served
   Big Island of Hawaii, Kauai, Maui & Oahu

Subscriber Information
   Average Subscriber Co-Payment:
      Home Health Care Max. Days/Visits Covered: Unlimited
      Nursing Home: Skilled nursing fac.
      Nursing Home Max. Days/Visits Covered: Skilled nursing fac.

Network Qualifications
   Pre-Admission Certification: No

Peer Review Type
   Utilization Review: Yes
   Case Management: Yes

Publishes and Distributes Report Card: Yes

Accreditation Certification
   NCQA
   TJC Accreditation, Medicare Approved, Utilization Review, State
   Licensure, Quality Assurance Program

Key Personnel
   Hawaii Region President . . . . Janet Liang
   Dir, Community Benefits . . . . Joy Barua
   Exec Medical Director . . . . Geoffrey S Sewell, MD
   Media Contact . . . . Laura M Lott
   808-432-5916
   laura.m.lott@kp.org

Specialty Managed Care Partners
   Enters into Contracts with Regional Business Coalitions: Yes

338 UnitedHealthCare of Hawaii

5757 Plaza Drive
Cypress, CA 90630
Toll-Free: 800-343-2608
www.uhc.com
Subsidiary of: UnitedHealth Group
For Profit Organization: Yes
Year Founded: 1986
Total Enrollment: 75,000,000
State Enrollment: 3,902

Healthplan and Services Defined
PLAN TYPE: HMO/PPO
Model Type: Network
Benefits Offered: Disease Management, Prescription, Wellness
Offers Demand Management Patient Information Service: Yes

Type of Coverage
Catastrophic Illness Benefit: Covered

Type of Payment Plans Offered
DFFS, Capitated

Geographic Areas Served
Statewide

Subscriber Information
Average Monthly Fee Per Subscriber
(Employee + Employer Contribution):
Employee Only (Self): $120.00
Employee & 1 Family Member: $240.00
Employee & 2 Family Members: $375.00
Average Annual Deductible Per Subscriber:
Employee & 2 Family Members: Varies
Average Subscriber Co-Payment:
Primary Care Physician: $5.00-10.00
Prescription Drugs: $5.00/10.00/25.00
Hospital ER: $50.00
Nursing Home Max. Days/Visits Covered: 120 per year

Publishes and Distributes Report Card: Yes

Accreditation Certification
NCQA
TJC Accreditation, Utilization Review, State Licensure

Key Personnel
Media Contact....................................Matt Yi
714-226-3842
matthew.yi@uhc.com

Specialty Managed Care Partners
Enters into Contracts with Regional Business Coalitions: Yes

339 University Health Alliance

700 Bishop Street
Suite 300, Bishop Street Tower
Honolulu, HI 96813-4100
Toll-Free: 800-458-4600
Phone: 808-532-4000
Fax: 866-572-4393
www.uhahealth.com
For Profit Organization: Yes
Year Founded: 1996
Total Enrollment: 36,505

Healthplan and Services Defined
PLAN TYPE: PPO
Benefits Offered: Dental, Prescription, Vision, Wellness

Type of Coverage
Commercial

Accreditation Certification
URAC, HUM

Key Personnel
President/CEO.........................Howard K F Lee, MD
EVP/Chief Operating Offic..................Lance Kaneshiro

EVP/Treasurer/CFO.........................Charles Murray
SVP/Secretary/CMO.........................Linda Kalahiki
SVP/Chief Medical Officer...........George O McPheeters, MD
Medical Director.......................Glenn Ishikawa, MD
SVP, Chief HR Officer........................Emily Weaver
SVP, Chief Info Officer...........................Chad Lee
SVP, Chief Sales Officer.....................Lance Kaneshiro

340 VSP: Vision Service Plan of Hawaii

1003 Bishop Street
Suite 890
Honolulu, HI 96813-6426
Phone: 808-532-1600
Fax: 808-533-0604
webmaster@vsp.com
www.vsp.com
Year Founded: 1955
Number of Primary Care Physicians: 28,000
Total Enrollment: 57,000,000

Healthplan and Services Defined
PLAN TYPE: Vision
Plan Specialty: Vision
Benefits Offered: Vision

Type of Payment Plans Offered
Capitated

Geographic Areas Served
Statewide

Network Qualifications
Pre-Admission Certification: Yes

Peer Review Type
Utilization Review: Yes

Accreditation Certification
Utilization Review, Quality Assurance Program

Key Personnel
Manager....................................Paula Palmer

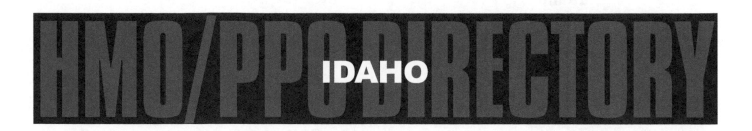
Health Insurance Coverage Status and Type of Coverage by Age

Category	All Persons		Under 18 years		Under 65 years		65 years and over	
	Number	%	Number	%	Number	%	Number	%
Total population	1,592	-	426	-	1,373	-	219	-
Covered by some type of health insurance	1,335 *(12)*	83.8 *(0.8)*	388 *(4)*	91.1 *(1.0)*	1,117 *(12)*	81.4 *(0.9)*	217 *(2)*	99.1 *(0.5)*
Covered by private health insurance	1,059 *(16)*	66.5 *(1.0)*	260 *(8)*	60.9 *(1.8)*	911 *(16)*	66.4 *(1.2)*	148 *(4)*	67.4 *(1.7)*
Employment based	818 *(17)*	51.4 *(1.1)*	218 *(9)*	51.3 *(2.0)*	755 *(17)*	55.0 *(1.2)*	62 *(4)*	28.5 *(1.7)*
Direct purchase	250 *(10)*	15.7 *(0.6)*	38 *(5)*	8.8 *(1.1)*	158 *(9)*	11.5 *(0.7)*	92 *(4)*	41.9 *(1.7)*
Covered by TRICARE	51 *(5)*	3.2 *(0.3)*	10 *(2)*	2.3 *(0.6)*	34 *(4)*	2.5 *(0.3)*	16 *(2)*	7.5 *(0.9)*
Covered by government health insurance	473 *(12)*	29.7 *(0.8)*	145 *(8)*	34.1 *(1.9)*	260 *(12)*	18.9 *(0.8)*	213 *(2)*	97.2 *(0.7)*
Covered by Medicaid	241 *(12)*	15.2 *(0.8)*	141 *(8)*	33.2 *(2.0)*	219 *(12)*	15.9 *(0.9)*	23 *(3)*	10.3 *(1.3)*
Also by private insurance	44 *(5)*	2.7 *(0.3)*	17 *(3)*	3.9 *(0.8)*	34 *(4)*	2.4 *(0.3)*	10 *(2)*	4.6 *(0.8)*
Covered by Medicare	250 *(3)*	15.7 *(0.2)*	2 *(1)*	0.4 *(0.2)*	38 *(3)*	2.7 *(0.2)*	213 *(2)*	97.0 *(0.8)*
Also by private insurance	155 *(4)*	9.7 *(0.3)*	Z *(Z)*	0.0 *(0.1)*	12 *(2)*	0.9 *(0.1)*	143 *(4)*	65.4 *(1.8)*
Also by Medicaid	41 *(3)*	2.6 *(0.2)*	1 *(Z)*	0.1 *(0.1)*	18 *(2)*	1.3 *(0.2)*	23 *(3)*	10.3 *(1.3)*
Covered by VA Care	49 *(4)*	3.1 *(0.2)*	3 *(2)*	0.6 *(0.5)*	25 *(4)*	1.8 *(0.3)*	24 *(2)*	10.8 *(0.9)*
Not covered at any time during the year	257 *(12)*	16.2 *(0.8)*	38 *(4)*	8.9 *(1.0)*	255 *(12)*	18.6 *(0.9)*	2 *(1)*	0.9 *(0.5)*

Note: Numbers in thousands; Figures cover 2013; Margin of error appears in parenthesis; A "Z" indicates that the value either represents or rounds to zero.
Source: U.S. Census Bureau, 2013 American Community Survey, Table HI05. Health Insurance Coverage Status and Type of Coverage by State and Age for All People: 2013

Idaho

341 Aetna Health of Idaho

151 Farmington Avenue
Hartford, CT 06156
Toll-Free: 800-872-3862
Phone: 860-273-0123
www.aetna.com
Partnered with: eHealthInsurance Services Inc.
For Profit Organization: Yes
Total Enrollment: 11,596,230

Healthplan and Services Defined
  PLAN TYPE: PPO
  Other Type: POS
  Plan Specialty: EPO
  Benefits Offered: Disease Management, Prescription, Wellness

Type of Coverage
  Commercial

Type of Payment Plans Offered
  POS, FFS

Geographic Areas Served
  Statewide

Key Personnel
  Chairman/CEO/President......................Mark T Bertolini
  EVP/General Counsel ....William J Casazza
  EVP/CFO ....Shawn M Guertin

342 Blue Cross of Idaho Health Service, Inc.

3000 East Pine Avenue
Meridian, ID 83642
Toll-Free: 800-274-4018
Phone: 208-345-4550
Fax: 208-331-7311
www.bcidaho.com
Mailing Address: PO Box 7408, Boise, ID 83707
Subsidiary of: Blue Cross and Blue Shield Association
Non-Profit Organization: Yes
Year Founded: 1945
Number of Affiliated Hospitals: 44
Number of Primary Care Physicians: 1,631
Total Enrollment: 563,000
State Enrollment: 563,000

Healthplan and Services Defined
  PLAN TYPE: HMO/PPO
  Model Type: IPA, Group, Network
  Plan Specialty: ASO, Chiropractic, Dental, Disease Management
  Benefits Offered: Chiropractic, Dental, Disease Management,
    Prescription, Vision, Wellness

Type of Coverage
  Commercial, Individual, Indemnity, Medicare, Supplemental
    Medicare

Type of Payment Plans Offered
  POS, DFFS, FFS

Geographic Areas Served
  Statewide

Subscriber Information
  Average Subscriber Co-Payment:
    Prescription Drugs: Varies
    Hospital ER: Varies
    Home Health Care: Varies
    Nursing Home: Varies

Network Qualifications
  Pre-Admission Certification: Yes

Peer Review Type
  Utilization Review: Yes

Case Management: Yes

Publishes and Distributes Report Card: Yes

Accreditation Certification
  TJC Accreditation, Pre-Admission Certification, State Licensure

Key Personnel
  President/CEO ....Zelda Geyer-Sylvia
  EVP/CFO ....Jack A. Myers
  VP Actuarial Services & U ....David J. Hutchins
  General Counsel/SVP, Lega ....Steve Tobiason
  SVP, Human Resources & Or ....Debra M Henry
  SVP, Marketing & Sales ....David Jeppesen
  Dir Pharmacy Management ....Stephen J Brocksome
  VP, Medicare & Medicaid P................Jeanie Phillilps, MD
  VP Benefits Management ....Drew S Forney
  VP Chief Information Offc ....Lance Hatfield
  VP Provider Services ....Jeff Crouch
  VP, Sales ....Rex Warwick
  Media Contact ....Josh Jordan
    208-331-7465
    jjordan@bcidaho.com
  Dir Human Resources.......................Doug Bullock

Specialty Managed Care Partners
  Wellpoint Pharmacy Management, Dental through Blue Cross of
    Idaho, Vision through VSP, Life Insurance, EAP through Business
    Psychology Associates
  Enters into Contracts with Regional Business Coalitions: No

343 CIGNA HealthCare of Idaho

3900 East Mexico Ave
#1100
Denver, CO 80210
Toll-Free: 866-438-2446
Phone: 303-782-1500
Fax: 303-691-3197
www.cigna.com
For Profit Organization: Yes
Total Enrollment: 27,000

Healthplan and Services Defined
  PLAN TYPE: PPO
  Model Type: Consumer Driven
  Benefits Offered: Behavioral Health, Dental, Prescription, Medical

Type of Coverage
  Commercial

Type of Payment Plans Offered
  POS, FFS

Geographic Areas Served
  Idaho

Network Qualifications
  Pre-Admission Certification: Yes

Key Personnel
  President & General Mgr ....Chris Blanton

344 Delta Dental of Idaho

555 East Parkcenter Boulevard
Boise, ID 83706
Toll-Free: 800-356-7586
Phone: 208-489-3580
customerservice@deltadentalid.com
www.deltadentalid.com
Mailing Address: PO Box 2870, Boise, ID 83701
Non-Profit Organization: Yes
Year Founded: 1971
Total Enrollment: 54,000,000

Healthplan and Services Defined
  PLAN TYPE: Dental
  Other Type: Dental PPO

Model Type: Network
Plan Specialty: Dental
Benefits Offered: Dental

Type of Coverage
Commercial

Type of Payment Plans Offered
DFFS

Geographic Areas Served
Statewide

Subscriber Information
Average Monthly Fee Per Subscriber
(Employee + Employer Contribution):
Employee Only (Self): $17
Employee & 2 Family Members: $50
Average Annual Deductible Per Subscriber:
Employee Only (Self): $150
Employee & 2 Family Members: $50
Average Subscriber Co-Payment:
Primary Care Physician: 80%
Non-Network Physician: 50%

Network Qualifications
Pre-Admission Certification: Yes

Publishes and Distributes Report Card: Yes

Key Personnel
Sales Manager . . . . .Joanna Ramer
jramer@deltadentalid.com
Dir/Media & Public Affair . . . . Elizabeth Risberg
415-972-8423

---

345   eHealthInsurance Services Inc.
11919 Foundation Place
Gold River, CA 95670
Toll-Free: 800-644-3491
webmaster@healthinsurance.com
www.e.healthinsurance.com
Year Founded: 1997

Healthplan and Services Defined
PLAN TYPE: HMO/PPO
Benefits Offered: Dental, Life, STD

Type of Coverage
Commercial, Individual, Medicare

Geographic Areas Served
All 50 states in the USA and District of Columbia

Key Personnel
Chairman & CEO . . . . .Gary L. Lauer
EVP/Business & Corp. Dev. .Bruce Telkamp
EVP/Chief Technology . . . . .Dr. Sheldon X. Wang
SVP & CFO . . . . .Stuart M. Huizinga
Pres. of eHealth Gov. Sys . . . . .Samuel C. Gibbs
SVP of Sales & Operations . . . . .Robert S. Hurley
Director Public Relations . . . . .Nate Purpura
650-210-3115

---

346   Humana Health Insurance of Idaho
1505 South Eagle Road
Suite 120
Meridian, ID 83642
Phone: 208-319-3400
Fax: 208-888-7298
www.humana.com
For Profit Organization: Yes

Healthplan and Services Defined
PLAN TYPE: HMO/PPO

Type of Coverage
Commercial, Individual

Accreditation Certification
URAC, NCQA, CORE

Key Personnel
Media Relations Manager . . . . .Ross McLerran
210-617-1771
rmclerran@humana.com

---

347   IHC: Intermountain Healthcare Health Plan
36 S. State Street
Salt Lake City, UT 84111
Toll-Free: 800-538-5038
Phone: 801-442-2000
Fax: 801-442-5183
www.intermountainhealthcare.org
Mailing Address: PO Box 30192, Salt Lake City, UT 84130-0192
Acquired by: SelectHealth
Non-Profit Organization: Yes
Year Founded: 1983
Number of Affiliated Hospitals: 19
Number of Primary Care Physicians: 1,167
Number of Referral/Specialty Physicians: 1,566
Total Enrollment: 456,719
State Enrollment: 296,175

Healthplan and Services Defined
PLAN TYPE: HMO
Benefits Offered: Chiropractic, Complementary Medicine, Dental,
Home Care, Inpatient SNF, Long-Term Care, Podiatry, Prescription,
Psychiatric, Transplant, Vision, Wellness, Worker's Compensation

Type of Coverage
Commercial, Individual, Medicare, Medicaid

Geographic Areas Served
Idaho: Bear Lake, Caribou, Cassia, Franklin, Oneida counties. Utah:
Beaver, Box Elder, Cache, Carbon, Daggett, Davis, Duschesne,
Emery, Garfield, Iron, Juab, Kane, Millard, Morgan, Piute, Rich, Salt
Lake, Sanpete, Sevier, summit, Tooele, Uintah, Utah, Wasatch,
Washigton, Wayne, Weber counties

Accreditation Certification
NCQA

Key Personnel
Chairman . . . . .A. Scott Anderson
President/CEO . . . . .Charles Sorenson, MD
President/CEO. . . . . .S. Neal Berube
Vice Chairman. . . . . .Bruce T. Reese
Medical Director . . . . .Richard Price, Md

---

348   Liberty Health Plan: Idaho
3501 E Overland Road
Meridian, ID 83642-6757
Toll-Free: 800-256-3853
Phone: 208-898-7621
Fax: 800-283-4456
customerservice.center@libertynorthwest.com
www.libertynorthwest.com
Mailing Address: PO Box 50098, Idaho Falls, ID 83405
Subsidiary of: Liberty Mutual Agency Corporation
For Profit Organization: Yes
Year Founded: 1983

Healthplan and Services Defined
PLAN TYPE: PPO
Model Type: Group
Plan Specialty: Worker's Compensation
Benefits Offered: Prescription

Type of Payment Plans Offered
POS, DFFS, FFS, Combination FFS & DFFS

Geographic Areas Served
Statewide

Network Qualifications
  Pre-Admission Certification: Yes

Peer Review Type
  Case Management: Yes

Publishes and Distributes Report Card: No

Specialty Managed Care Partners
  Enters into Contracts with Regional Business Coalitions: No

349 PacificSource Health Plans: Idaho

408 E. Parkcenter Blvd
Suite 100
Boise, ID 83706
Toll-Free: 800-624-6052
Phone: 208-342-3709
Fax: 208-342-4508
www.pacificsource.com
Secondary Address: 901 Pierview Drive, Suite 209, Idaho Falls, ID 83402, 208-522-1360
Non-Profit Organization: Yes
Year Founded: 1933
Number of Primary Care Physicians: 32,000
Total Enrollment: 280,000

Healthplan and Services Defined
  PLAN TYPE: HMO/PPO
  Benefits Offered: Dental, Disease Management, Prescription, Vision, Wellness

Type of Coverage
  Commercial, Individual

Type of Payment Plans Offered
  POS, Combination FFS & DFFS

Geographic Areas Served
  Oregon and Idaho

Key Personnel
  President & CEO . . . . Ken Provencher
  EVP/CFO . . . . Peter Davidson
  EVP/COO . . . . Sujata Sanghvi
  VP, Administration . . . . Paul Wyncoop
  VP, Finance & Controller . . . . Kari Patterson
  SVP, Govt. Programs . . . . Dan Stevens
  SVP, Marketing . . . . Dave Self
  EVP/Chief Medical Officer . . . . Tom Ewing, MD
  SVP/Chief Information Off . . . . Erick Doolen
  VP, Provider Network . . . . Peter McGarry
  SVP, Sales . . . . Troy Kirk
  Media Contact . . . . Colleen Thompson
    541-684-5453
    cthompson@pacificsource.com

Specialty Managed Care Partners
  Caremark Rx

350 Primary Health Plan

PO Box 191050
Boise, ID 83719
Toll-Free: 800-481-9777
Phone: 208-955-6470
Fax: 208-955-6501
information@primaryhealth.com
www.primaryhealth.com
Acquired by: PacificSource Health Plans
Year Founded: 1996
Number of Primary Care Physicians: 423
Number of Referral/Specialty Physicians: 487
Total Enrollment: 14,000

Healthplan and Services Defined
  PLAN TYPE: Multiple
  Model Type: IPA

Plan Specialty: ASO
Benefits Offered: Behavioral Health, Chiropractic, Dental, Disease Management, Home Care, Inpatient SNF, Physical Therapy, Podiatry, Prescription, Psychiatric, Transplant, Vision, Wellness, AD&D, Life

Type of Coverage
  Commercial, Individual, Indemnity

Type of Payment Plans Offered
  POS, DFFS

Accreditation Certification
  NCQA

Key Personnel
  CEO . . . . Ellwood Kleaver
  President, COO . . . . David Self
  Pres, ID Phys Network . . . . William Johankin
  Exec Dir, ID Phys Network . . . . Linda Duer
  Chief Medical Officer . . . . Robert Friedman, MD
  Dir, Information Tech . . . . Mike Hronek

351 Regence BlueShield of Idaho

1602 21st Avenue
PO Box 1106
Lewiston, ID 83501
Toll-Free: 800-632-2022
Phone: 208-746-2671
Fax: 208-798-2097
www.regence.com
Mailing Address: PO Box 1106, Lewiston, ID 83501
Non-Profit Organization: Yes
Total Enrollment: 2,200,000
State Enrollment: 2,200,000

Healthplan and Services Defined
  PLAN TYPE: Multiple
  Benefits Offered: Dental, Prescription, Vision, Life

Type of Coverage
  Commercial, Individual, Supplemental Medicare

Geographic Areas Served
  Idaho; Asotin and Garfield counties in Washington

Key Personnel
  President . . . . Scott Kreiling
  SVP, Govt Programs . . . . Lisa Brubaker
  SVP, Health Ins. Ops . . . . Scott Powers
  Media Contact . . . . Scott Thompson
    801-333-5905
    scott.thompson@regence.com

352 SelectHealth

5381 Green Street
Murray, ID 84123
Toll-Free: 800-538-5038
http://selecthealth.org
Subsidiary of: Intermountain Healthcare
Non-Profit Organization: Yes
Total Enrollment: 402,000

Healthplan and Services Defined
  PLAN TYPE: HMO

Type of Coverage
  Commercial, Individual

Accreditation Certification
  NCQA

Key Personnel
  President/CEO . . . . Patricia R Richards
  Media Contact . . . . Spencer Sutherland
    801-442-7960

353 UnitedHealthCare of Idaho

5757 Plaza Drive
Cypress, CA 90630
Toll-Free: 800-343-2608
www.uhc.com
Subsidiary of: UnitedHealth Group
For Profit Organization: Yes
Year Founded: 1986
Total Enrollment: 75,000,000
State Enrollment: 40,618

Healthplan and Services Defined
  PLAN TYPE: HMO/PPO
  Model Type: Network
  Benefits Offered: Disease Management, Prescription, Wellness
  Offers Demand Management Patient Information Service: Yes

Type of Coverage
  Catastrophic Illness Benefit: Covered

Type of Payment Plans Offered
  DFFS, Capitated

Geographic Areas Served
  Statewide

Subscriber Information
  Average Monthly Fee Per Subscriber
    (Employee + Employer Contribution):
      Employee Only (Self): $120.00
      Employee & 1 Family Member: $240.00
      Employee & 2 Family Members: $375.00
  Average Annual Deductible Per Subscriber:
    Employee & 2 Family Members: Varies
  Average Subscriber Co-Payment:
    Primary Care Physician: $5.00-10.00
    Prescription Drugs: $5.00/10.00/25.00
    Hospital ER: $50.00
    Nursing Home Max. Days/Visits Covered: 120 per year

Publishes and Distributes Report Card: Yes

Accreditation Certification
  NCQA
  TJC Accreditation, Utilization Review, State Licensure

Key Personnel
  Media Contact . . . . Kristen Hellmer
    602-255-8466
    kristen_hellmer@uhc.com

Specialty Managed Care Partners
  Enters into Contracts with Regional Business Coalitions: Yes

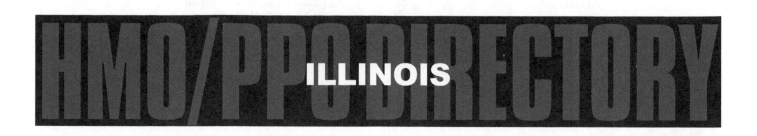

Health Insurance Coverage Status and Type of Coverage by Age

Category	All Persons		Under 18 years		Under 65 years		65 years and over	
	Number	%	Number	%	Number	%	Number	%
Total population	12,705	-	3,018	-	11,029	-	1,676	-
Covered by some type of health insurance	11,086 *(26)*	87.3 *(0.2)*	2,893 *(9)*	95.8 *(0.3)*	9,432 *(25)*	85.5 *(0.2)*	1,654 *(4)*	98.7 *(0.2)*
Covered by private health insurance	8,485 *(41)*	66.8 *(0.3)*	1,755 *(19)*	58.1 *(0.6)*	7,388 *(39)*	67.0 *(0.4)*	1,097 *(11)*	65.4 *(0.6)*
Employment based	7,241 *(42)*	57.0 *(0.3)*	1,596 *(21)*	52.9 *(0.7)*	6,633 *(41)*	60.1 *(0.4)*	608 *(10)*	36.3 *(0.6)*
Direct purchase	1,481 *(21)*	11.7 *(0.2)*	163 *(7)*	5.4 *(0.2)*	883 *(18)*	8.0 *(0.2)*	598 *(10)*	35.7 *(0.6)*
Covered by TRICARE	137 *(7)*	1.1 *(0.1)*	26 *(3)*	0.9 *(0.1)*	95 *(6)*	0.9 *(0.1)*	42 *(3)*	2.5 *(0.2)*
Covered by government health insurance	3,935 *(25)*	31.0 *(0.2)*	1,234 *(19)*	40.9 *(0.6)*	2,334 *(27)*	21.2 *(0.2)*	1,602 *(6)*	95.6 *(0.3)*
Covered by Medicaid	2,301 *(28)*	18.1 *(0.2)*	1,223 *(20)*	40.5 *(0.7)*	2,116 *(28)*	19.2 *(0.3)*	186 *(6)*	11.1 *(0.3)*
Also by private insurance	271 *(10)*	2.1 *(0.1)*	95 *(6)*	3.1 *(0.2)*	196 *(10)*	1.8 *(0.1)*	75 *(4)*	4.5 *(0.3)*
Covered by Medicare	1,862 *(10)*	14.7 *(0.1)*	17 *(3)*	0.6 *(0.1)*	263 *(9)*	2.4 *(0.1)*	1,599 *(6)*	95.4 *(0.3)*
Also by private insurance	1,112 *(11)*	8.8 *(0.1)*	1 *(Z)*	0.0 *(0.1)*	69 *(4)*	0.6 *(0.1)*	1,043 *(11)*	62.3 *(0.6)*
Also by Medicaid	302 *(8)*	2.4 *(0.1)*	8 *(2)*	0.3 *(0.1)*	116 *(6)*	1.1 *(0.1)*	186 *(6)*	11.1 *(0.3)*
Covered by VA Care	208 *(6)*	1.6 *(0.1)*	2 *(1)*	0.1 *(0.1)*	89 *(5)*	0.8 *(0.1)*	119 *(4)*	7.1 *(0.3)*
Not covered at any time during the year	1,618 *(27)*	12.7 *(0.2)*	125 *(8)*	4.2 *(0.3)*	1,596 *(26)*	14.5 *(0.2)*	22 *(3)*	1.3 *(0.2)*

Note: Numbers in thousands; Figures cover 2013; Margin of error appears in parenthesis; A "Z" indicates that the value either represents or rounds to zero.
Source: U.S. Census Bureau, 2013 American Community Survey, Table HI05. Health Insurance Coverage Status and Type of Coverage by State and Age for All People: 2013

Illinois

354 Aetna Health of Illinois
1 South Wacker Drive
Mail Stop F643
Chicago, IL 60606
Toll-Free: 866-582-9629
www.aetna.com
For Profit Organization: Yes
Total Enrollment: 45,014
State Enrollment: 45,014

Healthplan and Services Defined
  PLAN TYPE: HMO
  Other Type: POS
  Plan Specialty: EPO
  Benefits Offered: Dental, Disease Management, Long-Term Care,
    Prescription, Wellness, Life, LTD, STD

Type of Coverage
  Commercial, Individual

Type of Payment Plans Offered
  POS, FFS

Geographic Areas Served
  Statewide

355 Assurant Employee Benefits: Illinois
1 Tower Lane
Suite 2410
Oakbrook Terrace, IL 60181-4639
Phone: 630-954-5700
Fax: 630-954-1365
benefits@assurant.com
www.assurantemployeebenefits.com
Subsidiary of: Assurant, Inc
For Profit Organization: Yes
Number of Primary Care Physicians: 112,000
Total Enrollment: 47,000

Healthplan and Services Defined
  PLAN TYPE: Multiple
  Plan Specialty: Dental, Vision, Long & Short-Term Disability
  Benefits Offered: Dental, Vision, Wellness, AD&D, Life, LTD, STD

Type of Coverage
  Commercial, Indemnity, Individual Dental Plans

Geographic Areas Served
  Statewide

Subscriber Information
  Average Monthly Fee Per Subscriber
    (Employee + Employer Contribution):
      Employee Only (Self): Varies by plan

Key Personnel
  Business Manager..........................Paul Sweatman
  PR Specialist..............................Megan Hutchison
    816-556-7815
    megan.hutchison@assurant.com

356 Blue Cross & Blue Shield of Illinois
300 East Randolph Street
Chicago, IL 60601-5099
Toll-Free: 866-977-7378
www.bcbsil.com
Subsidiary of: Health Care Service Corporation
Non-Profit Organization: Yes
Year Founded: 1936
Total Enrollment: 7,000,000
State Enrollment: 7,000,000

Healthplan and Services Defined
  PLAN TYPE: HMO/PPO
  Benefits Offered: Disease Management, Physical Therapy,
    Prescription, Wellness

Type of Coverage
  Commercial, Individual, Supplemental Medicare, Medicaid

Type of Payment Plans Offered
  POS, FFS

Geographic Areas Served
  Illinois

Specialty Managed Care Partners
  Prime Therapeutics

357 Blue Cross and Blue Shield Association
225 North Michigan Avenue
BCBS Association Headquarters
Chicago, IL 60601
Toll-Free: 888-630-2583
BCBSWebmaster@bcbsa.com
www.bcbs.com/medicare
Secondary Address: 1310 G Street NW, Washington, DC 20005

Healthplan and Services Defined
  PLAN TYPE: Medicare
  Benefits Offered: Chiropractic, Disease Management, Home Care,
    Inpatient SNF, Physical Therapy, Podiatry, Prescription, Psychiatric,
    Wellness

Type of Coverage
  Individual, Medicare

Geographic Areas Served
  Available in multiple states. Go to Web/URL provided to view state by
  state availability of Medicare Plans which also provides direct Web
  links to state plans each with detailed information on coverages
  available and contact info for that state

Subscriber Information
  Average Monthly Fee Per Subscriber
    (Employee + Employer Contribution):
      Employee Only (Self): Varies
      Medicare: Varies
  Average Annual Deductible Per Subscriber:
      Employee Only (Self): Varies
      Medicare: Varies
  Average Subscriber Co-Payment:
      Primary Care Physician: Varies
      Non-Network Physician: Varies
      Prescription Drugs: Varies
      Hospital ER: Varies
      Home Health Care: Varies
      Home Health Care Max. Days/Visits Covered: Varies
      Nursing Home: Varies
      Nursing Home Max. Days/Visits Covered: Varies

Key Personnel
  President/CEO ....Scott P Serota
  VP, Venturing ....Paul F Brown
  SVP/Human Resources....................William A Colbourne
  VP, Operations & Prgms.......................Frank C Coyne
  VP/Federal Relations ....Jack Ericksen
  Legislation/Reg. Policy ....Alissa Fox
  VP, Government Prgms.....................William A Breskin
  SVP/Chief Medical Officer ....Allan M Korn, MD
  VP/Business Informatics.......................Shirley S Lady
  VP/Chief Tech Officer ....William B O'Loughlin
  SVP/Strategic Services ....Maureen E Sullivan
  SVP/Chief Info Officer ....Doug Porter
  General Counsel ....Roger G Wilson
  SVP/Chief Financial Offc.....................Robert Kolodgy
  VP, Marketing ....Jennifer Vachon
  VP, Strategic Commctns.......................Paul Gerrard

358 Catamaran Corporation

1600 McConnor Parkway
Schaumburg, IL 60173-6801
Toll-Free: 800-282-3232
Fax: 224-231-1901
www.catamaranrx.com

Healthplan and Services Defined
PLAN TYPE: Other
Other Type: PBM

Key Personnel
President & CEO .... Mark A Thierer
EVP, Operations .... Jeffrey Park
SVP/CFO .... Mike Shapiro
SVP, General Counsel .... Cliff Berman
SVP, Health Plans .... Michael Edwards
EVP, Pharmacy Operations .... Joel Saban
SVP, PBM Operations .... Kelly Kettlewell
EVP, Quality/Innovation .... John Romza

359 CIGNA HealthCare of Illinois

525 W Monroe Street
Suite 300
Chicago, IL 60661
Toll-Free: 800-832-3211
Phone: 312-648-2460
Fax: 312-648-3617
www.cigna.com
For Profit Organization: Yes
Year Founded: 1986
Total Enrollment: 18,588
State Enrollment: 18,588

Healthplan and Services Defined
PLAN TYPE: HMO
Other Type: POS
Model Type: IPA, Network
Plan Specialty: ASO, Behavioral Health, Dental
Benefits Offered: Behavioral Health, Complementary Medicine,
Dental, Disease Management, Prescription, Transplant, Vision,
Wellness

Type of Coverage
Commercial, Indemnity

Type of Payment Plans Offered
POS, DFFS, FFS

Geographic Areas Served
Illinois: Bureau, Coles, Cook, DuPage, Grundy, Kane, Kankakee,
Lake, LaSalle, Livingston, Madison, Massac, McHenry, Monroe,
Saint Clair, Shelby, Vermilion, Will counties

Network Qualifications
Pre-Admission Certification: Yes

Peer Review Type
Utilization Review: Yes

Publishes and Distributes Report Card: Yes

Accreditation Certification
NCQA
TJC Accreditation, Medicare Approved, Utilization Review,
Pre-Admission Certification, State Licensure, Quality Assurance
Program

Key Personnel
Midwest President & GM .... Sue Podbielski
Sales Manager .... Sue Povbielski

360 CNA Insurance Companies: Illinois

333 S Wabash
Chicago, IL 60604
Phone: 312-822-5000
jennifer.martinez-roth@cna.com
www.cna.com
Secondary Address: 801 Warrenville Road, Suite 700, Lisle, IL 60532,
630-719-3031
Year Founded: 1987
Owned by an Integrated Delivery Network (IDN): Yes
Number of Affiliated Hospitals: 57
Number of Primary Care Physicians: 3,400
Total Enrollment: 270,000

Healthplan and Services Defined
PLAN TYPE: PPO
Model Type: Network
Plan Specialty: Dental, Disease Management, Lab, MSO, Vision,
Radiology, Worker's Compensation, UR
Benefits Offered: Behavioral Health, Chiropractic, Dental, Disease
Management, Home Care, Inpatient SNF, Long-Term Care,
Physical Therapy, Podiatry, Prescription, Psychiatric, Transplant,
Vision, Wellness, Worker's Compensation, AD&D, Life, LTD, STD

Type of Coverage
Commercial, Individual, Indemnity, Medicaid, Catastrophic

Type of Payment Plans Offered
POS

Network Qualifications
Pre-Admission Certification: Yes

Peer Review Type
Utilization Review: Yes
Case Management: Yes

Publishes and Distributes Report Card: Yes

Accreditation Certification
URAC
TJC Accreditation, Pre-Admission Certification

Key Personnel
Chairman/CEO .... Thomas F Motamed
President/COO .... Bob Lindemann
EVP, Chief Actuary .... Larry A Haefner
EVP, Worldwide P&C Claim .... George R Fay
EVP, General Counsel .... Johathan D Kantor
EVP/CFO .... D Craig Mense
EVP, Chief Admin Officer .... Thomas Pontarelli
President, COO CNA Spec .... Peter W Wilson
President, Field Oper .... Tim Szerlong
SVP, CNA Select Risk .... John Angerami
SVP, Business Insurance .... Michael W Covne
Mid-Atlantic Zone Officer .... George Agven
Western Zone Officer .... Steve Stonehouse
Central Zone Officer .... Greg Vezzosi
Northern Zone Officer .... Steve Wachtel
Media Contact .... Katrina W Parker
312-822-5167

Specialty Managed Care Partners
Enters into Contracts with Regional Business Coalitions: Yes

361 CompBenefits: Illinois

200 W Jackson Blvd
9th Floor
Chicago, IL 60606
Toll-Free: 800-837-2341
Phone: 312-261-6200
Fax: 312-427-9665
www.compbenefits.com
Subsidiary of: Humana
Year Founded: 1978

Owned by an Integrated Delivery Network (IDN): Yes
Total Enrollment: 4,500,000

Healthplan and Services Defined
  PLAN TYPE: Multiple
  Model Type: Network, HMO, PPO, POS, TPA
  Plan Specialty: ASO, Dental, Vision
  Benefits Offered: Dental, Vision

Type of Coverage
  Commercial, Individual, Indemnity

Type of Payment Plans Offered
  DFFS, Capitated, FFS

Geographic Areas Served
  Alabama, Arkansas, Illinois, Indiana, Georgia, Florida, Mississippi, Missouri, Kentucky, Kansas, North Carolina, South Carolina, West Virginia, Texas, Tennessee, Ohio, Louisiana

Publishes and Distributes Report Card: Yes

Specialty Managed Care Partners
  Enters into Contracts with Regional Business Coalitions: Yes

362 CoreSource: Corporate Headquarters
400 Field Drive
Lake Forest, IL 60045
Toll-Free: 800-832-3332
Phone: 847-604-9200
www.coresource.com
Secondary Address: 18401 Maple Creek Drive, Suite 300, Tinley Park, IL 60477, 708-342-1237
Subsidiary of: Trustmark
Year Founded: 1980
Total Enrollment: 1,100,000

Healthplan and Services Defined
  PLAN TYPE: Multiple
  Other Type: TPA
  Model Type: Network
  Plan Specialty: Claims Administration, TPA
  Benefits Offered: Behavioral Health, Home Care, Prescription, Transplant

Type of Coverage
  Commercial

Geographic Areas Served
  Nationwide

Accreditation Certification
  Utilization Review, Pre-Admission Certification

Key Personnel
  President . . . . Nancy Eckrich
  VP, Chief Financial Offic. Clare Smith
  Chief Operating Officer . . . . Lloyd Sarrel
  VP, Product Management & . . . . Rob Corrigan
  VP, Healthcare Management. . . . . Donna Heiser
  VP, Marketing & Product D. . . . . Steve Horvath
  VP, Claims Operations. . . . . Pam Corso
  Media Contact. . . . . Cindy Gallaher
    847-283-4065
    cindy.gallaher@trustmark.com

363 Coventry Health Care of Illinois
2110 Fox Drive
Suite A
Champaign, IL 61820
Toll-Free: 800-431-1211
Fax: 217-366-5410
infochcil@cvty.com
www.chcillinois.com
Secondary Address: 4507 Sterling Avenue, Suite 205, Peoria, IL 61615
Subsidiary of: Coventry Health Care

For Profit Organization: Yes
Year Founded: 1984
Number of Affiliated Hospitals: 20
Number of Primary Care Physicians: 274
Number of Referral/Specialty Physicians: 711
Total Enrollment: 100,000
State Enrollment: 100,000

Healthplan and Services Defined
  PLAN TYPE: HMO
  Model Type: Network
  Plan Specialty: ASO
  Benefits Offered: Behavioral Health, Chiropractic, Disease Management, Home Care, Inpatient SNF, Physical Therapy, Podiatry, Prescription, Psychiatric, Transplant, Vision
  Offers Demand Management Patient Information Service: Yes

Type of Coverage
  Commercial, Individual, Supplemental Medicare

Type of Payment Plans Offered
  POS, DFFS, Capitated, FFS, Combination FFS & DFFS

Geographic Areas Served
  Bond, Boone, Calhoun, Champaign, Christian, Clark, Clinton, Coles, Crawford, Cumberland, DeWitt, Douglas, Edgar, Effingham, Fayette, Ford, Greene, Iroquois, Jasper, Jersey, Kankakee, LaSalle, Lee, Logan, Macon, Macoupin, Madison, Marshall, McLean, Menard, Monroe, Montgomery, Morgan, Moultrie, Ogle, Peoria, Piatt, Sangaman, Saint Clair, Shelby, Stark, Stephenson, Tazewell, Vermilion, Washington, Whiteside, Will, Winnebago, Woodford counties

Network Qualifications
  Pre-Admission Certification: Yes

Peer Review Type
  Utilization Review: Yes
  Second Surgical Opinion: Yes
  Case Management: Yes

Accreditation Certification
  NCQA
  TJC Accreditation, Medicare Approved, Utilization Review, Pre-Admission Certification, State Licensure, Quality Assurance Program

Key Personnel
  CEO . . . . Todd Petersen
  President . . . . Randy Hoffman
  Manager . . . . Mary Ellen Stinde
  Credentialing Manager . . . . Debbie Weiman
  Marketing Director . . . . Darcy Sementi
  Medical Director. . . . . Richard Grassy
  Member Relations. . . . . Toni Sauter
  Information Tech Manager . . . . Chuck Wallbaum
  Media Contact. . . . . Carrah Kalat
    630-737-7033
    cmkalat@cvty.com

Employer References
  Horace Mann, Verizon, Pepsi, Sarah Bush Lincoln Health, Walgreen's

364 Delta Dental of Illinois
111 Shuman Blvd
Naperville, IL 60563
Toll-Free: 800-323-1743
Phone: 630-718-4700
askdelta@deltadentalil.com
www.deltadentalil.com
Mailing Address: PO Box 5402, Lisle, IL 60532
Non-Profit Organization: Yes
Year Founded: 1967
Total Enrollment: 54,000,000
State Enrollment: 2,000,000

Healthplan and Services Defined
    PLAN TYPE: Dental
    Other Type: Dental PPO
    Model Type: Network
    Benefits Offered: Dental

Type of Coverage
    Commercial, Individual

Geographic Areas Served
    Statewide

Peer Review Type
    Utilization Review: Yes

Key Personnel
    President/CEO . . . . .Bernard Glossy
    CFO . . . . .David Behnke
    Chief Admin Officer. . . . . .Stacey Bonn
    VP Sales . . . . .Karyn Glogowski
    Dir, Community Relations . . . . .Lori Vitek
       630-718-4739
    Dir/Media & Public Affair . . . . .Elizabeth Risberg
       415-972-8423

365   Dental Network of America

701 E. 22nd Street
Suite 300
Lombard, IL 30148
Phone: 630-691-1133
general_inquiry@dnoa.com
www.dnoa.com
Subsidiary of: Health Care Service Corporation
For Profit Organization: Yes
Year Founded: 1985
Federally Qualified: Yes
Number of Primary Care Physicians: 80,000
Total Enrollment: 6,200,000

Healthplan and Services Defined
    PLAN TYPE: Dental
    Other Type: TPA, Dental PPO
    Plan Specialty: ASO, Dental, Dental, Fully Insured
    Benefits Offered: Dental

Type of Coverage
    Commercial, Individual, Indemnity, Group

Type of Payment Plans Offered
    Capitated

Geographic Areas Served
    Nationwide

Network Qualifications
    Pre-Admission Certification: Yes

Peer Review Type
    Utilization Review: Yes

366   eHealthInsurance Services Inc.

11919 Foundation Place
Gold River, CA 95670
Toll-Free: 800-644-3491
webmaster@healthinsurance.com
www.e.healthinsurance.com
Year Founded: 1997

Healthplan and Services Defined
    PLAN TYPE: HMO/PPO
    Benefits Offered: Dental, Life, STD

Type of Coverage
    Commercial, Individual, Medicare

Geographic Areas Served
    All 50 states in the USA and District of Columbia

Key Personnel
    Chairman & CEO . . . . .Gary L. Lauer
    EVP/Business & Corp. Dev. .Bruce Telkamp
    EVP/Chief Technology .Dr. Sheldon X. Wang
    SVP & CFO . . . . .Stuart M. Huizinga
    Pres. of eHealth Gov. Sys .Samuel C. Gibbs
    SVP of Sales & Operations . . . . .Robert S. Hurley
    Director Public Relations. . . . . .Nate Purpura
       650-210-3115

367   First Commonwealth

550 W Jackson
Suite 800
Chicago, IL 60661
Phone: 312-993-1000
Fax: 312-279-5140
www.firstcommonwealth.net
Subsidiary of: Guardian
Acquired by: Guardian Life Insurance Company
For Profit Organization: Yes
Year Founded: 1986
Number of Primary Care Physicians: 1,832
Number of Referral/Specialty Physicians: 594
Total Enrollment: 300,000

Healthplan and Services Defined
    PLAN TYPE: HMO
    Model Type: Network
    Plan Specialty: Dental
    Benefits Offered: Dental

Type of Coverage
    Commercial, Indemnity

Type of Payment Plans Offered
    POS, Capitated, FFS

Geographic Areas Served
    Illinois, Indiana, Michigan, Missouri, Wisconsin

Peer Review Type
    Utilization Review: Yes
    Second Surgical Opinion: Yes

Accreditation Certification
    Utilization Review, Quality Assurance Program

Key Personnel
    CFO . . . . .Scott B Sanders
    Network Contracting. . . . . .Ann Hunt
    Medical Affairs. . . . . .Paul Chaitkin, MD
    Information Systems. . . . . .Jon Helwig
    Provider Services . . . . .Greg Stobbe
    Sales . . . . .Paul Chaitkin, MD

368   First Health

, IL
Toll-Free: 800-226-5116
www.firsthealth.com
Subsidiary of: Coventry Health Care
For Profit Organization: Yes
Year Founded: 1984
Number of Affiliated Hospitals: 134
Number of Primary Care Physicians: 1,923
Number of Referral/Specialty Physicians: 5,744
Total Enrollment: 2,000,000
State Enrollment: 585,000

Healthplan and Services Defined
    PLAN TYPE: PPO
    Model Type: Network
    Benefits Offered: Disease Management, Wellness

Type of Payment Plans Offered
DFFS

Geographic Areas Served
State of Oklahoma and contiguous border cities of Missouri,
Arkansas, Kansas and Texas

Average Claim Compensation
Physician's Fees Charged: 72%
Hospital's Fees Charged: 62%

---

369   Great-West Healthcare Illinois
6250 River Road
Suite 7020
Rosemont, IL 60018
Toll-Free: 866-494-2111
Phone: 847-292-0024
eliginquiries@cigna.com
www.cignaforhealth.com
Subsidiary of: CIGNA HealthCare
Acquired by: CIGNA
For Profit Organization: Yes
Total Enrollment: 115,313
State Enrollment: 9,662

Healthplan and Services Defined
PLAN TYPE: HMO/PPO
Benefits Offered: Disease Management, Prescription, Wellness

Type of Coverage
Commercial

Type of Payment Plans Offered
POS, FFS

Geographic Areas Served
Illinois

Accreditation Certification
URAC

Specialty Managed Care Partners
Caremark Rx

---

370   Health Alliance Medical Plans
301 S Vine Street
Urbana, IL 61801
Toll-Free: 800-851-3379
Phone: 217-337-8000
Fax: 217-337-8093
www.healthalliance.org
For Profit Organization: Yes
Year Founded: 1980
Physician Owned Organization: Yes
Federally Qualified: Yes
Total Enrollment: 335,000

Healthplan and Services Defined
PLAN TYPE: HMO/PPO
Benefits Offered: Disease Management, Wellness

Type of Coverage
Medicare

Geographic Areas Served
Illinois and Central Iowa

Subscriber Information
Average Monthly Fee Per Subscriber
(Employee + Employer Contribution):
Employee Only (Self): $329.00
Employee & 2 Family Members: $1053.00
Average Subscriber Co-Payment:
Primary Care Physician: $20.00
Prescription Drugs: $10.00-15.00

Publishes and Distributes Report Card: Yes

Accreditation Certification
NCQA

Key Personnel
CEO . . . . .Jeffrey C Ingrum
CFO . . . . .Gordon Salm
Chief Medical Officer. . . . . .Robert Parker, MD
General Counsel . . . . .Lori Cowdrey
Marketing/Sales . . . . .Lori Rudd
Member Relations . . . . .Angela Beitelman
Pharmacy Director . . . . .Christina Barrington
Public Relations . . . . .Jane Hayes
Marketing/Sales. . . . . .Todd Hutchison
Communications Coord. . . . . .Nichole Evans
217-255-4694

---

371   Health Alliance Medicare
301 South Vine Street
Urbana, IL 61801
Toll-Free: 888-382-9771
memberservices@healthalliance.org
www.healthalliancemedicare.org
Secondary Address: 206 West Anthony Drive, Champaign, IL 61822
Year Founded: 1997
Number of Primary Care Physicians: 3,000
Total Enrollment: 255,494

Healthplan and Services Defined
PLAN TYPE: Medicare
Other Type: HMO/PPO
Benefits Offered: Prescription

Type of Coverage
Medicare, Supplemental Medicare

Accreditation Certification
NCQA

---

372   Health Care Service Corporation
300 East Randolph Street
Chicago, IL 60601-5099
Toll-Free: 800-654-7385
Phone: 312-653-6000
Fax: 312-819-1323
www.hcsc.com
Subsidiary of: A Mutual Legal Reserve Company
For Profit Organization: Yes
Year Founded: 1975
Owned by an Integrated Delivery Network (IDN): Yes
Total Enrollment: 13,000,000
State Enrollment: 13,000,000

Healthplan and Services Defined
PLAN TYPE: HMO/PPO
Other Type: POS, HSA, HCA
Model Type: Network
Plan Specialty: Chiropractic, Dental, Disease Management, Lab,
Vision, Radiology, UR
Benefits Offered: Chiropractic, Dental, Disease Management, Home
Care, Inpatient SNF, Physical Therapy, Podiatry, Prescription,
Psychiatric, Transplant, Vision, Wellness, AD&D, Life, LTD, STD

Type of Coverage
Commercial, Individual, Indemnity, Supplemental Medicare,
Catastrophic, Major Medical Plan

Type of Payment Plans Offered
Capitated

Geographic Areas Served
Illinois, New Mexico, Oklahoma, Texas

Peer Review Type
Second Surgical Opinion: Yes

Accreditation Certification
NCQA

Key Personnel

President/CEO	Patricia A Hemingway Hall
EVP, President Plan Oper	Martin G Foster
EVP/COO	Colleen Reitan
President, Ill. Division	Karen Atwood
Sr VP Chief Legal Officer	Deborah Dorman-Rodriguez
SVP, Human Resources	Nazneen Razi
SVP, Chief Financial Off	Kenneth Avner
EVP, Marketing	Paula A Steiner
Media Contact	Greg Thompson

312-653-7581
greg_thompson@hcsc.net

373 HealthSmart Preferred Care

222 West Las Colinas Boulevard
Suite 600N
Irving, IL 75039
info.cms@healthsmart.com
www.healthsmart.com
For Profit Organization: Yes
Year Founded: 1993
Number of Affiliated Hospitals: 63
Number of Primary Care Physicians: 400,000
Total Enrollment: 750,000

Healthplan and Services Defined
PLAN TYPE: PPO

Key Personnel

Chairman/President	Daniel D. Crowley
COO, Benefit Solutions	Loren W Claypool
COO/CFO	William Dembereckyj
EVP, Business Development	Todd E Archer
EVP, Network Solutions	Marty Sholder
Chief Information Officer	Jason Bielss
VP, Human Resources	Amy Willingham
Chief Marketing Officer	Mark Stadler

374 HealthSpring of Illinois

9701 W Higgins Road
Suite 360
Rosemont, IL 60018
Toll-Free: 888-588-4827
Phone: 847-318-8844
info@healthspringofillinois.com
www.healthspring.com
Year Founded: 2000
Physician Owned Organization: Yes

Healthplan and Services Defined
PLAN TYPE: Medicare

Type of Coverage
Medicare, Supplemental Medicare

Geographic Areas Served
Cook, DeKalb, DuPage, Kane, Kendall, Lake, McHenry, and Will counties

Key Personnel

President	Randy Fike
Corp Mgr, Media Relations	Graham Harrison

615-234-6710
graham.harrison@healthspring.com

375 Humana Benefit Plan of Illinois

800 NE Glen Oak Avenue
Peoria, IL 61603-3200
Phone: 309-655-2850
www.osfhealthcare.org

Secondary Address: 7915 Hale Avenue, Peoria, IL 61615, 309-683-6750
Subsidiary of: A Humana Afilliate
Year Founded: 1994

Healthplan and Services Defined
PLAN TYPE: Medicare

Type of Coverage
Medicare, Supplemental Medicare

Geographic Areas Served
CARE PREFERRED ONLY: Stephenson, Winnebago, Boone, Ogle, Whiteside, Lee, La Salle, Putnam, Bureau, Henry, Mercer, Warren, Hancock, McDonough, Fulton, Schuyler, Brown, Cass and De Witt; CARE PREFERRED & CARE ADVANTAGE: Knox, Stark, Marshall, Peoria, Woodford, Tazewell, McLean, and Livingston

Accreditation Certification
URAC, NCQA, CORE

Key Personnel

Marketing & Communication	James Farrell

309-655-2856
james.farrell@osfhealthcare.org

376 Humana Health Insurance of Illinois

2301 West 22nd Street
Suite 301
Oak Brook, IL 60523
Toll-Free: 800-569-2492
Phone: 630-794-5950
Fax: 630-794-0107
www.humana.com
Secondary Address: Chicago Guidtance CTR, 7945 South Harlem, Burbank, IL 60459, 708-430-9504
For Profit Organization: Yes
Year Founded: 1972
Number of Affiliated Hospitals: 437
Number of Primary Care Physicians: 21,070
Total Enrollment: 763,175
State Enrollment: 763,175

Healthplan and Services Defined
PLAN TYPE: HMO/PPO
Model Type: Network
Plan Specialty: Behavioral Health, Chiropractic, Dental, Disease Management, Lab, PBM, Vision, Worker's Compensation, UR
Benefits Offered: Behavioral Health, Chiropractic, Complementary Medicine, Dental, Disease Management, Home Care, Inpatient SNF, Long-Term Care, Physical Therapy, Prescription, Psychiatric, Transplant, Vision, Wellness, Worker's Compensation, AD&D, Life, LTD, STD

Type of Coverage
Commercial, Individual, Indemnity, Medicare, Supplemental Medicare, Medicaid, Catastrophic

Type of Payment Plans Offered
POS, DFFS, Capitated, FFS

Geographic Areas Served
18 States and Puerto Rico

Network Qualifications
Pre-Admission Certification: Yes

Peer Review Type
Utilization Review: Yes
Second Surgical Opinion: Yes
Case Management: Yes

Publishes and Distributes Report Card: Yes

Accreditation Certification
URAC, NCQA, CORE
TJC Accreditation, Medicare Approved, Utilization Review, Pre-Admission Certification, State Licensure, Quality Assurance Program

Key Personnel
President/CEO ....Mike McCallister
Sr VP Innovation Officer ....Jack Lord, MD
Sr VP/CFO....................................James Bloem
Sr VP Senior Products ....Douglas Carlisle
Sr VP General Counsel ....Art Hipwell
Sr VP Corporate Develop........................Tom Liston
VP Market Operations........................Stefen Brueckner
Sr VP Human Resources....................Bonnie Hathcock
COO Market/Business ....Jim Murray
Sr VP Government Relation ....Heidi Margulis
Sr VP Corporate Communica ....Tom Noland
Sr VP/CSO/CIO ....Bruce Goodman
Sr VP National Contracts ....Bruce Perkins
Sr VP Marketing Officer ....Steve Moya
Media Relations Manager......................Lindsey Minella
   312-441-5549
   lminella@humana.com

Specialty Managed Care Partners
Behavioral Health, Disease Management, PBM, Worker's
   Compensation
Enters into Contracts with Regional Business Coalitions: Yes
Midwest Business Group on Health, Mercer Coalition

377 Medical Associates Health Plan

1500 Associates Drive
Dubuque, IA 52002
Toll-Free: 800-648-6868
Phone: 563-584-3000
www.mahealthcare.com
Secondary Address: 100 Langworthy, Dubuque, IA 52002,
   563-584-3000
Non-Profit Organization: Yes
Year Founded: 1982
Physician Owned Organization: Yes
Total Enrollment: 45,000
State Enrollment: 37,792

Healthplan and Services Defined
PLAN TYPE: HMO
Other Type: EPO, POS
Plan Specialty: EPO, TPA
Benefits Offered: Behavioral Health, Chiropractic, Complementary
   Medicine, Home Care, Inpatient SNF, Physical Therapy, Podiatry,
   Prescription, Psychiatric, Transplant, Vision, Wellness

Type of Coverage
Commercial, Indemnity, Medicare, Supplemental Medicare

Type of Payment Plans Offered
POS

Geographic Areas Served
Illinois: Jo Daviess County. Iowa: Allamakee, Clayton, Delaware,
   Dubuque, Jackson, Jones counties

Peer Review Type
Utilization Review: Yes
Case Management: Yes

Accreditation Certification
NCQA
Pre-Admission Certification

Key Personnel
Executive Director.............................Tom O'Brien
CEO ....John Tallent

Specialty Managed Care Partners
Express Scripts

378 OSF Healthcare

800 NE Glen Oak Avenue
Peoria, IL 61603-3200
Phone: 309-655-2850
www.osfhealthcare.org
Subsidiary of: Sisters of the Third Order of St Francis
Non-Profit Organization: Yes
Number of Affiliated Hospitals: 8
Number of Primary Care Physicians: 210
Number of Referral/Specialty Physicians: 50
Total Enrollment: 1,500,000

Healthplan and Services Defined
PLAN TYPE: HMO
Model Type: Network
Plan Specialty: Integrated Healthcare Network of Facilities
Benefits Offered: Disease Management, Wellness

Geographic Areas Served
Illinois and Michigan

Key Personnel
CEO ....James Moore
SVP, Marketing/Comms......................James G Farrell
   309-655-2856
   james.g.farrell@osfhealthcare.org

379 OSF HealthPlans

7915 North Hale Avenue
Suite D
Peoria, IL 61615
Toll-Free: 800-673-4699
Phone: 309-677-8200
Fax: 309-677-8295
member@osfhealthcare.org
www.osfhealthplans.com
Secondary Address: 6957 Olde Creek Road, Suite 2300, Rockford, IL
   61114
Subsidiary of: A Humana Affiliate
For Profit Organization: Yes
Year Founded: 1995
Number of Affiliated Hospitals: 21
Number of Primary Care Physicians: 485
Number of Referral/Specialty Physicians: 1,133
Total Enrollment: 64,973
State Enrollment: 2,732

Healthplan and Services Defined
PLAN TYPE: PPO
Model Type: Network
Plan Specialty: ASO, Chiropractic, Dental, Disease Management,
   EPO, Lab, PBM, Vision, Radiology, UR
Benefits Offered: Chiropractic, Home Care, Inpatient SNF, Physical
   Therapy, Prescription, Psychiatric, Transplant, Wellness
Offers Demand Management Patient Information Service: Yes

Type of Coverage
Commercial, Medicare

Type of Payment Plans Offered
POS

Geographic Areas Served
Boone, Bureau, DeKalb, DeWitt, Fulton, Hancock, Henderson, Henry,
   Kane, Knox, LaSalle, Lee, Livingston, Marshall, McDonough,
   McHenry, McLean, Mercer, Ogle, Peoria, Putnam, Stark, Stephenson,
   Tazewell, Warren, Whiteside, Winnebago, Woodford counties

Publishes and Distributes Report Card: Yes

Accreditation Certification
NCQA

Key Personnel
Vice Chairperson & CEO ....James Moore
President & Director.........................Diane McGrew

VP Operations. . . . . Melody Berry
VP Chief Medical Officer . . . . Ralph Velazquez, MD

Specialty Managed Care Partners
McHelson

---

380 Preferred Network Access
1510 West 75th Street
Suite 250
Darien, IL 60561
Phone: 630-493-0905
www.pna-usa.com
For Profit Organization: Yes
Year Founded: 1995
Number of Affiliated Hospitals: 113
Number of Primary Care Physicians: 34,000
Number of Referral/Specialty Physicians: 250
Total Enrollment: 316,000
State Enrollment: 316,000

Healthplan and Services Defined
PLAN TYPE: PPO
Plan Specialty: Group, Health
Benefits Offered: Home Care, Physical Therapy, Wellness, Worker's
   Compensation, Occupational Health

Type of Coverage
Commercial

Geographic Areas Served
Illinois, Indiana, Iowa, Wisconsin

Key Personnel
President . . . . Joseph M Zerega

---

381 Trustmark Companies
400 Field Drive
Lake Forest, IL 60045
Phone: 847-615-1500
Fax: 847-615-3910
www.trustmarkcompanies.com
For Profit Organization: Yes
Year Founded: 1913
Federally Qualified: Yes
Total Enrollment: 475,000

Healthplan and Services Defined
PLAN TYPE: PPO
Other Type: Self-funded
Model Type: Network
Plan Specialty: Behavioral Health, Dental, Lab
Benefits Offered: Behavioral Health, Dental, Disease Management,
   Prescription, Wellness, AD&D, Life, LTD, STD, Major Medical,
   Nurse Line, Health Advocacy Service

Type of Coverage
Commercial, Indemnity

Type of Payment Plans Offered
FFS

Geographic Areas Served
Nationwide

Network Qualifications
Pre-Admission Certification: Yes

Peer Review Type
Utilization Review: Yes
Second Surgical Opinion: Yes

Accreditation Certification
TJC Accreditation, Utilization Review, State Licensure

Key Personnel
Chairman . . . . J Grover Thomas Jr., Jr
President, CEO . . . . Joseph L. Pray
SVP, CFO . . . . Phil Goss, CPA

SVP, Employer Medical . . . . John Anderson
Media Contact. . . . . Cindy Gallaher
   847-283-4065
   cindy.gallaher@trustmarkins.com

---

382 Unicare: Illinois
233 South Wacker Drive
Suite 3800
Chicago, IL 60607
Toll-Free: 800-618-6435
Fax: 888-882-0584
www.unicare.com
Subsidiary of: WellPoint
For Profit Organization: Yes
Year Founded: 1995
Number of Affiliated Hospitals: 30
Total Enrollment: 145,000

Healthplan and Services Defined
PLAN TYPE: HMO/PPO
Model Type: Network
Benefits Offered: Behavioral Health, Dental, Disease Management,
   Long-Term Care, Prescription, Vision, Wellness, Life, LTD, STD

Type of Coverage
Commercial, Individual, Medicare, Supplemental Medicare

Type of Payment Plans Offered
POS

Geographic Areas Served
Illinois: Cook, DuPage, Kane, Kankakee, Kendall, Lake, McHenry,
   Will counties. Indiana: Lake, Porter counties

Network Qualifications
Pre-Admission Certification: Yes

Peer Review Type
Utilization Review: Yes
Second Surgical Opinion: Yes

Accreditation Certification
NCQA
TJC Accreditation, State Licensure

Key Personnel
President/CEO . . . . David Fields
Sales Director . . . . Paul Nobile
   paul.nobile@wellpoint.com
Media Contact . . . . Tony Felts
   317-287-6036
   tony.felts@wellpoint.com

Specialty Managed Care Partners
Enters into Contracts with Regional Business Coalitions: Yes

---

383 UnitedHealthCare of Illinois
200 E. Randolph Street
Suite 5300
Chicago, IL 60601
Toll-Free: 800-627-0687
Phone: 312-803-5900
Fax: 888-311-4599
www.uhc.com
Subsidiary of: UnitedHealth Group
For Profit Organization: Yes
Total Enrollment: 75,000,000
State Enrollment: 646,192

Healthplan and Services Defined
PLAN TYPE: HMO/PPO

Geographic Areas Served
Statewide

Key Personnel
CEO . . . . Thomas Wiffler

Director...................................Julie Ward
Medical Director...........................David Stumpf
Media Contact ....Kevin Shermach
    312-453-0533
    kevin.shermach@uhc.com

384   VSP: Vision Service Plan of Illinois

222 S Riverside Plaza
#2210
Chicago, IL 60606-5808
Phone: 312-466-1601
Fax: 312-466-1733
webmaster@vsp.com
www.vsp.com
Year Founded: 1955
Number of Primary Care Physicians: 28,000
Total Enrollment: 57,000,000

Healthplan and Services Defined
   PLAN TYPE: Vision
   Plan Specialty: Vision
   Benefits Offered: Vision

Type of Payment Plans Offered
   Capitated

Geographic Areas Served
   Statewide

Network Qualifications
   Pre-Admission Certification: Yes

Peer Review Type
   Utilization Review: Yes

Accreditation Certification
   Utilization Review, Quality Assurance Program

Key Personnel
   President...................................Roger Valine
   Manager ....John Trybual

Health Insurance Coverage Status and Type of Coverage by Age

Category	All Persons		Under 18 years		Under 65 years		65 years and over	
	Number	%	Number	%	Number	%	Number	%
Total population	6,472	-	1,584	-	5,593	-	879	-
Covered by some type of health insurance	5,569 *(19)*	86.0 *(0.3)*	1,454 *(8)*	91.8 *(0.5)*	4,694 *(19)*	83.9 *(0.3)*	875 *(3)*	99.5 *(0.1)*
Covered by private health insurance	4,374 *(32)*	67.6 *(0.5)*	962 *(14)*	60.7 *(0.9)*	3,784 *(30)*	67.7 *(0.5)*	590 *(8)*	67.2 *(0.9)*
Employment based	3,722 *(31)*	57.5 *(0.5)*	881 *(14)*	55.6 *(0.9)*	3,416 *(30)*	61.1 *(0.5)*	305 *(7)*	34.7 *(0.8)*
Direct purchase	771 *(15)*	11.9 *(0.2)*	82 *(6)*	5.2 *(0.4)*	431 *(13)*	7.7 *(0.2)*	340 *(7)*	38.7 *(0.8)*
Covered by TRICARE	93 *(7)*	1.4 *(0.1)*	17 *(3)*	1.1 *(0.2)*	62 *(6)*	1.1 *(0.1)*	31 *(3)*	3.6 *(0.3)*
Covered by government health insurance	1,936 *(21)*	29.9 *(0.3)*	545 *(14)*	34.4 *(0.9)*	1,077 *(21)*	19.3 *(0.4)*	859 *(3)*	97.8 *(0.2)*
Covered by Medicaid	1,013 *(22)*	15.7 *(0.3)*	539 *(13)*	34.0 *(0.8)*	924 *(21)*	16.5 *(0.4)*	89 *(4)*	10.2 *(0.5)*
Also by private insurance	141 *(7)*	2.2 *(0.1)*	52 *(5)*	3.3 *(0.3)*	98 *(7)*	1.8 *(0.1)*	43 *(3)*	4.9 *(0.3)*
Covered by Medicare	1,040 *(9)*	16.1 *(0.1)*	9 *(2)*	0.6 *(0.1)*	181 *(8)*	3.2 *(0.1)*	858 *(3)*	97.7 *(0.2)*
Also by private insurance	624 *(9)*	9.6 *(0.1)*	1 *(1)*	0.1 *(0.1)*	50 *(4)*	0.9 *(0.1)*	574 *(8)*	65.4 *(0.9)*
Also by Medicaid	169 *(7)*	2.6 *(0.1)*	4 *(1)*	0.2 *(0.1)*	80 *(6)*	1.4 *(0.1)*	89 *(4)*	10.2 *(0.5)*
Covered by VA Care	148 *(5)*	2.3 *(0.1)*	2 *(1)*	0.1 *(0.1)*	69 *(4)*	1.2 *(0.1)*	80 *(4)*	9.1 *(0.4)*
Not covered at any time during the year	903 *(19)*	14.0 *(0.3)*	130 *(8)*	8.2 *(0.5)*	899 *(19)*	16.1 *(0.3)*	4 *(1)*	0.5 *(0.1)*

Note: Numbers in thousands; Figures cover 2013; Margin of error appears in parenthesis; A "Z" indicates that the value either represents or rounds to zero.
Source: U.S. Census Bureau, 2013 American Community Survey, Table HI05. Health Insurance Coverage Status and Type of Coverage by State and Age for All People: 2013

Indiana

385 Advantage Health Solutions

9045 River Road
Suite 200
Indianapolis, IN 46240
Toll-Free: 877-901-2237
v.perry@advantageplan.com
www.advantageplan.com
For Profit Organization: Yes
Year Founded: 2000
Number of Affiliated Hospitals: 37
Number of Primary Care Physicians: 754
Number of Referral/Specialty Physicians: 4,151
Total Enrollment: 86,000
State Enrollment: 61,064

Healthplan and Services Defined
PLAN TYPE: HMO
Benefits Offered: Behavioral Health, Chiropractic, Complementary
Medicine, Dental, Home Care, Inpatient SNF, Podiatry,
Prescription, Psychiatric, Transplant, Vision, Wellness

Type of Coverage
Commercial, Medicare

Accreditation Certification
NCQA

Key Personnel
President/CEO . . . . Vicki F Perry
317-573-6571
v.perry@advantageplan.com

Specialty Managed Care Partners
PharmaCare Management Services

386 Aetna Health of Indiana

1 South Wacker Drive
Mail Stop F643
Chicago, IL 60606
Toll-Free: 877-751-9310
www.aetna.com
Partnered with: eHealthInsurance Services Inc.
For Profit Organization: Yes
Year Founded: 1995
Total Enrollment: 45,014

Healthplan and Services Defined
PLAN TYPE: HMO
Other Type: POS
Plan Specialty: Dental, Vision
Benefits Offered: Chiropractic, Complementary Medicine, Dental,
Home Care, Inpatient SNF, Long-Term Care, Podiatry,
Prescription, Psychiatric, Transplant, Vision, Wellness

Type of Coverage
Commercial

Geographic Areas Served
Statewide

Subscriber Information
Average Monthly Fee Per Subscriber
(Employee + Employer Contribution):
Employee Only (Self): $94.38
Employee & 1 Family Member: $290.94
Average Subscriber Co-Payment:
Primary Care Physician: $20
Prescription Drugs: $10/$20

Key Personnel
Chairman . . . . John W Rowe, MD

387 American Health Network of Indiana

10689 North Pensylvannia Street
Suite 200
Indianapolis, IN 46280
Toll-Free: 888-255-2246
Phone: 317-580-6309
www.ahni.com
Secondary Address: 2500 Corporate Exchange, Suite 100, Columbus,
OH 43229, 614-794-4500
Year Founded: 1994
Number of Affiliated Hospitals: 70
Total Enrollment: 15,153

Healthplan and Services Defined
PLAN TYPE: PPO
Benefits Offered: Prescription

Type of Payment Plans Offered
Capitated

Geographic Areas Served
Indiana and Ohio

Subscriber Information
Average Annual Deductible Per Subscriber:
Employee Only (Self): $250
Average Subscriber Co-Payment:
Prescription Drugs: 100% post deductible
Home Health Care: 60% post deductible

Accreditation Certification
TJC Accreditation, State Licensure

388 Anthem Blue Cross & Blue Shield of Indiana

120 Monument Circle
Indianapolis, IN 46204
Toll-Free: 800-548-3394
Phone: 317-488-6000
Fax: 317-488-6028
www.anthem.com
Secondary Address: 1099 North Meridian Street, Indianapolis, IN
46204
For Profit Organization: Yes
Year Founded: 1988
Owned by an Integrated Delivery Network (IDN): Yes
Number of Affiliated Hospitals: 6
Number of Primary Care Physicians: 110
Number of Referral/Specialty Physicians: 363
Total Enrollment: 1,600,818
State Enrollment: 40,136

Healthplan and Services Defined
PLAN TYPE: HMO
Model Type: IPA
Plan Specialty: ASO, Behavioral Health, Chiropractic, Dental,
Disease Management, Lab, PBM, Vision, Radiology
Benefits Offered: Dental, Disease Management, Prescription, Vision,
Wellness, Life
Offers Demand Management Patient Information Service: Yes

Type of Coverage
Commercial, Individual, Medicare

Type of Payment Plans Offered
DFFS

Geographic Areas Served
Daviess, Dubois, Gibson, Knox, Martin, Perry, Pike, Posey, Spencer,
Vanderburgh, & Warrick

Subscriber Information
Average Subscriber Co-Payment:
Primary Care Physician: $10.00
Non-Network Physician: 20%
Prescription Drugs: $7.00
Hospital ER: $40.00

Home Health Care: 20%
Nursing Home: 20%

Network Qualifications
Pre-Admission Certification: Yes

Publishes and Distributes Report Card: Yes

Accreditation Certification
URAC, NCQA
Utilization Review, Quality Assurance Program

Key Personnel
CEO..Larry Glasscock
317-488-6000
President....................................Keith Faller
COO.....................................Jane Niederberger
CFO.......................................George Walker
Chief Medical Officer ....Samuel Cramer, MD
General Counsel ....Sandra H Miller
Provider Relations.........................Robert McIntire
Pharmacy Director ....John Klasner
Marketing/Sales ....Dennis Casey
Member Relations.........................Susan Cummins
Specialty Pharmacy ....Matt Totterdale
Public Relations ....Deborah New
Media Contact ....Tony Felts
317-287-6036
tony.felts@wellpoint.com

Specialty Managed Care Partners
Enters into Contracts with Regional Business Coalitions: No

---

389   Anthem Blue Cross & Blue Shield of Indiana
120 Monument Circle
Suite 200
Indianapolis, IN 46204
Toll-Free: 800-331-1476
Phone: 317-488-6000
Fax: 317-287-5582
anthem.corporate.communications@anthem.com
www.anthem.com
Secondary Address: 220 Virginia Avenue, Indianapolis, In 46204
Subsidiary of: WellPoint
For Profit Organization: Yes
Year Founded: 1990
Number of Affiliated Hospitals: 105
Number of Primary Care Physicians: 3,532
Number of Referral/Specialty Physicians: 8,475
Total Enrollment: 900,000

Healthplan and Services Defined
PLAN TYPE: HMO/PPO
Model Type: Network
Benefits Offered: Behavioral Health, Chiropractic, Complementary
Medicine, Dental, Disease Management, Home Care, Inpatient
SNF, Physical Therapy, Podiatry, Prescription, Psychiatric,
Transplant, Vision, Wellness

Type of Payment Plans Offered
DFFS, FFS, Combination FFS & DFFS

Geographic Areas Served
Statewide

Subscriber Information
Average Annual Deductible Per Subscriber:
Employee Only (Self): Varies $250-$5000
Employee & 2 Family Members: Varies $2500-$10000
Average Subscriber Co-Payment:
Primary Care Physician: Varies $25/20%
Non-Network Physician: 20%
Prescription Drugs: Varies $15/$30/$0
Hospital ER: 20%
Home Health Care: 20%
Home Health Care Max. Days/Visits Covered: 100 days

Nursing Home Max. Days/Visits Covered: 60 days

Network Qualifications
Pre-Admission Certification: Yes

Peer Review Type
Utilization Review: Yes
Second Surgical Opinion: No
Case Management: Yes

Publishes and Distributes Report Card: Yes

Accreditation Certification
URAC, NCQA
TJC Accreditation, Medicare Approved, Utilization Review,
Pre-Admission Certification, State Licensure, Quality Assurance
Program

Key Personnel
President..................................Dennis W Casey
Media Relations.................................Ed West
Media Relations.............................Deborah New
mediarelations@wellpoint.com
Media Relations ....James Kappel

---

390   Anthem Dental Services
120 Monument Circle
Indianapolis, IN 46204
Phone: 317-488-6000
www.anthem.com
Mailing Address: PO Box 37180, Dental Claims, Louisville, KY
40233-7180
Subsidiary of: Anthem Blue Cross & Blue Shield
For Profit Organization: Yes
Year Founded: 1972
Total Enrollment: 28,000,000

Healthplan and Services Defined
PLAN TYPE: Dental
Other Type: Dental PPO
Model Type: Network
Plan Specialty: Dental
Benefits Offered: Dental
Offers Demand Management Patient Information Service: Yes

Type of Payment Plans Offered
POS, Capitated, FFS

Geographic Areas Served
Colorado, Connecticut, Georgia, Indiana, Kentucky, Maine, Missouri,
Nevada, New Hampshire, Ohio, Virginia, Wisconsin

Network Qualifications
Pre-Admission Certification: Yes

Peer Review Type
Utilization Review: Yes
Second Surgical Opinion: Yes
Case Management: Yes

Publishes and Distributes Report Card: Yes

Accreditation Certification
Utilization Review, Pre-Admission Certification, State Licensure,
Quality Assurance Program

---

391   Arnett Health Plans
5165 McCarty Lane
Lafayette, IN 47905
Phone: 765-448-8000
patrefnurses@iuhealth.org
www.iuhealth.org/arnett/
Mailing Address: PO Box 5545, Lafayette, IN 47903-5545
Subsidiary of: Acquired by UnitedHealthcare
Acquired by: UnitedHealthCare
For Profit Organization: Yes
Year Founded: 1985
Owned by an Integrated Delivery Network (IDN): Yes

Number of Affiliated Hospitals: 6
Number of Primary Care Physicians: 300
Total Enrollment: 8,000
State Enrollment: 45,086

Healthplan and Services Defined
PLAN TYPE: HMO
Model Type: Group
Plan Specialty: Behavioral Health, Disease Management, Lab, PBM, Radiology
Benefits Offered: Behavioral Health, Disease Management, Home Care, Physical Therapy, Podiatry, Prescription, Psychiatric, Transplant, Wellness

Type of Coverage
Commercial, Individual, Medicare
Catastrophic Illness Benefit: Varies per case

Type of Payment Plans Offered
POS, Capitated, FFS

Geographic Areas Served
Central Indiana

Subscriber Information
Average Monthly Fee Per Subscriber
(Employee + Employer Contribution):
Employee Only (Self): $141.00
Medicare: $91.00
Average Annual Deductible Per Subscriber:
Employee Only (Self): $0
Medicare: $100.00
Average Subscriber Co-Payment:
Primary Care Physician: $15.00
Prescription Drugs: $5.00/15.00
Hospital ER: $80.00
Home Health Care: $0
Home Health Care Max. Days/Visits Covered: 60 days
Nursing Home: $0
Nursing Home Max. Days/Visits Covered: 120 days

Network Qualifications
Pre-Admission Certification: Yes

Peer Review Type
Utilization Review: Yes
Second Surgical Opinion: Yes
Case Management: Yes

Accreditation Certification
NCQA
Utilization Review, Quality Assurance Program

Key Personnel
CEO.....................................James A Brunnemer
CFO/COO...............................Robert S Paskowski
Claims Manager ....Betty Thomas
Member Services.................................Marci Hart

392   Avesis: Indiana

1493 Golfview Court
Lawrenceburg, IN 47025
Toll-Free: 800-522-0258
www.avesis.com
Year Founded: 1978
Number of Primary Care Physicians: 18,000
Total Enrollment: 2,000,000

Healthplan and Services Defined
PLAN TYPE: PPO
Other Type: Vision, Dental
Model Type: Network
Plan Specialty: Dental, Vision, Hearing
Benefits Offered: Dental, Vision

Type of Coverage
Commercial

Type of Payment Plans Offered
POS, Capitated, Combination FFS & DFFS

Geographic Areas Served
Nationwide and Puerto Rico

Publishes and Distributes Report Card: Yes

Accreditation Certification
AAAHC
TJC Accreditation

393   Cardinal Health Alliance

2401 W University Ave
Muncie, IN 47304
Phone: 765-741-1981
Fax: 765-751-3051
www.cardinalcare.com
For Profit Organization: Yes
Year Founded: 1996
Number of Affiliated Hospitals: 11
Number of Primary Care Physicians: 200
Number of Referral/Specialty Physicians: 215
Total Enrollment: 40,000

Healthplan and Services Defined
PLAN TYPE: HMO
Other Type: EPO
Model Type: Network
Plan Specialty: ASO, Disease Management, PBM, Worker's Compensation, UR
Benefits Offered: Behavioral Health, Disease Management, Home Care, Inpatient SNF, Physical Therapy, Podiatry, Prescription, Psychiatric, Wellness, Worker's Compensation

Type of Coverage
Commercial
Catastrophic Illness Benefit: Varies per case

Type of Payment Plans Offered
POS

Geographic Areas Served
11 counties in East Central Indiana

Peer Review Type
Utilization Review: Yes
Second Surgical Opinion: Yes
Case Management: Yes

Accreditation Certification
Utilization Review, State Licensure, Quality Assurance Program

Key Personnel
President and CEO ....Karen Popovich
CFO ....Kathy Edwards
Director ....Pam Livingston
Claims ....Tiffany Ridge
Network Contracting.........................Karen Popovich
Credentialing....................................Tiffany Ridge
In-House Formulary ....Mark Barnhart
Medical Affairs ....Charles Routh, MD
Provider Services ....Tiffany Ridge

Specialty Managed Care Partners
Enters into Contracts with Regional Business Coalitions: Yes

394   CIGNA HealthCare of Indiana

11595 North Meridian Street
Suite 500
Carmel, IN 46032
Toll-Free: 866-438-2446
Phone: 317-208-3230
Fax: 317-208-3241
www.cigna.com
Secondary Address: Great-West Healthcare, now part of CIGNA, 9025 North River Road, Suite 104, Indianapolis, IN 46240, 317-575-0022

For Profit Organization: Yes
Year Founded: 1993
Number of Affiliated Hospitals: 72
Number of Primary Care Physicians: 2,000
Number of Referral/Specialty Physicians: 2,000
Total Enrollment: 9,678
State Enrollment: 9,678

Healthplan and Services Defined
PLAN TYPE: HMO
Other Type: POS
Model Type: Network
Plan Specialty: ASO, Behavioral Health, Chiropractic, Dental, Disease Management, EPO, Lab, MSO, PBM, Vision, Radiology, UR
Benefits Offered: Behavioral Health, Dental, Disease Management, Prescription, Transplant, Vision, Wellness, Life, LTD, STD

Type of Coverage
Commercial

Geographic Areas Served
Adams, Allen, Boone, Cass, Clay, DeKalb, Grant, Hamilton, Hancock, Henricks, Howard, Huntington, Johnson, Kosciusko, Madison, Marion, Marshall, Miami, Montgomery, Morgan, Noble, Owen, Putnam, Saint Joseph, Shelby, Tipton, Wabash, Wells, Whitley, Michigan counties of Berrien, Cass and Van Buren

Network Qualifications
Pre-Admission Certification: Yes

Peer Review Type
Utilization Review: Yes

Publishes and Distributes Report Card: Yes

Accreditation Certification
NCQA
TJC Accreditation, Medicare Approved, Utilization Review, Pre-Admission Certification, State Licensure, Quality Assurance Program

Key Personnel
Chief Medical Officer....................... Aslam Khan, MD

Average Claim Compensation
Physician's Fees Charged: 82%
Hospital's Fees Charged: 85%

---

395   Deaconess Health Plans
350 W Columbia
Suite 400
Evansville, IN 47710
Toll-Free: 800-374-8993
Phone: 812-450-7265
Fax: 812-450-2030
www.deaconess.com
Subsidiary of: Deaconess Health System
Year Founded: 1985
Physician Owned Organization: Yes
Number of Affiliated Hospitals: 6
Number of Primary Care Physicians: 900
Number of Referral/Specialty Physicians: 555
Total Enrollment: 140,000
State Enrollment: 132,000

Healthplan and Services Defined
PLAN TYPE: PPO
Model Type: Network
Plan Specialty: Behavioral Health, Chiropractic
Benefits Offered: Disease Management, Wellness

Type of Coverage
Individual

Type of Payment Plans Offered
POS, FFS

Geographic Areas Served
Northwestern Kentucky, Southeastern Illinois, Southwestern Indiana

Network Qualifications
Pre-Admission Certification: Yes

Peer Review Type
Utilization Review: Yes
Second Surgical Opinion: No
Case Management: Yes

Accreditation Certification
TJC Accreditation, Medicare Approved, Utilization Review, Pre-Admission Certification, State Licensure, Quality Assurance Program

Key Personnel
CEO .... Joyce Hudson
joyce_hudson@deaconess.com
Provider Credentialing .... Mindi Alvey
Provider Credentialing.................... Jamie Montgomery
Provider Credentialing .... Laura Schilling
Marketing .... Tina Hazelip
Member Services .... Vicky Berneking
vicky_berneking@deaconess.com
Provider Relations .... Jolee Miller
Provider Relations......................... Sara Calverly
Sales .... Beth Deters

Average Claim Compensation
Physician's Fees Charged: 1%
Hospital's Fees Charged: 1%

---

396   Delta Dental of Michigan, Ohio and Indiana
225 S. East Street
Suite 358
Indianapolis, IN 46202
Toll-Free: 800-524-0149
www.deltadentalin.com
Subsidiary of: Delta Dental Plans Association
Total Enrollment: 54,000,000

Healthplan and Services Defined
PLAN TYPE: Dental
Other Type: Dental PPO
Plan Specialty: Dental
Benefits Offered: Dental

Type of Coverage
Commercial, Individual

Geographic Areas Served
Michigan, Ohio, Indiana

Key Personnel
President/CEO.......................... Laura L Czelada, CPA
VP/Chief Actuary .... Toby Hall
VP/Administration............................ Joadi Keck
SVP/CFO .... Goran Jurkovic, CPA
EVP/Chief of Staff....................... Nancy E Hostetier
Chief Science Officer .... Jed J Jacobson, DDS
VP/Sales .... Anthony Robinson
SVP/Marketing............................... Randy Tasco
Dir/Media & Public Affair .... Elizabeth Risberg
415-972-8423

---

397   eHealthInsurance Services Inc.
11919 Foundation Place
Gold River, CA 95670
Toll-Free: 800-644-3491
webmaster@healthinsurance.com
www.e.healthinsurance.com
Year Founded: 1997

Healthplan and Services Defined
PLAN TYPE: HMO/PPO

Benefits Offered: Dental, Life, STD

Type of Coverage
Commercial, Individual, Medicare

Geographic Areas Served
All 50 states in the USA and District of Columbia

Key Personnel
Chairman & CEO . . . . .Gary L. Lauer
EVP/Business & Corp. Dev. .Bruce Telkamp
EVP/Chief Technology. . . . . .Dr. Sheldon X. Wang
SVP & CFO . . . . .Stuart M. Huizinga
Pres. of eHealth Gov. Sys . . . . .Samuel C. Gibbs
SVP of Sales & Operations . . . . .Robert S. Hurley
Director Public Relations. . . . . .Nate Purpura
650-210-3115

398 Encircle Network

8520 Allison Pointe Blvd
Suite 200
Indianapolis, IN 46250-4299
Toll-Free: 888-574-8180
Phone: 317-621-4250
Fax: 317-621-2388
www.encoreconnect.com
Subsidiary of: Encore Connect, The HealthCare Group, LLC
For Profit Organization: Yes
Year Founded: 2003
Number of Affiliated Hospitals: 43
Number of Primary Care Physicians: 14,000

Healthplan and Services Defined
PLAN TYPE: Other
Other Type: EPO

Type of Coverage
Commercial, Individual

Geographic Areas Served
Select Indiana Markets

Key Personnel
President . . . . .Bruce Smiley
317-621-4253
bsmiley@encoreppo.com

399 Encore Health Network

8520 Allison Pointe Blvd
Suite 200
Indianapolis, IN 46250-4299
Toll-Free: 888-574-8180
Phone: 317-621-4250
Fax: 317-621-2388
www.encoreconnect.com
Subsidiary of: The Healthcare Group LLC
Year Founded: 1999
Number of Affiliated Hospitals: 176
Number of Primary Care Physicians: 29,000
Number of Referral/Specialty Physicians: 2,200
Total Enrollment: 664,318

Healthplan and Services Defined
PLAN TYPE: PPO
Model Type: Group
Plan Specialty: Medical PPO
Benefits Offered: Chiropractic, Complementary Medicine, Vision,
Wellness, Worker's Compensation, Alternative Heath Care
Management, Health Savings Plans, HealthyRoads

Type of Coverage
Fully insured & self-funded

Type of Payment Plans Offered
DFFS

Geographic Areas Served
All of Indiana, Chicago area, MI, IL & OH bordering couties &
northern KY

Peer Review Type
Utilization Review: Yes
Case Management: Yes

Key Personnel
President . . . . .Bruce Smiley
317-621-4253
bsmiley@encoreppo.com
Dir Sales & Marketing. . . . . .Shawn Gibbons
317-963-9733
sgibbons@encoreppo.com
Sales Account Executive . . . . .Rochelle Forrest, RN
317-963-9723
rforrest@encoreppo.com

Average Claim Compensation
Physician's Fees Charged: 36%
Hospital's Fees Charged: 29%

Specialty Managed Care Partners
Enters into Contracts with Regional Business Coalitions: Yes

Employer References
Marsh Supermarkets, Reid Hospital, Deaconness Development
Corporation, Suburu-Isuzu, Group Dekko/Multi-Kare

400 Great-West Healthcare Indiana

429 North Pennsylvania
Indianapolis, IN 46240
Toll-Free: 866-494-2111
Phone: 317-615-1200
eliginquiries@cigna.com
www.cignaforhealth.com
Subsidiary of: CIGNA HealthCare
Acquired by: CIGNA
For Profit Organization: Yes
Total Enrollment: 43,620
State Enrollment: 718

Healthplan and Services Defined
PLAN TYPE: HMO/PPO
Benefits Offered: Disease Management, Prescription, Wellness

Type of Coverage
Commercial

Type of Payment Plans Offered
POS, FFS

Geographic Areas Served
Indiana

Accreditation Certification
URAC

Specialty Managed Care Partners
Caremark Rx

401 Great-West Healthcare Indiana

9229 Delegates Row
Suite 260
Indianapolis, IN 46240
Toll-Free: 800-756-5530
Phone: 317-575-0022
eliginquiries@cigna.com
www.cignaforhealth.com
Subsidiary of: CIGNA HealthCare
Acquired by: CIGNA
For Profit Organization: Yes
Total Enrollment: 43,620
State Enrollment: 39,874

Healthplan and Services Defined
PLAN TYPE: HMO/PPO
Benefits Offered: Disease Management, Prescription, Wellness

Type of Coverage
Commercial

Type of Payment Plans Offered
POS, FFS

Geographic Areas Served
Indiana

Accreditation Certification
URAC

Specialty Managed Care Partners
Caremark Rx

402 Health Resources, Inc.
5010 Carriage Drive
PO Box 659
Evansville, IN 47704-0659
Toll-Free: 800-727-1444
Fax: 812-424-2096
info@hri-dho.com
www.hri-dho.com
For Profit Organization: Yes
Year Founded: 1986
Physician Owned Organization: Yes
Number of Primary Care Physicians: 1,800
Total Enrollment: 200,000

Healthplan and Services Defined
PLAN TYPE: Dental
Model Type: Network
Plan Specialty: Dental
Benefits Offered: Dental

Type of Payment Plans Offered
FFS

Geographic Areas Served
Northern, Southwest & Central Indiana, Western Kentucky

Subscriber Information
Average Annual Deductible Per Subscriber:
Employee Only (Self): $0
Employee & 1 Family Member: $0
Employee & 2 Family Members: $0

Network Qualifications
Pre-Admission Certification: No

Accreditation Certification
Utilization Review

Key Personnel
President/CEO . . . . .Allan Reid
COO . . . . .Cynthia Kuester
Marketing Director. . . . . .Chad Decker

Specialty Managed Care Partners
Dental

Employer References
University of Notre Dame, Old National Bank, University of
Southern Indiana, Integra

403 Healthy Indiana Plan
402 West Washington Street
PO Box 7083
Indianapolis, IN 46207-7083
Toll-Free: 877-438-4479
Phone: 317-655-3304
www.in.gov/fssa/hip
Subsidiary of: AmeriChoice, A UnitedHealth Group Company
Year Founded: 2007

Healthplan and Services Defined
PLAN TYPE: HMO
Benefits Offered: Behavioral Health, Disease Management, Home
Care, Inpatient SNF, Prescription, Wellness

Type of Coverage
Individual

Key Personnel
Media Contact. . . . . .Jeff Smith
952-931-5685
jeff.smith@uhc.com

404 Humana Health Insurance of Indiana
8888 Keystone Crossing
Suite 750
Indianapolis, IN 46240
Toll-Free: 866-355-6170
Phone: 317-841-1196
Fax: 317-816-9121
www.humana.com
Secondary Address: 6319 Mutual Drive, Fort Wayne, IN 46825
Non-Profit Organization: Yes
Year Founded: 1986
Total Enrollment: 102,506
State Enrollment: 900

Healthplan and Services Defined
PLAN TYPE: HMO/PPO
Model Type: IPA
Benefits Offered: Disease Management, Wellness

Type of Coverage
Commercial, Individual, Medicare, Medicaid

Geographic Areas Served
(Southern Indiana) Boone, Clark, Crawford, Delaware, Dubois, Floyd,
Gibson, Hamilton, Hancock, Harrison, Hendricks, Howard, Jackson,
Jefferson, Jennings, Johnson, Knox, Lake, LaPorte, Madison,
Marrion, Morgan, Orange, Pike, Porter, Posey, Scott, Shelby, Spencer,
Tipton, Vanderburgh, Warrick, Washington

Accreditation Certification
URAC, NCQA, CORE

Key Personnel
President/CEO . . . . .Bruce D. Broussard
EVP/Chief Operating Offic .James E. Murray
SVP/CFO/Treasurer . . . . .James H. Bloem
SVP/Chief HR Officer. . . . . .Tim Huval
SVP/Chief Medical Officer . . . . .Roy A. Beveridge
SVP, Chief Consumer Offic. .Jody Bilney
SVP/Chief Service & Inf. . . . . .Brian LeClaire
SVP, Public Affairs. . . . . .Heidi S. Margulis
Media Relations Manager . . . . .Jeff Blunt
513-826-7094
jblunt@humana.com

405 Magellan Health Services Indiana
9265 Counselor's Road
Suite 118
Indianapolis, IN 46240
Phone: 317-815-1356
www.magellanhealth.com
Secondary Address: Magellan RSC of The Northwest, 1501 Market
Street, Suite 200, Tacoma, WA 98411
For Profit Organization: Yes
Year Founded: 1986
Number of Affiliated Hospitals: 45
Total Enrollment: 36,500,000

Healthplan and Services Defined
PLAN TYPE: PPO
Model Type: Staff

Plan Specialty: Behavioral Health, Disease Management, EAP
Benefits Offered: Behavioral Health, Disease Management,
Prescription, Psychiatric, Wellness, EAP
Offers Demand Management Patient Information Service: Yes

Geographic Areas Served
Statewide

Network Qualifications
Pre-Admission Certification: Yes

Peer Review Type
Utilization Review: Yes
Second Surgical Opinion: Yes
Case Management: Yes

Publishes and Distributes Report Card: Yes

Accreditation Certification
URAC, NCQA
TJC Accreditation, Utilization Review, Pre-Admission Certification,
State Licensure

Key Personnel
Chairman/CEO . . . . .Rene Lerer, MD
CFO . . . . .Jonathan N Rubin
CIO . . . . .Gary D Anderson
General Counsel . . . . .Daniel N Gregoire
Chief Medical Officer . . . . .Anthony M Kotin, MD
Chief HR Officer. . . . . .Caskie Lewis-Clapper
Chief Marketing Officer . . . . .Ramon Soto
VP, Corporate Communs. . . . . .Tami Schmidt
Media Relations Manager. .Chris Pearsall
860-507-1923
cmpearsall@magellanhealth.com
Chief Commun Officer . . . . .David W Carter

Specialty Managed Care Partners
Enters into Contracts with Regional Business Coalitions: Yes

406 Meritain Health: Indiana
111 Southeast Third Street
Suite 101
Evansville, IN 47708
Toll-Free: 866-828-1338
sales@meritain.com
www.meritain.com
Secondary Address: 9254 N Meridian Street, Indianapolis, IN 46240,
800-624-8316
Subsidiary of: Aetna Company
For Profit Organization: Yes
Year Founded: 1983
Number of Affiliated Hospitals: 110
Number of Primary Care Physicians: 3,467
Number of Referral/Specialty Physicians: 5,720
Total Enrollment: 500,000
State Enrollment: 450,000

Healthplan and Services Defined
PLAN TYPE: PPO
Model Type: Network
Plan Specialty: Dental, Disease Management, Vision, Radiology, UR
Benefits Offered: Prescription
Offers Demand Management Patient Information Service: Yes

Type of Coverage
Commercial

Geographic Areas Served
Nationwide

Subscriber Information
Average Monthly Fee Per Subscriber
(Employee + Employer Contribution):
Employee Only (Self): Varies by plan

Accreditation Certification
URAC

TJC Accreditation, Medicare Approved, Utilization Review,
Pre-Admission Certification, State Licensure, Quality Assurance
Program

Key Personnel
Regional President . . . . .Chris Reef

Average Claim Compensation
Physician's Fees Charged: 78%
Hospital's Fees Charged: 90%

Specialty Managed Care Partners
Express Scripts, LabOne, Interactive Health Solutions

407 Parkview Total Health
10501 Corporate Drive
Fort Wayne, IN 46845
Toll-Free: 800-666-4449
Phone: 260-373-9100
Fax: 260-373-9004
signaturecarewebmaster@parkview.com
www.parkviewtotalhealth.com
Mailing Address: PO Box 5548, Fort Wayne, IN 46895-5548
Non-Profit Organization: Yes
Year Founded: 1992
Number of Affiliated Hospitals: 77
Number of Primary Care Physicians: 9,000
Total Enrollment: 90,000

Healthplan and Services Defined
PLAN TYPE: PPO
Other Type: EAP
Model Type: Network, IPA
Benefits Offered: Disease Management, Wellness

Type of Coverage
Commercial

Geographic Areas Served
Indiana & Northwestern Ohio

Network Qualifications
Pre-Admission Certification: Yes

Peer Review Type
Utilization Review: Yes
Second Surgical Opinion: No
Case Management: Yes

Accreditation Certification
TJC Accreditation, Medicare Approved, Utilization Review,
Pre-Admission Certification, State Licensure, Quality Assurance
Program

Employer References
Parkview Hospitals, East Allen County Schools, Guardian Industries,
Chore Timer Brook, Tomkins

408 Physicians Health Plan of Northern Indiana
8101 W Jefferson Boulevard
Fort Wayne, IN 46804-4163
Toll-Free: 800-982-6257
Phone: 260-432-6690
Fax: 260-432-0493
custsvc@phpni.com
www.phpni.com
Non-Profit Organization: Yes
Year Founded: 1983
Physician Owned Organization: Yes
Federally Qualified: Yes
Number of Affiliated Hospitals: 59
Number of Primary Care Physicians: 1,287
Number of Referral/Specialty Physicians: 5,873
Total Enrollment: 43,000
State Enrollment: 48,000

Healthplan and Services Defined
PLAN TYPE: HMO
Model Type: IPA, POS
Benefits Offered: Behavioral Health, Dental, Disease Management, Home Care, Physical Therapy, Podiatry, Prescription, Psychiatric, Transplant, Vision, Wellness, AD&D, Life, LTD, STD
Offers Demand Management Patient Information Service: Yes

Type of Coverage
Commercial, Individual
Catastrophic Illness Benefit: Unlimited

Type of Payment Plans Offered
POS, DFFS, FFS, Combination FFS & DFFS

Geographic Areas Served
Northern Indiana, Southwest Michigan, Northwest Ohio. counties covered include: Berrien, Cass, St. Joseph, Branch, La Porte, Elkhart, LaGrange, Steuben, Starke, Marshall, Kosciusko, Noble, DeKalb, Newton, Jasper, Pulaski, Fulton, Whitley, Allen, Benton, White, Cass, Miami, Wabash, Huntington, Wells, Adams, Benton, Carroll, Warren, Foundtain, Tippecanoe, Montgomery, Clinton, Boone, Howard, Tipton, Hamilton, Grant, Blackford, Jay, Delaware, Randolph, Defiance, Mercer

Subscriber Information
Average Monthly Fee Per Subscriber
(Employee + Employer Contribution):
Employee Only (Self): $210.25
Employee & 1 Family Member: $384.50
Employee & 2 Family Members: $610.74 family
Average Annual Deductible Per Subscriber:
Employee Only (Self): $250.00
Employee & 1 Family Member: $500.00
Employee & 2 Family Members: $500.00 family
Average Subscriber Co-Payment:
Primary Care Physician: $15.00
Non-Network Physician: Pos=20%
Prescription Drugs: $15.00
Hospital ER: $75.00
Home Health Care: 100%
Home Health Care Max. Days/Visits Covered: 60 per year
Nursing Home Max. Days/Visits Covered: 30 per year

Network Qualifications
Pre-Admission Certification: Yes

Peer Review Type
Utilization Review: Yes
Case Management: Yes

Publishes and Distributes Report Card: Yes

Accreditation Certification
Utilization Review, Pre-Admission Certification, State Licensure, Quality Assurance Program

Key Personnel
Director, Health Services . . . . .Carrie Marion
Credentialing Coordinator . . . . .Toni Roemer
Provider Relations. . . . . .Susan Werner
Community Relations Coor. . . . . .Carmen Parker
260-432-6690

Specialty Managed Care Partners
Enters into Contracts with Regional Business Coalitions: Yes

409   Sagamore Health Network
11555 N Meridian Street
Suite 400
Carmel, IN 46032
Toll-Free: 800-364-3469
Phone: 317-573-2886
mps@sagamorehn.com
www.sagamorehn.com
Subsidiary of: A CIGNA Company
Year Founded: 1985

Number of Affiliated Hospitals: 257
Number of Primary Care Physicians: 15,059
Number of Referral/Specialty Physicians: 39,212
Total Enrollment: 360,561

Healthplan and Services Defined
PLAN TYPE: PPO
Model Type: IPA

Geographic Areas Served
Entire state of Indiana, Kentucky, Illinois, Michigan and Ohio

Accreditation Certification
URAC
TJC Accreditation, Medicare Approved, Utilization Review, Pre-Admission Certification, State Licensure, Quality Assurance Program

Key Personnel
President . . . . .Ronald Vance

410   Southeastern Indiana Health Organization
417 Washington Street
PO Box 1787
Columbus, IN 47202-1787
Toll-Free: 800-443-2980
Phone: 812-378-7000
Fax: 812-378-7048
www.siho.org
Secondary Address: 222 South Walnut Street, Bloomington, IN 47404, 812-245-5200
Non-Profit Organization: Yes
Year Founded: 1987
Physician Owned Organization: Yes
Number of Affiliated Hospitals: 101
Number of Primary Care Physicians: 2,316
Number of Referral/Specialty Physicians: 4,722
Total Enrollment: 10,231
State Enrollment: 10,231

Healthplan and Services Defined
PLAN TYPE: HMO
Model Type: IPA, Network, POS
Plan Specialty: ASO, Dental, Disease Management, Vision
Benefits Offered: Behavioral Health, Chiropractic, Dental, Disease Management, Home Care, Inpatient SNF, Long-Term Care, Physical Therapy, Prescription, Transplant, Vision, Wellness, AD&D, Life, STD

Type of Coverage
Individual, Indemnity, Medicaid
Catastrophic Illness Benefit: Unlimited

Type of Payment Plans Offered
POS, DFFS, FFS

Geographic Areas Served
Bartholomew, Brown, Clark, Crawford, Davies, Decatur, Dubois, Gibson, Jackson, Jefferson, Jennings, Johnson, Knox, Lawrence, Martin, Monroe, Orange, Perry, Pike, Posey, Ripley, Scott, Shelby, Switzerland, Vanderburgh, Warrick, Washington

Subscriber Information
Average Subscriber Co-Payment:
Primary Care Physician: $15.00
Non-Network Physician: 40%
Prescription Drugs: $10/20/30
Hospital ER: $75.00

Network Qualifications
Pre-Admission Certification: Yes

Peer Review Type
Utilization Review: Yes
Case Management: Yes

Publishes and Distributes Report Card: Yes

Accreditation Certification
TJC Accreditation, Utilization Review, Pre-Admission Certification, State Licensure

Key Personnel
President / CEO ....David S Barker
812-378-7024
david.barker@siho.org
CFO ....Marc Rothbart, BSN
812-348-7458
COO.......................................Ronald Sewell
812-378-7021
VP Claims ....Jennifer Cutsinger
812-378-7030
Network Contracting...........................Randy Mills
812-378-7000
Medical Director ....Joseph Sheehy, MD
812-378-7067
Manager Member Services.......................Cathy Dykes
VP Information Services ....Mike Clancy
812-378-7052
Sales Representative...........................Mike Ketron
812-348-4575
mike.ketron@siho.org
Media Contact ....Chris Asher
812-378-7028
chris.asher@siho.org
Media Contact ....Alan Clark
812-348-4581
alan.clark@siho.org

Specialty Managed Care Partners
Caremark Rx
Enters into Contracts with Regional Business Coalitions: Yes

Employer References
Columbus Regional Hospital, Enkei America, Seymour Memorial Hospital, Seymour Tubing

411 UnitedHealthCare of Indiana
7440 Woodland Drive
Department 100
Indianapolis, IN 46278
Toll-Free: 800-382-5445
Fax: 317-405-3895
www.uhc.com
Secondary Address: 180 E Ocean Blvd, Suite 500, Long Beach, CA 90802, 888-283-9847
Subsidiary of: UnitedHealth Group
For Profit Organization: Yes
Year Founded: 1986
Number of Affiliated Hospitals: 66
Number of Primary Care Physicians: 1,208
Number of Referral/Specialty Physicians: 1,983
Total Enrollment: 75,000,000
State Enrollment: 244,441

Healthplan and Services Defined
PLAN TYPE: HMO/PPO
Model Type: IPA, Network
Benefits Offered: Chiropractic, Dental, Home Care, Inpatient SNF, Long-Term Care, Podiatry, Psychiatric, Transplant, Vision, Wellness

Type of Coverage
Commercial

Type of Payment Plans Offered
POS

Geographic Areas Served
Statewide

Subscriber Information
Average Monthly Fee Per Subscriber
(Employee + Employer Contribution):
Employee Only (Self): Varies per plan
Employee & 2 Family Members: Variers per plan
Average Annual Deductible Per Subscriber:
Employee Only (Self): Varies per plan
Employee & 2 Family Members: Varies per plan
Average Subscriber Co-Payment:
Primary Care Physician: Varies per plan

Accreditation Certification
TJC

Key Personnel
CEO ....Charles Price
Medical Director ....Alan Grimes, MD
Media Contact ....Jessica Kostner
952-979-5869
jessica_kostner@uhc.com

412 VSP: Vision Service Plan of Indiana
101 W Ohio Street
#875
Indianpolis, IN 46204-4207
Phone: 317-686-1066
Fax: 317-686-1140
webmaster@vsp.com
www.vsp.com
Year Founded: 1955
Number of Primary Care Physicians: 28,000
Total Enrollment: 57,000,000

Healthplan and Services Defined
PLAN TYPE: Vision
Plan Specialty: Vision
Benefits Offered: Vision

Type of Payment Plans Offered
Capitated

Geographic Areas Served
Statewide

Network Qualifications
Pre-Admission Certification: Yes

Peer Review Type
Utilization Review: Yes

Accreditation Certification
Utilization Review, Quality Assurance Program

Key Personnel
Administrator.................................Kathy Maxey
Senior Account Executive ....Linda Stevens

413 Welborn Health Plans
101 SE Third Street
Evansville, IN 47708
Toll-Free: 800-521-0265
Phone: 812-426-6600
Fax: 716-541-6335
memberservices@welbornhealthplans.com
www.welbornhealthplans.com
For Profit Organization: Yes
Year Founded: 1986
Physician Owned Organization: No
Number of Affiliated Hospitals: 27
Number of Primary Care Physicians: 300
Number of Referral/Specialty Physicians: 1,000
Total Enrollment: 38,515

Healthplan and Services Defined
PLAN TYPE: HMO
Model Type: Network

Plan Specialty: Health & Wellness, Diabetes, Hyperlipidemia,
    Hypertension, Heart Failure, Asthma, COPD, Migraine,
    Depression, Case Mgmt
Benefits Offered: HMO, POS/PPO-Type, Medicare Advantage
Offers Demand Management Patient Information Service: Yes

Type of Coverage
    Medicare, Group Health, Pharmacy
    Catastrophic Illness Benefit: Unlimited

Type of Payment Plans Offered
    POS, DFFS, Capitated, FFS

Geographic Areas Served
    IN counties: Vanderburgh, Posey, Warrick, Spencer, Perry, Gibson,
    Pike, Dubois, Knox, Daviess   KY counties: Henderson, Union,
    Daviess, Hancock, Breckinridge, Webster, McLean, Ohio, Hopkins,
    Muhlenberg, Crittenden, Caldwell, Butler, Edmonson, Livingston,
    Lyon, McCracken, Ballard, Carlisle, Hickman, Fulton, Graves,
    Marshall, Calloway, Trigg, Christian, Todd, Logan, Simpson, Allen,
    Warren, Barren, Metalfe, Monroe

Subscriber Information
    Average Annual Deductible Per Subscriber:
        Medicare: $90.00

Network Qualifications
    Pre-Admission Certification: Yes

Peer Review Type
    Utilization Review: Yes
    Second Surgical Opinion: Yes
    Case Management: Yes

Publishes and Distributes Report Card: Yes

Key Personnel
    Regional President, CEO . . . . Chris Reef
    Chief Financial Officer . . . . Debby Sidener
    COO, Evansville Ops Lead . . . . Claudia Winsett
    Director of Operations . . . . Heather Burns
    Pharmacy Tech . . . . Su Quinn
        812-773-0376
    Chief Marketing Officer . . . . Janet Burnett
    Chief Medical Director . . . . Roy Arnold, MD
    Director of Technology . . . . Jeremy Mathews

Average Claim Compensation
    Physician's Fees Charged: 75%
    Hospital's Fees Charged: 80%

Specialty Managed Care Partners
    Enters into Contracts with Regional Business Coalitions: Yes

414   WellPoint: Corporate Office
120 Monument Circle
Indianapolis, IN 46204
Phone: 317-532-6000
Fax: 317-488-6028
www.wellpoint.com
For Profit Organization: Yes
Year Founded: 2004
Total Enrollment: 35,000,000

Healthplan and Services Defined
    PLAN TYPE: HMO

Type of Coverage
    Commercial

Key Personnel
    Chief Executive Officer . . . . Joseph R. Swedish
    EVP/Chief Financial Offic . . . . Wayne DeVeydt
    EVP/Chief Admin Officer . . . . Gloria McCarthy
    EVP, Chief Strategy Offc . . . . Brad M Fluegel
    EVP/General Counsel/Chief . . . . John Cannon
    EVP, Health Solutions . . . . Harlan Levine, MD
    EVP/Chief HR Officer . . . . Randy Brown
    EVP/Chief Medical Officer . . . . Samuel Nussbaum
    EVP, IT . . . . Lori Beer

Media Contact . . . . Jill Becher
    jill.becher@wellpoint.com

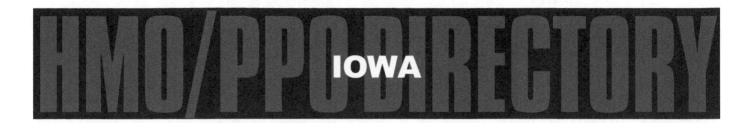

Health Insurance Coverage Status and Type of Coverage by Age

Category	All Persons		Under 18 years		Under 65 years		65 years and over	
	Number	%	Number	%	Number	%	Number	%
Total population	3,045	-	721	-	2,590	-	455	-
Covered by some type of health insurance	2,798 (9)	91.9 (0.3)	692 (4)	95.9 (0.5)	2,344 (8)	90.5 (0.3)	454 (2)	99.7 (0.1)
Covered by private health insurance	2,278 (15)	74.8 (0.5)	485 (7)	67.3 (1.0)	1,949 (14)	75.2 (0.5)	330 (4)	72.4 (1.0)
Employment based	1,834 (18)	60.2 (0.6)	433 (8)	60.1 (1.2)	1,706 (16)	65.9 (0.6)	128 (4)	28.1 (1.0)
Direct purchase	504 (11)	16.5 (0.4)	55 (4)	7.6 (0.6)	277 (9)	10.7 (0.4)	227 (5)	49.9 (1.1)
Covered by TRICARE	48 (4)	1.6 (0.1)	9 (2)	1.2 (0.3)	31 (4)	1.2 (0.1)	17 (2)	3.7 (0.4)
Covered by government health insurance	946 (12)	31.1 (0.4)	247 (7)	34.2 (1.0)	498 (12)	19.2 (0.5)	448 (2)	98.4 (0.3)
Covered by Medicaid	496 (12)	16.3 (0.4)	245 (7)	34.0 (1.0)	444 (12)	17.1 (0.5)	52 (2)	11.5 (0.5)
Also by private insurance	103 (6)	3.4 (0.2)	40 (4)	5.5 (0.6)	73 (6)	2.8 (0.2)	30 (2)	6.5 (0.4)
Covered by Medicare	516 (4)	16.9 (0.1)	4 (1)	0.5 (0.2)	68 (4)	2.6 (0.1)	448 (2)	98.3 (0.3)
Also by private insurance	344 (5)	11.3 (0.2)	1 (Z)	0.1 (0.1)	20 (2)	0.8 (0.1)	323 (4)	71.1 (1.0)
Also by Medicaid	92 (4)	3.0 (0.1)	2 (1)	0.3 (0.1)	39 (3)	1.5 (0.1)	52 (2)	11.5 (0.5)
Covered by VA Care	82 (4)	2.7 (0.1)	Z (Z)	0.0 (0.1)	33 (3)	1.3 (0.1)	49 (3)	10.8 (0.6)
Not covered at any time during the year	248 (9)	8.1 (0.3)	30 (4)	4.1 (0.5)	246 (9)	9.5 (0.3)	1 (1)	0.3 (0.1)

Note: Numbers in thousands; Figures cover 2013; Margin of error appears in parenthesis; A "Z" indicates that the value either represents or rounds to zero.
Source: U.S. Census Bureau, 2013 American Community Survey, Table HI05. Health Insurance Coverage Status and Type of Coverage by State and Age for All People: 2013

Iowa

415 Aetna Health of Iowa

151 Farmington Avenue
Hartford, CT 06156
Toll-Free: 800-872-3862
Phone: 860-273-0123
www.aetna.com
Partnered with: eHealthInsurance Services Inc.
For Profit Organization: Yes
Total Enrollment: 11,596,230

Healthplan and Services Defined
PLAN TYPE: PPO
Other Type: POS
Plan Specialty: EPO
Benefits Offered: Dental, Disease Management, Long-Term Care,
   Prescription, Wellness, Life, LTD, STD

Type of Coverage
Commercial, Individual

Type of Payment Plans Offered
POS, FFS

Geographic Areas Served
Statewide

Key Personnel
Chairman/CEO/President. . . . . Mark T Bertolini
EVP/General Counsel . . . . William J Casazza
EVP/CFO . . . . Shawn M Guertin

416 American Republic Insurance Company

P.O. Box 1
Des Moines, IA 50306-0001
Toll-Free: 800-247-2190
Fax: 515-247-2435
www.americanrepublic.com
For Profit Organization: Yes
Year Founded: 1929

Healthplan and Services Defined
PLAN TYPE: HMO

Type of Coverage
Commercial, Individual, Medicare

Geographic Areas Served
Alabama, Arizona, Arkansas, Colorado, Delaware, Florida, Georgia,
   Illinois, Indiana, Iowa, Kansas, Kentucky, Louisiana, Michigan,
   Mississippi, Missouri, Montana, Nebraska, Nevada, New Mexico,
   North Carolina, North Dakota, Ohio, Oklahoma, Pennsylvania, South
   Carolina, South Dakota, Tennessee, Virginia, West Virginia,
   Wisconsin, Wyoming

417 Avesis: Iowa

317 Sixth Avenue
Suite 1040
Des Moines, IA 50309
Phone: 515-244-6282
www.avesis.com
Year Founded: 1978
Number of Primary Care Physicians: 18,000
Total Enrollment: 2,000,000

Healthplan and Services Defined
PLAN TYPE: PPO
Other Type: Vision, Dental
Model Type: Network
Plan Specialty: Dental, Vision, Hearing
Benefits Offered: Dental, Vision

Type of Coverage
Commercial

Type of Payment Plans Offered
POS, Capitated, Combination FFS & DFFS

Geographic Areas Served
Nationwide and Puerto Rico

Publishes and Distributes Report Card: Yes

Accreditation Certification
AAAHC
TJC Accreditation

418 CIGNA HealthCare of Iowa

525 West Monroe Street
Suite 300
Chicago, IL 60661
Toll-Free: 800-832-3211
Phone: 312-648-2460
Fax: 312-648-3617
www.cigna.com
For Profit Organization: Yes
Total Enrollment: 34,284
State Enrollment: 28,259

Healthplan and Services Defined
PLAN TYPE: HMO
Benefits Offered: Disease Management, Prescription, Transplant,
   Wellness

Type of Coverage
Commercial

Type of Payment Plans Offered
POS, FFS

Geographic Areas Served
Iowa

Key Personnel
Vice President . . . . Sherry Husa
VP Network Services . . . . Thomas Golias
VP National Accounts . . . . Karen Weaver

419 Coventry Health Care of Iowa

4320 114th Street
Urbandale, IA 50322-5408
Toll-Free: 800-470-6352
Phone: 515-225-1234
http://chciowa.coventryhealthcare.com
Subsidiary of: Coventry Health Care Inc.
For Profit Organization: Yes
Year Founded: 1986
Number of Affiliated Hospitals: 152
Number of Primary Care Physicians: 3,500
Total Enrollment: 47,000
State Enrollment: 41,644

Healthplan and Services Defined
PLAN TYPE: HMO/PPO
Other Type: POS
Model Type: Group
Benefits Offered: Disease Management, Home Care, Inpatient SNF,
   Long-Term Care, Physical Therapy, Podiatry, Prescription,
   Psychiatric, Transplant, Vision, Wellness, Worker's Compensation

Type of Coverage
Commercial, Individual, Medicare, Supplemental Medicare, Medicaid

Type of Payment Plans Offered
POS

Geographic Areas Served
Sioux City, Waterloo/Cedar Falls, Cedar Rapids and Central Iowa

Peer Review Type
Utilization Review: Yes

Accreditation Certification
URAC

420 Delta Dental of Iowa

PO Box 9000
Johnson, IA 50131-9000
Toll-Free: 800-544-0718
Fax: 888-264-1440
claims@deltadentalia.com
www.deltadentalia.com
Mailing Address: PO Box 9010, Johnson, IA 50130-9010
Non-Profit Organization: Yes
Year Founded: 1970
Total Enrollment: 54,000,000
State Enrollment: 74,000

Healthplan and Services Defined
PLAN TYPE: Dental
Other Type: Dental PPO
Model Type: Network
Plan Specialty: Dental
Benefits Offered: Dental

Type of Coverage
Commercial

Type of Payment Plans Offered
DFFS

Geographic Areas Served
Statewide

Subscriber Information
Average Monthly Fee Per Subscriber
(Employee + Employer Contribution):
Employee Only (Self): $17
Employee & 2 Family Members: $50
Average Annual Deductible Per Subscriber:
Employee Only (Self): $150
Employee & 2 Family Members: $50
Average Subscriber Co-Payment:
Primary Care Physician: 80%
Non-Network Physician: 50%

Network Qualifications
Pre-Admission Certification: Yes

Publishes and Distributes Report Card: Yes

Key Personnel
President/CEO . . . . .Jeff Russell
VP & COO . . . . .Cheryl Harding
VP, Finance & Controller . . . . .Sherry Perkins
Dental Director . . . . .Ed Schooley, DDS
VP, Marketing & Business . . . . .Tami Rubino
VP, Public Affairs . . . . .Suzanne Heckenlaible
VP, Information Systems. . . . . .Tim Rolow
VP, Sales & Customer Rela . . . . .Greg Shireman
Corporate Comms Dir . . . . .Jill Hamilton
515-261-5526
jhamilton@deltadentalia.com

421 eHealthInsurance Services Inc.

11919 Foundation Place
Gold River, CA 95670
Toll-Free: 800-644-3491
webmaster@healthinsurance.com
www.e.healthinsurance.com
Year Founded: 1997

Healthplan and Services Defined
PLAN TYPE: HMO/PPO
Benefits Offered: Dental, Life, STD

Type of Coverage
Commercial, Individual, Medicare

Geographic Areas Served
All 50 states in the USA and District of Columbia

Key Personnel
Chairman & CEO . . . . .Gary L. Lauer
EVP/Business & Corp. Dev. .Bruce Telkamp
EVP/Chief Technology .Dr. Sheldon X. Wang
SVP & CFO . . . . .Stuart M. Huizinga
Pres. of eHealth Gov. Sys .Samuel C. Gibbs
SVP of Sales & Operations .Robert S. Hurley
Director Public Relations. . . . . .Nate Purpura
650-210-3115

422 Great-West Healthcare Iowa

525 West Monroe Street
Suite 300
Chicago, IL 60661
Toll-Free: 866-494-2111
Phone: 312-648-2460
eliginquiries@cigna.com
www.cignaforhealth.com
Subsidiary of: CIGNA HealthCare
Acquired by: CIGNA
For Profit Organization: Yes
Total Enrollment: 10,082
State Enrollment: 8,337

Healthplan and Services Defined
PLAN TYPE: HMO/PPO
Benefits Offered: Disease Management, Prescription, Wellness

Type of Coverage
Commercial

Type of Payment Plans Offered
POS, FFS

Geographic Areas Served
Iowa

Accreditation Certification
URAC

Specialty Managed Care Partners
Caremark Rx

423 Healthy & Well Kids in Iowa

PO Box 71336
Des Moines, IA 50325
Toll-Free: 800-257-8563
Fax: 877-457-7701
www.hawk-i.org
Subsidiary of: AmeriChoice, A UnitedHealth Group Company

Healthplan and Services Defined
PLAN TYPE: HMO

Key Personnel
Chairman . . . . .Kim Carson
Vice Chairman . . . . .Selden Spencer, MD

424 Humana Health Insurance of Iowa

1415 Kimberly Road
Bettendorf, IA 52722
Toll-Free: 866-653-7275
Phone: 563-388-7920
Fax: 563-388-6295
www.humana.com
For Profit Organization: Yes
Year Founded: 1961
Federally Qualified: Yes
Total Enrollment: 7,000,000

Healthplan and Services Defined
PLAN TYPE: HMO/PPO
Model Type: Staff
Plan Specialty: Dental

Benefits Offered: Behavioral Health, Chiropractic, Dental, Disease Management, Prescription, Psychiatric, Wellness, Worker's Compensation, Life, LTD, STD

Type of Coverage
Commercial, Individual, Supplemental Medicare

Geographic Areas Served
15 states and Puerto Rico

Accreditation Certification
URAC, NCQA, CORE

Key Personnel
Chairman.................................David A Jones, Jr
President/CEO ....Michael B McCallister
Sr VP Innovation Officer ....Jack Lord, MD
COO Market/Business ....Jim Murray
Sr VP/CFO.....................................James Bloem
Sr VP General Counsel ....Art Hipwell
Sr VP Human Resources.....................Bonnie Hathcock
Sr VP Corporate Dev...........................Tom Liston
Sr VP Gov't Relations.........................Hiedi Margulis
Sr VP/CSO/CIO ....Bruce Goodman
Sr VP Corporate Comm.........................Tom Noland
Sr VP Marketing Officer ....Steve Moya
Media Relations Manager....................Lindsey Minella
312-441-5549
lminella@humana.com

425 Medical Associates Health Plan: West

1500 Associates Drive
Dubuque, IA 52002
Toll-Free: 800-648-6868
Phone: 563-584-3000
Fax: 563-556-5134
www.mahealthcare.com
For Profit Organization: Yes
Year Founded: 1982
Physician Owned Organization: Yes
Federally Qualified: Yes
Total Enrollment: 45,000
State Enrollment: 14,412

Healthplan and Services Defined
PLAN TYPE: HMO
Other Type: EPO, POS
Model Type: Staff
Plan Specialty: Behavioral Health, Disease Management, Lab, MSO, Vision, Radiology, UR
Benefits Offered: Home Care, Inpatient SNF, Physical Therapy, Podiatry, Prescription, Psychiatric, Transplant, Vision, Wellness
Offers Demand Management Patient Information Service: Yes

Type of Coverage
Commercial, Indemnity, Medicare, Supplemental Medicare, Catastrophic
Catastrophic Illness Benefit: Varies per case

Type of Payment Plans Offered
POS

Geographic Areas Served
Iowa: Allamakee, Clayton, Delaware, Dubuque, Jackson, Jones counties. Illinois: JoDaviess County

Network Qualifications
Pre-Admission Certification: Yes

Peer Review Type
Utilization Review: Yes
Case Management: Yes

Publishes and Distributes Report Card: Yes

Accreditation Certification
NCQA

TJC Accreditation, Medicare Approved, Utilization Review, Pre-Admission Certification, State Licensure, Quality Assurance Program

Key Personnel
Executive Director ....Alan Avery
CEO ....John Tallent

Specialty Managed Care Partners
Enters into Contracts with Regional Business Coalitions: Yes

426 Mercy Health Network

1111 Sixth Avenue
Des Moines, IA 50314
Phone: 515-247-3121
nurse@mercydesmoines.org
www.mercyhealthnetwork.com
Subsidiary of: Catholic Health Initiatives, Trinity Health
Year Founded: 1998
Number of Affiliated Hospitals: 33

Healthplan and Services Defined
PLAN TYPE: HMO
Plan Specialty: Lab, Cardiac Care
Benefits Offered: Disease Management, Home Care, Physical Therapy, Prescription, Wellness

Type of Coverage
Individual

Geographic Areas Served
Clinton, Des Moines, Dubuque, North Iowa, Sioux City

Key Personnel
CEO..David Vellinga
Vice President ....Dave Hickman
Financial Services ....Steve Kukla
Planning ....Joe LeValley

427 Sanford Health Plan

300 Cherapa Place
Suite 201
Sioux Falls, SD 57103
Toll-Free: 877-305-5463
Phone: 605-328-6868
memberservices@sanfordhealth.org
www.sanfordhealthplan.com
Mailing Address: PO Box 91110, Sioux Falls, SD 57109-1110
Non-Profit Organization: Yes
Year Founded: 1996
Total Enrollment: 50,000

Healthplan and Services Defined
PLAN TYPE: HMO
Model Type: IPA
Plan Specialty: Commercial Group
Benefits Offered: Disease Management, Home Care, Long-Term Care, Prescription, Wellness

Type of Coverage
Commercial, Individual, Medicare, Supplemental Medicare, Sec 125, TPA, Individual, Lg Group

Geographic Areas Served
Northwest Iowa, Southwest Minnesota, South Dakota

Accreditation Certification
NCQA

Key Personnel
Executive Director ....Jerome Freeman, MD
Administrative Director ....Ellen Schellinger, MA
Director, Planning & Reg ....Lisa Carlson
605-328-6859
Media Strategy Manager ....Stacy Bauer Jones
605-328-7056
stacy.jones@sanfordhealth.org

428　UnitedHealthCare of Iowa

1089 Jordan Creek Parkway
Suite 320
West Des Moines, IA 50266
Toll-Free: 800-669-1830
www.uhc.com
Secondary Address: 2540 106th Street, Suite 201, Urbandale, IA
　50322, 800-669-1812
Subsidiary of: UnitedHealth Group
For Profit Organization: Yes
Year Founded: 1984
Number of Affiliated Hospitals: 4,500
Number of Primary Care Physicians: 470,000
Total Enrollment: 75,000,000

Healthplan and Services Defined
　PLAN TYPE: HMO/PPO
　Model Type: Network
　Plan Specialty: Dental, Vision
　Benefits Offered: Dental, Disease Management, Prescription, Vision,
　　Wellness, Life, LTD, STD

Type of Coverage
　Commercial, Individual, Indemnity

Type of Payment Plans Offered
　POS, DFFS, FFS

Geographic Areas Served
　Statewide

Network Qualifications
　Pre-Admission Certification: Yes

Peer Review Type
　Utilization Review: Yes
　Second Surgical Opinion: Yes
　Case Management: Yes

Publishes and Distributes Report Card: Yes

Accreditation Certification
　TJC Accreditation, Medicare Approved, Utilization Review,
　　Pre-Admission Certification, State Licensure, Quality Assurance
　　Program

Key Personnel
　President . . . . .Daniel Kuter
　Administrator . . . . .Julia Arnett
　Media Contact . . . . .Kevin Shermach
　　312-453-0533
　　kevin.shermach@uhc.com

429　Wellmark Blue Cross Blue Shield

1331 Grand Avenue
PO Box 9232
Des Moines, IA 50309-9232
Toll-Free: 800-524-9242
Phone: 515-245-4500
Fax: 515-245-5090
www.wellmark.com
Year Founded: 1939
Number of Affiliated Hospitals: 117
Number of Primary Care Physicians: 2,500
Total Enrollment: 250,000
State Enrollment: 250,000

Healthplan and Services Defined
　PLAN TYPE: HMO
　Model Type: IPA
　Plan Specialty: ASO, Chiropractic, Disease Management, Lab,
　　Vision, Radiology, UR
　Benefits Offered: Chiropractic, Disease Management, Home Care,
　　Inpatient SNF, Physical Therapy, Podiatry, Prescription,
　　Psychiatric, Transplant, Vision, Wellness
　Offers Demand Management Patient Information Service: Yes

Type of Coverage
　Commercial, Individual, Indemnity, Medicare, Supplemental
　　Medicare, Medicaid

Type of Payment Plans Offered
　POS, Capitated

Geographic Areas Served
　Statewide except Alamakee, Winneshiek, Fayette, Des Moines and
　　Dubuque counties

Network Qualifications
　Pre-Admission Certification: Yes

Peer Review Type
　Utilization Review: Yes

Publishes and Distributes Report Card: Yes

Accreditation Certification
　URAC, NCQA
　TJC Accreditation, Medicare Approved, Utilization Review,
　　Pre-Admission Certification, State Licensure, Quality Assurance
　　Program

Key Personnel
　Chairman/CEO . . . . .John Forsyth
　EVP/CFO. . . . . .David Brown
　VP Investments . . . . .Mike Crowley
　VP, Operations . . . . .Elaine Palmer
　Associate General Counsel .Michele Druker
　EVP Human Resources . . . . Marcelle Chickering
　VP Actuarial . . . . .Patricia Huffman
　EVP, Policy & Strategy . . . . .Laura Jackson
　VP, Chief Medical Offcr . . . . .Tim Gutshall
　EVP . . . . .Ellen J Gaucher
　EVP/CIO . . . . .Tim Peterson
　VP, Sales. . . . . .Scott Froyen
　Media Contact . . . . .Courtney Greene
　　515-376-4870
　　greenecm@wellmark.com

KANSAS

Health Insurance Coverage Status and Type of Coverage by Age

Category	All Persons		Under 18 years		Under 65 years		65 years and over	
	Number	%	Number	%	Number	%	Number	%
Total population	2,837	-	719	-	2,449	-	387	-
Covered by some type of health insurance	2,489 *(12)*	87.7 *(0.4)*	675 *(5)*	93.9 *(0.6)*	2,103 *(12)*	85.8 *(0.5)*	386 *(2)*	99.6 *(0.1)*
Covered by private health insurance	2,049 *(18)*	72.2 *(0.6)*	472 *(8)*	65.7 *(1.2)*	1,779 *(16)*	72.6 *(0.7)*	270 *(5)*	69.7 *(1.2)*
Employment based	1,609 *(19)*	56.7 *(0.7)*	395 *(10)*	54.9 *(1.4)*	1,508 *(18)*	61.6 *(0.7)*	101 *(5)*	26.0 *(1.2)*
Direct purchase	443 *(10)*	15.6 *(0.3)*	62 *(5)*	8.6 *(0.7)*	260 *(9)*	10.6 *(0.4)*	183 *(4)*	47.3 *(1.0)*
Covered by TRICARE	109 *(6)*	3.9 *(0.2)*	31 *(3)*	4.3 *(0.5)*	84 *(6)*	3.4 *(0.3)*	25 *(2)*	6.5 *(0.6)*
Covered by government health insurance	784 *(12)*	27.7 *(0.4)*	229 *(9)*	31.9 *(1.2)*	407 *(12)*	16.6 *(0.5)*	378 *(2)*	97.5 *(0.4)*
Covered by Medicaid	388 *(12)*	13.7 *(0.4)*	228 *(8)*	31.6 *(1.1)*	347 *(11)*	14.2 *(0.4)*	41 *(3)*	10.6 *(0.7)*
Also by private insurance	73 *(5)*	2.6 *(0.2)*	26 *(3)*	3.6 *(0.4)*	51 *(4)*	2.1 *(0.2)*	21 *(2)*	5.5 *(0.5)*
Covered by Medicare	442 *(5)*	15.6 *(0.2)*	3 *(1)*	0.4 *(0.1)*	64 *(5)*	2.6 *(0.2)*	377 *(2)*	97.4 *(0.4)*
Also by private insurance	282 *(5)*	9.9 *(0.2)*	Z *(Z)*	0.0 *(0.1)*	20 *(2)*	0.8 *(0.1)*	262 *(4)*	67.5 *(1.1)*
Also by Medicaid	71 *(4)*	2.5 *(0.1)*	1 *(1)*	0.2 *(0.1)*	29 *(3)*	1.2 *(0.1)*	41 *(3)*	10.6 *(0.7)*
Covered by VA Care	67 *(4)*	2.4 *(0.1)*	1 *(Z)*	0.1 *(0.1)*	31 *(3)*	1.3 *(0.1)*	36 *(2)*	9.3 *(0.5)*
Not covered at any time during the year	348 *(12)*	12.3 *(0.4)*	44 *(5)*	6.1 *(0.6)*	347 *(12)*	14.2 *(0.5)*	1 *(Z)*	0.4 *(0.1)*

Note: Numbers in thousands; Figures cover 2013; Margin of error appears in parenthesis; A "Z" indicates that the value either represents or rounds to zero.
Source: U.S. Census Bureau, 2013 American Community Survey, Table HI05. Health Insurance Coverage Status and Type of Coverage by State and Age for All People: 2013

Kansas

430 Advance Insurance Company of Kansas
1133 SW Topeka Blvd
Topeka, KS 66629
Toll-Free: 800-530-5989
Phone: 785-273-9804
Fax: 785-290-0727
csc-advance@advanceinsurance.com
www.advanceinsurance.com
Subsidiary of: Blue Cross & Blue Shield of Kansas
For Profit Organization: Yes
Total Enrollment: 135,000

Healthplan and Services Defined
PLAN TYPE: Multiple
Benefits Offered: Life, LTD, STD

Key Personnel
Chief Executive Officer . . . . Andrew C Corbin

431 Aetna Health of Kansas
151 Farmington Avenue
Hartford, CT 06156
Toll-Free: 800-872-3862
Phone: 860-273-0123
www.aetna.com
Partnered with: eHealthInsurance Services Inc.
For Profit Organization: Yes
Total Enrollment: 11,596,230

Healthplan and Services Defined
PLAN TYPE: PPO
Other Type: POS
Plan Specialty: EPO
Benefits Offered: Dental, Disease Management, Long-Term Care, Prescription, Wellness, Life, LTD, STD

Type of Coverage
Commercial, Individual

Type of Payment Plans Offered
POS, FFS

Geographic Areas Served
Statewide

Key Personnel
Chairman/CEO/President. Mark T Bertolini
EVP/General Counsel . . . . William J Casazza
EVP/CFO . . . . Shawn M Guertin

432 Assurant Employee Benefits: Kansas
8300 College Blvd
Suite 120
Shawnee Mission, KS 66210-2603
Phone: 913-469-8090
Fax: 913-469-8091
benefits@assurant.com
www.assurantemployeebenefits.com
Subsidiary of: Assurant, Inc
For Profit Organization: Yes
Number of Primary Care Physicians: 112,000
Total Enrollment: 47,000

Healthplan and Services Defined
PLAN TYPE: Multiple
Plan Specialty: Dental, Vision, Long & Short-Term Disability
Benefits Offered: Dental, Vision, Wellness, AD&D, Life, LTD, STD

Type of Coverage
Commercial, Indemnity, Individual Dental Plans

Geographic Areas Served
Statewide

Subscriber Information
Average Monthly Fee Per Subscriber
(Employee + Employer Contribution):
Employee Only (Self): Varies by plan

Key Personnel
Office Manager. . . . . Kristen Stine
PR Specialist. . . . . Megan Hutchison
816-556-7815
megan.hutchison@assurant.com

433 Blue Cross & Blue Shield of Kansas
1133 Southwest Topeka Boulevard
Topeka, KS 66629
Phone: 785-291-4180
Fax: 785-290-0754
www.bcbsks.com
For Profit Organization: Yes
Year Founded: 1941
Number of Affiliated Hospitals: 120
Total Enrollment: 898,111
State Enrollment: 680,466

Healthplan and Services Defined
PLAN TYPE: HMO
Model Type: Staff
Benefits Offered: Chiropractic, Disease Management, Inpatient SNF, Podiatry, Psychiatric, Wellness

Type of Coverage
Commercial, Individual

Geographic Areas Served
All Kansas counties except Johnson and Wyandotte

Subscriber Information
Average Annual Deductible Per Subscriber:
Employee Only (Self): $1,000
Employee & 2 Family Members: $2,000
Average Subscriber Co-Payment:
Primary Care Physician: $15.00
Prescription Drugs: $5.00
Hospital ER: $50.00

Accreditation Certification
TJC, URAC

Key Personnel
President/CEO. . . . . Andrew C. Corbin
Senior Vice President. . . . . Frederick D. Palenske
SVP/General Counsel . . . . Matthew D. All
VP, Medical Affairs . . . . Michael Atwood
VP, Information Services . . . . Julie Hinrichsen
VP, External Sales/Mktng . . . . Treena Mason
VP, Operations. . . . . Shelly Pittman
VP, Finance. . . . . Ron Simmons
VP, Human Development . . . . Bob Young
Mgr Corp Communications . . . . Mary Beth Chambers
785-291-8869
mary.beth.chambers@bcbsks.com

434 CIGNA HealthCare of Kansas
7400 West 110th Street
Suite 400
Overland Park, KS 66210
Toll-Free: 866-438-2446
Phone: 913-339-4700
Fax: 913-339-4705
www.cigna.com
For Profit Organization: Yes
Total Enrollment: 9,848

Healthplan and Services Defined
PLAN TYPE: HMO
Other Type: POS

Type of Coverage
Commercial

---

435 CoreSource: Kansas (FMH CoreSource)

13160 Foster Street
Suite 150
Overland Park, KS 66213
Toll-Free: 800-990-9058
Phone: 913-685-4740
www.coresource.com; www.f-m-h.com
Subsidiary of: Trustmark
Year Founded: 1996
Total Enrollment: 1,100,000

Healthplan and Services Defined
PLAN TYPE: Multiple
Other Type: TPA
Model Type: Network
Plan Specialty: Claims Administration, TPA
Benefits Offered: Behavioral Health, Home Care, Prescription,
Transplant

Type of Coverage
Commercial

Geographic Areas Served
Nationwide

Accreditation Certification
Utilization Review, Pre-Admission Certification

Key Personnel
President . . . . Nancy Eckrich
VP/Chief Financial Office . . . . Clare Smith
Chief Operations Officer. . . . . Lloyd Sarrel
VP, Product Management & . . . . Rob Corrigan
VP, Healthcare Management. Donna Heiser
VP, Client Management . . . . Kathy Hunt
VP, Marketing & Product D . . . . Steve Horvath

---

436 Coventry Health Care of Kansas

8535 East 21st Street N
Wichita, KS 67206
Toll-Free: 866-320-0697
www.chckansas.com
Secondary Address: 9401 Indian Creek Parkway, Suite 1300,
Overland Park, KS 66210, 800-969-3343
Subsidiary of: Coventry Health Care
For Profit Organization: Yes
Year Founded: 1988
Number of Affiliated Hospitals: 100
Number of Primary Care Physicians: 4,800
Number of Referral/Specialty Physicians: 731
Total Enrollment: 73,000
State Enrollment: 132,716

Healthplan and Services Defined
PLAN TYPE: HMO/PPO
Other Type: POS
Model Type: IPA
Benefits Offered: Complementary Medicine, Disease Management,
Prescription, Vision, Wellness, Alternative and complementary
care services include discounts on massage therapy, acupuncture
and chiropractic services.
Offers Demand Management Patient Information Service: Yes

Type of Coverage
Catastrophic Illness Benefit: Covered

Type of Payment Plans Offered
DFFS

Geographic Areas Served
Kansas, Missouri, Oklahoma

Subscriber Information
Average Monthly Fee Per Subscriber
(Employee + Employer Contribution):
Employee Only (Self): Varies
Average Annual Deductible Per Subscriber:
Employee & 2 Family Members: None
Average Subscriber Co-Payment:
Primary Care Physician: $10.00
Prescription Drugs: $5.00/15.00
Hospital ER: $50
Home Health Care: None
Nursing Home: None

Peer Review Type
Second Surgical Opinion: Yes
Case Management: Yes

Publishes and Distributes Report Card: Yes

Accreditation Certification
URAC, NCQA
Medicare Approved, Utilization Review, Pre-Admission Certification,
State Licensure, Quality Assurance Program

Key Personnel
President. . . . . Thomas P McDonough
CEO. . . . . Dale B Wolf
EVP. . . . . Harvey C DeMovick, Jr
EVP/Operations. . . . . Francis S Soistman, Jr
EVP/CFO. . . . . Richard Kleinner

Specialty Managed Care Partners
Enters into Contracts with Regional Business Coalitions: Yes

---

437 Delta Dental of Kansas

1619 North Waterfront Parkway
PO Box 789769
Wichita, KS 67278-9769
Toll-Free: 800-733-5823
Phone: 316-264-4511
Fax: 316-462-3393
moreinfo@deltadentalks.com
www.deltadentalks.com
Non-Profit Organization: Yes
Year Founded: 1972
Number of Primary Care Physicians: 1,200
Number of Referral/Specialty Physicians: 250
Total Enrollment: 54,000,000
State Enrollment: 880,000

Healthplan and Services Defined
PLAN TYPE: Dental
Other Type: Dental PPO
Model Type: Network
Plan Specialty: Dental
Benefits Offered: Dental

Type of Coverage
Commercial

Type of Payment Plans Offered
DFFS

Geographic Areas Served
Statewide

Subscriber Information
Average Monthly Fee Per Subscriber
(Employee + Employer Contribution):
Employee Only (Self): $17
Employee & 2 Family Members: $50
Average Annual Deductible Per Subscriber:
Employee Only (Self): $150
Employee & 2 Family Members: $50
Average Subscriber Co-Payment:

Primary Care Physician: 80%
Non-Network Physician: 50%

Network Qualifications
Pre-Admission Certification: Yes

Publishes and Distributes Report Card: Yes

Key Personnel
President/CEO..............................Michael Herbert
Managing Partner/EVP.........................Dean Newton
In-House Counsel........................Mindy McPheeters
Communications Coord......................Sarah Pritchard
  316-264-1099
  spritchard@deltadentalks.com
Dir/Media & Public Affair..................Elizabeth Risberg
  415-972-8423

438 eHealthInsurance Services Inc.
11919 Foundation Place
Gold River, CA 95670
Toll-Free: 800-644-3491
webmaster@healthinsurance.com
www.e.healthinsurance.com
Year Founded: 1997

Healthplan and Services Defined
PLAN TYPE: HMO/PPO
Benefits Offered: Dental, Life, STD

Type of Coverage
Commercial, Individual, Medicare

Geographic Areas Served
All 50 states in the USA and District of Columbia

Key Personnel
Chairman & CEO............................Gary L. Lauer
EVP/Business & Corp. Dev....................Bruce Telkamp
EVP/Chief Technology...................Dr. Sheldon X. Wang
SVP & CFO.........................Stuart M. Huizinga
Pres. of eHealth Gov. Sys.....................Samuel C. Gibbs
SVP of Sales & Operations...................Robert S. Hurley
Director Public Relations......................Nate Purpura
  650-210-3115

439 Great-West Healthcare Kansas
10851 Mastin
Building 82, Suite 200
Overland Park, KS 66210
Toll-Free: 866-494-2111
Phone: 913-491-9436
Fax: 913-317-8824
eliginquiries@cigna.com
www.cignaforhealth.com
Secondary Address: 7400 West 110th Street, Suite 400, Overland Park, KS 66210
Subsidiary of: CIGNA HealthCare
Acquired by: CIGNA
For Profit Organization: Yes
Total Enrollment: 21,580
State Enrollment: 17,258

Healthplan and Services Defined
PLAN TYPE: HMO/PPO
Benefits Offered: Disease Management, Prescription, Wellness

Type of Coverage
Commercial

Type of Payment Plans Offered
POS, FFS

Geographic Areas Served
Kansas

Accreditation Certification
URAC

Specialty Managed Care Partners
Caremark Rx

440 Health Partners of Kansas
550 North Lorraine Street
Wichita, KS 67214
Phone: 316-652-1327
www.hpkansas.com
For Profit Organization: Yes
Year Founded: 1987
Number of Affiliated Hospitals: 149
Number of Primary Care Physicians: 1,000
Number of Referral/Specialty Physicians: 6,000
Total Enrollment: 95,000
State Enrollment: 95,000

Healthplan and Services Defined
PLAN TYPE: PPO
Model Type: IPA, Network
Benefits Offered: Worker's Compensation, Network Rental, Provider Servicing, Provider Credentialing

Type of Coverage
Catastrophic Illness Benefit: Maximum $1M

Type of Payment Plans Offered
POS, DFFS, Capitated, FFS, Combination FFS & DFFS

Geographic Areas Served
Statewide

Network Qualifications
Pre-Admission Certification: Yes

Peer Review Type
Utilization Review: Yes
Second Surgical Opinion: Yes
Case Management: Yes

Key Personnel
President.......................................Gaylee Dolloff
  gaylee.dolloff@wesleymc.com

Specialty Managed Care Partners
Enters into Contracts with Regional Business Coalitions: No

441 Humana Health Insurance of Kansas
7311 W 132nd Street
Suite 200
Overland Park, MO 66213
Toll-Free: 800-842-6188
Phone: 913-217-3309
Fax: 913-217-3245
www.humana.com
Secondary Address: 601 South Greenwich Road, Suite 111, Wichita, KS 67207
For Profit Organization: Yes
Year Founded: 1985
Number of Affiliated Hospitals: 8
Number of Primary Care Physicians: 1,300
Total Enrollment: 84,841
State Enrollment: 40,800

Healthplan and Services Defined
PLAN TYPE: HMO/PPO
Model Type: IPA
Benefits Offered: Disease Management, Prescription, Wellness

Type of Coverage
Commercial, Individual

Geographic Areas Served
Kansas City metro area

Subscriber Information
Average Monthly Fee Per Subscriber
(Employee + Employer Contribution):

Employee Only (Self): $150.44
Employee & 1 Family Member: $354.06
Employee & 2 Family Members: $354.06
Medicare: $196.48
Average Subscriber Co-Payment:
Primary Care Physician: $5.00
Non-Network Physician: Not covered
Prescription Drugs: $5.00
Hospital ER: $25.00
Home Health Care: $0
Nursing Home: $0
Nursing Home Max. Days/Visits Covered: 60 days

Accreditation Certification
URAC, NCQA, CORE

Key Personnel
President/CEO . . . . Michael B McCallister
COO . . . . James E Murray
CFO . . . . James H Bloem
Chief Marketing Officer. . . . . Steven O Moya
Media Relations Manager . . . . Jeff Blunt
513-826-7094
jblunt@humana.com

Average Claim Compensation
Physician's Fees Charged: 70%
Hospital's Fees Charged: 60%

Specialty Managed Care Partners
Enters into Contracts with Regional Business Coalitions: Yes

---

442   Mercy Health Plans: Kansas
14528 South Outer 40
Suite 300
Chesterfield, MO 63017-5743
Toll-Free: 800-830-1918
Phone: 314-214-8100
Fax: 314-214-8101
Acquired by: Coventry Health Care
Non-Profit Organization: Yes
Total Enrollment: 73,000

Healthplan and Services Defined
PLAN TYPE: HMO

Type of Coverage
Commercial, Individual

Key Personnel
Interim CEO . . . . Chris Knackstedt
EVP, COO. . . . . Mike Treash
Executive Vice President . . . . Janet Pursley
CFO, Treasurer . . . . George Schneider
VP, General Counsel . . . . Charles Gilham
Chief Medical Officer . . . . Stephen Spurgeon, MD
VP, Human Resources . . . . Donna McDaniel
VP, Mission & Ethics . . . . Michael Doyle
VP, Sales & Service. . . . . Carl Schultz

---

443   PCC Preferred Chiropractic Care
555 North McLean Boulevard
Suite 200
Wichita, KS 67203
Toll-Free: 800-611-3048
Phone: 316-263-7800
Fax: 316-263-7814
providerrelations@pccnetwork.com
www.pccnetwork.com
For Profit Organization: Yes
Year Founded: 1984
Physician Owned Organization: No
Federally Qualified: No
Number of Primary Care Physicians: 3,500

Total Enrollment: 5,000,000

Healthplan and Services Defined
PLAN TYPE: PPO
Model Type: Network
Plan Specialty: Chiropractic
Benefits Offered: Chiropractic, Disease Management, Wellness, Worker's Compensation
Offers Demand Management Patient Information Service: Yes
DMPI Services Offered: Chiropractic, Physical Therapy

Type of Coverage
Medicaid

Type of Payment Plans Offered
POS, DFFS, Capitated, FFS, Combination FFS & DFFS

Geographic Areas Served
All continental states

Subscriber Information
Average Subscriber Co-Payment:
Primary Care Physician: 20%
Non-Network Physician: 50%

Network Qualifications
Pre-Admission Certification: No

Peer Review Type
Utilization Review: Yes
Second Surgical Opinion: Yes
Case Management: No

Publishes and Distributes Report Card: No

Accreditation Certification
URAC, NCQA

Key Personnel
President and CEO . . . . Brad Dopps, DC
CFO . . . . Mark Dopps, DC
COO. . . . . Robert Dopps, DC
Claims Manager . . . . Jacque Fox
316-263-7800
jfox@pccnetwork.com
Credentialing . . . . Kay Lukens
Marketing . . . . Beth Dauner
bdauner@pccnetwork.com
Member Services . . . . John Dopps, DC
Provider Services . . . . Kay Lukens
316-263-7800
kaylukens@pccnetwork.com

Average Claim Compensation
Physician's Fees Charged: 80%

Specialty Managed Care Partners
Enters into Contracts with Regional Business Coalitions: Yes

Employer References
Preferred Health Systems, fiserv, Health Partners of Kansas

---

444   Preferred Health Systems Insurance Company
8535 East 21st Street N
Wichita, KS 67206
Toll-Free: 866-320-0697
phsimail@phsystems.com
www.phsystems.com
Subsidiary of: A Coventry Health Care Plan
For Profit Organization: Yes
Year Founded: 1996
Number of Affiliated Hospitals: 140
Number of Primary Care Physicians: 1,386
Number of Referral/Specialty Physicians: 1,870
Total Enrollment: 33,153
State Enrollment: 31,453

Healthplan and Services Defined
PLAN TYPE: PPO

Model Type: Group
Plan Specialty: ASO, Behavioral Health, Chiropractic, Disease
Management, EPO, PBM, Vision, Radiology, UR, Medicare
Supplement
Benefits Offered: Behavioral Health, Chiropractic, Dental, Disease
Management, Home Care, Inpatient SNF, Physical Therapy,
Podiatry, Prescription, Psychiatric, Transplant, Vision, AD&D,
Life

Type of Coverage
Commercial, Supplemental Medicare
Catastrophic Illness Benefit: Maximum $2M

Type of Payment Plans Offered
FFS

Geographic Areas Served
Kansas: Statewide

Subscriber Information
Average Monthly Fee Per Subscriber
(Employee + Employer Contribution):
Employee Only (Self): $307.11
Employee & 1 Family Member: $625.79
Employee & 2 Family Members: $758.37
Average Annual Deductible Per Subscriber:
Employee Only (Self): $1151.20
Employee & 1 Family Member: $2302.40
Employee & 2 Family Members: $2302.40
Average Subscriber Co-Payment:
Primary Care Physician: $20.00
Non-Network Physician: Ded/coinsurance
Prescription Drugs: $10/30/50
Hospital ER: $150.00
Home Health Care: $0 up to $2500 max
Home Health Care Max. Days/Visits Covered: Varies
Nursing Home Max. Days/Visits Covered: Varies

Network Qualifications
Pre-Admission Certification: Yes

Peer Review Type
Utilization Review: Yes
Second Surgical Opinion: Yes
Case Management: Yes

Publishes and Distributes Report Card: No

Accreditation Certification
URAC
Utilization Review, Pre-Admission Certification, State Licensure,
Quality Assurance Program

Key Personnel
CFO . . . . .Todd Kasitz
COO. . . . . .Brad Clothier
Director . . . . .Robert Kenargy
Director. . . . . .Ken Griggs
Director. . . . . .George Fahnestock
Coord, Payer Relations . . . . .Tracy Biglow
Senior Marketing Exec . . . . .Jeremy Gilson
Senior Marketing Exec. . . . . .Jennifer Elliot
Mgr, Sales & Medicare . . . . .Dennis Manson
Medical Director . . . . .Paul Huser
Coord, Customer Service. . . . . .Ivy McCray
Human Resources Officer . . . . .Raedina Campbell
Mgr, Payer/Medicare Mktg . . . . .Dennis Manson
Director Sales & Mktg . . . . .Brian Rose
Administrative Specialist . . . . .Jessica Warren
316-609-2431
jwarren@phsystems.com

Average Claim Compensation
Physician's Fees Charged: 67%
Hospital's Fees Charged: 52%

Specialty Managed Care Partners
Express Scripts

Employer References
Royal Valley USD 337, Ark City USD 470, Chance Rides
Manufacturing, Butler Community College

---

445   Preferred Mental Health Management
401 East Douglas Avenue
Suite 505
Wichita, KS 67202
Toll-Free: 800-819-9571
Phone: 316-262-0444
providerrelations@pmhm.com
www.pmhm.com
Year Founded: 1987
Number of Affiliated Hospitals: 1,900
Number of Primary Care Physicians: 10,500
Number of Referral/Specialty Physicians: 4,000
Total Enrollment: 400,000

Healthplan and Services Defined
PLAN TYPE: Multiple
Model Type: Network
Plan Specialty: Mental Health
Benefits Offered: Behavioral Health, Prescription, Psychiatric
Offers Demand Management Patient Information Service: Yes

Type of Coverage
Work

Geographic Areas Served
All 50 states and Puerto Rico

Network Qualifications
Minimum Years of Practice: 6
Pre-Admission Certification: Yes

Peer Review Type
Utilization Review: Yes

Publishes and Distributes Report Card: Yes

Accreditation Certification
TJC Accreditation, Utilization Review, Pre-Admission Certification,
State Licensure, Quality Assurance Program

Key Personnel
President and CEO. . . . . .Les Ruthven, PhD
316-262-0444

Specialty Managed Care Partners
Enters into Contracts with Regional Business Coalitions: No

---

446   Preferred Plus of Kansas
8535 East 21st Street North
Wichita, KS 67206
Toll-Free: 800-660-8114
Phone: 316-609-2345
Fax: 316-609-2346
phsimail@phsystems.com
www.phsystems.com
Subsidiary of: Preferred Health Systems/A Coventry Health Care Plan
For Profit Organization: Yes
Year Founded: 1991
Physician Owned Organization: No
Federally Qualified: No
Number of Affiliated Hospitals: 34
Number of Primary Care Physicians: 416
Number of Referral/Specialty Physicians: 1,197
Total Enrollment: 83,151
State Enrollment: 82,778

Healthplan and Services Defined
PLAN TYPE: HMO
Model Type: IPA
Plan Specialty: Behavioral Health, Chiropractic, Disease
Management, Lab, PBM, Vision, Radiology, UR

Benefits Offered: Behavioral Health, Chiropractic, Dental, Disease Management, Home Care, Inpatient SNF, Physical Therapy, Podiatry, Prescription, Psychiatric, Transplant, Vision, Wellness, AD&D, Life
Offers Demand Management Patient Information Service: Yes
DMPI Services Offered: Diabetes, High Risk Pregnancy, Transplants, Catastrophic Case Management

Type of Coverage
Commercial
Catastrophic Illness Benefit: Maximum $2M

Type of Payment Plans Offered
DFFS, Capitated, FFS, Combination FFS & DFFS

Geographic Areas Served
Kansas: Butler, Chase, Chautauqua, Cowley, Dickenson, Elk, Greenwood, Harper, Harvey, Kingman, Marion, McPherson, Morris, Reno, Saline, Sedgwick and Sumner counties; Oklahoma: Kay county

Subscriber Information
Average Monthly Fee Per Subscriber
(Employee + Employer Contribution):
Employee Only (Self): $312.11
Employee & 1 Family Member: $674.23
Employee & 2 Family Members: $784.98
Average Annual Deductible Per Subscriber:
Employee Only (Self): $46.05
Employee & 1 Family Member: $92.09
Employee & 2 Family Members: $92.09
Average Subscriber Co-Payment:
Primary Care Physician: $19.64
Non-Network Physician: Not covered
Prescription Drugs: $10/30/50
Hospital ER: $127.15
Home Health Care: $0 up to $2500 max
Home Health Care Max. Days/Visits Covered: Varies
Nursing Home Max. Days/Visits Covered: Varies

Network Qualifications
Pre-Admission Certification: Yes

Peer Review Type
Utilization Review: Yes
Case Management: Yes

Publishes and Distributes Report Card: No

Accreditation Certification
URAC
TJC Accreditation, Medicare Approved, Utilization Review, Pre-Admission Certification, State Licensure, Quality Assurance Program

Key Personnel
CFO ....Todd Kasitz
COO...Brad Clothier
Director ....Robert Kenargy
Director..Ken Griggs
Director.................................George Fahnestock
Coord, Payer Relations ....Tracy Biglow
Senior Marketing Exec ....Jeremy Gilson
Senior Marketing Exec......................Jennifer Elliot
Mgr, Sales & Medicare ....Dennis Manson
Medical Director ....Paul Huser
Coord, Customer Service.......................Ivy McCray
Human Resources Officer ....Raedina Campbell
Mgr, Payer/Medicare Mktg ....Dennis Manson
Director Sales & Mktg ....Brian Rose
Administrative Specialist ....Jessica Warren
316-609-2431
jwarren@phsystems.com

Average Claim Compensation
Physician's Fees Charged: 61%
Hospital's Fees Charged: 36%

Specialty Managed Care Partners
Express Scripts

Enters into Contracts with Regional Business Coalitions: No
Employer References
Boeing, General Electric, Lear Jet, Spirit AeroSystems, ViaChrish Health System

447 Preferred Vision Care
PO Box 26025
Overland Park, KS 66225-6025
Phone: 913-451-1672
Fax: 913-451-1704
customerservice@preferredvisioncare.com
www.preferredvisioncare.com
For Profit Organization: Yes
Year Founded: 1987
Owned by an Integrated Delivery Network (IDN): Yes
Number of Primary Care Physicians: 10,000
Total Enrollment: 100,000
State Enrollment: 1,000,000

Healthplan and Services Defined
PLAN TYPE: Vision
Other Type: PPO
Model Type: Network
Plan Specialty: Vision
Benefits Offered: Vision

Type of Coverage
Commercial, Individual, Indemnity, Medicare, Supplemental Medicare, Medicaid, Catastrophic
Catastrophic Illness Benefit: Unlimited

Type of Payment Plans Offered
POS, DFFS

Geographic Areas Served
US, Puerto Rico, Guam, & VI

Subscriber Information
Average Monthly Fee Per Subscriber
(Employee + Employer Contribution):
Employee Only (Self): Varies
Employee & 1 Family Member: Varies
Employee & 2 Family Members: Varies

Network Qualifications
Pre-Admission Certification: No

Peer Review Type
Utilization Review: Yes
Second Surgical Opinion: Yes
Case Management: Yes

Publishes and Distributes Report Card: Yes

Accreditation Certification
URAC
Quality Assurance Program

Key Personnel
CEO...............................Michele G Disser, RN
Operations....................................E J Disser
Marketing ....P J Disser

Specialty Managed Care Partners
Enters into Contracts with Regional Business Coalitions: Yes

448 ProviDRs Care Network
1102 South Hillside
Wichita, KS 67211
Toll-Free: 800-801-9772
Phone: 316-683-4111
customerservice@providrscare.net
www.providrscare.net
Subsidiary of: Medical Society Medical Review Foundation
For Profit Organization: Yes
Year Founded: 1985
Physician Owned Organization: Yes

Number of Affiliated Hospitals: 139
Number of Primary Care Physicians: 4,500
Number of Referral/Specialty Physicians: 1,275
Total Enrollment: 152,000

Healthplan and Services Defined
PLAN TYPE: PPO
Model Type: Group
Benefits Offered: Behavioral Health, Chiropractic, Home Care, Physical Therapy, Podiatry, Psychiatric, Transplant, Worker's Compensation

Type of Coverage
Commercial, Individual

Type of Payment Plans Offered
POS

Geographic Areas Served
Kansas, Southwest Missouri; parts of Oklahoma and Nebraska; 1 county in Colorado

Subscriber Information
Average Monthly Fee Per Subscriber
(Employee + Employer Contribution):
Employee Only (Self): $3.00
Employee & 1 Family Member: $3.00
Employee & 2 Family Members: $3.00
Average Annual Deductible Per Subscriber:
Employee Only (Self): Varies
Employee & 1 Family Member: Varies
Average Subscriber Co-Payment:
Primary Care Physician: Varies
Non-Network Physician: Varies
Prescription Drugs: Varies
Hospital ER: Varies

Network Qualifications
Pre-Admission Certification: Yes

Peer Review Type
Utilization Review: Yes
Second Surgical Opinion: Yes
Case Management: No

Publishes and Distributes Report Card: No

Accreditation Certification
URAC
TJC Accreditation, Medicare Approved, Utilization Review, Pre-Admission Certification, State Licensure, Quality Assurance Program

Key Personnel
COO . . . . Karen Cox
karencox@providrscare.net
Operations Coordintaor . . . . Shari Rains
sharirains@providrscare.net
Dir, Care Utilization . . . . Shirley Sisco-Creed
Sr. Repricing Specialist . . . . Jeanne Hingst
jeannehingst@providrscare.net
Contracting/Networking . . . . Justin Leitzen
Credentialing Specialist . . . . Jeff Minson
jeffminson@providrscare.net
Claims & IS Administrator . . . . Nikki Sade
nikkisade@providrscare.net

Specialty Managed Care Partners
Enters into Contracts with Regional Business Coalitions: No

Employer References
Western Resources, Kansas Health Insurance Association, Medicalodges, County of Reno Kansas, National Cooperative of Refineries Association

---

449 Unicare: Kansas
825 Kansas Avenue
Suite 101
Topeka, KS 67214
Toll-Free: 877-864-2273
www.unicare.com
Secondary Address: 327 North Hillside Road, Wichita, KS 67214
Subsidiary of: WellPoint
For Profit Organization: Yes
Year Founded: 1995
Total Enrollment: 145,000

Healthplan and Services Defined
PLAN TYPE: HMO/PPO
Model Type: Network
Benefits Offered: Behavioral Health, Chiropractic, Complementary Medicine, Dental, Disease Management, Home Care, Inpatient SNF, Long-Term Care, Physical Therapy, Podiatry, Prescription, Psychiatric, Transplant, Vision, Wellness, Life, LTD, STD

Type of Coverage
Commercial, Individual, Medicare, Supplemental Medicare, Medicaid

Type of Payment Plans Offered
POS

Geographic Areas Served
Illinois: Cook, DuPage, Kane, Kankakee, Kendall, Lake, McHenry, Will counties. Indiana: Lake, Porter counties

Network Qualifications
Pre-Admission Certification: Yes

Peer Review Type
Utilization Review: Yes
Second Surgical Opinion: Yes
Case Management: Yes

Publishes and Distributes Report Card: Yes

Accreditation Certification
NCQA
TJC Accreditation, Utilization Review, Pre-Admission Certification, State Licensure, Quality Assurance Program

Key Personnel
CEO . . . . David Fields
Media Contact . . . . Tony Felts
317-287-6056
tony.felts@wellpoint.com

Specialty Managed Care Partners
WellPoint Pharmacy Management, WellPoint Dental Services, WellPoint Behavioral Health
Enters into Contracts with Regional Business Coalitions: Yes

---

450 UnitedHealthCare of Kansas
9900 West 109th Street
Suite 200
Overland Park, KS 66210
Toll-Free: 888-340-9716
Phone: 913-663-6500
kansas_pr_team@uhc.com
www.uhc.com
Secondary Address: 5901 Lincoln Dr, Edna, MN 55436, 800-842-3585
Subsidiary of: UnitedHealth Group
For Profit Organization: Yes
Total Enrollment: 75,000,000

Healthplan and Services Defined
PLAN TYPE: HMO/PPO

Geographic Areas Served
Statewide

Key Personnel
Media Contact . . . . Jessica Kostner
952-979-5869
jessica_kostner@uhc.com

451 **VSP: Vision Service Plan of Kansas**
9393 W 110th Street
Suite 500
Shawnee Mission, KS 66210-1464
Phone: 913-451-6730
Fax: 913-451-6976
webmaster@vsp.com
www.vsp.com
Year Founded: 1955
Number of Primary Care Physicians: 28,000
Total Enrollment: 57,000,000

Healthplan and Services Defined
PLAN TYPE: Vision
Plan Specialty: Vision
Benefits Offered: Vision

Type of Payment Plans Offered
Capitated

Geographic Areas Served
Statewide

Network Qualifications
Pre-Admission Certification: Yes

Peer Review Type
Utilization Review: Yes

Accreditation Certification
Utilization Review, Quality Assurance Program

Key Personnel
Manager . . . . .Susan Young

Health Insurance Coverage Status and Type of Coverage by Age

Category	All Persons		Under 18 years		Under 65 years		65 years and over	
	Number	%	Number	%	Number	%	Number	%
Total population	4,312	-	1,012	-	3,699	-	613	-
Covered by some type of health insurance	3,696 *(14)*	85.7 *(0.3)*	953 *(6)*	94.1 *(0.5)*	3,085 *(14)*	83.4 *(0.4)*	610 *(3)*	99.6 *(0.1)*
Covered by private health insurance	2,769 *(24)*	64.2 *(0.6)*	577 *(10)*	57.0 *(1.0)*	2,371 *(24)*	64.1 *(0.6)*	398 *(6)*	64.9 *(0.9)*
Employment based	2,329 *(22)*	54.0 *(0.5)*	511 *(9)*	50.5 *(0.9)*	2,101 *(21)*	56.8 *(0.6)*	228 *(5)*	37.2 *(0.8)*
Direct purchase	494 *(12)*	11.5 *(0.3)*	58 *(5)*	5.7 *(0.5)*	288 *(10)*	7.8 *(0.3)*	206 *(7)*	33.7 *(1.1)*
Covered by TRICARE	118 *(8)*	2.7 *(0.2)*	26 *(3)*	2.5 *(0.3)*	80 *(6)*	2.2 *(0.2)*	38 *(3)*	6.2 *(0.5)*
Covered by government health insurance	1,454 *(17)*	33.7 *(0.4)*	412 *(11)*	40.7 *(1.1)*	855 *(17)*	23.1 *(0.5)*	599 *(3)*	97.7 *(0.2)*
Covered by Medicaid	790 *(17)*	18.3 *(0.4)*	409 *(11)*	40.4 *(1.1)*	705 *(16)*	19.0 *(0.4)*	86 *(4)*	14.0 *(0.6)*
Also by private insurance	115 *(8)*	2.7 *(0.2)*	36 *(5)*	3.5 *(0.5)*	77 *(7)*	2.1 *(0.2)*	37 *(3)*	6.1 *(0.5)*
Covered by Medicare	770 *(7)*	17.9 *(0.2)*	6 *(1)*	0.6 *(0.1)*	172 *(7)*	4.6 *(0.2)*	598 *(3)*	97.6 *(0.3)*
Also by private insurance	434 *(7)*	10.1 *(0.2)*	Z *(Z)*	0.0 *(0.1)*	48 *(4)*	1.3 *(0.1)*	386 *(6)*	63.0 *(0.9)*
Also by Medicaid	154 *(5)*	3.6 *(0.1)*	3 *(1)*	0.3 *(0.1)*	68 *(4)*	1.8 *(0.1)*	86 *(4)*	14.0 *(0.6)*
Covered by VA Care	123 *(5)*	2.8 *(0.1)*	1 *(1)*	0.1 *(0.1)*	60 *(4)*	1.6 *(0.1)*	63 *(3)*	10.2 *(0.6)*
Not covered at any time during the year	616 *(14)*	14.3 *(0.3)*	60 *(5)*	5.9 *(0.5)*	614 *(14)*	16.6 *(0.4)*	2 *(1)*	0.4 *(0.1)*

Note: Numbers in thousands; Figures cover 2013; Margin of error appears in parenthesis; A "Z" indicates that the value either represents or rounds to zero.
Source: U.S. Census Bureau, 2013 American Community Survey, Table HI05. Health Insurance Coverage Status and Type of Coverage by State and Age for All People: 2013

Kentucky

452 Aetna Health of Kentucky

151 Farmington Avenue
Hartford, CT 06156
Toll-Free: 800-872-3862
Phone: 860-273-0123
www.aetna.com
Partnered with: eHealthInsurance Services Inc.
For Profit Organization: Yes
Total Enrollment: 11,596,230

Healthplan and Services Defined
PLAN TYPE: PPO
Other Type: POS
Plan Specialty: EPO
Benefits Offered: Dental, Disease Management, Long-Term Care, Prescription, Wellness, Life, LTD, STD

Type of Coverage
Commercial, Individual

Type of Payment Plans Offered
POS, FFS

Geographic Areas Served
Statewide

Key Personnel
Chairman/CEO/President......................Mark T Bertolini
EVP/General Counsel ....William J Casazza
EVP/CFO ....Shawn M Guertin

453 Anthem Blue Cross & Blue Shield of Kentucky

9901 Linn Station Road
Louisville, KY 40223
Toll-Free: 800-880-2583
Phone: 502-889-4600
www.anthem.com
Secondary Address: 1945 Scottsville Road, Bowling Green, KY 42104, 270-780-9916
Non-Profit Organization: Yes
Year Founded: 1999
Number of Affiliated Hospitals: 117
Number of Primary Care Physicians: 2,212
Number of Referral/Specialty Physicians: 3,952
Total Enrollment: 894,531
State Enrollment: 63,698

Healthplan and Services Defined
PLAN TYPE: HMO
Model Type: Network, PHO
Benefits Offered: Dental, Disease Management, Prescription, Vision, Wellness, Life

Type of Coverage
Individual, Medicare, Supplemental Medicare

Type of Payment Plans Offered
DFFS, FFS, Combination FFS & DFFS

Geographic Areas Served
Statewide

Subscriber Information
Average Annual Deductible Per Subscriber:
Employee Only (Self): $500
Employee & 2 Family Members: $1000
Average Subscriber Co-Payment:
Primary Care Physician: 30%
Non-Network Physician: 50%
Prescription Drugs: $15/$500 max annual
Hospital ER: 30%

Network Qualifications
Pre-Admission Certification: Yes

Peer Review Type
Utilization Review: Yes
Case Management: Yes

Publishes and Distributes Report Card: Yes

Accreditation Certification
URAC
TJC Accreditation, Medicare Approved, Utilization Review, Pre-Admission Certification, State Licensure, Quality Assurance Program

454 Bluegrass Family Health

651 Perimeter Drive
Suite 300
Lexington, KY 40517
Toll-Free: 800-787-2680
Phone: 859-269-4475
cservice@bgfh.com
www.bgfh.com
Secondary Address: 2630 Elm Hill Pike, Suite 110, Nashville, TN 37214, 615-872-8770
Subsidiary of: Baptist Health Care Systems
Non-Profit Organization: Yes
Year Founded: 1993
Number of Affiliated Hospitals: 40
Number of Primary Care Physicians: 764
Number of Referral/Specialty Physicians: 1,000
Total Enrollment: 136,472
State Enrollment: 65,428

Healthplan and Services Defined
PLAN TYPE: HMO/PPO
Other Type: POS
Model Type: Network
Plan Specialty: ASO, Behavioral Health, Dental, EPO, MSO, PBM, Vision
Benefits Offered: Chiropractic, Disease Management, Home Care, Physical Therapy, Podiatry, Prescription, Transplant, Wellness

Type of Coverage
Commercial

Type of Payment Plans Offered
POS, Combination FFS & DFFS

Geographic Areas Served
Kentucky & Southern Indiana (Clark, Crawford, Floyd, Harrison, Jefferson, Orange, Scott and Washington counties)

Peer Review Type
Second Surgical Opinion: Yes
Case Management: Yes

Publishes and Distributes Report Card: Yes

Accreditation Certification
TJC Accreditation, Medicare Approved, Utilization Review, Pre-Admission Certification, State Licensure, Quality Assurance Program

Key Personnel
President and CEO............................James S Fritz
859-269-4475

455 CHA Health

300 West Vine Street
16th Floor
Lexington, KY 40507
Toll-Free: 800-457-5683
Phone: 859-232-8686
Fax: 859-232-8525
www.cha-health.com
Mailing Address: PO Box 23468, Lexington, KY 40523

Subsidiary of: An Affilliate of Humana
Acquired by: Humana
For Profit Organization: Yes
Year Founded: 1991
Number of Primary Care Physicians: 15,000
Total Enrollment: 190,000
State Enrollment: 67,948

Healthplan and Services Defined
  PLAN TYPE: HMO
  Model Type: Group
  Benefits Offered: Prescription

Geographic Areas Served
  81 counties

Key Personnel
  CEO . . . . .Teresa Kline
  COO . . . . .Betty Chowning
  CFO . . . . .Tim Ryan
  Pharmacy Director . . . . .Phil Hanus
  Chief Medical Officer . . . . Timothy D Costrich, MD
  Member Services . . . . .Lesley Morgan
  Public Relations . . . . .Reagan Pruitt
  Provider Relations . . . . .Ryan Wilson

456   CIGNA HealthCare of Kentucky

1000 Corporate Center Drive
Suite 500
Franklin, TN 37067
Toll-Free: 866-438-2446
Phone: 615-595-3377
Fax: 615-595-3287
www.cigna.com
For Profit Organization: Yes
Total Enrollment: 75,000,000

Healthplan and Services Defined
  PLAN TYPE: HMO

Type of Coverage
  Commercial

Accreditation Certification
  URAC, NCQA

457   CoventryCares of Kentucky

9900 Corporate Campus Drive
Suite 1000
Louisville, KY 40223
Toll-Free: 855-300-5528
Phone: 502-719-8600
www.chcmedicaid-kentucky.coventryhealthcare.com
Mailing Address: PO Box 7812, London, KY 40742
Subsidiary of: Coventry Health & Life Insurance Co.
Non-Profit Organization: Yes

Healthplan and Services Defined
  PLAN TYPE: HMO/PPO
  Other Type: MCO, POS

Type of Coverage
  Medicare, Supplemental Medicare, Medicaid

Type of Payment Plans Offered
  FFS

Geographic Areas Served
  Kentucky

Subscriber Information
  Average Subscriber Co-Payment:
    Primary Care Physician: Varies
    Hospital ER: Varies
    Home Health Care: Varies
    Home Health Care Max. Days/Visits Covered: Varies
    Nursing Home: Varies

Nursing Home Max. Days/Visits Covered: Varies

458   Delta Dental of Kentucky

10100 Linn Station Rd
Suite 700
Louisville, KY 40223
Toll-Free: 800-955-2030
Fax: 877-224-0052
www.deltadentalky.com
Mailing Address: PO Box 242810, Louisville, KY 40224
Non-Profit Organization: Yes
Year Founded: 1966
Total Enrollment: 54,000,000
State Enrollment: 570,000

Healthplan and Services Defined
  PLAN TYPE: Dental
  Other Type: Dental PPO
  Model Type: IPA
  Plan Specialty: Dental
  Benefits Offered: Dental

Type of Coverage
  Commercial

Type of Payment Plans Offered
  DFFS

Geographic Areas Served
  Statewide

Subscriber Information
  Average Monthly Fee Per Subscriber
    (Employee + Employer Contribution):
      Employee Only (Self): $13.50
      Employee & 1 Family Member: $27.00
      Employee & 2 Family Members: $42.75
  Average Annual Deductible Per Subscriber:
      Employee Only (Self): $25.00
      Employee & 1 Family Member: $50.00
      Employee & 2 Family Members: $75.00

Network Qualifications
  Pre-Admission Certification: No

Peer Review Type
  Utilization Review: Yes
  Second Surgical Opinion: Yes
  Case Management: Yes

Publishes and Distributes Report Card: Yes

Key Personnel
  President/CEO .Clifford T. Maesaka Jr., DDS
  VP, Chief Marketing Offic . . . . .Stephen Day
  VP, Operations . . . . .Tammy York-Day
  Vp/General Counsel . . . . .John Weeks
  VP, IT & Professional Svc . . . . .Angie Zuvon Nenni
  VP, Finance . . . . .Russell Skaggs
  VP, Public & Govt Affairs . . . . .Jeff Album
    415-972-8418

Specialty Managed Care Partners
  Enters into Contracts with Regional Business Coalitions: Yes

459   eHealthInsurance Services Inc.

11919 Foundation Place
Gold River, CA 95670
Toll-Free: 800-644-3491
webmaster@healthinsurance.com
www.e.healthinsurance.com
Year Founded: 1997

Healthplan and Services Defined
  PLAN TYPE: HMO/PPO
  Benefits Offered: Dental, Life, STD

Type of Coverage
Commercial, Individual, Medicare

Geographic Areas Served
All 50 states in the USA and District of Columbia

Key Personnel
Chairman & CEO.............................Gary L. Lauer
EVP/Business & Corp. Dev......................Bruce Telkamp
EVP/Chief Technology....................Dr. Sheldon X. Wang
SVP & CFO ....Stuart M. Huizinga
Pres. of eHealth Gov. Sys ....Samuel C. Gibbs
SVP of Sales & Operations ....Robert S. Hurley
Director Public Relations.......................Nate Purpura
650-210-3115

460 Humana Health Insurance of Kentucky

101 East Main Street
Louisville, KY 40202
Toll-Free: 800-941-6172
Phone: 502-476-8605
Fax: 502-580-7633
www.humana.com
For Profit Organization: Yes

Healthplan and Services Defined
PLAN TYPE: HMO/PPO
Benefits Offered: Prescription

Type of Coverage
Commercial, Individual, Supplemental Medicare

Geographic Areas Served
Kentucky

Subscriber Information
Average Subscriber Co-Payment:
Prescription Drugs: $4.00-$30.00

Accreditation Certification
URAC, NCQA

Key Personnel
Chairman/President/CEO.................Michael B McCallister
COO ....James E Murray
SVP/CFO/Treasurer..........................James H Bloem
SVP/Chief Strategy Offc.....................Paul B Kusserow
SVP, Senior Products ....Thomas J Liston
SVP, Public Affairs ....Heidi S Marqulis
VP, Controller ....Steven E McCulley
SVP, General Counsel ....Christopher M Todoroff
SVP/Innovation & Mktg Ofc ....Raja Rajamannar
SVP/Ch Human Resources Of................Bonita C Hathcock
SVP/Ch Service & Info Ofc ....Brian LeClaire
Media Relations Manager ....Marvin Hill
502-476-0315
mhill1@humana.com

461 Humana Medicare Plan

Humana Corporate Headquarters
500 West Main Street
Louisville, KY 40202
Toll-Free: 800-645-7322
Phone: 502-580-3644
Fax: 502-580-3677
www.humana-medicare.com
For Profit Organization: Yes
Total Enrollment: 4,000,000

Healthplan and Services Defined
PLAN TYPE: Medicare
Benefits Offered: Chiropractic, Dental, Home Care, Inpatient SNF,
Physical Therapy, Podiatry, Prescription, Psychiatric, Vision,
Wellness

Type of Coverage
Commercial, Individual, Medicare

Geographic Areas Served
Available in multiple states

Subscriber Information
Average Monthly Fee Per Subscriber
(Employee + Employer Contribution):
Employee Only (Self): Varies
Medicare: Varies
Average Annual Deductible Per Subscriber:
Employee Only (Self): Varies
Medicare: Varies
Average Subscriber Co-Payment:
Primary Care Physician: Varies
Non-Network Physician: Varies
Prescription Drugs: Varies
Hospital ER: Varies
Home Health Care: Varies
Home Health Care Max. Days/Visits Covered: Varies
Nursing Home: Varies
Nursing Home Max. Days/Visits Covered: Varies

Accreditation Certification
URAC, NCQA, CORE

Key Personnel
President/CEO ....Michael B McCallister
Chief Operating Officer ....James E Murray
SVP/CFO and Treasurer ....James H Bloem
SVP/General Counsel ....Chistopher M Todoroff
SVP/CIO ....Brian LeClaire
SVP/Senior Products ....Thomas J Liston
SVP, Public Affairs ....Heidi S Margulis
SVP/Chief Mktg Officer.......................Paul Kusserow
SVP, Human Resources ....Bonita Hathcock
Corporate Communications ....Marvin Hill
502-476-0315
mhill1@humana.com

462 Meritain Health: Kentucky

1830 Destiny Lane
Suite 108
Bowling Green, KY 42104
Toll-Free: 800-570-6745
Phone: 270-745-0064
Fax: 800-646-9360
sales@meritain.com
www.meritain.com
Subsidiary of: Aetna
For Profit Organization: Yes
Year Founded: 1983
Number of Affiliated Hospitals: 110
Number of Primary Care Physicians: 3,467
Number of Referral/Specialty Physicians: 5,720
Total Enrollment: 500,000
State Enrollment: 450,000

Healthplan and Services Defined
PLAN TYPE: PPO
Model Type: Network
Plan Specialty: Dental, Disease Management, Vision, Radiology, UR
Benefits Offered: Prescription
Offers Demand Management Patient Information Service: Yes

Type of Coverage
Commercial

Geographic Areas Served
Nationwide

Subscriber Information
Average Monthly Fee Per Subscriber
(Employee + Employer Contribution):
Employee Only (Self): Varies by plan

Accreditation Certification
URAC
TJC Accreditation, Medicare Approved, Utilization Review, Pre-Admission Certification, State Licensure, Quality Assurance Program

Key Personnel
EVP, Chief Financial Offi.................... Vincent DiMura

Average Claim Compensation
Physician's Fees Charged: 78%
Hospital's Fees Charged: 90%

Specialty Managed Care Partners
Express Scripts, LabOne, Interactive Health Solutions

463   Passport Health Plan
5100 Commerce Crossings Drive
Louisville, KY 40229
Toll-Free: 800-578-0603
Phone: 502-585-7900
www.passporthealthplan.com
Subsidiary of: AmeriHealth Mercy Health Plan
Total Enrollment: 170,000
State Enrollment: 170,000

Healthplan and Services Defined
PLAN TYPE: HMO

Geographic Areas Served
Jefferson, Oldham, Trimble, Carroll, Henry, Shelby, Spencer, Bullitt, Nelson, Washington, Marion, Larue, Hardin, Grayson, Meade, Breckinridge counties

Accreditation Certification
NCQA

Key Personnel
Chief Executive Officer........................Mark B Carter
Chief Financial Officer ....David A. Stanley
VP/Chief Medical Officer............Stephen J. Houghland, MD
VP/Chief Communications......................Jill Joseph Bell
VP, Human Resources..........................Gary Bensing
VP, Clinical Operations ....Christie Spencer
VP, Public Affairs...............................Jill J Bell
   502-585-7983
   jill.bell@passporthealthplan.com

464   Preferred Health Plan Inc

, KY
Toll-Free: 800-832-8212
Phone: 502-339-7500
Fax: 502-339-8716
www.phpinc.com
For Profit Organization: Yes
Year Founded: 1983
Number of Affiliated Hospitals: 23
Number of Primary Care Physicians: 500
Number of Referral/Specialty Physicians: 1,500
Total Enrollment: 110,000
State Enrollment: 110,000

Healthplan and Services Defined
PLAN TYPE: PPO
Other Type: TPA
Model Type: Network
Plan Specialty: ASO, Dental, PBM, Vision, UR
Benefits Offered: TPA Services

Type of Coverage
Commercial

Type of Payment Plans Offered
DFFS

Geographic Areas Served
Nationwide

Network Qualifications
Pre-Admission Certification: Yes

Publishes and Distributes Report Card: No

Accreditation Certification
Medicare Approved, Utilization Review, Pre-Admission Certification, State Licensure, Quality Assurance Program

Specialty Managed Care Partners
Enters into Contracts with Regional Business Coalitions: No

465   Rural Carrier Benefit Plan
PO Box 7404
London, KY 40742
Toll-Free: 800-638-8432
www.rcbp.coventryhealthcare.com
Subsidiary of: Coventry Health Care

Healthplan and Services Defined
PLAN TYPE: PPO
Benefits Offered: Disease Management, Vision, Wellness, Cancer Treatment, Kidney Dialysis, 24-hour Nurse Line, Travel Assistance Program, Healthy Maternity, Lab One

Type of Coverage
Commercial, Individual

Type of Payment Plans Offered
Capitated, FFS

Geographic Areas Served
specific groups

Subscriber Information
Average Monthly Fee Per Subscriber
  (Employee + Employer Contribution):
    Employee Only (Self): $105.71
    Employee & 2 Family Members: $187.89
Average Annual Deductible Per Subscriber:
    Employee & 2 Family Members: $350.00
Average Subscriber Co-Payment:
    Primary Care Physician: 10%
    Prescription Drugs: $20 - $30
    Hospital ER: $0

466   UnitedHealthCare of Kentucky
230 Lexington Green Circle
Suite 400
Lexington, KY 40503
Toll-Free: 800-495-5285
Phone: 859-825-6132
Fax: 859-825-6174
www.uhc.com
Secondary Address: 301 North Hurtsbourne Parkway, Suite 100, Louisville, KY 40222, 800-307-4959
Subsidiary of: UnitedHealth Group
For Profit Organization: Yes
Year Founded: 1986
Number of Affiliated Hospitals: 66
Number of Primary Care Physicians: 1,208
Number of Referral/Specialty Physicians: 1,983
Total Enrollment: 75,000,000
State Enrollment: 135,106

Healthplan and Services Defined
PLAN TYPE: HMO/PPO
Model Type: IPA, Network
Plan Specialty: Dental, Vision
Benefits Offered: Chiropractic, Dental, Disease Management, Prescription, Vision, Wellness, Life, LTD, STD
Offers Demand Management Patient Information Service: Yes

Type of Coverage
Catastrophic Illness Benefit: Maximum $1M

Type of Payment Plans Offered
POS

Geographic Areas Served
Central Kentucky: 99 counties

Subscriber Information
Average Monthly Fee Per Subscriber
(Employee + Employer Contribution):
Employee Only (Self): $139.00
Employee & 1 Family Member: $282.00
Employee & 2 Family Members: $445.00
Medicare: $0
Average Annual Deductible Per Subscriber:
Employee Only (Self): $0
Employee & 1 Family Member: $0
Employee & 2 Family Members: $0
Average Subscriber Co-Payment:
Primary Care Physician: $10.00
Non-Network Physician: Not covered
Prescription Drugs: $7.00
Hospital ER: $50.00
Home Health Care: 20%
Nursing Home: Not covered

Network Qualifications
Pre-Admission Certification: Yes

Peer Review Type
Utilization Review: Yes
Second Surgical Opinion: No
Case Management: Yes

Publishes and Distributes Report Card: Yes

Accreditation Certification
TJC Accreditation, Utilization Review, Pre-Admission Certification,
State Licensure, Quality Assurance Program

Key Personnel
President . . . . Walter W Wakefield
CFO . . . . Richard Dunlop
Director Communications. . . . . Mark Lindsay
Media Contact . . . . Jessica Kostner
952-979-5869
jessica_kostner@uhc.com

Average Claim Compensation
Physician's Fees Charged: 1%
Hospital's Fees Charged: 1%

Specialty Managed Care Partners
Enters into Contracts with Regional Business Coalitions: Yes

Health Insurance Coverage Status and Type of Coverage by Age

Category	All Persons		Under 18 years		Under 65 years		65 years and over	
	Number	%	Number	%	Number	%	Number	%
Total population	4,523	-	1,111	-	3,936	-	587	-
Covered by some type of health insurance	3,772 (17)	83.4 (0.4)	1,048 (5)	94.3 (0.4)	3,190 (17)	81.1 (0.4)	581 (3)	99.0 (0.2)
Covered by private health insurance	2,673 (29)	59.1 (0.6)	549 (13)	49.4 (1.2)	2,331 (28)	59.2 (0.7)	343 (6)	58.4 (1.1)
Employment based	2,216 (31)	49.0 (0.7)	477 (13)	42.9 (1.2)	2,017 (29)	51.2 (0.8)	199 (6)	33.9 (1.0)
Direct purchase	500 (12)	11.1 (0.3)	63 (5)	5.7 (0.4)	333 (12)	8.4 (0.3)	168 (5)	28.6 (0.8)
Covered by TRICARE	115 (7)	2.5 (0.2)	27 (3)	2.4 (0.3)	82 (6)	2.1 (0.2)	33 (3)	5.7 (0.4)
Covered by government health insurance	1,558 (20)	34.5 (0.4)	543 (14)	48.9 (1.2)	996 (20)	25.3 (0.5)	562 (3)	95.8 (0.4)
Covered by Medicaid	987 (20)	21.8 (0.4)	539 (14)	48.5 (1.2)	885 (20)	22.5 (0.5)	102 (4)	17.4 (0.7)
Also by private insurance	130 (8)	2.9 (0.2)	45 (5)	4.0 (0.5)	92 (7)	2.3 (0.2)	38 (3)	6.5 (0.5)
Covered by Medicare	710 (7)	15.7 (0.2)	8 (2)	0.7 (0.1)	149 (7)	3.8 (0.2)	561 (3)	95.5 (0.5)
Also by private insurance	358 (6)	7.9 (0.1)	1 (1)	0.1 (0.1)	35 (3)	0.9 (0.1)	323 (6)	55.0 (1.0)
Also by Medicaid	179 (6)	4.0 (0.1)	4 (1)	0.4 (0.1)	77 (5)	2.0 (0.1)	102 (4)	17.4 (0.7)
Covered by VA Care	100 (5)	2.2 (0.1)	2 (1)	0.1 (0.1)	51 (4)	1.3 (0.1)	48 (3)	8.2 (0.4)
Not covered at any time during the year	751 (17)	16.6 (0.4)	63 (5)	5.7 (0.4)	746 (17)	18.9 (0.4)	6 (1)	1.0 (0.2)

Note: Numbers in thousands; Figures cover 2013; Margin of error appears in parenthesis; A "Z" indicates that the value either represents or rounds to zero.
Source: U.S. Census Bureau, 2013 American Community Survey, Table HI05. Health Insurance Coverage Status and Type of Coverage by State and Age for All People: 2013

Louisiana

467 Aetna Health of Louisiana

151 Farmington Avenue
Hartford, CT 06156
Toll-Free: 800-872-3862
Phone: 860-273-0123
www.aetna.com
Partnered with: eHealthInsurance Services Inc.
For Profit Organization: Yes
Total Enrollment: 11,596,230

Healthplan and Services Defined
PLAN TYPE: PPO
Other Type: POS
Plan Specialty: EPO
Benefits Offered: Dental, Disease Management, Long-Term Care,
   Prescription, Wellness, Life, LTD, STD

Type of Coverage
Commercial, Individual

Type of Payment Plans Offered
POS, FFS

Geographic Areas Served
Statewide

Key Personnel
Chairman/CEO/President.....................Mark T Bertolini
EVP/General Counsel ....William J Casazza
EVP/CFO ....Shawn M Guertin

468 Arcadian Community Care

Pierremont Office Park III
500 12th Street, Suite 350
Oakland, LA 94607
Toll-Free: 800-573-8597
Phone: 510-832-0311
Fax: 510-832-0170
www.arcadiancommunitycare.com
Subsidiary of: Arcadian Health Plans
Acquired by: Humana

Healthplan and Services Defined
PLAN TYPE: Medicare
Model Type: Network
Benefits Offered: Prescription

Type of Coverage
Medicare

Key Personnel
Chairman & CEO ....Robert Fahlman
Chief Financial Officer ....Les Granow
Chief Information Officer ....Prudence Kuai
SVP, General Counsel ....James Novella

469 Blue Cross & Blue Shield of Louisiana

5525 Reitz Avenue
PO Box 98029
Baton Rouge, LA 70809
Toll-Free: 800-599-2583
Phone: 225-295-3307
Fax: 225-295-2054
help@bcbsla.com
www.bcbsla.com
Mailing Address: P.O. Box 98029, Baton Rouge, LA 70898-9029
For Profit Organization: Yes
Year Founded: 1933
Number of Affiliated Hospitals: 39
Number of Primary Care Physicians: 962
Number of Referral/Specialty Physicians: 2,219

Total Enrollment: 1,172,000
State Enrollment: 1,172,000

Healthplan and Services Defined
PLAN TYPE: HMO/PPO
Model Type: Network
Benefits Offered: Disease Management, Prescription, Wellness

Type of Coverage
Catastrophic Illness Benefit: Maximum $2M

Geographic Areas Served
New Orleans, Baton Rouge and Shreveport Metropolitan areas

Subscriber Information
Average Subscriber Co-Payment:
   Primary Care Physician: 10%/20%
   Home Health Care: Varies

Network Qualifications
Pre-Admission Certification: Yes

Peer Review Type
Utilization Review: Yes

Publishes and Distributes Report Card: No

Accreditation Certification
URAC, NCQA
TJC Accreditation, Medicare Approved, Utilization Review,
   Pre-Admission Certification, State Licensure, Quality Assurance
   Program

Key Personnel
President & CEO................................Mike Reitz
Chairman....................................Thad Minaldi
Vice Chairman ....Dan Bourn,
Secretary ....Ann H. Knapp
SVP/General Counsel......................Michele Calandro
SVP, Human Resources....................Todd Schexnayder
EVP/COO......................................Peggy Scott
SVP, Business Development..........................Tej Shah
Chief Medical Examiner ....David Carmouche, MD

Specialty Managed Care Partners
Enters into Contracts with Regional Business Coalitions: Yes

470 Calais Health

5745 Essen Lane
Suite 220
Baton Rouge, LA 70810
Toll-Free: 800-572-6983
Phone: 225-765-6570
Fax: 225-765-9463
webmaster@calaishealth.com
www.calaishealth.com
Subsidiary of: Calais Health
For Profit Organization: Yes
Year Founded: 2000
Number of Affiliated Hospitals: 11
Number of Referral/Specialty Physicians: 99
Total Enrollment: 137,000

Healthplan and Services Defined
PLAN TYPE: Multiple
Model Type: Network
Plan Specialty: Behavioral Health, Worker's Compensation, UR
Benefits Offered: Behavioral Health, Disease Management,
   Psychiatric, EAP

Type of Payment Plans Offered
POS, Capitated, FFS

Geographic Areas Served
Louisiana, Oklahoma and Mississippi

Network Qualifications
Pre-Admission Certification: Yes

Peer Review Type
Utilization Review: Yes

Case Management: Yes

Accreditation Certification
State Licensure

Key Personnel
Mgr Information Services . . . . Ted Nguyen
225-765-6829
VP/ Health Services. . . . . Helen Granger
Director CCM/FMC. . . . . Laura Hebert
225-765-6882
Business Development . . . . Ann Sellars
CFO . . . . Michael Whittington
Human Resources Director . . . . Leslie Yander
225-765-6827

Employer References
City of East Baton Rouge Parish, East Baton Rouge Parish School
System, Our Lady of the Lake Hospital, The Advocate/Capitol
City Press, Woman's Hospital

471 CIGNA HealthCare of Louisiana

2700 Post Oak Blvd
Suite 700
Houston, TX 77056
Toll-Free: 866-438-2446
Phone: 713-576-4300
Fax: 866-530-3585
www.cigna.com
For Profit Organization: Yes
Total Enrollment: 75,000,000

Healthplan and Services Defined
PLAN TYPE: HMO

Type of Coverage
Commercial

Accreditation Certification
URAC, NCQA

472 Coventry Health Care of Louisiana

3838 North Causeway Blvd
Suite 3350
Metairie, LA 70002
Toll-Free: 800-341-6613
Phone: 504-834-0840
Fax: 504-828-6433
http://chclouisiana.coventryhealthcare.com
Secondary Address: 1720 South Sykes Drive, Bismarck, ND 58504
Subsidiary of: Coventry Health Care
For Profit Organization: Yes
Number of Primary Care Physicians: 2,000
Total Enrollment: 30,000
State Enrollment: 71,716

Healthplan and Services Defined
PLAN TYPE: HMO
Benefits Offered: Disease Management, Wellness

Geographic Areas Served
Louisiana

Accreditation Certification
URAC

Key Personnel
CMO . . . . Lynn Williamson, MD
Provider Relations . . . . Clay Bittner
Marketing. . . . . Carson Meehan
CFO. . . . . Angela Meoli

473 Delta Dental of Georgia

1130 Sanctuary Parkway
Suite 600
Alpharetta, GA 30004
Toll-Free: 800-521-2651
Fax: 770-641-5234
www.deltadentalins.com
Non-Profit Organization: Yes
Number of Primary Care Physicians: 198,000
Total Enrollment: 54,000,000

Healthplan and Services Defined
PLAN TYPE: Dental
Other Type: Dental PPO
Plan Specialty: Dental
Benefits Offered: Dental

Type of Coverage
Commercial

Type of Payment Plans Offered
POS, DFFS, FFS

Geographic Areas Served
Statewide

Key Personnel
CEO. . . . . Gary D Radine
VP, Public & Govt Affairs . . . . Jeff Album
415-972-8418
Dir/Media & Public Affair . . . . Elizabeth Risberg
415-972-8423

474 DINA Dental Plans

11969 Bricksome Avenue
Suite A
Baton Rouge, LA 70816
Toll-Free: 800-376-3462
Phone: 225-291-3172
Fax: 225-292-3075
info@dinadental.com
www.dinadental.com
For Profit Organization: Yes
Year Founded: 1978
Total Enrollment: 30,000

Healthplan and Services Defined
PLAN TYPE: Dental
Model Type: Group, Individual
Plan Specialty: Dental
Benefits Offered: Dental

Type of Coverage
Commercial, Individual

Geographic Areas Served
Statewide

Subscriber Information
Average Monthly Fee Per Subscriber
(Employee + Employer Contribution):
Employee Only (Self): $13.00-20.00
Employee & 1 Family Member: $21.00-38.00
Employee & 2 Family Members: $28.00-60.00
Medicare: $30.00
Average Annual Deductible Per Subscriber:
Employee Only (Self): $50.00
Employee & 1 Family Member: $50.00
Employee & 2 Family Members: $50.00

Network Qualifications
Pre-Admission Certification: Yes

Peer Review Type
Second Surgical Opinion: Yes

Publishes and Distributes Report Card: No

Key Personnel

President...James Taylor
CFO ....Patrick Stoner
COO...Rick Barrett

Specialty Managed Care Partners

Enters into Contracts with Regional Business Coalitions: No

---

475 eHealthInsurance Services Inc.

11919 Foundation Place
Gold River, CA 95670
Toll-Free: 800-644-3491
webmaster@healthinsurance.com
www.e.healthinsurance.com
Year Founded: 1997

Healthplan and Services Defined
PLAN TYPE: HMO/PPO
Benefits Offered: Dental, Life, STD

Type of Coverage
Commercial, Individual, Medicare

Geographic Areas Served
All 50 states in the USA and District of Columbia

Key Personnel

Chairman & CEO.............................Gary L. Lauer
EVP/Business & Corp. Dev....................Bruce Telkamp
EVP/Chief Technology....................Dr. Sheldon X. Wang
SVP & CFO ....Stuart M. Huizinga
Pres. of eHealth Gov. Sys ....Samuel C. Gibbs
SVP of Sales & Operations ....Robert S. Hurley
Director Public Relations.........................Nate Purpura
650-210-3115

---

476 Health Plus of Louisiana

2219 Line Avenue
Shreveport, LA 71104-2128
Toll-Free: 800-331-5055
Phone: 318-212-8800
Fax: 318-676-3372
webmaster@wkhealthplus.com
www.wkhealthplus.com
Mailing Address: PO Box 32625, Shreveport, LA 71130-2625
Subsidiary of: Willis-Knighton Health System
Non-Profit Organization: Yes
Year Founded: 1994
Physician Owned Organization: Yes
Number of Affiliated Hospitals: 1
Total Enrollment: 30,000
State Enrollment: 30,000

Healthplan and Services Defined
PLAN TYPE: HMO
Model Type: IPA
Benefits Offered: Dental, Prescription, Life, LTD, STD
Offers Demand Management Patient Information Service: Yes

Type of Payment Plans Offered
POS

Geographic Areas Served
Northern Louisiana

Subscriber Information
Average Monthly Fee Per Subscriber
(Employee + Employer Contribution):
Employee Only (Self): $0
Employee & 1 Family Member: $0
Employee & 2 Family Members: $0
Medicare: $0

Peer Review Type
Case Management: Yes

Accreditation Certification
TJC, NCQA

Key Personnel

President and CEO ....Patrick Bicknell
VP/CFO ....Larry Knighton
Business Office Director ....Patty Fuller
Claims/Operations Manager ....Sandy Brown
Compliance Director ....Jim Frantz
Business Office Assistant.......................Owen Rigby
Member Relations.................................Teri Graves
Human Resources Manager ....Debbie Forston
Dir, Sales & Marketing.........................Scott Johnson
VP, Chief Medical Officer ....Carey Allison
Medical Director ....Bendel Johnson
Director Medical Staff........................Marion Morrison
Credential Analyst ....Cynthia Blanchard
Credential Coordinator ....Camissa Decker
Peer Review Coordinator ....Joan Rigby

Specialty Managed Care Partners
Enters into Contracts with Regional Business Coalitions: Yes

---

477 Humana Health Insurance of Louisiana

1111 Veterans Boulevard
Suite 2B
Metairie, LA 70003
Phone: 504-833-1727
Fax: 504-219-5142
www.humana.com
Secondary Address: 910 Pierremont Road, Suite 410, Shreveport, LA 71106, 318-861-8609
For Profit Organization: Yes
Year Founded: 1985
Physician Owned Organization: Yes
Federally Qualified: Yes
Number of Affiliated Hospitals: 60
Number of Primary Care Physicians: 3,500
Number of Referral/Specialty Physicians: 2,427
Total Enrollment: 142,000
State Enrollment: 155,722

Healthplan and Services Defined
PLAN TYPE: HMO/PPO
Model Type: IPA, mixed
Benefits Offered: Behavioral Health, Chiropractic, Disease Management, Home Care, Inpatient SNF, Physical Therapy, Podiatry, Prescription, Psychiatric, Transplant, Vision, Wellness

Type of Coverage
Commercial, Individual, Indemnity, Medicare
Catastrophic Illness Benefit: Unlimited

Type of Payment Plans Offered
POS, Combination FFS & DFFS

Geographic Areas Served
Louisiana, excluding Monroe

Subscriber Information
Average Monthly Fee Per Subscriber
(Employee + Employer Contribution):
Employee Only (Self): $189.31
Employee & 1 Family Member: $378.62
Employee & 2 Family Members: $530.07
Average Subscriber Co-Payment:
Primary Care Physician: $15.00
Prescription Drugs: $10/$25/$40
Home Health Care Max. Days/Visits Covered: 60 days

Network Qualifications
Pre-Admission Certification: Yes

Peer Review Type
Utilization Review: Yes
Second Surgical Opinion: Yes
Case Management: Yes

Publishes and Distributes Report Card: Yes

Accreditation Certification
URAC, NCQA, CORE
Medicare Approved, Utilization Review, Pre-Admission
Certification, State Licensure, Quality Assurance Program

Key Personnel
President and CEO . . . . .Hassan Rifaat
Media Relations Manager . . . . .Mitch Lubitz
813-287-6180
mlubitz@humana.com

Specialty Managed Care Partners
CMS Healthcare, Medimpact
Enters into Contracts with Regional Business Coalitions: Yes
Chamber of Commerce

Employer References
State Of Louisiana, Exxon-Mobil, Shell, Chevron, Sears

---

478 Meritain Health: Louisiana

920 Pierremont Road
Suite 308
Shreveport, LA 71106
Toll-Free: 800-256-2657
Fax: 318-424-9702
sales@meritain.com
www.meritain.com
Subsidiary of: Aetna
For Profit Organization: Yes
Year Founded: 1983
Number of Affiliated Hospitals: 110
Number of Primary Care Physicians: 3,467
Number of Referral/Specialty Physicians: 5,720
Total Enrollment: 500,000
State Enrollment: 450,000

Healthplan and Services Defined
PLAN TYPE: PPO
Model Type: Network
Plan Specialty: Dental, Disease Management, Vision, Radiology, UR
Benefits Offered: Prescription
Offers Demand Management Patient Information Service: Yes

Type of Coverage
Commercial

Geographic Areas Served
Nationwide

Subscriber Information
Average Monthly Fee Per Subscriber
(Employee + Employer Contribution):
Employee Only (Self): Varies by plan

Accreditation Certification
URAC
TJC Accreditation, Medicare Approved, Utilization Review,
Pre-Admission Certification, State Licensure, Quality Assurance
Program

Key Personnel
Regional President. . . . . .Margie Mann
Regional VP Sales. . . . . .Jack Groseclose

Average Claim Compensation
Physician's Fees Charged: 78%
Hospital's Fees Charged: 90%

Specialty Managed Care Partners
Express Scripts, LabOne, Interactive Health Solutions

---

479 Peoples Health

Chase Riverside Tower North
450 Laurel Street, Suite 1101
Baton Rouge, LA 70801
Toll-Free: 800-222-8600
Phone: 225-346-5704
www.peopleshealth.com
For Profit Organization: Yes
Total Enrollment: 41,000
State Enrollment: 4,707

Healthplan and Services Defined
PLAN TYPE: HMO
Plan Specialty: Lab, Radiology
Benefits Offered: Dental, Disease Management, Home Care,
Prescription, Wellness

Type of Coverage
Commercial, Medicare

Geographic Areas Served
Louisiana

Key Personnel
Chief Executive Officer . . . . .Carol Solomon
Chief Operating Officer . . . . .Warren Murrell
Chief Financial Officer . . . . .Kim Eller
Chief Information Officer . . . . .Colin Hulin
Chief Marketing Officer . . . . .Mike Putiak
General Counsel . . . . .Donna Klein
VP, Health Services . . . . .Barbara Guerard
VP, Human Resources. . . . . .Greg Ruppert
VP, Finance/Controller . . . . .Emmet Geary
VP, Clinic Operations . . . . .Jeffrey Friedman
VP, Network Development. .Macon Moore
VP, Medical Affairs . . . . .Kevin J. Roache
SVP, Network Development. . . . . .Janice Ortego
SVP, Internal Audit. . . . . .Michael J. Robert

---

480 Peoples Health

3838 North Causeway Blvd
Suite 2200, Three Lakeway Center
Metairie, LA 70002
Toll-Free: 800-631-8443
Phone: 504-849-4500
Fax: 504-464-1015
www.peopleshealth.com
Year Founded: 1994
Physician Owned Organization: Yes
Total Enrollment: 42,000
State Enrollment: 50,000

Healthplan and Services Defined
PLAN TYPE: Medicare
Other Type: HMO-POS

Type of Coverage
Medicare, Supplemental Medicare

Geographic Areas Served
Choices 65 (HMO): Jefferson, Orleans, Plaquemines, St. Tammany;
Choices Plus (HMO-POS): Ascension, East Baton Rouge, Livingston,
St. Bernard, St. Charles, St. James, St. John, West Baton Rouge;
Choice Select (HMO-POS): Tangipahoa, Washington; SecureHealth
(HMO SNP): Ascension, East Baton Rouge, Jefferson, Livingston,
Orleans, Plaquemines, St. Bernard, St. Charles, St. James, St. John, St.
Tammany, Tangipahoa, Washington, West Baton Rouge

Accreditation Certification
URAC

Key Personnel
Chief Executive Officer . . . . .Carol A Solomon
Chief Operating Officer . . . . .Warren Murrell
Chief Financial Officer . . . . .Kim Eller

VP, Network Development . . . . Macon Moore
SVP, Network Development . . . . Janice Ortega
VP, Audit & Compliance . . . . Michael J Robert
Asst VP, Decision Support . . . . Kristie Marino
Chief Marketing Officer . . . . Mike Putiak
Medical Director Benefits . . . . Frank N Deus, MD
VP, Medical Affairs . . . . Kevin J Roache, MD
Director, Human Resources . . . . Greg Ruppert
Chief Information Officer . . . . Colin Hulin
VP, Sales & Marketing . . . . John Van Wart
Director, Communications . . . . Suzanne M Whitaker, APR
　　504-681-8978
　　suzanne.whitaker@peopleshealth.com

481　UnitedHealthCare of Louisiana

3838 N. Causeway Boulevard
Suite 2600
Metairie, LA 70002
Toll-Free: 800-826-1981
www.uhc.com
Subsidiary of: UnitedHealth Group
For Profit Organization: Yes
Year Founded: 1986
Number of Affiliated Hospitals: 42
Number of Primary Care Physicians: 356
Number of Referral/Specialty Physicians: 877
Total Enrollment: 75,000,000
State Enrollment: 272,972

Healthplan and Services Defined
　PLAN TYPE: HMO/PPO
　Model Type: IPA
　Benefits Offered: Disease Management, Prescription, Wellness

Geographic Areas Served
　Ascension, Assumption, East Baton Rouge, East Feliciana, Iberville,
　Jefferson, LaFourche, Livingston, Orleans, Plaquemines, Point
　Coupee, St. Bernard, St. Charles, St. Helena, St. James, St. Tammany,
　Tangipahoa, Terrabona, West Baton Rouge, West Feliciana

Subscriber Information
　Average Monthly Fee Per Subscriber
　　(Employee + Employer Contribution):
　　　Employee Only (Self): $129.45
　　　Employee & 1 Family Member: $261.04
　　　Employee & 2 Family Members: $422.40
　Average Annual Deductible Per Subscriber:
　　　Employee Only (Self): $5.00
　Average Subscriber Co-Payment:
　　　Primary Care Physician: $10.00
　　　Prescription Drugs: $10.00
　　　Hospital ER: $50.00

Network Qualifications
　Pre-Admission Certification: Yes

Peer Review Type
　Utilization Review: Yes

Publishes and Distributes Report Card: No

Accreditation Certification
　TJC Accreditation, Medicare Approved, Utilization Review,
　　Pre-Admission Certification, State Licensure, Quality Assurance
　　Program

Key Personnel
　CFO . . . . Steve Cunningham
　Marketing . . . . Glen Golemi
　Medical Affairs . . . . Debbie Bates, MD
　Member Services . . . . Kathy Magby
　Information Systems . . . . Heidi Chapman
　Provider Services . . . . Charles Brewer
　Media Contact . . . . Liz Calzadilla-Fiallo
　　954-378-0537
　　elizabeth.calzadilla-fiallo@uhc.com

Specialty Managed Care Partners
　Enters into Contracts with Regional Business Coalitions: No

482　Vantage Health Plan

130 DeSiard Street
Suite 300
Monroe, LA 71201
Toll-Free: 888-823-1910
Phone: 318-361-0900
Fax: 318-361-2159
www.vhpla.com
Secondary Address: 855 Pierremont Road, Suite 109, Shreveport, LA
　71106, 318-678-0008
For Profit Organization: Yes
Year Founded: 1994
Number of Affiliated Hospitals: 4
Total Enrollment: 14,000
State Enrollment: 14,000

Healthplan and Services Defined
　PLAN TYPE: HMO
　Plan Specialty: Lab, Radiology
　Benefits Offered: Behavioral Health, Chiropractic, Disease
　　Management, Home Care, Inpatient SNF, Physical Therapy,
　　Prescription, Wellness, Durable Medical Equipment

Type of Coverage
　Commercial

Geographic Areas Served
　Louisiana

Network Qualifications
　Pre-Admission Certification: Yes

Key Personnel
　CEO . . . . P Gary Jones, MD
　COO . . . . Wendy Poe, RN
　CFO . . . . Mike Briard
　Provider Relations . . . . Annette Napier
　Marketing . . . . Billy Justice

Specialty Managed Care Partners
　Caremark Rx

483　Vantage Medicare Advantage

130 DeSiard Street
Suite 300
Monroe, LA 71201
Toll-Free: 888-823-1910
Phone: 318-361-0900
www.vhp-medicare.com
Secondary Address: 855 Pierremont Road, Suite 109, Shreveport, LA
　71106, 318-678-0008
Year Founded: 1994
Total Enrollment: 14,000

Healthplan and Services Defined
　PLAN TYPE: Medicare
　Other Type: Medicare PPO
　Benefits Offered: Home Care, Inpatient SNF, Prescription

Type of Coverage
　Medicare, Supplemental Medicare

Geographic Areas Served
　Bossier, Caddo, Caldwell, Jackson, Lincoln, Morehouse, Rapides,
　Ouachita, richland, and Union Parishes

Health Insurance Coverage Status and Type of Coverage by Age

Category	All Persons		Under 18 years		Under 65 years		65 years and over	
	Number	%	Number	%	Number	%	Number	%
Total population	1,314	-	260	-	1,085	-	229	-
Covered by some type of health insurance	1,167 *(7)*	88.8 *(0.5)*	244 *(3)*	94.1 *(1.0)*	939 *(7)*	86.5 *(0.7)*	228 *(1)*	99.8 *(0.1)*
Covered by private health insurance	853 *(12)*	64.9 *(0.9)*	156 *(5)*	59.9 *(2.0)*	704 *(11)*	64.8 *(1.0)*	149 *(4)*	65.1 *(1.7)*
Employment based	698 *(13)*	53.1 *(1.0)*	139 *(6)*	53.3 *(2.2)*	622 *(12)*	57.3 *(1.1)*	76 *(4)*	33.1 *(1.7)*
Direct purchase	157 *(6)*	11.9 *(0.5)*	13 *(2)*	5.1 *(0.7)*	79 *(5)*	7.3 *(0.5)*	77 *(3)*	33.8 *(1.5)*
Covered by TRICARE	45 *(4)*	3.4 *(0.3)*	7 *(2)*	2.8 *(0.7)*	26 *(4)*	2.4 *(0.3)*	19 *(2)*	8.4 *(0.9)*
Covered by government health insurance	509 *(10)*	38.8 *(0.7)*	106 *(5)*	40.9 *(2.0)*	287 *(10)*	26.4 *(0.9)*	223 *(1)*	97.3 *(0.5)*
Covered by Medicaid	296 *(10)*	22.5 *(0.7)*	106 *(5)*	40.7 *(2.0)*	255 *(9)*	23.5 *(0.9)*	40 *(3)*	17.5 *(1.3)*
Also by private insurance	53 *(5)*	4.0 *(0.4)*	17 *(3)*	6.6 *(1.1)*	36 *(4)*	3.4 *(0.4)*	17 *(2)*	7.2 *(0.9)*
Covered by Medicare	270 *(4)*	20.5 *(0.3)*	1 *(1)*	0.5 *(0.2)*	48 *(3)*	4.4 *(0.3)*	222 *(1)*	97.1 *(0.5)*
Also by private insurance	153 *(4)*	11.6 *(0.3)*	Z *(Z)*	0.1 *(0.1)*	10 *(1)*	0.9 *(0.1)*	143 *(4)*	62.4 *(1.7)*
Also by Medicaid	71 *(4)*	5.4 *(0.3)*	1 *(1)*	0.3 *(0.2)*	31 *(3)*	2.9 *(0.2)*	40 *(3)*	17.5 *(1.3)*
Covered by VA Care	45 *(2)*	3.4 *(0.2)*	Z *(Z)*	0.1 *(0.1)*	20 *(2)*	1.8 *(0.2)*	26 *(2)*	11.2 *(0.7)*
Not covered at any time during the year	147 *(7)*	11.2 *(0.5)*	15 *(3)*	5.9 *(1.0)*	147 *(7)*	13.5 *(0.7)*	Z *(Z)*	0.2 *(0.1)*

Note: Numbers in thousands; Figures cover 2013; Margin of error appears in parenthesis; A "Z" indicates that the value either represents or rounds to zero.
Source: U.S. Census Bureau, 2013 American Community Survey, Table HI05. Health Insurance Coverage Status and Type of Coverage by State and Age for All People: 2013

Maine

484   Aetna Health of Maine

151 Farmington Avenue
Hartford, CT 06156
Toll-Free: 800-872-3862
Phone: 860-273-0123
www.aetna.com
For Profit Organization: Yes
Year Founded: 1996
Federally Qualified: Yes
Total Enrollment: 22,417
State Enrollment: 22,417

Healthplan and Services Defined
  PLAN TYPE: HMO
  Other Type: POS
  Model Type: Network
  Plan Specialty: PBM
  Benefits Offered: Chiropractic, Home Care, Prescription, Psychiatric,
    Vision, Wellness

Type of Coverage
  Commercial, Individual

Geographic Areas Served
  Statewide

Subscriber Information
  Average Monthly Fee Per Subscriber
    (Employee + Employer Contribution):
      Employee Only (Self): $73.42
      Employee & 1 Family Member: $168.89

Key Personnel
  Chairman/CEO/President . . . . Mark T Bertolini
  EVP/General Counsel . . . . William J Casazza
  EVP/CFO . . . . Shawn M Guertin

485   Anthem Blue Cross & Blue Shield of Maine

2 Gannett Dr.
S. Portland, ME 04106
Toll-Free: 800-585-0099
Phone: 207-822-7000
www.anthem.com
Secondary Address: One Merchants Plaza, Bangor, ME 04401
For Profit Organization: Yes
Year Founded: 1985
Number of Affiliated Hospitals: 42
Number of Primary Care Physicians: 971
Number of Referral/Specialty Physicians: 1,604
Total Enrollment: 545,610
State Enrollment: 85,917

Healthplan and Services Defined
  PLAN TYPE: HMO/PPO
  Model Type: Staff
  Plan Specialty: ASO, Behavioral Health, Chiropractic, Disease
    Management, Lab, PBM, Vision, Radiology, Worker's
    Compensation, UR
  Benefits Offered: Behavioral Health, Chiropractic, Dental, Disease
    Management, Home Care, Inpatient SNF, Physical Therapy,
    Podiatry, Prescription, Psychiatric, Transplant, Vision, Wellness,
    Worker's Compensation, Life

Type of Coverage
  Commercial, Individual, Supplemental Medicare

Type of Payment Plans Offered
  POS, DFFS, Capitated, FFS

Geographic Areas Served
  Statewide

Network Qualifications
  Pre-Admission Certification: Yes

Peer Review Type
  Utilization Review: Yes
  Second Surgical Opinion: Yes
  Case Management: Yes

Publishes and Distributes Report Card: Yes

Accreditation Certification
  NCQA
  TJC Accreditation, Medicare Approved, Utilization Review,
    Pre-Admission Certification, State Licensure, Quality Assurance
    Program

Key Personnel
  CEO . . . . John Cannon
  CFO . . . . Wayne Deveyolt
  Pharmacy Director . . . . James Lang
  Chief Medical Officer . . . . Samuel Nussbaum, MD
  Member Relations . . . . Karen Andrews
  Public Relations . . . . Deborah New
  Sales Executive . . . . James Parker
  Media Contact . . . . Chris Dugan
  603-695-7202
  chris.dugan@anthem.com

Specialty Managed Care Partners
  Green Spring Health Service

Employer References
  Maine Education Association, State of Maine Employees Benefits
    Trust, Sappi Fine Paper, Maine Medical Center, Maine General
    Health

486   CIGNA HealthCare of Maine

500 Southborough Drive
Suite 302, Rtg 596
South Portland, ME 04106
Toll-Free: 866-438-2446
Phone: 207-828-9700
Fax: 207-728-9717
www.cigna.com
For Profit Organization: Yes
Year Founded: 1986
Owned by an Integrated Delivery Network (IDN): Yes
Number of Affiliated Hospitals: 39
Number of Primary Care Physicians: 900
Number of Referral/Specialty Physicians: 1,200
Total Enrollment: 6,343
State Enrollment: 6,343

Healthplan and Services Defined
  PLAN TYPE: HMO
  Other Type: POS
  Model Type: IPA
  Plan Specialty: Dental, Vision
  Benefits Offered: Behavioral Health, Chiropractic, Disease
    Management, Home Care, Inpatient SNF, Long-Term Care,
    Physical Therapy, Podiatry, Prescription, Transplant, Vision,
    Wellness
  Offers Demand Management Patient Information Service: Yes

Type of Coverage
  Commercial

Type of Payment Plans Offered
  POS, DFFS

Geographic Areas Served
  CIGNA @ Maine serves the counties of Aroostook, Cumberland,
    Hancock, Kennebec, Knox, Penobscot, Piscataquis, Somerset, Waldo,
    and York

Subscriber Information
  Average Annual Deductible Per Subscriber:
    Employee Only (Self): $0
    Employee & 1 Family Member: $0
    Employee & 2 Family Members: $0

Average Subscriber Co-Payment:
>> Primary Care Physician: $10.00
>> Prescription Drugs: $5.00/10.00/20.00
>> Hospital ER: $25.00

Network Qualifications
Pre-Admission Certification: Yes

Peer Review Type
Utilization Review: Yes
Second Surgical Opinion: Yes
Case Management: Yes

Publishes and Distributes Report Card: Yes

Accreditation Certification
NCQA
TJC Accreditation, Medicare Approved, Utilization Review,
Pre-Admission Certification, State Licensure, Quality Assurance
Program

Key Personnel
Chairman and CEO . . . . .David Cordini
215-762-6002
CFO . . . . .Mark Boxer
Chief Medical Officer . . . . .Alan Muney
Chief Counsel . . . . .Nicole Jones
Chief Marketing Officer .Robert G Romasco
Human Resources . . . . .Donald M Levinson
Chief Information Officer . . . . .Andrea Anania

Specialty Managed Care Partners
CIGNA Behavioral Health

Employer References
BIW, UNUM

---

487   eHealthInsurance Services Inc.
11919 Foundation Place
Gold River, CA 95670
Toll-Free: 800-644-3491
webmaster@healthinsurance.com
www.e.healthinsurance.com
Year Founded: 1997

Healthplan and Services Defined
PLAN TYPE: HMO/PPO
Benefits Offered: Dental, Life, STD

Type of Coverage
Commercial, Individual, Medicare

Geographic Areas Served
All 50 states in the USA and District of Columbia

Key Personnel
Chairman & CEO . . . . .Gary L. Lauer
EVP/Business & Corp. Dev. .Bruce Telkamp
EVP/Chief Technology . . . . .Dr. Sheldon X. Wang
SVP & CFO . . . . .Stuart M. Huizinga
Pres. of eHealth Gov. Sys . . . . .Samuel C. Gibbs
SVP of Sales & Operations . . . . .Robert S. Hurley
Director Public Relations . . . . .Nate Purpura
650-210-3115

---

488   Great-West Healthcare Maine
500 Southborough Drive
Suite 302
South Portland, ME 04106-6903
Toll-Free: 866-494-2111
Phone: 207-828-5084
eliginquiries@cigna.com
www.cignaforhealth.com
Secondary Address: 6 Fundy Road, Suite 300, Falmouth, ME 04105
Subsidiary of: CIGNA HealthCare
Acquired by: CIGNA
For Profit Organization: Yes

Total Enrollment: 8,184
State Enrollment: 8,078

Healthplan and Services Defined
PLAN TYPE: HMO/PPO
Benefits Offered: Disease Management, Prescription, Wellness

Type of Coverage
Commercial

Type of Payment Plans Offered
POS, FFS

Geographic Areas Served
Maine

Accreditation Certification
URAC

Key Personnel
Manager . . . . .Tom Griffin

Specialty Managed Care Partners
Caremark Rx

---

489   Harvard Pilgrim Health Care: Maine
1 Market Street
3rd Floor
Portland, ME 04101
Toll-Free: 888-888-4742
www.harvardpilgrim.org
Non-Profit Organization: Yes
Year Founded: 1977
Number of Affiliated Hospitals: 135
Number of Primary Care Physicians: 28,000
Total Enrollment: 1,100,000
State Enrollment: 67,000

Healthplan and Services Defined
PLAN TYPE: Multiple
Model Type: Network
Plan Specialty: ASO, Behavioral Health, Chiropractic, Dental,
Disease Management, EPO, Lab, MSO, PBM, Vision, Radiology,
Worker's Compensation, UR
Benefits Offered: Behavioral Health, Chiropractic, Disease
Management, Home Care, Inpatient SNF, Long-Term Care,
Physical Therapy, Podiatry, Prescription, Psychiatric, Transplant,
Vision, Wellness
Offers Demand Management Patient Information Service: Yes
DMPI Services Offered: Clinical Program, Specialty On-Line, Case
Management, Cybernurse, On-Line A-Z

Type of Coverage
Commercial, Individual, Indemnity, Medicare, Supplemental
Medicare, Medicaid

Type of Payment Plans Offered
POS, Combination FFS & DFFS

Geographic Areas Served
Mass.: All counties; Rhode Island: All counties; New Hampshire:
Sullivan, Belknap, Merrimack, Strafford, Cheshire, Hillsborough,
Rockingham counties, parts of Coos, Grafton and Carroll counties;
Vermont: Windham, Windsor and Caledonia county

Subscriber Information
Average Monthly Fee Per Subscriber
(Employee + Employer Contribution):
Employee Only (Self): $5.50
Average Annual Deductible Per Subscriber:
Employee Only (Self): $1000.00
Employee & 1 Family Member: $2000.00
Employee & 2 Family Members: $2000.00
Average Subscriber Co-Payment:
Primary Care Physician: $20.00
Non-Network Physician: 20%
Prescription Drugs: $10.00
Hospital ER: $50.00-50.00
Home Health Care: $0

Home Health Care Max. Days/Visits Covered: Subject to review
Nursing Home: $0
Nursing Home Max. Days/Visits Covered: 60 days

Network Qualifications
Pre-Admission Certification: Yes

Peer Review Type
Utilization Review: Yes
Second Surgical Opinion: Yes
Case Management: Yes

Publishes and Distributes Report Card: Yes

Accreditation Certification
NCQA
TJC Accreditation, Medicare Approved, Utilization Review,
Pre-Admission Certification, State Licensure, Quality Assurance
Program

Key Personnel
Executive Director ....Karen Voci

Average Claim Compensation
Physician's Fees Charged: 51%
Hospital's Fees Charged: 40%

Specialty Managed Care Partners
Mass General, Brigham And Women Hospital, Boston Medical,
Value Options, MedImpact
Enters into Contracts with Regional Business Coalitions: No

Employer References
Commonwealth of Massachusetts, City of Boston, Harvard
University

---

490 Martin's Point HealthCare

331 Veranda Street
Building 6
Portland, ME 04104
Phone: 207-828-2402
Fax: 207-828-2433
www.martinspoint.org
Non-Profit Organization: Yes
Year Founded: 1981
Total Enrollment: 85,000

Healthplan and Services Defined
PLAN TYPE: Multiple
Benefits Offered: Disease Management, Prescription, Wellness, No
co-pay for: routine physical exams/hearing tests/eye
exams/mammograms/prostrate & pap exams/bone mass/flu
vaccines.

Type of Coverage
Commercial, Medicare, Military

Geographic Areas Served
Maine, New Hampshire, Vermont, northeastern New York

Subscriber Information
Average Monthly Fee Per Subscriber
(Employee + Employer Contribution):
Employee Only (Self): Varies
Medicare: Varies
Average Annual Deductible Per Subscriber:
Employee Only (Self): Varies
Medicare: Varies
Average Subscriber Co-Payment:
Primary Care Physician: Varies
Prescription Drugs: Varies
Hospital ER: Varies

Key Personnel
President/CEO ....David Howes, MD
Chief Financial Officer ....Dale Bradford
Chief Operating Officer.........................Larry Henry
Chief Organizational Effe ....Sandra Monfiletto
Chief Medical Officer ....Jonathan Harvey, MD

491 Northeast Community Care

49 Atlantic Place
South Portland, ME 04106-2316
Toll-Free: 800-998-3056
Phone: 207-773-3920
Fax: 207-773-3990
www.northeastcommunitycare.com
Subsidiary of: Arcadian Health Plans

Healthplan and Services Defined
PLAN TYPE: Medicare

Type of Coverage
Medicare

---

492 UnitedHealthCare of Maine

9700 Health Care Lane
Minnetonka, MN 55343
Toll-Free: 800-842-3585
www.uhc.com
Subsidiary of: UnitedHealth Group
Year Founded: 1977
Number of Affiliated Hospitals: 4,200
Number of Primary Care Physicians: 460,000
Total Enrollment: 75,000,000

Healthplan and Services Defined
PLAN TYPE: HMO/PPO
Model Type: IPA, Group, Network
Plan Specialty: Lab, Radiology
Benefits Offered: Chiropractic, Dental, Physical Therapy,
Prescription, Wellness, AD&D, Life, LTD, STD
Offers Demand Management Patient Information Service: Yes

Type of Coverage
Commercial, Individual, Indemnity, Medicare

Geographic Areas Served
Statewide

Network Qualifications
Pre-Admission Certification: Yes

Peer Review Type
Utilization Review: Yes
Second Surgical Opinion: Yes
Case Management: Yes

Publishes and Distributes Report Card: Yes

Accreditation Certification
TJC, NCQA

Specialty Managed Care Partners
Enters into Contracts with Regional Business Coalitions: Yes

Health Insurance Coverage Status and Type of Coverage by Age

Category	All Persons		Under 18 years		Under 65 years		65 years and over	
	Number	%	Number	%	Number	%	Number	%
Total population	5,834	-	1,343	-	5,065	-	769	-
Covered by some type of health insurance	5,241 *(18)*	89.8 *(0.3)*	1,284 *(6)*	95.6 *(0.4)*	4,483 *(18)*	88.5 *(0.3)*	758 *(3)*	98.6 *(0.2)*
Covered by private health insurance	4,292 *(26)*	73.6 *(0.5)*	896 *(13)*	66.7 *(0.9)*	3,733 *(25)*	73.7 *(0.5)*	559 *(6)*	72.7 *(0.7)*
Employment based	3,699 *(31)*	63.4 *(0.5)*	790 *(13)*	58.8 *(1.0)*	3,310 *(29)*	65.3 *(0.6)*	389 *(7)*	50.6 *(0.9)*
Direct purchase	671 *(19)*	11.5 *(0.3)*	87 *(6)*	6.4 *(0.5)*	439 *(16)*	8.7 *(0.3)*	232 *(6)*	30.2 *(0.8)*
Covered by TRICARE	222 *(9)*	3.8 *(0.2)*	51 *(4)*	3.8 *(0.3)*	166 *(8)*	3.3 *(0.2)*	56 *(4)*	7.3 *(0.5)*
Covered by government health insurance	1,644 *(19)*	28.2 *(0.3)*	432 *(12)*	32.1 *(0.9)*	919 *(19)*	18.1 *(0.4)*	725 *(3)*	94.4 *(0.4)*
Covered by Medicaid	892 *(19)*	15.3 *(0.3)*	427 *(12)*	31.8 *(0.9)*	803 *(19)*	15.9 *(0.4)*	89 *(5)*	11.6 *(0.6)*
Also by private insurance	150 *(8)*	2.6 *(0.1)*	43 *(5)*	3.2 *(0.4)*	105 *(7)*	2.1 *(0.1)*	45 *(3)*	5.9 *(0.3)*
Covered by Medicare	839 *(8)*	14.4 *(0.1)*	9 *(2)*	0.7 *(0.2)*	114 *(7)*	2.3 *(0.1)*	725 *(3)*	94.3 *(0.4)*
Also by private insurance	562 *(7)*	9.6 *(0.1)*	1 *(Z)*	0.1 *(0.1)*	37 *(3)*	0.7 *(0.1)*	526 *(6)*	68.4 *(0.8)*
Also by Medicaid	140 *(7)*	2.4 *(0.1)*	6 *(2)*	0.4 *(0.2)*	51 *(5)*	1.0 *(0.1)*	89 *(5)*	11.6 *(0.6)*
Covered by VA Care	110 *(4)*	1.9 *(0.1)*	1 *(1)*	0.1 *(0.1)*	61 *(4)*	1.2 *(0.1)*	49 *(2)*	6.4 *(0.3)*
Not covered at any time during the year	593 *(17)*	10.2 *(0.3)*	59 *(6)*	4.4 *(0.4)*	582 *(17)*	11.5 *(0.3)*	11 *(1)*	1.4 *(0.2)*

Note: Numbers in thousands; Figures cover 2013; Margin of error appears in parenthesis; A "Z" indicates that the value either represents or rounds to zero.
Source: U.S. Census Bureau, 2013 American Community Survey, Table HI05. Health Insurance Coverage Status and Type of Coverage by State and Age for All People: 2013

Maryland

493 Aetna Health of Maryland

151 Farmington Avenue
Hartford, CT 06156
Toll-Free: 800-872-3862
Phone: 860-273-0123
www.aetna.com
For Profit Organization: Yes
Year Founded: 1987
Number of Affiliated Hospitals: 50
Number of Primary Care Physicians: 10,032
Total Enrollment: 211,156

Healthplan and Services Defined
  PLAN TYPE: HMO
  Other Type: POS
  Model Type: Network
  Plan Specialty: EPO
  Benefits Offered: Behavioral Health, Dental, Disease Management,
    Prescription, Vision
  Offers Demand Management Patient Information Service: Yes

Type of Coverage
  Commercial, Individual, Medicare

Type of Payment Plans Offered
  Capitated, FFS

Geographic Areas Served
  Statewide

Subscriber Information
  Average Monthly Fee Per Subscriber
    (Employee + Employer Contribution):
      Employee Only (Self): $67.32
      Employee & 1 Family Member: $157.54

Network Qualifications
  Pre-Admission Certification: Yes

Peer Review Type
  Utilization Review: Yes

Publishes and Distributes Report Card: Yes

Accreditation Certification
  NCQA

Key Personnel
  Chairman/CEO/President.....................Mark T Bertolini
  EVP/General Counsel ....William J Casazza
  EVP/CFO ....Shawn M Guertin

Specialty Managed Care Partners
  Enters into Contracts with Regional Business Coalitions: Yes

494 American Postal Workers Union (APWU) Health Plan

799 Cromwell Park Drive
Suite K-Z
Glen Burnie, MD 21061
Toll-Free: 800-222-2798
www.apwuhp.com
Subsidiary of: American Postal Workers Union / AFL-CIO
Year Founded: 1960
Number of Affiliated Hospitals: 6,000
Number of Primary Care Physicians: 600,000
Total Enrollment: 141,000

Healthplan and Services Defined
  PLAN TYPE: HMO/PPO
  Benefits Offered: Disease Management, Wellness
  Offers Demand Management Patient Information Service: Yes
  DMPI Services Offered: 24 Hour Nurse Advisory Line

Type of Payment Plans Offered
  FFS

Geographic Areas Served
  Nationwide - APWU/The American Postal Workers Union Health
  Plan is health insurance for federal employees and retirees

Subscriber Information
  Average Monthly Fee Per Subscriber
    (Employee + Employer Contribution):
      Employee Only (Self): $36.80-177.20 varies
      Employee & 2 Family Members: $82.80-398.66 varies
  Average Annual Deductible Per Subscriber:
    Employee Only (Self): $250
  Average Subscriber Co-Payment:
    Primary Care Physician: 15%
    Prescription Drugs: 25%
    Hospital ER: 15% - 30%
    Home Health Care Max. Days/Visits Covered: 10 - 30%

Key Personnel
  Director.............................William J. Kaczor, Jr.

495 Amerigroup Maryland

7550 Teague Road
Suite 500
Hanover, MD 21076
Toll-Free: 800-977-7388
Phone: 410-859-5800
www.realsolutions.com
For Profit Organization: Yes
Year Founded: 1999
Total Enrollment: 1,900,000

Healthplan and Services Defined
  PLAN TYPE: HMO

Type of Coverage
  Medicare, Medicaid, SCHIP, SSI

Key Personnel
  Chief Financial Officer.........................Scott Anglin
  SVP, Chief Information Of....................Timothy Skeen
  Chief Compliance Officer ....Georgia Dodds Foley
  EVP/Huma Resources ....Linda Whitley
  Chief Operating Officer......................Richard Zoretic

496 Avesis: Maryland

10324 S Dolfiled Road
Owings Mills, MD 21117
Toll-Free: 800-643-1132
www.avesis.com
Year Founded: 1978
Number of Primary Care Physicians: 18,000
Total Enrollment: 2,000,000

Healthplan and Services Defined
  PLAN TYPE: PPO
  Other Type: Vision, Dental
  Model Type: Network
  Plan Specialty: Dental, Vision, Hearing
  Benefits Offered: Dental, Vision

Type of Coverage
  Commercial

Type of Payment Plans Offered
  POS, Capitated, Combination FFS & DFFS

Geographic Areas Served
  Nationwide and Puerto Rico

Publishes and Distributes Report Card: Yes

Accreditation Certification
  AAAHC
  TJC Accreditation

497   Block Vision

939 Elkridge Landing Road
Suite 200
Linthicum, MD 21090
Toll-Free: 800-243-1401
Phone: 410-752-0121
Fax: 410-752-8969
www.blockvision.com
Secondary Address: 6737 West Washington Street, Suite 2202, P.O.
    Box 44077, Milwaukee, WI 53213-7077, 800-883-5747
Subsidiary of: Block Vision Holdings Corporation
For Profit Organization: Yes
Year Founded: 1990
Number of Primary Care Physicians: 18,000
Total Enrollment: 3,000,000

Healthplan and Services Defined
PLAN TYPE: Vision
Plan Specialty: Vision
Benefits Offered: Vision

Type of Coverage
Commercial, Medicare, Medicaid

Key Personnel
President/CEO . . . . Andrew Alcorn
Sr VP/COO/CFO . . . . Ernest A Viscuso
Sr VP/General Counsel . . . . Audrey M Weinstein
SVP, Business Development. . . . . Stephanie Lucas
    slucas@blockvision.com
Sr VP/Clinical Director . . . . Howard Levin, OD
VP, Group Sales . . . . Steven Fleischer
    866-246-9589
    sfleischer@blockvision.com
VP, Sales . . . . Mark Wallner
    800-883-5747
    mwallner@visionplans.com

498   Catalyst Health Solutions Inc

800 King Farm Boulevard
Rockville, MD 20850
Toll-Free: 800-323-6640
Phone: 301-548-2900
Fax: 301-548-2991
rxcsinfo@catalystrx.com
www.catalysthealthsolutions.com
For Profit Organization: Yes
Year Founded: 1986
Owned by an Integrated Delivery Network (IDN): Yes
Number of Primary Care Physicians: 54,000
Total Enrollment: 3,000,000

Healthplan and Services Defined
PLAN TYPE: HMO
Model Type: Group
Plan Specialty: PBM
Benefits Offered: Prescription, Worker's Compensation

Type of Coverage
Commercial, Medicare, Supplemental Medicare, Catastrophic
Catastrophic Illness Benefit: Varies per case

Type of Payment Plans Offered
POS

Geographic Areas Served
Nationwide with concentration in Southeast

Network Qualifications
Pre-Admission Certification: Yes

Peer Review Type
Utilization Review: Yes
Second Surgical Opinion: No
Case Management: No

Publishes and Distributes Report Card: Yes

Accreditation Certification
TJC Accreditation, Utilization Review, State Licensure

Key Personnel
Chief Executive Officer . . . . David T Blair
President/COO . . . . Richard Bates
Treasurer/CFO. . . . . Hai Tran
General Counsel . . . . Bruce Metge
Chief Financial Officer . . . . Hai Tran
    301-548-2900
    htran@chsi.com

Specialty Managed Care Partners
Catalyst Rx
Enters into Contracts with Regional Business Coalitions: Yes

499   Cigna Health-Spring

3601 O'Donnell Street
Baltimore, MD 21224
Toll-Free: 800-668-3813
www.cignahealthspring.com
Subsidiary of: Health Springs
Year Founded: 1996
Number of Primary Care Physicians: 30,000
Total Enrollment: 360,000

Healthplan and Services Defined
PLAN TYPE: Medicare

Type of Coverage
Medicare, Supplemental Medicare

Geographic Areas Served
Delaware, Maryland, Pennslyvania, Texas, Washington DC, New
Jersey

Key Personnel
Media Contact. . . . . Lisa Trapani
    410-245-0094
    ltrapani@rosecomm.com
SVP, Chief Compliance Ofc . . . . Ena Authur Pierce

500   CIGNA HealthCare of the Mid-Atlantic

9700 Patuxent Woods Drive
Columbia, MD 20146
Toll-Free: 866-438-2446
Phone: 410-837-4005
www.cigna.com
Secondary Address: Great-West Healthcare, now part of CIGNA, 6701
    Democracy Blvd, Suite 401, Bethesda, MD 20817, 301-841-0950
For Profit Organization: Yes
Year Founded: 1984
Physician Owned Organization: No
Number of Affiliated Hospitals: 54
Number of Primary Care Physicians: 2,032
Number of Referral/Specialty Physicians: 5,028
Total Enrollment: 109,186

Healthplan and Services Defined
PLAN TYPE: HMO/PPO
Model Type: IPA
Benefits Offered: Disease Management, Prescription, Transplant,
    Wellness
Offers Demand Management Patient Information Service: Yes

Type of Coverage
Commercial

Type of Payment Plans Offered
Combination FFS & DFFS

Geographic Areas Served
District of Columbia, Maryland, Virginia

Network Qualifications
Pre-Admission Certification: Yes

Peer Review Type
Utilization Review: Yes
Second Surgical Opinion: Yes
Case Management: Yes

Publishes and Distributes Report Card: Yes

Accreditation Certification
NCQA

Key Personnel
President.....................................Mike Triplett
Government Affairs ....Katie Wade
Medical Director ....Nicholas Gettas, MD
Sales.......................................Ron Vance Jr
Provider Relations ....Yvonne Van Lowe

Specialty Managed Care Partners
CIGNA Dental, CIGNA Behavioral Health
Enters into Contracts with Regional Business Coalitions: No

501 CoreSource: Maryland

4940 Campbell Blvd
Suite 200
Baltimore, MD 21236
Toll-Free: 800-624-7130
Phone: 410-931-5060
inquiries@coresource.com
www.coresource.com
Subsidiary of: Trustmark
Year Founded: 1980
Total Enrollment: 1,100,000

Healthplan and Services Defined
PLAN TYPE: Multiple
Other Type: TPA
Model Type: Network
Plan Specialty: Claims Administration, TPA
Benefits Offered: Behavioral Health, Home Care, Prescription,
Transplant

Type of Coverage
Commercial

Geographic Areas Served
Nationwide

Accreditation Certification
Utilization Review, Pre-Admission Certification

Key Personnel
President ....Nancy Eckrich
Chief Operating Officer ....Lloyd Sarrel
VP, Product Management ....Rob Corrigan
VP/CFO ....Clare Smith
VP, Product Marketing.........................Steve Horvath

502 Coventry Health Care: Corporate Headquarters

6720 - B Rockledge Drive
Suite 700
Bethesda, MD 20817
Phone: 301-581-0600
www.coventryhealthcare.com
For Profit Organization: Yes
Year Founded: 1987
Total Enrollment: 5,000,000

Healthplan and Services Defined
PLAN TYPE: HMO/PPO
Other Type: POS, ASO
Model Type: IPA
Plan Specialty: Behavioral Health, Dental, Disease Management,
Worker's Compensation
Benefits Offered: Behavioral Health, Dental, Disease Management,
Prescription, Wellness, Worker's Compensation

Type of Coverage
Commercial, Individual, Medicare, Supplemental Medicare, Medicaid

Type of Payment Plans Offered
POS, DFFS, Capitated, FFS, Combination FFS & DFFS

Geographic Areas Served
Nationwide

Subscriber Information
Average Annual Deductible Per Subscriber:
Employee Only (Self): Varies
Employee & 1 Family Member: Varies
Employee & 2 Family Members: Varies
Medicare: Varies
Average Subscriber Co-Payment:
Primary Care Physician: $10.00
Non-Network Physician: Varies
Prescription Drugs: $5.00
Hospital ER: Varies
Home Health Care: Varies
Nursing Home: Varies
Nursing Home Max. Days/Visits Covered: Varies

Network Qualifications
Pre-Admission Certification: Yes

Peer Review Type
Utilization Review: Yes
Second Surgical Opinion: Yes
Case Management: Yes

Publishes and Distributes Report Card: No

Accreditation Certification
NCQA
TJC Accreditation, Utilization Review, Pre-Admission Certification,
State Licensure, Quality Assurance Program

Specialty Managed Care Partners
Enters into Contracts with Regional Business Coalitions: No

503 Delta Dental of the Mid-Atlantic

One Delta Drive
Mechanicsburg, PA 17055-6999
Toll-Free: 800-932-0783
Fax: 717-766-8719
www.deltadentalins.com
Non-Profit Organization: Yes
Total Enrollment: 54,000,000

Healthplan and Services Defined
PLAN TYPE: Dental
Other Type: Dental PPO

Type of Coverage
Commercial

Geographic Areas Served
Statewide

Key Personnel
President/CEO..............................Gary D Radine
VP, Public & Govt Affairs ....Jeff Album
415-972-8418
Dir/Media & Public Affair ....Elizabeth Risberg
415-972-8423

504 Denta-Chek of Maryland

10400 Little Patuxet Parkway
Suite 260
Columbia, MD 21044
Toll-Free: 888-478-8833
Phone: 410-997-3300
Fax: 410-997-3796
info@dentachek.com
www.dentachek.com

Secondary Address: One Delta Drive, Mechanicsburg, PA 17055, 800-422-4234

Non-Profit Organization: Yes

Year Founded: 1981

Number of Primary Care Physicians: 300

Number of Referral/Specialty Physicians: 200

Total Enrollment: 10,000

Healthplan and Services Defined
PLAN TYPE: Multiple
Model Type: IPA
Plan Specialty: Dental
Benefits Offered: Dental

Type of Coverage
Catastrophic Illness Benefit: None

Type of Payment Plans Offered
POS, Combination FFS & DFFS

Geographic Areas Served
Statewide

Subscriber Information
Average Monthly Fee Per Subscriber
(Employee + Employer Contribution):
Employee Only (Self): $16.00
Employee & 1 Family Member: $22.00
Employee & 2 Family Members: $28.00
Medicare: $0
Average Annual Deductible Per Subscriber:
Employee Only (Self): $0
Employee & 1 Family Member: $0
Employee & 2 Family Members: $0
Medicare: $0
Average Subscriber Co-Payment:
Primary Care Physician: $5.00
Non-Network Physician: $0
Prescription Drugs: $0
Hospital ER: $0
Home Health Care: $0
Nursing Home: $0

Network Qualifications
Pre-Admission Certification: Yes

Peer Review Type
Utilization Review: Yes
Second Surgical Opinion: Yes
Case Management: Yes

Publishes and Distributes Report Card: No

Accreditation Certification
State Licensure, Quality Assurance Program

Specialty Managed Care Partners
Enters into Contracts with Regional Business Coalitions: No

505 Dental Benefit Providers

6220 Old Dobbin Lane
Columbia, MD 21045
Toll-Free: 800-638-3895
www.dbp.com
Secondary Address: 425 Market Street, 12th Floor, Mail Route CA035-1200, San Francisco, CA 94105, 415-778-3800
For Profit Organization: Yes
Year Founded: 1984
Number of Primary Care Physicians: 125,000
Total Enrollment: 6,600,000

Healthplan and Services Defined
PLAN TYPE: Dental
Model Type: IPA
Plan Specialty: ASO, Dental, EPO, DHMO, PPO, CSO, Preventive, Claims Repricing and Network Access
Benefits Offered: Dental

Type of Coverage
Indemnity, Medicare, Medicaid

Type of Payment Plans Offered
POS, DFFS, Capitated, FFS

Geographic Areas Served
48 states including District of Columbia, Puerto Rico and Virgin Islands

Accreditation Certification
NCQA

Key Personnel
CEO . . . . .Dawn Owens
President & COO . . . . .Ralph Foxman
COO . . . . .Kevin Ruth
VP . . . . .Ben Davis
CEO . . . . .David Hall
COO . . . . .Karen Schievelbein

506 eHealthInsurance Services Inc.

11919 Foundation Place
Gold River, CA 95670
Toll-Free: 800-644-3491
webmaster@healthinsurance.com
www.e.healthinsurance.com
Year Founded: 1997

Healthplan and Services Defined
PLAN TYPE: HMO/PPO
Benefits Offered: Dental, Life, STD

Type of Coverage
Commercial, Individual, Medicare

Geographic Areas Served
All 50 states in the USA and District of Columbia

Key Personnel
Chairman & CEO . . . . .Gary L. Lauer
EVP/Business & Corp. Dev. . . . . .Bruce Telkamp
EVP/Chief Technology .Dr. Sheldon X. Wang
SVP & CFO . . . . .Stuart M. Huizinga
Pres. of eHealth Gov. Sys .Samuel C. Gibbs
SVP of Sales & Operations .Robert S. Hurley
Director Public Relations . . . . .Nate Purpura
650-210-3115

507 Graphic Arts Benefit Corporation

64 11 Ivy Lane
Suite 700
Greenbelt, MD 20770-1411
Phone: 301-474-7950
Fax: 301-474-3197
gtoner@gabchealth.org
www.gabchealth.org
Non-Profit Organization: Yes
Total Enrollment: 8,000

Healthplan and Services Defined
PLAN TYPE: HMO/PPO
Benefits Offered: Dental, Prescription, Vision, AD&D, Life, STD

Type of Coverage
Commercial, Individual

Geographic Areas Served
Maryland, Virginia, District of Columbia

Key Personnel
President . . . . .Jerry McGeehan
Principal . . . . .Gerard J. McGeehan

508 Humana Health Insurance of Maryland

1 International Blvd
Suite 400
Mahwah, NJ 07495
Toll-Free: 800-967-2370
Phone: 201-512-8818
www.humana.com
For Profit Organization: Yes

Healthplan and Services Defined
PLAN TYPE: HMO/PPO

Type of Coverage
Commercial, Individual

Accreditation Certification
URAC, NCQA, CORE

509 Kaiser Permanente Health Plan of the Mid-Atlantic States

2101 E Jefferson Street
Rockville, MD 20852
Toll-Free: 888-777-5536
www.kaiserpermanente.org
Non-Profit Organization: Yes
Year Founded: 1980
Number of Affiliated Hospitals: 35
Number of Primary Care Physicians: 15,129
Total Enrollment: 471,360
State Enrollment: 471,360

Healthplan and Services Defined
PLAN TYPE: HMO
Model Type: Group
Benefits Offered: Disease Management, Prescription, Wellness
Offers Demand Management Patient Information Service: Yes

Type of Payment Plans Offered
POS, DFFS, FFS, Combination FFS & DFFS

Geographic Areas Served
Metro Baltimore & Metro Washington

Subscriber Information
Average Annual Deductible Per Subscriber:
Employee Only (Self): $0
Employee & 1 Family Member: $0
Employee & 2 Family Members: $0
Medicare: $0

Peer Review Type
Case Management: Yes

Publishes and Distributes Report Card: Yes

Accreditation Certification
NCQA
Medicare Approved, Quality Assurance Program

Key Personnel
Pres/CEO, Mid-Atlantic . . . . Robert M Pearl, MD
Media Contact . . . . Beverlie Brinson
301-816-6264
beverlie.brinson@kp.org

Specialty Managed Care Partners
Enters into Contracts with Regional Business Coalitions: Yes

510 Magellan Health Services: Corporate Headquarters

6950 Columbia Gateway Drive
Columbia, MD 21046
Toll-Free: 800-410-8312
Phone: 410-953-1000
Fax: 410-953-5200
www.magellanhealth.com

Non-Profit Organization: Yes
Year Founded: 1998
Owned by an Integrated Delivery Network (IDN): Yes
Number of Affiliated Hospitals: 5,000
Number of Primary Care Physicians: 67,000
Number of Referral/Specialty Physicians: 45,000
Total Enrollment: 36,500,000

Healthplan and Services Defined
PLAN TYPE: Multiple
Model Type: Network
Plan Specialty: Behavioral Health
Benefits Offered: Behavioral Health, Psychiatric
Offers Demand Management Patient Information Service: Yes
DMPI Services Offered: Behavioral Health Managment, EAP

Type of Coverage
Behavioral Health

Geographic Areas Served
National

Peer Review Type
Utilization Review: Yes
Case Management: Yes

Accreditation Certification
AAAHC, URAC, NCQA

Key Personnel
Chairman & CEO . . . . Rene Lerer, MD
Pres, Health Services . . . . Karen S Rohan
Chief Financial Officer . . . . Jonathan N Rubin
CEO, Natl Imaging Assoc . . . . Tina Blasi
Chief Oper & Finance Offc . . . . Edward J Christie
General Counsel . . . . Daniel N Gregoire
SVP, Comm Behav Health . . . . Suzanne Kunis
President, ICORE . . . . Alan M Lotvin, MD
SVP, Marketing & Comm . . . . David W Carter
SVP, Public Sector. . . . . Anne M McCabe
Chief Medical Officer . . . . Anthony M Kotin, MD
Chief Human Res Officer . . . . Caskie Lewis-Clapper
Chief Information Offc. . . . . Gary D Anderson
Pres, Medicaid Adminstr . . . . Tim Nolan
Chief Corp Dev Officer. . . . . Prakash R Patel, MD

511 Mid Atlantic Medical Services: Corporate Office

4 Taft Court
Rockville, MD 20850
Toll-Free: 800-884-5188
Phone: 301-762-8205
Fax: 301-545-5380
masales99@uhc.com
www.mamsiunitedhealthcare.com
Secondary Address: 6095 Marshalee Drive South, Suite 200, Baltimore, MD 21075
Subsidiary of: United HealthGroup
For Profit Organization: Yes
Year Founded: 1979
Number of Affiliated Hospitals: 342
Number of Primary Care Physicians: 3,276
Total Enrollment: 180,000

Healthplan and Services Defined
PLAN TYPE: HMO/PPO
Other Type: POS
Model Type: IPA
Benefits Offered: Dental, Disease Management, Home Care, Prescription, Vision, Wellness, Life, STD

Type of Coverage
Catastrophic Illness Benefit: Varies per case

Type of Payment Plans Offered
POS, FFS, Combination FFS & DFFS

Geographic Areas Served
Delaware, Washington DC, Maryland and Virginia

Subscriber Information
Average Monthly Fee Per Subscriber
(Employee + Employer Contribution):
Employee Only (Self): $129.03
Employee & 1 Family Member: $245.15
Employee & 2 Family Members: $390.96
Average Annual Deductible Per Subscriber:
Employee Only (Self): $0
Employee & 1 Family Member: $0
Employee & 2 Family Members: $0
Medicare: $0
Average Subscriber Co-Payment:
Primary Care Physician: $10.00
Prescription Drugs: $10.00/20.00
Hospital ER: $50.00
Home Health Care Max. Days/Visits Covered: Varies
Nursing Home Max. Days/Visits Covered: 60 days

Network Qualifications
Pre-Admission Certification: Yes

Peer Review Type
Utilization Review: Yes
Second Surgical Opinion: Yes
Case Management: Yes

Publishes and Distributes Report Card: Yes

Accreditation Certification
NCQA
TJC Accreditation, Medicare Approved, Utilization Review,
Pre-Admission Certification, State Licensure, Quality Assurance
Program

Key Personnel
SVP, Controller . . . . .Christopher Mackail
Senior Vice President . . . . .Debbie Hulen
Vice President. . . . . .Wayne Monroe

Specialty Managed Care Partners
Enters into Contracts with Regional Business Coalitions: Yes

---

512   OneNet PPO
800 King Farm Boulevard
6th Floor
Rockville, MD
Toll-Free: 800-884-5188
Fax: 866-563-6609
www.onenetppo.com
Mailing Address: PO Box 934, Frederick, MA 21705
Subsidiary of: United Health Care Insurance Co.
For Profit Organization: Yes
Year Founded: 1988
Number of Affiliated Hospitals: 26
Number of Primary Care Physicians: 950
Total Enrollment: 970,000

Healthplan and Services Defined
PLAN TYPE: PPO
Model Type: Network
Benefits Offered: Prescription

Type of Payment Plans Offered
POS

Geographic Areas Served
Southwestern Pennsylvania, Delaware, Washington DC, Maryland,
West Virginia, Virginia, Central North Carolina

Subscriber Information
Average Monthly Fee Per Subscriber
(Employee + Employer Contribution):
Employee Only (Self): $2.00
Average Annual Deductible Per Subscriber:
Employee Only (Self): $100.00

Employee & 1 Family Member: $200.00
Employee & 2 Family Members: $200.00
Average Subscriber Co-Payment:
Primary Care Physician: Varies
Non-Network Physician: Varies

Publishes and Distributes Report Card: Yes

Key Personnel
President/CEO . . . . .Jerry Alonge
Marketing . . . . .Mike Ebert

---

513   OneNet PPO
800 King Farm Boulevard
6th Floor
Rockville, MD 20850
Toll-Free: 800-884-5188
Fax: 866-563-6609
www.onenetppo.com
Mailing Address: P.O. Box 934, Frederick, MD 21705
For Profit Organization: Yes
Year Founded: 1988
Number of Affiliated Hospitals: 350
Number of Primary Care Physicians: 57,000
Total Enrollment: 960,000

Healthplan and Services Defined
PLAN TYPE: PPO
Model Type: IPA
Plan Specialty: Behavioral Health, Worker's Compensation
Benefits Offered: Behavioral Health, Dental, Prescription, Vision,
Worker's Compensation, Life, STD, Accident, Disability
Offers Demand Management Patient Information Service: Yes

Type of Payment Plans Offered
Capitated

Geographic Areas Served
Delaware, Maryland, North Carolina, Virginia, Pennsylvania, West
Virginia, & Washington, DC

Subscriber Information
Average Monthly Fee Per Subscriber
(Employee + Employer Contribution):
Employee Only (Self): $4.25
Average Subscriber Co-Payment:
Primary Care Physician: $15.00

Network Qualifications
Minimum Years of Practice: 2
Pre-Admission Certification: Yes

Peer Review Type
Utilization Review: Yes
Second Surgical Opinion: Yes
Case Management: Yes

Publishes and Distributes Report Card: Yes

Accreditation Certification
Quality Assurance Program

Specialty Managed Care Partners
Enters into Contracts with Regional Business Coalitions: Yes

---

514   Optimum Choice
4 Taft Court
Rockville, MD 20850
Toll-Free: 800-447-6267
Phone: 301-762-8205
Fax: 301-838-5682
masales99@uhc.com
www.mamsiunitedhealthcare.com
Subsidiary of: United Healthcare / United Health Group
Acquired by: UnitedHealthcare
For Profit Organization: Yes
Year Founded: 1988

Number of Affiliated Hospitals: 340
Number of Primary Care Physicians: 3,276
Total Enrollment: 151,000

Healthplan and Services Defined
PLAN TYPE: HMO
Model Type: IPA
Benefits Offered: Prescription

Type of Coverage
Catastrophic Illness Benefit: Varies per case

Type of Payment Plans Offered
POS, FFS, Combination FFS & DFFS

Geographic Areas Served
Maryland, Virginia, Delaware, West Virginia, North Carolina

Subscriber Information
Average Subscriber Co-Payment:
Primary Care Physician: $10.00
Prescription Drugs: $10.00/20.00

Network Qualifications
Pre-Admission Certification: Yes

Peer Review Type
Utilization Review: Yes
Second Surgical Opinion: Yes
Case Management: Yes

Publishes and Distributes Report Card: Yes

Accreditation Certification
NCQA
TJC Accreditation, Medicare Approved, Utilization Review, Pre-Admission Certification, State Licensure, Quality Assurance Program

Key Personnel
President/CEO . . . . Thomas P Barbera
SEVP/CFO . . . . Robert E Foss
EVP/CIO . . . . R Larry Mauzy

Specialty Managed Care Partners
Enters into Contracts with Regional Business Coalitions: No

515   Priority Partners Health Plans

6704 Curtis Court
Glen Burnie, MD 21060-9949
Toll-Free: 800-654-9728
ppcustomerservice@jhhc.com
www.hopkinsmedicine.org/priority_partners
Subsidiary of: John Hopkins HealthCare LLC/Maryland Community Health System
Non-Profit Organization: Yes
Year Founded: 1996
Total Enrollment: 185,000
State Enrollment: 185,000

Healthplan and Services Defined
PLAN TYPE: HMO

Type of Coverage
Medicaid

Type of Payment Plans Offered
Capitated, FFS

Peer Review Type
Second Surgical Opinion: Yes

Publishes and Distributes Report Card: Yes

Accreditation Certification
TJC, NCQA, JACHO, HMO

Key Personnel
COO . . . . Jeff Joy
President. . . . . Patricia M.C. Brown
Medical Director . . . . Chester Schmidt, MD
Chief Medical Officer . . . . Chet Schmidt
Chief Financial Officer. . . . . Mike Larson

Communications Dept . . . . Deb Chase
dchase@jhhc.com

516   Spectera

6220 Old Dobbin Lane
Liberty 6, Suite 200
Columbia, MD 21045
Toll-Free: 800-638-3120
www.spectera.com
Mailing Address: PO Box 30978, Salt Lake City, UT 84130
Subsidiary of: United Health Group
For Profit Organization: Yes
Year Founded: 1964
Number of Primary Care Physicians: 24,000
Total Enrollment: 17,000,000

Healthplan and Services Defined
PLAN TYPE: Multiple
Model Type: Network
Plan Specialty: Vision
Benefits Offered: Disease Management, Vision

Type of Coverage
Commercial, Individual

Type of Payment Plans Offered
POS, DFFS, Capitated

Geographic Areas Served
Continental United States

Subscriber Information
Average Monthly Fee Per Subscriber
(Employee + Employer Contribution):
Employee Only (Self): Varies
Average Annual Deductible Per Subscriber:
Employee & 2 Family Members: Varies
Average Subscriber Co-Payment:
Primary Care Physician: Varies

Network Qualifications
Pre-Admission Certification: Yes

Publishes and Distributes Report Card: Yes

Key Personnel
CEO . . . . Paul Gaulstrand
COO . . . . Tom Rekart
CFO . . . . Kyle Stern
General Counsel . . . . Jennifer Lewis
SVP, Marketing. . . . . Susan E Cox
800-638-3895
susan_cox@uhc.com
Chief Sales Officer. . . . . Laurida Mackenzie
Media Contact . . . . Susan Cox
800-638-3895
susan_cox@uhc.com

Specialty Managed Care Partners
United Heath Group
Enters into Contracts with Regional Business Coalitions: No

517   United Concordia: Maryland

Longview Executive Park
309 International Circle, Suite 130
Hunt Valley, MD 21030
Toll-Free: 800-272-8865
Phone: 443-866-9500
Fax: 443-886-9525
ucproducer@ucci.com
www.secure.ucci.com
For Profit Organization: Yes
Year Founded: 1971
Number of Primary Care Physicians: 111,000
Total Enrollment: 8,000,000

Healthplan and Services Defined
  PLAN TYPE: Dental
  Plan Specialty: Dental
  Benefits Offered: Dental

Type of Coverage
  Commercial, Individual

Geographic Areas Served
  Military personnel and their families, nationwide

---

518   UnitedHealthCare of the Mid-Atlantic
6300 Security Blvd
Baltimore, MD 21207-5102
Toll-Free: 800-307-7820
Phone: 410-379-3402
Fax: 410-379-3446
midatlantic_pr_team@uhc.com
www.uhc.com
Subsidiary of: UnitedHealth Group
Non-Profit Organization: Yes
Year Founded: 1976
Number of Affiliated Hospitals: 58
Number of Primary Care Physicians: 2,559
Number of Referral/Specialty Physicians: 8,300
Total Enrollment: 75,000,000
State Enrollment: 176,000

Healthplan and Services Defined
  PLAN TYPE: HMO/PPO
  Model Type: Network
  Benefits Offered: Disease Management, Prescription, Wellness
  Offers Demand Management Patient Information Service: Yes

Geographic Areas Served
  Baltimore Metro Area, Washington DC Metro Area, Eastern Shore, Southern Maryland, Western Maryland

Subscriber Information
  Average Monthly Fee Per Subscriber
    (Employee + Employer Contribution):
      Employee Only (Self): $104.00-135.00
      Employee & 1 Family Member: $143.00-184.00
      Employee & 2 Family Members: $331.00-440.00
      Medicare: $112.00-156.00
  Average Annual Deductible Per Subscriber:
      Employee Only (Self): $100.00-250.00
      Employee & 1 Family Member: $500.00-1500.00
      Employee & 2 Family Members: $200.00-500.00
      Medicare: $0
  Average Subscriber Co-Payment:
      Primary Care Physician: $5.00/10.00
      Non-Network Physician: Deductible
      Prescription Drugs: $5.00/10.00
      Hospital ER: $25.00/50.00
      Home Health Care: $5.00/10.00

Network Qualifications
  Pre-Admission Certification: Yes

Peer Review Type
  Utilization Review: Yes
  Second Surgical Opinion: Yes
  Case Management: Yes

Publishes and Distributes Report Card: Yes

Accreditation Certification
  TJC Accreditation, Medicare Approved, Utilization Review, Pre-Admission Certification, State Licensure, Quality Assurance Program

Key Personnel
  President and CEO...........................Richard Zoretic
  CFO.......................................John Dell Erba
  Network Contracting.......................Marie Carpenter
  Marketing............................David Yalowitz, MD

Member Services.......................Laverne Smith-boykin
Provider Services...........................Theresa Farasce
Media Contact ....Debora Spano
  401-732-7374
  debora_m_spano@uhc.com

Specialty Managed Care Partners
  Enters into Contracts with Regional Business Coalitions: Yes

Health Insurance Coverage Status and Type of Coverage by Age

Category	All Persons		Under 18 years		Under 65 years		65 years and over	
	Number	%	Number	%	Number	%	Number	%
Total population	6,614	-	1,389	-	5,662	-	952	-
Covered by some type of health insurance	6,367 (11)	96.3 (0.2)	1,368 (3)	98.5 (0.2)	5,419 (11)	95.7 (0.2)	948 (2)	99.6 (0.1)
Covered by private health insurance	4,926 (28)	74.5 (0.4)	972 (12)	70.0 (0.9)	4,293 (25)	75.8 (0.4)	633 (7)	66.6 (0.7)
Employment based	4,275 (30)	64.6 (0.5)	901 (13)	64.8 (1.0)	3,876 (28)	68.5 (0.5)	400 (8)	42.0 (0.8)
Direct purchase	815 (16)	12.3 (0.2)	80 (6)	5.8 (0.4)	514 (15)	9.1 (0.3)	301 (7)	31.6 (0.7)
Covered by TRICARE	72 (5)	1.1 (0.1)	10 (2)	0.7 (0.1)	43 (4)	0.8 (0.1)	30 (3)	3.1 (0.3)
Covered by government health insurance	2,246 (25)	34.0 (0.4)	462 (13)	33.2 (0.9)	1,339 (25)	23.7 (0.4)	906 (3)	95.2 (0.3)
Covered by Medicaid	1,432 (25)	21.7 (0.4)	458 (13)	33.0 (0.9)	1,261 (25)	22.3 (0.4)	171 (6)	18.0 (0.7)
Also by private insurance	236 (9)	3.6 (0.1)	64 (5)	4.6 (0.4)	170 (9)	3.0 (0.2)	66 (4)	6.9 (0.4)
Covered by Medicare	1,049 (8)	15.9 (0.1)	6 (2)	0.5 (0.1)	144 (7)	2.5 (0.1)	905 (3)	95.1 (0.3)
Also by private insurance	636 (9)	9.6 (0.1)	2 (1)	0.2 (0.1)	45 (4)	0.8 (0.1)	591 (8)	62.1 (0.8)
Also by Medicaid	261 (8)	3.9 (0.1)	4 (1)	0.3 (0.1)	89 (5)	1.6 (0.1)	171 (6)	18.0 (0.7)
Covered by VA Care	96 (4)	1.4 (0.1)	1 (1)	0.1 (0.1)	35 (3)	0.6 (0.1)	60 (3)	6.3 (0.3)
Not covered at any time during the year	247 (10)	3.7 (0.2)	21 (3)	1.5 (0.2)	243 (10)	4.3 (0.2)	4 (1)	0.4 (0.1)

Note: Numbers in thousands; Figures cover 2013; Margin of error appears in parenthesis; A "Z" indicates that the value either represents or rounds to zero.
Source: U.S. Census Bureau, 2013 American Community Survey, Table HI05. Health Insurance Coverage Status and Type of Coverage by State and Age for All People: 2013

Massachusetts

519 Aetna Health of Massachusetts
151 Farmington Avenue
Hartford, CT 06156
Toll-Free: 800-872-3862
Phone: 860-273-0123
www.aetna.com
Partnered with: eHealthInsurance Services Inc.
For Profit Organization: Yes
Year Founded: 1987
Number of Affiliated Hospitals: 58
Number of Primary Care Physicians: 7,500
Total Enrollment: 11,121
State Enrollment: 11,121

Healthplan and Services Defined
PLAN TYPE: HMO
Other Type: POS
Model Type: IPA
Plan Specialty: Dental
Benefits Offered: Behavioral Health, Dental, Disease Management, Prescription, Vision

Type of Coverage
Commercial, Individual
Catastrophic Illness Benefit: Covered

Geographic Areas Served
Statewide

Subscriber Information
Average Monthly Fee Per Subscriber
(Employee + Employer Contribution):
Employee Only (Self): $73.42
Employee & 1 Family Member: $168.89
Medicare: Zero premium

Peer Review Type
Second Surgical Opinion: Yes
Case Management: Yes

Publishes and Distributes Report Card: Yes

Accreditation Certification
NCQA

Key Personnel
Chairman/CEO/President. .Mark T Bertolini
EVP/General Counsel . . . . .William J Casazza
EVP/CFO . . . . .Shawn M Guertin

520 Assurant Employee Benefits: Massachusetts
33 Boston Post Road West
#590
Marlborough, MA 01752-1867
Phone: 508-870-2200
Fax: 508-382-3750
benefits@assurant.com
www.assurantemployeebenefits.com
Subsidiary of: Assurant, Inc
For Profit Organization: Yes
Number of Primary Care Physicians: 112,000
Total Enrollment: 47,000

Healthplan and Services Defined
PLAN TYPE: Multiple
Plan Specialty: Dental, Vision, Long & Short-Term Disability
Benefits Offered: Dental, Vision, Wellness, AD&D, Life, LTD, STD

Type of Coverage
Commercial, Indemnity, Individual Dental Plans

Geographic Areas Served
Statewide

Subscriber Information
Average Monthly Fee Per Subscriber
(Employee + Employer Contribution):
Employee Only (Self): Varies by plan

Key Personnel
President . . . . .Michael Germain
Regional Sales Manager. . . . . .David Fraser
PR Specialist. . . . . .Megan Hutchison
816-556-7815
megan.hutchison@assurant.com

521 Avesis: Massachusetts
790 Turnpike Street
Suite 202
North Andover, MA 01845
Toll-Free: 800-522-4834
www.avesis.com
Year Founded: 1978
Number of Primary Care Physicians: 18,000
Total Enrollment: 2,000,000

Healthplan and Services Defined
PLAN TYPE: PPO
Other Type: Vision, Dental
Model Type: Network
Plan Specialty: Dental, Vision, Hearing
Benefits Offered: Dental, Vision

Type of Coverage
Commercial

Type of Payment Plans Offered
POS, Capitated, Combination FFS & DFFS

Geographic Areas Served
Nationwide and Puerto Rico

Publishes and Distributes Report Card: Yes

Accreditation Certification
AAAHC
TJC Accreditation

522 Blue Cross & Blue Shield of Massachusetts
Landmark Center
401 Park Drive
Boston, MA 02215-3326
Toll-Free: 800-262-2583
www.bcbsma.com
Non-Profit Organization: Yes
Year Founded: 1937
Number of Affiliated Hospitals: 77
Number of Primary Care Physicians: 20,266
Total Enrollment: 3,000,000
State Enrollment: 3,000,000

Healthplan and Services Defined
PLAN TYPE: HMO
Model Type: Network
Plan Specialty: Dental, Group Medical
Benefits Offered: Behavioral Health, Chiropractic, Complementary Medicine, Dental, Disease Management, Home Care, Inpatient SNF, Long-Term Care, Physical Therapy, Podiatry, Prescription, Psychiatric, Transplant, Vision, Wellness, AD&D, Life, LTD, STD
Offers Demand Management Patient Information Service: Yes
DMPI Services Offered: 24-Hour Nurse Care Line

Type of Coverage
Group Insurance

Type of Payment Plans Offered
FFS

Geographic Areas Served
Massachusetts & Southern New Hampshire

Subscriber Information
Average Monthly Fee Per Subscriber
(Employee + Employer Contribution):
Employee Only (Self): Varies by plan
Average Annual Deductible Per Subscriber:
Employee Only (Self): $0
Employee & 1 Family Member: $0
Employee & 2 Family Members: $0
Average Subscriber Co-Payment:
Primary Care Physician: $10.00
Non-Network Physician: 20%
Prescription Drugs: $5.00/10.00
Hospital ER: $25.00
Nursing Home: Not covered

Network Qualifications
Pre-Admission Certification: Yes

Peer Review Type
Utilization Review: Yes

Accreditation Certification
NCQA
TJC Accreditation, Medicare Approved, Utilization Review,
Pre-Admission Certification, State Licensure

Key Personnel
President & CEO . . . . .Andrew Dreyfus
COO. . . . . .Bruce Bullen
EVP, CFO . . . . .Allen P Maltz
SVP/Chief Physician Exec . . . . .John Fallon, MD
SVP/General Counsel . . . . .Stephanie Lovell
Chief Strategy Officer . . . . .Sarah Iselin
SVP, Corp Communications . . . . .Jay McQuaide
SVP, Sales Division . . . . .Tim O'Brien
Chief HR Officer . . . . .Jason Robart

Specialty Managed Care Partners
Express Scripts

---

523 Boston Medical Center Healthnet Plan

, MA
Toll-Free: 888-566-0010
memberquestions@bmchp.org
www.bmchp.org
Year Founded: 1997
Number of Affiliated Hospitals: 60
Number of Primary Care Physicians: 3,000
Number of Referral/Specialty Physicians: 12,000
Total Enrollment: 240,890
State Enrollment: 240,890

Healthplan and Services Defined
PLAN TYPE: HMO
Benefits Offered: Disease Management, Prescription, Wellness

Type of Coverage
Individual

Key Personnel
Interim President. . . . . .Susan Coakley
Chief Financial Officer . . . . .Laurie Doran
Chief Operating Officer . . . . .Eric Hunter
Chief Information Officer. . . . . .Kim Sinclair
Chief Medical Officer . . . . .Karen Boudreau, MD
Chief, Marketing & Sales . . . . .Kevin Klein

---

524 CIGNA HealthCare of Massachusetts

Three Newton Executive Park
2223 Washington Street, Suite 200
Newton, MA 02462
Toll-Free: 866-438-2446
Phone: 617-630-4300
Fax: 617-630-4383
www.cigna.com
Secondary Address: Great-West Healthcare, now part of CIGNA, 130
Turner Street, Bldg 3, Suite 610, Waltham, MA 02453, 781-893-0370
For Profit Organization: Yes
Total Enrollment: 10,315
State Enrollment: 10,315

Healthplan and Services Defined
PLAN TYPE: PPO
Benefits Offered: Disease Management, Prescription, Transplant,
Wellness

Type of Coverage
Commercial

Type of Payment Plans Offered
POS, FFS

Geographic Areas Served
Massachusetts

Key Personnel
President. . . . . .Donald M Curry
CMO . . . . .Dr Rob Hockmuth

---

525 ConnectiCare of Massachusetts

175 Scott Swamp Road
PO Box 4050
Farmington, CT 06034-4050
Toll-Free: 800-251-7772
Phone: 860-574-5757
info@connecticare.com
www.connecticare.com
Mailing Address: PO Box 416191, Boston, MA 02241-6191
For Profit Organization: Yes
Year Founded: 1981
Number of Affiliated Hospitals: 126
Number of Primary Care Physicians: 22,000
Total Enrollment: 240,000
State Enrollment: 9,000

Healthplan and Services Defined
PLAN TYPE: HMO/PPO
Other Type: POS
Plan Specialty: Lab, Radiology
Benefits Offered: Dental, Disease Management, Physical Therapy,
Prescription, Wellness

Type of Coverage
Commercial, Individual, Medicare

Type of Payment Plans Offered
POS

Geographic Areas Served
Massachusetts

Key Personnel
President . . . . .Michael Wise
COO . . . . .Ida Schnipper
CFO. . . . . .Tom Tran
CMO . . . . .Paul Bluestein, MD
General Counsel . . . . .Gail Bogossian
Marketing . . . . .Paul Philpott
Pharmacy Director. . . . . .Jeff Casberg
Public Relations. . . . . .Deb Hoyt
Media Contact. . . . . .Stephen Jewett
publicrelations@connecticare.com

Specialty Managed Care Partners
Express Scripts

526 Dentaquest

465 Medford Street
Boston, MA 02129-1454
Toll-Free: 800-417-7140
learnmore@dentaquest.com
www.dentaquest.com
Subsidiary of: DentaQuest Ventures
Year Founded: 1980
Number of Primary Care Physicians: 750
Total Enrollment: 14,000,000

Healthplan and Services Defined
PLAN TYPE: Dental
Plan Specialty: Dental
Benefits Offered: Dental

Geographic Areas Served
District of Columbia, Florida, Maryland, Virginia

Key Personnel
President & CEO.............................Fay Donohue
Chief Financial Officer.........................James Collins
Chief Operating Officer ....Steve Pollock
SVP, HR & Admin Services ....Sheryl Traylor
SVP, Market Development ....Bob Lynn
Chief Mission Officer ....Ralph Fuccillo
Chief Dental Officer ....John Luther
SVP/General Counsel ....David Abelman
CEO, Healthcare Delivery....................Jeffrey A. Parker
SVP, IT.....................................Ken Erdelt
SVP, Chief Sales Officer......................Dennis Leonard
Director, Marketing/PR ....Jill Tobacco
617-886-1652
jill.tobacco@greatdentalplans.com

527 eHealthInsurance Services Inc.

11919 Foundation Place
Gold River, CA 95670
Toll-Free: 800-644-3491
webmaster@healthinsurance.com
www.e.healthinsurance.com
Year Founded: 1997

Healthplan and Services Defined
PLAN TYPE: HMO/PPO
Benefits Offered: Dental, Life, STD

Type of Coverage
Commercial, Individual, Medicare

Geographic Areas Served
All 50 states in the USA and District of Columbia

Key Personnel
Chairman & CEO.............................Gary L. Lauer
EVP/Business & Corp. Dev....................Bruce Telkamp
EVP/Chief Technology..................Dr. Sheldon X. Wang
SVP & CFO ....Stuart M. Huizinga
Pres. of eHealth Gov. Sys ....Samuel C. Gibbs
SVP of Sales & Operations ....Robert S. Hurley
Director Public Relations.......................Nate Purpura
650-210-3115

528 Fallon Community Health Plan

10 Chestnut Street
Worcester, MA 01608
Toll-Free: 800-333-2535
Phone: 508-799-2100
Fax: 508-368-9953
contactcustomerservice@fchp.org

www.fchp.org
Mailing Address: P.O. Box 15121, Worcester, MA 01615
Non-Profit Organization: Yes
Year Founded: 1977
Federally Qualified: Yes
Number of Affiliated Hospitals: 57
Number of Primary Care Physicians: 1,291
Number of Referral/Specialty Physicians: 3,504
Total Enrollment: 178,000
State Enrollment: 135,581

Healthplan and Services Defined
PLAN TYPE: HMO/PPO
Model Type: Network
Plan Specialty: ASO, Behavioral Health, Chiropractic, Dental, Disease Management, Lab, PBM, Vision, Worker's Compensation, HMO, PPO, POS
Benefits Offered: Behavioral Health, Chiropractic, Complementary Medicine, Dental, Disease Management, Home Care, Inpatient SNF, Physical Therapy, Podiatry, Prescription, Psychiatric, Transplant, Vision, Wellness

Type of Coverage
Commercial, Individual, Indemnity, Medicare, Medicaid
Catastrophic Illness Benefit: Covered

Type of Payment Plans Offered
POS, DFFS, Capitated, FFS, Combination FFS & DFFS

Geographic Areas Served
Worcester, Norfolk, Plymouth, Hampshire, Middlesex, Bristol, Franklin, Essex, Suffolk and Hampden counties

Subscriber Information
Average Monthly Fee Per Subscriber
(Employee + Employer Contribution):
Employee Only (Self): $306.00
Employee & 1 Family Member: $623.00
Employee & 2 Family Members: $802.00
Medicare: $223.00
Average Annual Deductible Per Subscriber:
Employee Only (Self): $316.00
Employee & 1 Family Member: $633.00
Employee & 2 Family Members: $561.00
Medicare: $512.00
Average Subscriber Co-Payment:
Primary Care Physician: $12.97
Non-Network Physician: $10.00
Prescription Drugs: $14.83
Hospital ER: $51.00
Home Health Care: $0
Nursing Home: $0
Nursing Home Max. Days/Visits Covered: 100days/year

Peer Review Type
Utilization Review: Yes
Second Surgical Opinion: Yes
Case Management: Yes

Publishes and Distributes Report Card: Yes

Accreditation Certification
NCQA
Medicare Approved, Utilization Review, Pre-Admission Certification, State Licensure, Quality Assurance Program

Key Personnel
President/CEO ....Patrick Hughes
SVP/Chief Medical Officer................Sarika Aggarwal, MD
Chief Compliance Officer ....Richard P. Burke
Chief Legal Counsel ....Jesse Caplan, Esq.
SVP/Chief, Communications ....Christine Cassidy
SVP/COO...............................Richard Commander
SVP, Sales/Marketing.......................David Przesiek
Chief Strategy Officer ....Mary Ritter
SVP/Chief HR Officer........................Linda St. John
EVP/CFO...............................R. Scott Walker

Average Claim Compensation
Physician's Fees Charged: 125%

Specialty Managed Care Partners
American Specialty Health Networks, Beacon Health Strategies, Pharma Care, Dental Benefits
Enters into Contracts with Regional Business Coalitions: Yes
West Suburban Health Group, Reserves Management Inc, Minuteman Nashoba Health Group, Municipalities of Regional Effectiveness(MORE)

Employer References
Federal Employees Benefit Program, Commonwealth of Massachusetts, City of Worcester, Wyman Gordon, National Grid

529 Fallon Community Medicare Plan

10 Chestnut Street
Worcester, MA 01608
Toll-Free: 800-868-5200
Phone: 508-799-2100
Fax: 508-797-9621
seniorplan@fchp.org
www.fchp.org
Non-Profit Organization: Yes
Year Founded: 1977

Healthplan and Services Defined
PLAN TYPE: Medicare
Benefits Offered: Chiropractic, Dental, Disease Management, Home Care, Inpatient SNF, Physical Therapy, Podiatry, Prescription, Psychiatric, Vision, Wellness

Type of Coverage
Individual, Medicare

Geographic Areas Served
Available for Massachusetts only

Subscriber Information
Average Monthly Fee Per Subscriber
(Employee + Employer Contribution):
Employee Only (Self): Varies
Medicare: Varies
Average Annual Deductible Per Subscriber:
Employee Only (Self): Varies
Medicare: Varies
Average Subscriber Co-Payment:
Primary Care Physician: Varies
Non-Network Physician: Varies
Prescription Drugs: Varies
Hospital ER: Varies
Home Health Care: Varies
Home Health Care Max. Days/Visits Covered: Varies
Nursing Home: Varies
Nursing Home Max. Days/Visits Covered: Varies

Key Personnel
President/CEO . . . . Patrick Hughes
patrick.hughes@fchp.org
EVP/CFO . . . . R Scott Walker
charles.goheen@fchp.org
Div Pres, Senior Care . . . . Richard Commander
Div Pres, Health Plan Op. . . . . W Patrick Hughes
EVP/Chief Compliance Offc . . . . Richard P. Burke
Chiel Legal Counsel . . . . Jesse Caplan, Esq
Chief Communications Offi . . . . Christine Cassidy
VP, Strategy & Business D . . . . Patricia Forts
VP, Marketing. . . . . Janis Liepins
EVP, Interim CMO . . . . Russell Munson, MD
SVP, Chief HR Officer. . . . . Linda St. John
EVP, Human Resources . . . . Teena Osgood
VP, Sales . . . . David Przesiek
Public Relations . . . . Christine Cassidy
508-368-9502
mediainfo@fchp.org

530 Great-West Healthcare of Massachusetts

130 Turner St, Stoneybrook Office Park
Building 3, Suite 610
Waltham, MA 02453
Toll-Free: 800-234-2040
Phone: 508-650-9590
eliginquiries@cigna.com
www.cignaforhealth.com
Secondary Address: Three Newton Executive Park, 2223 Washington Street, Suite 200, Newton, MA 02462
Subsidiary of: CIGNA HealthCare
Acquired by: CIGNA
For Profit Organization: Yes
Total Enrollment: 2,000,000
State Enrollment: 19,053

Healthplan and Services Defined
PLAN TYPE: HMO/PPO
Model Type: Staff

Type of Coverage
Commercial

Type of Payment Plans Offered
DFFS, FFS

Subscriber Information
Average Monthly Fee Per Subscriber
(Employee + Employer Contribution):
Employee & 2 Family Members: Varies per plan
Average Annual Deductible Per Subscriber:
Employee Only (Self): Varies per plan
Employee & 2 Family Members: Varies per plan
Average Subscriber Co-Payment:
Primary Care Physician: Varies per plan
Prescription Drugs: Varies per plan

Publishes and Distributes Report Card: Yes

Accreditation Certification
URAC

Key Personnel
EVP . . . . Richard F Rivers
SVP US Markets. . . . . Mark Stadler
SVP Healthcare Operations . . . . Donna Goldin
SVP Healthcare Management . . . . Chris Knackstedt
Chief Medical Officer . . . . Terry Fouts, MD
VP Product Development . . . . Cindy Donohoe
VP Specialty Risk. . . . . Kent Boyer

531 Harvard Pilgrim Health Care

93 Worcester Street
Wellesley, MA 02481
Toll-Free: 888-888-4742
Phone: 617-745-1000
Fax: 617-509-0049
www.harvardpilgrim.org
Secondary Address: 1600 Crown Colony Drive, Quincy, MA 02169
Non-Profit Organization: Yes
Year Founded: 1977
Number of Affiliated Hospitals: 135
Number of Primary Care Physicians: 28,000
Total Enrollment: 1,079,674
State Enrollment: 65,000

Healthplan and Services Defined
PLAN TYPE: Multiple
Model Type: Network
Plan Specialty: ASO, Behavioral Health, Chiropractic, Dental, Disease Management, EPO, Lab, MSO, PBM, Vision, Radiology, Worker's Compensation, UR
Benefits Offered: Behavioral Health, Chiropractic, Disease Management, Home Care, Inpatient SNF, Long-Term Care,

Physical Therapy, Podiatry, Prescription, Psychiatric, Transplant, Vision, Wellness

Offers Demand Management Patient Information Service: Yes

DMPI Services Offered: Clinical Program, Specialty On-Line, Case Management, Cybernurse, On-Line A-Z

Type of Coverage
Commercial, Individual, Indemnity, Medicare, Supplemental Medicare, Medicaid

Type of Payment Plans Offered
POS, Combination FFS & DFFS

Geographic Areas Served
Mass.: All counties; Rhode Island: All counties; New Hampshire: Sullivan, Belknap, Merrimack, Strafford, Cheshire, Hillsborough, Rockingham counties, parts of Coos, Grafton and Carroll counties; Vermont: Windham, Windsor and Caledonia county

Subscriber Information
Average Monthly Fee Per Subscriber
  (Employee + Employer Contribution):
    Employee Only (Self): $5.50
Average Annual Deductible Per Subscriber:
    Employee Only (Self): $1000.00
    Employee & 1 Family Member: $2000.00
    Employee & 2 Family Members: $2000.00
Average Subscriber Co-Payment:
    Primary Care Physician: $20.00
    Non-Network Physician: 20%
    Prescription Drugs: $10.00
    Hospital ER: $50.00-50.00
    Home Health Care: $0
    Home Health Care Max. Days/Visits Covered: Subject to review
    Nursing Home: $0
    Nursing Home Max. Days/Visits Covered: 60 days

Network Qualifications
Pre-Admission Certification: Yes

Peer Review Type
Utilization Review: Yes
Second Surgical Opinion: Yes
Case Management: Yes

Publishes and Distributes Report Card: Yes

Accreditation Certification
NCQA
TJC Accreditation, Medicare Approved, Utilization Review, Pre-Admission Certification, State Licensure, Quality Assurance Program

Key Personnel
President/CEO . . . . Eric Schultz
  888-333-4742
CFO . . . . James DuCharme
COO/Chief Medical Officer . . . . Roberta Herman
SVP Sales & Cust Service . . . . Vincent Capozzi
Chief Human Resources Ofc. . . . . Jack Lane
Manager Regional Claims . . . . Barbara Chapman
Medical Director . . . . Carolyn Langer
Chief Legal Officer . . . . Laura S Peabody
VP, Marketing . . . . Dana Rashti
VP, Policy & Govt Affairs . . . . William J Graham
SVP Provider Network . . . . Rick Weisblatt, PhD
VP, Customer Service . . . . Lynn Bowman
  lynn_bowman@hphc.org
Chief Information Officer . . . . Deborah Norton
SVP, Actuarial Services . . . . Gary H Lin
Media Contact. . . . . Sharon Torgerson
  617-509-7458
  sharon_torgerson@hphc.org

Average Claim Compensation
Physician's Fees Charged: 51%
Hospital's Fees Charged: 40%

Specialty Managed Care Partners
Mass General, Brigham And Women Hospital, Boston Medical, Value Options, MedImpact
Enters into Contracts with Regional Business Coalitions: No

Employer References
Commonwealth of Massachusetts, City of Boston, Harvard University

---

532 Harvard University Group Health Plan
75 Mount Auburn Street
First Floor
Cambridge, MA 02138
Phone: 617-495-2008
Fax: 617-496-6125
mservices@uhs.harvard.edu
www.hughp.harvard.edu
Non-Profit Organization: Yes
Year Founded: 1973
Number of Affiliated Hospitals: 4
Number of Primary Care Physicians: 430
Number of Referral/Specialty Physicians: 60
Total Enrollment: 6,443

Healthplan and Services Defined
PLAN TYPE: HMO
Other Type: POS
Model Type: Staff
Benefits Offered: Prescription

Type of Payment Plans Offered
POS

Geographic Areas Served
Harvard University faculty, staff and their families

Subscriber Information
Average Annual Deductible Per Subscriber:
    Employee Only (Self): $0
Average Subscriber Co-Payment:
    Primary Care Physician: $10.00
    Prescription Drugs: $10/$20/$35
    Hospital ER: $0
    Home Health Care: $0
    Nursing Home: $0

Network Qualifications
Pre-Admission Certification: Yes

Peer Review Type
Utilization Review: Yes
Second Surgical Opinion: No
Case Management: Yes

Publishes and Distributes Report Card: No

Accreditation Certification
TJC Accreditation, Medicare Approved, Utilization Review, Pre-Admission Certification, State Licensure, Quality Assurance Program

Key Personnel
Director. . . . . David S Rosenthal, MD
CFO . . . . Marc Pollack
Director of Health Plan . . . . Paula Fiore
In House Formulary. . . . . Maureen McCarthy
Marketing . . . . Catherine Lukas
Materials Management . . . . Art Strauss
Medical Affairs . . . . Christopher Coley, MD
Director of Health Plan. . . . . Paula Fiore
Information Systems . . . . Marc Pollack
Director of Health Plan. . . . . Paula Fiore

Specialty Managed Care Partners
Enters into Contracts with Regional Business Coalitions: No

533 Health New England

One Monarch Place
Suite 1500
Springfield, MA 01144-1500
Toll-Free: 800-842-4464
Phone: 413-787-4000
Fax: 413-734-3356
jcampbell@hne.com
www.hne.com
For Profit Organization: Yes
Year Founded: 1985
Number of Affiliated Hospitals: 14
Number of Primary Care Physicians: 4,310
Number of Referral/Specialty Physicians: 3,000
Total Enrollment: 106,000
State Enrollment: 106,000

Healthplan and Services Defined
   PLAN TYPE: HMO
   Model Type: IPA
   Plan Specialty: ASO, Disease Management
   Benefits Offered: Behavioral Health, Chiropractic, Complementary
      Medicine, Dental, Disease Management, Home Care, Inpatient
      SNF, Physical Therapy, Podiatry, Prescription, Psychiatric,
      Transplant, Vision, Wellness

Type of Coverage
   Commercial, Catastrophic, HMO Unlimited
   Catastrophic Illness Benefit: Maximum $1M

Type of Payment Plans Offered
   POS

Geographic Areas Served
   Western Massachusetts (Berkshire, Franklin, Hampden, and
   Hampshire counties as well as parts of Worcester county)

Subscriber Information
   Average Subscriber Co-Payment:
      Primary Care Physician: $15.00
      Non-Network Physician: Not covered
      Prescription Drugs: $15.00/25.00/45.00
      Hospital ER: $50.00
      Nursing Home Max. Days/Visits Covered: 100 days

Network Qualifications
   Pre-Admission Certification: Yes

Peer Review Type
   Utilization Review: Yes
   Second Surgical Opinion: Yes
   Case Management: Yes

Publishes and Distributes Report Card: Yes

Accreditation Certification
   NCQA
   TJC Accreditation, Medicare Approved, Utilization Review,
      Pre-Admission Certification, State Licensure, Quality Assurance
      Program

Key Personnel
   President/CEO...............................Peter F Straley
   VP Finance/CFO...........................Robert A Kosior
   VP, General Counsel...........................James Kessler
   VP Marketing..............................Maura McCaffrey
   Chief Medical Officer ....Thomas H Ebert, MD
   VP, Human Resources ....Amy Trombley
   VP Information Technology ....Philip M Lacombe
   VP Sales..................................Juan A Campbell
   RFP Analyst..............................Laurie Beebe
      413-233-3244
      lbeebe@hne.com

Average Claim Compensation
   Physician's Fees Charged: 59%
   Hospital's Fees Charged: 49%

Specialty Managed Care Partners
   Enters into Contracts with Regional Business Coalitions: No

534 Health Plan of New York: Massachusetts

55 Water Street
New York, NY 10041
Toll-Free: 800-447-8255
Phone: 646-447-5900
Fax: 646-447-3011
www.hipusa.com
Subsidiary of: An Emblem Health Company
Total Enrollment: 1,200,000

Healthplan and Services Defined
   PLAN TYPE: HMO/PPO
   Other Type: POS, EPO, ASO
   Benefits Offered: Chiropractic, Dental, Disease Management, Home
      Care, Inpatient SNF, Physical Therapy, Podiatry, Prescription,
      Psychiatric, Vision, Wellness

Type of Coverage
   Individual, Medicare

Geographic Areas Served
   New York, Connecticut, Massachusetts

Subscriber Information
   Average Monthly Fee Per Subscriber
      (Employee + Employer Contribution):
         Employee Only (Self): Varies
         Medicare: Varies
   Average Annual Deductible Per Subscriber:
         Employee Only (Self): Varies
         Medicare: Varies
   Average Subscriber Co-Payment:
         Primary Care Physician: Varies
         Non-Network Physician: Varies
         Prescription Drugs: Varies
         Hospital ER: Varies
         Home Health Care: Varies
         Home Health Care Max. Days/Visits Covered: Varies
         Nursing Home: Varies
         Nursing Home Max. Days/Visits Covered: Varies

535 Health Plans, Inc.

1500 West Park Drive
Suite 330, PO Box 5199
Westborough, MA 01581
Toll-Free: 800-532-7575
Phone: 508-752-2480
Fax: 508-754-9664
info@healthplansinc.com
www.healthplansinc.com
Secondary Address: 300 TradeCenter, Suite 2500, Woburn, MA 01801
Subsidiary of: A Harvard Pilgrim Company
For Profit Organization: Yes
Year Founded: 1981
Number of Affiliated Hospitals: 12
Number of Primary Care Physicians: 1,700
Total Enrollment: 12,000

Healthplan and Services Defined
   PLAN TYPE: Other
   Other Type: TPA
   Model Type: Network
   Plan Specialty: ASO, Behavioral Health, Chiropractic, Dental,
      Disease Management, EPO, Lab, PBM, Vision, Radiology, UR
   Benefits Offered: Home Care, Inpatient SNF, Long-Term Care,
      Physical Therapy, Podiatry, Prescription, Psychiatric, Transplant,
      Vision, Wellness, Worker's Compensation, AD&D, Life, LTD, STD

Type of Coverage
   Employer Self Funded

Geographic Areas Served
Statewide

Subscriber Information
Average Monthly Fee Per Subscriber
(Employee + Employer Contribution):
Employee Only (Self): $2.00
Employee & 1 Family Member: $2.00
Employee & 2 Family Members: $2.00
Average Subscriber Co-Payment:
Primary Care Physician: $5.00
Non-Network Physician: $250.00
Prescription Drugs: $4.00
Hospital ER: $25.00
Home Health Care: $0
Nursing Home: $250.00

Accreditation Certification
TJC Accreditation, Pre-Admission Certification

Key Personnel
President/CEO........................William R Breidenbach
Marketing..............................Debra Hovagimian
Medical Affairs.........................Michael Galica, MD
Sales.....................................Deb Hoges

Specialty Managed Care Partners
Care Management Service

536 Humana Health Insurance of Massachusetts
One International Boulevard
Suite 904
Mahwah, NJ 07495
Toll-Free: 800-967-2370
Fax: 201-934-1369
www.humana.com
For Profit Organization: Yes

Healthplan and Services Defined
PLAN TYPE: HMO/PPO

Type of Coverage
Commercial, Individual

Accreditation Certification
URAC, NCQA, CORE

537 Neighborhood Health Plan
253 Summer Street
Boston, MA 02210
Toll-Free: 800-433-5556
Phone: 617-772-5500
MemberServices@nhp.org
www.nhp.org
Non-Profit Organization: Yes
Year Founded: 1986
Owned by an Integrated Delivery Network (IDN): Yes
Number of Affiliated Hospitals: 41
Number of Primary Care Physicians: 2,800
Number of Referral/Specialty Physicians: 10,400
Total Enrollment: 186,000
State Enrollment: 25,804

Healthplan and Services Defined
PLAN TYPE: HMO
Model Type: Network
Plan Specialty: ASO, Behavioral Health, Disease Management,
Medicaid Focus
Benefits Offered: Behavioral Health, Complementary Medicine,
Disease Management, Home Care, Prescription, Vision, Wellness

Type of Coverage
Commercial, Medicaid
Catastrophic Illness Benefit: Covered

Geographic Areas Served
Most of Massachusetts counties

Subscriber Information
Average Subscriber Co-Payment:
Primary Care Physician: $0
Prescription Drugs: $5.00
Hospital ER: $0
Home Health Care: $0

Network Qualifications
Pre-Admission Certification: Yes

Peer Review Type
Utilization Review: Yes
Second Surgical Opinion: Yes
Case Management: Yes

Publishes and Distributes Report Card: Yes

Accreditation Certification
State Of Ma
TJC Accreditation, Medicare Approved, Utilization Review,
Pre-Admission Certification, State Licensure, Quality Assurance
Program

Key Personnel
President/CEO............................Deborah C Enos
VP Strategic Partnerships......................Carla Bettano
Chief Medical Officer........................Paul Mendis, MD
Chief Financial Officer..........................Garrett Parker
Chief Information Officer....................Marilyn Daly
VP, Operations.............................Katie Catlender
Chief Operating Officer........................David Segal
Chief, Stategy/Marketing.........................Dana Rashti
VP, Provider Network Mgmt...............Jennifer Kent Weiner
Director, Marketing...........................Rhian Gregory
617-772-5660

Specialty Managed Care Partners
Beacon Health Strategies
Enters into Contracts with Regional Business Coalitions: No

538 Tufts Health Medicare Plan
705 Mt Auburn Street
Watertown, MA 02472
Toll-Free: 800-462-0024
Phone: 617-972-9400
www.tuftshealthplan.com
Secondary Address: 1441 Main Street, 9th Floor, Springfield, MA
01103
Year Founded: 1979

Healthplan and Services Defined
PLAN TYPE: Medicare
Benefits Offered: Chiropractic, Dental, Disease Management, Home
Care, Inpatient SNF, Physical Therapy, Podiatry, Prescription,
Psychiatric, Vision, Wellness

Type of Coverage
Individual, Medicare

Geographic Areas Served
Available within Massachusetts, Connecticut, New Hampshire, Rhode
Island and Vermont

Subscriber Information
Average Monthly Fee Per Subscriber
(Employee + Employer Contribution):
Employee Only (Self): Varies
Medicare: Varies
Average Annual Deductible Per Subscriber:
Employee Only (Self): Varies
Medicare: Varies
Average Subscriber Co-Payment:
Primary Care Physician: Varies
Non-Network Physician: Varies
Prescription Drugs: Varies

Hospital ER: Varies
Home Health Care: Varies
Home Health Care Max. Days/Visits Covered: Varies
Nursing Home: Varies
Nursing Home Max. Days/Visits Covered: Varies

Key Personnel
President and CEO . . . . James Roosevelt Jr., Jr
COO. . . . . .Thomas A Croswell
SVP/CIO. . . . . .Tricia Trebino
SVP/Senior Products . . . . .Patty Blake
SVP/Human Resources. . . . . .Lois Dehls Cornell
SVP/Marketing . . . . .Rob Egan
Chief Medical Officer. . . . . Pual Kasuba, MD
SVP/CFO . . . . .Umesh Kurpad
SVP/Sales & Client Svcs .Brian P Pagliaro

539 Tufts Health Plan

705 Mt Auburn Street
Watertown, MA 02472
Toll-Free: 800-462-0224
Phone: 617-972-9400
www.tuftshealthplan.com
Secondary Address: 1441 Main Street, 9th Floor, Springfield, MA
   02201, 413-746-8200
Non-Profit Organization: Yes
Year Founded: 1979
Number of Affiliated Hospitals: 90
Number of Primary Care Physicians: 25,000
Number of Referral/Specialty Physicians: 12,500
Total Enrollment: 737,411

Healthplan and Services Defined
PLAN TYPE: HMO/PPO
Other Type: POS
Model Type: IPA
Plan Specialty: ASO, Behavioral Health, Chiropractic, Disease
   Management, EPO, Lab, PBM, Vision, Radiology, UR, Pharmacy
Benefits Offered: Behavioral Health, Chiropractic, Complementary
   Medicine, Disease Management, Home Care, Inpatient SNF,
   Physical Therapy, Podiatry, Prescription, Psychiatric, Transplant,
   Vision, Wellness

Type of Coverage
Commercial, Individual, Medicare, Supplemental Medicare, HSA,
   HRA

Type of Payment Plans Offered
POS, DFFS, FFS, Combination FFS & DFFS

Geographic Areas Served
Massachusetts, New Hampshire and Rhode Island

Subscriber Information
Average Monthly Fee Per Subscriber
   (Employee + Employer Contribution):
      Employee Only (Self): $190.00-220.00
      Employee & 2 Family Members: $800.00-950.00
      Medicare: $150.00
Average Annual Deductible Per Subscriber:
      Employee Only (Self): $1000.00
      Employee & 1 Family Member: $500.00
      Employee & 2 Family Members: $3000.00
Average Subscriber Co-Payment:
      Primary Care Physician: $10.00
      Non-Network Physician: 20%
      Prescription Drugs: $10/20/35
      Hospital ER: $50.00
      Home Health Care: $0
      Home Health Care Max. Days/Visits Covered: 120 days
      Nursing Home: $0
      Nursing Home Max. Days/Visits Covered: 120 days

Network Qualifications
Pre-Admission Certification: No

Peer Review Type
Utilization Review: Yes
Case Management: Yes

Publishes and Distributes Report Card: Yes

Accreditation Certification
TJC, AAPI, NCQA

Key Personnel
CEO. . . . . .James Roosevelt Jr., Jr
President/COO . . . . .Thomas A Croswell
SVP/CIO. . . . . .Tricia Trebino
President, Sr. Products . . . . .Patty Blake
General Counsel . . . . .Lois Dehls Cornell
Chief Medical Officer. . . . . Pual Kasuba, MD
SVP/CFO . . . . .Umesh Kurpad
SVP/Sales & Client Svcs .Brian P Pagliaro

Average Claim Compensation
Physician's Fees Charged: 75%
Hospital's Fees Charged: 70%

Specialty Managed Care Partners
Advance PCS, Private Healthe Care Systems

Employer References
Commonwealth of Massachuestts, Fleet Boston, Roman Catholic
   Archdiocese of Boston, City of Boston, State Street Corporation

540 Unicare: Massachusetts

681 Main Campus Dr#3
Waltham, MA 01810-0916
Toll-Free: 800-862-9988
Phone: 781-642-6869
Fax: 978-247-6599
www.unicare.com
Year Founded: 1985
Number of Affiliated Hospitals: 102
Number of Primary Care Physicians: 3,500
Number of Referral/Specialty Physicians: 8,000
Total Enrollment: 80,000

Healthplan and Services Defined
PLAN TYPE: HMO/PPO
Model Type: Network
Benefits Offered: Chiropractic, Physical Therapy, Prescription

Geographic Areas Served
Massachusetts, Southern New Hampshire & Rhode Island

Subscriber Information
Average Monthly Fee Per Subscriber
   (Employee + Employer Contribution):
      Employee Only (Self): Varies
      Employee & 1 Family Member: Varies
      Employee & 2 Family Members: Varies
      Medicare: Varies
Average Annual Deductible Per Subscriber:
      Employee Only (Self): Varies
      Employee & 1 Family Member: Varies
      Employee & 2 Family Members: Varies
      Medicare: Varies
Average Subscriber Co-Payment:
      Primary Care Physician: Varies
      Non-Network Physician: Varies
      Prescription Drugs: Varies
      Hospital ER: Varies
      Home Health Care: Varies
      Home Health Care Max. Days/Visits Covered: Varies
      Nursing Home: Varies
      Nursing Home Max. Days/Visits Covered: Varies

Network Qualifications
Pre-Admission Certification: Yes

Peer Review Type
Utilization Review: Yes

Second Surgical Opinion: Yes
Case Management: Yes

Publishes and Distributes Report Card: No

Accreditation Certification
TJC Accreditation, Medicare Approved, Utilization Review, Pre-Admission Certification, State Licensure, Quality Assurance Program

Key Personnel
CEO and President..........................David W Fields
Sales Director ....Cynthia L Paralta
   cynthia.paralta@wellpoint.com
Media Contact ....Tony Felts
   317-287-6036
   tony.felts@wellpoint.com

541   UnitedHealthCare of Massachusetts

475 Kilvert Street
Warwick, RI 02886
Toll-Free: 888-735-5842
www.uhc.com
Secondary Address: 950 Winter Street, Suite 1700, Waltham, MA 02451, 800-444-7855
For Profit Organization: Yes
Number of Affiliated Hospitals: 5,609
Number of Primary Care Physicians: 726,537
Total Enrollment: 70,000,000

Healthplan and Services Defined
PLAN TYPE: HMO/PPO
Model Type: Network
Benefits Offered: Disease Management, Prescription, Wellness
Offers Demand Management Patient Information Service: Yes

Type of Coverage
Catastrophic Illness Benefit: None

Type of Payment Plans Offered
POS, FFS

Geographic Areas Served
Connecticut, Massachusetts, Maine, New Hampshire, Rhode Island

Subscriber Information
Average Monthly Fee Per Subscriber
   (Employee + Employer Contribution):
      Employee Only (Self): $150.00
      Employee & 2 Family Members: $300.00

Network Qualifications
Pre-Admission Certification: Yes

Peer Review Type
Utilization Review: Yes
Second Surgical Opinion: Yes
Case Management: Yes

Publishes and Distributes Report Card: Yes

Accreditation Certification
AAPI, NCQA
TJC Accreditation, Medicare Approved, Utilization Review, Pre-Admission Certification, State Licensure, Quality Assurance Program

Key Personnel
President/CEO.................................Amy Knapp
CFO...Donald Powers
Marketing....................................Mark Butler
Medical Affairs ....Tony Kazlauskas
Sales..James Moniz
Media Contact ....Debora Spano
   401-732-7374
   debora_m_spano@uhc.com

Average Claim Compensation
Physician's Fees Charged: 70%
Hospital's Fees Charged: 80%

Specialty Managed Care Partners
Enters into Contracts with Regional Business Coalitions: Yes

542   VSP: Vision Service Plan of Massachusetts

8 Faneuil Hall Market Place
Boston, MA 02109-6114
Phone: 617-854-7471
webmaster@vsp.com
www.vsp.com
Year Founded: 1955
Number of Primary Care Physicians: 26,000
Total Enrollment: 55,000,000

Healthplan and Services Defined
PLAN TYPE: Vision
Plan Specialty: Vision
Benefits Offered: Vision

Type of Payment Plans Offered
Capitated

Geographic Areas Served
Statewide

Network Qualifications
Pre-Admission Certification: Yes

Peer Review Type
Utilization Review: Yes

Accreditation Certification
Utilization Review, Quality Assurance Program

Health Insurance Coverage Status and Type of Coverage by Age

Category	All Persons		Under 18 years		Under 65 years		65 years and over	
	Number	%	Number	%	Number	%	Number	%
Total population	9,784	-	2,240	-	8,337	-	1,448	-
Covered by some type of health insurance	8,713 *(19)*	89.0 *(0.2)*	2,150 *(6)*	96.0 *(0.3)*	7,273 *(19)*	87.2 *(0.2)*	1,440 *(3)*	99.5 *(0.1)*
Covered by private health insurance	6,760 *(32)*	69.1 *(0.3)*	1,374 *(14)*	61.3 *(0.7)*	5,666 *(30)*	68.0 *(0.4)*	1,094 *(8)*	75.5 *(0.5)*
Employment based	5,815 *(35)*	59.4 *(0.4)*	1,268 *(15)*	56.6 *(0.7)*	5,096 *(33)*	61.1 *(0.4)*	720 *(9)*	49.7 *(0.6)*
Direct purchase	1,166 *(18)*	11.9 *(0.2)*	112 *(7)*	5.0 *(0.3)*	660 *(15)*	7.9 *(0.2)*	506 *(8)*	34.9 *(0.6)*
Covered by TRICARE	117 *(6)*	1.2 *(0.1)*	20 *(3)*	0.9 *(0.1)*	78 *(6)*	0.9 *(0.1)*	39 *(3)*	2.7 *(0.2)*
Covered by government health insurance	3,376 *(26)*	34.5 *(0.3)*	894 *(15)*	39.9 *(0.7)*	1,959 *(26)*	23.5 *(0.3)*	1,418 *(4)*	97.9 *(0.2)*
Covered by Medicaid	1,922 *(28)*	19.6 *(0.3)*	890 *(15)*	39.7 *(0.7)*	1,749 *(27)*	21.0 *(0.3)*	174 *(7)*	12.0 *(0.4)*
Also by private insurance	331 *(12)*	3.4 *(0.1)*	116 *(7)*	5.2 *(0.3)*	241 *(11)*	2.9 *(0.1)*	91 *(4)*	6.3 *(0.3)*
Covered by Medicare	1,717 *(8)*	17.6 *(0.1)*	9 *(2)*	0.4 *(0.1)*	301 *(7)*	3.6 *(0.1)*	1,416 *(4)*	97.8 *(0.2)*
Also by private insurance	1,173 *(9)*	12.0 *(0.1)*	2 *(1)*	0.1 *(0.1)*	103 *(4)*	1.2 *(0.1)*	1,070 *(8)*	73.9 *(0.5)*
Also by Medicaid	328 *(9)*	3.3 *(0.1)*	6 *(2)*	0.3 *(0.1)*	154 *(6)*	1.8 *(0.1)*	174 *(7)*	12.0 *(0.4)*
Covered by VA Care	188 *(6)*	1.9 *(0.1)*	2 *(1)*	0.1 *(0.1)*	88 *(4)*	1.1 *(0.1)*	100 *(3)*	6.9 *(0.2)*
Not covered at any time during the year	1,072 *(19)*	11.0 *(0.2)*	90 *(6)*	4.0 *(0.3)*	1,064 *(19)*	12.8 *(0.2)*	8 *(2)*	0.5 *(0.1)*

Note: Numbers in thousands; Figures cover 2013; Margin of error appears in parenthesis; A "Z" indicates that the value either represents or rounds to zero.
Source: U.S. Census Bureau, 2013 American Community Survey, Table HI05. Health Insurance Coverage Status and Type of Coverage by State and Age for All People: 2013

Michigan

543 Aetna Health of Michigan
151 Farmington Avenue
Hartford, CT 06156
Toll-Free: 800-872-3862
Phone: 860-273-0123
www.aetna.com
For Profit Organization: Yes
Year Founded: 1988
Total Enrollment: 11,596,230

Healthplan and Services Defined
 PLAN TYPE: PPO
 Other Type: POS
 Plan Specialty: PBM
 Benefits Offered: Behavioral Health, Dental, Disease Management,
  Prescription, Vision
 Offers Demand Management Patient Information Service: Yes

Type of Payment Plans Offered
 DFFS

Geographic Areas Served
 Statewide

Subscriber Information
 Average Monthly Fee Per Subscriber
  (Employee + Employer Contribution):
   Employee Only (Self): $73.42
   Employee & 1 Family Member: $168.89

Network Qualifications
 Pre-Admission Certification: Yes

Peer Review Type
 Utilization Review: Yes

Publishes and Distributes Report Card: Yes

Key Personnel
 Chairman/CEO/President . . . . Mark T Bertolini
 EVP/General Counsel . . . . William J Casazza
 EVP/CFO . . . . Shawn M Guertin

544 American Community Mutual Insurance Company
PO Box 530459
Livonia, MI 48153
Phone: 734-591-9000
Fax: 734-591-8104
www.american-community.com
Partnered with: Security Life
Non-Profit Organization: Yes
Year Founded: 1938
Total Enrollment: 185,000

Healthplan and Services Defined
 PLAN TYPE: PPO

Key Personnel
 President/CEO . . . . Michael E Tobin
 CFO . . . . Steven N Clarren
 SVP, General Counsel . . . . Francis P Dempsey
 SVP & CIO . . . . Beth McCrohan
 VP, Corp Communications. Ellen Downey
  734-591-4694
  edowney@american-community.com

545 Assurant Employee Benefits: Michigan
3001 W Big Beaver Road
#330
Troy, MI 48084-3101
Phone: 248-649-4410
Fax: 248-643-7626
benefits@assurant.com
www.assurantemployeebenefits.com
Subsidiary of: Assurant, Inc
For Profit Organization: Yes
Number of Primary Care Physicians: 112,000
Total Enrollment: 47,000

Healthplan and Services Defined
 PLAN TYPE: Multiple
 Plan Specialty: Dental, Vision, Long & Short-Term Disability
 Benefits Offered: Dental, Vision, Wellness, AD&D, Life, LTD, STD

Type of Coverage
 Commercial, Indemnity, Individual Dental Plans

Geographic Areas Served
 Statewide

Subscriber Information
 Average Monthly Fee Per Subscriber
  (Employee + Employer Contribution):
   Employee Only (Self): Varies by plan

Key Personnel
 Sales Manager . . . . Molly Dunn
 Manager . . . . Dave Braff
 PR Specialist. . . . . Megan Hutchison
  816-556-7815
  megan.hutchison@assurant.com

546 Blue Care Network of Michigan: Corporate Headquarters
20500 Civic Center Drive
The Commons
Southfield, MI 48076
Toll-Free: 800-662-6667
Fax: 248-799-6327
www.mibcn.com
Mailing Address: PO Box 5184, Southfield, MI 48086
Subsidiary of: Blue Cross Blue Shield
Non-Profit Organization: Yes
Year Founded: 1998
Federally Qualified: Yes
Number of Affiliated Hospitals: 116
Number of Primary Care Physicians: 4,500
Number of Referral/Specialty Physicians: 13,500
Total Enrollment: 620,000
State Enrollment: 620,000

Healthplan and Services Defined
 PLAN TYPE: HMO
 Model Type: IPA, Network
 Plan Specialty: Lab, Radiology
 Benefits Offered: Behavioral Health, Disease Management,
  Prescription, Psychiatric, Wellness
 Offers Demand Management Patient Information Service: Yes

Type of Coverage
 Commercial, Individual, Supplemental Medicare
 Catastrophic Illness Benefit: Covered

Type of Payment Plans Offered
 POS

Geographic Areas Served
 Statewide

Subscriber Information
 Average Monthly Fee Per Subscriber
  (Employee + Employer Contribution):

Employee Only (Self): Varies
Employee & 1 Family Member: Varies
Employee & 2 Family Members: Varies
Medicare: Varies

Network Qualifications
Pre-Admission Certification: Yes

Peer Review Type
Case Management: Yes

Publishes and Distributes Report Card: Yes

Accreditation Certification
NCQA

Key Personnel
President/CEO . . . . Kevin L Klobucar
SVP, CFO . . . . Susan Kluge
SVP, Chief Medical Offc . . . . Marc Keshishian, MD
General Counsel . . . . Lisa S DeMoss
Chief Information Officer . . . . William P Smith

Specialty Managed Care Partners
Enters into Contracts with Regional Business Coalitions: Yes

Employer References
General Motors, Ford Motor Company, State of Michigan, Federal
Employee Program, Daimler Chrysler

---

547   Blue Care Network of Michigan: Medicare
P.O. Box 68767
Grand Rapids, MI 48086-5043
Toll-Free: 800-662-6667
Fax: 248-799-6327
www.mibcn.com

Healthplan and Services Defined
PLAN TYPE: Medicare
Benefits Offered: Chiropractic, Disease Management, Home Care,
Inpatient SNF, Physical Therapy, Podiatry, Prescription,
Psychiatric, Wellness

Type of Coverage
Individual, Medicare

Geographic Areas Served
Available in Michigan within specific counties - contact Blue Care
Network of Michigan for further information

Subscriber Information
Average Monthly Fee Per Subscriber
(Employee + Employer Contribution):
Employee Only (Self): Varies
Medicare: Varies
Average Annual Deductible Per Subscriber:
Employee Only (Self): Varies
Medicare: Varies
Average Subscriber Co-Payment:
Primary Care Physician: Varies
Non-Network Physician: Varies
Prescription Drugs: Varies
Hospital ER: Varies
Home Health Care: Varies
Home Health Care Max. Days/Visits Covered: Varies
Nursing Home: Varies
Nursing Home Max. Days/Visits Covered: Varies

Key Personnel
President/CEO Blue Care . . . . Kevin J. Klobucar
EVP/CFO . . . . Mark R. Bartlett
EVP, Operations . . . . Darrell E. Middleton
EVP, Group Business . . . . Kenneth R. Dallafor
SVP, Subsidiary Ops. . . . . Elizabeth R. Haar
EVP, Strategy . . . . Lynda M. Rossi
SVP/Corporate Secretary . . . . Tricia A. Keith
SVP/General Auditor . . . . Michele A. Samuels
SVP, Value Partnershps . . . . David A. Share, MD
SVP/Chief Medical Officer . . . . Thomas L. Simmer, MD

VP/Treasurer . . . . Carolynn Walton

---

548   Blue Care Network: Ann Arbor
2311 Green Road
Ann Arbor, MI 48507
Toll-Free: 800-428-7361
Fax: 517-322-4315
www.mibcn.com
Non-Profit Organization: Yes
Year Founded: 1975
Federally Qualified: Yes
Number of Affiliated Hospitals: 116
Number of Primary Care Physicians: 4,500
Number of Referral/Specialty Physicians: 13,500
Total Enrollment: 620,000
State Enrollment: 620,000

Healthplan and Services Defined
PLAN TYPE: HMO
Model Type: Staff
Plan Specialty: Lab, Radiology
Benefits Offered: Behavioral Health, Dental, Disease Management,
Prescription, Psychiatric, Wellness
Offers Demand Management Patient Information Service: Yes

Type of Coverage
Commercial, Individual, Supplemental Medicare
Catastrophic Illness Benefit: Varies per case

Type of Payment Plans Offered
POS, DFFS, Capitated, FFS, Combination FFS & DFFS

Geographic Areas Served
Clinton, Eaton, Ingham, Ionia, Jackson, Livingston, Shiawassee
counties

Subscriber Information
Average Monthly Fee Per Subscriber
(Employee + Employer Contribution):
Employee Only (Self): Varies by plan
Employee & 1 Family Member: $365.40
Average Annual Deductible Per Subscriber:
Employee Only (Self): $0
Employee & 1 Family Member: $0
Employee & 2 Family Members: $0
Medicare: $0
Average Subscriber Co-Payment:
Primary Care Physician: $0
Home Health Care: $0
Home Health Care Max. Days/Visits Covered: Unlimited
Nursing Home: $0
Nursing Home Max. Days/Visits Covered: 45 days

Network Qualifications
Pre-Admission Certification: Yes

Peer Review Type
Utilization Review: Yes
Second Surgical Opinion: Yes
Case Management: Yes

Publishes and Distributes Report Card: Yes

Accreditation Certification
AAAHC, URAC, AAPI, NCQA
TJC Accreditation, Medicare Approved, Utilization Review,
Pre-Admission Certification, State Licensure, Quality Assurance
Program

Key Personnel
President/CEO BCBSMi . . . . Richard E Whitmer
President/CEO Blue Care . . . . Kevin L Seitz
CFO . . . . Mark R Bartlett
Chief Medical Officer . . . . Thomas L Simmer, MD
Chief Information Officer . . . . William P Smith

Average Claim Compensation
Physician's Fees Charged: 1%

Specialty Managed Care Partners
Enters into Contracts with Regional Business Coalitions: Yes

---

549 Blue Care Network: Flint

4520 Linden Creek Parkway
Suite A
Flint, MI 48507
Toll-Free: 800-654-3708
Phone: 810-720-6715
Fax: 810-720-6778
www.micbn.com
Subsidiary of: Blue Cross Blue Shield
Non-Profit Organization: Yes
Number of Affiliated Hospitals: 116
Number of Primary Care Physicians: 4,500
Number of Referral/Specialty Physicians: 13,500
Total Enrollment: 620,000
State Enrollment: 620,000

Healthplan and Services Defined
PLAN TYPE: HMO
Plan Specialty: Lab, Radiology
Benefits Offered: Behavioral Health, Disease Management,
Prescription, Psychiatric, Wellness

Type of Coverage
Commercial, Individual, Indemnity, Supplemental Medicare

Type of Payment Plans Offered
DFFS, Capitated

Publishes and Distributes Report Card: Yes

Key Personnel
Chief Executive Officer . . . . Richard E Whitmer
President/CEO Blue Care . . . . Kevin L Seitz
Chief Financial Officer . . . . Mark R Bartlett
Chief Medical Officer . . . . Thomas L Simmer, MD
General Counsel . . . . Lisa S DeMoss
Chief Information Officer . . . . William P Smith

---

550 Blue Care Network: Great Lakes, Muskegon Heights

611 Cascade W Parkway SE
Grand Rapids, MI 49546
Phone: 616-389-2060
Fax: 616-389-2115
www.mibcn.com
Non-Profit Organization: Yes
Year Founded: 1984
Federally Qualified: Yes
Number of Affiliated Hospitals: 116
Number of Primary Care Physicians: 4,500
Number of Referral/Specialty Physicians: 13,500
Total Enrollment: 620,000
State Enrollment: 620,000

Healthplan and Services Defined
PLAN TYPE: HMO
Model Type: IPA
Plan Specialty: Lab, Radiology
Benefits Offered: Behavioral Health, Dental, Disease Management,
Physical Therapy, Prescription, Psychiatric, Vision, Wellness

Type of Coverage
Commercial, Individual
Catastrophic Illness Benefit: Varies per case

Type of Payment Plans Offered
POS, Capitated, Combination FFS & DFFS

Geographic Areas Served
Muskegon, Newago, Oceana & Ottawa counties

Subscriber Information
Average Monthly Fee Per Subscriber
(Employee + Employer Contribution):
Employee Only (Self): Varies
Employee & 1 Family Member: Varies
Employee & 2 Family Members: Varies
Medicare: Varies
Average Annual Deductible Per Subscriber:
Employee Only (Self): $0
Employee & 1 Family Member: $0
Employee & 2 Family Members: $0
Medicare: $0
Average Subscriber Co-Payment:
Primary Care Physician: Varies
Non-Network Physician: Varies
Prescription Drugs: Varies
Hospital ER: Varies
Home Health Care: Varies
Nursing Home: Varies

Network Qualifications
Pre-Admission Certification: Yes

Peer Review Type
Utilization Review: Yes
Second Surgical Opinion: Yes

Publishes and Distributes Report Card: Yes

Key Personnel
President and CEO . . . . Kevin L Seitz
General Counsel . . . . Lisa S DeMoss
Chief Medical Officer . . . . Thomas L Simmer, MD
Chief Information Officer . . . . William P Smith

---

551 Blue Cross Blue Shield of Michigan

600 E Lafayette Blvd
Detroit, MI 48226-2998
Toll-Free: 877-469-2583
Phone: 313-225-9000
Fax: 313-225-6764
www.bcbsm.com
Non-Profit Organization: Yes
Number of Affiliated Hospitals: 159
Number of Primary Care Physicians: 30,000
Total Enrollment: 4,300,000
State Enrollment: 4,300,000

Healthplan and Services Defined
PLAN TYPE: PPO
Other Type: Major Medical
Model Type: IPA
Plan Specialty: Lab, Radiology
Benefits Offered: Behavioral Health, Disease Management, Home
Care, Prescription, Psychiatric, Wellness, Pharmacy

Type of Coverage
Commercial, Individual, Indemnity
Catastrophic Illness Benefit: Varies per case

Geographic Areas Served
Statewide/Michigan

Subscriber Information
Average Monthly Fee Per Subscriber
(Employee + Employer Contribution):
Employee Only (Self): Varies
Employee & 1 Family Member: Varies
Employee & 2 Family Members: Varies
Average Annual Deductible Per Subscriber:
Employee Only (Self): Varies

Network Qualifications
Pre-Admission Certification: Yes

Peer Review Type
Utilization Review: Yes

Second Surgical Opinion: No
Case Management: Yes

Publishes and Distributes Report Card: Yes

Accreditation Certification

TJC Accreditation, Medicare Approved, Utilization Review, Pre-Admission Certification, State Licensure, Quality Assurance Program

Key Personnel

President & CEO	Daniel J Loepp
EVP, CFO	Mark R Bartlett
SVP, Health Care Value	Susan L Barkell
SVP, Group Sales	Kenneth R Dallafior
SVP, Subsidiary Operation	Elizabeth R Harr
VP, Corporate Secretary	Tricia A Keith
SVP, Business Efficiency	Darrell E Middleton
VP, Treasurer	Carolynn Walton
Chief Medical Officer	Thomas L Simmer, MD
Chief Information Officer	Joseph H Hohner

Specialty Managed Care Partners

Enters into Contracts with Regional Business Coalitions: Yes

552 Care Choices

34505 West Twelve Mile Road
Farmington Hills, MI 48331-3263
Toll-Free: 800-942-0954
Phone: 248-489-6365
www.carechoices.com
Subsidiary of: Priority Health
Acquired by: Priority Health
Year Founded: 1985
Number of Affiliated Hospitals: 89
Number of Primary Care Physicians: 11,500
State Enrollment: 102,752

Healthplan and Services Defined

PLAN TYPE: HMO

Plan Specialty: Lab

Benefits Offered: Behavioral Health, Disease Management, Prescription, Psychiatric, Wellness, Massage therapy

Offers Demand Management Patient Information Service: Yes

DMPI Services Offered: Health Library, Health Education Classes

Type of Coverage

Commercial

Geographic Areas Served

Livingston, Macomb, Oakland, St. Clair, Washtenaw & Wayne counties

Publishes and Distributes Report Card: Yes

Accreditation Certification

NCQA

Key Personnel

Manager	Mike Koziara
COO	Laurie Westfall
248-489-6944	
westfall@trinity-health.org	
CIO	Tammy Rupp
248-489-6915	
ruppt@trinity-health.org	
Medical Director	Gilbert Burgos, MD
248-489-6216	
burgosg@trinity-health.org	
Disease Management	Alice Albu
248-489-5181	
albua@trinity-health.org	
Provider Services	Carole Mroue
248-489-5170	
Public Relations	Ellen M Downey
248-489-6358	
downeye@trinity-health.org	

Legal Counsel	Jeanne Dunk
248-489-6707	
dunkj@trinity-health.org	
Quality Improvement	Edwin Tuller
248-489-6304	
tullere@trinity-health.org	
Human Resources	Jene Wynn
248-489-6454	
wynnj@trinity-health.org	
Marketing	Pamela Henderson
248-489-5080	
henderp@trinity-health.org	
Provider Credentialling	Lois McKinley
248-489-6271	
mckinlel@trinity-health.org	
Manager Customer Service	Miriam Bielski
248-489-5107	
bielskim@trinity-health.org	
Medical Management	Rachel Godwin
248-489-5017	
godwinr@trinity-health.org	

Specialty Managed Care Partners

Express Scripts

553 CareSource: Michigan

2900 West Road
Suite 201
East Lansing, MI 48823
Toll-Free: 800-390-7102
Phone: 517-349-9922
Fax: 517-349-5343
www.caresource-michigan.com
Non-Profit Organization: Yes
Year Founded: 1996
Number of Primary Care Physicians: 588
Number of Referral/Specialty Physicians: 3,983
Total Enrollment: 50,000
State Enrollment: 50,000

Healthplan and Services Defined

PLAN TYPE: HMO

Model Type: Network

Benefits Offered: Disease Management, Prescription, Wellness

Offers Demand Management Patient Information Service: Yes

DMPI Services Offered: 24-Hour Nurse Advice Line

Type of Coverage

Medicaid

Catastrophic Illness Benefit: Covered

Type of Payment Plans Offered

POS, DFFS, FFS, Combination FFS & DFFS

Geographic Areas Served

39 counties in Michigan

Subscriber Information

Average Subscriber Co-Payment:

Home Health Care Max. Days/Visits Covered: As necessary with pc

Nursing Home Max. Days/Visits Covered: 100/year

Network Qualifications

Pre-Admission Certification: Yes

Peer Review Type

Utilization Review: Yes

Publishes and Distributes Report Card: Yes

Accreditation Certification

TJC Accreditation, Medicare Approved, Utilization Review, Pre-Admission Certification, State Licensure, Quality Assurance Program

Key Personnel

President & CEO	Pamela Morris

Chief Operating Officer . . . . Bobby Jones
EVP, External Affairs . . . . Janet Grant
Chief Financial Officer . . . . Tarlton Thomas, III
EVP, General Counsel. . . . . Mark Chilson
Chief Technical Officerr. . . . . Paul Stoddard
Chief Medical Officer. . . . . Craig Thiele, MD

Average Claim Compensation
Physician's Fees Charged: 40%
Hospital's Fees Charged: 35%

Specialty Managed Care Partners
Enters into Contracts with Regional Business Coalitions: Yes

---

554   CIGNA HealthCare of Michigan
400 Galleria Officenter
Suite 500
Southfield, MI 48034
Toll-Free: 866-438-2446
Phone: 248-226-9400
Fax: 248-226-9425
www.cigna.com
For Profit Organization: Yes

Healthplan and Services Defined
PLAN TYPE: PPO

Type of Coverage
Commercial

---

555   Cofinity
28588 Northwestern Highway
Southfield, MI 48034
Toll-Free: 800-831-1166
Fax: 888-499-3957
www.cofinity.net
Subsidiary of: Division of Aetna
For Profit Organization: Yes
Year Founded: 1979
Physician Owned Organization: Yes
Total Enrollment: 2,500,000

Healthplan and Services Defined
PLAN TYPE: PPO
Other Type: TPA
Model Type: Network
Plan Specialty: Behavioral Health, Chiropractic, Disease
Management, EPO, Lab, Vision, Radiology, Worker's
Compensation, UR, Medical Management, Medical Networks,
Out-of-Network Claims Mgmt, Fraud & Abuse Mgmt,
Credentialing Services
Benefits Offered: Dental, Prescription, Transplant, Worker's
Compensation

Type of Coverage
Catastrophic Illness Benefit: Varies per case

Type of Payment Plans Offered
FFS

Geographic Areas Served
Statewide

Subscriber Information
Average Monthly Fee Per Subscriber
(Employee + Employer Contribution):
Employee Only (Self): $4.00
Employee & 1 Family Member: $4.00
Employee & 2 Family Members: $4.00
Average Subscriber Co-Payment:
Primary Care Physician: $15.00
Hospital ER: $50.00-75.00

Network Qualifications
Pre-Admission Certification: Yes

Peer Review Type
Utilization Review: Yes
Second Surgical Opinion: Yes
Case Management: Yes

Publishes and Distributes Report Card: No

Accreditation Certification
TJC Accreditation, Medicare Approved, Utilization Review,
Pre-Admission Certification, State Licensure, Quality Assurance
Program

Key Personnel
President. . . . . Kelly Wright
Products & Partnerships. . . . . Kathy Edelman
Sales. . . . . Doug Wilson

Average Claim Compensation
Physician's Fees Charged: 1%
Hospital's Fees Charged: 1%

Specialty Managed Care Partners
Gentiva
Enters into Contracts with Regional Business Coalitions: No

---

556   ConnectCare
4009 Orchard Drive
Suite 3021
Midland, MI 48640
Toll-Free: 888-646-2429
Phone: 989-839-1629
info@connectcare.com
www.connectcare.com
Subsidiary of: MidMichigan Health Network LLC
Non-Profit Organization: Yes
Year Founded: 1993
Physician Owned Organization: Yes
Owned by an Integrated Delivery Network (IDN): Yes
Federally Qualified: No
Number of Affiliated Hospitals: 4
Number of Primary Care Physicians: 113
Number of Referral/Specialty Physicians: 273
Total Enrollment: 17,000
State Enrollment: 36,000

Healthplan and Services Defined
PLAN TYPE: PPO
Model Type: Network
Benefits Offered: Behavioral Health, Dental, Home Care, Inpatient
SNF, Long-Term Care, Physical Therapy, Podiatry, Prescription,
Psychiatric, Wellness

Type of Coverage
Commercial, Indemnity

Type of Payment Plans Offered
POS, DFFS

Geographic Areas Served
Domiciled in central Michigan, with primary counties served
including Clare, Gladwin, Gratiot, Isabella, Midland, Montcalm and
Roscommon. Arrangement with national PPO's for coverage of
downstate and those enrollees residing outside of Michigan

Subscriber Information
Average Annual Deductible Per Subscriber:
Employee Only (Self): $275.00
Employee & 2 Family Members: $550.00

Network Qualifications
Pre-Admission Certification: Yes

Peer Review Type
Utilization Review: Yes
Second Surgical Opinion: Yes
Case Management: Yes

Accreditation Certification
NCQA

Quality Assurance Program

557   CoreSource: Michigan (NGS CoreSource)

19800 Hall Road
Clinton Township, MI 48038
Toll-Free: 800-521-1555
Phone: 586-779-7676
Fax: 586-416-3001
www.ngs.com
Mailing Address: PO Box 2310, Mt. Clemens, MI 48046
Subsidiary of: Trustmark
Year Founded: 1980
Total Enrollment: 1,100,000

Healthplan and Services Defined
  PLAN TYPE: Multiple
  Other Type: TPA
  Model Type: Network
  Plan Specialty: Claims Administration, TPA
  Benefits Offered: Behavioral Health, Home Care, Prescription,
    Transplant

Type of Coverage
  Commercial

Geographic Areas Served
  Nationwide

Accreditation Certification
  Utilization Review, Pre-Admission Certification

558   Delta Dental: Corporate Headquarters

4100 Okemos Road
Okemos, MI 48864
Toll-Free: 800-524-0149
www.deltadentalmi.com
Secondary Address: 27500 Stansbury, Farmington Hills, MI 48334
Non-Profit Organization: Yes
Year Founded: 1957
Total Enrollment: 54,000,000

Healthplan and Services Defined
  PLAN TYPE: Dental
  Other Type: Dental PPO
  Model Type: Group
  Plan Specialty: Dental
  Benefits Offered: Dental

Type of Coverage
  Commercial

Type of Payment Plans Offered
  POS, Capitated, FFS

Geographic Areas Served
  Nationwide

Network Qualifications
  Pre-Admission Certification: Yes

Peer Review Type
  Utilization Review: Yes

Publishes and Distributes Report Card: Yes

Key Personnel
  President & CEO . . . . Laura Czelada, CPA
  Enterprise Application . . . . Wael Awad
  SVP/Chief Relationships . . . . Lu Battaglieri
  VP, Quality Assurance . . . . Karen M. Green
  VP/General Counsel . . . . Jonathan S. Groat, Esq.
  SVP/Chief Actuary . . . . Toby Hall, FSA
  SVP/Chief of Staff . . . . Nancy E. Hostetler
  SVP/Chief Science Officer. . . . . Jed J. Jacobson, DDS, MS
  SVP/CFO . . . . Goran Jurkovic, CPA
  VP, HR/Administration . . . . Joadi Keck
  VP, Sales/Acct. Mgmt. . . . . Anthony Robinson
  VP, E-Commerce Support . . . . Bradley Ross

SVP/Chief, Marketing . . . . Randy A. Tasco
Specialty Managed Care Partners
  Enters into Contracts with Regional Business Coalitions: No

Employer References
  General Motors Corp, State of Michigan, Michigan Public School
    Employee Retirement System, Daimler Chrysler Corp, Dow
    Chemical Company

559   Dencap Dental Plans

45 E Milwaukee Avenue
Detroit, MI 48202
Toll-Free: 888-988-3384
Phone: 313-972-1400
Fax: 313-972-4662
sales@dencap.com
www.dencap.com
Year Founded: 1984
Number of Primary Care Physicians: 200
State Enrollment: 20,000

Healthplan and Services Defined
  PLAN TYPE: Dental
  Model Type: Network
  Plan Specialty: Dental
  Benefits Offered: Dental

Type of Coverage
  Commercial, Individual

Type of Payment Plans Offered
  DFFS, FFS

Geographic Areas Served
  Southeastern Michigan

Subscriber Information
  Average Monthly Fee Per Subscriber
    (Employee + Employer Contribution):
      Employee Only (Self): Varies
  Average Annual Deductible Per Subscriber:
    Employee Only (Self): $0
    Employee & 1 Family Member: $0
    Employee & 2 Family Members: $0
  Average Subscriber Co-Payment:
    Primary Care Physician: 25%

Peer Review Type
  Case Management: Yes

Publishes and Distributes Report Card: Yes

Accreditation Certification
  Utilization Review, Quality Assurance Program

Key Personnel
  Provider Relations Dir. . . . . Frank Berge
    fberge@dencap.com
  Director, Marketing . . . . Roger Roberts
    rroberts@dencap.com
  Account Executive . . . . Precious Stigall
    pstigall@dencap.com

Specialty Managed Care Partners
  Midwest and Dentals, Great Expression

560   DenteMax

25925 Telegraph Road
Suite 400
Southfield, MI 48033
Toll-Free: 800-752-1547
Fax: 888-586-0296
customerservices@dentemax.com
www.dentemax.com
Subsidiary of: Blue Cross/Blue Shield of Michigan
For Profit Organization: Yes

Year Founded: 1985
Number of Primary Care Physicians: 113,000
Total Enrollment: 4,500,000

Healthplan and Services Defined
PLAN TYPE: Dental
Other Type: Dental PPO
Plan Specialty: Dental
Benefits Offered: Dental

Type of Coverage
Commercial, Individual
Catastrophic Illness Benefit: None

Type of Payment Plans Offered
DFFS

Geographic Areas Served
Nationwide

Subscriber Information
Average Monthly Fee Per Subscriber
(Employee + Employer Contribution):
Employee Only (Self): Varies by plan

Network Qualifications
Pre-Admission Certification: No

Peer Review Type
Utilization Review: Yes

Accreditation Certification
Quality Assurance Program

Key Personnel
President/CEO..............................Melissa Wagner
Dental Director........................Timothy Custer, MD
Manager, Leasing Sales ....Cathy Francis
Network Operations ....Andrea Garrett
Network Support ....Quincy Glass
Regulatory ....Kathy Larking
VP, Dental Networks ....Mike Miller
Network Development ....Ignacio Quiaro von Thun
Marketing/Communications ....Kim Sharbatz
Network Development.........................James Thomas
Professional Services........................Neil Valenzuela

561 eHealthInsurance Services Inc.
11919 Foundation Place
Gold River, CA 95670
Toll-Free: 800-644-3491
webmaster@healthinsurance.com
www.e.healthinsurance.com
Year Founded: 1997

Healthplan and Services Defined
PLAN TYPE: HMO/PPO
Benefits Offered: Dental, Life, STD

Type of Coverage
Commercial, Individual, Medicare

Geographic Areas Served
All 50 states in the USA and District of Columbia

Key Personnel
Chairman & CEO..............................Gary L. Lauer
EVP/Business & Corp. Dev.....................Bruce Telkamp
EVP/Chief Technology....................Dr. Sheldon X. Wang
SVP & CFO ....Stuart M. Huizinga
Pres. of eHealth Gov. Sys ....Samuel C. Gibbs
SVP of Sales & Operations ....Robert S. Hurley
Director Public Relations.......................Nate Purpura
650-210-3115

562 Golden Dental Plans
29377 Hoover Road
Warren, MI 48093
Toll-Free: 800-451-5918
Phone: 586-573-8118
Fax: 586-573-8720
www.goldendentalplans.com
Secondary Address: 5671 Trumbell St., Detroit, MI 48208
Year Founded: 1984
Number of Primary Care Physicians: 3,200
Total Enrollment: 130,000

Healthplan and Services Defined
PLAN TYPE: Dental
Other Type: Dental HMO
Model Type: Network
Plan Specialty: Dental
Benefits Offered: Dental

Type of Payment Plans Offered
DFFS

Geographic Areas Served
Michigan, Illinois, Kentucky, Washington, DC, Maryland and Virginia

Accreditation Certification
Utilization Review, Pre-Admission Certification

563 Grand Valley Health Plan
829 Forest Hill Avenue SE
Grand Rapids, MI 49546
Phone: 616-949-2410
info@gvhp.com
www.gvhp.com
For Profit Organization: Yes
Year Founded: 1982
Number of Affiliated Hospitals: 7
Total Enrollment: 8,000
State Enrollment: 26,599

Healthplan and Services Defined
PLAN TYPE: HMO
Model Type: Staff
Plan Specialty: Radiology
Benefits Offered: Behavioral Health, Chiropractic, Disease
Management, Physical Therapy, Podiatry, Prescription, Transplant,
Vision, Wellness
Offers Demand Management Patient Information Service: Yes

Type of Coverage
Commercial

Type of Payment Plans Offered
POS

Network Qualifications
Pre-Admission Certification: Yes

Peer Review Type
Utilization Review: Yes
Second Surgical Opinion: Yes
Case Management: Yes

Publishes and Distributes Report Card: Yes

Accreditation Certification
NCQA
TJC Accreditation

Specialty Managed Care Partners
Enters into Contracts with Regional Business Coalitions: Yes

564   Great Lakes Health Plan

26957 Northwestern Highway
Suite 400
Southfield, MI 48033
Toll-Free: 800-903-5253
Phone: 248-331-4296
Fax: 248-559-4640
info@glhp.com
www.glhp.com
Subsidiary of: United Healthcare
For Profit Organization: Yes
Year Founded: 1994
Number of Affiliated Hospitals: 7
Number of Primary Care Physicians: 1,622
Number of Referral/Specialty Physicians: 4,928
Total Enrollment: 215,000
State Enrollment: 215,000

Healthplan and Services Defined
  PLAN TYPE: HMO
  Plan Specialty: Case Management
  Benefits Offered: Disease Management, Home Care, Prescription

Type of Coverage
  Medicare, Medicaid, MIChild

Type of Payment Plans Offered
  DFFS, Capitated

Geographic Areas Served
  Medicaid: Wayne, Oakland, Macomb, Washtenaw, Livingston, Lenawee, Calhoun, Hillsdale, Jackson, Berrien, Cass, Van Buren, Kalamazoo, St. Clair, Lapeer, Sanilac, Arenac, Huron, Tuscola, Saginaw, Alger, Baraga, Chippewa, Delta, Dickinson, Gogebic, Iron, Keweenaw, Houghton, Luce, Mackinac, Menominee, Marquette, Ontonogon, Schoolcraft. Commercial: Wayne, Oakland, Macomb, Washtenaw, Lapeer, Genesee, Calhoun, Jackson, Kalamazoo

Subscriber Information
  Average Monthly Fee Per Subscriber
    (Employee + Employer Contribution):
      Employee Only (Self): Varies by plan
  Average Subscriber Co-Payment:
    Home Health Care: $0
    Home Health Care Max. Days/Visits Covered: 180 days
    Nursing Home: 10%
    Nursing Home Max. Days/Visits Covered: Unlimited

Network Qualifications
  Pre-Admission Certification: Yes

Publishes and Distributes Report Card: No

Accreditation Certification
  TJC
  Utilization Review

Key Personnel
  President . . . . David Livingston
  Chief Financial Officer . . . . Guy Gauthier
  EVP . . . . Michele Oliveto Hill
  Chief Medical Director . . . . David Siegel, MD
  Legal Counsel . . . . Eric J Wexler, Esq
    248-331-4264
    ewexler@glhp.com
  Disease Management . . . . Janice Prewitt, RN/CPHQ
    248-331-4368
    jprewitt@glhp.com
  Provider Services. . . . . Sue Tomba
  Human Resources . . . . Aimee Taube
    248-331-4226
    atauve@glho.com
  VP, Health Services . . . . Rachel Godwin
  VP, Customer Operations . . . . Lisa Gray
  Marketing Director . . . . Dawn Siggett

Media Contact. . . . . Jeff Smith
  952-931-5685
  jeff.smith@uhc.com

Specialty Managed Care Partners
  Rx America
  Enters into Contracts with Regional Business Coalitions: No

565   Great-West Healthcare Michigan

26100 Northwestern Highway
Southfield, MI 48076
Toll-Free: 866-494-2111
Phone: 248-355-3919
eliginquiries@cigna.com
www.cignaforhealth.com
Secondary Address: 400 Galleria Officenter, Suite 500, Southfield, MI 48034
Subsidiary of: CIGNA HealthCare
Acquired by: CIGNA
For Profit Organization: Yes
Total Enrollment: 35,992
State Enrollment: 31,314

Healthplan and Services Defined
  PLAN TYPE: HMO/PPO
  Benefits Offered: Disease Management, Prescription, Wellness

Type of Coverage
  Commercial

Type of Payment Plans Offered
  POS, FFS

Geographic Areas Served
  Michigan

Accreditation Certification
  URAC

Specialty Managed Care Partners
  Caremark Rx

566   Health Alliance Medicare

2850 West Grand Boulevard
Detroit, MI 48202
Toll-Free: 800-801-1770
msweb1@hap.org
www.hap.org/medicare
For Profit Organization: Yes
Total Enrollment: 383,000

Healthplan and Services Defined
  PLAN TYPE: Medicare
  Other Type: HMO/PPO, POS
  Benefits Offered: Chiropractic, Dental, Home Care, Inpatient SNF, Physical Therapy, Podiatry, Prescription, Psychiatric, Wellness, Worldwide Emergency, Fitness Benefits, Hearing Exams, Preventive Services, Eye Exams & Eyeglasses, Urgent Care, Hosp

Type of Coverage
  Individual, Medicare, Group Medicare Plans

Geographic Areas Served
  Michigan statewide

Subscriber Information
  Average Monthly Fee Per Subscriber
    (Employee + Employer Contribution):
      Employee Only (Self): Varies
      Medicare: Varies
  Average Annual Deductible Per Subscriber:
    Employee Only (Self): Varies
    Medicare: Varies
  Average Subscriber Co-Payment:
    Primary Care Physician: Varies
    Non-Network Physician: Varies
    Prescription Drugs: Varies

Hospital ER: Varies
Home Health Care: Varies
Home Health Care Max. Days/Visits Covered: Varies
Nursing Home: Varies
Nursing Home Max. Days/Visits Covered: Varies

Key Personnel
President/CEO . . . . .William R. Alvin
SVP/Chief Operating Offic .Christopher Pike
SVP/Chief Medical Officer . . . . .Naim Munir
VP, Compliance & Legislat . . . . .Jeanne Dunk
Deputy General Counsel .Dan E. Champney
VP, Human Resources . . . . .Derick Adams
SVP/Chief Marketing Offic . . . . .Mary Ann Tournoux
VP, Corporate Initiatives .H. Michael Flasch

567 Health Alliance Plan

2850 West Grand Boulevard
Detroit, MI 48202
Toll-Free: 888-999-4347
Phone: 313-664-7010
Fax: 248-443-4424
msweb1@hap.org
www.hap.org
Non-Profit Organization: Yes
Year Founded: 1979
Number of Affiliated Hospitals: 157
Number of Primary Care Physicians: 18,000
Number of Referral/Specialty Physicians: 1,000
Total Enrollment: 500,000
State Enrollment: 500,000

Healthplan and Services Defined
PLAN TYPE: HMO/PPO
Other Type: EPO
Model Type: Staff
Benefits Offered: Disease Management, Prescription, Vision,
Wellness, Alternative Medicine
Offers Demand Management Patient Information Service: Yes
DMPI Services Offered: Health Education Classes

Type of Coverage
Commercial, Individual, Medicare

Type of Payment Plans Offered
POS, Capitated, FFS, Combination FFS & DFFS

Geographic Areas Served
Macomb, Monroe, Oakland, St Clair, Washtenaw & Wayne counties;
Genesse, Livingston, Laper

Network Qualifications
Pre-Admission Certification: Yes

Peer Review Type
Utilization Review: Yes
Second Surgical Opinion: No
Case Management: Yes

Publishes and Distributes Report Card: Yes

Accreditation Certification
NCQA
TJC Accreditation, Medicare Approved, Utilization Review,
Pre-Admission Certification, State Licensure, Quality Assurance
Program

Key Personnel
President/CEO . . . . .James Connelly
SVP/Chief, Medical . . . . .Naim Munir, MD
SVP/Chief, Marketing .Mary Ann Tournoux
VP, IT/CIO . . . . .Annette Marcath
Deputy General Counsel .Dan E. Champney
Chief Compliance Officer . . . . .Dawn Geisert
VP, Human Resources . . . . .Derick Adams

Specialty Managed Care Partners
Enters into Contracts with Regional Business Coalitions: Yes

568 Health Plan of Michigan

777 Woodward Avenue
Suite 600
Detroit, MI 48226
Toll-Free: 888-437-0606
Fax: 313-202-0007
memberservices.mi@mhplan.com
www.hpmich.com
Total Enrollment: 290,000
State Enrollment: 250,863

Healthplan and Services Defined
PLAN TYPE: HMO

Accreditation Certification
URAC, NCQA

569 HealthPlus of Michigan: Flint

2050 S Linden Road
Flint Township, MI 48532
Toll-Free: 800-332-9161
Phone: 810-230-2000
www.healthplus.org
Non-Profit Organization: Yes
Year Founded: 1977
Federally Qualified: Yes
Number of Affiliated Hospitals: 29
Number of Primary Care Physicians: 900
Number of Referral/Specialty Physicians: 1,800
Total Enrollment: 200,000
State Enrollment: 200,000

Healthplan and Services Defined
PLAN TYPE: HMO
Model Type: Network
Plan Specialty: Lab, Radiology
Benefits Offered: Behavioral Health, Chiropractic, Complementary
Medicine, Disease Management, Home Care, Inpatient SNF,
Long-Term Care, Physical Therapy, Podiatry, Prescription,
Psychiatric, Transplant, Vision, Wellness, Women's Health
Offers Demand Management Patient Information Service: Yes

Type of Coverage
Commercial, Individual, Medicare, Supplemental Medicare,
Medicaid, Catastrophic, TPA
Catastrophic Illness Benefit: Unlimited

Type of Payment Plans Offered
POS, DFFS, Capitated, Combination FFS & DFFS

Geographic Areas Served
Commercial Product: Bay, Genesee, Huron, Lapeer, Livingston,
Midland, Northern Oakland counties, Saginaw, Sanilac, Shiawassee,
Tuscola. Full counties: Arenac, Sanilac and St Clair

Subscriber Information
Average Monthly Fee Per Subscriber
(Employee + Employer Contribution):
Employee Only (Self): Varies by plan
Average Subscriber Co-Payment:
Nursing Home Max. Days/Visits Covered: 730 days

Network Qualifications
Pre-Admission Certification: Yes

Peer Review Type
Utilization Review: Yes
Second Surgical Opinion: Yes
Case Management: Yes

Publishes and Distributes Report Card: Yes

Accreditation Certification
NCQA
TJC Accreditation, Medicare Approved, Utilization Review,
Pre-Admission Certification, State Licensure, Quality Assurance
Program

Key Personnel
President and CEO . . . . .David Crosby
810-230-2132
dcrosby@healthplus.com
VP Finance/Operations. . . . . .Matthew Mendrygal
810-230-2179
mmendryg@healthplus.com
General Counsel . . . . .Dan E Champney, Esq
810-230-2170
dchampne@healthplus.com
CIO . . . . .Julie Boyer
810-230-2061
jboyer@healthplus.com
Medical Director. . . . . .John J Saalwaechter, MD
810-230-2027
jsaalwae@healthplus.com
Pharmacy Director. . . . . .Carrie Germain, RPh
810-230-2027
cgermain@healthplus.com
Provider Services . . . . .Elyse Berry
810-230-2001
eberry@healthplus.com
Public Relations . . . . .Richard Swenson
810-230-2196
rswenson@healthplus.com
Compliance Officer. . . . . .Theresa Schurman
tschurma@healthplus.com
Quality Improvement. . . . . .Laraine Yapo
810-230-2167
lyapo@healthplus.com
Human Resources . . . . .April Williamson
810-230-2215
awilliam@healthplus.com
Marketing. . . . . .Nancy Jenkins
810-230-2183
njenkins@healthplus.com
Health Promotions . . . . .Randy Jones
810-230-2037
rjones@healthplus.com
VP/Government Programs. . . . . .Christine Tomcala
810-230-2173
ctomcala@healthplus.com
Sr Director/UR . . . . .Meg Pointon
800-345-9956
mpointon@healthplus.com

Specialty Managed Care Partners
American Healthways
Enters into Contracts with Regional Business Coalitions: No

Employer References
General Motors, Delphi, Covenant Health Partners

---

570 **HealthPlus of Michigan: Saginaw**
5454 Hampton Place
Saginaw, MI 48604
Toll-Free: 800-942-8816
Phone: 989-797-4000
www.healthplus.org
Non-Profit Organization: Yes
Number of Affiliated Hospitals: 29
Number of Primary Care Physicians: 900
Number of Referral/Specialty Physicians: 1,800
Total Enrollment: 200,000
State Enrollment: 200,000

Healthplan and Services Defined
PLAN TYPE: HMO
Model Type: IPA
Plan Specialty: Lab, Radiology
Benefits Offered: Behavioral Health, Disease Management,
Prescription, Psychiatric, Wellness, Women's Health

Type of Coverage
Commercial, Individual, MIChild
Catastrophic Illness Benefit: Covered

Type of Payment Plans Offered
POS, Capitated, Combination FFS & DFFS

Geographic Areas Served
Bay City, Saginaw & Tuscola counties

Network Qualifications
Pre-Admission Certification: Yes

Publishes and Distributes Report Card: Yes

Accreditation Certification
NCQA

Key Personnel
CEO . . . . .David P Crosby
810-230-2132
dcrosby@healthplus.com
CFO . . . . .Matthew Mendrygal
810-230-2179
mmendryg@healthplus.com
CIO . . . . .Julie Boyer
810-230-2061
jboyer@healthplu.com
Medical Director. . . . . .John J Saalwaechter, MD
810-230-2027
jsaalwae@healthplus.com
Pharmacy Director. .Carrie Germain, RPh
810-230-2027
cgermain@healthplus.com
Legal Counsel . . . . .Dan E Champney, Esq
810-230-2170
dchampne@healthplus.com
Public Relations . . . . .Richard Swenson
810-230-2196
rswenson@healthplus.com
Compliance Officer. . . . . .Theresa Schurman
tschurman@healthplus.com
Quality Improvement. . . . . .Laraine Yapo
810-230-2167
lyapo@healthplus.com
Human Resources . . . . .April Williamson
810-230-2215
awilliam@healthplus.com
Marketing. . . . . .Nancy Jenkins
810-230-2183
njenkins@healthplus.com
Health Promotions . . . . .Randy Jones
810-230-2037
rjones@healthplus.com
VP/Government Programs. . . . . .Christine Tomcala
810-230-2173
ctomcala@healthplus.com
Sr Director/UR . . . . .Meg Pointon
800-345-9956
mpointon@healthplus.com

---

571 **HealthPlus of Michigan: Troy**
101 West Big Beaver Road
Suite 1400
Troy, MI 48084
Toll-Free: 800-332-9161
Phone: 248-687-1420
www.healthplus.org
Non-Profit Organization: Yes

Healthplan and Services Defined
PLAN TYPE: HMO

572 HealthPlus of Michigan: Troy

101 W Big Beaver Road
Suite 1400
Troy, MI 48084
Toll-Free: 800-332-9161
Phone: 248-687-1420
customerservice@healthplus.org
www.healthplus.org
Non-Profit Organization: Yes
Number of Affiliated Hospitals: 29
Number of Primary Care Physicians: 900
Number of Referral/Specialty Physicians: 1,800
Total Enrollment: 200,000
State Enrollment: 200,000

Healthplan and Services Defined
  PLAN TYPE: HMO
  Model Type: IPA
  Plan Specialty: Lab, Radiology
  Benefits Offered: Behavioral Health, Disease Management,
    Prescription, Psychiatric, Wellness, Women's Health

Type of Coverage
  Commercial, Individual, Medicare, MIChild
  Catastrophic Illness Benefit: Covered

Type of Payment Plans Offered
  POS, Capitated, Combination FFS & DFFS

Geographic Areas Served
  Bay City, Saginaw & Tuscola counties

Publishes and Distributes Report Card: Yes

Accreditation Certification
  NCQA

573 HealthPlus Senior Medicare Plan

5454 Hampton Place
Saginaw, MI 48604
Toll-Free: 800-942-8816
Phone: 989-797-4000
customerservice@healthplus.org
www.healthplus.org
Non-Profit Organization: Yes
Number of Affiliated Hospitals: 29
Number of Primary Care Physicians: 900
Number of Referral/Specialty Physicians: 1,800
Total Enrollment: 14,000
State Enrollment: 14,000

Healthplan and Services Defined
  PLAN TYPE: Medicare
  Benefits Offered: Chiropractic, Disease Management, Home Care,
    Inpatient SNF, Physical Therapy, Podiatry, Prescription,
    Psychiatric, Vision, Wellness

Type of Coverage
  Individual, Medicare, MIChild

Geographic Areas Served
  Health Plus Senior Medicare Coverage Plans available only within
  Michigan

Subscriber Information
  Average Monthly Fee Per Subscriber
    (Employee + Employer Contribution):
      Employee Only (Self): Varies
      Medicare: Varies
  Average Annual Deductible Per Subscriber:
      Employee Only (Self): Varies
      Medicare: Varies
  Average Subscriber Co-Payment:
      Primary Care Physician: Varies
      Non-Network Physician: Varies
      Prescription Drugs: Varies

  Hospital ER: Varies
  Home Health Care: Varies
  Home Health Care Max. Days/Visits Covered: Varies
  Nursing Home: Varies
  Nursing Home Max. Days/Visits Covered: Varies

Key Personnel
  President/CEO . . . . .David Crosby
  Communications Director . . . . .Rich Swenson
  VP Health Care Services . . . . .Laraine Yapo

574 Humana Health Insurance of Michigan

5555 Glenwood Hills Parkway
Suite 150
Grand Rapids, MI 49512
Toll-Free: 800-649-0059
Phone: 616-942-6701
Fax: 616-940-3655
www.humana.com
For Profit Organization: Yes
Total Enrollment: 112,011
State Enrollment: 47,400

Healthplan and Services Defined
  PLAN TYPE: HMO/PPO
  Plan Specialty: ASO
  Benefits Offered: Disease Management, Prescription, Wellness

Type of Coverage
  Commercial, Individual

Geographic Areas Served
  Michigan

Accreditation Certification
  URAC, NCQA, CORE

Key Personnel
  President/CEO . . . . .Bruce D. Broussard
  EVP/Chief Operating Offic. . . . . .James E Murray
  SVP/CFO/Treasurer . . . . .James H. Bloem
  SVP/General Counsel . . . . .Christopher M. Todoroff

Specialty Managed Care Partners
  Caremark Rx

Employer References
  Tricare

575 M-Care

2311 Green Rd
Suite C
Ann Arbor, MI 48105-2955
Toll-Free: 877-469-2583
Phone: 734-747-8700
Fax: 734-747-7152
custserv@mcare.org
www.bcbsm.com
Subsidiary of: University of Michigan
Acquired by: Blue Care Network of Michigan
Non-Profit Organization: Yes
Year Founded: 1986
Owned by an Integrated Delivery Network (IDN): Yes
Number of Affiliated Hospitals: 30
Number of Primary Care Physicians: 5,000
Number of Referral/Specialty Physicians: 3,884
Total Enrollment: 220,000
State Enrollment: 3,944

Healthplan and Services Defined
  PLAN TYPE: PPO
  Model Type: Network
  Benefits Offered: Disease Management, Prescription, Wellness
  Offers Demand Management Patient Information Service: Yes

DMPI Services Offered: HouseCall Newsletter, Health Education Classes, Health Education Resource Center, Health Related Books & Videos

Type of Coverage
Commercial, Medicaid
Catastrophic Illness Benefit: Covered

Type of Payment Plans Offered
POS, Combination FFS & DFFS

Geographic Areas Served
Ann Arbor, Clinton, Dearborn, Eaton, Genesee, Hillsdale, Howell, Ingham, Jackson, Lapeer, Livingston, Macomb, Monroe, Mt Clemens, Oakland, Pontiac, Saginaw, Shiawasee, St Clair, Washtenaw, Wayne and Wyandotte

Subscriber Information
Average Subscriber Co-Payment:
  Hospital ER: $50.00
  Nursing Home: $0
  Nursing Home Max. Days/Visits Covered: 100

Network Qualifications
Pre-Admission Certification: Yes

Peer Review Type
Second Surgical Opinion: Yes
Case Management: Yes

Accreditation Certification
NCQA
Pre-Admission Certification

Key Personnel
President . . . . Thomas Rennell
Vice President/CIO . . . . Dolph Courchaine
CFO. . . . . Gregory Hawkins
Marketing . . . . Timothy George
  734-332-2266
  tgeorge@mcare.med.umich.edu
Health Promotions . . . . Betsy Nota-Kirby
  734-332-2782
  bnotakir@mcare.med.umich.edu
Director Government Prog. . . . . Richard Nowakowski
  734-332-2314
  ricknow@mcare.med.umich.edu

Specialty Managed Care Partners
Ford Motor Company, General Motors, Pfizer, The State of Michigan, University of Michigan
Enters into Contracts with Regional Business Coalitions: Yes

576   Meritain Health: Michigan

2370 Science Parkway
Okemos, MI 48864
Toll-Free: 800-748-0003
sales@meritain.com
www.meritain.com
For Profit Organization: Yes
Year Founded: 1983
Number of Affiliated Hospitals: 110
Number of Primary Care Physicians: 3,467
Number of Referral/Specialty Physicians: 5,720
Total Enrollment: 500,000
State Enrollment: 450,000

Healthplan and Services Defined
  PLAN TYPE: PPO
  Model Type: Network
  Plan Specialty: Dental, Disease Management, Vision, Radiology, UR
  Benefits Offered: Prescription
  Offers Demand Management Patient Information Service: Yes

Type of Coverage
Commercial

Geographic Areas Served
Nationwide

Subscriber Information
Average Monthly Fee Per Subscriber
  (Employee + Employer Contribution):
    Employee Only (Self): Varies by plan

Accreditation Certification
URAC
TJC Accreditation, Medicare Approved, Utilization Review, Pre-Admission Certification, State Licensure, Quality Assurance Program

Average Claim Compensation
Physician's Fees Charged: 78%
Hospital's Fees Charged: 90%

Specialty Managed Care Partners
Express Scripts, LabOne, Interactive Health Solutions

577   Molina Healthcare: Michigan

100 West Big Beaver Road
Suite 600
Troy, MI 48084
Toll-Free: 888-898-7969
Phone: 248-925-1700
www.molinahealthcare.com
For Profit Organization: Yes
Year Founded: 1980
Physician Owned Organization: Yes
Number of Affiliated Hospitals: 84
Number of Primary Care Physicians: 2,167
Number of Referral/Specialty Physicians: 6,184
Total Enrollment: 1,400,000

Healthplan and Services Defined
  PLAN TYPE: HMO
  Model Type: Network
  Benefits Offered: Chiropractic, Dental, Home Care, Inpatient SNF, Long-Term Care, Podiatry, Vision

Type of Coverage
Commercial, Medicare, Supplemental Medicare, Medicaid

Accreditation Certification
URAC, NCQA

Key Personnel
President/CEO. . . . . J. Mario Molina
Chief Financial Officer . . . . John C. Molina, JD
Chief Operating Officer . . . . Terry Bayer, JD, MPH
EVP, R&D . . . . Martha Molina Bernadett, MD

578   OmniCare: A Coventry Health Care Plan

1333 Gratiot Avenue
Suite 400
Detroit, MI 48207
Toll-Free: 866-316-3784
Phone: 313-465-1500
www.omnicarehealthplan.com
Mailing Address: PO Box 7150, Claims Department, London, KY 10742
Subsidiary of: Coventry Health Plans
Non-Profit Organization: Yes
Year Founded: 1973
Number of Affiliated Hospitals: 37
Number of Primary Care Physicians: 3,076
Total Enrollment: 50,000
State Enrollment: 50,000

Healthplan and Services Defined
  PLAN TYPE: HMO
  Model Type: IPA
  Benefits Offered: Disease Management, Prescription, Wellness
  Offers Demand Management Patient Information Service: Yes
  DMPI Services Offered: Foreign Language Service, Newsletter

Type of Coverage
Commercial, Individual, Medicaid
Catastrophic Illness Benefit: Varies per case

Type of Payment Plans Offered
POS, DFFS, Capitated, FFS, Combination FFS & DFFS

Geographic Areas Served
Macomb, Monroe, Oakland, Wayne, Washtenaw counties

Subscriber Information
Average Monthly Fee Per Subscriber
(Employee + Employer Contribution):
Employee Only (Self): Varies by plan
Average Annual Deductible Per Subscriber:
Employee Only (Self): $0
Employee & 1 Family Member: $0
Employee & 2 Family Members: $0
Medicare: $0
Average Subscriber Co-Payment:
Home Health Care: $0
Home Health Care Max. Days/Visits Covered: Unlimited
Nursing Home: $0
Nursing Home Max. Days/Visits Covered: 30 days

Network Qualifications
Pre-Admission Certification: Yes

Peer Review Type
Utilization Review: Yes
Second Surgical Opinion: Yes
Case Management: Yes

Publishes and Distributes Report Card: Yes

Accreditation Certification
NCQA
TJC Accreditation, Medicare Approved, Utilization Review,
Pre-Admission Certification, State Licensure, Quality Assurance
Program

Key Personnel
President/CEO . . . . .Beverly Allen
CFO . . . . .Kenyata Rogers
SVP, Medicaid . . . . .Bobby Jones
Network Contracting .Marshall Katz, MD
In House Formulary . . . . .Esther Rose, RPh
Marketing . . . . .Velina Glass
Materials Management. . . . . .Solomon Payne
Medical Affairs . . . . .Robert Levine, MD
Member Services. . . . . .Marshall Howard
Provider Services . . . . .Sandra Hooks
Sales . . . . .Velina Glass

Average Claim Compensation
Physician's Fees Charged: 1%
Hospital's Fees Charged: 1%

Specialty Managed Care Partners
Enters into Contracts with Regional Business Coalitions: Yes

---

579 **Paramount Care of Michigan**

106 Park Place
Dundee, MI 48131
Toll-Free: 888-241-5604
Phone: 734-529-7800
www.paramounthealthcare.com
Subsidiary of: ProMedica Health System
For Profit Organization: Yes
Year Founded: 1988
Number of Affiliated Hospitals: 34
Number of Primary Care Physicians: 1,900
Total Enrollment: 187,000

Healthplan and Services Defined
PLAN TYPE: HMO/PPO
Benefits Offered: Disease Management, Prescription, Wellness

Type of Coverage
Commercial, Medicare

Geographic Areas Served
Southeast Michigan

Accreditation Certification
NCQA

Specialty Managed Care Partners
Express Scripts

---

580 **Physicians Health Plan of Mid-Michigan**

1400 East Michigan Avenue
Lansing, MI 48912
Toll-Free: 800-562-6197
Phone: 517-364-8400
Fax: 517-364-8460
www.phpmichigan.com
Mailing Address: PO Box 30377, Lansing, MI 48909-7877
Subsidiary of: Sparrow Health System
Non-Profit Organization: Yes
Year Founded: 1980
Owned by an Integrated Delivery Network (IDN): Yes
Number of Affiliated Hospitals: 38
Number of Primary Care Physicians: 1,063
Number of Referral/Specialty Physicians: 1,781
Total Enrollment: 68,942
State Enrollment: 68,942

Healthplan and Services Defined
PLAN TYPE: HMO
Model Type: IPA
Plan Specialty: Behavioral Health, Chiropractic, Dental, Disease
Management, Lab, PBM, Vision, Radiology, UR
Benefits Offered: Behavioral Health, Chiropractic, Dental, Disease
Management, Home Care, Inpatient SNF, Physical Therapy,
Podiatry, Prescription, Psychiatric, Transplant, Vision, Wellness,
AD&D, Life, STD, FSA

Type of Coverage
Commercial, Medicaid, Catastrophic, PPO, TPA
Catastrophic Illness Benefit: Unlimited

Type of Payment Plans Offered
POS, DFFS

Geographic Areas Served
Clinton, Eaton, Gratiot, Ionia, Ingham, Isabella, Montcalm, Saginaw
and Shiawassee counties

Subscriber Information
Average Subscriber Co-Payment:
Primary Care Physician: $10.00
Non-Network Physician: 20%
Prescription Drugs: $10.00/25.00/40.00
Hospital ER: $50.00
Home Health Care: $0
Nursing Home: $0
Nursing Home Max. Days/Visits Covered: 100

Network Qualifications
Pre-Admission Certification: Yes

Peer Review Type
Utilization Review: Yes
Second Surgical Opinion: Yes
Case Management: Yes

Publishes and Distributes Report Card: No

Accreditation Certification
URAC, NCQA
Medicare Approved, Utilization Review, Pre-Admission Certification,
State Licensure, Quality Assurance Program

Key Personnel

President/CEO . . . . Scott Wilkerson
  517-364-8400
  scott.wilkerson@phpmm.org
CFO . . . . David Vis
  517-364-8370
  david.vis@phpmm.org
Pharmacy Management . . . . Ann Hunt-Fugate
  517-364-8428
  ann.hunt@phpmm.org
VP, Sales & Marketing . . . . Kevin Kaplan
  517-364-8331
  kevin.kaplan@phpmm.org
Advertising . . . . Connie Scarpone
  517-364-8266
  connie.scarpone@phpmm.org
Medical Director . . . . Howard Burgess
  howard.burgess@phpmm.org
Community Services . . . . Larry Smith
  517-364-8263
Provider Services . . . . Gary Gonzales
  517-364-8461
  gary.gonzales@phpmm.org
Sales Administrative Assi . . . . Molly Rutan
  517-364-8273
  molly.rutan@phpmm.org

Specialty Managed Care Partners
United Behavioral Health
Enters into Contracts with Regional Business Coalitions: No

---

581 Priority Health

34505 West Twelve Mile Road
Farmington Hills, MI 48331
Toll-Free: 800-942-0954
Phone: 616-942-1820
Fax: 616-957-2529
ph-salessbd@priorityhealth.com
www.priorityhealth.com
Secondary Address: 250 East Eighth Street, Holland, MI 49423
Non-Profit Organization: Yes
Year Founded: 1986
Owned by an Integrated Delivery Network (IDN): Yes
Number of Affiliated Hospitals: 100
Number of Primary Care Physicians: 12,000
Number of Referral/Specialty Physicians: 12,000
State Enrollment: 146,000

Healthplan and Services Defined
  PLAN TYPE: HMO/PPO
  Other Type: POS
  Model Type: Network
  Plan Specialty: ASO, Behavioral Health, Chiropractic, Dental,
    Disease Management, EPO, Lab, MSO, PBM, Vision, Radiology
  Benefits Offered: Behavioral Health, Chiropractic, Complementary
    Medicine, Dental, Disease Management, Home Care, Inpatient
    SNF, Long-Term Care, Physical Therapy, Podiatry, Prescription,
    Psychiatric, Transplant, Vision, Wellness, AD&D, Life, LTD, STD
  Offers Demand Management Patient Information Service: Yes
  DMPI Services Offered: Health Library

Type of Coverage
  Commercial, Individual, Medicare, Medicaid

Type of Payment Plans Offered
  POS, DFFS, Capitated, FFS, Combination FFS & DFFS

Publishes and Distributes Report Card: Yes

Accreditation Certification
  URAC, NCQA

Key Personnel
  President & CEO . . . . Michael P. Freed
  Vice President, Chief Fin . . . . Mary Anne Jones

VP, Government Programs . . . . Leon Lamoreaux
Claims . . . . Barry Cofield
VP, Network Strategy . . . . Michael Koziara
Chief Admin Officer . . . . Deborah Phillips
Chief Marketing Officer . . . . Joan Budden
Chief Medical Officer . . . . James F Byrne, MD
VP, Medical Operations . . . . Kim Suarez
CIO & VP, Enterprise Oper . . . . James S Slubowski
VP, Sales . . . . Mark J Zickel
Media Relations . . . . Amy Miller
  616-464-8571
  amy.miller@priorityhealth.com

Specialty Managed Care Partners
Principal, Fortis Time, Secure 1, US Life and Health
Enters into Contracts with Regional Business Coalitions: Yes

---

582 Priority Health: Corporate Headquarters

1231 E Beltline NE
Grand Rapids, MI 49525-4501
Toll-Free: 800-942-0954
Phone: 616-942-0954
Fax: 616-942-5651
rob.pocock@priorityhealth.com
www.priorityhealth.com
Non-Profit Organization: Yes
Year Founded: 1986
Physician Owned Organization: Yes
Owned by an Integrated Delivery Network (IDN): Yes
Federally Qualified: No
Number of Affiliated Hospitals: 5,000
Number of Referral/Specialty Physicians: 617,000
Total Enrollment: 596,220

Healthplan and Services Defined
  PLAN TYPE: HMO
  Model Type: IPA
  Plan Specialty: ASO, Behavioral Health, Chiropractic, Dental,
    Disease Management, EPO, Lab, MSO, PBM, Vision, Radiology,
    UR
  Benefits Offered: Behavioral Health, Chiropractic, Complementary
    Medicine, Dental, Disease Management, Home Care, Inpatient
    SNF, Long-Term Care, Physical Therapy, Podiatry, Prescription,
    Psychiatric, Transplant, Vision, Wellness, AD&D, Life, LTD, STD
  Offers Demand Management Patient Information Service: No

Type of Coverage
  Commercial, Individual, Indemnity, Medicare, Medicaid
  Catastrophic Illness Benefit: Varies per case

Type of Payment Plans Offered
  DFFS, Capitated, FFS, Combination FFS & DFFS

Geographic Areas Served
  69 counties in Michigan

Subscriber Information
  Average Monthly Fee Per Subscriber
    (Employee + Employer Contribution):
      Employee Only (Self): Varies
      Employee & 1 Family Member: Varies
      Employee & 2 Family Members: Varies
      Medicare: Varies
  Average Annual Deductible Per Subscriber:
      Employee Only (Self): Varies
      Employee & 1 Family Member: Varies
      Employee & 2 Family Members: Varies
      Medicare: Varies
  Average Subscriber Co-Payment:
      Primary Care Physician: Varies
      Non-Network Physician: Varies
      Prescription Drugs: Varies
      Hospital ER: Varies
      Home Health Care: Varies

Home Health Care Max. Days/Visits Covered: Varies
Nursing Home: Varies
Nursing Home Max. Days/Visits Covered: Varies

Network Qualifications
Pre-Admission Certification: No

Peer Review Type
Utilization Review: Yes
Case Management: Yes

Publishes and Distributes Report Card: No

Accreditation Certification
NCQA
Utilization Review, Pre-Admission Certification, State Licensure,
Quality Assurance Program

Key Personnel
President and CEO . . . . .Michael P. Freed
Chief Financial Officer . . . . .Mary Anne Jones
Chief Administrative Off. . . . . .Deborah Phillips
General Counsel . . . . .Kimberly Thomas
Chief Information Officer . . . . .Krischa Winright
Dir, Pharmacy Programs . . . . .Steven Marciniak
Chief Marketing Officer . . . . .Joan Budden
Director Communications .Robert Pocock
Chief Medical Officer/VP . . . . .James F Byrne, MD
VP Sales/Client Services . . . . .Don Whitford

Specialty Managed Care Partners
Enters into Contracts with Regional Business Coalitions: Yes
National Federation of Independent Business

583   PriorityHealth Medicare Plans
1231 East Beltline Northeast
Grand Rapids, MI 49525
Toll-Free: 800-942-0954
Phone: 616-942-0954
amy.miller@priorityhealth.com
www.priorityhealth.com/medicare
Subsidiary of: PriorityHealth

Healthplan and Services Defined
PLAN TYPE: Medicare
Benefits Offered: Chiropractic, Dental, Disease Management, Home
Care, Inpatient SNF, Physical Therapy, Podiatry, Prescription,
Psychiatric, Vision, Wellness

Type of Coverage
Individual, Medicare

Geographic Areas Served
Medicare Plans available within Michigan only

Subscriber Information
Average Monthly Fee Per Subscriber
(Employee + Employer Contribution):
Employee Only (Self): Varies
Medicare: Varies
Average Annual Deductible Per Subscriber:
Employee Only (Self): Varies
Medicare: Varies
Average Subscriber Co-Payment:
Primary Care Physician: Varies
Non-Network Physician: Varies
Prescription Drugs: Varies
Hospital ER: Varies
Home Health Care: Varies
Home Health Care Max. Days/Visits Covered: Varies
Nursing Home: Varies
Nursing Home Max. Days/Visits Covered: Varies

Accreditation Certification
NCQA

Key Personnel
President and CEO . . . . .Michael P. Freed
616-942-0954

Vice President, Chief Fin .Mary Anne Jones
Chief Operating Officer . . . . .Michael Koziara
VP/General Counsel . . . . .Kimberly Thomas
Chief Medical Officer . . . . .Jay LaBine, MD

584   SVS Vision
140 Macomb Place
Mount Clemens, MI 48043
Toll-Free: 800-787-4600
Phone: 586-468-7612
customerservice@svsvision.com
www.svsvision.com
For Profit Organization: Yes
Year Founded: 1974
Number of Primary Care Physicians: 1,135
Total Enrollment: 390,000

Healthplan and Services Defined
PLAN TYPE: Vision
Other Type: Vision Plan
Plan Specialty: Vision
Benefits Offered: Disease Management, Vision, Wellness, Services
limited to vision care

Type of Payment Plans Offered
DFFS

Geographic Areas Served
Michigan; Illinois: Chicago; Indiana: Indianpolis; Kentucky:
Louisville; Tennessee: Nashville; Missouri: Kansas City & St. Louis;
Georgia: Atlanta; New York: Buffalo; Minnesota: St. Paul; Virginia:
Norfolk

Subscriber Information
Average Monthly Fee Per Subscriber
(Employee + Employer Contribution):
Employee Only (Self): Varies by plan

Network Qualifications
Pre-Admission Certification: Yes

Peer Review Type
Utilization Review: Yes
Second Surgical Opinion: Yes
Case Management: Yes

Key Personnel
President/CEO . . . . .Ronald Dooley
CFO . . . . .Janice Gonzales-Basile
VP, Sales & Marketing . . . . .Catherine Walker
586-464-1573
cwalker@svsvision.com
Medical Affairs . . . . .Robert G Farrell, Jr
Media Contact . . . . .Catherine Walker
586-464-1573
cwalker@svsvision.com

585   Total Health Care
3011 W Grand Boulevard
Suite 1600
Detroit, MI 48202
Toll-Free: 800-826-2862
Phone: 313-871-2000
thc@thc-online.com
www.totalhealthcareonline.com
Non-Profit Organization: Yes
Year Founded: 1973
Owned by an Integrated Delivery Network (IDN): Yes
Number of Affiliated Hospitals: 45
Number of Primary Care Physicians: 600
Number of Referral/Specialty Physicians: 1,500
Total Enrollment: 90,000
State Enrollment: 90,000

Healthplan and Services Defined
PLAN TYPE: HMO
Other Type: PPN, POS
Model Type: Staff
Plan Specialty: Lab, Radiology
Benefits Offered: Behavioral Health, Chiropractic, Complementary
    Medicine, Disease Management, Home Care, Inpatient SNF,
    Long-Term Care, Physical Therapy, Podiatry, Prescription,
    Psychiatric, Transplant, Vision, Wellness, Worker's Compensation,
    Alternative Treatments, Dur
Offers Demand Management Patient Information Service: Yes
DMPI Services Offered: Educational Classes and Programs, 24 hour
    nurse line

Type of Coverage
Commercial, Individual, Medicare, Medicaid

Type of Payment Plans Offered
Combination FFS & DFFS

Geographic Areas Served
Wayne, Oakland, Macomb and Genesee counties

Subscriber Information
Average Monthly Fee Per Subscriber
    (Employee + Employer Contribution):
        Employee Only (Self): $67.12
        Employee & 2 Family Members: $164.88
Average Subscriber Co-Payment:
        Primary Care Physician: $10.00
        Hospital ER: $40.00

Accreditation Certification
TJC, NCQA

Key Personnel
Executive Director . . . . Lyle Algate
CFO. . . . . Brian Efrusy
COO . . . . Randy Narowitz
Claims Manager . . . . Nancy Kowal
Compliance Officer. . . . . Karen Connolly
Pharmacy Director . . . . Karen Bunio
Marketing Manager . . . . Steven Slaga
Contracting Manager . . . . Gary Francis
Medical Director. . . . . Robyn James Arrington Jr, MD
Supervisor, Member Svcs. . . . . Natalie Burke
Chief Information Officer . . . . Sean Bumstead

Specialty Managed Care Partners
RxAmerica

Employer References
Federal Government, State of Michigan, American Airlines, Detroit
    Board of Education, Wayne County Employees

---

586   Unicare: Michigan
3200 Greenfield Road
Dearborn, MI 48120
Phone: 313-336-5550
www.unicare.com
Subsidiary of: WellPoint Health Networks
For Profit Organization: Yes
Year Founded: 1995
Total Enrollment: 1,700,000

Healthplan and Services Defined
PLAN TYPE: HMO
Model Type: Network
Benefits Offered: Behavioral Health, Chiropractic, Complementary
    Medicine, Dental, Disease Management, Home Care, Inpatient
    SNF, Long-Term Care, Physical Therapy, Podiatry, Prescription,
    Psychiatric, Transplant, Vision, Wellness, Life

Type of Coverage
Commercial, Individual, Supplemental Medicare, Medicaid

Geographic Areas Served
Illinois, Indiana, Kentucky, Ohio, Oklahoma, Michigan, Texas,
    Nevada, Massachusetts, Virginia, and Wasington DC

Network Qualifications
Pre-Admission Certification: Yes

Peer Review Type
Utilization Review: Yes
Second Surgical Opinion: Yes
Case Management: Yes

Publishes and Distributes Report Card: Yes

Accreditation Certification
NCQA
TJC Accreditation, Utilization Review, Pre-Admission Certification,
    State Licensure, Quality Assurance Program

Key Personnel
President. . . . . Mark Weinberg
Media Contact . . . . Tony Felts
    317-287-6037
    tony.felts@wellpoint.com

Specialty Managed Care Partners
WellPoint Pharmacy Management, WellPoint Dental Services,
    WellPoint Behavioral Health
Enters into Contracts with Regional Business Coalitions: Yes

---

587   United Concordia: Michigan
Fifth Avenue Place
120 5th Avenue, Suite P2503
Pittsburgh, MI 15222
Phone: 412-544-2426
ucproducer@ucci.com
www.secure.ucci.com
For Profit Organization: Yes
Year Founded: 1971
Number of Primary Care Physicians: 111,000
Total Enrollment: 8,000,000

Healthplan and Services Defined
PLAN TYPE: Dental
Plan Specialty: Dental
Benefits Offered: Dental

Type of Coverage
Commercial, Individual

Geographic Areas Served
Military personnel and their families, nationwide

---

588   UnitedHealthCare of Michigan
26957 Northwestern Highway
Suite 400
Southfield, MI 48034
Toll-Free: 800-842-3585
Fax: 248-936-1231
www.uhc.com
Subsidiary of: UnitedHealth Group
Year Founded: 1977
Number of Affiliated Hospitals: 4,200
Number of Primary Care Physicians: 460,000
Total Enrollment: 75,000,000
State Enrollment: 207,319

Healthplan and Services Defined
PLAN TYPE: HMO/PPO
Model Type: IPA, Group, Network
Plan Specialty: Lab, Radiology
Benefits Offered: Chiropractic, Dental, Physical Therapy,
    Prescription, Wellness, AD&D, Life, LTD, STD
Offers Demand Management Patient Information Service: Yes

Type of Coverage
Commercial, Individual, Indemnity, Medicare

Geographic Areas Served
Statewide

Network Qualifications
Pre-Admission Certification: Yes

Peer Review Type
Utilization Review: Yes
Second Surgical Opinion: Yes
Case Management: Yes

Publishes and Distributes Report Card: Yes

Accreditation Certification
TJC, NCQA

Key Personnel
Media Contact.............................Tracey Lempner

Specialty Managed Care Partners
Enters into Contracts with Regional Business Coalitions: Yes

589 Upper Peninsula Health Plan

228 West Washington Street
Marquette, MI 49855
Toll-Free: 800-835-2556
Phone: 906-225-7500
Fax: 906-225-7690
uphpcsw@uphp.com
www.uphp.com
Total Enrollment: 25,278
State Enrollment: 25,278

Healthplan and Services Defined
PLAN TYPE: HMO

Type of Coverage
Medicaid

Accreditation Certification
NCQA

Key Personnel
Owner ....Cynthia Nyquist
Chief Financial Officer ....Greg Gustafson

590 VSP: Vision Service Plan of Michigan

2000 Town Center
Suite 1790
Southfield, MI 48075-1254
Phone: 248-350-2082
Fax: 248-350-1645
webmaster@vsp.com
www.vsp.com
Year Founded: 1955
Number of Primary Care Physicians: 26,000
Total Enrollment: 55,000,000

Healthplan and Services Defined
PLAN TYPE: Vision
Plan Specialty: Vision
Benefits Offered: Vision

Type of Payment Plans Offered
Capitated

Geographic Areas Served
Statewide

Network Qualifications
Pre-Admission Certification: Yes

Peer Review Type
Utilization Review: Yes

Accreditation Certification
Utilization Review, Quality Assurance Program

Key Personnel
President....................................Bob Koval
CEO ....Jay Alix

Health Insurance Coverage Status and Type of Coverage by Age

Category	All Persons		Under 18 years		Under 65 years		65 years and over	
	Number	%	Number	%	Number	%	Number	%
Total population	5,363	-	1,280	-	4,637	-	725	-
Covered by some type of health insurance	4,923 *(14)*	91.8 *(0.3)*	1,208 *(6)*	94.4 *(0.4)*	4,201 *(14)*	90.6 *(0.3)*	722 *(2)*	99.5 *(0.2)*
Covered by private health insurance	4,081 *(22)*	76.1 *(0.4)*	929 *(11)*	72.6 *(0.8)*	3,545 *(22)*	76.5 *(0.5)*	535 *(5)*	73.8 *(0.7)*
Employment based	3,339 *(25)*	62.3 *(0.5)*	833 *(11)*	65.1 *(0.9)*	3,130 *(24)*	67.5 *(0.5)*	210 *(6)*	28.9 *(0.9)*
Direct purchase	840 *(15)*	15.7 *(0.3)*	101 *(6)*	7.9 *(0.5)*	467 *(14)*	10.1 *(0.3)*	374 *(7)*	51.5 *(1.0)*
Covered by TRICARE	75 *(5)*	1.4 *(0.1)*	12 *(2)*	1.0 *(0.2)*	48 *(5)*	1.0 *(0.1)*	27 *(2)*	3.8 *(0.3)*
Covered by government health insurance	1,506 *(19)*	28.1 *(0.4)*	331 *(12)*	25.9 *(0.9)*	802 *(20)*	17.3 *(0.4)*	704 *(3)*	97.1 *(0.3)*
Covered by Medicaid	779 *(20)*	14.5 *(0.4)*	329 *(12)*	25.7 *(0.9)*	708 *(20)*	15.3 *(0.4)*	71 *(4)*	9.8 *(0.5)*
Also by private insurance	132 *(6)*	2.5 *(0.1)*	51 *(5)*	4.0 *(0.4)*	95 *(6)*	2.1 *(0.1)*	36 *(2)*	5.0 *(0.3)*
Covered by Medicare	801 *(5)*	14.9 *(0.1)*	4 *(1)*	0.3 *(0.1)*	98 *(5)*	2.1 *(0.1)*	703 *(3)*	96.9 *(0.3)*
Also by private insurance	548 *(6)*	10.2 *(0.1)*	1 *(Z)*	0.1 *(0.1)*	31 *(2)*	0.7 *(0.1)*	517 *(6)*	71.3 *(0.7)*
Also by Medicaid	118 *(5)*	2.2 *(0.1)*	3 *(1)*	0.2 *(0.1)*	47 *(4)*	1.0 *(0.1)*	71 *(4)*	9.8 *(0.5)*
Covered by VA Care	132 *(5)*	2.5 *(0.1)*	2 *(1)*	0.2 *(0.1)*	54 *(4)*	1.2 *(0.1)*	78 *(3)*	10.8 *(0.4)*
Not covered at any time during the year	440 *(14)*	8.2 *(0.3)*	72 *(5)*	5.6 *(0.4)*	436 *(14)*	9.4 *(0.3)*	4 *(1)*	0.5 *(0.2)*

Note: Numbers in thousands; Figures cover 2013; Margin of error appears in parenthesis; A "Z" indicates that the value either represents or rounds to zero.
Source: U.S. Census Bureau, 2013 American Community Survey, Table HI05. Health Insurance Coverage Status and Type of Coverage by State and Age for All People: 2013

Minnesota

591 Aetna Health of Minnesota
151 Farmington Avenue
Hartford, CT 06156
Toll-Free: 800-872-3862
Phone: 860-273-0123
www.aetna.com
Partnered with: eHealthInsurance Services Inc.
For Profit Organization: Yes
Year Founded: 1987
Number of Affiliated Hospitals: 22
Number of Primary Care Physicians: 670
Total Enrollment: 11,596,230

Healthplan and Services Defined
PLAN TYPE: PPO
Other Type: POS
Model Type: IPA
Benefits Offered: Behavioral Health, Dental, Disease Management, Prescription, Vision

Type of Coverage
Commercial, Individual

Type of Payment Plans Offered
POS, DFFS, Combination FFS & DFFS

Geographic Areas Served
Statewide

Peer Review Type
Second Surgical Opinion: Yes
Case Management: Yes

Accreditation Certification
AAAHC, URAC
TJC Accreditation

Key Personnel
Chairman/CEO/President.....................Mark T Bertolini
EVP/General Counsel ....William J Casazza
EVP/CFO ....Shawn M Guertin

592 Araz Group
7201 West 78th Street
Bloomington, MN 55439
Toll-Free: 800-444-3005
info@araz.com
www.araz.com
Subsidiary of: America's PPO, HealthEZ
For Profit Organization: Yes
Year Founded: 1982
Number of Affiliated Hospitals: 260
Number of Primary Care Physicians: 18,000
Total Enrollment: 250,000
State Enrollment: 160,000

Healthplan and Services Defined
PLAN TYPE: PPO
Plan Specialty: UR
Benefits Offered: Behavioral Health, Disease Management, Prescription, Worker's Compensation, AD&D, LTD, STD

Type of Coverage
Commercial, Medicare

Geographic Areas Served
Nationwide

Accreditation Certification
Pre-Admission Certification

Key Personnel
President/CEO ....Nazie Eftekhari
CFO..Josh Kutzler

Specialty Managed Care Partners
Intracorp

593 Assurant Employee Benefits: Minnesota
6600 France Ave South
Suite 314
Minneapolis, MN 55435-1803
Toll-Free: 800-328-0153
Phone: 952-920-8990
Fax: 952-920-8218
minneapolis.rfp@assurant.com
www.assurantemployeebenefits.com
Subsidiary of: Assurant, Inc
For Profit Organization: Yes
Number of Primary Care Physicians: 112,000
Total Enrollment: 47,000

Healthplan and Services Defined
PLAN TYPE: Multiple
Plan Specialty: Dental, Vision, Long & Short-Term Disability
Benefits Offered: Dental, Vision, Wellness, AD&D, Life, LTD, STD

Type of Coverage
Commercial, Indemnity, Individual Dental Plans

Geographic Areas Served
Statewide

Subscriber Information
Average Monthly Fee Per Subscriber
(Employee + Employer Contribution):
Employee Only (Self): Varies by plan

Key Personnel
Principal....................................Amie Benson
President and Chief Execu.....................John S. Roberts
Vice President and Corpor...................Richard J. Lauria
PR Specialist...............................Megan Hutchison
816-556-7815
megan.hutchison@assurant.com

594 Avesis: Minnesota
904 Oak Pond Court
Sartell, MN 56377
Toll-Free: 888-363-1377
www.avesis.com
Year Founded: 1978
Number of Primary Care Physicians: 18,000
Total Enrollment: 2,000,000

Healthplan and Services Defined
PLAN TYPE: PPO
Other Type: Vision, Dental
Model Type: Network
Plan Specialty: Dental, Vision, Hearing
Benefits Offered: Dental, Vision

Type of Coverage
Commercial

Type of Payment Plans Offered
POS, Capitated, Combination FFS & DFFS

Geographic Areas Served
Nationwide and Puerto Rico

Publishes and Distributes Report Card: Yes

Accreditation Certification
AAAHC
TJC Accreditation

Key Personnel
CEO ....Alan Cohn
CFO..Joel Alperstein
Chief Operation Officer ....Linda Chirichella
Chief Marketing Officer.....................Michael Reamer
Chief Information Officer....................Laura Gill

595   Blue Cross & Blue Shield of Minnesota

PO Box 64560
St. Paul, MN 55164-0560
Toll-Free: 800-382-2000
Phone: 651-662-8000
www.bluecrossmn.com
Secondary Address: 3535 Blue Cross Road, Eagan, MN 55122-1154
Subsidiary of: Blue Cross Blue Shield
Non-Profit Organization: Yes
Year Founded: 1933
Owned by an Integrated Delivery Network (IDN): Yes
Number of Affiliated Hospitals: 30
Number of Primary Care Physicians: 8,000
Total Enrollment: 2,700,000
State Enrollment: 2,700,000

Healthplan and Services Defined
PLAN TYPE: HMO
Model Type: Network
Plan Specialty: Medical
Benefits Offered: Disease Management, Prescription, Wellness, Life

Type of Coverage
Individual, Medicare, Supplemental Medicare

Geographic Areas Served
Statewide

Network Qualifications
Pre-Admission Certification: Yes

Peer Review Type
Utilization Review: Yes
Second Surgical Opinion: Yes

Publishes and Distributes Report Card: Yes

Accreditation Certification
URAC, NCQA

Key Personnel
President & CEO . . . . Patricia Geraghty
SVP, Health Management . . . . James Eppel
SVP, Chief Legal Officer . . . . Scott Lynch
SVP, Public & Health Aff. . . . . Kathleen Mock
SVP, Corp Operations . . . . Patricia Riley
SVP, Chief Financial Offc . . . . Pamela Sedmak
VP, Community Relations . . . . Marsha Shotley
SVP, Chief Innovation Ofc. MaryAnn Stump
SVP, Human Resources . . . . Colleen Connors
SVP, Chief Info Officer . . . . Jay Levine

Specialty Managed Care Partners
Enters into Contracts with Regional Business Coalitions: No

Employer References
General Mills/Pillsbury, Northwest Airlines, Target

596   CIGNA HealthCare of Minnesota

11095 Viking Drive
Suite 520
Eden Prairie, MN 55344
Toll-Free: 866-438-2446
Phone: 952-996-2144
Fax: 952-996-2158
www.cigna.com
For Profit Organization: Yes
Total Enrollment: 64,977
State Enrollment: 53,490

Healthplan and Services Defined
PLAN TYPE: HMO
Benefits Offered: Disease Management, Prescription, Transplant, Wellness

Type of Coverage
Commercial

Type of Payment Plans Offered
POS, FFS

Geographic Areas Served
Minnesota

Key Personnel
President . . . . David Cordani
Chief Financial Officer . . . . Ralph Nicoletti
Executive Vice President . . . . Lisa Bacus
Chief Medical Officer . . . . Alan Muney, MD, MHA
Executive Vice President . . . . Mark Boxer

597   Delta Dental of Minnesota

NW 5772
PO Box 1450
Minneapolis, MN 55485-5772
Toll-Free: 800-906-4702
Phone: 651-406-5902
Fax: 651-406-5934
www.deltadentalmn.org
Non-Profit Organization: Yes
Year Founded: 1969
Number of Primary Care Physicians: 1,500
Total Enrollment: 54,000,000
State Enrollment: 3,500,000

Healthplan and Services Defined
PLAN TYPE: Dental
Other Type: Dental PPO
Model Type: Network
Plan Specialty: ASO, Dental
Benefits Offered: Dental

Type of Coverage
Commercial, Individual, Group
Catastrophic Illness Benefit: None

Geographic Areas Served
Minnesota, North Dakota

Subscriber Information
Average Monthly Fee Per Subscriber
(Employee + Employer Contribution):
Employee Only (Self): Varies
Employee & 1 Family Member: Varies
Employee & 2 Family Members: Varies
Average Annual Deductible Per Subscriber:
Employee Only (Self): Varies
Employee & 1 Family Member: Varies
Employee & 2 Family Members: Varies
Average Subscriber Co-Payment:
Prescription Drugs: $0
Home Health Care: $0
Nursing Home: $0

Key Personnel
President/CEO . . . . Rodney Young
Board Vice Chair . . . . Douglas A. Alger

598   eHealthInsurance Services Inc.

11919 Foundation Place
Gold River, CA 95670
Toll-Free: 800-644-3491
webmaster@healthinsurance.com
www.e.healthinsurance.com
Year Founded: 1997

Healthplan and Services Defined
PLAN TYPE: HMO/PPO
Benefits Offered: Dental, Life, STD

Type of Coverage
Commercial, Individual, Medicare

Geographic Areas Served
All 50 states in the USA and District of Columbia

Key Personnel
Chairman & CEO . . . . Gary L. Lauer
EVP/Business & Corp. Dev. . . . . Bruce Telkamp
EVP/Chief Technology . . . . Dr. Sheldon X. Wang
SVP & CFO . . . . Stuart M. Huizinga
Pres. of eHealth Gov. Sys . . . . Samuel C. Gibbs
SVP of Sales & Operations . . . . Robert S. Hurley
Director Public Relations . . . . Nate Purpura
650-210-3115

599   Evercare Health Plans
2920 Oakes Avenue
Anacortes, MN 98221
Toll-Free: 800-905-8671
Phone: 952-936-1300
Fax: 952-936-6902
www.evercareonline.com
Subsidiary of: Ovations/UnitedHealthcare Community Plan
Year Founded: 1987
Total Enrollment: 3,971
State Enrollment: 3,971

Healthplan and Services Defined
PLAN TYPE: Medicare

Type of Coverage
Medicare

Key Personnel
President . . . . Wayne Cook
EVP/Field Operations . . . . William Pastore
Chief Financial Officer . . . . Scott Fries

600   Great-West Healthcare Minnesota
11095 Viking Drive
Suite 300
Eden Prairie, MN 55344
Toll-Free: 866-494-2111
Phone: 952-942-7565
eliginquiries@cigna.com
www.cignaforhealth.com
Acquired by: CIGNA
For Profit Organization: Yes
Total Enrollment: 18,556
State Enrollment: 17,322

Healthplan and Services Defined
PLAN TYPE: HMO/PPO
Benefits Offered: Disease Management, Prescription, Wellness

Type of Coverage
Commercial

Type of Payment Plans Offered
POS, FFS

Geographic Areas Served
Minnesota

Specialty Managed Care Partners
Caremark Rx

601   Health Partners Medicare Plan
8170 33rd Avenue South
Bloomington, MN 55425
Toll-Free: 800-883-2177
Phone: 952-883-5000
http://medicare.healthpartners.com
Mailing Address: PO Box 1309, Bloomington, MN 55440-1309

Healthplan and Services Defined
PLAN TYPE: Medicare

Benefits Offered: Chiropractic, Dental, Disease Management, Home
Care, Inpatient SNF, Physical Therapy, Podiatry, Prescription,
Psychiatric, Vision, Wellness

Type of Coverage
Individual, Medicare

Geographic Areas Served
Available only within Minnesota

Subscriber Information
Average Monthly Fee Per Subscriber
(Employee + Employer Contribution):
Employee Only (Self): Varies
Medicare: Varies
Average Annual Deductible Per Subscriber:
Employee Only (Self): Varies
Medicare: Varies
Average Subscriber Co-Payment:
Primary Care Physician: Varies
Non-Network Physician: Varies
Prescription Drugs: Varies
Hospital ER: Varies
Home Health Care: Varies
Home Health Care Max. Days/Visits Covered: Varies
Nursing Home: Varies
Nursing Home Max. Days/Visits Covered: Varies

Key Personnel
President/CEO . . . . Mary Brainerd
EVP, Chief Admin Officer . . . . Kathy Cooney
SVP, General Counsel . . . . Barb Tretheway
CEO, Regions Hospital . . . . Brock Nelson
EVP, Chief Marketing Offc . . . . Andrea Walsh
Medical Director . . . . George Isham
Dir, Corp Communications . . . . Amy von Walter
952-883-5274
amy.e.vonwalter@healthpartners.com

602   HealthPartners
8170 33rd Avenue S
Bloomington, MN 55425
Toll-Free: 800-883-2177
Phone: 952-883-5000
www.healthpartners.com
Non-Profit Organization: Yes
Year Founded: 1957
Owned by an Integrated Delivery Network (IDN): Yes
Number of Affiliated Hospitals: 200
Number of Primary Care Physicians: 36,000
Number of Referral/Specialty Physicians: 650,000
Total Enrollment: 1,250,000
State Enrollment: 349,070

Healthplan and Services Defined
PLAN TYPE: HMO
Model Type: Staff, Network
Benefits Offered: Behavioral Health, Chiropractic, Dental, Disease
Management, Home Care, Inpatient SNF, Physical Therapy,
Prescription, Psychiatric, Transplant, Vision, Worker's
Compensation, Durable Medical Equipment
Offers Demand Management Patient Information Service: Yes
DMPI Services Offered: HealthPartners Nurse Navigators, CareLine,
BabyLine, Personalized Assistance Line

Type of Coverage
Commercial, Individual, Indemnity, Medicare, Supplemental
Medicare, Medicaid
Catastrophic Illness Benefit: Unlimited

Type of Payment Plans Offered
POS, Combination FFS & DFFS

Geographic Areas Served
Iowa: Allamakee, Dickinson, Emmet, Howard, Osceola counties;
Minnesota: most counties

Subscriber Information
Average Monthly Fee Per Subscriber
(Employee + Employer Contribution):
Employee Only (Self): Varies by plan
Average Annual Deductible Per Subscriber:
Employee Only (Self): $150
Average Subscriber Co-Payment:
Primary Care Physician: $10.00-20

Peer Review Type
Utilization Review: Yes
Case Management: Yes

Accreditation Certification
URAC, NCQA

Key Personnel
President/CEO................................Mary Brainerd
EVP, Chief Admin Officer.....................Kathy Cooney
SVP, General Counsel........................Barb Tretheway
CEO, Regions Hospital........................Brock Nelson
EVP, Chief Marketing Offc.....................Andrea Walsh
Medical Director.............................George Isham
Dir, Corp Communications....................Amy von Walter
952-883-5274
amy.e.vonwalter@healthpartners.com

Specialty Managed Care Partners
Alere, Accordant, RMS
Enters into Contracts with Regional Business Coalitions: Yes

Employer References
University of MN, St Paul Public Schools, The College of St
Catherine

603   HSM: Healthcare Cost Management

7805 Hudson Road
Suite 190
St Paul, MN 55125
Toll-Free: 800-432-3640
Phone: 651-501-9635
Fax: 651-501-9644
info@hsminc.com
www.hsminc.com
For Profit Organization: Yes
Year Founded: 1985
Number of Referral/Specialty Physicians: 4,000

Healthplan and Services Defined
PLAN TYPE: PPO
Model Type: Network
Plan Specialty: Chiropractic, Disease Management
Benefits Offered: Chiropractic, Complementary Medicine, Disease
Management, Physical Therapy, Accupuncture, Massage therapy,
OT, Speech

Type of Coverage
Commercial, Indemnity, Medicare, Medicaid

Type of Payment Plans Offered
POS, DFFS, Capitated, FFS, Combination FFS & DFFS

Geographic Areas Served
North Dakota, South Dakota, Minnesota, Wisconsin, Illinois,
Indiana, Ohio, Michigan, Kentucky, Iowa, Missouri, Montana, Idaho,
Nebraska, Tennessee, Kansas, Oklahoma, Utah, Arkansas, Arizona,
Georgia, Texas, Alabama

Peer Review Type
Utilization Review: Yes

Publishes and Distributes Report Card: Yes

Accreditation Certification
TJC, NCQA

Key Personnel
President/CEO................................David Olsen
Claims......................................Steve Oberg

Marketing...................................Jim Wieland
Clinical Services.........................Rick Branson, DC
CIO...Jim Cassell
Clinical Management........................Karen Froyum

Specialty Managed Care Partners
Enters into Contracts with Regional Business Coalitions: Yes

604   Humana Health Insurance of Minnesota

11010 Prairie Lake Drive
Suite 175
Eden Prairie, MN 55344
Toll-Free: 877-367-6990
Phone: 952-253-3540
Fax: 952-944-6364
www.humana.com
For Profit Organization: Yes

Healthplan and Services Defined
PLAN TYPE: HMO/PPO

Type of Coverage
Commercial, Individual

Accreditation Certification
URAC, NCQA, CORE

605   Medica Health - Medicare Plan

401 Carlson Parkway
PO Box 9310
Minnetonka, MN 55440-9310
Toll-Free: 800-234-8819
Phone: 952-992-2345
centerforhealthyaging@medica.com
http://member.medica.com/C0/medicare/default.aspx

Healthplan and Services Defined
PLAN TYPE: Medicare
Benefits Offered: Chiropractic, Dental, Disease Management, Home
Care, Inpatient SNF, Physical Therapy, Podiatry, Prescription,
Psychiatric, Vision, Wellness

Type of Coverage
Individual, Medicare

Geographic Areas Served
Available within multiple states

Subscriber Information
Average Monthly Fee Per Subscriber
(Employee + Employer Contribution):
Employee Only (Self): Varies
Medicare: Varies
Average Annual Deductible Per Subscriber:
Employee Only (Self): Varies
Medicare: Varies
Average Subscriber Co-Payment:
Primary Care Physician: Varies
Non-Network Physician: Varies
Prescription Drugs: Varies
Hospital ER: Varies
Home Health Care: Varies
Home Health Care Max. Days/Visits Covered: Varies
Nursing Home: Varies
Nursing Home Max. Days/Visits Covered: Varies

Key Personnel
President/CEO................................David Tilford
EVP/CFO/CAO................................Aaron Reynolds
SVP/Operations.............................Jana L Johnson
SVP/Medical Officer.......................Charles Faxio, MD
SVP/General Counsel.........................Jim Jacobson
SVP/Communications........................Rob Longendyke
SVP/CIO......................................Scott Boher
SVP/Government Programs....................Glenn E Andis

SVP/Healthcare Economics . . . . Mark Baird

606 Medica: Corporate Office

401 Carlson Parkway
Minnetonka, MN 55305
Toll-Free: 800-952-3455
Phone: 952-992-2900
Fax: 952-992-3700
www.medica.com
Secondary Address: 878 2nd Street South, Suite 160, Waite Park, MN 56387
Non-Profit Organization: Yes
Year Founded: 1975
Number of Affiliated Hospitals: 158
Number of Primary Care Physicians: 27,000
Total Enrollment: 1,600,000

Healthplan and Services Defined
  PLAN TYPE: PPO
  Model Type: IPA
  Benefits Offered: Behavioral Health, Chiropractic, Disease
    Management, Prescription

Type of Coverage
  Commercial, Individual, Medicare

Type of Payment Plans Offered
  FFS

Geographic Areas Served
  Aitkin, Anoka, Becker, Beltrami, Benton, Blue Earth, Brown,
  Carlton, Carver, Cass, Chisago, Clay, Clearwater, Cottonwood, Crow
  Wing, Dakota, Dodge, Douglas, Fillmore, Goodhue, Grant,
  Hennepin, Hubbard, Isanti, Itasca, Jackson, Kanabec, Koochiching,
  Lac Qui Parle, Lake, Le Sueur, Lincoln, Lyon, Mahnomen, McLeod,
  Meeker, Mille Lacs, Minneapolis, Morrison, Murray, Nicollet,
  Norman, Olmsted, Otter Tail, Pine, Polk, Pope, Ramsey, Renville,
  Rice, Rock, Scott

Subscriber Information
  Average Monthly Fee Per Subscriber
    (Employee + Employer Contribution):
      Employee Only (Self): Varies by plan
  Average Subscriber Co-Payment:
      Primary Care Physician: $15.00
      Non-Network Physician: Deductible + 20%
      Hospital ER: $60.00
      Home Health Care: 20%
      Home Health Care Max. Days/Visits Covered: 180 visits/yr.
      Nursing Home: 20%
      Nursing Home Max. Days/Visits Covered: 120/yr.

Network Qualifications
  Pre-Admission Certification: Yes

Peer Review Type
  Utilization Review: Yes
  Second Surgical Opinion: Yes
  Case Management: Yes

Publishes and Distributes Report Card: Yes

Accreditation Certification
  NCQA
  TJC Accreditation, Medicare Approved, Utilization Review,
    Pre-Admission Certification, State Licensure, Quality Assurance
    Program

Key Personnel
  President/CEO . . . . David Tilford
  CFO/CAO/EVP . . . . Aaron Reynolds
  SVP, Government Programs . . . . Glenn E Andis
  SVP, Finance & Healthcare . . . . Mark Baird
  SVP/Chief Information Off. . . . . Tim Thull
  SVP, Communications & Mar. . . . . Rob Longendyke, MD
  SVP/Commercial Markets . . . . John Naylor
  SVP/General Counsel . . . . Jim Jacobson

SVP/Operations . . . . Jana L Johnson
SVP/Human Resources . . . . Deb Knutson
Average Claim Compensation
  Physician's Fees Charged: 65%
  Hospital's Fees Charged: 60%

607 Meritain Health: Minnesota

1405 Xenium Lane
Minneapolis, MN 55441
Toll-Free: 800-925-2272
Phone: 763-557-7283
Fax: 952-593-3750
sales@meritain.com
www.meritain.com
For Profit Organization: Yes
Year Founded: 1983
Number of Affiliated Hospitals: 110
Number of Primary Care Physicians: 3,467
Number of Referral/Specialty Physicians: 5,720
Total Enrollment: 500,000
State Enrollment: 450,000

Healthplan and Services Defined
  PLAN TYPE: PPO
  Model Type: Network
  Plan Specialty: Dental, Disease Management, Vision, Radiology, UR
  Benefits Offered: Prescription
  Offers Demand Management Patient Information Service: Yes

Type of Coverage
  Commercial

Geographic Areas Served
  Nationwide

Subscriber Information
  Average Monthly Fee Per Subscriber
    (Employee + Employer Contribution):
      Employee Only (Self): Varies by plan

Accreditation Certification
  URAC
  TJC Accreditation, Medicare Approved, Utilization Review,
    Pre-Admission Certification, State Licensure, Quality Assurance
    Program

Key Personnel
  EVP/Chief Financial Offic . . . . Vincent DiMura

Average Claim Compensation
  Physician's Fees Charged: 78%
  Hospital's Fees Charged: 90%

Specialty Managed Care Partners
  Express Scripts, LabOne, Interactive Health Solutions

608 Metropolitan Health Plan

400 South 4th Street
Suite 201
Minneapolis, MN 55415
Toll-Free: 800-647-0550
Phone: 612-348-3000
Fax: 612-904-4264
mhp@co.hennepin.mn.us
www.mhp4life.org
Subsidiary of: Hennepin County
Non-Profit Organization: Yes
Year Founded: 1983
Number of Affiliated Hospitals: 8
Number of Primary Care Physicians: 200
Number of Referral/Specialty Physicians: 275
Total Enrollment: 21,000

Healthplan and Services Defined
  PLAN TYPE: HMO

Model Type: Network
Benefits Offered: Behavioral Health, Chiropractic, Disease
Management, Home Care, Inpatient SNF, Long-Term Care,
Physical Therapy, Podiatry, Prescription, Psychiatric, Transplant,
Vision
Offers Demand Management Patient Information Service: Yes
DMPI Services Offered: C.A.R.S. (Children Are Riding Safely)
carseat prog, Interpretive Services, Cell Phone Program,
Transportation Program, HealthConnection Nurse Line

Type of Coverage
Medicaid

Type of Payment Plans Offered
Combination FFS & DFFS

Geographic Areas Served
Anoka, Carver, Hennepin, Mower, Polk and Scott counties

Subscriber Information
Average Subscriber Co-Payment:
Primary Care Physician: $0
Non-Network Physician: $0
Home Health Care: $0
Nursing Home: $0

Peer Review Type
Utilization Review: Yes
Case Management: Yes

Key Personnel
Executive Director . . . . Sue Zuidema
Chief Operating Officer . . . . Cynthia MacDonald
Chief Financial Officer . . . . Tim Schultz
Compliance Officer. . . . . Christine Reiten
Medical Director . . . . Joseph C Horozaniecki, MD
Chief Information Officer. . . . . Sandy Hvizdos

Specialty Managed Care Partners
United Behavioral Health, Delta Dental, Carcmark Rx

Employer References
Hennepin County

609 MHP North Star Plans
Grain Exchange Building
400 South Fourth Street, Suite 201
Minneapolis, MN 55415
Toll-Free: 888-562-8000
Phone: 612-347-8557
Fax: 612-904-4267
mhp@co.hennepin.mn.us
www.mhpnorthstarplans.org
Healthplan and Services Defined
PLAN TYPE: Medicare
Other Type: HMO/POS
Benefits Offered: Chiropractic, Dental, Disease Management, Home
Care, Inpatient SNF, Physical Therapy, Podiatry, Prescription,
Psychiatric, Vision, Wellness

Type of Coverage
Medicare, Supplemental Medicare

Geographic Areas Served
Anoka, Carver, Dakota, Hennepin, Ramsey, Scott and Washington
counties

Subscriber Information
Average Monthly Fee Per Subscriber
(Employee + Employer Contribution):
Employee Only (Self): Varies
Medicare: Varies
Average Annual Deductible Per Subscriber:
Employee Only (Self): Varies
Medicare: Varies
Average Subscriber Co-Payment:
Primary Care Physician: Varies
Non-Network Physician: Varies

Prescription Drugs: Varies
Hospital ER: Varies
Home Health Care: Varies
Home Health Care Max. Days/Visits Covered: Varies
Nursing Home: Varies
Nursing Home Max. Days/Visits Covered: Varies

Key Personnel
Executive Director. . . . . David R Johnson

610 OptumHealth Care Solutions: Physical Health
6300 Olson Memorial Highway
Golden Valley, MN 55427
Toll-Free: 866-427-6845
Phone: 763-595-3200
Fax: 763-595-3333
engage@optumhealth.com
www.optumhealth.com
For Profit Organization: Yes
Year Founded: 1987
Number of Primary Care Physicians: 29,000
Number of Referral/Specialty Physicians: 40,000
Total Enrollment: 60,000,000

Healthplan and Services Defined
PLAN TYPE: Multiple
Model Type: Network
Plan Specialty: Behavioral Health, Chiropractic, Dental, Vision,
Worker's Compensation
Benefits Offered: Behavioral Health, Chiropractic, Complementary
Medicine, Dental, Physical Therapy, Vision, Worker's
Compensation, Alternative Medicine

Type of Coverage
Commercial, Medicare, Medicaid, Workers' Compensation, HSA

Type of Payment Plans Offered
POS, Capitated, FFS

Geographic Areas Served
Nationwide

Network Qualifications
Pre-Admission Certification: Yes

Peer Review Type
Utilization Review: Yes
Case Management: Yes

Publishes and Distributes Report Card: Yes

Accreditation Certification
URAC
Utilization Review, Quality Assurance Program

Key Personnel
Chief Financial Officer . . . . Paul Emerson
Chief Information Officer . . . . Kelly Clark
General Counsel . . . . Timothy F. Ryan
Chief Marketing Office. . . . . W. Thomas McEnery
thomas.mcenery@optumhealth.com
Sr Human Capital Partner . . . . David Sparkman
david.sparkman@optumhealth.com
Chief Medical Offier . . . . Miles Snowden, MD
miles.snowden@optumhealth.com
Chief Client Officer . . . . Russ Johannesson
russ.johannesson@optumhealth.com
Media Relations . . . . Brian Kane
763-797-2229
brian.kane@optumhealth.com

Specialty Managed Care Partners
Enters into Contracts with Regional Business Coalitions: Yes

611 Patient Choice

401 Carlson Parkway
CP 217
Minnetonka, MN 55305
Toll-Free: 800-254-6254
Phone: 952-992-1700
Fax: 952-992-1730
info@pchealthcare.com
www.patientchoicehealthcare.com
Year Founded: 1997
Number of Affiliated Hospitals: 142
Total Enrollment: 80,000

Healthplan and Services Defined
PLAN TYPE: PPO
Model Type: Network
Plan Specialty: Tiering health care delivery networks

Type of Coverage
Commercial

Geographic Areas Served
Minnesota, North Dakota, South Dakota

Publishes and Distributes Report Card: Yes

Key Personnel
Dir, Health Plan Analysis . . . . Gunnar Nelson
Director, Data Services . . . . Christopher Passauer
Provider Value Management . . . . Lisa Spann
Communications Manager . . . . Michelle Nied
952-992-1700
mnied@pchealthcare.com

Specialty Managed Care Partners
American Care Partner
Enters into Contracts with Regional Business Coalitions: Yes

612 PreferredOne

6105 Golden Hills Drive
Golden Valley, MN 55416
Toll-Free: 800-940-5049
Phone: 763-847-4000
Fax: 763-847-4010
www.preferredone.com
Mailing Address: PO Box 59052, Minneapolis, MN 55459-0052
For Profit Organization: Yes
Year Founded: 1984
Number of Affiliated Hospitals: 284
Number of Primary Care Physicians: 9,200
Number of Referral/Specialty Physicians: 11,350
Total Enrollment: 97,800
State Enrollment: 216,150

Healthplan and Services Defined
PLAN TYPE: HMO/PPO
Model Type: Network
Benefits Offered: Inpatient SNF, Physical Therapy, Podiatry,
Prescription, Psychiatric, Transplant, Vision, Wellness, Durable
Medical Equipment

Type of Coverage
Commercial, Individual
Catastrophic Illness Benefit: Varies per case

Type of Payment Plans Offered
Combination FFS & DFFS

Geographic Areas Served
Minnesota

Peer Review Type
Second Surgical Opinion: No

Accreditation Certification
URAC

Key Personnel
President/CEO . . . . Marcus Merz
EVP/Chief Marketing Off . . . . Paul Geiwitz
EVP/Chief Medical Officer . . . . John Frederick, MD
Marketing Director . . . . Dennis S. Fenster
763-847-3355
dennis.fenster@preferredone.com

613 Security Life Insurance Company of America

10901 Red Circle Drive
Minnetonka, MN 55343
Toll-Free: 800-328-4667
Phone: 952-544-2121
Fax: 952-945-3419
sales@securitylife.com
www.securitylife.com
For Profit Organization: Yes
Total Enrollment: 55,000,000

Healthplan and Services Defined
PLAN TYPE: Multiple
Other Type: Dental, Vision
Plan Specialty: Dental, Vision
Benefits Offered: Dental, Vision

Type of Coverage
Commercial, Individual

Key Personnel
Chairman . . . . Stephen Beckman
Co-Chairman . . . . JS Beckman
Executive Vice President . . . . Stuart L Sorensen

614 UCare Medicare Plan

500 Stinson Blvd NE
Minneapolis, MN 55413
Toll-Free: 877-523-1518
Phone: 612-676-3500
conact@ucare.org
www.ucare.org/members/healthplans/ufs.html
Mailing Address: PO Box 52, Minneapolis, MN 55440-0052
Number of Primary Care Physicians: 16,000
Total Enrollment: 75,000

Healthplan and Services Defined
PLAN TYPE: Medicare
Benefits Offered: Chiropractic, Dental, Disease Management, Home
Care, Inpatient SNF, Physical Therapy, Podiatry, Prescription,
Psychiatric, Vision, Wellness

Type of Coverage
Individual, Medicare

Geographic Areas Served
Available only within Minnesota

Subscriber Information
Average Monthly Fee Per Subscriber
(Employee + Employer Contribution):
Employee Only (Self): Varies
Medicare: Varies
Average Annual Deductible Per Subscriber:
Employee Only (Self): Varies
Medicare: Varies
Average Subscriber Co-Payment:
Primary Care Physician: Varies
Non-Network Physician: Varies
Prescription Drugs: Varies
Hospital ER: Varies
Home Health Care: Varies
Home Health Care Max. Days/Visits Covered: Varies
Nursing Home: Varies
Nursing Home Max. Days/Visits Covered: Varies

Key Personnel

President and CEO.............................Nancy Feldman
SVP/Chief Financial Offic ....Beth Monsrud, MD
SVP/Chief Admin Officer................Hilary Marden-Resnik
SVP, Chief Medical Office ....Russel J Kuzel, MD
SVP/General Counsel..........................Mark Traynor
SVP/Strategy & Product Mg ....Thomas Mahowald
SVP, Marketing...........................Ghita Worcester
Product Management.........................Patricia Ball
Information Systems....................Robert G Beauchamp
Health Care Economics.......................Jamie Carsello
Clinical & Quality Mgmt ....R Craig Christianson, MD
Business Services ....Renae Froemming
Sales ....Brian Eck

---

615   UCare Minnesota

500 Stinson Blvd NE
Minneapolis, MN 55413
Toll-Free: 866-457-7144
Phone: 612-676-6500
contact@ucare.org
www.ucare.org
Mailing Address: PO Box 52, Minneapolis, MN 55440-0052
Non-Profit Organization: Yes
Year Founded: 1984
Owned by an Integrated Delivery Network (IDN): Yes
Number of Affiliated Hospitals: 164
Number of Primary Care Physicians: 16,000
Number of Referral/Specialty Physicians: 9,367
Total Enrollment: 200,000

Healthplan and Services Defined
PLAN TYPE: HMO/PPO
Model Type: Network
Benefits Offered: Behavioral Health, Chiropractic, Dental, Disease
  Management, Home Care, Inpatient SNF, Physical Therapy,
  Podiatry, Prescription, Psychiatric, Transplant, Vision, Wellness,
  Durable Medical Equipment

Type of Coverage
Medicare, Supplemental Medicare, Medicaid, MinnesotaCare
Catastrophic Illness Benefit: Unlimited

Type of Payment Plans Offered
POS

Geographic Areas Served
Minnestota & western Wisconsin

Subscriber Information
Average Subscriber Co-Payment:
    Home Health Care Max. Days/Visits Covered: Unlimited
    Nursing Home Max. Days/Visits Covered: 100 days

Network Qualifications
Pre-Admission Certification: Yes

Peer Review Type
Utilization Review: Yes
Second Surgical Opinion: Yes
Case Management: Yes

Publishes and Distributes Report Card: Yes

Accreditation Certification
Medicare Approved, Utilization Review, Pre-Admission
  Certification, State Licensure, Quality Assurance Program

Key Personnel
President and CEO.............................Nancy Feldman
SVP/Chief Financial Offic ....Beth Monsrud, MD
SVP/Chief Admin Officer................Hilary Marden-Resnik
SVP, Chief Medical Office ....Russel J Kuzel, MD
SVP/General Counsel..........................Mark Traynor
SVP/Strategy & Product Mg ....Thomas Mahowald
SVP, Marketing...........................Ghita Worcester
Product Management.........................Patricia Ball

Information Systems....................Robert G Beauchamp
Health Care Economics.......................Jamie Carsello
Clinical & Quality Mgmt ....R Craig Christianson, MD
Business Services ....Renae Froemming
Sales ....Brian Eck

Specialty Managed Care Partners
Doral Dental, Chriocare, ProCare Rx, BHP
Enters into Contracts with Regional Business Coalitions: Yes

Employer References
Xcel Energy, State of Minnesota, City of Minneapolis, University of
  Minnesota, Pentair

---

616   UnitedHealthCare of Minnesota

9700 Health Care Lane
Minnetonka, MN 55343
Toll-Free: 800-842-3585
www.uhc.com
Subsidiary of: UnitedHealth Group
Year Founded: 1977
Number of Affiliated Hospitals: 4,200
Number of Primary Care Physicians: 460,000
Total Enrollment: 75,000,000

Healthplan and Services Defined
PLAN TYPE: HMO/PPO
Model Type: IPA, Group, Network
Plan Specialty: Lab, Radiology
Benefits Offered: Chiropractic, Dental, Physical Therapy,
  Prescription, Wellness, AD&D, Life, LTD, STD
Offers Demand Management Patient Information Service: Yes

Type of Coverage
Commercial, Individual, Indemnity, Medicare

Geographic Areas Served
Nationwide and Puerto Rico

Network Qualifications
Pre-Admission Certification: Yes

Peer Review Type
Utilization Review: Yes
Second Surgical Opinion: Yes
Case Management: Yes

Publishes and Distributes Report Card: Yes

Accreditation Certification
TJC, NCQA

Key Personnel
CEO ....William W McGuire, MD
President/COO ....Stephen J Hemsley
Chief Exec Officer-UHC ....Robert J Sheehy
Senior Vice Preisdent.......................David S Wichmann
General Counsel ....David J Lubben

Specialty Managed Care Partners
Enters into Contracts with Regional Business Coalitions: Yes

---

617   UnitedHealthCare of Minnesota

9700 Health Care Lane
Minnetonka, MN 55343
Toll-Free: 800-842-3585
www.uhc.com
Subsidiary of: UnitedHealth Group
For Profit Organization: Yes
Total Enrollment: 75,000,000
State Enrollment: 283,106

Healthplan and Services Defined
PLAN TYPE: HMO/PPO
Benefits Offered: Disease Management, Wellness

Type of Payment Plans Offered
DFFS

Geographic Areas Served
Statewide

Publishes and Distributes Report Card: Yes

Key Personnel
Marketing . . . . Elliot Holtz
Media Contact . . . . Mary McElrath-Jones
914-467-2039
mary_r_mcelrath-jones@uhc.com

618 UnitedHealthCare of Pennsylvania
5901 Lincoln Drive
Edina, MN 55436
www.uhc.com
Secondary Address: 6095 Marshalee Drive, Suite 200, Elkridge, MD
21075, 800-307-7820
For Profit Organization: Yes
Number of Affiliated Hospitals: 5
Number of Primary Care Physicians: 726,537
Total Enrollment: 70,000,000
State Enrollment: 283,106

Healthplan and Services Defined
PLAN TYPE: HMO/PPO
Benefits Offered: Disease Management, Wellness

Type of Payment Plans Offered
DFFS

Geographic Areas Served
Statewide

Publishes and Distributes Report Card: Yes

Accreditation Certification
AAPI, NCQA

Key Personnel
Contact . . . . Tracey Lempner
770-300-3573
tracey.lempner@uhc.com

619 UnitedHealthCare of Wisconsin: Central
9700 Health Care Lane
Minnetonka, MN 55343
Toll-Free: 800-842-3585
www.uhc.com
Secondary Address: 10701 W Research Drive, Milwaukee, WI 53226,
800-879-0071
Subsidiary of: UnitedHealth Group
For Profit Organization: Yes
Total Enrollment: 75,000,000
State Enrollment: 392,782

Healthplan and Services Defined
PLAN TYPE: HMO/PPO
Benefits Offered: Disease Management, Prescription, Wellness

Type of Coverage
Commercial, Medicare, Medicaid

Geographic Areas Served
Statewide

Key Personnel
CEO . . . . William Felsing
CFO . . . . Glen Reinhard
Media Contact . . . . Greg Thompson
312-424-6913
gregory_a_thompson@uhc.com

620 VSP: Vision Service Plan of Minnesota
8400 Normandale Lake Blvd
#920
Minneapolis, MN 55437-1085
Phone: 952-921-2360
Fax: 952-921-2383
webmaster@vsp.com
www.vsp.com
Year Founded: 1955
Number of Primary Care Physicians: 26,000
Total Enrollment: 55,000,000

Healthplan and Services Defined
PLAN TYPE: Vision
Plan Specialty: Vision
Benefits Offered: Vision

Type of Payment Plans Offered
Capitated

Geographic Areas Served
Statewide

Network Qualifications
Pre-Admission Certification: Yes

Peer Review Type
Utilization Review: Yes

Accreditation Certification
Utilization Review, Quality Assurance Program

Key Personnel
Manager . . . . Theresa Callanan

Health Insurance Coverage Status and Type of Coverage by Age

Category	All Persons		Under 18 years		Under 65 years		65 years and over	
	Number	%	Number	%	Number	%	Number	%
Total population	2,925	-	734	-	2,525	-	400	-
Covered by some type of health insurance	2,425 *(16)*	82.9 *(0.5)*	678 *(7)*	92.4 *(0.9)*	2,026 *(16)*	80.2 *(0.6)*	399 *(2)*	99.8 *(0.1)*
Covered by private health insurance	1,637 *(21)*	56.0 *(0.7)*	323 *(10)*	44.0 *(1.4)*	1,416 *(20)*	56.1 *(0.8)*	221 *(5)*	55.2 *(1.3)*
Employment based	1,317 *(19)*	45.0 *(0.6)*	272 *(9)*	37.1 *(1.3)*	1,219 *(18)*	48.3 *(0.7)*	98 *(5)*	24.5 *(1.1)*
Direct purchase	323 *(12)*	11.0 *(0.4)*	43 *(5)*	5.9 *(0.7)*	194 *(8)*	7.7 *(0.3)*	129 *(7)*	32.1 *(1.7)*
Covered by TRICARE	112 *(8)*	3.8 *(0.3)*	21 *(3)*	2.9 *(0.5)*	78 *(7)*	3.1 *(0.3)*	34 *(3)*	8.5 *(0.8)*
Covered by government health insurance	1,102 *(16)*	37.7 *(0.6)*	381 *(9)*	51.9 *(1.3)*	710 *(17)*	28.1 *(0.7)*	392 *(2)*	98.0 *(0.4)*
Covered by Medicaid	701 *(16)*	24.0 *(0.5)*	377 *(10)*	51.4 *(1.3)*	621 *(15)*	24.6 *(0.6)*	81 *(4)*	20.1 *(1.0)*
Also by private insurance	87 *(6)*	3.0 *(0.2)*	26 *(4)*	3.5 *(0.5)*	63 *(6)*	2.5 *(0.2)*	24 *(2)*	6.1 *(0.6)*
Covered by Medicare	511 *(7)*	17.5 *(0.2)*	6 *(2)*	0.8 *(0.2)*	119 *(7)*	4.7 *(0.3)*	392 *(2)*	97.9 *(0.4)*
Also by private insurance	243 *(6)*	8.3 *(0.2)*	1 *(Z)*	0.1 *(0.1)*	29 *(4)*	1.2 *(0.1)*	214 *(6)*	53.4 *(1.4)*
Also by Medicaid	140 *(6)*	4.8 *(0.2)*	3 *(1)*	0.4 *(0.1)*	59 *(5)*	2.3 *(0.2)*	81 *(4)*	20.1 *(1.0)*
Covered by VA Care	77 *(4)*	2.6 *(0.1)*	1 *(1)*	0.2 *(0.1)*	40 *(3)*	1.6 *(0.1)*	37 *(3)*	9.2 *(0.6)*
Not covered at any time during the year	500 *(16)*	17.1 *(0.5)*	56 *(6)*	7.6 *(0.9)*	499 *(16)*	19.8 *(0.6)*	1 *(Z)*	0.2 *(0.1)*

Note: Numbers in thousands; Figures cover 2013; Margin of error appears in parenthesis; A "Z" indicates that the value either represents or rounds to zero.
Source: U.S. Census Bureau, 2013 American Community Survey, Table HI05. Health Insurance Coverage Status and Type of Coverage by State and Age for All People: 2013

Mississippi

621 Aetna Health of Mississippi

151 Farmington Avenue
Hartford, CT 06156
Toll-Free: 800-872-3862
Phone: 860-273-0123
www.aetna.com
Partnered with: eHealthInsurance Services Inc.
For Profit Organization: Yes
Total Enrollment: 11,596,230

Healthplan and Services Defined
PLAN TYPE: PPO
Other Type: POS
Plan Specialty: EPO
Benefits Offered: Dental, Disease Management, Long-Term Care, Prescription, Wellness, Life, LTD, STD

Type of Coverage
Commercial, Individual

Type of Payment Plans Offered
POS, FFS

Geographic Areas Served
Statewide

Key Personnel
Chairman/CEO/President.....................Mark T Bertolini
EVP, General Counsel ....William J Casazza
EVP/CFO ....Shawn M Guertin
SVP, Marketing............................Robert E Mead
Chief Medical Officer ....Lonny Reisman, MD
SVP, Human Resources......................Elease E Wright
SVP, CIO..................................Meg McCarthy

622 CIGNA HealthCare of Mississippi

3400 Players Club Pkwy
Suite 140
Memphis, TN 38125
Toll-Free: 866-438-2446
Phone: 901-748-4100
Fax: 901-748-4104
www.cigna.com
For Profit Organization: Yes
Year Founded: 1993
Total Enrollment: 75,000,000
State Enrollment: 53,490

Healthplan and Services Defined
PLAN TYPE: HMO
Model Type: IPA
Benefits Offered: Disease Management, Prescription, Transplant, Vision, Wellness
Offers Demand Management Patient Information Service: Yes

Type of Coverage
Commercial, Individual
Catastrophic Illness Benefit: Varies per case

Type of Payment Plans Offered
POS

Geographic Areas Served
Bolivar, Calhoun, Carroll, Chickasaw, Coahoma, Grenada, Leflore, Monroe, Montgomery, Tallahatchie, Tate, Tunica, Webster, Yalobusha counties

Publishes and Distributes Report Card: Yes

Accreditation Certification
URAC, NCQA
TJC Accreditation, Medicare Approved

Key Personnel
President/CEO..............................David Mathis

CFO ....Stuart Wright
Medical Affairs...........................Frederick Buckwold
Member Services ....Chuck Utterbeck

623 Delta Dental Insurance Company

1130 Sanctuary Parkway
Suite 600
Alpharetta, GA 30004
Toll-Free: 888-858-5252
Phone: 770-645-8700
Fax: 770-518-4757
4gasales@delta.org
www.deltadentalins.com
Mailing Address: PO Box 1809, Alpharetta, GA 30023-1809
Non-Profit Organization: Yes
Number of Primary Care Physicians: 198,000
Total Enrollment: 54,000,000

Healthplan and Services Defined
PLAN TYPE: Dental
Other Type: Dental PPO
Plan Specialty: Dental
Benefits Offered: Dental

Type of Coverage
Commercial

Type of Payment Plans Offered
POS, DFFS, FFS

Geographic Areas Served
Statewide

Key Personnel
CEO.......................................Gary D Radine
VP, Public & Govt Affairs ....Jeff Album
415-972-8418
Dir/Media & Public Affair ....Elizabeth Risberg
415-972-8423

624 eHealthInsurance Services Inc.

11919 Foundation Place
Gold River, CA 95670
Toll-Free: 800-644-3491
webmaster@healthinsurance.com
www.e.healthinsurance.com
Year Founded: 1997

Healthplan and Services Defined
PLAN TYPE: HMO/PPO
Benefits Offered: Dental, Life, STD

Type of Coverage
Commercial, Individual, Medicare

Geographic Areas Served
All 50 states in the USA and District of Columbia

Key Personnel
Chairman & CEO ....Gary L. Lauer
EVP/Business & Corp. Dev..................Bruce Telkamp
EVP/Chief Technology......................Dr. Sheldon X. Wang
SVP & CFO ....Stuart M. Huizinga
Pres. of eHealth Gov. Sys ....Samuel C. Gibbs
SVP of Sales & Operations ....Robert S. Hurley
Director Public Relations.................Nate Purpura
650-210-3115

625 Health Link PPO

808 Varsity Drive
Tupelo, MS 38801
Toll-Free: 888-855-2740
Phone: 662-377-3868
Fax: 662-377-7599
www.healthlinkppo.com
Non-Profit Organization: Yes
Year Founded: 1986
Number of Affiliated Hospitals: 30
Number of Primary Care Physicians: 1,500
Total Enrollment: 155,070

Healthplan and Services Defined
  PLAN TYPE: PPO
  Benefits Offered: Dental, Prescription, Transplant, Vision, Life, LTD, STD, Major Medical

Type of Coverage
  Commercial, Individual

Geographic Areas Served
  33 counties in Mississippi & Western Alabama

Accreditation Certification
  NCQA
  Medicare Approved, Utilization Review, Pre-Admission Certification, State Licensure, Quality Assurance Program

Key Personnel
  Vice President . . . . .Wally Davis
  Health Link Manager . . . . .Rose Harvey
  Marketing . . . . .Len Grice
  Medical Affairs . . . . .Homer Horton, MD
  Information Services . . . . .Faye Perry

626 Humana Health Insurance of Mississippi

772 Lake Harbour Drive
Suite #3
Ridgeland, MS 39157
Toll-Free: 800-224-4171
Phone: 601-956-8247
Fax: 601-956-1351
www.humana.com
For Profit Organization: Yes
Total Enrollment: 78,600
State Enrollment: 2,900

Healthplan and Services Defined
  PLAN TYPE: HMO/PPO
  Plan Specialty: ASO
  Benefits Offered: Disease Management, Prescription, Wellness

Type of Coverage
  Commercial, Individual, Medicare

Geographic Areas Served
  Alabama, Mississippi

Accreditation Certification
  URAC, NCQA

Key Personnel
  CEO . . . . .Rick Remmers

Specialty Managed Care Partners
  Caremark Rx

Employer References
  Tricare

627 UnitedHealthCare of Mississippi

32 Milbranch Road
Suite 30
Hattiesburg, MS 39402
Toll-Free: 800-345-1520
mississippi_pr_team@uhc.com
www.uhc.com
Subsidiary of: UnitedHealth Group
For Profit Organization: Yes
Year Founded: 1992
Number of Affiliated Hospitals: 44
Number of Primary Care Physicians: 452
Total Enrollment: 75,000,000

Healthplan and Services Defined
  PLAN TYPE: HMO/PPO
  Model Type: IPA
  Benefits Offered: Dental, Disease Management, Prescription, Vision, Wellness, LTD, STD

Type of Coverage
  Commercial, Individual, Indemnity

Type of Payment Plans Offered
  FFS

Geographic Areas Served
  Statewide

Network Qualifications
  Pre-Admission Certification: Yes

Peer Review Type
  Utilization Review: Yes
  Second Surgical Opinion: Yes
  Case Management: Yes

Publishes and Distributes Report Card: Yes

Accreditation Certification
  NCQA
  TJC Accreditation, Medicare Approved, Utilization Review, Pre-Admission Certification, State Licensure, Quality Assurance Program

Key Personnel
  Chairman/CEO . . . . .William McGuire, MD
  President . . . . .Kim Dukes
  Media Contact . . . . .Roger Rollman
    roger_f_rollman@uhc.com

Specialty Managed Care Partners
  Enters into Contracts with Regional Business Coalitions: Yes

628 Universal Health Care Group: Mississippi

100 Central Ave
Suite 200
St. Petersburg, MS 33701
Toll-Free: 866-690-4872
Phone: 727-329-0640
www.univhc.com

Healthplan and Services Defined
  PLAN TYPE: Medicare

Type of Coverage
  Individual, Medicare, Supplemental Medicare, Medicaid

Health Insurance Coverage Status and Type of Coverage by Age

Category	All Persons		Under 18 years		Under 65 years		65 years and over	
	Number	%	Number	%	Number	%	Number	%
Total population	5,931	-	1,395	-	5,061	-	870	-
Covered by some type of health insurance	5,158 *(18)*	87.0 *(0.3)*	1,297 *(9)*	93.0 *(0.6)*	4,292 *(18)*	84.8 *(0.4)*	866 *(3)*	99.5 *(0.1)*
Covered by private health insurance	4,056 *(27)*	68.4 *(0.4)*	873 *(12)*	62.6 *(0.9)*	3,496 *(24)*	69.1 *(0.5)*	560 *(8)*	64.3 *(0.9)*
Employment based	3,327 *(26)*	56.1 *(0.4)*	757 *(12)*	54.3 *(0.9)*	3,046 *(24)*	60.2 *(0.5)*	280 *(7)*	32.2 *(0.8)*
Direct purchase	789 *(17)*	13.3 *(0.3)*	102 *(6)*	7.3 *(0.4)*	472 *(13)*	9.3 *(0.3)*	318 *(7)*	36.5 *(0.8)*
Covered by TRICARE	154 *(9)*	2.6 *(0.2)*	34 *(4)*	2.4 *(0.3)*	109 *(8)*	2.2 *(0.2)*	45 *(4)*	5.2 *(0.4)*
Covered by government health insurance	1,813 *(20)*	30.6 *(0.3)*	472 *(15)*	33.8 *(1.0)*	965 *(20)*	19.1 *(0.4)*	848 *(4)*	97.5 *(0.3)*
Covered by Medicaid	879 *(20)*	14.8 *(0.3)*	467 *(15)*	33.5 *(1.0)*	796 *(19)*	15.7 *(0.4)*	83 *(4)*	9.6 *(0.5)*
Also by private insurance	125 *(7)*	2.1 *(0.1)*	47 *(5)*	3.4 *(0.4)*	91 *(7)*	1.8 *(0.1)*	34 *(2)*	4.0 *(0.3)*
Covered by Medicare	1,032 *(9)*	17.4 *(0.1)*	6 *(2)*	0.4 *(0.1)*	185 *(7)*	3.7 *(0.1)*	847 *(4)*	97.4 *(0.3)*
Also by private insurance	596 *(8)*	10.1 *(0.1)*	1 *(Z)*	0.1 *(0.1)*	55 *(4)*	1.1 *(0.1)*	542 *(8)*	62.3 *(0.8)*
Also by Medicaid	162 *(5)*	2.7 *(0.1)*	3 *(1)*	0.2 *(0.1)*	78 *(4)*	1.5 *(0.1)*	83 *(4)*	9.6 *(0.5)*
Covered by VA Care	167 *(6)*	2.8 *(0.1)*	2 *(1)*	0.2 *(0.1)*	80 *(5)*	1.6 *(0.1)*	87 *(4)*	10.0 *(0.5)*
Not covered at any time during the year	773 *(18)*	13.0 *(0.3)*	98 *(8)*	7.0 *(0.6)*	768 *(18)*	15.2 *(0.4)*	4 *(1)*	0.5 *(0.1)*

Note: Numbers in thousands; Figures cover 2013; Margin of error appears in parenthesis; A "Z" indicates that the value either represents or rounds to zero.
Source: U.S. Census Bureau, 2013 American Community Survey, Table HI05. Health Insurance Coverage Status and Type of Coverage by State and Age for All People: 2013

Missouri

629 Aetna Health of Missouri

1 South Wacker Drive
Mail Stop F643
Chicago, IL 60606
Toll-Free: 866-582-9629
www.aetna.com
For Profit Organization: Yes
Year Founded: 1996
Federally Qualified: Yes
Total Enrollment: 10,885
State Enrollment: 10,885

Healthplan and Services Defined
PLAN TYPE: HMO
Other Type: POS
Model Type: Mixed
Benefits Offered: Behavioral Health, Chiropractic, Complementary Medicine, Dental, Home Care, Inpatient SNF, Long-Term Care, Physical Therapy, Podiatry, Prescription, Psychiatric, Transplant, Vision, Wellness

Type of Coverage
Commercial, Medicare

Geographic Areas Served
Statewide

Accreditation Certification
NCQA

Key Personnel
President . . . . Allan Ira Greenberg
CFO . . . . Joan Barnicle
CMO . . . . Haydee Muse
Pharmacy. . . . . Eric Elliot

630 American Health Care Alliance

9229 Ward Parkway
Suite 300
Kansas City, MO 64114
Toll-Free: 800-870-6252
Fax: 816-523-1098
customerservice@ahappo.com
www.ahappo.com
Mailing Address: PO Box 8530, Kansas City, MO 64114-0530
Year Founded: 1990
Number of Affiliated Hospitals: 5,745
Number of Primary Care Physicians: 190,736
Number of Referral/Specialty Physicians: 285,353
Total Enrollment: 942,000
State Enrollment: 860,000

Healthplan and Services Defined
PLAN TYPE: PPO
Model Type: Network of PPOs
Benefits Offered: Behavioral Health, Chiropractic, Complementary Medicine, Dental, Home Care, Physical Therapy, Podiatry, Prescription, Psychiatric, Vision, Wellness
Offers Demand Management Patient Information Service: Yes

Geographic Areas Served
Nationwide

Subscriber Information
Average Annual Deductible Per Subscriber:
Employee Only (Self): Varies
Employee & 1 Family Member: Varies
Employee & 2 Family Members: Varies
Medicare: Varies
Average Subscriber Co-Payment:
Primary Care Physician: Varies
Non-Network Physician: Varies

Prescription Drugs: Varies
Hospital ER: Varies
Home Health Care: Varies
Nursing Home: Varies

Publishes and Distributes Report Card: Yes

Accreditation Certification
AAAHC, URAC, AAPI, NCQA
TJC Accreditation, Medicare Approved, Utilization Review, Pre-Admission Certification, State Licensure

Key Personnel
Executive Vice President . . . . Phil Mehelic
pmehelic@ahappo.com
Director Claims. . . . . Rochelle Barrett
Director Client Service . . . . Lisa Enslinger

631 Anthem Blue Cross & Blue Shield of Missouri

1831 Chestnut Street
Saint Louis, MO 63103
Toll-Free: 800-392-8740
Phone: 314-923-4444
moreinfo@bcbsmo.com
www.anthem.com
Secondary Address: 1000 W Nifong, Columbia, MO 65203
Subsidiary of: WellPoint
For Profit Organization: Yes
Year Founded: 1985
Owned by an Integrated Delivery Network (IDN): Yes
Number of Affiliated Hospitals: 35
Number of Primary Care Physicians: 4,000
Total Enrollment: 1,100,000
State Enrollment: 900,000

Healthplan and Services Defined
PLAN TYPE: PPO
Model Type: Group
Plan Specialty: Behavioral Health, Chiropractic, Disease Management, Lab, PBM, Vision, Radiology, UR
Benefits Offered: Behavioral Health, Chiropractic, Disease Management, Home Care, Inpatient SNF, Long-Term Care, Physical Therapy, Podiatry, Prescription, Psychiatric, Transplant, Wellness, AD&D

Type of Coverage
Individual, Indemnity, Medicare, Supplemental Medicare

Type of Payment Plans Offered
POS

Geographic Areas Served
St Louis City & County; 68 other counties

Subscriber Information
Average Annual Deductible Per Subscriber:
Employee Only (Self): $200.00
Employee & 1 Family Member: $400.00
Employee & 2 Family Members: $400.00
Medicare: $0
Average Subscriber Co-Payment:
Primary Care Physician: $0
Non-Network Physician: $0
Prescription Drugs: $7.00
Hospital ER: $0
Home Health Care: $0
Home Health Care Max. Days/Visits Covered: 100 visits/yr.
Nursing Home: $0
Nursing Home Max. Days/Visits Covered: 70/yr.

Network Qualifications
Pre-Admission Certification: Yes

Peer Review Type
Utilization Review: Yes
Second Surgical Opinion: Yes

Case Management: Yes

Accreditation Certification
NCQA
TJC Accreditation, Medicare Approved, Utilization Review,
Pre-Admission Certification, State Licensure, Quality Assurance
Program

Key Personnel
President.....................................Angela Braly
CFO.......................................Sandra Van Trease
Medical Affairs............................Joseph Hughenot
Information Systems...........................Tom Ogdon
Provider Services...........................Eleanor Bencic
Sales.......................................Ed Tenholder

Average Claim Compensation
Physician's Fees Charged: 1%
Hospital's Fees Charged: 65%

---

632 Assurant Employee Benefits: Corporate Headquarters

1 Chase Manhattan Plz
#41
New York, NY 10005
Toll-Free: 800-325-8385
Phone: 212-859-7000
Fax: 816-881-8996
benefits@assurant.com
www.assurantemployeebenefits.com
Subsidiary of: Assurant, Inc
For Profit Organization: Yes
Number of Primary Care Physicians: 112,000
Total Enrollment: 47,000

Healthplan and Services Defined
PLAN TYPE: Multiple
Other Type: Benefits Insurance
Plan Specialty: Dental, Vision, Long & Short-Term Disability
Benefits Offered: Dental, Vision, Wellness, AD&D, Life, LTD, STD

Type of Coverage
Commercial, Indemnity, Individual Dental Plans

Geographic Areas Served
Nationwide

Subscriber Information
Average Monthly Fee Per Subscriber
(Employee + Employer Contribution):
Employee Only (Self): Varies by plan

Key Personnel
Interim President & CEO.....................John S. Roberts
VP & General Counsel......................Kenneth D Bowen
SVP, Risk...................................Dianna D Duvall
Vice President, Claims......................Sheryle L Ohme
SVP & CFO....................................Miles B Yakre
VP, Marketing.............................Joseph A Sevcik
SVP, Human Resources.......................Sylvia Wagner
SVP & Chief Info Officer...................Karla J Schacht
Sr VP, Sales..............................J Marc Warrington
PR Specialist.............................Megan Hutchison
  816-556-7815
  megan.hutison@assurant.com
SVP, Investor Relations.......................Melissa Kivett
  212-859-7029
  melissa.kivett@assurant.com

633 Blue Cross & Blue Shield of Kansas City

2301 Main Street
One Pershing Square
Kansas City, MO 64108
Toll-Free: 888-989-8842
Phone: 816-395-3558
Fax: 816-395-2035
www.bluekc.com
Non-Profit Organization: Yes
Year Founded: 1982
Number of Affiliated Hospitals: 56
Number of Primary Care Physicians: 1,189
Number of Referral/Specialty Physicians: 1,386
Total Enrollment: 1,000,000
State Enrollment: 1,000,000

Healthplan and Services Defined
PLAN TYPE: PPO
Model Type: Network
Benefits Offered: Behavioral Health, Chiropractic, Dental, Physical
Therapy, Podiatry, Prescription, Psychiatric

Type of Coverage
Commercial, Individual, Medicare, Supplemental Medicare
Catastrophic Illness Benefit: Maximum $2M

Type of Payment Plans Offered
POS, FFS

Geographic Areas Served
32 counties in greater Kansas City, northwest Missouri and Johnson
and Wyandotte counties in Kansas

Subscriber Information
Average Subscriber Co-Payment:
  Primary Care Physician: $10.00
  Non-Network Physician: Ded/coins.
  Prescription Drugs: $10.00/20.00/10.00
  Hospital ER: $50.00

Network Qualifications
Pre-Admission Certification: Yes

Peer Review Type
Utilization Review: Yes

Publishes and Distributes Report Card: No

Accreditation Certification
URAC, NCQA

Key Personnel
President & CEO.............................David Gentile
Group Ex, Financial & Int...................Bryan Camerlinck
Group Ex, Legal & Legisla....................Rick Kastner
CEO, Blue KC Subsidiaries..................John W Kennedy
EVP, Chief Mktg Officer....................Roger Foreman
Medical Affairs.............................Frank DiTorro
Information Services...........................Judy Bond
Media Contact..................................Sue Johnson
  816-395-3566
  susan.johnson@bluekc.com

Specialty Managed Care Partners
Enters into Contracts with Regional Business Coalitions: Yes

---

634 BlueChoice

1831 Chestnut Street
St. Louis, MO 63103
Toll-Free: 800-634-4395
Phone: 314-923-7700
www.bcbsmo.com
Subsidiary of: Bell Point
Acquired by: Anthem Blue Cross & Blue Shield
For Profit Organization: Yes
Year Founded: 1987
Owned by an Integrated Delivery Network (IDN): Yes

Number of Affiliated Hospitals: 44
Number of Primary Care Physicians: 535
Number of Referral/Specialty Physicians: 2,000
Total Enrollment: 1,159,875
State Enrollment: 68,070

Healthplan and Services Defined
PLAN TYPE: HMO
Model Type: Network
Plan Specialty: ASO, Behavioral Health, Chiropractic, Disease
Management, Lab, Vision, Radiology
Benefits Offered: Prescription

Type of Coverage
Commercial, Individual, Medicare

Type of Payment Plans Offered
POS

Geographic Areas Served
Boone, Camden, Crawford, Franklin, Gasconade, Howard, Jefferson,
Madison, Maries, Miller, Moniteau, Morgan, Osage, Phelps, Pike, St.
Charles, St. Claire, St. Louis, Warren

Network Qualifications
Pre-Admission Certification: Yes

Peer Review Type
Utilization Review: Yes
Second Surgical Opinion: No
Case Management: Yes

Publishes and Distributes Report Card: No

Accreditation Certification
NCQA
TJC Accreditation, Medicare Approved, Utilization Review, State
Licensure, Quality Assurance Program

Specialty Managed Care Partners
Well Point
Enters into Contracts with Regional Business Coalitions: No

---

635 Centene Corporation

7700 Forsyth Blvd
Centene Plaza
Saint Louis, MO 63105
Phone: 314-725-4477
hr@centene.com
www.centene.com
For Profit Organization: Yes
Year Founded: 1984
Number of Affiliated Hospitals: 23
Number of Primary Care Physicians: 1,700
Total Enrollment: 1,450,000

Healthplan and Services Defined
PLAN TYPE: HMO
Benefits Offered: Behavioral Health, Disease Management,
Long-Term Care, Prescription, Psychiatric, Vision, Wellness
Offers Demand Management Patient Information Service: Yes
DMPI Services Offered: 24/7 Nurse Line

Type of Coverage
Medicaid, SCHIP

Geographic Areas Served
Arizona, Florida, Georgia, Indiana, Massachusetts, Ohio, South
Carolina, Texas, Wisonsin

Accreditation Certification
TJC Accreditation, Medicare Approved, Utilization Review,
Pre-Admission Certification, State Licensure, Quality Assurance
Program

Key Personnel
Chairman, President, CEO . . . . Michael F Neidorff
EVP, CFO & Treasurer . . . . William N. Scheffel
EVP, Chief Admin Officer . . . . Carol E. Goldman
EVP, Corp. Secretary & Ge . . . . Keith H. Williamson

Sr VP/Medical Affairs . . . . Robert C Packman, MD
SVP, Specialty Business . . . . Jason M Harrold
SVP, New Business Integra . . . . Karen A. Bedell
EVP, Chief Info Officer . . . . Donald G Imholz
SVP, Investor Relations . . . . Edmund E Kroll
EVP, Health Plans . . . . Robert T. Hitchcock
SVP, Chief Tech Officer . . . . Glendon A Schuster
SVP, Public Affairs . . . . Toni Simonetti

---

636 Children's Mercy Pediatric Care Network

2400 Pershing Road
Suite 125
Kansas City, MO 64141
Toll-Free: 888-670-7261
www.fhp.org
Mailing Address: P.O. Box 411596, Kansas City, MO 64141
Subsidiary of: Children's Mercy Pediatric Care Network
Non-Profit Organization: Yes
Year Founded: 1996
Owned by an Integrated Delivery Network (IDN): Yes
Number of Affiliated Hospitals: 31
Number of Primary Care Physicians: 200
Number of Referral/Specialty Physicians: 2,400
Total Enrollment: 49,976
State Enrollment: 49,976

Healthplan and Services Defined
PLAN TYPE: HMO
Model Type: Network, Medicaid
Benefits Offered: Behavioral Health, Dental, Disease Management,
Home Care, Inpatient SNF, Physical Therapy, Podiatry,
Prescription, Psychiatric, Vision, Wellness

Type of Coverage
Medicaid
Catastrophic Illness Benefit: None

Geographic Areas Served
Cass, Clay, Henry, Jackson, Johnson, Lafayette, Platte, Ray, St. Claire
counties in Missouri

Subscriber Information
Average Monthly Fee Per Subscriber
(Employee + Employer Contribution):
Employee Only (Self): $0.00
Employee & 1 Family Member: $0.00
Employee & 2 Family Members: $0.00

Peer Review Type
Utilization Review: Yes
Second Surgical Opinion: Yes
Case Management: Yes

Publishes and Distributes Report Card: Yes

Key Personnel
VP/Executive Director . . . . Bob Finuf
Director, IT . . . . Bob Clark
Director, Finance . . . . Suzie Dunaway
Associate Medical Dir . . . . Michelle Haley, MD
Provider Relations Dir . . . . Pamela MK Johnson
Medical Director . . . . Timothy Johnson, DO, MMM
Dir., Medical Economics . . . . Kent Pack
Director, Clinical Svcs. . . . . Ma'ata Touslee, RN, MBA

Average Claim Compensation
Physician's Fees Charged: 50%
Hospital's Fees Charged: 60%

Specialty Managed Care Partners
Enters into Contracts with Regional Business Coalitions: Yes

Employer References
State of Missouri, Division of Medical Services, State of Kansas, SRS

637 CIGNA HealthCare of St. Louis

231 S Bemiston Avenue
Suite 500
Clayton, MO 63105
Toll-Free: 866-438-2446
Phone: 314-290-7300
Fax: 314-290-7303
www.cigna.com
For Profit Organization: Yes
Year Founded: 1984
Number of Affiliated Hospitals: 27
Total Enrollment: 8,049
State Enrollment: 8,049

Healthplan and Services Defined
  PLAN TYPE: HMO
  Other Type: POS
  Model Type: IPA
  Benefits Offered: Behavioral Health, Chiropractic, Dental, Physical
    Therapy, Podiatry, Prescription, Psychiatric, Vision
  Offers Demand Management Patient Information Service: Yes

Type of Coverage
  Commercial
  Catastrophic Illness Benefit: Varies per case

Type of Payment Plans Offered
  POS, FFS

Geographic Areas Served
  Franklin, Jefferson, Madison, Monroe, St. Charles, St. Clair, St.
  Louis counties

Subscriber Information
  Average Monthly Fee Per Subscriber
    (Employee + Employer Contribution):
      Employee Only (Self): Varies on plan
  Average Annual Deductible Per Subscriber:
    Employee Only (Self): $200.00
    Employee & 1 Family Member: $200.00
    Employee & 2 Family Members: $200.00
  Average Subscriber Co-Payment:
    Primary Care Physician: $10.00
    Prescription Drugs: $5.00-10.00
    Hospital ER: $50.00
    Home Health Care: $0
    Home Health Care Max. Days/Visits Covered: 60-120 days
    Nursing Home: $0
    Nursing Home Max. Days/Visits Covered: 60-120 days

Network Qualifications
  Pre-Admission Certification: Yes

Peer Review Type
  Utilization Review: Yes
  Second Surgical Opinion: Yes
  Case Management: Yes

Publishes and Distributes Report Card: Yes

Accreditation Certification
  NCQA

Key Personnel
  President & CEO . . . . David Cordani
  EVP/Global Chief Mkt Offi . . . . Lisa Bacus
  EVP/Global Chief Inf. Off. . . . . Mark Boxer
  Director Network Development . . . . David Bird
  Medical Affairs. . . . . Debbie Zimmerman, MD
  Information Services . . . . Jeff Robertson

Average Claim Compensation
  Physician's Fees Charged: 85%
  Hospital's Fees Charged: 75%

Specialty Managed Care Partners
  Enters into Contracts with Regional Business Coalitions: Yes

638 Community Health Improvement Solutions

Heartland Health Business Plaza
137 N Belt Highway
Saint Joseph, MO 64506
Toll-Free: 800-990-9247
Phone: 816-271-1247
Fax: 816-271-1266
www.mychp.com
Subsidiary of: Aetna
Non-Profit Organization: Yes
Year Founded: 1995
Federally Qualified: Yes
Number of Affiliated Hospitals: 34
Number of Primary Care Physicians: 578
Number of Referral/Specialty Physicians: 2,203
Total Enrollment: 7,000
State Enrollment: 25,335

Healthplan and Services Defined
  PLAN TYPE: HMO
  Model Type: Group
  Plan Specialty: ASO, Behavioral Health, Chiropractic, Disease
    Management, EPO, Lab, MSO, PBM, Vision, Radiology, Worker's
    Compensation, UR
  Benefits Offered: Behavioral Health, Chiropractic, Complementary
    Medicine, Disease Management, Home Care, Inpatient SNF,
    Long-Term Care, Physical Therapy, Podiatry, Prescription,
    Psychiatric, Transplant, Vision, Wellness, Worker's Compensation,
    Life
  Offers Demand Management Patient Information Service: Yes

Type of Coverage
  Commercial, Individual, Indemnity, Catastrophic
  Catastrophic Illness Benefit: Varies per case

Type of Payment Plans Offered
  FFS, Combination FFS & DFFS

Geographic Areas Served
  Northwest Missouri and Northeast Kansas

Publishes and Distributes Report Card: Yes

Accreditation Certification
  NCQA
  Medicare Approved, Utilization Review, State Licensure, Quality
    Assurance Program

Key Personnel
  Plan Admin . . . . Linda Bahrke
  CFO. . . . . Stan Vaughan
  Claims . . . . Marci Gillis
  Marketing/Sales. . . . . Ricard Pugh
  Medical Affairs. . . . . Robert Chabon, MD
  Provider Services. . . . . Audrey Shanley

Specialty Managed Care Partners
  Heartland Regional Medical Centre, American Family
  Enters into Contracts with Regional Business Coalitions: Yes

639 Cox Healthplans

Kelly Plaza
3200 S National, Building B
Springfield, MO 65807
Toll-Free: 800-664-1244
Phone: 417-269-4679
Fax: 417-269-4667
grouphealth@coxhealthplans.com
www.coxhealthplans.com
Mailing Address: PO Box 5750, Springfield, MO 65801-5750
Subsidiary of: CoxHealth
For Profit Organization: Yes
Number of Primary Care Physicians: 1,000
Number of Referral/Specialty Physicians: 5,000

Total Enrollment: 5,000
State Enrollment: 1,964

Healthplan and Services Defined
 PLAN TYPE: HMO/PPO
 Benefits Offered: Disease Management, Prescription, Wellness

Type of Coverage
 Commercial, Individual

Type of Payment Plans Offered
 POS

Geographic Areas Served
 Missouri

Key Personnel
 President & CEO...................................Jeff Bond
 Chief Financial Officer ....John Gamble
 Chief Operating Officer ....Matthew Aug
 Sr. Director, MIS ....Susan Butts

Specialty Managed Care Partners
 Caremark Rx

640 Delta Dental of Missouri

12399 Gravois Road
Saint Louis, MO 63127-1702
Toll-Free: 800-392-1167
Phone: 314-656-3000
Fax: 314-656-2900
service@ddpmo.org
www.deltadentalmo.com
Mailing Address: PO Box 8690, Saint Louis, MO 63126-0690
Subsidiary of: Delta Dental Plans Association
Non-Profit Organization: Yes
Year Founded: 1958
Owned by an Integrated Delivery Network (IDN): Yes
Number of Primary Care Physicians: 3,000
Total Enrollment: 54,000,000
State Enrollment: 1,400,000

Healthplan and Services Defined
 PLAN TYPE: Dental
 Other Type: Dental PPO
 Model Type: Group
 Plan Specialty: Dental
 Benefits Offered: Dental

Type of Coverage
 Commercial

Geographic Areas Served
 Statewide

Subscriber Information
 Average Monthly Fee Per Subscriber
  (Employee + Employer Contribution):
   Employee Only (Self): Varies
   Employee & 1 Family Member: Varies
   Employee & 2 Family Members: Varies
   Medicare: Varies
 Average Annual Deductible Per Subscriber:
   Employee Only (Self): Varies
   Employee & 1 Family Member: Varies
   Employee & 2 Family Members: Varies
   Medicare: Varies
 Average Subscriber Co-Payment:
   Primary Care Physician: Varies
   Non-Network Physician: Varies
   Prescription Drugs: Varies
   Hospital ER: Varies
   Home Health Care: Varies
   Home Health Care Max. Days/Visits Covered: Varies
   Nursing Home: Varies
   Nursing Home Max. Days/Visits Covered: Varies

Network Qualifications
 Pre-Admission Certification: Yes

Publishes and Distributes Report Card: No

Key Personnel
 Chief Financial Officer.........................David Haynes
 SVP, COO ....Pamela Martin
 VP, Act & Underwriting ....Rob Goren
 VP, Board Relations............................Janice M Lees
 VP, Dental Affairs ....Alcides O Martinez
 Chief Marketing/Sales ....Richard W Klassen
 Chief Information Officer......................Karl A Mudra
 Dir/Media & Public Affair ....Elizabeth Risberg
  415-972-8423

Specialty Managed Care Partners
 Enters into Contracts with Regional Business Coalitions: No

641 Dental Health Alliance

2323 Grand Boulevard
Kansas City, MO 64108
Toll-Free: 800-522-1313
dha@assurant.com
www.dha.com
Subsidiary of: Union Security Insurance Company, Assurant Employee
 Benefits
Year Founded: 1994
Number of Primary Care Physicians: 74,000
Total Enrollment: 1,700,000

Healthplan and Services Defined
 PLAN TYPE: Dental
 Other Type: Dental PPO Network
 Model Type: Network, Dental PPO Network
 Plan Specialty: Dental
 Benefits Offered: Dental

Type of Coverage
 Commercial

Type of Payment Plans Offered
 POS, FFS, Combination FFS & DFFS

Geographic Areas Served
 Nationwide

Network Qualifications
 Pre-Admission Certification: No

Peer Review Type
 Utilization Review: Yes

Key Personnel
 President ....Stacia Alnequist

642 eHealthInsurance Services Inc.

11919 Foundation Place
Gold River, CA 95670
Toll-Free: 800-644-3491
webmaster@healthinsurance.com
www.e.healthinsurance.com
Year Founded: 1997

Healthplan and Services Defined
 PLAN TYPE: HMO/PPO
 Benefits Offered: Dental, Life, STD

Type of Coverage
 Commercial, Individual, Medicare

Geographic Areas Served
 All 50 states in the USA and District of Columbia

Key Personnel
 Chairman & CEO ....Gary L. Lauer
 EVP/Business & Corp. Dev.....................Bruce Telkamp
 EVP/Chief Technology..................Dr. Sheldon X. Wang
 SVP & CFO ....Stuart M. Huizinga

Pres. of eHealth Gov. Sys . . . . Samuel C. Gibbs
SVP of Sales & Operations . . . . Robert S. Hurley
Director Public Relations. . . . . Nate Purpura
650-210-3115

---

643 Essence Healthcare

13900 Riverport Drive
Maryland Heights, MO 63043
Toll-Free: 866-597-9560
Phone: 314-209-2700
Fax: 314-770-6096
customerservice@essencehealthcare.com
www.essencehealthcare.com
Mailing Address: PO Box 12488, St. Louis, MO 63132
Subsidiary of: EGHC

Healthplan and Services Defined
PLAN TYPE: Medicare
Benefits Offered: Chiropractic, Dental, Disease Management, Home
Care, Inpatient SNF, Physical Therapy, Podiatry, Prescription,
Psychiatric, Vision, Wellness

Type of Coverage
Individual, Medicare

Geographic Areas Served
Available within select counties in Missouri and Illinois only

Subscriber Information
Average Monthly Fee Per Subscriber
(Employee + Employer Contribution):
Employee Only (Self): Varies
Medicare: Varies
Average Annual Deductible Per Subscriber:
Employee Only (Self): Varies
Medicare: Varies
Average Subscriber Co-Payment:
Primary Care Physician: Varies
Non-Network Physician: Varies
Prescription Drugs: Varies
Hospital ER: Varies
Home Health Care: Varies
Home Health Care Max. Days/Visits Covered: Varies
Nursing Home: Varies
Nursing Home Max. Days/Visits Covered: Varies

Key Personnel
Chairmain & CEO. . . . . Frank Ingari
Executive Vice President . . . . Debra Gribble, RN
VP, Chief Operating Offc . . . . Martha Butler, RN, MPH
Chief Medical Officer . . . . Deborah Zimmerman, MD
VP, Human Resources. . . . . Tom Murrill
Chief Technology Officer . . . . Tony Butler
Media Contact . . . . Andrew Shea
314-209-2865
ashea@essencecorp.com

---

644 GEHA-Government Employees Hospital Association

PO Box 4665
17306 E 24 Highway
Independence, MO 64051-4665
Toll-Free: 800-821-6136
Phone: 816-257-5500
Fax: 816-257-3333
cs.geha@geha.com
www.geha.com
Non-Profit Organization: Yes
Year Founded: 1939
Total Enrollment: 900,000

Healthplan and Services Defined
PLAN TYPE: Multiple

Benefits Offered: Dental, Disease Management, Prescription, Vision,
Wellness
Offers Demand Management Patient Information Service: Yes
DMPI Services Offered: 24-Hour Health Advice Line

Type of Coverage
Commercial, Medicare
Catastrophic Illness Maximum Benefit: $5,000

Type of Payment Plans Offered
FFS

Geographic Areas Served
Nationwide

Subscriber Information
Average Monthly Fee Per Subscriber
(Employee + Employer Contribution):
Employee Only (Self): $109.25
Employee & 2 Family Members: $221.78
Average Annual Deductible Per Subscriber:
Employee Only (Self): $450.00
Average Subscriber Co-Payment:
Primary Care Physician: $10.00
Non-Network Physician: $25.00
Prescription Drugs: $5.00

Network Qualifications
Pre-Admission Certification: Yes

Key Personnel
President. . . . . Richard Miles

Average Claim Compensation
Hospital's Fees Charged: 85%

---

645 GHP Coventry Health Plan

550 Maryville Center Drive
Suite 300
St. Louis, MO 63141
Toll-Free: 800-755-3901
marketingchcmo@cvty.com
http://chcmissouri.coventryhealthcare.com
Non-Profit Organization: Yes
Year Founded: 1978
Number of Affiliated Hospitals: 100
Number of Primary Care Physicians: 4,000
Number of Referral/Specialty Physicians: 8,000
Total Enrollment: 330,000
State Enrollment: 330,000

Healthplan and Services Defined
PLAN TYPE: HMO/PPO
Other Type: POS
Model Type: IPA
Benefits Offered: Behavioral Health, Chiropractic, Dental, Disease
Management, Home Care, Inpatient SNF, Physical Therapy,
Podiatry, Prescription, Psychiatric, Transplant, Vision, Wellness

Type of Coverage
Commercial, Individual, Advantage

Geographic Areas Served
St. Louis/Metro East Area, Mid-Missouri and Central and Southern
Illinois

Accreditation Certification
URAC

Key Personnel
President & CEO . . . . Roman Kulich
VP, Medical Affairs . . . . Scott Spradlin
VP, Medicare. . . . . Thor Anderson

646 Great-West Healthcare Missouri

1000 Great West Drive
Kennett, MO 63857
Toll-Free: 800-663-8081
Phone: 314-569-3232
eliginquiries@cigna.com
www.cignaforhealth.com
Secondary Address: 231 S Bemiston Avenue, Suite 500, St. Louis, MO 63105-7300
Subsidiary of: CIGNA HealthCare
Acquired by: CIGNA
For Profit Organization: Yes
Total Enrollment: 67,308
State Enrollment: 47,367

Healthplan and Services Defined
PLAN TYPE: HMO/PPO
Benefits Offered: Disease Management, Prescription, Wellness

Type of Coverage
Commercial

Type of Payment Plans Offered
POS, FFS

Geographic Areas Served
Missouri

Accreditation Certification
URAC

Specialty Managed Care Partners
Caremark Rx

647 Healthcare USA of Missouri

2420 Hyde Park Road
Jefferson City, MO 65109
Toll-Free: 800-566-6444
Phone: 573-761-0544
Fax: 314-241-8010
smwijkowski@cvty.com
http://chcmedicaid-missouri.coventryhealthcare.com
Secondary Address: 2420 Hyde Park Road, Suite B, Provider Services Department, Jefferson City, MO 65109
Subsidiary of: Coventry Health Care
For Profit Organization: Yes
Year Founded: 1995
Total Enrollment: 185,375
State Enrollment: 185,375

Healthplan and Services Defined
PLAN TYPE: HMO
Model Type: Network
Benefits Offered: Prescription
Offers Demand Management Patient Information Service: Yes

Type of Coverage
Medicaid

Type of Payment Plans Offered
Combination FFS & DFFS

Geographic Areas Served
Eastern, Central and Western Missouri

Network Qualifications
Pre-Admission Certification: Yes

Peer Review Type
Utilization Review: Yes
Second Surgical Opinion: Yes
Case Management: Yes

Publishes and Distributes Report Card: Yes

Accreditation Certification
TJC Accreditation, Medicare Approved, Utilization Review, Pre-Admission Certification, State Licensure, Quality Assurance Program

Key Personnel
President/CFO . . . . .Claudia Bjerre
Secretary . . . . .Jennifer Handshy
Executive Director. . . . . .Ancelmo Lopes
Director . . . . .Becky Pierce
Chief Medical Officer .Mary Mason, MD

Specialty Managed Care Partners
Enters into Contracts with Regional Business Coalitions: No

648 HealthLink HMO

12443 Olive Boulevard
St Louis, MO 63141
Toll-Free: 800-624-2356
Phone: 314-989-6000
www.healthlink.com
Subsidiary of: Wellpoint Health Networks
For Profit Organization: Yes
Year Founded: 1993
Number of Affiliated Hospitals: 129
Number of Primary Care Physicians: 2,705
Number of Referral/Specialty Physicians: 6,984
Total Enrollment: 1,000,000
State Enrollment: 395,996

Healthplan and Services Defined
PLAN TYPE: HMO
Model Type: IPA
Plan Specialty: ASO, UR
Benefits Offered: Behavioral Health, Chiropractic, Disease Management, Home Care, Physical Therapy, Podiatry, Prescription, Psychiatric, Transplant, Vision, Wellness
Offers Demand Management Patient Information Service: Yes
DMPI Services Offered: Heart Disease, Nurse Triage

Type of Coverage
Commercial
Catastrophic Illness Benefit: Varies per case

Type of Payment Plans Offered
POS, DFFS, Combination FFS & DFFS

Geographic Areas Served
Missouri, Illinois, Indiana, Arkansas, Kentucky, West Virginia

Subscriber Information
Average Subscriber Co-Payment:
Primary Care Physician: $10.00
Prescription Drugs: $10/15/25
Hospital ER: $50.00

Network Qualifications
Pre-Admission Certification: Yes

Peer Review Type
Utilization Review: Yes
Second Surgical Opinion: No
Case Management: Yes

Accreditation Certification
URAC
Utilization Review, Pre-Admission Certification, Quality Assurance Program

Key Personnel
President/CEO. . . . . .David Ott
877-284-0101
DOTT@healthlink.com
General Manager . . . . .Bruce Gosser
877-284-0101
bgosser@healthlink.com
VP Sales/Network Devel. .Donna Geringer
877-284-0101
dgeringer@healthlink.com
Vice President/Marketing . . . . .Courtney Walter

Chief Medical Officer....................John Seidenfeld, MD
877-284-0101
seidenfj@healthlink.com
Vice President/Planning ....Art Stengol
Regional/VP Sales..........................Donna Geringer
877-284-0101
dgeringer@healthlink.com
Media Contact ....Jon Mills
jon.mills@wellpoint.com
Media Contact ....Jill Becher
jill.becher@wellpoint.com

Specialty Managed Care Partners
WellPoint Pharmacy Management, Cigna Behavioral Health, Vision
Service Plan
Enters into Contracts with Regional Business Coalitions: Yes
Gateway Purchases

Employer References
Local fifty benefits service trust, Jefferson City Public Schools,
ConAgra

---

649 Humana Health Insurance of Missouri
909 E Montclair
Suite 108
Springfield, MO 65807
Toll-Free: 800-951-0128
Phone: 417-882-3020
Fax: 417-882-2015
www.humana.com
For Profit Organization: Yes

Healthplan and Services Defined
PLAN TYPE: HMO/PPO

Type of Coverage
Commercial, Individual

Accreditation Certification
URAC, NCQA, CORE

---

650 Med-Pay
1650 Battlefield
Suite 300
Springfield, MO 65804-3706
Toll-Free: 800-777-9087
Phone: 417-886-6886
Fax: 417-886-2276
apinegar@med-pay.com
www.med-pay.com
Year Founded: 1983
State Enrollment: 26,000

Healthplan and Services Defined
PLAN TYPE: Other
Other Type: TPA, HSA, HRA
Model Type: Network
Plan Specialty: ASO, Behavioral Health, Chiropractic, Dental,
Disease Management, Lab, MSO, PBM, Vision, Radiology
Benefits Offered: Behavioral Health, Chiropractic, Dental, Disease
Management, Home Care, Inpatient SNF, Long-Term Care,
Physical Therapy, Prescription, Transplant, Vision
Offers Demand Management Patient Information Service: Yes

Type of Coverage
Commercial, Individual

Accreditation Certification
State of MO
Utilization Review

Key Personnel
President.....................................Gordon Kinne
Director Claims ....Pam Mathis
Director Client Services.....................Megan Broemmer

Specialty Managed Care Partners
HCC, BCBS, Healthlink
Enters into Contracts with Regional Business Coalitions: Yes

---

651 Mercy Health Medicare Plan
14528 South Outer 40
Suite 300
Chesterfield, MO 63017-5743
Toll-Free: 800-830-1918
Phone: 314-214-8100
Fax: 314-214-8101
www.mercyhealthplans.com
Non-Profit Organization: Yes

Healthplan and Services Defined
PLAN TYPE: Medicare
Benefits Offered: Chiropractic, Dental, Disease Management, Home
Care, Inpatient SNF, Physical Therapy, Podiatry, Prescription,
Psychiatric, Vision, Wellness

Type of Coverage
Individual, Medicare

Geographic Areas Served
Available within multiple states

Subscriber Information
Average Monthly Fee Per Subscriber
(Employee + Employer Contribution):
Employee Only (Self): Varies
Medicare: Varies
Average Annual Deductible Per Subscriber:
Employee Only (Self): Varies
Medicare: Varies
Average Subscriber Co-Payment:
Primary Care Physician: Varies
Non-Network Physician: Varies
Prescription Drugs: Varies
Hospital ER: Varies
Home Health Care: Varies
Home Health Care Max. Days/Visits Covered: Varies
Nursing Home: Varies
Nursing Home Max. Days/Visits Covered: Varies

Key Personnel
Interim CEO ....Chris Knackstedt
EVP, COO...................................Mike Treash
Executive Vice President.......................Janet Pursley
CFO, Treasurer..........................George Schneider
VP, General Counsel ....Charles Gilham
Chief Medical Officer ....Stephen Spurgeon, MD
VP, Human Resources.....................Donna McDaniel
VP, Mission & Ethics ....Michael Doyle
VP, Sales & Service............................Carl Schultz

---

652 Mercy Health Plans: Corporate Office
14528 South Outer 40
Suite 300
Chesterfield, MO 63017-5705
Toll-Free: 800-830-1918
Phone: 314-214-8100
Fax: 314-214-8101
www.mercyhealthplans.com
Secondary Address: 4520 South National, Springfield, MO 65810,
417-836-0450
Non-Profit Organization: Yes
Year Founded: 1994
Number of Primary Care Physicians: 8,500
Total Enrollment: 73,000

Healthplan and Services Defined
PLAN TYPE: HMO
Model Type: IPA

Benefits Offered: Behavioral Health, Chiropractic, Physical Therapy, Prescription, Vision

Type of Coverage
Commercial, Individual, Medicare, Supplemental Medicare, Medicaid

Geographic Areas Served
Eastern Central Missouri, Southwest Missouri, South Texas

Subscriber Information
Average Monthly Fee Per Subscriber
(Employee + Employer Contribution):
Employee Only (Self): Varies by plan
Average Annual Deductible Per Subscriber:
Employee Only (Self): $1000.00
Average Subscriber Co-Payment:
Primary Care Physician: $10.00
Non-Network Physician: $30.00
Prescription Drugs: $7-$12

Key Personnel
Interim CEO . . . . .Chris Knackstedt
EVP, COO. . . . . .Mike Treash
Executive Vice President. . . . . .Janet Pursley
CFO, Treasurer. . . . . .George Schneider
VP, General Counsel . . . . .Charles Gilham
Chief Medical Officer . . . . .Stephen Spurgeon, MD
VP, Human Resources. . . . . .Donna McDaniel
VP, Mission & Ethics . . . . .Michael Doyle
VP, Sales & Service. . . . . .Carl Schultz

653   Meritain Health: Missouri
9201 Watson Road
St. Louis, MO 63126
Toll-Free: 800-776-2452
Phone: 314-889-2100
Fax: 314-918-3535
sales@meritain.com
www.meritain.com
For Profit Organization: Yes
Year Founded: 1983
Number of Affiliated Hospitals: 110
Number of Primary Care Physicians: 3,467
Number of Referral/Specialty Physicians: 5,720
Total Enrollment: 500,000
State Enrollment: 450,000

Healthplan and Services Defined
PLAN TYPE: PPO
Model Type: Network
Plan Specialty: Dental, Disease Management, Vision, Radiology, UR
Benefits Offered: Prescription
Offers Demand Management Patient Information Service: Yes

Type of Coverage
Commercial

Geographic Areas Served
Nationwide

Subscriber Information
Average Monthly Fee Per Subscriber
(Employee + Employer Contribution):
Employee Only (Self): Varies by plan

Accreditation Certification
URAC
TJC Accreditation, Medicare Approved, Utilization Review, Pre-Admission Certification, State Licensure, Quality Assurance Program

Key Personnel
EVP/Chief Financial Offic . . . . Vincent DiMura

Average Claim Compensation
Physician's Fees Charged: 78%
Hospital's Fees Charged: 90%

Specialty Managed Care Partners
Express Scripts, LabOne, Interactive Health Solutions

654   Mid America Health
8320 Ward Parkway
Kansas City, MO 64114
Toll-Free: 800-468-1442
Phone: 816-221-8400
Fax: 816-221-1870
www.chckansascity.com
Secondary Address: 8301 East 21st Street North, Suite 300, Wichita, KS 67206
Subsidiary of: Coventry
Acquired by: Coventry Health Care of Kansas
Year Founded: 1994
Owned by an Integrated Delivery Network (IDN): Yes
Number of Affiliated Hospitals: 30
Number of Primary Care Physicians: 2,000
Number of Referral/Specialty Physicians: 2,070
Total Enrollment: 119,600

Healthplan and Services Defined
PLAN TYPE: HMO/PPO
Model Type: IPA
Plan Specialty: ASO, Behavioral Health, Chiropractic, Dental, Disease Management, EPO, Lab, MSO, PBM, Vision, Radiology, UR
Benefits Offered: Prescription

Type of Coverage
Commercial, Medicare

Type of Payment Plans Offered
DFFS

Geographic Areas Served
Kansa, Missouri, Oklahoma

Network Qualifications
Pre-Admission Certification: Yes

Peer Review Type
Utilization Review: No
Second Surgical Opinion: No
Case Management: No

Publishes and Distributes Report Card: Yes

Accreditation Certification
URAC
TJC Accreditation, Medicare Approved, Utilization Review, Pre-Admission Certification, State Licensure, Quality Assurance Program

Key Personnel
President and CEO . . . . .Jan Stalmeyer
CFO. . . . . .Joe Stasi
Medical Affairs . . . . .Milton Thomas, MD
Information Services . . . . .Kevin Sparks

Specialty Managed Care Partners
Yellow
Enters into Contracts with Regional Business Coalitions: Yes

655   Molina Healthcare: Missouri
12400 Olive Blvd Creve Couer
St. Louis, MO 63141
Toll-Free: 800-875-0679
Phone: 314-819-5300
www.molinahealthcare.com
For Profit Organization: Yes
Year Founded: 1980
Physician Owned Organization: Yes
Number of Affiliated Hospitals: 84
Number of Primary Care Physicians: 2,167
Number of Referral/Specialty Physicians: 6,184

Total Enrollment: 1,400,000

Healthplan and Services Defined
PLAN TYPE: HMO
Model Type: Network
Benefits Offered: Chiropractic, Dental, Home Care, Inpatient SNF, Long-Term Care, Podiatry, Vision

Type of Coverage
Commercial, Medicare, Supplemental Medicare, Medicaid

Accreditation Certification
URAC, NCQA

656 Ozark Health Plan

3335 E Ridgeview Street
Springfield, MO 65804
Toll-Free: 800-658-3518
Phone: 417-823-3910
Fax: 417-823-3706
www.ozarkhealthplan.com
Subsidiary of: Arcadian Health Plans

Healthplan and Services Defined
PLAN TYPE: Medicare

Type of Coverage
Medicare

Key Personnel
Chairman & CEO . . . . Robert Fahlman
Chief Financial Officer . . . . Les Granow
Chief Information Officer . . . . Prudence Kuai
SVP, General Counsel . . . . James Novello

657 Preferred Care Blue

2301 Main Street
One Pershing Square
Kansas City, MO 64108
Toll-Free: 888-989-8842
Phone: 816-395-3558
www.bluekc.com
Acquired by: BlueCross BlueShield of Kansas City
Non-Profit Organization: Yes
Year Founded: 1983
Number of Affiliated Hospitals: 49
Number of Primary Care Physicians: 1,119
Total Enrollment: 238,976

Healthplan and Services Defined
PLAN TYPE: PPO
Model Type: IPA, Group
Benefits Offered: Disease Management, Prescription, Wellness

Type of Coverage
Catastrophic Illness Benefit: Maximum $2M

Geographic Areas Served
Kansas City, Metropolitan & Northwestern Missouri (32 counties)

Subscriber Information
Average Subscriber Co-Payment:
Primary Care Physician: $10.00
Non-Network Physician: Ded/coins
Prescription Drugs: $10.00/20.00/40.00
Hospital ER: $50.00 copay
Home Health Care: Ded/coins
Home Health Care Max. Days/Visits Covered: 60 days
Nursing Home: $0
Nursing Home Max. Days/Visits Covered: 60 days

Network Qualifications
Pre-Admission Certification: Yes

Peer Review Type
Utilization Review: Yes

Accreditation Certification
AAAHC
TJC Accreditation, Medicare Approved, Utilization Review, Pre-Admission Certification, State Licensure, Quality Assurance Program

Key Personnel
President & CEO . . . . David Gentile
Group Ex, Financial & Int . . . . Bryan Camerlinck
Group Ex, Legal & Legisla . . . . Rick Kastner

Specialty Managed Care Partners
Enters into Contracts with Regional Business Coalitions: Yes

658 UnitedHealthCare of Missouri

13655 Riverport Drive
Maryland Heights, MO 63043
Toll-Free: 800-627-0687
Phone: 314-592-7000
www.uhc.com
Subsidiary of: UnitedHealth Group
For Profit Organization: Yes
Total Enrollment: 75,000,000
State Enrollment: 60,000

Healthplan and Services Defined
PLAN TYPE: HMO/PPO

Geographic Areas Served
Statewide

Key Personnel
Media Contact . . . . Greg Thompson
312-424-6913
gregory_a_thompson@uhc.com

Health Insurance Coverage Status and Type of Coverage by Age

Category	All Persons		Under 18 years		Under 65 years		65 years and over	
	Number	%	Number	%	Number	%	Number	%
Total population	999	-	223	-	839	-	160	-
Covered by some type of health insurance	835 *(8)*	83.5 *(0.8)*	201 *(4)*	89.9 *(1.4)*	675 *(8)*	80.5 *(0.9)*	160 *(1)*	99.6 *(0.2)*
Covered by private health insurance	650 *(10)*	65.1 *(1.0)*	125 *(4)*	56.1 *(1.9)*	546 *(9)*	65.1 *(1.0)*	104 *(3)*	65.1 *(1.9)*
Employment based	492 *(10)*	49.2 *(1.0)*	103 *(5)*	46.0 *(2.2)*	450 *(10)*	53.6 *(1.2)*	42 *(3)*	26.5 *(1.8)*
Direct purchase	167 *(7)*	16.7 *(0.7)*	20 *(3)*	9.1 *(1.2)*	99 *(6)*	11.8 *(0.7)*	67 *(4)*	42.1 *(2.3)*
Covered by TRICARE	32 *(4)*	3.2 *(0.4)*	7 *(2)*	3.1 *(0.7)*	23 *(3)*	2.7 *(0.4)*	10 *(2)*	6.0 *(1.0)*
Covered by government health insurance	318 *(7)*	31.9 *(0.7)*	84 *(5)*	37.8 *(2.2)*	162 *(7)*	19.2 *(0.8)*	157 *(1)*	97.9 *(0.4)*
Covered by Medicaid	148 *(6)*	14.8 *(0.6)*	83 *(5)*	37.2 *(2.1)*	133 *(6)*	15.9 *(0.8)*	15 *(1)*	9.4 *(0.9)*
Also by private insurance	24 *(3)*	2.4 *(0.3)*	8 *(2)*	3.7 *(0.7)*	18 *(3)*	2.2 *(0.3)*	6 *(1)*	3.8 *(0.7)*
Covered by Medicare	181 *(2)*	18.1 *(0.2)*	1 *(1)*	0.5 *(0.3)*	24 *(2)*	2.8 *(0.3)*	157 *(1)*	97.9 *(0.4)*
Also by private insurance	109 *(3)*	10.9 *(0.3)*	1 *(1)*	0.3 *(0.2)*	8 *(1)*	0.9 *(0.2)*	102 *(3)*	63.4 *(2.0)*
Also by Medicaid	25 *(2)*	2.5 *(0.2)*	Z *(Z)*	0.0 *(0.1)*	10 *(2)*	1.2 *(0.2)*	15 *(1)*	9.4 *(0.9)*
Covered by VA Care	38 *(3)*	3.8 *(0.3)*	Z *(Z)*	0.2 *(0.1)*	17 *(2)*	2.1 *(0.2)*	21 *(1)*	13.0 *(0.9)*
Not covered at any time during the year	165 *(8)*	16.5 *(0.8)*	22 *(3)*	10.1 *(1.4)*	164 *(8)*	19.5 *(0.9)*	1 *(Z)*	0.4 *(0.2)*

Note: Numbers in thousands; Figures cover 2013; Margin of error appears in parenthesis; A "Z" indicates that the value either represents or rounds to zero.
Source: U.S. Census Bureau, 2013 American Community Survey, Table HI05. Health Insurance Coverage Status and Type of Coverage by State and Age for All People: 2013

Montana

659 Aetna Health of Montana
151 Farmington Avenue
Hartford, CT 06156
Toll-Free: 800-872-3862
Phone: 860-273-0123
www.aetna.com
Partnered with: eHealthInsurance Services Inc.
For Profit Organization: Yes
Total Enrollment: 11,596,230

Healthplan and Services Defined
  PLAN TYPE: PPO
  Other Type: POS
  Plan Specialty: EPO
  Benefits Offered: Dental, Disease Management, Long-Term Care,
    Prescription, Wellness, Life, LTD, STD

Type of Coverage
  Commercial, Individual

Type of Payment Plans Offered
  POS, FFS

Geographic Areas Served
  Statewide

Key Personnel
  Chairman/CEO/President. . . . . .Mark T Bertolini
  EVP, General Counsel . . . . .William J Casazza
  EVP/CFO . . . . .Shawn M Guertin

660 Allegiance Life & Health Insurance Company
2806 South Garfield Street
PO Box 3018
Missoula, MT 59806-3018
Toll-Free: 800-877-1122
Phone: 406-721-2222
inquire@askallegiance.com
www.allegiancelifeandhealth.com
For Profit Organization: Yes
Year Founded: 2006

Healthplan and Services Defined
  PLAN TYPE: HMO
  Benefits Offered: Dental, Vision, Wellness, Pharmacy

Type of Coverage
  Commercial, Individual

Geographic Areas Served
  Montana

Key Personnel
  Chairman. . . . . .Dirk Visser

661 Blue Cross & Blue Shield of Montana
560 N Park Avenue
PO Box 4309
Helena, MT 59605-4309
Toll-Free: 800-447-7828
Phone: 406-437-5000
john_doran@bcbsmt.com
www.bcbsmt.com
Subsidiary of: Blue Cross Blue Shield Association
Non-Profit Organization: Yes
Year Founded: 1986
Owned by an Integrated Delivery Network (IDN): Yes
Federally Qualified: Yes
Number of Affiliated Hospitals: 58
Number of Primary Care Physicians: 1,900

Number of Referral/Specialty Physicians: 2,800
Total Enrollment: 236,000
State Enrollment: 236,000

Healthplan and Services Defined
  PLAN TYPE: HMO
  Model Type: Network
  Plan Specialty: ASO, Behavioral Health, Chiropractic, Dental,
    Disease Management, EPO, Lab, MSO, PBM, Vision, Radiology,
    Worker's Compensation, UR
  Benefits Offered: Behavioral Health, Chiropractic, Complementary
    Medicine, Dental, Disease Management, Home Care, Inpatient
    SNF, Long-Term Care, Physical Therapy, Podiatry, Prescription,
    Psychiatric, Transplant, Vision, Wellness, Worker's Compensation,
    AD&D, Life, LTD, ST
  Offers Demand Management Patient Information Service: Yes

Type of Coverage
  Commercial, Individual, Indemnity, Medicare, Supplemental
    Medicare, Catastrophic
  Catastrophic Illness Benefit: Varies per case

Type of Payment Plans Offered
  POS, DFFS, Capitated

Geographic Areas Served
  Beaverhead, Big Horn, Blaine, Broadwater, Carbon, Carter, Cascade,
    Choteau, Custer, Deer Lodge, Flathead, Glacier, Hill, Jefferson, Lake,
    Lewis and Clark, Liberty, Lincoln, Madison, McCone, Meagher,
    Mineral, Missoula, Musselshell, Pondera, Ravalli, Sanders, Silver
    Bow, Stillwater, Sweet Grass, Teton, Wheatland, Yellowstone

Subscriber Information
  Average Subscriber Co-Payment:
      Primary Care Physician: $15
      Non-Network Physician: Deductible
      Hospital ER: $75.00
      Home Health Care: No deductible
      Home Health Care Max. Days/Visits Covered: 180 days
      Nursing Home: $300 per admit co-pay
      Nursing Home Max. Days/Visits Covered: 60 days

Network Qualifications
  Pre-Admission Certification: Yes

Peer Review Type
  Utilization Review: Yes
  Second Surgical Opinion: Yes
  Case Management: Yes

Publishes and Distributes Report Card: Yes

Key Personnel
  President & CEO . . . . .Michael Frank
  Chief Financial Officer . . . . .Mark Burzynski
  Chief Information Officer . . . . .Patrick Law
  Chief Marketing Officer. . . . . .Shannon Marsden
  EVP Internal Operations . . . . .Fred Olson, MD
  Corp Communications . . . . .Tim Warner
    406-431-4366
    tim_warner@bcbsmt.com

Specialty Managed Care Partners
  Behavioral Health, Chiropractic, Dental, Disease Management, Home
    Care, Inpatient SNF, and more
  Enters into Contracts with Regional Business Coalitions: Yes

Employer References
  Montana University System, Evening Post Publishing Company,
    Costco Wholesale, State of Montana, Huntley Project Schools

662 CIGNA HealthCare of Montana

3900 East Mexico Avenue
Suite 1100
Denver, CO 80210
Toll-Free: 800-832-3211
Phone: 303-782-1500
Fax: 303-691-3197
www.cigna.com
For Profit Organization: Yes
Total Enrollment: 7,642
State Enrollment: 5,008

Healthplan and Services Defined
PLAN TYPE: HMO
Plan Specialty: Behavioral Health, Dental, Vision
Benefits Offered: Behavioral Health, Dental, Disease Management, Prescription, Transplant, Vision, Wellness, Life

Type of Coverage
Commercial

Type of Payment Plans Offered
POS, FFS

Geographic Areas Served
Montana

Key Personnel
Director At Cigna . . . . Sallie Vanasdale
VP Provider Relations . . . . William Cetti
VP Client Relations . . . . Gregg Prussing

663 Delta Dental of Montana

55 West 14th Street
Suite 101
Helena, MT 59601
Toll-Free: 800-547-1986
Phone: 406-449-0255
Fax: 406-495-0322
mtsales@delta.org
www.deltadentalins.com
Non-Profit Organization: Yes
Total Enrollment: 54,000,000

Healthplan and Services Defined
PLAN TYPE: Dental
Other Type: Dental PPO

Type of Coverage
Commercial

Geographic Areas Served
Statewide

Key Personnel
Chief Executive Officer . . . . Gary D. Radine
VP, Public & Govt Affairs . . . . Jeff Album
   415-972-8418
Dir/Media & Public Affair . . . . Elizabeth Risberg
   415-972-8423

664 eHealthInsurance Services Inc.

11919 Foundation Place
Gold River, CA 95670
Toll-Free: 800-644-3491
webmaster@healthinsurance.com
www.e.healthinsurance.com
Year Founded: 1997

Healthplan and Services Defined
PLAN TYPE: HMO/PPO
Benefits Offered: Dental, Life, STD

Type of Coverage
Commercial, Individual, Medicare

Geographic Areas Served
All 50 states in the USA and District of Columbia

Key Personnel
Chairman & CEO . . . . Gary L. Lauer
EVP/Business & Corp. Dev. Bruce Telkamp
EVP/Chief Technology . . . . Dr. Sheldon X. Wang
SVP & CFO . . . . Stuart M. Huizinga
Pres. of eHealth Gov. Sys . . . . Samuel C. Gibbs
SVP of Sales & Operations . . . . Robert S. Hurley
Director Public Relations . . . . Nate Purpura
   650-210-3115

665 Great-West Healthcare Montana

155 108th Avenue NE
Suite 800
Bellevue, WA 98004
Toll-Free: 866-860-2225
Phone: 425-803-9030
eliginquiries@cigna.com
www.cignaforhealth.com
Subsidiary of: CIGNA HealthCare
Acquired by: CIGNA
For Profit Organization: Yes
Total Enrollment: 4,970
State Enrollment: 3,405

Healthplan and Services Defined
PLAN TYPE: HMO/PPO
Benefits Offered: Disease Management, Prescription, Wellness

Type of Coverage
Commercial

Type of Payment Plans Offered
POS, FFS

Geographic Areas Served
Montana

Accreditation Certification
URAC

Specialty Managed Care Partners
Caremark Rx

666 Health InfoNet

PO Box 20559
Billings, MT 59104
Fax: 406-256-9466
jmcglone@fchn.com
www.healthinfonetmt.com
Subsidiary of: Paradigm Group
For Profit Organization: Yes
Number of Affiliated Hospitals: 94
Number of Primary Care Physicians: 980
Number of Referral/Specialty Physicians: 1,793
Total Enrollment: 80,000
State Enrollment: 56,000

Healthplan and Services Defined
PLAN TYPE: PPO
Model Type: Open Panel & GeoExclusive
Benefits Offered: Wellness, Provider Network Access

Type of Coverage
Commercial, Individual, Private & Public Plans, Geo-specifi

Geographic Areas Served
Montana, Wyoming, Colorado, North Dakota, South Dakota

Key Personnel
CEO . . . . Robert L Hunter
Principal, CIO . . . . Jim McInerney
CFO . . . . Michael W Young
CMO . . . . Lionel Tapia, MD
Provider Relations . . . . John Larson

Credentialing Specialist . . . . Jen McGone
PPO Services Director . . . . Melody Heide
Wellness & Disease Mgmt. . . . . Tabatha Elsberry

Specialty Managed Care Partners
Enters into Contracts with Regional Business Coalitions: Yes
First Choice Health Network (Pacific NW)

667 Humana Health Insurance of Montana
1611 Alderson Avenue
Billings, MT 59102
Toll-Free: 800-967-2308
Phone: 406-238-7130
Fax: 406-238-0131
www.humana.com
For Profit Organization: Yes

Healthplan and Services Defined
PLAN TYPE: HMO/PPO

Type of Coverage
Commercial, Individual

Accreditation Certification
URAC, NCQA, CORE

668 Liberty Health Plan: Montana
55 W 14th Street
Suite 202
Helena, MT 59601-3312
Toll-Free: 888-937-3944
Phone: 406-457-5360
Fax: 406-457-5364
customerservice.center@libertynorthwest.com
www.libertynorthwest.com
Secondary Address: 614 Ferguson Avenue, Suite 5, Bozeman, MT
59718-6415
For Profit Organization: Yes
Year Founded: 1983

Healthplan and Services Defined
PLAN TYPE: PPO
Model Type: Group
Plan Specialty: Worker's Compensation
Benefits Offered: Prescription

Type of Payment Plans Offered
POS, DFFS, FFS, Combination FFS & DFFS

Geographic Areas Served
Statewide

Network Qualifications
Pre-Admission Certification: Yes

Peer Review Type
Case Management: Yes

Publishes and Distributes Report Card: No

Specialty Managed Care Partners
Enters into Contracts with Regional Business Coalitions: No

669 New West Health Services
2132 Broadwate Avenue
Unit A-1
Billings, MT 59102
Toll-Free: 888-873-8049
Phone: 406-255-0186
customerservice@nwhp.com
www.newwesthealth.com
Secondary Address: 1203 Highway 2 West, Suite 45, Kalispell, MT
59901-6071
Non-Profit Organization: Yes
Year Founded: 1998

Number of Affiliated Hospitals: 6
Number of Primary Care Physicians: 3,300
Total Enrollment: 43,000
State Enrollment: 43,000

Healthplan and Services Defined
PLAN TYPE: HMO/PPO
Plan Specialty: ASO
Benefits Offered: Prescription, Wellness

Type of Coverage
Commercial, Individual, Indemnity, Medicare, Supplemental
Medicare

Type of Payment Plans Offered
FFS

Geographic Areas Served
Montana

Key Personnel
President/CEO . . . . Leon Lamoreaux
CFO. . . . . Angela Huschka
Medical Director . . . . JP Pujol, MD
Director Medical Services . . . . Erin DeBorde
Chief Medical Officer . . . . Dorothy Fisher, Dr.
Director Sales/Marketing . . . . Ryan O'Connell

Specialty Managed Care Partners
Caremark Rx

670 New West Medicare Plan
130 Neill Avenue
Helena, MT 59601
Toll-Free: 888-873-8044
Phone: 406-457-2200
www.newwesthealth.com
Total Enrollment: 43,000
State Enrollment: 43,000

Healthplan and Services Defined
PLAN TYPE: Medicare
Other Type: PPO
Benefits Offered: Chiropractic, Dental, Disease Management, Home
Care, Inpatient SNF, Physical Therapy, Podiatry, Prescription,
Psychiatric, Vision, Wellness

Type of Coverage
Individual, Medicare

Geographic Areas Served
Available within Montana only

Subscriber Information
Average Monthly Fee Per Subscriber
(Employee + Employer Contribution):
Employee Only (Self): Varies
Medicare: Varies
Average Annual Deductible Per Subscriber:
Employee Only (Self): Varies
Medicare: Varies
Average Subscriber Co-Payment:
Primary Care Physician: Varies
Non-Network Physician: Varies
Prescription Drugs: Varies
Hospital ER: Varies
Home Health Care: Varies
Home Health Care Max. Days/Visits Covered: Varies
Nursing Home: Varies
Nursing Home Max. Days/Visits Covered: Varies

Key Personnel
President/CEO . . . . Leon Lamoreaux
CFO. . . . . Angela Huschka
Medical Director . . . . JP Pujol, MD
Chief Medical Officer . . . . Dorothy Fisher, Dr.
Director Medical Services . . . . Erin DeBorde
Director, Sales/Marketing . . . . Ryan O'Connell

671   UnitedHealthCare of Montana

6465 S Greenwood Plaza Boulevard
Suite 300
Centennial, CO 80111
Toll-Free: 866-574-6088
www.uhc.com
Subsidiary of: UnitedHealth Group
For Profit Organization: Yes
Year Founded: 1986
Number of Affiliated Hospitals: 47
Number of Primary Care Physicians: 1,600
Number of Referral/Specialty Physicians: 3,500
Total Enrollment: 75,000,000
State Enrollment: 17,853

Healthplan and Services Defined
   PLAN TYPE: HMO/PPO
   Model Type: Mixed Model
   Plan Specialty: MSO
   Benefits Offered: Behavioral Health, Chiropractic, Complementary
      Medicine, Dental, Disease Management, Home Care, Inpatient
      SNF, Long-Term Care, Physical Therapy, Podiatry, Prescription,
      Psychiatric, Transplant, Vision, Wellness, AD&D, Life

Type of Coverage
   Commercial, Individual, Medicaid, Commercial Group

Type of Payment Plans Offered
   DFFS, FFS, Combination FFS & DFFS

Geographic Areas Served
   Statewide

Subscriber Information
   Average Monthly Fee Per Subscriber
      (Employee + Employer Contribution):
         Employee Only (Self): Varies
   Average Subscriber Co-Payment:
         Primary Care Physician: $10
         Prescription Drugs: $10/15/30
         Hospital ER: $50

Network Qualifications
   Pre-Admission Certification: Yes

Peer Review Type
   Case Management: Yes

Publishes and Distributes Report Card: Yes

Accreditation Certification
   URAC, NCQA
   State Licensure, Quality Assurance Program

Average Claim Compensation
   Physician's Fees Charged: 70%
   Hospital's Fees Charged: 55%

Specialty Managed Care Partners
   United Behavioral Health
   Enters into Contracts with Regional Business Coalitions: No

Health Insurance Coverage Status and Type of Coverage by Age

Category	All Persons		Under 18 years		Under 65 years		65 years and over	
	Number	%	Number	%	Number	%	Number	%
Total population	1,841	-	463	-	1,588	-	253	-
Covered by some type of health insurance	1,632 (9)	88.7 (0.5)	437 (3)	94.5 (0.7)	1,381 (9)	87.0 (0.6)	251 (1)	99.3 (0.3)
Covered by private health insurance	1,356 (13)	73.7 (0.7)	312 (7)	67.5 (1.4)	1,184 (13)	74.5 (0.8)	172 (3)	68.2 (1.3)
Employment based	1,066 (14)	57.9 (0.7)	267 (7)	57.8 (1.4)	1,002 (13)	63.1 (0.8)	64 (3)	25.3 (1.3)
Direct purchase	311 (8)	16.9 (0.5)	43 (3)	9.2 (0.7)	195 (7)	12.3 (0.5)	116 (4)	45.9 (1.4)
Covered by TRICARE	60 (5)	3.2 (0.3)	14 (2)	3.0 (0.5)	43 (5)	2.7 (0.3)	16 (2)	6.4 (0.7)
Covered by government health insurance	492 (8)	26.8 (0.4)	140 (6)	30.3 (1.4)	247 (8)	15.6 (0.5)	245 (2)	97.1 (0.5)
Covered by Medicaid	240 (9)	13.0 (0.5)	138 (7)	29.9 (1.4)	212 (8)	13.3 (0.5)	28 (2)	11.1 (0.8)
Also by private insurance	47 (4)	2.5 (0.2)	15 (3)	3.3 (0.5)	31 (3)	2.0 (0.2)	15 (2)	6.1 (0.6)
Covered by Medicare	279 (3)	15.2 (0.2)	2 (1)	0.5 (0.3)	35 (3)	2.2 (0.2)	245 (2)	96.9 (0.5)
Also by private insurance	176 (4)	9.6 (0.2)	Z (Z)	0.0 (0.1)	10 (1)	0.6 (0.1)	166 (3)	65.8 (1.3)
Also by Medicaid	44 (2)	2.4 (0.1)	1 (Z)	0.1 (0.1)	16 (2)	1.0 (0.1)	28 (2)	11.1 (0.8)
Covered by VA Care	51 (3)	2.8 (0.2)	Z (Z)	0.0 (0.1)	21 (2)	1.3 (0.1)	30 (2)	11.9 (0.8)
Not covered at any time during the year	209 (9)	11.3 (0.5)	25 (3)	5.5 (0.7)	207 (9)	13.0 (0.6)	2 (1)	0.7 (0.3)

Note: Numbers in thousands; Figures cover 2013; Margin of error appears in parenthesis; A "Z" indicates that the value either represents or rounds to zero.
Source: U.S. Census Bureau, 2013 American Community Survey, Table HI05. Health Insurance Coverage Status and Type of Coverage by State and Age for All People: 2013

Nebraska

672 Aetna Health of Nebraska
151 Farmington Avenue
Hartford, CT 06156
Toll-Free: 800-872-3862
Phone: 860-273-0123
www.aetna.com
Partnered with: eHealthInsurance Services Inc.
For Profit Organization: Yes
Total Enrollment: 11,596,230

Healthplan and Services Defined
PLAN TYPE: PPO
Other Type: POS
Plan Specialty: EPO
Benefits Offered: Dental, Disease Management, Long-Term Care, Prescription, Wellness, Life, LTD, STD

Type of Coverage
Commercial, Individual

Type of Payment Plans Offered
POS, FFS

Geographic Areas Served
Statewide

Key Personnel
Chairman/CEO/President.....................Mark T Bertolini
EVP, General Counsel.....................William J Casazza
EVP/CFO.................................Shawn M Guertin

673 Ameritas Group
PO Box 81889
Lincoln, NE 68501
Toll-Free: 800-659-2223
Fax: 402-467-7338
adminserv@employeebenefitservice.com
www.ameritasgroup.com
For Profit Organization: Yes
Year Founded: 1990
Number of Primary Care Physicians: 49,256
Number of Referral/Specialty Physicians: 16,508
Total Enrollment: 2,543,705
State Enrollment: 818,531

Healthplan and Services Defined
PLAN TYPE: Dental
Model Type: Staff
Plan Specialty: ASO, Dental, Vision
Benefits Offered: Dental, Vision

Type of Coverage
Commercial, Individual

Type of Payment Plans Offered
POS, DFFS, Capitated, Combination FFS & DFFS

Geographic Areas Served
Nationwide

Peer Review Type
Utilization Review: Yes
Second Surgical Opinion: Yes
Case Management: Yes

Publishes and Distributes Report Card: Yes

Accreditation Certification
Medicare Approved

Key Personnel
Chairman..................................Lawrence J Arth
President & CEO...........................JoAnn M Martin
SVP, Group Marketing.......................Karen Gustin

674 Blue Cross & Blue Shield of Nebraska
1919 Aksarben Drive
PO Box 3248
Omaha, NE 68180
Toll-Free: 800-622-2763
Phone: 402-982-7000
sales@nebraskablue.com
www.nebraskablue.com
Secondary Address: 1233 Lincoln Mall, Lincoln, NE 68508, 402-458-4800
Non-Profit Organization: Yes
Year Founded: 1974
Total Enrollment: 717,000
State Enrollment: 717,000

Healthplan and Services Defined
PLAN TYPE: PPO
Model Type: Network
Benefits Offered: Behavioral Health, Chiropractic, Dental, Disease Management, Home Care, Inpatient SNF, Long-Term Care, Physical Therapy, Podiatry, Prescription, Psychiatric, Vision

Type of Coverage
Commercial, Individual, Medicare, Supplemental Medicare

Publishes and Distributes Report Card: No

Key Personnel
President/CEO.............................Steve S Martin
402-982-7000
EVP/CFO/Treasurer.....................Lewis E Trowbridge
EVP/COO..............................Steven H Grandfield
VP/Ethical Practices.......................Sarah Waldman
Dir, Corp Communications....................Andy Williams
402-982-7779
andy.williams@bcbsne.com
Public Relations Spec........................Nate Odgaard
402-982-6528
nathan.odgaard@bcbsne.com

675 CIGNA HealthCare of Nebraska
7400 West 110th Street
Suite 400
Overland Park, KS 66210
Toll-Free: 866-438-2446
Phone: 913-339-4700
www.cigna.com
For Profit Organization: Yes
Total Enrollment: 18,322
State Enrollment: 15,405

Healthplan and Services Defined
PLAN TYPE: PPO
Benefits Offered: Disease Management, Prescription, Transplant, Wellness

Type of Coverage
Commercial

Type of Payment Plans Offered
POS, FFS

Geographic Areas Served
Nebraska

676 Coventry Health Care of Nebraska
15950 West Dodge Road
Omaha, NE 68118
Toll-Free: 800-471-0240
Phone: 402-498-9030
http://chcnebraska.coventryhealthcare.com
Secondary Address: 6720 B Rockledge Drive, Suite 700, Bethesda, MD 20817, 301-581-0600
Subsidiary of: Coventry Health Care Inc.

For Profit Organization: Yes
Year Founded: 1985
Number of Affiliated Hospitals: 120
Number of Primary Care Physicians: 1,500
Number of Referral/Specialty Physicians: 3,500
Total Enrollment: 54,000
State Enrollment: 63,000

Healthplan and Services Defined
  PLAN TYPE: HMO/PPO
  Other Type: POS
  Model Type: IPA
  Benefits Offered: Behavioral Health, Chiropractic, Complementary
    Medicine, Dental, Disease Management, Home Care, Inpatient
    SNF, Long-Term Care, Physical Therapy, Podiatry, Prescription,
    Psychiatric, Transplant, Vision, Wellness

Type of Coverage
  Commercial

Type of Payment Plans Offered
  POS

Accreditation Certification
  URAC

Key Personnel
  Chief Executive Officer . . . . Allen F Wise
  Chief Operating Officer. . . . . Michael D Bahr
  EVP . . . . Harvey C Demovick Jr
  EVP/CFO. . . . . Randy Giles
  EVP/Government Programs . . . . Timothy Nolan
  General Counsel . . . . Thomas Zielinski
  Director of Sales. . . . . Mike Nelson
  Medical Director. . . . . Joseph Blount

---

677   Delta Dental of Nebraska
11235 Davenport Street
Suite 113
Omaha, NE 68154
Toll-Free: 800-736-0710
Phone: 402-397-4878
www.deltadentalne.org
Non-Profit Organization: Yes
Year Founded: 1969
Total Enrollment: 54,000,000

Healthplan and Services Defined
  PLAN TYPE: Dental
  Other Type: Dental PPO
  Model Type: Network
  Plan Specialty: ASO, Dental
  Benefits Offered: Dental

Type of Coverage
  Commercial, Individual, Group
  Catastrophic Illness Benefit: None

Geographic Areas Served
  Statewide

Subscriber Information
  Average Monthly Fee Per Subscriber
    (Employee + Employer Contribution):
      Employee Only (Self): Varies
      Employee & 1 Family Member: Varies
      Employee & 2 Family Members: Varies
  Average Annual Deductible Per Subscriber:
      Employee Only (Self): Varies
      Employee & 1 Family Member: Varies
      Employee & 2 Family Members: Varies
  Average Subscriber Co-Payment:
      Prescription Drugs: $0
      Home Health Care: $0
      Nursing Home: $0

Key Personnel
  Dental Director . . . . Richard Hastreiter
  Chief Sales Officer . . . . Chris Earl
  Media Contact . . . . Barb Jensen
    402-397-4878
    bjensen@deltadentalne.org
  Director Public Affairs . . . . Elizabeth Risberg
    415-972-8423

---

678   eHealthInsurance Services Inc.
11919 Foundation Place
Gold River, CA 95670
Toll-Free: 800-644-3491
webmaster@healthinsurance.com
www.e.healthinsurance.com
Year Founded: 1997

Healthplan and Services Defined
  PLAN TYPE: HMO/PPO
  Benefits Offered: Dental, Life, STD

Type of Coverage
  Commercial, Individual, Medicare

Geographic Areas Served
  All 50 states in the USA and District of Columbia

Key Personnel
  Chairman & CEO . . . . Gary L. Lauer
  EVP/Business & Corp. Dev. . . . . Bruce Telkamp
  EVP/Chief Technology . . . . Dr. Sheldon X. Wang
  SVP & CFO . . . . Stuart M. Huizinga
  Pres. of eHealth Gov. Sys . . . . Samuel C. Gibbs
  SVP of Sales & Operations . . . . Robert S. Hurley
  Director Public Relations. . . . . Nate Purpura
    650-210-3115

---

679   Humana Health Insurance of Nebraska
11420 Blondo Street
Suite 102
Omaha, NE 68164
Toll-Free: 800-941-1182
Phone: 402-496-3388
Fax: 402-498-2850
www.humana.com
For Profit Organization: Yes

Healthplan and Services Defined
  PLAN TYPE: HMO/PPO

Type of Coverage
  Commercial, Individual

Accreditation Certification
  URAC, NCQA, CORE

Key Personnel
  CEO/Chairman. . . . . Michael McCallister
  President. . . . . Bruce Brousard
  Chief Operating Officer . . . . James Murray
  SVP/CFO . . . . James Bloem
  SVP/ Chief HR Manager . . . . Bonita Hathcock

---

680   Midlands Choice
8420 W Dodge Road
Suite 210
Omaha, NE 68114-3492
Toll-Free: 800-605-8259
Phone: 402-390-8233
Fax: 402-390-7210
www.midlandschoice.com
Mailing Address: PO Box 5809, Troy, MI 48007-5809
For Profit Organization: Yes

Year Founded: 1993
Physician Owned Organization: Yes
Number of Affiliated Hospitals: 320
Number of Primary Care Physicians: 20,000
Total Enrollment: 615,000

Healthplan and Services Defined
 PLAN TYPE: PPO
 Model Type: PPO Network

Geographic Areas Served
 Iowa, Nebraska, eastern South Dakota and portions of Colorado, Wyoming, Kansas, Missouri, Illinois, Wisconsin and Minnesota

Accreditation Certification
 URAC

Key Personnel
 President/CEO . . . . Thomas E Press
  402-390-7245
 VP/Provider Relations . . . . Greta Vaught
  402-390-8394
 Dir., Medical Economics . . . . Daniel R. McCulley
 Dir., Professional Svcs. . . . . Sharon K. Rasmussen
 Director, IT . . . . Matthew G Dill
  402-390-8392

Specialty Managed Care Partners
 Enters into Contracts with Regional Business Coalitions: No

681 Mutual of Omaha DentaBenefits

Mutual of Omaha Plaza
S-3
Omaha, NE 68175
Toll-Free: 800-775-6000
Phone: 402-351-4255
Fax: 402-351-2999
corporatesecretary@mutualofomaha.com
www.mutualofomaha.com
Subsidiary of: Mutual of Omaha
For Profit Organization: Yes
Year Founded: 1985
Number of Affiliated Hospitals: 3,999
Number of Primary Care Physicians: 216,781
Number of Referral/Specialty Physicians: 414,227
State Enrollment: 602,578

Healthplan and Services Defined
 PLAN TYPE: Dental
 Other Type: PPO
 Model Type: Network
 Benefits Offered: Behavioral Health, Chiropractic, Complementary Medicine, Dental, Disease Management, Home Care, Inpatient SNF, Long-Term Care, Physical Therapy, Podiatry, Prescription, Psychiatric, Transplant, Vision, Wellness

Type of Coverage
 Commercial, Individual

Type of Payment Plans Offered
 Combination FFS & DFFS

Geographic Areas Served
 All 50 States and DC except for Hawaii, Vermont and Wyoming

Network Qualifications
 Pre-Admission Certification: Yes

Peer Review Type
 Utilization Review: Yes
 Second Surgical Opinion: Yes
 Case Management: Yes

Publishes and Distributes Report Card: Yes

Accreditation Certification
 TJC Accreditation, Medicare Approved, Utilization Review, Pre-Admission Certification, State Licensure, Quality Assurance Program

Key Personnel
 Chairman/CEO . . . . Daniel P Neary
 EVP, General Counsel . . . . Richard C Anderi
 EVP, CFO . . . . David A Diamond
 EVP, Group Benefits . . . . Daniel P Martin
 EVP, Customer Service . . . . Madeline R Rucker
 EVP, Corporate Services . . . . Stacy A Scholtz
 EVP, Chief Investment Ofc. . . . . Richard A Witt
 EVP, Information Services . . . . James T Blackledge

Specialty Managed Care Partners
 Enters into Contracts with Regional Business Coalitions: No

Employer References
 National Rural Letter Carrier, Harrah's Entertainment, Sandia National Labs, Bechtel Nevada, Creighton University

682 Mutual of Omaha Health Plans

Mutual of Omaha Plaza
Omaha, NE 68175
webmaster@mutualofomaha.com
www.mutualofomaha.com
For Profit Organization: Yes
Year Founded: 1988
Number of Affiliated Hospitals: 43
Number of Primary Care Physicians: 673
Number of Referral/Specialty Physicians: 1,718
Total Enrollment: 54,418
State Enrollment: 28,978

Healthplan and Services Defined
 PLAN TYPE: HMO/PPO
 Other Type: POS
 Model Type: IPA
 Plan Specialty: ASO, Behavioral Health, Chiropractic, Disease Management, Lab, Vision, Radiology, UR
 Benefits Offered: Behavioral Health, Chiropractic, Disease Management, Home Care, Inpatient SNF, Long-Term Care, Physical Therapy, Podiatry, Prescription, Psychiatric, Transplant, Vision, Wellness, AD&D, Life, LTD, STD, Critical Illness, EAP

Type of Coverage
 Commercial, Individual, Indemnity, Medicare, Supplemental Medicare, Medicaid
 Catastrophic Illness Benefit: Covered

Type of Payment Plans Offered
 POS, Combination FFS & DFFS

Geographic Areas Served
 Iowa: Harrison, Mills & Pottawattamie counties; Nebraska: Burt, Butler, Cass, Colfas, Cuming, Oakota, Dixon, Filmore, Johnson, Lancaster, Madison, Otoe, Salone, Saunders, Seuard, Stanton, Dodge, Douglas, Sampy, Washington counties

Subscriber Information
 Average Monthly Fee Per Subscriber
  (Employee + Employer Contribution):
   Employee Only (Self): Varies by plan
 Average Annual Deductible Per Subscriber:
   Employee Only (Self): $0.00
 Average Subscriber Co-Payment:
   Primary Care Physician: $15.00
   Prescription Drugs: $15.00
   Hospital ER: $50.00
   Home Health Care: $25.00
   Home Health Care Max. Days/Visits Covered: Unlimited
   Nursing Home: $0.00
   Nursing Home Max. Days/Visits Covered: 100 days

Network Qualifications
 Pre-Admission Certification: Yes

Peer Review Type
 Utilization Review: Yes
 Second Surgical Opinion: No
 Case Management: Yes

Publishes and Distributes Report Card: Yes

Accreditation Certification
URAC, NCQA
TJC Accreditation, Utilization Review, Pre-Admission Certification, State Licensure, Quality Assurance Program

Key Personnel
President . . . . .Daniel P Neary
EVP, General Counsel . . . . .Richard C Anderi
EVP, CFO. . . . . .David A Diamond
EVP, Group Benefits . . . . .Daniel P Martin
EVP, Customer Service .Madeline R Rucker
EVP, Corporate Services .Stacy A Scholtz
EVP, Chief Investment Ofc. . . . . .Richard A Witt
EVP, Information Services . . . . .James T Blackledge

Average Claim Compensation
Physician's Fees Charged: 75%
Hospital's Fees Charged: 60%

Specialty Managed Care Partners
Enters into Contracts with Regional Business Coalitions: No

Employer References
Mutual of Omaha, Forest National Bank, Nebraska Furniture Mart, Saint Joseph Hospital

---

683   UnitedHealthCare of Nebraska

2717 N 118th Street
Suite 300
Omaha, NE 68164
Toll-Free: 800-284-0626
Phone: 402-445-5400
Fax: 402-445-5575
Nebraska_PR_Team@uhc.com
www.uhc.com
Secondary Address: 8101 O Street, Lincoln, NE 68510, 800-284-0626
Subsidiary of: UnitedHealth Group
For Profit Organization: Yes
Year Founded: 1984
Number of Affiliated Hospitals: 41
Number of Primary Care Physicians: 516
Number of Referral/Specialty Physicians: 994
Total Enrollment: 75,000,000
State Enrollment: 44,000

Healthplan and Services Defined
PLAN TYPE: HMO/PPO
Model Type: Network
Plan Specialty: ASO, Behavioral Health, Chiropractic, Dental, Disease Management, Lab, MSO, PBM, Vision, Radiology
Benefits Offered: Disease Management, Prescription, Wellness

Type of Coverage
Commercial, Medicare, Medicaid

Type of Payment Plans Offered
POS, DFFS, FFS

Geographic Areas Served
Iowa: Cass, Fremont, Harrison, Mills, Mononas, Page, Pottawattsmie, Shelby, Woodbury counties; Nebraska: Buffalo, Burt, Butler, Dodge, Douglas, Gage, Hale, Jefferson, Johnson, Lancaster, Madison, Nemaha, Otoe, Pierce, Platte, Saline, Sarpy, Seward, & Washington counties

Subscriber Information
Average Subscriber Co-Payment:
Primary Care Physician: $10.00
Non-Network Physician: Deductible
Prescription Drugs: $10.00
Hospital ER: $50.00

Network Qualifications
Pre-Admission Certification: Yes

Peer Review Type
Utilization Review: Yes

Second Surgical Opinion: Yes
Case Management: Yes

Publishes and Distributes Report Card: Yes

Accreditation Certification
TJC Accreditation, Medicare Approved, Utilization Review, Pre-Admission Certification, State Licensure, Quality Assurance Program

Key Personnel
President/CEO . . . . .Stephen J. Hemsley
EVP. . . . . .Gail K. Boudreaux
VP/Chief Marketing Office. . . . . .Barbara Anason
VP/Physician Services . . . . .Robert Browne
VP/Performance. . . . . .Julie Cerese
Marketing . . . . .Sherry Helmke
Medical Affairs. . . . . .Deb Esser, MD
Member Services . . . . .Shelly Wedergren
Provider Services . . . . .Bob Starman
Sales. . . . . .Dorinda Card
Media Contact. . . . . .Greg Thompson
312-424-6913
gregory_a_thompson@uhc.com

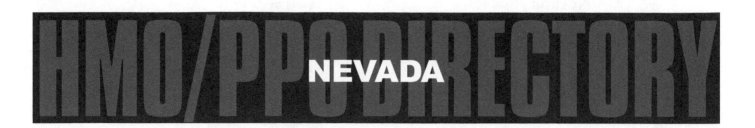

Health Insurance Coverage Status and Type of Coverage by Age

Category	All Persons		Under 18 years		Under 65 years		65 years and over	
	Number	%	Number	%	Number	%	Number	%
Total population	2,757	-	661	-	2,381	-	376	-
Covered by some type of health insurance	2,187 *(17)*	79.3 *(0.6)*	563 *(8)*	85.1 *(1.2)*	1,819 *(17)*	76.4 *(0.7)*	368 *(2)*	97.9 *(0.5)*
Covered by private health insurance	1,717 *(23)*	62.3 *(0.8)*	394 *(11)*	59.5 *(1.6)*	1,515 *(22)*	63.6 *(0.9)*	203 *(5)*	53.9 *(1.4)*
Employment based	1,471 *(24)*	53.4 *(0.9)*	353 *(12)*	53.4 *(1.8)*	1,355 *(24)*	56.9 *(1.0)*	117 *(4)*	31.0 *(1.1)*
Direct purchase	250 *(10)*	9.1 *(0.3)*	36 *(4)*	5.5 *(0.6)*	165 *(9)*	6.9 *(0.4)*	86 *(4)*	22.8 *(1.1)*
Covered by TRICARE	95 *(6)*	3.5 *(0.2)*	18 *(3)*	2.7 *(0.5)*	63 *(6)*	2.6 *(0.2)*	32 *(3)*	8.6 *(0.7)*
Covered by government health insurance	727 *(16)*	26.4 *(0.6)*	188 *(11)*	28.5 *(1.7)*	373 *(16)*	15.7 *(0.7)*	354 *(3)*	94.2 *(0.6)*
Covered by Medicaid	351 *(16)*	12.7 *(0.6)*	186 *(11)*	28.1 *(1.7)*	304 *(15)*	12.8 *(0.6)*	47 *(3)*	12.4 *(0.8)*
Also by private insurance	55 *(5)*	2.0 *(0.2)*	19 *(3)*	2.9 *(0.4)*	38 *(4)*	1.6 *(0.2)*	17 *(2)*	4.6 *(0.5)*
Covered by Medicare	412 *(5)*	14.9 *(0.2)*	2 *(1)*	0.4 *(0.2)*	59 *(4)*	2.5 *(0.2)*	354 *(3)*	94.0 *(0.6)*
Also by private insurance	203 *(5)*	7.4 *(0.2)*	Z *(Z)*	0.0 *(0.1)*	15 *(2)*	0.6 *(0.1)*	189 *(5)*	50.1 *(1.4)*
Also by Medicaid	72 *(4)*	2.6 *(0.2)*	1 *(1)*	0.1 *(0.1)*	25 *(3)*	1.0 *(0.1)*	47 *(3)*	12.4 *(0.8)*
Covered by VA Care	83 *(5)*	3.0 *(0.2)*	1 *(1)*	0.1 *(0.1)*	42 *(4)*	1.8 *(0.2)*	40 *(2)*	10.7 *(0.6)*
Not covered at any time during the year	570 *(17)*	20.7 *(0.6)*	99 *(8)*	14.9 *(1.2)*	562 *(17)*	23.6 *(0.7)*	8 *(2)*	2.1 *(0.5)*

Note: Numbers in thousands; Figures cover 2013; Margin of error appears in parenthesis; A "Z" indicates that the value either represents or rounds to zero.
Source: U.S. Census Bureau, 2013 American Community Survey, Table HI05. Health Insurance Coverage Status and Type of Coverage by State and Age for All People: 2013

Nevada

684 Aetna Health of Nevada
151 Farmington Avenue
Hartford, CT 06156
Toll-Free: 800-872-3862
Phone: 860-273-0123
www.aetna.com
For Profit Organization: Yes
Total Enrollment: 109,089

Healthplan and Services Defined
PLAN TYPE: HMO
Other Type: POS
Model Type: Network
Benefits Offered: Behavioral Health, Dental, Disease Management, Wellness

Geographic Areas Served
Statewide

Subscriber Information
Average Monthly Fee Per Subscriber
(Employee + Employer Contribution):
Employee Only (Self): $85.87
Employee & 1 Family Member: $213.80

Peer Review Type
Second Surgical Opinion: Yes

Key Personnel
Chairman/CEO/President . . . . Mark J Bertolini
EVP/General Counsel . . . . William J Casazza
EVP/CFO . . . . Shawn M Guertin

685 Amerigroup Nevada
7251 West Lake Mead Blvd
Suite 104
Las Vegas, NV 89128
Toll-Free: 800-600-4441
Phone: 702-486-5000
www.realsolutions.com
For Profit Organization: Yes
Year Founded: 2009
Total Enrollment: 85,000

Healthplan and Services Defined
PLAN TYPE: HMO

Type of Coverage
Medicaid, Nevada Child Health Assurance & Sta

Key Personnel
Chairman/President . . . . James Carlson
EVP/External Affairs . . . . John E Littel
EVP/Chief Medical Officer . . . . Mary T McCluskey
EVP/General Counsel . . . . Nicholas Pace
EVP/CFO . . . . James Truess

686 Behavioral Healthcare Options, Inc.
2716-5 North Tenaya Way
Las Vegas, NV 89128
Toll-Free: 800-873-2246
Phone: 702-242-5864
Fax: 702-242-5864
www.behavioralhealthcareoptions.com
Subsidiary of: UnitedHealthcare
Year Founded: 1991
Number of Primary Care Physicians: 250
Total Enrollment: 600,000
State Enrollment: 600,000

Healthplan and Services Defined
PLAN TYPE: HMO/PPO

Model Type: Group
Plan Specialty: Behavioral Health
Benefits Offered: Behavioral Health, Psychiatric, Mental Health, Substance Abuse, EAP, Worklife Enhancement, Gambling Treatment

Type of Payment Plans Offered
POS, Capitated, FFS

Network Qualifications
Pre-Admission Certification: Yes

Accreditation Certification
TJC, URAC, NCQA
Utilization Review, Pre-Admission Certification

Key Personnel
President and CEO . . . . Michael R Adams
Director Finance . . . . Brad Ellerman
VP/COO . . . . Carole A Fisher
Claims Supervisor . . . . Tracey Toothcare
Director, Member Services . . . . Pam Smith
Director of New Business . . . . Harry Baut
Marketing . . . . Carole A Fisher
Medical Director . . . . George Westerman, MD
Sr Systems Analyst . . . . Albert Wu

687 CIGNA HealthCare of Nevada
PO Box 34886
6795 Edmond Street
Las Vegas, NV 89133-4886
Toll-Free: 866-438-2446
Fax: 602-861-8333
www.cigna.com
For Profit Organization: Yes

Healthplan and Services Defined
PLAN TYPE: PPO

Type of Coverage
Commercial

Key Personnel
President/CEO . . . . David Cordani
EVP/Global Chief Officer . . . . Mark Boxer
Chief Financial Officer . . . . Ralph Nicoletti
Regional Operations . . . . Matt Manders
Chief Medical Officer . . . . Alan Muney

688 eHealthInsurance Services Inc.
11919 Foundation Place
Gold River, CA 95670
Toll-Free: 800-644-3491
webmaster@healthinsurance.com
www.e.healthinsurance.com
Year Founded: 1997

Healthplan and Services Defined
PLAN TYPE: HMO/PPO
Benefits Offered: Dental, Life, STD

Type of Coverage
Commercial, Individual, Medicare

Geographic Areas Served
All 50 states in the USA and District of Columbia

Key Personnel
Chairman & CEO . . . . Gary L. Lauer
EVP/Business & Corp. Dev. . . . . Bruce Telkamp
EVP/Chief Technology . . . . Dr. Sheldon X. Wang
SVP & CFO . . . . Stuart M. Huizinga
Pres. of eHealth Gov. Sys . . . . Samuel C. Gibbs
SVP of Sales & Operations . . . . Robert S. Hurley
Director Public Relations . . . . Nate Purpura
650-210-3115

689   Health Plan of Nevada

2720 N Tenaya Way
Las Vegas, NV 89128
Toll-Free: 800-777-1840
Phone: 702-242-7300
Fax: 702-242-7960
www.healthplanofnevada.com
Subsidiary of: AmeriChoice, A UnitedHealth Group Company
For Profit Organization: Yes
Year Founded: 1982
Total Enrollment: 418,000
State Enrollment: 25,576

Healthplan and Services Defined
  PLAN TYPE: HMO/PPO
  Other Type: POS, Medicare
  Benefits Offered: Disease Management, Prescription, Wellness

Type of Coverage
  Commercial, Individual, Medicare, Supplemental Medicare,
  Medicaid

Geographic Areas Served
  Mohave County

Accreditation Certification
  NCQA

Key Personnel
  President/CEO . . . . .Jonathan W Bunker
  Director Claims and Procedures . . . . .Corrine Spaeth
    cspaeth@sierraheath.com
  Chief Information Offc . . . . .Robert Schaich
    rschaich@sierrahealth.com
  Quality Improvemnt . . . . .Deborah Wheeler
  VP Member Services . . . . .Sonya Winter
    swinter@sierrahealth.com
  VP Network Development . . . . .Scott Cassano
    scassono@sierrahealth.com
  Media Contact . . . . .Jeff Smith
    952-931-5685
    jeff.smith@uhc.com

Specialty Managed Care Partners
  Express Scripts

690   Hometown Health Plan

830 Harvard Way
Reno, NV 89502
Toll-Free: 800-336-0123
Phone: 775-982-3232
Fax: 775-982-3741
customer_Service@hometownhealth.com
www.hometownhealth.com
Subsidiary of: Renown Health
Non-Profit Organization: Yes
Year Founded: 1988
Owned by an Integrated Delivery Network (IDN): Yes
Number of Affiliated Hospitals: 19
Number of Primary Care Physicians: 256
Number of Referral/Specialty Physicians: 8,917
Total Enrollment: 32,000
State Enrollment: 10,000

Healthplan and Services Defined
  PLAN TYPE: Multiple
  Model Type: Network
  Plan Specialty: ASO, Behavioral Health, Chiropractic, Dental,
    Disease Management, EPO, Lab, PBM, Vision, Radiology,
    Worker's Compensation, UR
  Benefits Offered: Behavioral Health, Chiropractic, Complementary
    Medicine, Dental, Disease Management, Home Care, Inpatient
    SNF, Physical Therapy, Podiatry, Prescription, Psychiatric,

Transplant, Vision, Wellness, Worker's Compensation, AD&D,
    Life, LTD, STD, Accupuncture
  Offers Demand Management Patient Information Service: Yes

Type of Coverage
  Commercial, Medicare, Supplemental Medicare

Geographic Areas Served
  Statewide

Subscriber Information
  Average Monthly Fee Per Subscriber
    (Employee + Employer Contribution):
      Employee Only (Self): Varies
      Employee & 1 Family Member: Varies
      Employee & 2 Family Members: Varies
      Medicare: Varies
  Average Annual Deductible Per Subscriber:
      Employee Only (Self): Varies
      Employee & 1 Family Member: Varies
      Employee & 2 Family Members: Varies
      Medicare: Varies
  Average Subscriber Co-Payment:
      Primary Care Physician: Varies
      Non-Network Physician: Varies
      Prescription Drugs: Varies
      Hospital ER: Varies
      Home Health Care: Varies
      Home Health Care Max. Days/Visits Covered: Varies
      Nursing Home: Varies
      Nursing Home Max. Days/Visits Covered: Varies

Accreditation Certification
  TJC

Key Personnel
  President/CEO . . . . .Jim Miller
  VP . . . . .Troy Smith
  Director Of Finance . . . . .Jeff Brutcher
  Marketing Director . . . . .Ty Windfeldt
  Medical Director . . . . .Linda Ash-Jackson
  Customer Service Manager .John Ormond
  IR Director . . . . .Bob Farrer
  Health Service Director . . . . .Linda Keenan
  COO . . . . .Patrick Kluna

691   Humana Health Insurance of Nevada

770 E Warm Springs Road
Suite 340
Las Vegas, NV 89119
Phone: 702-837-4401
Fax: 702-562-0134
www.humana.com
For Profit Organization: Yes

Healthplan and Services Defined
  PLAN TYPE: HMO/PPO

Type of Coverage
  Commercial, Individual

Accreditation Certification
  URAC, NCQA, CORE

Key Personnel
  Chairman/CEO . . . . .Michael McCallister
  President . . . . .Bruce Broussard
  Chief Operating Officer .James E Murray
  SVP/CFO . . . . .James Bloem

692   Liberty Dental Plan of Nevada

6385 S. Rainbow Blvd
Suite 200
Las Vegas, NV 89118
Toll-Free: 888-401-1128
www.libertydentalplan.com/nv

For Profit Organization: Yes

Healthplan and Services Defined
  PLAN TYPE: Dental
  Other Type: Dental HMO
  Plan Specialty: Dental
  Benefits Offered: Dental

Type of Coverage
  Commercial

Key Personnel
  President/CEO .... Amir Neshat, DDS
  EVP .... John Carvelli
  Chief Financial Officer .... Maja Kapic
  Dental Director .... Richard Hague, DMD
  National Dental Director .... Gary Dougan, DDS
  VP, Client Services .... Marsha Hazlewood
  VP, Business Development .... Hugh Hazlewood
  SVP/Professional Services .... Kay Kabarsky, DMD
  SVP/Govt. Health Programs .... Dave Meadows
  VP, Account Management .... Lynda Bull

693 Nevada Preferred Healthcare Providers

639 Isbell Road
Suite 400
Las Vegas, NV 89509
Toll-Free: 800-776-6959
Phone: 775-356-1159
Fax: 775-356-5746
info@nevadapreferred.com
www.nvpp.com
Subsidiary of: Universal Health Network/Catholic Healthcare West
For Profit Organization: Yes
Year Founded: 1983
Owned by an Integrated Delivery Network (IDN): Yes
Number of Primary Care Physicians: 1,253
Number of Referral/Specialty Physicians: 2,162
Total Enrollment: 150,000
State Enrollment: 150,000

Healthplan and Services Defined
  PLAN TYPE: PPO
  Model Type: Network

Type of Payment Plans Offered
  Capitated, FFS, Combination FFS & DFFS

Geographic Areas Served
  Statewide

Network Qualifications
  Pre-Admission Certification: Yes

Peer Review Type
  Utilization Review: Yes
  Second Surgical Opinion: Yes
  Case Management: Yes

Publishes and Distributes Report Card: No

Accreditation Certification
  Utilization Review, Pre-Admission Certification, State Licensure, Quality Assurance Program

Average Claim Compensation
  Physician's Fees Charged: 60%
  Hospital's Fees Charged: 55%

Specialty Managed Care Partners
  Enters into Contracts with Regional Business Coalitions: No

694 Nevada Preferred Healthcare Providers

639 Isbell Road
Suite 400
Reno, NV 89509
Toll-Free: 800-776-6959
Phone: 775-356-1159
Fax: 775-356-5746
info@nevadapreferred.com
www.universalhealthnet.com
Subsidiary of: Universal Health Network
Year Founded: 1991
Number of Affiliated Hospitals: 80
Number of Primary Care Physicians: 4,483
Total Enrollment: 150,000
State Enrollment: 150,000

Healthplan and Services Defined
  PLAN TYPE: HMO/PPO
  Other Type: EPO
  Model Type: Network
  Plan Specialty: EPO, Worker's Compensation
  Benefits Offered: Behavioral Health, Chiropractic, Home Care, Physical Therapy, Podiatry, Psychiatric, Transplant, Wellness, Worker's Compensation

Type of Payment Plans Offered
  POS, DFFS, FFS, Combination FFS & DFFS

Geographic Areas Served
  Comprehensive coverage for California, Louisiana, Nevada, South Carolina, Texas, Utah, Georgia, Washington, DC

Network Qualifications
  Pre-Admission Certification: Yes

Peer Review Type
  Utilization Review: Yes
  Second Surgical Opinion: Yes
  Case Management: Yes

Publishes and Distributes Report Card: No

Specialty Managed Care Partners
  Enters into Contracts with Regional Business Coalitions: Yes

Employer References
  State of Nevada, CCN, PPO USA GEHA, Valley Health System, Pepperpill

695 NevadaCare

1210 S Valley View
Suite 104
Las Vegas, NV 89102
Toll-Free: 800-447-9834
Phone: 702-668-4200
nevadacare@imxinc.com
www.nevadacare.com
Mailing Address: PO Box 379020, Las Vegas, NV 89137
Subsidiary of: Imxinc
For Profit Organization: Yes
Year Founded: 1991
Number of Primary Care Physicians: 4,000
Number of Referral/Specialty Physicians: 2,900
Total Enrollment: 3,000
State Enrollment: 19,642

Healthplan and Services Defined
  PLAN TYPE: HMO
  Model Type: Network
  Benefits Offered: Prescription

Type of Payment Plans Offered
  Combination FFS & DFFS

Geographic Areas Served
  Clark county and Reno/Sparks in Washoe counties

Network Qualifications
Pre-Admission Certification: Yes

Peer Review Type
Utilization Review: Yes

Publishes and Distributes Report Card: No

Accreditation Certification
TJC Accreditation, Medicare Approved, Utilization Review, Pre-Admission Certification, State Licensure, Quality Assurance Program

Key Personnel
President . . . . Todd Meek
Public Affairs . . . . Larry Frank
480-921-8944
lawrencef@imxinc.com

---

696 PacifiCare of Nevada
700 E Warm Springs Road
#200
Las Vegas, NV 89119
Phone: 702-269-7500
www.pacificare.com
Secondary Address: 5190 Neil Road, #420, Reno, NV 89502
Subsidiary of: UnitedHealthCare
Non-Profit Organization: Yes
Year Founded: 1992
Number of Affiliated Hospitals: 11
Number of Primary Care Physicians: 267
Number of Referral/Specialty Physicians: 805
Total Enrollment: 26,000
State Enrollment: 28,591

Healthplan and Services Defined
PLAN TYPE: HMO
Model Type: IPA, Network
Plan Specialty: Behavioral Health, Chiropractic, Dental, Lab, Vision, Radiology
Benefits Offered: Behavioral Health, Chiropractic, Dental, Inpatient SNF, Physical Therapy, Prescription, Vision
Offers Demand Management Patient Information Service: Yes

Type of Coverage
Commercial, Individual, Indemnity, Medicare, Supplemental Medicare
Catastrophic Illness Benefit: Maximum $2M

Type of Payment Plans Offered
Capitated, FFS

Accreditation Certification
NCQA

Key Personnel
President . . . . Howard G. Phanstiel
CFO . . . . Gregory W Scott
President . . . . Brad Bowlus
Executive Vice President . . . . Jacqueline Kosecoff, PhD
Director of Sales . . . . Bruce Huxghue

Employer References
350 businesses in Nevada

---

697 Saint Mary's Health Plans
1510 Meadow Wood Lane
Reno, NV 89502
Toll-Free: 800-433-3077
Phone: 775-770-6000
www.saintmaryshealthplans.com
Secondary Address: 2475 Village View Drive, Suite 100, Henderson, NV 89074
Subsidiary of: CHW
For Profit Organization: Yes
Year Founded: 1983

Number of Affiliated Hospitals: 21
Number of Primary Care Physicians: 4,000
Number of Referral/Specialty Physicians: 1,500
Total Enrollment: 15,000

Healthplan and Services Defined
PLAN TYPE: HMO
Other Type: POS
Model Type: Group, Network
Plan Specialty: ASO, Behavioral Health, Chiropractic, Dental, Disease Management, EPO, MSO, PBM, Vision, Radiology, Worker's Compensation
Benefits Offered: Behavioral Health, Chiropractic, Complementary Medicine, Dental, Disease Management, Home Care, Inpatient SNF, Long-Term Care, Physical Therapy, Podiatry, Prescription, Psychiatric, Transplant, Vision, Wellness, Worker's Compensation, Routine PE, pre and

Type of Payment Plans Offered
POS, DFFS, FFS, Combination FFS & DFFS

Geographic Areas Served
Nevada and border communities in California and Arizona

Subscriber Information
Average Monthly Fee Per Subscriber
(Employee + Employer Contribution):
Employee Only (Self): Varies by plan
Average Subscriber Co-Payment:
Nursing Home: Varies

Network Qualifications
Pre-Admission Certification: Yes

Peer Review Type
Utilization Review: Yes
Second Surgical Opinion: Yes
Case Management: Yes

Accreditation Certification
NCQA
TJC Accreditation, Medicare Approved, Pre-Admission Certification

Key Personnel
President/CEO . . . . M Donald Kowitz
VP, Chief Financial Offic . . . . Dave Challis
VP, CDS Group Health . . . . Rayne Niehaus
VP, Sales/Marketing . . . . Glen Padula

---

698 UnitedHealthcare Nevada
2700 North Tenaya Way
Las Vegas, NV 89128
Phone: 702-242-7000
Fax: 702-242-7920
w3_hpnsd_sl@sierrahealth.com
www.uhcnevada.com
Mailing Address: PO Box 15645, Las Vegas, NV 89114-5645
For Profit Organization: Yes
Year Founded: 1984
Number of Affiliated Hospitals: 6
Number of Primary Care Physicians: 161
Total Enrollment: 580,000
State Enrollment: 107,963

Healthplan and Services Defined
PLAN TYPE: HMO/PPO
Other Type: POS
Model Type: Network
Benefits Offered: Prescription
Offers Demand Management Patient Information Service: Yes

Type of Payment Plans Offered
POS, DFFS, Capitated, FFS

Geographic Areas Served
Clark County

Subscriber Information

Average Monthly Fee Per Subscriber
(Employee + Employer Contribution):
Employee Only (Self): $39.00

Average Annual Deductible Per Subscriber:
Employee Only (Self): $0
Employee & 1 Family Member: $0
Employee & 2 Family Members: $0
Medicare: $0

Average Subscriber Co-Payment:
Primary Care Physician: $0.00
Prescription Drugs: $10.00
Hospital ER: $50.00
Home Health Care: Varies
Home Health Care Max. Days/Visits Covered: Unlimited
Nursing Home: Varies
Nursing Home Max. Days/Visits Covered: 100 days

Peer Review Type

Case Management: Yes

Publishes and Distributes Report Card: Yes

Key Personnel

Market CEO . . . . Donald J Giancursio
Sr VP/CFO/Treasurer. . . . . Paul Palmer
Executive VP/Administrat . . . . William Godfrey
Vice President, PR . . . . Peter O'Neill
Sr VP/Program Office . . . . Larry Howard
President, Managed Health . . . . Jonathan Bunker
COO . . . . Ray Summerson
VP/Customer Service. . . . . Mike Montalvo
VP/Human Resources . . . . Daniel Kruger
CMO/VP Medical Affairs . . . . Christine Peterson, MD
Sr VP/Legal & Administ. . . . . Frank Collins
VP/Information Technology. Robert Schaich
VP/Healthcare Quality/Ed . . . . Allan Ebbin, MD, MPH
Executive VP/Special Proj . . . . Marie Soldo
SVP, Public Relations . . . . Peter O'Neill
702-242-7156
peter.oneill@uhc.com
Manager, Public Relations . . . . Amanda Penn
702-242-7784
amanda.penn@uhc.com

Health Insurance Coverage Status and Type of Coverage by Age

Category	All Persons		Under 18 years		Under 65 years		65 years and over	
	Number	%	Number	%	Number	%	Number	%
Total population	1,309	-	271	-	1,114	-	195	-
Covered by some type of health insurance	1,168 (7)	89.3 (0.5)	260 (2)	96.2 (0.7)	973 (7)	87.4 (0.6)	195 (1)	99.9 (0.1)
Covered by private health insurance	979 (10)	74.8 (0.8)	189 (6)	69.7 (2.0)	839 (10)	75.3 (0.9)	141 (3)	72.1 (1.7)
Employment based	841 (10)	64.3 (0.8)	174 (5)	64.2 (2.0)	759 (10)	68.2 (0.9)	82 (4)	42.0 (1.8)
Direct purchase	150 (7)	11.5 (0.5)	14 (2)	5.2 (0.9)	85 (5)	7.6 (0.5)	66 (3)	33.7 (1.7)
Covered by TRICARE	30 (4)	2.3 (0.3)	4 (1)	1.3 (0.5)	16 (3)	1.4 (0.3)	14 (2)	7.0 (0.8)
Covered by government health insurance	354 (9)	27.0 (0.7)	81 (6)	29.7 (2.3)	165 (9)	14.9 (0.8)	188 (2)	96.4 (0.6)
Covered by Medicaid	148 (8)	11.3 (0.6)	80 (6)	29.6 (2.3)	134 (8)	12.0 (0.7)	14 (2)	7.0 (0.9)
Also by private insurance	22 (3)	1.7 (0.2)	9 (2)	3.2 (0.8)	16 (3)	1.4 (0.3)	7 (1)	3.4 (0.6)
Covered by Medicare	222 (4)	17.0 (0.3)	1 (Z)	0.2 (0.2)	34 (3)	3.1 (0.3)	188 (2)	96.2 (0.6)
Also by private insurance	144 (4)	11.0 (0.3)	Z (Z)	0.1 (0.1)	10 (2)	0.9 (0.2)	134 (4)	68.5 (1.8)
Also by Medicaid	27 (3)	2.1 (0.2)	Z (Z)	0.1 (0.1)	14 (2)	1.2 (0.2)	14 (2)	7.0 (0.9)
Covered by VA Care	32 (2)	2.4 (0.2)	Z (Z)	0.0 (0.1)	13 (2)	1.2 (0.2)	19 (1)	9.5 (0.8)
Not covered at any time during the year	140 (7)	10.7 (0.5)	10 (2)	3.8 (0.7)	140 (7)	12.6 (0.6)	Z (Z)	0.1 (0.1)

Note: Numbers in thousands; Figures cover 2013; Margin of error appears in parenthesis; A "Z" indicates that the value either represents or rounds to zero.
Source: U.S. Census Bureau, 2013 American Community Survey, Table HI05. Health Insurance Coverage Status and Type of Coverage by State and Age for All People: 2013

New Hampshire

699 Aetna Health of New Hampshire

151 Farmington Avenue
Hartford, CT 06156
Toll-Free: 800-872-3862
Phone: 860-273-0123
www.aetna.com
Partnered with: eHealthInsurance Services Inc.
For Profit Organization: Yes
Total Enrollment: 11,596,230

Healthplan and Services Defined
PLAN TYPE: PPO
Other Type: POS
Plan Specialty: EPO
Benefits Offered: Dental, Disease Management, Long-Term Care, Prescription, Wellness, Life, LTD, STD

Type of Coverage
Commercial, Individual

Type of Payment Plans Offered
POS, FFS

Geographic Areas Served
Statewide

Key Personnel
Chairman/CEO/President . . . . Mark T Bertolini
EVP, General Counsel . . . . William J Casazza
EVP/CFO . . . . Shawn M Guertin

700 Anthem Blue Cross & Blue Shield of New Hampshire

3000 Goffs Falls Road
Manchester, NH 03103
Phone: 603-695-7000
www.anthem.com
Year Founded: 1942
Owned by an Integrated Delivery Network (IDN): Yes
Number of Affiliated Hospitals: 26
Number of Primary Care Physicians: 90
Number of Referral/Specialty Physicians: 3,608
Total Enrollment: 560,000
State Enrollment: 400,000

Healthplan and Services Defined
PLAN TYPE: HMO
Model Type: IPA, TPA
Plan Specialty: ASO, Behavioral Health, Chiropractic, Dental, Disease Management, EPO, Lab, MSO, PBM, Vision
Benefits Offered: Behavioral Health, Chiropractic, Dental, Disease Management, Home Care, Inpatient SNF, Physical Therapy, Prescription, Psychiatric, Transplant, Wellness, Life
Offers Demand Management Patient Information Service: Yes
DMPI Services Offered: Asthma, Diabetes, Cardiovascular, Healthy Babies, Lifestyle

Type of Coverage
Commercial, Individual

Geographic Areas Served
Maine, New Hampshire, Connecticut

Subscriber Information
Average Subscriber Co-Payment:
Nursing Home: Varies

Network Qualifications
Pre-Admission Certification: Yes

Peer Review Type
Utilization Review: Yes
Case Management: Yes

Publishes and Distributes Report Card: Yes
Accreditation Certification
NCQA
Utilization Review, Quality Assurance Program

Key Personnel
President/GM . . . . Lisa M Guertin
Dir, Commun & Comm Relat . . . . Chris Dugan
Director, Govt Affairs . . . . Paula Rogers
SVP . . . . Dennis Casey
Provider Network Manager . . . . Lance Milner
Media Contact . . . . Chris Dugan
603-695-7202
chris.dugan@anthem.com

701 CIGNA HealthCare of New Hampshire

Two College Park Drive
Suite 250
Hooksett, NH 03106
Toll-Free: 800-531-4584
Phone: 603-268-7839
Fax: 603-268-7981
www.cigna.com
For Profit Organization: Yes
Year Founded: 1985
Physician Owned Organization: Yes
Owned by an Integrated Delivery Network (IDN): Yes
Federally Qualified: Yes
Number of Affiliated Hospitals: 26
Number of Primary Care Physicians: 1,055
Number of Referral/Specialty Physicians: 3,129
Total Enrollment: 23,559
State Enrollment: 23,559

Healthplan and Services Defined
PLAN TYPE: HMO
Other Type: POS
Model Type: Network
Plan Specialty: General Medical
Benefits Offered: Behavioral Health, Chiropractic, Complementary Medicine, Disease Management, Home Care, Inpatient SNF, Physical Therapy, Podiatry, Prescription, Psychiatric, Transplant, Vision, Wellness, Healthy babies, women's health, men's health
Offers Demand Management Patient Information Service: Yes

Type of Coverage
Commercial, Small Groups HMO All Network
Catastrophic Illness Benefit: Varies per case

Type of Payment Plans Offered
DFFS, Capitated, FFS, Combination FFS & DFFS

Geographic Areas Served
State of New Hampshire, all counties

Subscriber Information
Average Monthly Fee Per Subscriber
(Employee + Employer Contribution):
Employee Only (Self): Varies by plan
Average Subscriber Co-Payment:
Primary Care Physician: $10.00
Non-Network Physician: Not covered
Prescription Drugs: $5/15/35
Hospital ER: $50.00
Home Health Care Max. Days/Visits Covered: Unlimited
Nursing Home Max. Days/Visits Covered: 60 days per year

Network Qualifications
Pre-Admission Certification: Yes

Peer Review Type
Utilization Review: Yes
Second Surgical Opinion: Yes
Case Management: Yes

Publishes and Distributes Report Card: Yes

Accreditation Certification
TJC Accreditation, Medicare Approved, Utilization Review,
Pre-Admission Certification, State Licensure, Quality Assurance
Program

Key Personnel
President/CEO . . . . .David Cordani
EVP/Global Chief Mkt Offi . . . . .Lisa Bacus
EVP/Global Chief Info Off . . . . .Mark Boxer
Claims . . . . .Ellie St Pierre
Credentialing . . . . .Edna York
In-House Formulary . . . . .Jim Demosthenes
Marketing. . . . . .Deborah Wing
Medical Affairs . . . . .Rob Hockmuth, MD
Provider Services . . . . .Kathy Smith
Sales . . . . .Karynlee Harrington

---

702   Delta Dental of New Hampshire

One Delta Drive
PO Box 2002
Concord, NH 03302
Toll-Free: 800-537-1715
Phone: 603-223-1000
Fax: 603-223-1199
nedelta@nedelta.com
www.nedelta.com
Non-Profit Organization: Yes
Year Founded: 1961
Total Enrollment: 745,000
State Enrollment: 700,000

Healthplan and Services Defined
PLAN TYPE: Dental
Other Type: Dental PPO
Model Type: Network
Plan Specialty: ASO, Dental
Benefits Offered: Dental

Type of Coverage
Commercial, Individual, Group
Catastrophic Illness Benefit: None

Geographic Areas Served
Statewide

Subscriber Information
Average Monthly Fee Per Subscriber
(Employee + Employer Contribution):
Employee Only (Self): Varies
Employee & 1 Family Member: Varies
Employee & 2 Family Members: Varies
Average Annual Deductible Per Subscriber:
Employee Only (Self): Varies
Employee & 1 Family Member: Varies
Employee & 2 Family Members: Varies
Average Subscriber Co-Payment:
Prescription Drugs: $0
Home Health Care: $0
Nursing Home: $0

Key Personnel
President/CEO. . . . . .Thomas Raffio
Chairman . . . . .Terence Wardrop
VP, Information Systems. . . . . .Michael D Bourbeau
Strategy Management. . . . . .Linda J Roche
General Counsel . . . . .Kenneth L Robinson, Jr
VP, Marketing . . . . .Gene R Emery
VP, Human Resources . . . . .Connie M Roy-Czyzowski, SHPR
Dir, Corporate Relations . . . . .Barbara A McLaughlin
SVP, Finance . . . . .Helen T Biglin
Dir, Actuarial & Research . . . . .Laurence R Weissbrot, FSA
VP, Professional Relation. . . . . .Shannon E Mills, DDS
Chief Dental Officer . . . . .Michael E Couret, DDS

---

703   eHealthInsurance Services Inc.

11919 Foundation Place
Gold River, CA 95670
Toll-Free: 800-644-3491
webmaster@healthinsurance.com
www.e.healthinsurance.com
Year Founded: 1997

Healthplan and Services Defined
PLAN TYPE: HMO/PPO
Benefits Offered: Dental, Life, STD

Type of Coverage
Commercial, Individual, Medicare

Geographic Areas Served
All 50 states in the USA and District of Columbia

Key Personnel
Chairman & CEO . . . . .Gary L. Lauer
EVP/Business & Corp. Dev. . . . . .Bruce Telkamp
EVP/Chief Technology . . . . .Dr. Sheldon X. Wang
SVP & CFO . . . . .Stuart M. Huizinga
Pres. of eHealth Gov. Sys . . . . .Samuel C. Gibbs
SVP of Sales & Operations . . . . .Robert S. Hurley
Director Public Relations. .Nate Purpura
650-210-3115

---

704   Harvard Pilgrim Health Care of New England

650 Elm Street
Suite 700
Manchester, NH 03101-2596
Toll-Free: 888-888-4742
www.harvardpilgrim.org
Non-Profit Organization: Yes
Year Founded: 1977
Number of Affiliated Hospitals: 135
Number of Primary Care Physicians: 28,000
Total Enrollment: 1,100,000
State Enrollment: 139,000

Healthplan and Services Defined
PLAN TYPE: Multiple
Model Type: Mixed

Geographic Areas Served
Massachusetts, New Hampshire and Maine

Accreditation Certification
NCQA

Key Personnel
Executive Director . . . . .Karen Voci

---

705   Humana Health Insurance of New Hampshire

1 New Hampshire Ave
Suite 125
Portsmouth, NH 03801
Toll-Free: 800-967-2370
www.humana.com
For Profit Organization: Yes

Healthplan and Services Defined
PLAN TYPE: HMO/PPO

Type of Coverage
Commercial, Individual

Accreditation Certification
URAC, NCQA, CORE

Key Personnel
Chairman . . . . .Michael R McCallister
President. . . . . .Bruce Broussard

Chief Operating Officer . . . . James Murray
SVP/CFO . . . . James Bloem

706 MVP Health Care: New Hampshire

33 South Commercial Street
Suite 303
Manchester, NH 03101
Toll-Free: 888-656-5695
Phone: 603-647-7181
Fax: 603-647-9607
www.mvphealthcare.com
Non-Profit Organization: Yes
Year Founded: 1983
Number of Primary Care Physicians: 24,000
Total Enrollment: 750,000

Healthplan and Services Defined
PLAN TYPE: HMO/PPO
Model Type: IPA
Benefits Offered: Behavioral Health, Chiropractic, Complementary
Medicine, Dental, Disease Management, Home Care, Inpatient
SNF, Physical Therapy, Podiatry, Prescription, Psychiatric,
Transplant, Vision, Wellness, Worker's Compensation, Online
Health Library

Type of Coverage
Commercial, Individual, Indemnity

Type of Payment Plans Offered
POS, DFFS, Capitated, FFS, Combination FFS & DFFS

Subscriber Information
Average Monthly Fee Per Subscriber
(Employee + Employer Contribution):
Employee Only (Self): Varies by plan
Average Annual Deductible Per Subscriber:
Employee Only (Self): Varies by plan

Accreditation Certification
NCQA

Key Personnel
President/CEO . . . . David Oliker
EVP/COO . . . . Chris Henchey
EVP/Rochester Operations . . . . Lisa A Brubaker
EVP/Network Management . . . . Mark Fish
EVP/Planning . . . . Alfred Gatti
EVP/Chief Legal Officer . . . . Denise Gonick, Esq
EVP/Human Resources . . . . James Morrill

707 Northeast Community Care

49 Atlantic Place
South Portland, ME 04106-2316
Toll-Free: 800-998-3056
Phone: 207-773-3920
Fax: 207-773-3990
www.northeastcommunitycare.com
Subsidiary of: Arcadian Health Plans

Healthplan and Services Defined
PLAN TYPE: Medicare

Type of Coverage
Medicare

708 UnitedHealthCare of New Hampshire

One Research Drive
Westborough, MA 01581
Toll-Free: 800-444-7855
www.uhc.com
Subsidiary of: UnitedHealth Group
For Profit Organization: Yes
Year Founded: 1986

Number of Affiliated Hospitals: 47
Number of Primary Care Physicians: 1,600
Number of Referral/Specialty Physicians: 3,500
Total Enrollment: 75,000,000

Healthplan and Services Defined
PLAN TYPE: HMO/PPO
Model Type: Mixed Model
Plan Specialty: MSO
Benefits Offered: Behavioral Health, Chiropractic, Complementary
Medicine, Dental, Disease Management, Home Care, Inpatient
SNF, Long-Term Care, Physical Therapy, Podiatry, Prescription,
Psychiatric, Transplant, Vision, Wellness, AD&D, Life

Type of Coverage
Commercial, Individual, Medicaid, Commercial Group

Type of Payment Plans Offered
DFFS, FFS, Combination FFS & DFFS

Geographic Areas Served
Statewide

Subscriber Information
Average Monthly Fee Per Subscriber
(Employee + Employer Contribution):
Employee Only (Self): Varies
Average Subscriber Co-Payment:
Primary Care Physician: $10
Prescription Drugs: $10/15/30
Hospital ER: $50

Network Qualifications
Pre-Admission Certification: Yes

Peer Review Type
Case Management: Yes

Publishes and Distributes Report Card: Yes

Accreditation Certification
URAC, NCQA
State Licensure, Quality Assurance Program

Average Claim Compensation
Physician's Fees Charged: 70%
Hospital's Fees Charged: 55%

Specialty Managed Care Partners
United Behavioral Health
Enters into Contracts with Regional Business Coalitions: No

Health Insurance Coverage Status and Type of Coverage by Age

Category	All Persons		Under 18 years		Under 65 years		65 years and over	
	Number	%	Number	%	Number	%	Number	%
Total population	8,792	-	2,018	-	7,547	-	1,245	-
Covered by some type of health insurance	7,631 (21)	86.8 (0.2)	1,906 (8)	94.4 (0.4)	6,406 (21)	84.9 (0.3)	1,226 (3)	98.4 (0.2)
Covered by private health insurance	6,156 (30)	70.0 (0.3)	1,349 (13)	66.9 (0.7)	5,368 (27)	71.1 (0.4)	788 (9)	63.3 (0.7)
Employment based	5,434 (29)	61.8 (0.3)	1,239 (14)	61.4 (0.7)	4,923 (27)	65.2 (0.4)	511 (9)	41.1 (0.7)
Direct purchase	901 (19)	10.2 (0.2)	121 (7)	6.0 (0.3)	540 (14)	7.2 (0.2)	361 (10)	29.0 (0.8)
Covered by TRICARE	84 (6)	1.0 (0.1)	18 (3)	0.9 (0.1)	55 (6)	0.7 (0.1)	29 (2)	2.3 (0.2)
Covered by government health insurance	2,389 (23)	27.2 (0.3)	606 (13)	30.0 (0.6)	1,210 (22)	16.0 (0.3)	1,180 (4)	94.8 (0.3)
Covered by Medicaid	1,238 (23)	14.1 (0.3)	600 (13)	29.8 (0.6)	1,083 (22)	14.3 (0.3)	156 (6)	12.5 (0.5)
Also by private insurance	177 (8)	2.0 (0.1)	48 (4)	2.4 (0.2)	117 (7)	1.5 (0.1)	61 (3)	4.9 (0.3)
Covered by Medicare	1,357 (10)	15.4 (0.1)	9 (2)	0.5 (0.1)	178 (8)	2.4 (0.1)	1,179 (4)	94.7 (0.3)
Also by private insurance	796 (10)	9.1 (0.1)	2 (1)	0.1 (0.1)	54 (3)	0.7 (0.1)	741 (9)	59.5 (0.7)
Also by Medicaid	233 (9)	2.7 (0.1)	5 (1)	0.2 (0.1)	77 (6)	1.0 (0.1)	156 (6)	12.5 (0.5)
Covered by VA Care	95 (4)	1.1 (0.1)	1 (1)	0.1 (0.1)	34 (3)	0.4 (0.1)	62 (3)	5.0 (0.3)
Not covered at any time during the year	1,160 (22)	13.2 (0.2)	112 (8)	5.6 (0.4)	1,141 (21)	15.1 (0.3)	19 (3)	1.6 (0.2)

Note: Numbers in thousands; Figures cover 2013; Margin of error appears in parenthesis; A "Z" indicates that the value either represents or rounds to zero.
Source: U.S. Census Bureau, 2013 American Community Survey, Table HI05. Health Insurance Coverage Status and Type of Coverage by State and Age for All People: 2013

New Jersey

709 Aetna Health of New Jersey
151 Farmington Avenue
Hartford, CT 06156
Toll-Free: 800-872-3862
Phone: 860-273-0123
www.aetna.com
For Profit Organization: Yes
Year Founded: 1981
Number of Affiliated Hospitals: 4,135
Number of Primary Care Physicians: 405,000
Number of Referral/Specialty Physicians: 684,000
Total Enrollment: 5,183,333
State Enrollment: 518,333

Healthplan and Services Defined
PLAN TYPE: HMO
Other Type: POS
Model Type: Network
Plan Specialty: ASO, Behavioral Health, Chiropractic, Dental, Disease Management, Vision, Radiology, Worker's Compensation
Benefits Offered: Behavioral Health, Chiropractic, Complementary Medicine, Dental, Disease Management, Home Care, Prescription, Vision, Worker's Compensation
Offers Demand Management Patient Information Service: Yes

Type of Coverage
Commercial, Medicare

Type of Payment Plans Offered
POS, DFFS, Capitated, FFS, Combination FFS & DFFS

Geographic Areas Served
Statewide

Peer Review Type
Case Management: No

Publishes and Distributes Report Card: Yes

Key Personnel
Chairman/President/CEO.....................Mark T Bertolini
EVP/General Counsel ....William J Casazza
EVP/CFO ....Shawn M Guertin

710 AmeriChoice by UnitedHealthCare
Four Gateway Center
4th Floor
Newark, NJ 07102
Toll-Free: 800-941-4647
Phone: 973-297-5500
www.americhoice.com
Subsidiary of: A UnitedHealth Group Company
For Profit Organization: Yes
Year Founded: 1989
Total Enrollment: 200,871
State Enrollment: 199,018

Healthplan and Services Defined
PLAN TYPE: HMO

Type of Coverage
Medicare, Medicaid, NJ Family Care

Geographic Areas Served
16 state area

Key Personnel
Chief Operating Officer ....Carolyn Magill
Finance Director...........................Phillip Franz
Chief Medical Officer ....Ebben Smith, MD
Member Services ....Dorothy Ward
Media Contact...............................Jeff Smith
952-931-5685
jeff.smith@uhc.com

711 AmeriChoice New Jersey
Four Gateway Center
4th Floor
Newark, NJ 07102
Toll-Free: 800-941-4647
Phone: 973-297-5500
www.americhoice.com

Healthplan and Services Defined
PLAN TYPE: Other

712 Amerigroup New Jersey
4425 Corporation Lane
Suite 400
Virginia Beach, VA 23462
Toll-Free: 800-231-8076
Phone: 732-452-6000
info@amerigroupcorp.com
www.amerigroupcorp.com
For Profit Organization: Yes
Year Founded: 1996
Total Enrollment: 1,900,000
State Enrollment: 105,000

Healthplan and Services Defined
PLAN TYPE: HMO

Type of Payment Plans Offered
Capitated

Geographic Areas Served
20 of the 21 counties in New Jersey

Accreditation Certification
Quality Assurance Program

Key Personnel
President/CEO...........................Peter Haytaian
SVP/Chief Medical Officer..............Mary T McCluskey, MD
CFO.......................................Scott Anglin
Staff VP, Communications....................Cindy Wakefield
404-788-8957

713 AmeriHealth HMO
259 Prospect Plains Road
Bldg M
Cranbury, NJ 08512
Phone: 609-662-2400
Fax: 856-778-6551
www.amerihealth.com
Secondary Address: 485C US Highway 1 South, Suite 300, Iselin, NJ 08830-3052
For Profit Organization: Yes
Year Founded: 1995
Number of Affiliated Hospitals: 230
Number of Primary Care Physicians: 37,000
Number of Referral/Specialty Physicians: 36,496
Total Enrollment: 265,000
State Enrollment: 77,761

Healthplan and Services Defined
PLAN TYPE: HMO/PPO
Other Type: POS
Model Type: IPA, PPO
Benefits Offered: Dental, Disease Management, Prescription, Vision, Wellness

Type of Coverage
Commercial, Individual, Medicare, Supplemental Medicare, Medicaid

Type of Payment Plans Offered
POS, DFFS, FFS

Geographic Areas Served
New Jersey, Delaware, Pennsylvania counties: Berks, Bucks, Chester, Delaware, Lancaster, Lehigh, Montgomery, Northhampton, Philadelphia

Subscriber Information
Average Monthly Fee Per Subscriber
(Employee + Employer Contribution):
Employee Only (Self): $190 per mo and up

Accreditation Certification
TJC, NCQA

Key Personnel
President and CEO . . . . .William F Haggett
Media Contact . . . . .Kate Wilhelmi
856-778-6552

Specialty Managed Care Partners
Enters into Contracts with Regional Business Coalitions: Yes

---

714 Assurant Employee Benefits: New Jersey
10 Lanidex Plaza W
Parsippany, NJ 07054-4412
Phone: 973-428-8445
benefits@assurant.com
www.assurantemployeebenefits.com
Subsidiary of: Assurant, Inc
For Profit Organization: Yes
Number of Primary Care Physicians: 112,000
Total Enrollment: 47,000

Healthplan and Services Defined
PLAN TYPE: Multiple
Plan Specialty: Dental, Vision, Long & Short-Term Disability
Benefits Offered: Dental, Vision, Wellness, AD&D, Life, LTD, STD

Type of Coverage
Commercial, Indemnity, Individual Dental Plans

Geographic Areas Served
Statewide

Subscriber Information
Average Monthly Fee Per Subscriber
(Employee + Employer Contribution):
Employee Only (Self): Varies by plan

Key Personnel
President/CEO. . . . . .John S Roberts
VP/General Counsel . . . . .Kenneth Bowen
SVP/Underwriting . . . . .Dianna Duvall
SVP/Claims . . . . .Sheryle Ohme
SVP/Chief Info Officer. . . . . .Karla Schacht
PR Specialist. . . . . .Megan Hutchison
816-556-7815
megan.hutchison@assurant.com

---

715 Atlanticare Health Plans
2500 English Creek Avenue
Egg Harbor Township, NJ 08234
Phone: 609-407-2300
www.atlanticare.org
Non-Profit Organization: Yes
Year Founded: 1993
Number of Affiliated Hospitals: 36
Number of Primary Care Physicians: 15,009
Number of Referral/Specialty Physicians: 4,000
Total Enrollment: 150,000
State Enrollment: 150,000

Healthplan and Services Defined
PLAN TYPE: HMO/PPO
Model Type: IPA
Plan Specialty: ASO, Behavioral Health, Worker's Compensation, UR

Type of Payment Plans Offered
Combination FFS & DFFS

Geographic Areas Served
Southeastern New Jersey

Subscriber Information
Average Subscriber Co-Payment:
Primary Care Physician: $10.00
Non-Network Physician: $20.00
Prescription Drugs: $15.00
Hospital ER: $50.00
Home Health Care: $60
Nursing Home: $120

Network Qualifications
Pre-Admission Certification: Yes

Peer Review Type
Utilization Review: Yes
Second Surgical Opinion: Yes
Case Management: Yes

Accreditation Certification
TJC, URAC, NCQA

Key Personnel
President . . . . .George F Lynn

Specialty Managed Care Partners
Horizon BC/BS of NJ

---

716 Block Vision of New Jersey
325 Columbia Turnpike
Suite 303
Florham Park, NJ 21090
Toll-Free: 866-246-9589
www.blockvision.com
Year Founded: 1986
Number of Primary Care Physicians: 18,000
Total Enrollment: 300,000

Healthplan and Services Defined
PLAN TYPE: Vision
Model Type: Network
Plan Specialty: Vision
Benefits Offered: Vision
Offers Demand Management Patient Information Service: Yes

Type of Payment Plans Offered
Capitated

Geographic Areas Served
Nationwide

Key Personnel
President/CEO . . . . .Andrew Alcorn
VP/Group Sales . . . . .Steven Fleischer
Business Development . . . . .Jackie Threadgill
Member Services. . . . . .Ilana Stone
Account Executive. . . . . .Stacey Fiorina
866-246-9589
sfiorina@blockvision.com

---

717 CHN PPO
300 American Metro Boulevard
Suite 170
Hamilton, NJ 08619
Toll-Free: 800-225-4246
marketing@conservgrp.com
www.csg-inc.net
Secondary Address: Towamencin Corporate Center, Building 1, 1555 Bustard Road, Suite 100, Lansdale, PA 19446, 215-661-0500
Subsidiary of: Consolidated Services Group
For Profit Organization: Yes
Year Founded: 1986
Number of Affiliated Hospitals: 165

Number of Primary Care Physicians: 116,000
Number of Referral/Specialty Physicians: 57,550
Total Enrollment: 975,000

Healthplan and Services Defined
PLAN TYPE: PPO
Model Type: Network
Plan Specialty: Behavioral Health, Chiropractic, EPO, Lab, Vision, Radiology, Worker's Compensation, UR
Benefits Offered: Behavioral Health, Chiropractic, Disease Management, Home Care, Inpatient SNF, Long-Term Care, Physical Therapy, Podiatry, Psychiatric, Transplant, Vision, Wellness, Worker's Compensation

Type of Coverage
Catastrophic Illness Benefit: Varies per case

Type of Payment Plans Offered
POS, DFFS, FFS

Geographic Areas Served
Connecticut, New Jersey & New York

Subscriber Information
Average Monthly Fee Per Subscriber
(Employee + Employer Contribution):
Employee Only (Self): Varies
Employee & 1 Family Member: Varies
Employee & 2 Family Members: Varies
Medicare: Varies
Average Annual Deductible Per Subscriber:
Employee Only (Self): Varies
Employee & 1 Family Member: Varies
Employee & 2 Family Members: Varies
Medicare: Varies
Average Subscriber Co-Payment:
Primary Care Physician: Varies
Non-Network Physician: Varies
Prescription Drugs: Varies
Hospital ER: Varies
Home Health Care: Varies
Home Health Care Max. Days/Visits Covered: Varies
Nursing Home: Varies
Nursing Home Max. Days/Visits Covered: Varies

Network Qualifications
Pre-Admission Certification: Yes

Peer Review Type
Utilization Review: Yes
Second Surgical Opinion: Yes
Case Management: Yes

Accreditation Certification
URAC, AAPI
TJC Accreditation, Medicare Approved, Utilization Review, Pre-Admission Certification, State Licensure, Quality Assurance Program

Key Personnel
President/CEO . . . . Michael A Morrone
Executive VP/COO . . . . Craig Goldstein
SVP, Financial Operations . . . . Lee Ann Iannelli
Chief Medical Officer . . . . William P. Anthony, MD
Medical Director . . . . Robert A. Ericksen, PhD
SVP, Medical Case Mgmt. . . . . Maria Longworth
SVP, Network Operations . . . . Cara Ianniello
VP Strategic Partnerships . . . . Missy Pudimott
VP, New Jersey Sales . . . . Steve Armenti
SVP, Chief Info Officer . . . . Stan Tomasevich

Average Claim Compensation
Physician's Fees Charged: 33%
Hospital's Fees Charged: 40%

Specialty Managed Care Partners
Enters into Contracts with Regional Business Coalitions: Yes

718 CIGNA HealthCare of New Jersey
499 Washington Boulevard
Suite 526
Jersey City, NJ 07310
Toll-Free: 866-438-2446
Phone: 201-533-7000
Fax: 201-533-7164
www.cigna.com
Secondary Address: Great-West Healthcare, now part of CIGNA, 1 Centennial Ave, 1st Floor, Piscataway, NJ 08855, 732-357-2900
For Profit Organization: Yes
Year Founded: 1978
Number of Affiliated Hospitals: 82
Number of Primary Care Physicians: 5,250
Number of Referral/Specialty Physicians: 12,240
Total Enrollment: 68,935
State Enrollment: 68,935

Healthplan and Services Defined
PLAN TYPE: HMO
Other Type: POS
Model Type: Network, PPO, POS
Plan Specialty: ASO, Behavioral Health, Dental, Disease Management
Benefits Offered: Behavioral Health, Chiropractic, Dental, Disease Management, Home Care, Physical Therapy, Podiatry, Prescription, Psychiatric, Transplant, Vision, Wellness, Worker's Compensation

Type of Coverage
Commercial
Catastrophic Illness Benefit: Varies per case

Type of Payment Plans Offered
POS, FFS

Geographic Areas Served
Bergen, Essex, Hudson, Hunterdon, Middlesex, Monmouth, Morris, Passaic, Somerset, Sussex, Union, Warren, Atlantic. Burlington, Camden, Cape May, Cumberland, Gloucester, Ocean and Mercer counties

Subscriber Information
Average Monthly Fee Per Subscriber
(Employee + Employer Contribution):
Employee Only (Self): Varies by plan
Average Subscriber Co-Payment:
Primary Care Physician: $10/15/20

Network Qualifications
Pre-Admission Certification: Yes

Peer Review Type
Utilization Review: Yes
Second Surgical Opinion: Yes
Case Management: Yes

Accreditation Certification
NCQA

Key Personnel
President . . . . Charles Catalano
CFO . . . . Michael Wise
Director/Sales/Marketing . . . . John Gumkowski
VP Sales/Marketing . . . . Steven Fleisher
VP Network . . . . Thomas Garvey
VP Medical Executive . . . . Don Nicoll, MD
Director Provider Services . . . . Ann Marie Castro
VP Sales . . . . Mike Mascolo

Specialty Managed Care Partners
Enters into Contracts with Regional Business Coalitions: Yes

719 Delta Dental of New Jersey & Connecticut

Delta Dental Plaza
1639 Route 10
Parsippany, NJ 07054
Toll-Free: 800-452-9310
Fax: 973-285-4141
service@deltadentalnj.com
www.deltadentalnj.com
Non-Profit Organization: Yes
Year Founded: 1969
Total Enrollment: 54,000,000

Healthplan and Services Defined
　PLAN TYPE: Dental
　Other Type: Dental HMO/PPO/POS
　Model Type: Staff
　Plan Specialty: Dental
　Benefits Offered: Dental

Type of Coverage
　Commercial

Type of Payment Plans Offered
　POS, DFFS, Capitated, FFS, Combination FFS & DFFS

Geographic Areas Served
　New Jersey and Connecticut

Key Personnel
　President/CEO . . . . Walter VenBrunt
　CFO. . . . . James Suleski
　Senior Vice President . . . . Bruce Silverman
　Vice President . . . . Scott Navarro, DDS
　Vice President . . . . Mark Nadeau
　Dir/Media & Public Affair . . . . Elizabeth Risberg
　　415-972-8423

720 eHealthInsurance Services Inc.

11919 Foundation Place
Gold River, CA 95670
Toll-Free: 800-644-3491
webmaster@healthinsurance.com
www.e.healthinsurance.com
Year Founded: 1997

Healthplan and Services Defined
　PLAN TYPE: HMO/PPO
　Benefits Offered: Dental, Life, STD

Type of Coverage
　Commercial, Individual, Medicare

Geographic Areas Served
　All 50 states in the USA and District of Columbia

Key Personnel
　Chairman & CEO . . . . Gary L. Lauer
　EVP/Business & Corp. Dev. . . . . Bruce Telkamp
　EVP/Chief Technology . . . . Dr. Sheldon X. Wang
　SVP & CFO . . . . Stuart M. Huizinga
　Pres. of eHealth Gov. Sys . . . . Samuel C. Gibbs
　SVP of Sales & Operations . . . . Robert S. Hurley
　Director Public Relations. . . . . Nate Purpura
　　650-210-3115

721 Family Choice Health Alliance

401 Hackensack Avenue
9th Floor
Hackensack, NJ 07601-6402
Toll-Free: 800-732-7892
Phone: 201-487-6002
customerservice@familychoicehealth.com
www.familychoicehealth.com
For Profit Organization: Yes

Year Founded: 1991
Number of Affiliated Hospitals: 51
Number of Primary Care Physicians: 10,000
State Enrollment: 115,000

Healthplan and Services Defined
　PLAN TYPE: PPO
　Model Type: Network
　Benefits Offered: Chiropractic, Dental, Disease Management, Home
　　Care, Vision, Wellness

Type of Coverage
　Commercial, Individual

Type of Payment Plans Offered
　Combination FFS & DFFS

Geographic Areas Served
　Statewide

Subscriber Information
　Average Monthly Fee Per Subscriber
　　(Employee + Employer Contribution):
　　　Employee Only (Self): Varies by plan
　Average Annual Deductible Per Subscriber:
　　　Employee Only (Self): $250.00
　Average Subscriber Co-Payment:
　　　Primary Care Physician: $10.00

Network Qualifications
　Pre-Admission Certification: No

Peer Review Type
　Utilization Review: Yes
　Second Surgical Opinion: No
　Case Management: No

Accreditation Certification
　TJC Accreditation, Medicare Approved, Utilization Review,
　　Pre-Admission Certification, State Licensure, Quality Assurance
　　Program

Key Personnel
　President/CEO . . . . Andrew H Baker
　CFO. . . . . Jim Giacobello
　Marketing. . . . . Karen Piotti
　Medical Affairs . . . . Sheldon Ashley
　Provider Services . . . . Jo-carol Leonard
　Sales . . . . Karen Piotti

Specialty Managed Care Partners
　Enters into Contracts with Regional Business Coalitions: Yes

722 FC Diagnostic

401 Hackensack Avenue
Hackensack, NJ 07601
Toll-Free: 800-833-2132
Phone: 201-487-6001
customerservice@fcdiagnostic.com
www.fcdiagnostic.com
Year Founded: 1989
Number of Primary Care Physicians: 6,000

Healthplan and Services Defined
　PLAN TYPE: PPO
　Model Type: Network
　Plan Specialty: Lab, Radiology
　Benefits Offered: Physical Therapy, Diagnostic Imaging,
　　Laboratories, Rehabilitation

Geographic Areas Served
　Nationwide

Accreditation Certification
　Quality Assurance Program

Key Personnel
　President/CEO . . . . Andrew H Baker
　CFO. . . . . Jim Giacobello
　Marketing. . . . . Karen Piotti

Provider Services . . . . Jo-carol Leonard
Sales . . . . Karen Piotti

723 HealthFirst New Jersey Medicare Plan
821 Alexander Road
Suite 140
Princeton, NJ 08540
Toll-Free: 877-237-1308
www.healthfirstnj.org
Non-Profit Organization: Yes
Number of Affiliated Hospitals: 26
Total Enrollment: 500,000
State Enrollment: 500,000

Healthplan and Services Defined
　PLAN TYPE: Medicare

Type of Coverage
　Medicare

Key Personnel
President . . . . Terence L. Byrd, JD
EVP/COO . . . . Daniel McCarthy
SVP, Corporate Finance . . . . Marybeth Tita
Director, Operations . . . . Sean McBride
SVP, General Counsel . . . . Elizabeth St. Clair, Esq
Dir, NJ Network Mgmt . . . . Jessica Gamzon
SVP, Business Development. . . . . Paul Portsmore
Chief Marketing Officer. . . . . John Cheng
VP, Medical Director. . . . . Deborah Hammond, MD

724 Horizon Blue Cross & Blue Shield of New Jersey
975 Raymond Blvd
Newark, NJ 07105
Toll-Free: 800-355-2583
Phone: 973-466-4000
www.horizonblue.com
Secondary Address: 33 Washington Street, Newark, NJ 07102
Non-Profit Organization: Yes
Year Founded: 1932
Number of Affiliated Hospitals: 65
Number of Primary Care Physicians: 961
Total Enrollment: 3,600,000
State Enrollment: 3,600,000

Healthplan and Services Defined
　PLAN TYPE: HMO/PPO
　Other Type: POS
　Model Type: Staff, Network
　Benefits Offered: Behavioral Health, Dental, Prescription,
　　Psychiatric, Worker's Compensation
　Offers Demand Management Patient Information Service: Yes

Type of Coverage
　Commercial, Individual, Indemnity, Medicare
　Catastrophic Illness Benefit: None

Type of Payment Plans Offered
　POS, Combination FFS & DFFS

Geographic Areas Served
　All of North, Central and Southern New Jersey

Subscriber Information
　Average Monthly Fee Per Subscriber
　　(Employee + Employer Contribution):
　　　Employee Only (Self): Varies by plan
　Average Subscriber Co-Payment:
　　　Primary Care Physician: 100% in network/70%
　　　Non-Network Physician: Not covered
　　　Prescription Drugs: $3.00/6.00
　　　Hospital ER: $35.00
　　　Home Health Care: $0

Nursing Home: $0

Network Qualifications
　Pre-Admission Certification: Yes

Peer Review Type
　Utilization Review: Yes
　Second Surgical Opinion: Yes
　Case Management: Yes

Accreditation Certification
　AAAHC, URAC, NCQA
　TJC Accreditation, Medicare Approved, Utilization Review,
　　Pre-Admission Certification, State Licensure, Quality Assurance
　　Program

Key Personnel
President/CEO . . . . Robert A. Marino
SVP. . . . . Mark Barnard
SVP/Chief Information Off . . . . Douglas E. Blackwell
EVP, COO . . . . Robert A Marino
SVP, Service . . . . Mark Barnard
SVP/Market Business Units . . . . Christopher M Lepre
Pres\CEO, Horiz Health NJ . . . . Christy W Bell
Dir, Public Affairs. Thomas W Rubino, Esq
　973-468-8755
　trubino@horizonblue.com
Mgr, Public Relations. . . . . Thomas Vincz
　973-466-6625
　thomas_vincz@horizonblue.com

Specialty Managed Care Partners
　Enters into Contracts with Regional Business Coalitions: Yes

Employer References
　Lesnevich & Marzano-Lesnevich

725 Horizon Healthcare of New Jersey
3 Penn Plaza East
PO Box 820
Newark, NJ 07105
Toll-Free: 800-355-2583
www.horizon-healthcare.com
Secondary Address: 33 Washington Street, Newark, NJ 07102
Subsidiary of: Blue Cross Blue Shield
Acquired by: Horizon Blue Cross & Blue Shield
Non-Profit Organization: Yes
Year Founded: 1932
Number of Affiliated Hospitals: 71
Number of Primary Care Physicians: 4,465
Total Enrollment: 3,600,000
State Enrollment: 3,000,000

Healthplan and Services Defined
　PLAN TYPE: HMO/PPO
　Model Type: IPA
　Plan Specialty: EPO
　Benefits Offered: Behavioral Health, Chiropractic, Complementary
　　Medicine, Dental, Disease Management, Home Care, Physical
　　Therapy, Podiatry, Prescription, Psychiatric, Transplant, Vision,
　　Wellness
　Offers Demand Management Patient Information Service: Yes

Type of Coverage
　Commercial, Individual, Indemnity, Medicare, Supplemental
　　Medicare, Medicaid
　Catastrophic Illness Benefit: None

Type of Payment Plans Offered
　Capitated, FFS

Geographic Areas Served
　New Jersey

Subscriber Information
　Average Annual Deductible Per Subscriber:
　　　Employee Only (Self): None
　　　Employee & 1 Family Member: None

Employee & 2 Family Members: None
Medicare: None
Average Subscriber Co-Payment:
Primary Care Physician: $15.00
Non-Network Physician: Not covered
Prescription Drugs: $5/12/25
Hospital ER: $50.00
Home Health Care: None
Home Health Care Max. Days/Visits Covered: 100 days

Network Qualifications
Pre-Admission Certification: No

Peer Review Type
Utilization Review: Yes
Second Surgical Opinion: No
Case Management: Yes

Publishes and Distributes Report Card: Yes

Accreditation Certification
NCQA
TJC Accreditation, Medicare Approved, Utilization Review,
Pre-Admission Certification, State Licensure, Quality Assurance
Program

Key Personnel
President/CEO . . . . Robert Marino
CFO . . . . Robert Pures
SVP/Service . . . . Mark Barnard
SVP/Chief Info Officer. . . . . Douglas Blackwell
SVp/Administration . . . . David Huber
Member Services. . . . . Jackie Jennifer
Information Services . . . . Charles Emory, PhD
Dir, Public Affairs. Thomas M Rubino, Esq
973-466-8755
trubino@horizonblue.com
Mgr, Public Relations . . . . Dan Emmer
973-466-4805
daniel_emmer@horizonblue.com

Average Claim Compensation
Physician's Fees Charged: 43%

Specialty Managed Care Partners
Magellan, LabCorp, Advance PCS
Enters into Contracts with Regional Business Coalitions: Yes

Employer References
AT&T, Pharmacia, Chubb & Son, Dunn & Bradstreet, American
Standard

---

726 Horizon NJ Health
210 Silvia Street
West Trenton, NJ 08628
Toll-Free: 800-682-9094
www.horizonnjhealth.com
Subsidiary of: Horizon Blue Cross Blue Shield of NJ
Year Founded: 1993
Total Enrollment: 467,000
State Enrollment: 467,000

Healthplan and Services Defined
PLAN TYPE: PPO
Model Type: Network
Benefits Offered: Dental, Disease Management, Prescription, Vision,
Wellness

Type of Coverage
Individual, Medicaid

Geographic Areas Served
All 21 New Jersey counties

Accreditation Certification
URAC

Key Personnel
President & COO . . . . Karen L Clark
Controller . . . . James D'Alessio

Dir, Marketing & Comm . . . . Len Kudgis
Chief Medical Officer. . . . . Philip M Bonaparte, MD
Media Contact . . . . Carol Chernack
609-718-9290
carol_chernack@horizonnjhealth.com

---

727 Humana Health Insurance of New Jersey
One International Boulevard
Suite 904
Mahwah, NJ 07495
Toll-Free: 800-967-2370
Fax: 201-934-1369
www.humana.com
For Profit Organization: Yes

Healthplan and Services Defined
PLAN TYPE: HMO/PPO

Type of Coverage
Commercial, Individual

Accreditation Certification
URAC, NCQA, CORE

---

728 Managed Healthcare Systems of New Jersey
2 Gateway Center
13th Floor
Newark, NJ 07102-5003
Phone: 973-622-8476
Fax: 973-297-5599
Subsidiary of: Americhoice of New Jersey
Acquired by: Americhoice of New Jersey
For Profit Organization: Yes
Year Founded: 1995
State Enrollment: 30,000

Healthplan and Services Defined
PLAN TYPE: HMO
Model Type: IPA

Type of Payment Plans Offered
FFS

Geographic Areas Served
Statewide

Publishes and Distributes Report Card: Yes

Key Personnel
President/CEO . . . . Karen Clark
CFO . . . . Ronald Arfin
Marketing . . . . Steve Manobianco
Medical Affairs. . . . . Kathleen VanClees

---

729 National Health Plan Corporation
PO Box 33
Bayonne, NJ 07002
Toll-Free: 800-647-2677
Phone: 212-279-3232
Fax: 212-629-0749
dkonigsberg@nationalhealthplan.com
www.nationalhealthplan.com
For Profit Organization: Yes
Year Founded: 1975
Number of Affiliated Hospitals: 2,500
Number of Primary Care Physicians: 250,000
Number of Referral/Specialty Physicians: 5,000
State Enrollment: 200,000

Healthplan and Services Defined
PLAN TYPE: PPO
Model Type: IPA, Group

Plan Specialty: ASO, Behavioral Health, Chiropractic, Dental, Disease Management, EPO, Lab, MSO, PBM, Vision, Radiology, Worker's Compensation
Benefits Offered: Prescription

Type of Coverage
Individual, Indemnity, Supplemental Medicare

Type of Payment Plans Offered
DFFS, FFS, Combination FFS & DFFS

Geographic Areas Served
Connecticut, New Jersey, New York & Pennsylvania; Prescriptions nationwide

Subscriber Information
Average Monthly Fee Per Subscriber
(Employee + Employer Contribution):
Employee & 2 Family Members: $8.00
Medicare: $6.25
Average Annual Deductible Per Subscriber:
Employee Only (Self): $0
Employee & 1 Family Member: $0
Employee & 2 Family Members: $0
Medicare: $0
Average Subscriber Co-Payment:
Primary Care Physician: $0
Non-Network Physician: Varies
Prescription Drugs: $1.00-5.00
Home Health Care: $0

Network Qualifications
Pre-Admission Certification: Yes

Peer Review Type
Utilization Review: Yes
Second Surgical Opinion: Yes
Case Management: Yes

Publishes and Distributes Report Card: No

Accreditation Certification
TJC Accreditation, Pre-Admission Certification

Key Personnel
President and CEO........................David Konigsberg
EVP......................................David H. Zaback
VP, Operations...........................Jamie Konigsberg
Director Claims..........................Sharon Weinberg
VP/Operations............................Jamie Konigsberg
Sales....................................David Konigsberg

Average Claim Compensation
Physician's Fees Charged: 10%
Hospital's Fees Charged: 10%

Specialty Managed Care Partners
Enters into Contracts with Regional Business Coalitions: No

730 One Call Medical

20 Waterview Boulevard
PO Box 614
Parsippany, NJ 07054
Toll-Free: 800-872-2875
Phone: 973-257-1000
Fax: 973-257-9284
webqcustomerservice@onecallmedical.com
www.onecallmedical.com
For Profit Organization: Yes
Year Founded: 1993

Healthplan and Services Defined
PLAN TYPE: PPO
Model Type: Network
Benefits Offered: Worker's Compensation, Group Health

Type of Payment Plans Offered
POS, DFFS, FFS, Combination FFS & DFFS

Geographic Areas Served
Nationwide

Network Qualifications
Pre-Admission Certification: Yes

Publishes and Distributes Report Card: No

Accreditation Certification
Utilization Review, Quality Assurance Program

Key Personnel
Chairman.................................Don Duford
President................................Jim Phifer
Chief Financial Officer..................Warren Green
VP, Business Development..................Bob Zeccardi
610-453-5910
Business Development......................Lori Lentz
803-749-4101
Chief Legal Officer......................Steven Davis
Chief Sales/Marketing....................John Baxter

Specialty Managed Care Partners
Enters into Contracts with Regional Business Coalitions: No

731 Oxford Health Plans: New Jersey

111 Woods Avenue
Suite 2
Iselin, NJ 08830
Toll-Free: 800-201-6920
Phone: 732-623-1000
www.oxhp.com
For Profit Organization: Yes
Year Founded: 1985
Total Enrollment: 332,840
State Enrollment: 59,800

Healthplan and Services Defined
PLAN TYPE: HMO
Model Type: IPA
Benefits Offered: Disease Management, Prescription, Wellness

Type of Coverage
Commercial, Medicare

Type of Payment Plans Offered
Capitated

Geographic Areas Served
Sussex, Passaic, Bergen, Morris, Warren, Essex, Hudson, Union, Hunterdon, Somerset, Middlesex, Mercer, Monmouth, Ocean, Burlington, Camden, Gloucester, Salem, Cumberland, Atlantic, Cape May counties

Key Personnel
President/CEO............................Charles G Berg
COO.....................................Steven H Black
CFO.....................................Kurt B Thompson
CMO.....................................Alan M Muney
General Counsel.........................Daniel N Gregoire
Provider Relations......................Paul Conlin
Sales/Marketing.........................Kevin R Hill
Member Relations........................Kevin Appleton
Pharmacy Director.......................Burton Orland
Public Relations........................Maria Gordon Shydlo

732 QualCare

30 Knightbridge Road
Piscataway, NJ 08854
Toll-Free: 800-992-6613
Phone: 732-562-0833
info@qualcareinc.com
www.qualcareinc.com
For Profit Organization: Yes
Year Founded: 1993
Federally Qualified: Yes

Number of Affiliated Hospitals: 75
Number of Primary Care Physicians: 9,000
Number of Referral/Specialty Physicians: 14,000
Total Enrollment: 750,000
State Enrollment: 750,000

Healthplan and Services Defined
  PLAN TYPE: HMO/PPO
  Other Type: POS
  Model Type: Network
  Plan Specialty: ASO, Behavioral Health, Chiropractic, Dental,
    Disease Management, EPO, Lab, MSO, PBM, Vision, Radiology,
    Worker's Compensation, UR
  Benefits Offered: Behavioral Health, Chiropractic, Complementary
    Medicine, Dental, Disease Management, Home Care, Inpatient
    SNF, Long-Term Care, Physical Therapy, Podiatry, Prescription,
    Psychiatric, Transplant, Vision, Wellness, Worker's Compensation,
    AD&D, Life, LTD, ST
  Offers Demand Management Patient Information Service: Yes

Type of Coverage
  Commercial

Type of Payment Plans Offered
  FFS

Geographic Areas Served
  Statewide

Peer Review Type
  Utilization Review: Yes
  Second Surgical Opinion: Yes
  Case Management: Yes

Publishes and Distributes Report Card: Yes

Accreditation Certification
  AAAHC, TJC, AAPI, NCQA
  Medicare Approved, Utilization Review, State Licensure, Quality
    Assurance Program

Key Personnel
  CEO. . . . . .Annette Catino
  President. . . . . .Sharon Seitzman
  EVP, COO & CIO . . . . .Karthick Ganesh
  EVP/Corporate CFO . . . . .John J. McSorley
  VP Network/Delivery . . . . .Kevin Joyce
  EVP. . . . . .Tim Ford
  VP, Insurance Services . . . . .Dawn Wright

Specialty Managed Care Partners
  Multiplan

---

733   Rayant Insurance Company
3 Penn Plaza East
PP03C
Newark, NJ 07105
Toll-Free: 888-667-4547
life@horizonblue.com
www.rayant.com
Subsidiary of: Horizon Healthcare Services
For Profit Organization: Yes
Total Enrollment: 21,000

Healthplan and Services Defined
  PLAN TYPE: Dental
  Plan Specialty: Dental
  Benefits Offered: Dental

Geographic Areas Served
  New York and Pennsylvania

Key Personnel
  Chairman/President/CEO . . . . .William J Marino
  EVP/COO . . . . .Robert A Marino
  SVP Admin, CFO, Treasurer. . . . . .Robert J Pures
  SVP/Information Tech . . . . .Mark Barnard
  VP, Chief Actuary. . . . . .Edward M Mailander
  VP, Chief Medical Officer. . . . . .Richard G Popiel

VP, Chief Pharmacy Offc. . . . . .Margaret M Johnson
SVP, General Counsel . . . . .Linda A Willett

---

734   UnitedHealthCare of New Jersey
170 Wood Avenue South
3rd Floor
Iselin, NJ 08830
Toll-Free: 866-223-5802
Phone: 732-623-1000
www.uhc.com
For Profit Organization: Yes
Total Enrollment: 75,000,000
State Enrollment: 431,833

Healthplan and Services Defined
  PLAN TYPE: HMO/PPO

Geographic Areas Served
  Statewide

---

735   VSP: Vision Service Plan of New Jersey
1 Gatehall Drive
Suite 303
Parsippany, NJ 07054
Phone: 973-538-2626
Fax: 973-538-0368
webmaster@vsp.com
www.vsp.com
Year Founded: 1955
Number of Primary Care Physicians: 26,000
Total Enrollment: 55,000,000

Healthplan and Services Defined
  PLAN TYPE: Vision
  Plan Specialty: Vision
  Benefits Offered: Vision

Type of Payment Plans Offered
  Capitated

Geographic Areas Served
  Statewide

Network Qualifications
  Pre-Admission Certification: Yes

Peer Review Type
  Utilization Review: Yes

Accreditation Certification
  Utilization Review, Quality Assurance Program

Key Personnel
  President/CEO. . . . . .Robert Lynch
  Director/Media . . . . .Pat McNeil

---

736   WellChoice
120 Wood Avenue S
Suite 200
Iselin, NJ 08830
Toll-Free: 888-476-8069
Phone: 732-635-7112
Fax: 888-592-3154
www.wellchoicenj.com
Subsidiary of: Wellpoint
For Profit Organization: Yes
Year Founded: 1998
Number of Affiliated Hospitals: 231
Number of Primary Care Physicians: 92,000
Total Enrollment: 12,317
State Enrollment: 12,317

Healthplan and Services Defined
  PLAN TYPE: HMO

Geographic Areas Served
Northern and central New Jersey

Subscriber Information
Average Subscriber Co-Payment:
Primary Care Physician: $5.00 to 50.00

Key Personnel
President . . . . .Dan McCarthy
Vice President/Sales . . . . .Christopher Fallon

HMO/PPO DIRECTORY

Health Insurance Coverage Status and Type of Coverage by Age

Category	All Persons		Under 18 years		Under 65 years		65 years and over	
	Number	%	Number	%	Number	%	Number	%
Total population	2,052	-	507	-	1,750	-	302	-
Covered by some type of health insurance	1,669 *(13)*	81.4 *(0.6)*	464 *(5)*	91.5 *(1.0)*	1,373 *(13)*	78.4 *(0.8)*	297 *(2)*	98.4 *(0.4)*
Covered by private health insurance	1,097 *(17)*	53.5 *(0.8)*	213 *(7)*	42.1 *(1.4)*	927 *(16)*	53.0 *(0.9)*	170 *(5)*	56.3 *(1.6)*
Employment based	894 *(17)*	43.6 *(0.8)*	187 *(7)*	36.9 *(1.4)*	790 *(16)*	45.1 *(0.9)*	104 *(4)*	34.6 *(1.3)*
Direct purchase	186 *(9)*	9.1 *(0.4)*	17 *(3)*	3.3 *(0.6)*	121 *(8)*	6.9 *(0.5)*	66 *(4)*	21.8 *(1.3)*
Covered by TRICARE	85 *(6)*	4.2 *(0.3)*	17 *(3)*	3.4 *(0.6)*	59 *(6)*	3.4 *(0.3)*	26 *(2)*	8.8 *(0.8)*
Covered by government health insurance	806 *(13)*	39.3 *(0.6)*	272 *(7)*	53.7 *(1.3)*	516 *(13)*	29.5 *(0.7)*	290 *(2)*	96.0 *(0.6)*
Covered by Medicaid	504 *(12)*	24.6 *(0.6)*	267 *(7)*	52.6 *(1.3)*	457 *(12)*	26.1 *(0.7)*	48 *(3)*	15.8 *(0.9)*
Also by private insurance	62 *(6)*	3.0 *(0.3)*	21 *(4)*	4.1 *(0.7)*	46 *(5)*	2.6 *(0.3)*	16 *(2)*	5.3 *(0.7)*
Covered by Medicare	356 *(5)*	17.3 *(0.2)*	7 *(2)*	1.4 *(0.4)*	67 *(4)*	3.8 *(0.2)*	289 *(3)*	95.9 *(0.6)*
Also by private insurance	177 *(5)*	8.6 *(0.3)*	1 *(Z)*	0.1 *(0.1)*	14 *(2)*	0.8 *(0.1)*	162 *(5)*	53.8 *(1.6)*
Also by Medicaid	79 *(4)*	3.9 *(0.2)*	2 *(1)*	0.5 *(0.2)*	32 *(3)*	1.8 *(0.2)*	48 *(3)*	15.8 *(0.9)*
Covered by VA Care	63 *(5)*	3.1 *(0.2)*	1 *(1)*	0.2 *(0.2)*	31 *(3)*	1.8 *(0.2)*	32 *(2)*	10.6 *(0.8)*
Not covered at any time during the year	382 *(13)*	18.6 *(0.6)*	43 *(5)*	8.5 *(1.0)*	378 *(13)*	21.6 *(0.8)*	5 *(1)*	1.6 *(0.4)*

Note: Numbers in thousands; Figures cover 2013; Margin of error appears in parenthesis; A "Z" indicates that the value either represents or rounds to zero.
Source: U.S. Census Bureau, 2013 American Community Survey, Table HI05. Health Insurance Coverage Status and Type of Coverage by State and Age for All People: 2013

New Mexico

737 Aetna Health of New Mexico

151 Farmington Avenue
Hartford, CT 06156
Toll-Free: 800-872-3862
Phone: 860-273-0123
www.aetna.com
Partnered with: eHealthInsurance Services Inc.
For Profit Organization: Yes
Total Enrollment: 11,596,230

Healthplan and Services Defined
PLAN TYPE: PPO
Other Type: POS
Plan Specialty: EPO
Benefits Offered: Dental, Disease Management, Long-Term Care,
    Prescription, Wellness, Life, LTD, STD

Type of Coverage
Commercial, Individual

Type of Payment Plans Offered
POS, FFS

Geographic Areas Served
Statewide

Key Personnel
Chairman/CEO/President. .Mark T Bertolini
EVP, General Counsel . . . . .William J Casazza
EVP/CFO . . . . Shawn M Guertin

738 Amerigroup New Mexico

6565 Americas Parkway NE
Albuquerque, NM 87110
Toll-Free: 888-997-2583
Phone: 505-875-4320
www.realsolutions.com
For Profit Organization: Yes
Year Founded: 2008
Total Enrollment: 1,900,000

Healthplan and Services Defined
PLAN TYPE: HMO

Type of Coverage
Medicare, Coordiation of Long Term Care Svcs.

739 Blue Cross & Blue Shield of New Mexico

5701 Balloon Fiesta Parkway NE
Albuquerque, NM 87113
Toll-Free: 800-835-8699
Phone: 505-291-3500
www.bcbsnm.com
Mailing Address: PO Box 27630, Albuquerque, NM 87125-7630
Subsidiary of: Health Care Service Corporation
Non-Profit Organization: Yes
Year Founded: 1940
Owned by an Integrated Delivery Network (IDN): Yes
Number of Affiliated Hospitals: 54
Number of Primary Care Physicians: 3,322
Number of Referral/Specialty Physicians: 6,742
Total Enrollment: 367,000
State Enrollment: 367,000

Healthplan and Services Defined
PLAN TYPE: HMO/PPO
Other Type: EPO, CDHP
Model Type: Network
Plan Specialty: ASO, Behavioral Health
Benefits Offered: Dental, Disease Management, Vision, Wellness,
    Medical, Case Management

Offers Demand Management Patient Information Service: Yes
DMPI Services Offered: Fully Insured

Type of Coverage
Commercial, Individual, Indemnity, Supplemental Medicare

Geographic Areas Served
Statewide

Network Qualifications
Pre-Admission Certification: Yes

Peer Review Type
Utilization Review: Yes
Second Surgical Opinion: Yes

Publishes and Distributes Report Card: Yes

Accreditation Certification
NCQA

Key Personnel
President/CEO . . . . .Patricia Hemingway Hall
EVP/Plan Operations. . . . . .Martin Foster
EVP/COO . . . . .Colleen Reitan
VP Subscriber Services . . . . .Linda Amburn
VP Health Care Management .Tom Maclean
Marketing . . . . .Bette Bolton
Materials Management. . . . . .Liz Carrillo
VP, Sales . . . . .Jeff Newland
Media Contact . . . . .Becky Kenny
    505-816-2012
    becky_kenny@bcbsnm.com

Specialty Managed Care Partners
Pharmacy Manager, Prime Theraputics

740 CIGNA HealthCare of New Mexico

6565 Americas Parkway
Suite 150
Albuquerque, NM 87110
Toll-Free: 888-244-6264
Fax: 505-872-2946
www.cigna.com
For Profit Organization: Yes
Year Founded: 1981
Owned by an Integrated Delivery Network (IDN): Yes

Healthplan and Services Defined
PLAN TYPE: HMO
Other Type: POS
Model Type: IPA
Plan Specialty: ASO, Behavioral Health, Chiropractic, Dental,
    Disease Management, EPO, Lab, MSO, PBM, Vision, Radiology,
    UR
Benefits Offered: Behavioral Health, Chiropractic, Dental, Disease
    Management, Home Care, Inpatient SNF, Physical Therapy,
    Podiatry, Prescription, Psychiatric, Transplant, Vision, Wellness,
    Life

Type of Coverage
Commercial

Type of Payment Plans Offered
FFS, Combination FFS & DFFS

Geographic Areas Served
Atlanta & Metro Area

Subscriber Information
Average Annual Deductible Per Subscriber:
    Employee Only (Self): $0
    Employee & 1 Family Member: $0
    Employee & 2 Family Members: $0
Average Subscriber Co-Payment:
    Primary Care Physician: $15.00
    Non-Network Physician: Varies
    Prescription Drugs: $10.00
    Hospital ER: $50.00
    Home Health Care: $0

Network Qualifications
Pre-Admission Certification: Yes

Peer Review Type
Utilization Review: Yes
Second Surgical Opinion: Yes
Case Management: Yes

Publishes and Distributes Report Card: Yes

Accreditation Certification
NCQA
TJC Accreditation, Utilization Review, Pre-Admission Certification, State Licensure, Quality Assurance Program

Specialty Managed Care Partners
Enters into Contracts with Regional Business Coalitions: No

---

741 Delta Dental of New Mexico

2500 Louisiana Boulevard NE
Suite 600
Albuquerque, NM 87110
Toll-Free: 877-395-9420
Phone: 505-884-4777
Fax: 505-883-7444
www.deltadentalnm.com
Non-Profit Organization: Yes
Year Founded: 1973
Number of Primary Care Physicians: 1,186
Total Enrollment: 54,000,000
State Enrollment: 200,000

Healthplan and Services Defined
PLAN TYPE: Dental
Other Type: Dental PPO
Model Type: Group
Plan Specialty: ASO, Dental, Vision
Benefits Offered: Dental, Vision
Offers Demand Management Patient Information Service: Yes

Type of Coverage
Commercial

Geographic Areas Served
Statewide

Network Qualifications
Pre-Admission Certification: Yes

Publishes and Distributes Report Card: Yes

Key Personnel
Chief Executive Officer . . . . Walter S Bolic
Chief Financial Officer . . . . Goran Jurkovic
Chief Operating Officer . . . . Sara Limon
VP, Sales & Account Mgmt . . . . Frank Amaro
VP Marketing . . . . Gail Davalos
Chief Dental Officer . . . . Jesus Galvan
VP, Public & Govt Affairs . . . . Jeff Album
415-972-8418

Specialty Managed Care Partners
Enters into Contracts with Regional Business Coalitions: Yes

---

742 eHealthInsurance Services Inc.

11919 Foundation Place
Gold River, CA 95670
Toll-Free: 800-644-3491
webmaster@healthinsurance.com
www.e.healthinsurance.com
Year Founded: 1997

Healthplan and Services Defined
PLAN TYPE: HMO/PPO
Benefits Offered: Dental, Life, STD

Type of Coverage
Commercial, Individual, Medicare

Geographic Areas Served
All 50 states in the USA and District of Columbia

Key Personnel
Chairman & CEO . . . . Gary L. Lauer
EVP/Business & Corp. Dev . . . . Bruce Telkamp
EVP/Chief Technology . . . . Dr. Sheldon X. Wang
SVP & CFO . . . . Stuart M. Huizinga
Pres. of eHealth Gov. Sys . . . . Samuel C. Gibbs
SVP of Sales & Operations . . . . Robert S. Hurley
Director Public Relations . . . . Nate Purpura
650-210-3115

---

743 Great-West Healthcare New Mexico

6909 East Greenway Parkway
Suite 180
Scottsdale, AZ 85254
Toll-Free: 866-494-2111
Phone: 480-922-6508
eliginquiries@cigna.com
www.cignaforhealth.com
Subsidiary of: CIGNA HealthCare
Acquired by: CIGNA
For Profit Organization: Yes
Total Enrollment: 10,816
State Enrollment: 7,417

Healthplan and Services Defined
PLAN TYPE: HMO/PPO
Benefits Offered: Disease Management, Prescription, Wellness

Type of Coverage
Commercial

Type of Payment Plans Offered
POS, FFS

Geographic Areas Served
New Mexico

Accreditation Certification
URAC

Specialty Managed Care Partners
Caremark Rx

---

744 Humana Health Insurance of New Mexico

4904 Alameda Blvd NE
Suite A
Albuquerque, NM 87113
Toll-Free: 800-681-0680
Phone: 505-468-0500
Fax: 505-468-0554
www.humana.com
For Profit Organization: Yes

Healthplan and Services Defined
PLAN TYPE: HMO/PPO

Type of Coverage
Commercial, Individual

Accreditation Certification
URAC, NCQA, CORE

Key Personnel
Chairman/CEO . . . . Michael McCallister
President . . . . Bruce Broussard
SVP/CFO . . . . James Bloem
SVP/Corporate Development . . . . Paul Kusserow

745 Lovelace Health Plan

4101 Indian School Road NE
Altura Office Complex
Albuquerque, NM 87110
Toll-Free: 800-808-7363
Phone: 505-727-5500
Fax: 505-262-7307
www.lovelacehealthplan.com
Mailing Address: PO Box 27107
Subsidiary of: Ardent
For Profit Organization: Yes
Year Founded: 1973
Owned by an Integrated Delivery Network (IDN): Yes
Number of Affiliated Hospitals: 39
Number of Primary Care Physicians: 7,000
Number of Referral/Specialty Physicians: 5,000
Total Enrollment: 163,000
State Enrollment: 68,674

Healthplan and Services Defined
  PLAN TYPE: HMO
  Model Type: Network
  Plan Specialty: ASO, Behavioral Health, Chiropractic, Disease
    Management, EPO, Lab, MSO, PBM, Vision, Radiology, UR
  Benefits Offered: Behavioral Health, Chiropractic, Complementary
    Medicine, Disease Management, Home Care, Inpatient SNF,
    Long-Term Care, Physical Therapy, Podiatry, Prescription,
    Psychiatric, Transplant, Vision, Wellness

Type of Coverage
  Commercial, Medicare
  Catastrophic Illness Benefit: Covered

Type of Payment Plans Offered
  POS, DFFS, FFS

Geographic Areas Served
  Statewide

Network Qualifications
  Pre-Admission Certification: No

Peer Review Type
  Utilization Review: Yes
  Second Surgical Opinion: No
  Case Management: Yes

Accreditation Certification
  NCQA
  TJC Accreditation, Medicare Approved, Utilization Review,
    Pre-Admission Certification, State Licensure, Quality Assurance
    Program

Key Personnel
  Chief Executive Officer . . . . Terri Chinn
  Chief Operating Officer . . . . Karen Eskridge
  VP & General Cousel. . . . . Phil Bisesi
  VP/Communications . . . . Tyra Palmer
  Asst VP, Underwriting. . . . . Carole Henry
  Asst VP, Quality Health . . . . Linda Hubbard
  Chief Medical Officer . . . . John Cruickshank, MD
  Director, Human Resources . . . . Patricia Harris
  Asst VP, Info Services. . . . . Bob Skinner
  Compliance Officer . . . . Ann Greenberg
  Chief Sales Officer . . . . Marlene Baca
  Media Contact . . . . Susan Wilson
    505-727-4440
    susan.wilson@lovelace.com

Specialty Managed Care Partners
  CIGNA Behavioral Health

746 Lovelace Medicare Health Plan

4101 Indian School Road Northeast
Suite 110
Albuquerque, NM 87110
Toll-Free: 800-808-7363
Phone: 505-727-LOVE
serena.lyons@lovelace.com
www.lovelacehealthplan.com
Number of Affiliated Hospitals: 40
Number of Referral/Specialty Physicians: 7,000
Total Enrollment: 200,000

Healthplan and Services Defined
  PLAN TYPE: HMO/PPO
  Plan Specialty: Medicare, Medicaid
  Benefits Offered: Chiropractic, Dental, Disease Management, Home
    Care, Inpatient SNF, Physical Therapy, Podiatry, Prescription,
    Psychiatric, Vision, Wellness

Type of Coverage
  Individual, Medicare

Geographic Areas Served
  Available witin New Mexico only

Subscriber Information
  Average Monthly Fee Per Subscriber
    (Employee + Employer Contribution):
      Employee Only (Self): Varies
      Medicare: Varies
  Average Annual Deductible Per Subscriber:
      Employee Only (Self): Varies
      Medicare: Varies
  Average Subscriber Co-Payment:
      Primary Care Physician: Varies
      Non-Network Physician: Varies
      Prescription Drugs: Varies
      Hospital ER: Varies
      Home Health Care: Varies
      Home Health Care Max. Days/Visits Covered: Varies
      Nursing Home: Varies
      Nursing Home Max. Days/Visits Covered: Varies

Key Personnel
  Chief Executive Officer . . . . Terri Chinn
  Chief Operating Officer . . . . Karen Eskridge
  VP & General Cousel. . . . . Phil Bisesi
  AVP, Commercial Sales . . . . Douglas Gullino
  Asst VP, Underwriting. . . . . Carole Henry
  Asst VP, Quality Health . . . . Linda Hubbard
  Marketing. . . . . Serena Lyons
  Chief Medical Officer . . . . John Cruickshank, MD
  Dir, Human Resources. . . . . Patricia Harris
  Asst VP, Info Services. . . . . Bob Skinner
  VP Legal Operations . . . . Angela Martinez
  Chief Sales & Service Ofc . . . . Marlene Baca

747 Molina Healthcare: New Mexico

8801 Horizon Boulevard NE
P.O. Box 3887
Albuquerque, NM 87113
Toll-Free: 800-377-9594
Phone: 505-342-4660
www.molinahealthcare.com
For Profit Organization: Yes
Number of Affiliated Hospitals: 60
Number of Primary Care Physicians: 1,511
Number of Referral/Specialty Physicians: 5,799
Total Enrollment: 1,400,000
State Enrollment: 83,000

Healthplan and Services Defined
  PLAN TYPE: HMO

Benefits Offered: Disease Management, Wellness

Type of Coverage
Commercial, Medicare, Supplemental Medicare, Medicaid

Accreditation Certification
URAC, NCQA

Key Personnel
President/CEO . . . . .J Mario Molina, MD
   888-562-5442
Chief Financial Officer. . . . . .John C. Molina
Chief Operating Officer . . . . .Terry P. Bayer
SVP/General Counsel. . . . . .Jeff Barlow
Accounting Officer . . . . .Joseph White
Chief Medical Officer . . . . .Eugene Sun, MD
   505-342-4660
   eugene.sun@molinahealthcare.com

748   Presbyterian Health Plan

9521 San Mateo Boulevard NE
Albuquerque, NM 87106-4260
Toll-Free: 800-356-2219
Phone: 505-923-5700
info@phs.org
www.phs.org
Non-Profit Organization: Yes
Year Founded: 1985
Number of Affiliated Hospitals: 28
Number of Primary Care Physicians: 1,200
Number of Referral/Specialty Physicians: 4,850
Total Enrollment: 400,000
State Enrollment: 400,000

Healthplan and Services Defined
  PLAN TYPE: HMO
  Other Type: POS
  Model Type: Contracted Network

Type of Coverage
Commercial, Medicare, Medicaid

Type of Payment Plans Offered
POS, DFFS, Capitated, FFS

Geographic Areas Served
State of New Mexico

Subscriber Information
Average Monthly Fee Per Subscriber
  (Employee + Employer Contribution):
    Employee Only (Self): Varies by plan
Average Subscriber Co-Payment:
    Primary Care Physician: $10.00
    Prescription Drugs: $0
    Hospital ER: $50.00

Accreditation Certification
NCQA

Key Personnel
President . . . . .Dennis Batey, MD
Chief Financial Officer. . . . . .Lisa Farrell
VP, Chief Service Officer. . . . . .Jana Burdick
VP, Government Programs . . . . .Mary Eden
Exed Dir, Health Info . . . . .Cesar Goulart
VP, Chief Medical Officer. . . . . .Chuck Baumgart, MD
VP, Sales & Marketing . . . . .Neal Spero

Employer References
State of New Mexico, Albuquerque Public Schools, Intel Corporation

749   Presbyterian Medicare Plans

PO Box 27489
Albuquerque, NM 87125-7489
Toll-Free: 800-347-4766
Phone: 505-841-1234
info@phs.org
www.phs.org

Healthplan and Services Defined
  PLAN TYPE: Medicare
  Benefits Offered: Chiropractic, Dental, Disease Management, Home
    Care, Inpatient SNF, Physical Therapy, Podiatry, Prescription,
    Psychiatric, Vision, Wellness

Type of Coverage
Individual, Medicare, Employer Group

Geographic Areas Served
Available within New Mexico only

Subscriber Information
Average Monthly Fee Per Subscriber
  (Employee + Employer Contribution):
    Employee Only (Self): Varies
    Medicare: Varies
Average Annual Deductible Per Subscriber:
    Employee Only (Self): Varies
    Medicare: Varies
Average Subscriber Co-Payment:
    Primary Care Physician: Varies
    Non-Network Physician: Varies
    Prescription Drugs: Varies
    Hospital ER: Varies
    Home Health Care: Varies
    Home Health Care Max. Days/Visits Covered: Varies
    Nursing Home: Varies
    Nursing Home Max. Days/Visits Covered: Varies

Key Personnel
President . . . . .Dennis Batey, MD
Chief Financial Officer. . . . . .Lisa Farrell
VP, Chief Service Officer. . . . . .David Field
VP, Government Programs . . . . .Mary Eden
Exed Dir, Health Info . . . . .Cesar Goulart
VP, Chief Medical Officer. . . . . .Chuck Baumgart, MD
VP, Sales & Marketing . . . . .Neal Spero

750   United Concordia: New Mexico

4401 Deer Path Road
Harrisbury, NM 17110
Toll-Free: 877-654-2124
Phone: 717-260-6800
Fax: 505-563-5867
ucproducer@ucci.com
www.secure.ucci.com
For Profit Organization: Yes
Year Founded: 1971
Number of Primary Care Physicians: 111,000
Total Enrollment: 8,000,000

Healthplan and Services Defined
  PLAN TYPE: Dental
  Plan Specialty: Dental
  Benefits Offered: Dental

Type of Coverage
Commercial, Individual

Geographic Areas Served
Military personnel and their families, nationwide

Key Personnel
Chairman/CEO . . . . .Daniel Lebish
President/COO. . . . . .F G Chip Merkel
Innovation Manager . . . . .John Glindeman

751 UnitedHealthCare of New Mexico
170 Wood Avenue South
3rd Floor
Iselin, NM 08830
Toll-Free: 866-573-2458
Phone: 732-623-1000
Fax: 505-449-4140
Colorado_PR_Team@uhc.com
www.uhc.com
Subsidiary of: UnitedHealth Group
For Profit Organization: Yes
Total Enrollment: 75,000,000
State Enrollment: 120,937

Healthplan and Services Defined
 PLAN TYPE: HMO/PPO

Geographic Areas Served
 Statewide

Key Personnel
 Media Contact . . . . Will Shanley
  will.shanley@uhc.com

Health Insurance Coverage Status and Type of Coverage by Age

Category	All Persons		Under 18 years		Under 65 years		65 years and over	
	Number	%	Number	%	Number	%	Number	%
Total population	19,400	-	4,231	-	16,671	-	2,729	-
Covered by some type of health insurance	17,331 *(31)*	89.3 *(0.2)*	4,060 *(10)*	96.0 *(0.2)*	14,629 *(31)*	87.7 *(0.2)*	2,702 *(4)*	99.0 *(0.1)*
Covered by private health insurance	12,619 *(55)*	65.0 *(0.3)*	2,546 *(25)*	60.2 *(0.6)*	11,002 *(53)*	66.0 *(0.3)*	1,617 *(14)*	59.2 *(0.5)*
Employment based	10,955 *(51)*	56.5 *(0.3)*	2,232 *(23)*	52.8 *(0.5)*	9,851 *(49)*	59.1 *(0.3)*	1,104 *(12)*	40.4 *(0.5)*
Direct purchase	2,086 *(29)*	10.8 *(0.1)*	346 *(14)*	8.2 *(0.3)*	1,399 *(26)*	8.4 *(0.2)*	687 *(13)*	25.2 *(0.5)*
Covered by TRICARE	167 *(8)*	0.9 *(0.1)*	34 *(4)*	0.8 *(0.1)*	115 *(8)*	0.7 *(0.1)*	52 *(3)*	1.9 *(0.1)*
Covered by government health insurance	6,834 *(46)*	35.2 *(0.2)*	1,717 *(22)*	40.6 *(0.5)*	4,223 *(46)*	25.3 *(0.3)*	2,611 *(6)*	95.7 *(0.2)*
Covered by Medicaid	4,416 *(48)*	22.8 *(0.2)*	1,700 *(22)*	40.2 *(0.5)*	3,905 *(44)*	23.4 *(0.3)*	511 *(11)*	18.7 *(0.4)*
Also by private insurance	585 *(17)*	3.0 *(0.1)*	200 *(10)*	4.7 *(0.2)*	452 *(15)*	2.7 *(0.1)*	133 *(5)*	4.9 *(0.2)*
Covered by Medicare	3,075 *(17)*	15.9 *(0.1)*	29 *(7)*	0.7 *(0.2)*	467 *(16)*	2.8 *(0.1)*	2,609 *(6)*	95.6 *(0.2)*
Also by private insurance	1,653 *(15)*	8.5 *(0.1)*	4 *(1)*	0.1 *(0.1)*	128 *(6)*	0.8 *(0.1)*	1,525 *(14)*	55.9 *(0.5)*
Also by Medicaid	746 *(15)*	3.8 *(0.1)*	13 *(2)*	0.3 *(0.1)*	235 *(9)*	1.4 *(0.1)*	511 *(11)*	18.7 *(0.4)*
Covered by VA Care	274 *(7)*	1.4 *(0.1)*	2 *(1)*	0.1 *(0.1)*	115 *(5)*	0.7 *(0.1)*	158 *(5)*	5.8 *(0.2)*
Not covered at any time during the year	2,070 *(30)*	10.7 *(0.2)*	171 *(9)*	4.0 *(0.2)*	2,042 *(30)*	12.3 *(0.2)*	27 *(3)*	1.0 *(0.1)*

Note: Numbers in thousands; Figures cover 2013; Margin of error appears in parenthesis; A "Z" indicates that the value either represents or rounds to zero.
Source: U.S. Census Bureau, 2013 American Community Survey, Table HI05. Health Insurance Coverage Status and Type of Coverage by State and Age for All People: 2013

New York

752 Aetna Health of New York
151 Farmington Avenue
Hartford, CT 06156
Toll-Free: 866-582-9629
www.aetna.com
Year Founded: 1986
Number of Affiliated Hospitals: 61
Number of Primary Care Physicians: 2,691
Total Enrollment: 154,162
State Enrollment: 154,162

Healthplan and Services Defined
PLAN TYPE: PPO
Model Type: IPA, Network
Benefits Offered: Disease Management, Prescription, Wellness
Offers Demand Management Patient Information Service: Yes

Type of Coverage
Catastrophic Illness Benefit: Varies per case

Type of Payment Plans Offered
POS, Capitated

Geographic Areas Served
Statewide

Subscriber Information
Average Subscriber Co-Payment:
Primary Care Physician: $2.00/5.00/10.00
Non-Network Physician: Deductible
Prescription Drugs: $2.00/5.00/10.00
Hospital ER: $35.00

Network Qualifications
Pre-Admission Certification: Yes

Peer Review Type
Utilization Review: Yes
Second Surgical Opinion: No
Case Management: Yes

Publishes and Distributes Report Card: Yes

Accreditation Certification
NCQA
TJC Accreditation, Medicare Approved, Utilization Review, Pre-Admission Certification, State Licensure, Quality Assurance Program

Key Personnel
CEO .... Ronald A Williams
President .... Mark T Bertolini
SVP, General Counsel .... William J Casazza
EVP, CFO .... Joseph M Zubretsky
Head, M&A Integration .... Kay Mooney
SVP, Marketing .... Robert E Mead
Chief Medical Officer .... Lonny Reisman, MD
SVP, Human Resources .... Elease E Wright
SVP, CIO .... Meg McCarthy

Specialty Managed Care Partners
Enters into Contracts with Regional Business Coalitions: Yes

753 Affinity Health Plan
2500 Halsey Street
#2
Bronx, NY 10461
Toll-Free: 866-206-1775
Phone: 718-794-7700
Fax: 718-794-7800
mainoffice@affinityplan.org
www.affinityplan.org
Non-Profit Organization: Yes
Year Founded: 1986

Number of Affiliated Hospitals: 60
Number of Primary Care Physicians: 1,400
Number of Referral/Specialty Physicians: 5,000
Total Enrollment: 134,837
State Enrollment: 134,837

Healthplan and Services Defined
PLAN TYPE: HMO
Model Type: Staff

Type of Coverage
Medicaid

Geographic Areas Served
NY Metropolitan Area

Accreditation Certification
TJC Accreditation, Medicare Approved, Utilization Review, State Licensure

Key Personnel
President/CEO .... Bertram Scott
EVP/Chief of Operations .... Bob Allen
SVP/Chief of Marketing .... Abenaa Udochi
SVP/Chief Medical Officer ..... Munish Khaneja, MD, MPH
VP, Human Resource Svcs. ...... Ann M. Van Etten
SVP/Compliance Officer .... Caron Cullen
VP, Sales & Retention .... Dewitt Smith
VP/General Counsel .... Claire Dematteis

754 AmeriChoice by UnitedHealthCare
7 Hanover Square
#5
New York, NY 10004-2674
Toll-Free: 800-493-4647
Phone: 212-509-5999
Fax: 347-438-3019
www.americhoice.com
Secondary Address: 1083 Coney Island Avenue, Brooklyn, NY 11230
Subsidiary of: UnitedHealth Group
For Profit Organization: Yes
Total Enrollment: 107,387

Healthplan and Services Defined
PLAN TYPE: HMO

Type of Coverage
Medicare, Medicaid

Key Personnel
Manager .... Ernesto Monfitletto
Network Contracting .... Lilli Brillstein
Marketing Director .... Jill Tobin
Sales Director .... Jill Tobin
Media Contact .... Jeff Smith
952-931-5685
jeff.smith@uhc.com

755 Amerigroup New York
360 West 31st Street
5th Floor
New York, NY 10001
Toll-Free: 877-472-8411
Phone: 212-372-6900
www.realsolutions.com
Secondary Address: 47 Mott Street, New York, NY 10013
For Profit Organization: Yes
Year Founded: 2005
Total Enrollment: 1,900,000

Healthplan and Services Defined
PLAN TYPE: HMO

Type of Coverage
Medicare, Medicaid, Expanded Medicaid, SCHIP, Managed L

Geographic Areas Served
New York City, boroughs of Brooklyn, Bronx, Manhattan, Queens, and Staten Island, and Putnam County

---

756   Blue Cross & Blue Shield of Western New York

257 West Genesee Street
Buffalo, NY 14202-2657
Toll-Free: 800-544-2583
Phone: 716-887-6900
Fax: 716-887-8993
snyder.julie@bcbswny.com
www.bcbswny.com
Mailing Address: PO Box 80, Buffalo, NY 14240-0080
Non-Profit Organization: Yes
Year Founded: 1936
Total Enrollment: 555,405
State Enrollment: 197,194

Healthplan and Services Defined
PLAN TYPE: HMO/PPO
Other Type: POS, EPO
Plan Specialty: Lab
Benefits Offered: Dental, Disease Management, Prescription, Wellness

Type of Coverage
Commercial, Medicare, Supplemental Medicare, Medicaid

Geographic Areas Served
New York

Key Personnel
CEO . . . . Alphonso O'Neil-White
COO . . . . Stephen G Jepson
CFO. . . . . James Cardone
CMO . . . . John Gillsepie, MD
General Counsel . . . . Kenneth Sodaro
Provider Relations . . . . Lisa Meyers-Alessi
Member Relations. . . . . Pauline Cataldi
Pharmacy Director . . . . Renee Fleming
Public Relations . . . . Laura Perry
SVP, Chief Medical Offc . . . . Cynthia Ambres
VP, Information Systems . . . . Paul Stoddard
Public Relations. . . . . John F. Pitts
716-887-8825
pitts.john@bcbswny.com

Specialty Managed Care Partners
Wellpoint Pharmacy Management

---

757   BlueShield of Northeastern New York

30 Century Hill Drive
Latham, NY 12110
Toll-Free: 800-459-7587
Phone: 518-220-5800
www.bsneny.com
Mailing Address: PO Box 15013, Albany, NY 12212
Non-Profit Organization: Yes
Year Founded: 1946
Total Enrollment: 193,498
State Enrollment: 72,563

Healthplan and Services Defined
PLAN TYPE: HMO/PPO
Other Type: POS, EPO
Benefits Offered: Disease Management, Prescription, Wellness

Type of Coverage
Commercial, Medicare, Supplemental Medicare, Medicaid

Type of Payment Plans Offered
POS, FFS

Geographic Areas Served
Albany, Clinton, Columbia, Essex, Fulton, Green, Montgomery, Schoharie, Schenectedy, Warren and Washington counties

Accreditation Certification
NCQA

Key Personnel
Public Relations . . . . : . . . . Kyle Rodgers
518-220-4805
rogers.kyle@bsneny.com

Specialty Managed Care Partners
Wellpoint Pharmacy Management

---

758   CDPHP Medicare Plan

500 Patroon Creek Boulevard
Albany, NY 12206-1057
Toll-Free: 888-248-6522
Phone: 518-641-3950
www.cdphp.com
Year Founded: 1984
Total Enrollment: 400,000

Healthplan and Services Defined
PLAN TYPE: Medicare
Benefits Offered: Chiropractic, Dental, Disease Management, Home Care, Inpatient SNF, Physical Therapy, Podiatry, Prescription, Psychiatric, Vision, Wellness

Type of Coverage
Individual, Medicare

Geographic Areas Served
Available within New York state only

Subscriber Information
Average Monthly Fee Per Subscriber
(Employee + Employer Contribution):
Employee Only (Self): Varies
Medicare: Varies
Average Annual Deductible Per Subscriber:
Employee Only (Self): Varies
Medicare: Varies
Average Subscriber Co-Payment:
Primary Care Physician: Varies
Non-Network Physician: Varies
Prescription Drugs: Varies
Hospital ER: Varies
Home Health Care: Varies
Home Health Care Max. Days/Visits Covered: Varies
Nursing Home: Varies
Nursing Home Max. Days/Visits Covered: Varies

Key Personnel
President/CEO . . . . John D Bennett, MD
SVP, Corp Admin/COO . . . . Barbara A Downs, RN
SVP, Legal Affairs . . . . Frederick B Galt
SVP, Sales . . . . Brian O'Grady
Chief Strategy Officer . . . . Robert R. Hinckley
SVP, Human Capital Mgmt. . . . . Scott Klenk
Chief Marketing Officer . . . . Brian J. Morrissey
Chief Medical Officer . . . . Bruce D. Nash, MD, MBA
Chief Information Officer . . . . Neil Brandmaier
Chief Financial Officer . . . . Bethany R. Smith, CPA

---

759   CDPHP: Capital District Physicians' Health Plan

500 Patroon Creek Boulevard
Albany, NY 12206-1057
Toll-Free: 800-777-2273
Phone: 518-641-3700
www.cdphp.com
Non-Profit Organization: Yes

Year Founded: 1984
Number of Primary Care Physicians: 5,000
Total Enrollment: 350,000
State Enrollment: 350,000

Healthplan and Services Defined
 PLAN TYPE: HMO/PPO
 Other Type: POS, ASO
 Model Type: IPA
 Benefits Offered: Dental, Disease Management, Prescription,
  Wellness

Type of Coverage
 Commercial, Individual, Medicare, Medicaid

Geographic Areas Served
 Albany, Broome, Chenango, Columbia, Delaware, Dutchess, Essex,
 Fulton, Greene, Hamilton, Herkimer, Madison, Montgomery, Oneida,
 Orange, Ostego, Rensselaer, Saratoga, Schenectady, Schoharie,
 Tioga, Ulster, Warren, and Washington counties

Subscriber Information
 Average Monthly Fee Per Subscriber
  (Employee + Employer Contribution):
   Employee Only (Self): $64.41
   Employee & 2 Family Members: $175.47
 Average Subscriber Co-Payment:
   Primary Care Physician: $10
   Prescription Drugs: $5-20

Accreditation Certification
 NCQA

Key Personnel
 President/CEO . . . . John D Bennett, MD
 SVP, Corp Admin, COO . . . . Barbara A Downs, RN
 SVP, Legal Affairs, Gener . . . . Frederick B Galt
 SVP, Govt Relations, CSO . . . . Robert R Hinckley
 SVP, Finance/CFO . . . . Bethany R. Smith, CMA
 SVP, Human Capital Mgmt . . . . Scott Klenk
 SVP, Medical Affairs, CMO . . . . Bruce D. Nash, MD
 SVP, Marketing . . . . Brian J Morrissey
 Public Realtions Manager . . . . Kristin C Marshall
  518-641-5031
  kmarshall@cdphp.com
 Public Realtions Spec . . . . Julie K Tracy
  518-641-5126
  jtracy@cdphp.com

760   CIGNA HealthCare of New York

111 John Street
#2500
New York, NY 10038-3107
Toll-Free: 866-438-2446
Phone: 212-285-2100
Fax: 201-533-7000
www.cigna.com
Secondary Address: Great-West Healthcare, now part of CIGNA, 50
 Main Street, 9th Floor, White Plains, NY 10606, 914-682-0159
For Profit Organization: Yes
Total Enrollment: 40,319
State Enrollment: 40,319

Healthplan and Services Defined
 PLAN TYPE: HMO
 Other Type: POS

Type of Coverage
 Commercial

Key Personnel
 Chief Medical Officer . . . . Dr Nicholas Gettas
 Regional Medical Director . . . . Dan Niccolli

761   Coalition America's National Preferred Provider Network

419 E Main Street
Middletown, NY 10940
Toll-Free: 800-557-1656
Phone: 845-343-1600
Fax: 845-344-3233
clientservices@coalitionamerica.com
www.nppn.com
For Profit Organization: Yes
Year Founded: 1993
Number of Affiliated Hospitals: 4,000
Number of Primary Care Physicians: 550,000
Number of Referral/Specialty Physicians: 90,000
Total Enrollment: 4,450,116
State Enrollment: 76,753

Healthplan and Services Defined
 PLAN TYPE: PPO
 Model Type: Network
 Benefits Offered: Prescription

Type of Payment Plans Offered
 DFFS, Capitated

Geographic Areas Served
 Nationwide

Subscriber Information
 Average Monthly Fee Per Subscriber
  (Employee + Employer Contribution):
   Employee Only (Self): Varies
   Employee & 1 Family Member: Varies
   Employee & 2 Family Members: Varies
   Medicare: Varies
 Average Annual Deductible Per Subscriber:
   Employee Only (Self): Varies
   Employee & 1 Family Member: Varies
   Employee & 2 Family Members: Varies
   Medicare: Varies
 Average Subscriber Co-Payment:
   Primary Care Physician: Varies
   Non-Network Physician: Varies
   Prescription Drugs: Varies
   Hospital ER: Varies
   Home Health Care: Varies
   Home Health Care Max. Days/Visits Covered: Varies
   Nursing Home: Varies
   Nursing Home Max. Days/Visits Covered: Varies

Publishes and Distributes Report Card: Yes

Accreditation Certification
 TJC Accreditation, Medicare Approved, Utilization Review,
  Pre-Admission Certification, State Licensure, Quality Assurance
  Program

Key Personnel
 Chairman . . . . Sean Smith
  813-353-2300
 CEO . . . . Scott Smith
 President . . . . Mollie Brown
 CFO . . . . Anthony R Levinson
 COO . . . . Tina Ellex
 Vice President . . . . Larry Madlem
 CIO . . . . Greg Comrie
 Director, Marketing . . . . Libby Ricks
  404-459-7201
  libbyricks@coalitionamerica.com

Average Claim Compensation
 Physician's Fees Charged: 1%
 Hospital's Fees Charged: 1%

762 ConnectiCare of New York

175 Scott Swamp Road
P.O. Box 4050
Farmington, NY 06034-4050
info@connecticare.com
www.connecticare.com
For Profit Organization: Yes
Year Founded: 1981
Number of Affiliated Hospitals: 126
Number of Primary Care Physicians: 22,000
Total Enrollment: 240,000

Healthplan and Services Defined
  PLAN TYPE: HMO/PPO
  Other Type: POS
  Benefits Offered: Dental

Type of Coverage
  Commercial, Individual, Medicare

Key Personnel
  President . . . . .Michael Wise
  Media Contact . . . . .Stephen Jewett
    publicrelations@connecticare.com

763 Davis Vision

Capital Region Health Park, Suite 301
711 Troy-Schenectady Road
Latham, NY 12110
Toll-Free: 800-999-5431
www.davisvision.com
Subsidiary of: HVHC Inc.
For Profit Organization: Yes
Year Founded: 1964
Number of Primary Care Physicians: 30,000
Total Enrollment: 55,000,000

Healthplan and Services Defined
  PLAN TYPE: Vision
  Model Type: Network
  Plan Specialty: Vision
  Benefits Offered: Vision
  Offers Demand Management Patient Information Service: Yes

Type of Payment Plans Offered
  DFFS, Capitated, FFS

Geographic Areas Served
  National & Puerto Rico, Guam, Saipan, Dominican Republic

Subscriber Information
  Average Monthly Fee Per Subscriber
    (Employee + Employer Contribution):
      Employee Only (Self): Varies by plan
      Medicare: Varies

Network Qualifications
  Pre-Admission Certification: No

Peer Review Type
  Utilization Review: Yes
  Second Surgical Opinion: Yes
  Case Management: Yes

Publishes and Distributes Report Card: Yes

Accreditation Certification
  NCQA, COLTS Certification
  TJC Accreditation

Key Personnel
  President . . . . .Steven Holden
  COO/CFO . . . . .Lawrence Gabel
  EVP/CMO . . . . .Tom Davis
  Contracting Manager . . . . .Heather Reynolds
  Chief Marketing Officer . . . . .Dale Paustian
  Manager . . . . .Michael O'Connor
  Chief Information Officer . . . . .Michael Thibdeau

SVP Provider Affairs . . . . .Joseph Wende, OD
VP Business Development . . . . .Robert Elsas

Average Claim Compensation
  Physician's Fees Charged: 75%

Specialty Managed Care Partners
  Enters into Contracts with Regional Business Coalitions: Yes

764 Delta Dental of the Mid-Atlantic

One Delta Drive
Mechanicsburg, PA 17055-6999
Toll-Free: 800-932-0783
Fax: 717-766-8719
www.deltadentalins.com
Non-Profit Organization: Yes
Total Enrollment: 54,000,000

Healthplan and Services Defined
  PLAN TYPE: Dental
  Other Type: Dental PPO

Type of Coverage
  Commercial

Geographic Areas Served
  Statewide

Key Personnel
  President/CEO . . . . .Gary D Radine
  VP, Public & Govt Affairs . . . . .Jeff Album
    415-972-8418
  Dir/Media & Public Affair .Elizabeth Risberg
    415-972-8423

765 Dentcare Delivery Systems

333 Earle Ovington Boulevard
Uniondale, NY 11553
Toll-Free: 800-468-0608
Phone: 516-542-2200
Fax: 516-794-3186
www.dentcaredeliverysystems.org
Non-Profit Organization: Yes
Year Founded: 1978
Number of Primary Care Physicians: 267
Number of Referral/Specialty Physicians: 175
State Enrollment: 295,841

Healthplan and Services Defined
  PLAN TYPE: Dental
  Model Type: IPA
  Plan Specialty: Dental
  Benefits Offered: Dental

Type of Coverage
  Commercial, Individual
  Catastrophic Illness Benefit: None

Type of Payment Plans Offered
  FFS

Geographic Areas Served
  Statewide

Subscriber Information
  Average Annual Deductible Per Subscriber:
    Employee Only (Self): $0
    Employee & 1 Family Member: $0
    Employee & 2 Family Members: $0
    Medicare: $0

Accreditation Certification
  NCQA
  Utilization Review, Quality Assurance Program

Key Personnel
  President . . . . .Glenn J Sobel
    516-794-3000

Treasurer.....................................Mary J Kelly
Secretary.............................Nicole Mastantuono
Marketing.................................Bruce H Safran

766   Easy Choice Health Plan

45 Broadway
Suite 300
New York, NY 10006
Toll-Free: 888-300-9320
Fax: 212-747-0843
www.easychoiceny.com
For Profit Organization: Yes
Year Founded: 1995
Total Enrollment: 30,000
State Enrollment: 30,000

Healthplan and Services Defined
   PLAN TYPE: HMO

Type of Coverage
   Commercial

767   eHealthInsurance Services Inc.

11919 Foundation Place
Gold River, CA 95670
Toll-Free: 800-644-3491
webmaster@healthinsurance.com
www.e.healthinsurance.com
Year Founded: 1997

Healthplan and Services Defined
   PLAN TYPE: HMO/PPO
   Benefits Offered: Dental, Life, STD

Type of Coverage
   Commercial, Individual, Medicare

Geographic Areas Served
   All 50 states in the USA and District of Columbia

Key Personnel
   Chairman & CEO...............................Gary L. Lauer
   EVP/Business & Corp. Dev......................Bruce Telkamp
   EVP/Chief Technology....................Dr. Sheldon X. Wang
   SVP & CFO ....Stuart M. Huizinga
   Pres. of eHealth Gov. Sys ....Samuel C. Gibbs
   SVP of Sales & Operations ....Robert S. Hurley
   Director Public Relations.......................Nate Purpura
      650-210-3115

768   Elderplan

6323 Seventh Avenue
Brooklyn, NY 11220
Toll-Free: 800-353-3765
Phone: 718-921-7979
info@elderplan.org
www.elderplan.org
Non-Profit Organization: Yes
Year Founded: 1985
Number of Affiliated Hospitals: 35
Number of Primary Care Physicians: 1,200
Number of Referral/Specialty Physicians: 3,800
Total Enrollment: 16,000
State Enrollment: 15,000

Healthplan and Services Defined
   PLAN TYPE: Medicare
   Other Type: Medicare Advantage
   Model Type: Network
   Plan Specialty: ASO, Behavioral Health, Chiropractic, Dental,
      Disease Management, EPO, Lab, Vision, Radiology
   Benefits Offered: Behavioral Health, Chiropractic, Complementary
      Medicine, Dental, Disease Management, Home Care, Inpatient

SNF, Long-Term Care, Physical Therapy, Podiatry, Prescription,
   Psychiatric, Transplant, Vision

Type of Coverage
   Medicare

Type of Payment Plans Offered
   FFS

Geographic Areas Served
   Brooklyn, Bronx, Manhattan, Queens and Staten Island

Subscriber Information
   Average Monthly Fee Per Subscriber
      (Employee + Employer Contribution):
         Medicare: No premium
   Average Annual Deductible Per Subscriber:
      Medicare: $0.00
   Average Subscriber Co-Payment:
      Primary Care Physician: $0.00 co-pay
      Prescription Drugs: $5.00/9.00
      Hospital ER: $50.00
      Home Health Care: $0.00
      Home Health Care Max. Days/Visits Covered: 365 days
      Nursing Home Max. Days/Visits Covered: 200 days

Network Qualifications
   Pre-Admission Certification: Yes

Peer Review Type
   Utilization Review: Yes
   Second Surgical Opinion: Yes
   Case Management: Yes

Publishes and Distributes Report Card: No

Accreditation Certification
   TJC Accreditation, Medicare Approved, Utilization Review, State
      Licensure, Quality Assurance Program

Key Personnel
   President/CEO ....Eli S Feldman
   CFO ....Joe Pinho
   VP/Corporate Marketing/PR....................Janet Rothman
   Medical Affairs ....Herbert Segal
   Provider Services ....Jim Berg
   Dir, Public Relations ....Audrey O Waters
      718-759-4677
      media@elderplan.org

Specialty Managed Care Partners
   Health Plex, Maxore
   Enters into Contracts with Regional Business Coalitions: Yes

769   Empire Blue Cross & Blue Shield

One Liberty Avenue
New York, NY 10006
www.empireblue.com
Subsidiary of: A Subsidiary of Wellpoint
Non-Profit Organization: Yes
Year Founded: 1934
Owned by an Integrated Delivery Network (IDN): Yes
Number of Affiliated Hospitals: 200
Number of Primary Care Physicians: 66,000
Number of Referral/Specialty Physicians: 62,000
Total Enrollment: 171,028

Healthplan and Services Defined
   PLAN TYPE: HMO/PPO
   Other Type: EPO, POS
   Model Type: Network
   Plan Specialty: Behavioral Health, Vision, Radiology, Worker's
      Compensation
   Benefits Offered: Behavioral Health, Dental, Disease Management,
      Prescription, Psychiatric, Transplant, Vision, Wellness, Maternity
   Offers Demand Management Patient Information Service: Yes

Type of Coverage
   Individual, Medicare

Catastrophic Illness Benefit: Varies per case

Type of Payment Plans Offered
POS, DFFS

Geographic Areas Served
28 eastern counties of New York

Network Qualifications
Pre-Admission Certification: Yes

Peer Review Type
Utilization Review: Yes
Second Surgical Opinion: Yes
Case Management: Yes

Publishes and Distributes Report Card: Yes

Accreditation Certification
NCQA
TJC Accreditation, State Licensure

Key Personnel
Public Relations Director........................Sally Kweskin
303-831-5899
sally.kweskin@anthem.com

Specialty Managed Care Partners
Enters into Contracts with Regional Business Coalitions: Yes

770 Excellus Blue Cross Blue Shield: Central New York

333 Butternut Drive
Syracuse, NY 13214-1803
Toll-Free: 800-919-8809
Phone: 315-671-6400
www.excellusbcbs.com
Subsidiary of: Lifetime Healthcare Companies
Non-Profit Organization: Yes
Year Founded: 1985
Number of Affiliated Hospitals: 14
Number of Primary Care Physicians: 290
Number of Referral/Specialty Physicians: 677
Total Enrollment: 1,700,000
State Enrollment: 1,700,000

Healthplan and Services Defined
PLAN TYPE: HMO
Model Type: Network
Plan Specialty: ASO, Behavioral Health, Chiropractic, Dental, Disease Management
Benefits Offered: Behavioral Health, Chiropractic, Dental, Disease Management, Physical Therapy, Podiatry, Prescription, Psychiatric, Vision, Wellness

Type of Coverage
Indemnity, Medicare, Supplemental Medicare

Type of Payment Plans Offered
Capitated

Geographic Areas Served
St. Lawrence, Jefferson, Lewis, Oswego, Onondaga, Cayuga, Tompkins, Courtland, Chenango, Broome, Tioga, Chemung, Schuyler and Steuben counties

Subscriber Information
Average Monthly Fee Per Subscriber
(Employee + Employer Contribution):
Employee Only (Self): Varies by plan
Average Subscriber Co-Payment:
Primary Care Physician: $10.00
Prescription Drugs: $10.00

Peer Review Type
Second Surgical Opinion: No
Case Management: Yes

Publishes and Distributes Report Card: Yes

Accreditation Certification
NCQA
TJC Accreditation, Medicare Approved, Utilization Review, State Licensure

Key Personnel
President................................Arthur Vercillo, MD
Sr Deputy General Counsel.............Margaret M Cassady, Esq
VP, Contracting.........................Antonio V Vitagliano
VP, Communications ....Elizabeth Martin
VP, Sales...................................Todd Muscatello
VP, Human Resources ....Ellen Wilson

Specialty Managed Care Partners
Enters into Contracts with Regional Business Coalitions: Yes

771 Excellus Blue Cross Blue Shield: Rochester Region

165 Court Street
Rochester, NY 14647
www.excellusbcbs.com
Mailing Address: PO Box 22999, Rochester, NY 14692
Subsidiary of: Lifetime Healthcare Companies
Non-Profit Organization: Yes
Year Founded: 1985
Number of Affiliated Hospitals: 18
Number of Primary Care Physicians: 1,035
Number of Referral/Specialty Physicians: 2,082
Total Enrollment: 1,700,000
State Enrollment: 1,700,000

Healthplan and Services Defined
PLAN TYPE: HMO
Model Type: IPA
Benefits Offered: Disease Management, Prescription, Wellness
Offers Demand Management Patient Information Service: Yes

Type of Payment Plans Offered
POS, Combination FFS & DFFS

Geographic Areas Served
Livingston, Monroe, Ontario, Seneca, Wayne & Yates counties

Subscriber Information
Average Monthly Fee Per Subscriber
(Employee + Employer Contribution):
Employee Only (Self): $73.78
Employee & 1 Family Member: $365.24
Employee & 2 Family Members: $232.09
Medicare: $113.54
Average Annual Deductible Per Subscriber:
Employee Only (Self): $0
Employee & 1 Family Member: $0
Employee & 2 Family Members: $0
Medicare: $0
Average Subscriber Co-Payment:
Primary Care Physician: $15.00
Non-Network Physician: $0
Prescription Drugs: $0
Hospital ER: $50.00
Home Health Care: $0
Home Health Care Max. Days/Visits Covered: Unlimited
Nursing Home: $0
Nursing Home Max. Days/Visits Covered: 120-360 days

Publishes and Distributes Report Card: Yes

Accreditation Certification
NCQA
TJC Accreditation, Medicare Approved, Utilization Review, State Licensure, Quality Assurance Program

Key Personnel
President................................Arthur Vercillo, MD
VP/Chief Medical Officer ....Marybeth McCall, MD

VP, Human Resources . . . . Ellen Wilson
VP, Communications . . . . Elizabeth Martin
VP, Sales. . . . . Todd Muscatello

772 Excellus Blue Cross Blue Shield: Utica Region

12 Rhoads Drive
Utica, NY 13502
Toll-Free: 877-757-3850
www.excellusbcbs.com
Mailing Address: PO Box 22999, Rochester, NY 14692
Subsidiary of: Lifetime Healthcare Companies
Non-Profit Organization: Yes
Total Enrollment: 1,700,000
State Enrollment: 1,700,000

Healthplan and Services Defined
PLAN TYPE: HMO
Benefits Offered: Disease Management, Wellness

Type of Coverage
Commercial, Medicare, Medicaid

Type of Payment Plans Offered
POS

Geographic Areas Served
Franklin, Cliton, Essex, Hamilton, Herkimer, Fulton, Oneida, Madison, Montgomery, Ostego and Delaware counties

Key Personnel
President . . . . Eve Van de Wal
Sr Deputy General Counsel . . . . Margaret M Cassady, Esq
VP, Communications. . . . . Stephanie Davis
VP, Chief Medical Officer . . . . Mary Beth McCall, MD
VP, Provider Relations . . . . Kathy Horn
VP, Sales. . . . . Todd Muscatello

773 Fidelis Care

95-25 Queens Boulevard
Rego Park, NY 11374
Toll-Free: 888-343-3547
Phone: 718-896-6500
Fax: 718-896-1910
www.fideliscare.org
Secondary Address: 8 Southwoods Blvd, Albany, NY 12211
For Profit Organization: Yes
Year Founded: 1993
Number of Primary Care Physicians: 42,000
Total Enrollment: 625,000
State Enrollment: 625,000

Healthplan and Services Defined
PLAN TYPE: Multiple
Benefits Offered: Chiropractic, Dental, Disease Management, Home Care, Inpatient SNF, Physical Therapy, Podiatry, Prescription, Psychiatric, Vision, Wellness

Type of Coverage
Individual, Medicare, Medicaid

Geographic Areas Served
53 counties in New York State

Subscriber Information
Average Monthly Fee Per Subscriber
(Employee + Employer Contribution):
Employee Only (Self): Varies
Medicare: Varies
Average Annual Deductible Per Subscriber:
Employee Only (Self): Varies
Medicare: Varies
Average Subscriber Co-Payment:
Primary Care Physician: Varies
Non-Network Physician: Varies

Prescription Drugs: Varies
Hospital ER: Varies
Home Health Care: Varies
Home Health Care Max. Days/Visits Covered: Varies
Nursing Home: Varies
Nursing Home Max. Days/Visits Covered: Varies

Key Personnel
Interim CEO. . . . . Patrick Frawley
SVP/Provider Relations. . . . . David Thomas
Chief Information Officer . . . . Patrick Garland
VP/Information Technology . . . . John Olearczyk
Director Financial Ops . . . . Irene Amican
Director Info Technology. . . . . Don Martin
Network/Telecommunication . . . . Gary Crane
Chief Medical Officer. . . . . Edward Anselm, MD
Director, Communications . . . . Darla Shattenkirk
518-445-3918
dshattenkirk@fideliscare.org
Public Relations Coord . . . . Jayson R White
518-445-3923
jwhite@fideliscare.org

774 GHI

441 Ninth Avenue
New York, NY 10001
Toll-Free: 800-611-8454
Phone: 212-615-0000
www.emblemhealth.com
Mailing Address: PO Box 3000, New York, NY 10116-3000
Subsidiary of: EmblemHealth
Non-Profit Organization: Yes
Year Founded: 1937
Number of Affiliated Hospitals: 230
Number of Primary Care Physicians: 15,529
Number of Referral/Specialty Physicians: 25,173
Total Enrollment: 1,601,000
State Enrollment: 2,475,666

Healthplan and Services Defined
PLAN TYPE: HMO/PPO
Model Type: Network
Plan Specialty: ASO, Behavioral Health, Dental, EPO
Benefits Offered: Behavioral Health, Chiropractic, Complementary Medicine, Dental, Disease Management, Home Care, Inpatient SNF, Physical Therapy, Podiatry, Prescription, Psychiatric, Transplant, Vision, Wellness

Type of Coverage
Commercial, Individual, Indemnity, Medicare, Supplemental Medicare, Medicaid

Type of Payment Plans Offered
DFFS

Geographic Areas Served
GHI operates statewide in New York. GHI HMO serves 26 eastern New York counties, including five New York City boroughs

Subscriber Information
Average Monthly Fee Per Subscriber
(Employee + Employer Contribution):
Employee Only (Self): $69.44
Average Annual Deductible Per Subscriber:
Employee & 2 Family Members: $214.30
Average Subscriber Co-Payment:
Primary Care Physician: $10.00
Prescription Drugs: $10.00/20.00/30.00

Peer Review Type
Utilization Review: Yes
Second Surgical Opinion: Yes
Case Management: Yes

Accreditation Certification
NCQA

Key Personnel
Chairman/CEO . . . . Frank J Branchini
Chief Financial Officer . . . . Arthur J. Byrd
General Counsel . . . . Nicholas P. Kambolis
SVP, Underwriting . . . . George Babitsch
SVP/Deputy General Couns. . . . . Jeffrey D. Chansler
VP, Human Resources . . . . Mariann E. Drohan
SVP, Government Programs. . . . . Shawn M. Fitzgibbon
Chief Medical Officer . . . . William A. Gillespie, MD
EVP, Corporate Operations . . . . William C. Lamoreaux
Chief Marketing Officer. . . . . Charlene A. Maher
Chief Actuary . . . . Edward Mailander
SVP/Deputy General Couns. . . . . William Mastro
SVP, Finance . . . . Michael Palmateer
Chief Compliance Officer . . . . Valerie A. Reardon

Specialty Managed Care Partners
Value Options, Express Scrips, Davis Vision, New York Medical
Imaging, Multi-Plan, CCN

775 GHI Medicare Plan
441 Ninth Avenue
New York, NY 10001
Toll-Free: 800-611-8454
Phone: 212-615-0000
www.emblemhealth.com
Mailing Address: PO Box 3000, New York, NY 10116-3000
Subsidiary of: EmblemHealth
Year Founded: 1931
Total Enrollment: 53,000

Healthplan and Services Defined
PLAN TYPE: Medicare
Benefits Offered: Chiropractic, Dental, Disease Management, Home
Care, Inpatient SNF, Physical Therapy, Podiatry, Prescription,
Psychiatric, Vision, Wellness

Type of Coverage
Individual, Medicare

Geographic Areas Served
Available within New York state only

Subscriber Information
Average Monthly Fee Per Subscriber
(Employee + Employer Contribution):
Employee Only (Self): Varies
Medicare: Varies
Average Annual Deductible Per Subscriber:
Employee Only (Self): Varies
Medicare: Varies
Average Subscriber Co-Payment:
Primary Care Physician: Varies
Non-Network Physician: Varies
Prescription Drugs: Varies
Hospital ER: Varies
Home Health Care: Varies
Home Health Care Max. Days/Visits Covered: Varies
Nursing Home: Varies
Nursing Home Max. Days/Visits Covered: Varies

Key Personnel
Chairman/CEO . . . . Frank J. Branchini
Chief Financial Officer . . . . Arthur J. Byrd
General Counsel . . . . Nicholas P. Kambolis
SVP, Underwriting . . . . George Babitsch
SVP/Deputy General Couns. . . . . Jeffrey D. Chansler
VP, Human Resources . . . . Mariann E. Drohan
SVP, Government Programs. . . . . Shawn M. Fitzgibbon
Chief Medical Officer . . . . William A. Gillespie, MD
EVP, Corporate Operations . . . . William C. Lamoreaux
Chief Marketing Officer. . . . . Charlene A. Maher
Chief Actuary . . . . Edward Mailander
SVP/Deputy General Couns. . . . . William Mastro
SVP, Finance . . . . Michael Palmateer

Chief Compliance Officer . . . . Valerie A. Reardon

776 Great-West Healthcare New York
475 Park Ave
New York, NY 10022
Toll-Free: 866-494-2111
Phone: 212-685-5999
eliginquiries@cigna.com
www.cignaforhealth.com
Secondary Address: 330 Motor Parkway, Suite 206, Hauppauge, NY
11788
Subsidiary of: CIGNA HealthCare
Acquired by: CIGNA
For Profit Organization: Yes
Total Enrollment: 28,785
State Enrollment: 24,502

Healthplan and Services Defined
PLAN TYPE: HMO/PPO
Benefits Offered: Disease Management, Prescription, Wellness

Type of Coverage
Commercial

Type of Payment Plans Offered
POS, FFS

Geographic Areas Served
New York

Accreditation Certification
URAC

Specialty Managed Care Partners
Caremark Rx

777 Guardian Life Insurance Company of America
7 Hanover Square
H-6-D
New York, NY 10004
Toll-Free: 888-482-7342
Phone: 212-598-8000
marketcc@glic.com
www.guardianlife.com
Subsidiary of: Guardian
For Profit Organization: Yes
Year Founded: 1860
Owned by an Integrated Delivery Network (IDN): Yes
Number of Affiliated Hospitals: 2,966
Number of Primary Care Physicians: 121,815
Number of Referral/Specialty Physicians: 193,137
Total Enrollment: 205,677

Healthplan and Services Defined
PLAN TYPE: HMO/PPO
Model Type: Network
Plan Specialty: Chiropractic, Dental, Disease Management, Lab,
PBM, Vision, Radiology, UR
Benefits Offered: Behavioral Health, Chiropractic, Complementary
Medicine, Dental, Disease Management, Home Care, Physical
Therapy, Podiatry, Prescription, Psychiatric, Vision, Wellness,
AD&D, Life, LTD, STD

Type of Coverage
Commercial, Indemnity

Type of Payment Plans Offered
Combination FFS & DFFS

Geographic Areas Served
Nationwide

Subscriber Information
Average Monthly Fee Per Subscriber
(Employee + Employer Contribution):

Employee Only (Self): Varies by plan

Peer Review Type
Utilization Review: Yes
Second Surgical Opinion: Yes
Case Management: Yes

Publishes and Distributes Report Card: Yes

Accreditation Certification
URAC, NCQA

Key Personnel
EVP, Chief Financial Offi . . . . Robert E. Broatch
Chief Operating Officer . . . . Scott Dolfi
President/CEO . . . . Deanna M. Mulligan
Chief Actuary . . . . Armand M De Palo
Risk Management Products . . . . Gary B Lenderink
Chief Investment Officer . . . . Thomas G Sorell
Sr VP/Individual Markets . . . . David W Allen
Sr VP/Corporate Secretary . . . . Joseph A Caruso
Sr VP/Human Resources . . . . Brad Thomas
Sr VP/Corporate Marketing . . . . Nancy F Rogers
Sr VP/Group Insurance . . . . Richard A White
Sr VP/General Counsel . . . . John Peluso
VP/Reinsurance . . . . Jeremy Starr
EVP/COO . . . . K Rone Baldwin
Public Relations . . . . Richard Jones
richard_jones@glic.com

Specialty Managed Care Partners
Health Net
Enters into Contracts with Regional Business Coalitions: Yes

778 Health Plan of New York

55 Water Street
New York, NY 10041
Toll-Free: 800-447-8255
Phone: 646-447-5900
Fax: 646-447-3011
www.hipusa.com
Subsidiary of: An Emblem Health Company
Total Enrollment: 1,200,000

Healthplan and Services Defined
PLAN TYPE: HMO/PPO
Other Type: POS, EPO, ASO
Benefits Offered: Chiropractic, Dental, Disease Management, Home
Care, Inpatient SNF, Physical Therapy, Podiatry, Prescription,
Psychiatric, Vision, Wellness

Type of Coverage
Individual, Medicare

Geographic Areas Served
New York, Connecticut, Massachusetts

Subscriber Information
Average Monthly Fee Per Subscriber
(Employee + Employer Contribution):
Employee Only (Self): Varies
Medicare: Varies
Average Annual Deductible Per Subscriber:
Employee Only (Self): Varies
Medicare: Varies
Average Subscriber Co-Payment:
Primary Care Physician: Varies
Non-Network Physician: Varies
Prescription Drugs: Varies
Hospital ER: Varies
Home Health Care: Varies
Home Health Care Max. Days/Visits Covered: Varies
Nursing Home: Varies
Nursing Home Max. Days/Visits Covered: Varies

Key Personnel
Chairman/CEO . . . . Anthony L Watson

President/COO . . . . Frank J Branchini
SVP, Customer Service . . . . Marilyn DeQuatro
SVP, Operations . . . . Thomas K Dwyer
SVP, Network Mgmt . . . . Shawn M Fitzgibbon
SVP, Govt Relations . . . . David S Abernathy
EVP, CFO . . . . Michael D Fullwood
SVP, Govt Programs . . . . William C Lamoreaux
SVP, Sales & Marketing . . . . Charlene Maher
SVP, Dep General Counsel . . . . William Mastro
SVP, Chief Medical Offc . . . . William A Gillespie, MD
SVP . . . . Fred Blickman
EVP, Chief Info Officer . . . . John H Steber
SVP, Human Resources . . . . Thomas A Nemeth
SVP, Sales & Acct Mgmt . . . . George Babitsch
SVP, Public Affairs . . . . Ilene D Margolin
SVP, Finance . . . . Michael Palmaterr

779 HealthNow New York - Emblem Health

1901 Main Street
Buffalo, NY 14240
Toll-Free: 800-856-0480
Phone: 716-887-6900
Fax: 716-887-8981
www.healthnowny.com
Mailing Address: PO Box 15013, Albany, NY 12212-5013
Non-Profit Organization: Yes
Year Founded: 1936
Number of Affiliated Hospitals: 33
Number of Primary Care Physicians: 927
Number of Referral/Specialty Physicians: 2,059
Total Enrollment: 553,000
State Enrollment: 553,000

Healthplan and Services Defined
PLAN TYPE: HMO
Model Type: IPA
Benefits Offered: Behavioral Health, Chiropractic, Disease
Management, Home Care, Inpatient SNF, Physical Therapy,
Podiatry, Prescription, Psychiatric, Transplant, Vision, Wellness

Type of Coverage
Commercial, Individual, Indemnity, Medicare, Supplemental
Medicare, Medicaid

Type of Payment Plans Offered
Capitated, FFS

Geographic Areas Served
Broome, Cayuga, Chenango, Cortland, Delaware, Franklin, Hamilton,
Herkimer, Jefferson, Lewis, Madison, Oneida, Onondaga, Oswego,
Otsego, St Lawrence and Tioga counties

Network Qualifications
Pre-Admission Certification: Yes

Peer Review Type
Utilization Review: Yes
Second Surgical Opinion: Yes
Case Management: Yes

Publishes and Distributes Report Card: Yes

Accreditation Certification
NCQA
Utilization Review, Pre-Admission Certification, State Licensure,
Quality Assurance Program

Key Personnel
Chairman/CEO . . . . Anthony Watson
President/COO . . . . Frank Branchini
Executive Vice President . . . . Daniel Fink
Chief Financial Officer . . . . Arthur Byrd
General Counsel . . . . Nicholas Kambolis
SVP/Governement Relations . . . . David Abernathy
Sales Manager . . . . Brian Beaton
716-887-7993
beaton.brian@healthnow.org

Dir, Public Relations . . . . Karen Merkel-Liberatore
716-887-8811
merkel-liberatore.karen@healthnow.org

Specialty Managed Care Partners
Integra, Quest Diagnostics, Prism, Alterna Health

---

780 Healthplex

333 Earle Ovington Boulevard
Suite 300
Uniondale, NY 11553
Toll-Free: 800-468-0608
info@healthplex.com
www.healthplex.com
For Profit Organization: Yes
Year Founded: 1977
Number of Primary Care Physicians: 2,855
Number of Referral/Specialty Physicians: 448
Total Enrollment: 2,000,000

Healthplan and Services Defined
 PLAN TYPE: Dental
 Other Type: Dental HMO/PPO
 Model Type: IPA
 Plan Specialty: Dental
 Benefits Offered: Dental

Type of Coverage
 Commercial, Individual, Indemnity

Type of Payment Plans Offered
 POS, DFFS, Capitated, FFS, Combination FFS & DFFS

Geographic Areas Served
 New Jersey & New York

Subscriber Information
 Average Monthly Fee Per Subscriber
  (Employee + Employer Contribution):
   Employee Only (Self): $159.00
   Employee & 1 Family Member: $264.00
   Employee & 2 Family Members: $350.00
 Average Annual Deductible Per Subscriber:
   Employee Only (Self): $0
   Employee & 1 Family Member: $0
   Employee & 2 Family Members: $0

Network Qualifications
 Pre-Admission Certification: No

Peer Review Type
 Utilization Review: Yes
 Second Surgical Opinion: Yes
 Case Management: Yes

Accreditation Certification
 NCQA
 Utilization Review, Quality Assurance Program

Specialty Managed Care Partners
 Enters into Contracts with Regional Business Coalitions: Yes

---

781 Humana Health Insurance of New York

125 Wolf Road
Suite 501
Albany, NY 12205
Toll-Free: 800-967-2370
Fax: 518-435-0412
www.humana.com
Secondary Address: 160 Linden Oaks, Rochester, NY 14625
For Profit Organization: Yes
Total Enrollment: 81,000

Healthplan and Services Defined
 PLAN TYPE: HMO/PPO

Type of Coverage
 Commercial, Individual

Accreditation Certification
 URAC, NCQA, CORE

---

782 Independent Health

511 Farber Lakes Drive
Buffalo, NY 14221
Toll-Free: 800-501-3439
Phone: 716-631-3001
www.independenthealth.com
Non-Profit Organization: Yes
Year Founded: 1980
Number of Affiliated Hospitals: 35
Number of Primary Care Physicians: 1,125
Number of Referral/Specialty Physicians: 1,626
Total Enrollment: 365,000
State Enrollment: 365,000

Healthplan and Services Defined
 PLAN TYPE: HMO
 Model Type: IPA
 Plan Specialty: EPO
 Benefits Offered: Behavioral Health, Chiropractic, Dental, Disease
  Management, Home Care, Inpatient SNF, Physical Therapy,
  Podiatry, Prescription, Psychiatric, Transplant, Vision, Wellness

Type of Coverage
 Commercial, Individual, Indemnity, Medicaid, Choice
 Catastrophic Illness Benefit: Varies per case

Type of Payment Plans Offered
 POS, Combination FFS & DFFS

Geographic Areas Served
 Allegany, Cattaraugus, Chautauqua, Erie, Genesee, Niagara, Orleans
 & Wyoming counties of western New York

Subscriber Information
 Average Monthly Fee Per Subscriber
  (Employee + Employer Contribution):
   Employee Only (Self): Varies by plan
 Average Subscriber Co-Payment:
   Primary Care Physician: $10.00
   Prescription Drugs: $7.00
   Hospital ER: $35.00
   Home Health Care: $10.00
   Home Health Care Max. Days/Visits Covered: 365 days
   Nursing Home: $0
   Nursing Home Max. Days/Visits Covered: 45 days

Network Qualifications
 Pre-Admission Certification: Yes

Peer Review Type
 Utilization Review: Yes
 Second Surgical Opinion: Yes
 Case Management: Yes

Publishes and Distributes Report Card: No

Accreditation Certification
 TJC, NCQA
 Utilization Review, Pre-Admission Certification, State Licensure,
  Quality Assurance Program

Key Personnel
 President and CEO . . . . Michael W Cropp, MD
  mcropp@independenthealth.com
 EVP/COO . . . . John Rodgers
 EVP/Chief Medical Officer . . . . Thomas Foels
 EVP, Chief of Servicing . . . . Jill Syracuse
 SVP, Human Resources . . . . Patricia Clabeaux
 EVP/CFO . . . . Mark Johnson
 SVP/General Counsel . . . . John Mineo

Specialty Managed Care Partners
 Enters into Contracts with Regional Business Coalitions: No

783 Independent Health Medicare Plan

511 Farber Lakes Drive
Buffalo, NY 14221
Toll-Free: 800-501-3439
Phone: 716-631-3001
www.independenthealth.com

Healthplan and Services Defined
  PLAN TYPE: Medicare
  Benefits Offered: Chiropractic, Dental, Disease Management, Home
    Care, Inpatient SNF, Physical Therapy, Podiatry, Prescription,
    Psychiatric, Vision, Wellness

Type of Coverage
  Individual, Medicare

Geographic Areas Served
  Available within New York state only

Subscriber Information
  Average Monthly Fee Per Subscriber
    (Employee + Employer Contribution):
      Employee Only (Self): Varies
      Medicare: Varies
  Average Annual Deductible Per Subscriber:
      Employee Only (Self): Varies
      Medicare: Varies
  Average Subscriber Co-Payment:
      Primary Care Physician: Varies
      Non-Network Physician: Varies
      Prescription Drugs: Varies
      Hospital ER: Varies
      Home Health Care: Varies
      Home Health Care Max. Days/Visits Covered: Varies
      Nursing Home: Varies
      Nursing Home Max. Days/Visits Covered: Varies

Key Personnel
  President and CEO . . . . Michael W Cropp, MD
    mcropp@independenthealth.com
  Exec Dir, IH Foundation . . . . Carrie Meyer
  Dir, Health Promotion . . . . Peggy Davis , RN
  SVP, HR & Org Development . . . . Gord Cumming
  SVP, Member Services . . . . Jill Syracuse
  Dir, Pharmacy Services . . . . Martin Burruano, RPh
  EVP, Chief Marketing Offc . . . . John Rodgers
  Chief Medical Officer . . . . Thomas J Foels, MD
  Assoc Medical Director . . . . Kathleen Mylotte, MD
  Assoc Medical Director . . . . Judith Feld, MD
  Dir, Public Relations . . . . Frank Sava
    716-635-3885
    fsava@independenthealth.com

784 Island Group Administration, Inc.

3 Toilsome Lane
East Hampton, NY 11937
Toll-Free: 800-926-2306
Phone: 631-324-2306
Fax: 631-324-7021
lrkaplan@optonline.net
www.islandgroupadmin.com
For Profit Organization: Yes
Year Founded: 1990
Owned by an Integrated Delivery Network (IDN): No
Federally Qualified: No
Number of Affiliated Hospitals: 9,055
Number of Primary Care Physicians: 21,010
Total Enrollment: 52,000

Healthplan and Services Defined
  PLAN TYPE: Multiple
  Model Type: TPA

Plan Specialty: Dental, Vision, Radiology, Worker's Compensation,
    UR, Medical
  Benefits Offered: Chiropractic, Dental, Disease Management, Home
    Care, Podiatry, Prescription, Psychiatric, Transplant, Vision,
    Wellness, Worker's Compensation, Medical, Hospital

Type of Coverage
  Varies

Geographic Areas Served
  Nationwide

Subscriber Information
  Average Monthly Fee Per Subscriber
    (Employee + Employer Contribution):
      Employee Only (Self): Varies by plan

Peer Review Type
  Utilization Review: Yes
  Second Surgical Opinion: Yes
  Case Management: Yes

Accreditation Certification
  Utilization Review, Pre-Admission Certification, State Licensure

Key Personnel
  President . . . . Alan Kaplan
  VP, Operations . . . . Rosemarie Nuzzi
  EVP & Provider Relations . . . . Lynn Kaplan
  Claims Supervisor . . . . Cindy Bacon, RN
  Case Review . . . . Lucille Dunn

Specialty Managed Care Partners
  Standard Security; CareMark PBM

785 Liberty Health Advantage Medicare Plan

1 Huntington Quadrangle
Suite 3N01
Melville, NY 11747
Toll-Free: 866-542-4269
Fax: 631-227-3484
www.libertyhealthadvantage.com

Healthplan and Services Defined
  PLAN TYPE: Medicare
  Other Type: HMO
  Benefits Offered: Chiropractic, Dental, Disease Management, Home
    Care, Inpatient SNF, Physical Therapy, Podiatry, Prescription,
    Psychiatric, Vision, Wellness

Type of Coverage
  Individual, Medicare

Geographic Areas Served
  Available within New York state only

Subscriber Information
  Average Monthly Fee Per Subscriber
    (Employee + Employer Contribution):
      Employee Only (Self): Varies
      Medicare: Varies
  Average Annual Deductible Per Subscriber:
      Employee Only (Self): Varies
      Medicare: Varies
  Average Subscriber Co-Payment:
      Primary Care Physician: Varies
      Non-Network Physician: Varies
      Prescription Drugs: Varies
      Hospital ER: Varies
      Home Health Care: Varies
      Home Health Care Max. Days/Visits Covered: Varies
      Nursing Home: Varies
      Nursing Home Max. Days/Visits Covered: Varies

Key Personnel
  President/CEO . . . . Kevin M Grace
  VP/Operations . . . . Lucy Oliva
  VP/Behavioral Health . . . . Jim McCreath
  VP/Client Services . . . . Cindy Waterman

Office Manager. . . . . Stacey Carroll

786 MagnaCare

One Penn Plaza
46th Floor
New York, NY 10119
Toll-Free: 800-235-7267
Phone: 516-282-8000
providerrelations@magnacare.com
www.magnacare.com
Secondary Address: 1600 Stewart Avenue, Suite 700, Westbury, NY
  11590
For Profit Organization: Yes
Year Founded: 1990
Number of Affiliated Hospitals: 260
Number of Primary Care Physicians: 70,000
Number of Referral/Specialty Physicians: 58,000
Total Enrollment: 1,326,000
State Enrollment: 928,200

Healthplan and Services Defined
  PLAN TYPE: PPO
  Model Type: Network
  Plan Specialty: ASO, Behavioral Health, Chiropractic, Dental, Lab,
    Radiology, Worker's Compensation, UR
  Benefits Offered: Behavioral Health, Chiropractic, Dental, Home
    Care, Inpatient SNF, Physical Therapy, Podiatry, Prescription,
    Psychiatric, Worker's Compensation

Type of Coverage
  Leased Network Arrangement

Type of Payment Plans Offered
  DFFS

Geographic Areas Served
  New Jersey and New York

Subscriber Information
  Average Monthly Fee Per Subscriber
    (Employee + Employer Contribution):
      Employee Only (Self): Varies
  Average Subscriber Co-Payment:
    Primary Care Physician: $15.00
    Prescription Drugs: $10.00/20.00
    Home Health Care: Varies
    Home Health Care Max. Days/Visits Covered: Varies
    Nursing Home: Varies
    Nursing Home Max. Days/Visits Covered: Varies

Network Qualifications
  Pre-Admission Certification: Yes

Peer Review Type
  Utilization Review: Yes
  Second Surgical Opinion: No
  Case Management: Yes

Accreditation Certification
  TJC Accreditation, Utilization Review, Pre-Admission Certification,
    State Licensure, Quality Assurance Program

Key Personnel
  President/CEO. . . . . Joseph Berardo, Jr
  EVP, Operations. . . . . Terry Beach
  SVP, CFO . . . . Jim Cusumano
  COO . . . . Thomas Considine
  VP, General Counsel. . . . . Craig B Greenfield
  SVP, Marketing. . . . . Robert Post
  VP, Business Development . . . . Derek Moore
  SVP, Chief Medical Offc . . . . Catherine Marino, MD
  VP, Human Resources . . . . Julie Bank
  SVP, Information Systems. . . . . Arun Bhatia
  SVP, Sales & Acct Mgmt. . . . . Michael Jordan

Average Claim Compensation
  Physician's Fees Charged: 50%

  Hospital's Fees Charged: 60%

Specialty Managed Care Partners
  American Psych Systems, Intra State Choice Management
    Chiropractic

Employer References
  Local 947, District Council of Painters #9

787 Meritain Health: Corporate Headquarters

300 Corporate Parkway
Amherst, NY 14226
Toll-Free: 800-242-6922
Phone: 716-319-5725
sales@meritain.com
www.meritain.com
For Profit Organization: Yes
Year Founded: 1983
Number of Affiliated Hospitals: 110
Number of Primary Care Physicians: 3,467
Number of Referral/Specialty Physicians: 5,720
Total Enrollment: 500,000
State Enrollment: 450,000

Healthplan and Services Defined
  PLAN TYPE: PPO
  Model Type: Network
  Plan Specialty: Dental, Disease Management, Vision, Radiology, UR
  Benefits Offered: Prescription
  Offers Demand Management Patient Information Service: Yes

Type of Coverage
  Commercial

Geographic Areas Served
  Nationwide

Subscriber Information
  Average Monthly Fee Per Subscriber
    (Employee + Employer Contribution):
      Employee Only (Self): Varies by plan

Accreditation Certification
  URAC
  TJC Accreditation, Medicare Approved, Utilization Review,
    Pre-Admission Certification, State Licensure, Quality Assurance
    Program

Key Personnel
  CEO. . . . . Elliot Cooperstone
    ecooperstone@prodigyhealthgroup.com
  EVP/CFO. . . . . Vincent DiMura, CPA
    vince.dimura@meritain.com
  Regional President . . . . Melissa Ellwood
    melissa.ellwood@meritain.com
  Regional President . . . . Stephen H Heck
    steve.heck@meritain.com
  Regional President. . . . . Margie Mann
    margie.degrace@meritain.com
  SVP, Cost Management . . . . Dale N Lyman
    dale.lyman@meritain.com
  Chief Medical Officer. Larry J Lutter, MD
    larry.lutter@meritain.com
  Regional President . . . . Chris Reef
    reefc@wellbornhealthplans.com
  SVP/CIO. . . . . Peter Fianu
    peter.fianu@meritain.com
  Regional President . . . . David Smith
    david.smith@meritain.com
  SVP, Sales. . . . . David C Parker
    dave.parker@mertain.com
  SVP, Corp Development . . . . Todd Squilanti
    todd.squilanti@meritain.com
  SVP, Underwriting. . . . . John T Sullivan
    john.sullivan@meritain.com

Average Claim Compensation
Physician's Fees Charged: 78%
Hospital's Fees Charged: 90%

Specialty Managed Care Partners
Express Scripts, LabOne, Interactive Health Solutions

---

788 MetroPlus Health Plan

160 Water Street
3rd Floor
New York, NY 10038
Toll-Free: 800-303-9626
Phone: 212-908-8600
Fax: 212-908-8601
www.metroplus.org
Subsidiary of: New York City Health Hospitals Corporation
Non-Profit Organization: Yes
Year Founded: 1985
Owned by an Integrated Delivery Network (IDN): Yes
Number of Affiliated Hospitals: 11
Number of Primary Care Physicians: 12,000
Total Enrollment: 332,128
State Enrollment: 332,128

Healthplan and Services Defined
  PLAN TYPE: HMO
  Model Type: Network
  Benefits Offered: Disease Management, Prescription, Wellness,
    Nurse management line, TeleHealth

Type of Coverage
  Medicaid, Child Health Plus, Family Health Pl

Geographic Areas Served
  Brooklyn, Bronx, Manhattan and Queens

Accreditation Certification
  TJC Accreditation

Key Personnel
  Chairman of the Board . . . . Bernard Rosen
  Executive Director . . . . Arnold Saperstein, MD
  Medical Affairs . . . . Van Dunn, MD
  CIO . . . . Michael Mattola
  Provider Services . . . . Joseph Dicks

Specialty Managed Care Partners
  Enters into Contracts with Regional Business Coalitions: Yes

---

789 MultiPlan, Inc.

115 Fifth Avenue
New York, NY 10003
Toll-Free: 800-677-1098
sales@multiplan.com
www.multiplan.com
For Profit Organization: Yes
Year Founded: 1980
Physician Owned Organization: No
Owned by an Integrated Delivery Network (IDN): No
Federally Qualified: No
Number of Affiliated Hospitals: 5,000
Number of Primary Care Physicians: 772,000
Number of Referral/Specialty Physicians: 772,000
Total Enrollment: 19,000,000

Healthplan and Services Defined
  PLAN TYPE: PPO
  Model Type: Network
  Plan Specialty: Primary PPO Network
  Offers Demand Management Patient Information Service: No

Geographic Areas Served
  Nationwide

Accreditation Certification
  URAC, NCQA

Key Personnel
  Chief Executive Officer . . . . Mark Tabak
  EVP, CFO . . . . David Redmond
    800-279-9776
  EVP, COO . . . . Michael Ferrante
    800-279-9776
  EVP, Chief Marketing Off . . . . Warren Handelman
    800-279-9776
  VP, Corporate Medical Dir . . . . Paul Goldstein, MD
    800-279-9776
  EVP, Sales & Acct Mgmt . . . . Dale White
    800-279-9776
  Dir, Marketing & Comm . . . . Pamela Walker
    800-253-4417
    pamela.walker@muliplan.com

---

790 MVP Health Care Medicare Plan

625 State Street
PO Box 2207
Schenectady, NY 12301-2207
Toll-Free: 800-777-4793
Phone: 518-370-4793
Fax: 518-370-0830
www.mvphealthcare.com
Non-Profit Organization: Yes

Healthplan and Services Defined
  PLAN TYPE: Medicare
  Benefits Offered: Chiropractic, Dental, Disease Management, Home
    Care, Inpatient SNF, Physical Therapy, Podiatry, Prescription,
    Psychiatric, Vision, Wellness

Type of Coverage
  Commercial, Individual, Medicare

Geographic Areas Served
  Available witin New York state only

Subscriber Information
  Average Monthly Fee Per Subscriber
    (Employee + Employer Contribution):
      Employee Only (Self): Varies
      Medicare: Varies
  Average Annual Deductible Per Subscriber:
      Employee Only (Self): Varies
      Medicare: Varies
  Average Subscriber Co-Payment:
      Primary Care Physician: Varies
      Non-Network Physician: Varies
      Prescription Drugs: Varies
      Hospital ER: Varies
      Home Health Care: Varies
      Home Health Care Max. Days/Visits Covered: Varies
      Nursing Home: Varies
      Nursing Home Max. Days/Visits Covered: Varies

Accreditation Certification
  NCQA

Key Personnel
  President/CEO . . . . David Oliker
  EVP/COO . . . . Chris Henchey
  EVP/Rochester Operations . . . . Lisa A Brubaker
  EVP/Network Management . . . . Mark Fish
  EVP/Planning . . . . Alfred Gatti
  EVP/Chief Legal Officer . . . . Denise Gonick, Esq
  EVP/Human Resources . . . . James Morrill

791 MVP Health Care: Buffalo Region

6255 Sheridan Drive
Buffalo, NY 14221
Phone: 716-839-1366
Fax: 716-839-1795
www.mvphealthcare.com
Non-Profit Organization: Yes
Total Enrollment: 750,000

Healthplan and Services Defined
PLAN TYPE: HMO/PPO

Type of Coverage
Commercial, Individual

Accreditation Certification
NCQA

Key Personnel
President/CEO . . . . David Oliker
EVP/COO . . . . Chris Henchey
EVP/Rochester Operations . . . . Lisa A Brubaker
EVP/Network Management . . . . Mark Fish
EVP/Planning. . . . . Alfred Gatti
EVP/Chief Legal Officer. . . . . Denise Gonick, Esq
EVP/Human Resources. . . . . James Morrill

792 MVP Health Care: Central New York

421 Broad Street
Utica, NY 13501
Toll-Free: 800-888-9635
Phone: 315-736-1625
Fax: 315-736-7002
www.mvphealthcare.com
Non-Profit Organization: Yes
Year Founded: 1983
Owned by an Integrated Delivery Network (IDN): Yes
Number of Affiliated Hospitals: 115
Number of Primary Care Physicians: 12,000
Number of Referral/Specialty Physicians: 7,371
Total Enrollment: 750,000

Healthplan and Services Defined
PLAN TYPE: HMO/PPO
Model Type: IPA
Plan Specialty: ASO
Benefits Offered: Behavioral Health, Chiropractic, Complementary
   Medicine, Dental, Disease Management, Home Care, Inpatient
   SNF, Physical Therapy, Podiatry, Prescription, Psychiatric,
   Transplant, Vision, Wellness, Worker's Compensation
DMPI Services Offered: After Hours Phone Line, Health Central
   (Library), Little Footprints Prenatal Program, Health Risk
   Assestments, Adult and Childhood Immunizations

Type of Coverage
Commercial, Individual, Indemnity, Self Funded, Administrative
   Service
Catastrophic Illness Benefit: Covered

Type of Payment Plans Offered
POS, DFFS, Capitated, FFS, Combination FFS & DFFS

Geographic Areas Served
In New York State: Albany, Broome, Cayuga, Chenango, Columbia,
   Cortland, Oswego, Delaware, Dutchess, Fulton, Greene, Hamilton,
   Herkimer, Lewis, Madison, Montgomery, Oneida, Onondaga,
   Orange, Ostego, Putnam, Rensselaer, Saratoga, Schenectady,
   Schoharie, Tioga, Ulster, Warren, Washington counties. In Vermont:
   Addison, Bennington, Caledonia, Chittenden, Essex, Franklin, Gran
   Isle, Lamoille, Orange, Rutland, Washington, Windham, Windsor

Subscriber Information
Average Monthly Fee Per Subscriber
   (Employee + Employer Contribution):
      Employee Only (Self): Varies by plan
      Employee & 2 Family Members: $0

Average Annual Deductible Per Subscriber:
   Employee Only (Self): $200
   Employee & 1 Family Member: $200
   Employee & 2 Family Members: $200 ind./500 family
Average Subscriber Co-Payment:
   Primary Care Physician: $20.00
   Non-Network Physician: $20.00
   Prescription Drugs: $5.00/10.00
   Hospital ER: $50.00
   Home Health Care Max. Days/Visits Covered: Unlimited
   Nursing Home Max. Days/Visits Covered: 45 days

Network Qualifications
Pre-Admission Certification: Yes

Peer Review Type
Utilization Review: Yes
Case Management: Yes

Publishes and Distributes Report Card: Yes

Accreditation Certification
NCQA
TJC Accreditation, Medicare Approved, Utilization Review,
   Pre-Admission Certification, State Licensure, Quality Assurance
   Program

Key Personnel
President/CEO . . . . Denise Gonick, Esq.
EVP, Commercial Business. David P. Crosby
EVP/Chief Medical Officer . . . . Allen J. Hinkle, MD
EVP, Networks/Contracting . . . . Karla A. Austen
EVP, Government Programs . . . . Patrick J. Glavey
VP/CIO. . . . . James H. Poole, III

Average Claim Compensation
Physician's Fees Charged: 75%
Hospital's Fees Charged: 65%

793 MVP Health Care: Corporate Office

625 State Street
PO Box 2207
Schenectady, NY 12301-2207
Toll-Free: 800-777-4793
Phone: 518-370-4793
Fax: 518-370-0830
www.mvphealthcare.com
Non-Profit Organization: Yes
Year Founded: 1983
Owned by an Integrated Delivery Network (IDN): Yes
Federally Qualified: Yes
Number of Affiliated Hospitals: 115
Number of Primary Care Physicians: 13,840
Number of Referral/Specialty Physicians: 7,371
Total Enrollment: 750,000

Healthplan and Services Defined
PLAN TYPE: HMO/PPO
Model Type: IPA
Plan Specialty: ASO
Benefits Offered: Behavioral Health, Chiropractic, Complementary
   Medicine, Dental, Disease Management, Home Care, Inpatient
   SNF, Physical Therapy, Podiatry, Prescription, Psychiatric,
   Transplant, Vision, Wellness, Worker's Compensation
DMPI Services Offered: After Hours Phone Line, Health Central
   (Library), Little Footprints Prenatal Program, Health Risk
   Assestments, Adult and Childhood Immunizations

Type of Coverage
Commercial, Individual, Indemnity, Self Funded, Administrative
   Service
Catastrophic Illness Benefit: Covered

Type of Payment Plans Offered
POS, DFFS, Capitated, FFS, Combination FFS & DFFS

Geographic Areas Served

In New York State: Albany, Cayuga, Cortland, Oswego, Columbia, Delaware, Dutchess, Fulton, Greene, Herkimer, Lewis, Madison, Montgomery, Oneida, Onondaga, Ostego, Putnam, Rensselaer, Rockland, Saratoga, Schenectady, Schoharie, Sullivan, Ulster, Warren, Westchwester counties. In Vermont: Addison, Bennington, Caledonia, Chittenden, Essex, Franklin, Gran Isle, Lamoille, Orange, Orleans, Rutland, Washington, Windham, Windsor counties

Subscriber Information

Average Monthly Fee Per Subscriber
 (Employee + Employer Contribution):
   Employee Only (Self): Varies by plan
   Employee & 2 Family Members: $0
Average Annual Deductible Per Subscriber:
   Employee Only (Self): $200
   Employee & 1 Family Member: $200
   Employee & 2 Family Members: $200 ind/500 family
Average Subscriber Co-Payment:
   Primary Care Physician: $20.00
   Non-Network Physician: $20.00
   Prescription Drugs: $5.00/10.00
   Hospital ER: $50.00
   Home Health Care Max. Days/Visits Covered: Unlimited
   Nursing Home Max. Days/Visits Covered: 45 days

Network Qualifications

Pre-Admission Certification: Yes

Peer Review Type

Utilization Review: Yes
Case Management: Yes

Publishes and Distributes Report Card: Yes

Accreditation Certification

NCQA
TJC Accreditation, Medicare Approved, Utilization Review, Pre-Admission Certification, State Licensure, Quality Assurance Program

Key Personnel

President/CEO . . . . Denise Gonick, Esq.
EVP, Networks/Contracting . . . . Karla A. Austen
EVP, Commercial Business. David P. Crosby
EVP, Government Programs. . . . . Patrick J. Glavey
EVP/Chief Medical Officer . . . . Allen J. Hinkle, MD
VP/CIO. . . . . James H. Poole, III

Average Claim Compensation

Physician's Fees Charged: 75%
Hospital's Fees Charged: 65%

794 MVP Health Care: Mid-State Region

120 Madison Street
AXA Tower 2, Suite 1000
Syracuse, NY 13202
Toll-Free: 800-568-3668
Phone: 315-436-3701
Fax: 315-426-3799
www.mvphealthcare.com
Non-Profit Organization: Yes
Total Enrollment: 750,000

Healthplan and Services Defined

PLAN TYPE: HMO/PPO

Type of Coverage

Commercial, Individual

Accreditation Certification

NCQA

Key Personnel

President/CEO . . . . David Oliker
EVP/COO . . . . Chris Henchey
EVP/Rochester Operations. . . . . Lisa A Brubaker
EVP/Network Management . . . . Mark Fish

EVP/Planning. . . . . Alfred Gatti
EVP/Chief Legal Officer. . . . . Denise Gonick, Esq
EVP/Human Resources. . . . . James Morrill

795 MVP Health Care: Western New York

325 State Street
Schenectady, NY 12305
Toll-Free: 800-777-4793
Fax: 518-386-7800
www.mvphealthcare.com
Non-Profit Organization: Yes
Year Founded: 1979
Owned by an Integrated Delivery Network (IDN): Yes
Federally Qualified: Yes
Number of Affiliated Hospitals: 20
Number of Primary Care Physicians: 1,091
Number of Referral/Specialty Physicians: 4,500
Total Enrollment: 750,000

Healthplan and Services Defined

PLAN TYPE: HMO/PPO
Model Type: IPA
Plan Specialty: ASO, Behavioral Health, Chiropractic, Disease Management, Vision
Benefits Offered: Behavioral Health, Chiropractic, Dental, Disease Management, Home Care, Inpatient SNF, Physical Therapy, Podiatry, Prescription, Psychiatric, Transplant, Vision, Wellness
Offers Demand Management Patient Information Service: Yes
DMPI Services Offered: Diabetes, CHF, Cancer

Type of Coverage

Commercial, Individual, Medicare, Medicaid
Catastrophic Illness Benefit: Covered

Type of Payment Plans Offered

POS, DFFS, Capitated, FFS

Geographic Areas Served

Genesee, Livingston, Monroe, Ontario, Orleans, Seneca, Wayne, Wyoming, & Yates counties

Subscriber Information

Average Monthly Fee Per Subscriber
 (Employee + Employer Contribution):
   Employee Only (Self): Varies by plan
Average Annual Deductible Per Subscriber:
   Employee Only (Self): $0
   Employee & 1 Family Member: $0
   Employee & 2 Family Members: $0
   Medicare: $0
Average Subscriber Co-Payment:
   Primary Care Physician: $5.00/10.00/15.00
   Non-Network Physician: Not covered
   Prescription Drugs: $10.00/20.00/35.00
   Hospital ER: $50.00-100.00
   Home Health Care: $10/day
   Home Health Care Max. Days/Visits Covered: Varies
   Nursing Home Max. Days/Visits Covered: 120/yr

Network Qualifications

Pre-Admission Certification: Yes

Peer Review Type

Utilization Review: Yes
Second Surgical Opinion: Yes
Case Management: Yes

Publishes and Distributes Report Card: Yes

Accreditation Certification

NCQA, HEDIS
TJC Accreditation

Key Personnel

President/CEO . . . . David Oliker
EVP/COO . . . . Chris Henchey
EVP/Rochester Operations. . . . . Lisa A Brubaker

EVP/Network Management . . . . Karla Austen
Chief Financial Officer . . . . Mark Fish
EVP/Planning . . . . Alfred Gatti
EVP/Chief Legal Officer . . . . Denise Gonick, Esq
Chief Medical Officer . . . . Dennis Allen
EVP/Human Resources . . . . James Morrill
Dir, Public Relations . . . . Gary Hughes
  800-777-4793
  hughesg@mvphealthcare.com

Average Claim Compensation
  Physician's Fees Charged: 1%

Specialty Managed Care Partners
  MH, LandMark

Employer References
  Eastman Kodak, Xerox, Federal Government, Monroe County
    Employees, New York State Employees

796 National Medical Health Card
2441 Warrenville Road
Suite 610
Lisle, NY 60532
Toll-Free: 800-282-3232
Phone: 630-577-3100
Fax: 630-577-3101
www.informedrx.com
Subsidiary of: Acquired by SXC Health Solutions Corp.
Acquired by: SXC Health Solutions
For Profit Organization: Yes
Year Founded: 1985
Total Enrollment: 1,850,000

Healthplan and Services Defined
  PLAN TYPE: Multiple
  Plan Specialty: PBM
  Benefits Offered: Prescription, MedIntelligence Products and
    Services.

Type of Coverage
  Commercial, Medicaid

Type of Payment Plans Offered
  FFS

Geographic Areas Served
  Nationwide

Network Qualifications
  Pre-Admission Certification: Yes

Peer Review Type
  Utilization Review: Yes
  Case Management: Yes

Publishes and Distributes Report Card: No

Key Personnel
  President/CEO . . . . James F Smith
  CFO . . . . Stuart F Fleischer
  Chief Marketing Officer . . . . Tery Baskin, PharmD
  Chief Clinical Officer . . . . Robert Kordella
  Chief Information Officer . . . . Bill Masters

Specialty Managed Care Partners
  Enters into Contracts with Regional Business Coalitions: No

797 Northeast Community Care
100 Elwood Davis Road
North Syracuse, NY 13212
Toll-Free: 866-395-4754
Phone: 315-461-4790
Fax: 315-461-4798
www.northeastcommunitycare.com
Subsidiary of: Arcadian Health Plans

Healthplan and Services Defined
  PLAN TYPE: Medicare

Type of Coverage
  Medicare

798 NOVA Healthcare Administrators
511 Farber Lakes Drive
Buffalo, NY 14221
Phone: 716-631-3001
Fax: 716-773-1276
sales@novahealthcare.com
www.novahealthcare.com
Subsidiary of: Acquired by Azeros Health Plans
For Profit Organization: Yes
Year Founded: 1982
Number of Affiliated Hospitals: 60
Number of Primary Care Physicians: 3,000
Total Enrollment: 80,000
State Enrollment: 100,000

Healthplan and Services Defined
  PLAN TYPE: Other
  Other Type: TPA
  Plan Specialty: ASO, Dental
  Benefits Offered: Dental, Disease Management, Prescription,
    Wellness

Type of Coverage
  Commercial, Indemnity

Geographic Areas Served
  Nationwide

Network Qualifications
  Pre-Admission Certification: Yes

Peer Review Type
  Utilization Review: Yes
  Second Surgical Opinion: Yes
  Case Management: Yes

Key Personnel
  President . . . . Larry Thompson
  Vice President . . . . Kristy Long

Specialty Managed Care Partners
  Express Scripts

799 Oxford Health Plans: New York
202 Canal Street
6th Floor
New York, NY 10013
Phone: 212-437-1200
Fax: 212-805-3020
www.oxhp.com
Subsidiary of: UnitedHealthCare
For Profit Organization: Yes
Number of Affiliated Hospitals: 218
Number of Primary Care Physicians: 50,000
Total Enrollment: 1,500,000

Healthplan and Services Defined
  PLAN TYPE: HMO
  Benefits Offered: Behavioral Health, Chiropractic, Disease
    Management, Inpatient SNF, Physical Therapy, Podiatry,
    Psychiatric

Type of Coverage
  Commercial, Medicare

Type of Payment Plans Offered
  POS

Geographic Areas Served
Sullivan, Ulster, Dutchess, Putman, Orange, Rockland, Westchester, Bergen, Bronx, Kings, Richmond, Queens, Nassau and Suffolk counties

Subscriber Information
Average Monthly Fee Per Subscriber
(Employee + Employer Contribution):
Employee Only (Self): Varies by plan

Peer Review Type
Case Management: Yes

Publishes and Distributes Report Card: Yes

Accreditation Certification
NCQA

Key Personnel
Chairman and CEO . . . . .Charles G Berg
Public Relations . . . . .Maria Gordon Shydlo
Executive VP/CFO. . . . . .Kurt B Thompson
VP Claims. . . . . .Micheal Santoro
Executive VP Sales/Marketing. . . . . .Kevin R Hill
Exec. VP/Chief Medical. . . . . .Alan M Muney, MD
Sr VP Chief Info Officer . . . . .Arthur L Gonzalez
VP Operations . . . . .Kevin Appleton
Sales . . . . .Kevin R Hill

800 Perfect Health Insurance Company

1200 South Ave
Staten Island, NY 10314
Toll-Free: 866-472-9447
Phone: 718-370-5380
Fax: 718-370-6098
www.perfectny.com
Subsidiary of: WellPoint
Acquired by: GHI
Year Founded: 1997
Number of Affiliated Hospitals: 200
Number of Primary Care Physicians: 60,000
Number of Referral/Specialty Physicians: 3,276
Total Enrollment: 9,000
State Enrollment: 3,000

Healthplan and Services Defined
PLAN TYPE: PPO
Model Type: Multi Plan Network
Plan Specialty: ASO, Behavioral Health, Chiropractic, Dental, Disease Management, Lab, MSO, PBM, Radiology, UR, Prescriptions
Benefits Offered: Prescription

Type of Coverage
Major Medical
Catastrophic Illness Benefit: Unlimited

Geographic Areas Served
Orange, Putnam, Queens, Richmond, Rockland, Suffolk, Westchester, Bronx, Kings, Nassau, New York counties; Fairfield, Connecticut; Sussex, Passiac, Bergen, Warren, Morris, Essex, Hunterdon, Union, Somerset, Middlesex, Mercer, Monmouth counties, in New Jersey

Subscriber Information
Average Monthly Fee Per Subscriber
(Employee + Employer Contribution):
Employee Only (Self): $155.03
Employee & 1 Family Member: $324.83
Employee & 2 Family Members: $457.71
Average Annual Deductible Per Subscriber:
Employee Only (Self): $10000
Employee & 2 Family Members: $20000
Average Subscriber Co-Payment:
Primary Care Physician: 20%
Non-Network Physician: 30%
Hospital ER: $25.00

Home Health Care: $0
Home Health Care Max. Days/Visits Covered: Unlimited
Nursing Home: $120.00 in network

Network Qualifications
Pre-Admission Certification: Yes

Peer Review Type
Utilization Review: Yes
Second Surgical Opinion: Yes
Case Management: Yes

Publishes and Distributes Report Card: No

Accreditation Certification
State Of Ny
TJC Accreditation, Medicare Approved, Utilization Review, Pre-Admission Certification, State Licensure, Quality Assurance Program

Key Personnel
President . . . . .DeWitt Smith
646-447-6980
dsmith@emblemhealth.com
Chief Administrative Off . . . . .Linda Farren
646-447-4466
lfarren@emblemhealth.com
Director/HSA Services .Antoinette Lapetina
646-447-4467
alapetina@perfectny.com
Vice President/Regulatory . . . . .Adeline Gallagher
646-447-4496
agallagher@emblemhealth.com
Director, HSA Sales/Mktg .Arthur DiMarco

Average Claim Compensation
Physician's Fees Charged: 60%
Hospital's Fees Charged: 60%

Specialty Managed Care Partners
Multi Plans, GHI Hospitals, Health Advocate, Express Scripts, First HAS
Enters into Contracts with Regional Business Coalitions: No

801 Quality Health Plans

2805 Veterans Memorial Highway
Suite 17
Ronkonkoma, NY 11779
Toll-Free: 877-233-7058
Phone: 727-945-8400
Fax: 877-817-1008
www.qualityhealthplans.com
Year Founded: 2003
Physician Owned Organization: Yes
Total Enrollment: 19,000

Healthplan and Services Defined
PLAN TYPE: Medicare

Type of Coverage
Supplemental Medicare

Geographic Areas Served
13 counties in Florida

Key Personnel
President . . . . .Haider A Khan, MD
Chief Financial Officer .Stacy L. Martin, MD
Medical Director . . . . .Michael Yanuck, MBA
Medical Director . . . . .Richard Bonanna, MS MMM
Reg Mgr, Network Services . . . . .Dawn R Smith
Director, Finance . . . . .David A Sherwin
Corp Services Manager . . . . .Farrah Sanabria, PHR
Director, Medical Affairs . . . . .Lisa Cierpka, RN
Dir, Business Development . . . . .Amber R Clements
Dir, Compliance. . . . . .Angela Hart
Medical Director. . . . . .Michael Yanuck, MD
Medical Director. . . . . .Richard Bonanno, MD

Media Contact . . . . Mike Worley
866-747-2700
mworley@qualityhealthplans.comm

---

802   Quality Health Plans of New York

2805 Veterans Memorial Highway
Suite 17
Ronkonkoma, NY 11779
Toll-Free: 877-233-7058
compliancemail@qualityhealthplansny.com
www.qualityhealthplans.com
Year Founded: 2003
Physician Owned Organization: Yes
Total Enrollment: 19,000

Healthplan and Services Defined
   PLAN TYPE: Medicare

Type of Coverage
   Supplemental Medicare

Geographic Areas Served
   13 counties in Florida

Key Personnel
President . . . . Haider A Khan, MD
CEO & CMO . . . . Nazeer H Khan, MD
COO . . . . Sabiha Khan, MBA
Medical Director . . . . Trevor A Rose, MD, MS MMM
Reg Mgr, Network Services . . . . Dawn R Smith
Director, Finance . . . . David A Sherwin
Corp Services Manager . . . . Farrah Sanabria, PHR
Director, Medical Affairs . . . . Lisa Cierpka, RN
Dir, Business Development . . . . Amber R Clements
Dir, Compliance. . . . . Angela Hart
Medical Director. . . . . Michael Yanuck, MD
Medical Director. . . . . Richard Bonanno, MD
Media Contact . . . . Mike Worley
866-747-2700
mworley@qualityhealthplans.comm

---

803   Touchstone Health HMO

Church Street Station
PO Box 1265
White Plains, NY 10602
Toll-Free: 877-805-3629
information@touchstoneh.com
www.touchstoneh.com
Year Founded: 1980
Total Enrollment: 11,000

Healthplan and Services Defined
   PLAN TYPE: Medicare
   Benefits Offered: Chiropractic, Dental, Disease Management, Home
     Care, Inpatient SNF, Physical Therapy, Podiatry, Prescription,
     Psychiatric, Vision, Wellness

Type of Coverage
   Individual, Medicare, Supplemental Medicare

Geographic Areas Served
   New York state only

Subscriber Information
   Average Monthly Fee Per Subscriber
     (Employee + Employer Contribution):
       Employee Only (Self): Varies
       Medicare: Varies
   Average Annual Deductible Per Subscriber:
       Employee Only (Self): Varies
       Medicare: Varies
   Average Subscriber Co-Payment:
       Primary Care Physician: Varies
       Non-Network Physician: Varies
       Prescription Drugs: Varies

Hospital ER: Varies
Home Health Care: Varies
Home Health Care Max. Days/Visits Covered: Varies
Nursing Home: Varies
Nursing Home Max. Days/Visits Covered: Varies

Key Personnel
Chief Operating Officer . . . . Vicki Cleary
Chief Compliance Officer . . . . Lisa Mingione
Chief Executive Officer . . . . Edward C Fargis
Chief Medical Officer . . . . Mitchell Strand, MD
Chief Information Officer . . . . Michael Richmond
Chief Marketing Officer . . . . Steven V Calabrese
Chief Medical Officer . . . . Roger London, MD

---

804   United Concordia: New York

4401 Deer Path Road
Harrisbury, NY 17110
Toll-Free: 800-235-6753
Phone: 717-260-6800
Fax: 212-921-0539
nysales@ucci.com
www.secure.ucci.com
Secondary Address: 159 Express Street, Plainview, NY 11803,
   516-827-6720
For Profit Organization: Yes
Year Founded: 1971
Number of Primary Care Physicians: 111,000
Total Enrollment: 8,000,000

Healthplan and Services Defined
   PLAN TYPE: Dental
   Plan Specialty: Dental
   Benefits Offered: Dental

Type of Coverage
   Commercial, Individual

Geographic Areas Served
   Military personnel and their families, nationwide

---

805   UnitedHealthCare of New York

1 Pensylvannia Plaza
New York, NY 10119
Toll-Free: 800-339-5380
Phone: 212-216-6400
www.uhc.com
Secondary Address: 2 Penn Plaza, 7th Floor, New York, NY 10121,
   212-216-6400
Subsidiary of: UnitedHealth Group
For Profit Organization: Yes
Year Founded: 1987
Federally Qualified: Yes
Number of Affiliated Hospitals: 170
Number of Primary Care Physicians: 8,500
Number of Referral/Specialty Physicians: 2,225
Total Enrollment: 75,000,000
State Enrollment: 222,000

Healthplan and Services Defined
   PLAN TYPE: HMO/PPO
   Model Type: IPA
   Benefits Offered: Disease Management, Prescription, Wellness
   Offers Demand Management Patient Information Service: Yes

Type of Payment Plans Offered
   DFFS, Capitated

Geographic Areas Served
   New York, New Jersey & Fairfield County, Connecticut

Network Qualifications
   Pre-Admission Certification: Yes

Peer Review Type
Utilization Review: Yes
Second Surgical Opinion: Yes
Case Management: Yes

Publishes and Distributes Report Card: Yes

Accreditation Certification
TJC Accreditation, Medicare Approved, Utilization Review, Pre-Admission Certification, State Licensure, Quality Assurance Program

Key Personnel
President..................................Sharon Seitzman
CFO......................................Dan Gollman
In House Formulary.......................Ann Marie O'Brien
Marketing.................................Barbara Willis
Medical Affairs...........................Lillian Grillo
Member Services..........................Timothy Stover
Provider Services........................William Lamoreux
Sales....................................Gregory Choy
Media Contact...........................Mary McElrath-Jones
914-467-2039
mary_r_mcelrath-jones@uhc.com

Specialty Managed Care Partners
Enters into Contracts with Regional Business Coalitions: Yes

806 Univera Healthcare
205 Park Club Lane
Buffalo, NY 14221
Toll-Free: 800-427-8490
www.univerahealthcare.com
Mailing Address: PO Box 23000, Rochester, NY 14692
Subsidiary of: The Lifetime Healthcare Companies
Non-Profit Organization: Yes
Number of Affiliated Hospitals: 35
Number of Primary Care Physicians: 5,700
Total Enrollment: 1,700,000
State Enrollment: 1,700,000

Healthplan and Services Defined
PLAN TYPE: HMO
Model Type: Network
Plan Specialty: ASO, Behavioral Health, Chiropractic, Dental, Disease Management, EPO, Lab, MSO, PBM, Vision, Radiology, Worker's Compensation, UR
Benefits Offered: Behavioral Health, Chiropractic, Complementary Medicine, Dental, Disease Management, Home Care, Inpatient SNF, Long-Term Care, Physical Therapy, Podiatry, Prescription, Psychiatric, Transplant, Vision, Wellness, Worker's Compensation, Life

Type of Coverage
Commercial, Individual, Medicare

Geographic Areas Served
Allegany, Cattaraugus, Chautauqua, Erie, Genesee, Niagara, Orleans and Wyoming counties

Subscriber Information
Average Monthly Fee Per Subscriber
(Employee + Employer Contribution):
Employee Only (Self): Varies by plan
Average Subscriber Co-Payment:
Primary Care Physician: Varies
Prescription Drugs: Varies

Publishes and Distributes Report Card: Yes

Accreditation Certification
NCQA

Key Personnel
President..................................Arthur Wingerter
Chief Executive Officer......................David H Klein
Chief Financial Officer.....................Emil D Duda
VP Network Contracting..................Lisa Meyers-Alessi

VP, Chief Medical Officer...................Robert Holzhauer
Regional Medical Officer..................Richard Vienne, DO
VP, Sales................................Pamela J Pawenski
VP, Communications.........................Peter B Kates
716-857-4495
peter.kates@univerahealthcare.com

807 Universal American Medicare Plans
44 South Boradway
Suite 1200
White Plains, NY 10601-4411
Phone: 914-934-5200
Fax: 914-934-0700
www.universalamerican.com
Total Enrollment: 2,000,000

Healthplan and Services Defined
PLAN TYPE: Medicare
Benefits Offered: Prescription

Type of Coverage
Individual, Medicare

Geographic Areas Served
Available in multiple states

Subscriber Information
Average Monthly Fee Per Subscriber
(Employee + Employer Contribution):
Employee Only (Self): Varies
Medicare: Varies
Average Annual Deductible Per Subscriber:
Employee Only (Self): Varies
Medicare: Varies
Average Subscriber Co-Payment:
Primary Care Physician: Varies
Non-Network Physician: Varies
Prescription Drugs: Varies
Hospital ER: Varies

Key Personnel
Chairman & CEO.........................Richard A Barasch
EVP, Chief Financial Offc.............Robert A Waegelein, CPA
SVP, Corporate Developmnt....................Gary M Jacobs
Chief Operating Officer.......................Jason J Israel
Pres, Medicare Advantage.............Theodore M Carpenter, Jr
Pres, Medicare Part D...........................John Wardle
SVP, Health Quality..........................Robert M Hayes

808 Vytra Health Plans
395 N Service Road
PO Box 9091
Melville, NY 11747-9091
Toll-Free: 800-406-0806
Phone: 631-694-4000
Fax: 631-719-0911
memberservices@vytra.com
www.vytra.com
Subsidiary of: HIP Health Plan
Non-Profit Organization: Yes
Year Founded: 1985
Number of Affiliated Hospitals: 38
Number of Primary Care Physicians: 1,500
Number of Referral/Specialty Physicians: 10,000
Total Enrollment: 200,000
State Enrollment: 76,213

Healthplan and Services Defined
PLAN TYPE: HMO/PPO
Other Type: POS
Model Type: IPA
Plan Specialty: ASO, Chiropractic, Dental, Disease Management, EPO, Vision, Radiology

Benefits Offered: Behavioral Health, Chiropractic, Complementary
   Medicine, Dental, Disease Management, Home Care, Inpatient
   SNF, Physical Therapy, Podiatry, Prescription, Psychiatric,
   Transplant, Vision, Wellness

Type of Payment Plans Offered
   Capitated

Geographic Areas Served
   Nassau, Queens, Suffolk counties and Long Island

Subscriber Information
   Average Monthly Fee Per Subscriber
      (Employee + Employer Contribution):
         Employee Only (Self): Varies by plan
   Average Subscriber Co-Payment:
         Primary Care Physician: $10.00
         Non-Network Physician: 25%
         Prescription Drugs: $5.00
         Hospital ER: $25.00
         Nursing Home: $0.00
         Nursing Home Max. Days/Visits Covered: 45 days

Accreditation Certification
   URAC, NCQA
   TJC Accreditation, Medicare Approved, Utilization Review,
      Pre-Admission Certification, State Licensure, Quality Assurance
      Program

Key Personnel
   President/CEO . . . . Tom McAteer, Jr
   COO . . . . Michael G Murphy
   CFO. . . . . Roy Goldman
   Marketing . . . . William A Bennett
   Chief Medical Officer . . . . Jerry Royer, MD, MBA
   Human Resources . . . . Donna McDaniel
   Information Services. . . . . Garth Womack
   SVP, Public Affairs . . . . Ilene Margolin
      646-447-0098
      imargolin@emblemhealth.com

Specialty Managed Care Partners
   Health Care, Multi Plan

Health Insurance Coverage Status and Type of Coverage by Age

Category	All Persons		Under 18 years		Under 65 years		65 years and over	
	Number	%	Number	%	Number	%	Number	%
Total population	9,645	-	2,281	-	8,281	-	1,365	-
Covered by some type of health insurance	8,136 *(26)*	84.4 *(0.3)*	2,136 *(10)*	93.7 *(0.4)*	6,780 *(26)*	81.9 *(0.3)*	1,357 *(4)*	99.4 *(0.1)*
Covered by private health insurance	6,104 *(36)*	63.3 *(0.4)*	1,229 *(18)*	53.9 *(0.8)*	5,235 *(34)*	63.2 *(0.4)*	869 *(11)*	63.7 *(0.8)*
Employment based	4,786 *(34)*	49.6 *(0.4)*	983 *(17)*	43.1 *(0.8)*	4,327 *(32)*	52.3 *(0.4)*	459 *(9)*	33.6 *(0.7)*
Direct purchase	1,300 *(23)*	13.5 *(0.2)*	174 *(8)*	7.6 *(0.4)*	834 *(19)*	10.1 *(0.2)*	467 *(11)*	34.2 *(0.8)*
Covered by TRICARE	422 *(12)*	4.4 *(0.1)*	109 *(6)*	4.8 *(0.3)*	307 *(11)*	3.7 *(0.1)*	115 *(5)*	8.4 *(0.4)*
Covered by government health insurance	3,153 *(25)*	32.7 *(0.3)*	974 *(19)*	42.7 *(0.8)*	1,819 *(25)*	22.0 *(0.3)*	1,334 *(5)*	97.7 *(0.2)*
Covered by Medicaid	1,729 *(28)*	17.9 *(0.3)*	966 *(20)*	42.4 *(0.8)*	1,554 *(27)*	18.8 *(0.3)*	175 *(6)*	12.8 *(0.5)*
Also by private insurance	217 *(10)*	2.3 *(0.1)*	65 *(6)*	2.9 *(0.3)*	148 *(9)*	1.8 *(0.1)*	69 *(4)*	5.1 *(0.3)*
Covered by Medicare	1,619 *(10)*	16.8 *(0.1)*	11 *(2)*	0.5 *(0.1)*	286 *(9)*	3.5 *(0.1)*	1,333 *(5)*	97.7 *(0.2)*
Also by private insurance	929 *(12)*	9.6 *(0.1)*	1 *(1)*	0.1 *(0.1)*	84 *(5)*	1.0 *(0.1)*	845 *(11)*	61.9 *(0.8)*
Also by Medicaid	300 *(8)*	3.1 *(0.1)*	5 *(2)*	0.2 *(0.1)*	126 *(6)*	1.5 *(0.1)*	175 *(6)*	12.8 *(0.5)*
Covered by VA Care	253 *(9)*	2.6 *(0.1)*	3 *(1)*	0.1 *(0.1)*	129 *(7)*	1.6 *(0.1)*	124 *(5)*	9.1 *(0.3)*
Not covered at any time during the year	1,509 *(26)*	15.6 *(0.3)*	144 *(9)*	6.3 *(0.4)*	1,501 *(26)*	18.1 *(0.3)*	8 *(2)*	0.6 *(0.1)*

Note: Numbers in thousands; Figures cover 2013; Margin of error appears in parenthesis; A "Z" indicates that the value either represents or rounds to zero.
Source: U.S. Census Bureau, 2013 American Community Survey, Table HI05. Health Insurance Coverage Status and Type of Coverage by State and Age for All People: 2013

North Carolina

809 Aetna Health of the Carolinas

11675 Great Oaks Way
Suite 330
Alpharetta, GA 30022
Toll-Free: 866-582-9629
www.aetna.com
For Profit Organization: Yes
Year Founded: 1995
Total Enrollment: 18,960

Healthplan and Services Defined
 PLAN TYPE: HMO
 Other Type: POS
 Benefits Offered: Prescription

Type of Coverage
 Commercial, Individual

Type of Payment Plans Offered
 POS, DFFS, FFS

Geographic Areas Served
 Statewide

Peer Review Type
 Case Management: Yes

Accreditation Certification
 NCQA

Key Personnel
 President/CEO . . . . .William H Donaldson
 General Manager . . . . .Rick Kelly
 Sales. . . . . .Brian O'Shields

Employer References
 NC Baptist Hospital

810 Assurant Employee Benefits: North Carolina

7621 Little Avenue
Suite 400
Charlotte, NC 28226
Phone: 704-553-7609
Fax: 704-553-7821
benefits@assurant.com
www.assurantemployeebenefits.com
Subsidiary of: Assurant, Inc
For Profit Organization: Yes
Number of Primary Care Physicians: 112,000
Total Enrollment: 47,000

Healthplan and Services Defined
 PLAN TYPE: Multiple
 Plan Specialty: Dental, Vision, Long & Short-Term Disability
 Benefits Offered: Dental, Vision, Wellness, AD&D, Life, LTD, STD

Type of Coverage
 Commercial, Indemnity, Individual Dental Plans

Geographic Areas Served
 Statewide

Subscriber Information
 Average Monthly Fee Per Subscriber
  (Employee + Employer Contribution):
   Employee Only (Self): Varies by plan

Key Personnel
 President & CEO . . . . .Robert B. Pollock
 EVP/Chief Financial Offic . . . . .Michael J. Peninger
 EVP/Treasurer . . . . .Christopher J. Pagano
 PR Specialist. . . . . .Megan Hutchison
  816-556-7815
  megan.hutchison@assurant.com

811 Blue Cross & Blue Shield of North Carolina

5901 Chapel Hill Road
Durham, NC 27707
Toll-Free: 800-324-4973
Phone: 919-765-7347
Fax: 919-765-7288
www.bcbsnc.com
Mailing Address: PO Box 2291, Durham, NC 27702-2291
Non-Profit Organization: Yes
Year Founded: 1933
Number of Affiliated Hospitals: 113
Number of Primary Care Physicians: 5,200
Number of Referral/Specialty Physicians: 20,000
Total Enrollment: 3,718,355
State Enrollment: 3,718,355

Healthplan and Services Defined
 PLAN TYPE: HMO/PPO
 Model Type: Network
 Plan Specialty: ASO, Behavioral Health, Chiropractic, Dental,
  Disease Management, Lab, PBM, Vision, Radiology, UR
 Benefits Offered: Behavioral Health, Chiropractic, Complementary
  Medicine, Dental, Disease Management, Home Care, Inpatient
  SNF, Long-Term Care, Physical Therapy, Podiatry, Prescription,
  Psychiatric, Transplant, Vision, Wellness, AD&D, Life, LTD, STD
 Offers Demand Management Patient Information Service: Yes
 DMPI Services Offered: Health Line Blue Nurseline, VitaBlue, Optic
  Blue, Atl Med Blue, Active Blue Magazine

Type of Coverage
 Commercial, Individual, Supplemental Medicare

Type of Payment Plans Offered
 POS, DFFS, FFS, Combination FFS & DFFS

Geographic Areas Served
 Blue Cross and Blue Shield of North Carolina is licensed to do
 business in all 100 counties in North Carolina

Subscriber Information
 Average Monthly Fee Per Subscriber
  (Employee + Employer Contribution):
   Employee Only (Self): Varies by plan
 Average Annual Deductible Per Subscriber:
   Employee Only (Self): $250.00
   Employee & 1 Family Member: $500.00
   Employee & 2 Family Members: $500.00
 Average Subscriber Co-Payment:
   Primary Care Physician: $15.00
   Prescription Drugs: $10.00/20.00/30.00
   Hospital ER: $100.00
   Home Health Care: 10%
   Home Health Care Max. Days/Visits Covered: 20 days
   Nursing Home: 10%
   Nursing Home Max. Days/Visits Covered: 60 days

Network Qualifications
 Pre-Admission Certification: Yes

Peer Review Type
 Utilization Review: Yes
 Second Surgical Opinion: Yes
 Case Management: Yes

Accreditation Certification
 NCQA
 State Licensure

Key Personnel
 President & CEO. . . . . .J Bradley Wilson
 Chief Financial Officer. . . . . .Gerald Petkau
 EVP/General Counsel .Maureen K O'Connor
 SVP/Chief Info Officer . . . . .Alan Hughes
 SVP/Human Resources Offc . . . . .Fara M Palumbo
 Sr VP Sales/Marketing . . . . .John T Roos
  john.roos@bcbsnc.com
 SVP/Chief Medical Officer . . . . .Don W Bradley, MD

Average Claim Compensation
Physician's Fees Charged: 43%
Hospital's Fees Charged: 35%

Specialty Managed Care Partners
Magellan Behavioral Health (MH), Health Dialog (24-hour nurseline), Merck-Medco (pharmacy), Ceridian Benefits Services (COBRA), Chiropractic Network of the Carolinas, OptiCare Eye Health Network (vision)

812 Catalyst RX

4020 Wake Forest Road
Suite 102
Raleigh, NC 27609
Toll-Free: 800-323-6640
Phone: 301-548-2900
rxcsinfo@catalystrx.com
www.catalystrx.com
Subsidiary of: Catalyst Health Solutions
For Profit Organization: Yes
Year Founded: 1994
Total Enrollment: 5,000,000
State Enrollment: 325,000

Healthplan and Services Defined
PLAN TYPE: PPO
Model Type: Network
Plan Specialty: PBM
Benefits Offered: Prescription

Geographic Areas Served
Nationwide

Subscriber Information
Average Subscriber Co-Payment:
Prescription Drugs: $12.00

Accreditation Certification
Utilization Review, State Licensure

Key Personnel
Chief Executive Officer . . . . .David T Blair
301-548-2901
President & COO . . . . .Richard Bates
Treasurer & CFO. . . . . .Hai Tran
htran@chsi.com
General Counsel . . . . .Bruce Metge
Mgr, Sales Administration .Ronelle Rondon
301-548-2900
media@catalysthealthsolutions.com

Employer References
Progress Energy, BB&T, SC Local Government Assurance Group, General Shale, Hickory Springs Manufacturing

813 CIGNA HealthCare of North Carolina

11016 Rushmore Drive
Suite 300
Charlotte, NC 28277
Toll-Free: 800-888-4973
Phone: 704-586-0708
Fax: 704-586-7181
www.cigna.com
Secondary Address: 701 Corporate Center Drive, Raleigh, NC 27607, 919-854-7000
For Profit Organization: Yes
Year Founded: 1992
Number of Primary Care Physicians: 20,100
Number of Referral/Specialty Physicians: 9,000
Total Enrollment: 29,583
State Enrollment: 29,583

Healthplan and Services Defined
PLAN TYPE: HMO

Other Type: POS
Model Type: IPA, Network
Benefits Offered: Behavioral Health, Chiropractic, Complementary Medicine, Dental, Disease Management, Home Care, Physical Therapy, Podiatry, Prescription, Psychiatric, Transplant, Vision, Wellness
DMPI Services Offered: 24 hour Health Information Line, Health Information Library, Automated ReferralLine

Type of Coverage
Commercial

Type of Payment Plans Offered
POS

Geographic Areas Served
Buncombe, Cabarrus, Caldwell, Catawba, Cleveland, Gaston, Henderson, Lincoln, Mecklenburg, Rowan, Stanly and Union counties

Subscriber Information
Average Monthly Fee Per Subscriber
(Employee + Employer Contribution):
Employee Only (Self): Varies by plan

Network Qualifications
Pre-Admission Certification: Yes

Peer Review Type
Utilization Review: Yes
Second Surgical Opinion: Yes
Case Management: Yes

Publishes and Distributes Report Card: Yes

Accreditation Certification
NCQA

Key Personnel
President . . . . .David M Cordani
EVP/Chief Info Officer . . . . .Mark Boxer
Communications Officer .Maggie Fitzpatrick
President/Healthspring . . . . .Herb Fritch
Sr VP/Chief Underwriting . . . . .Jonathan Rubin
Executive VP/Operations . . . . .Scott A Storrer
President, Southeast Reg. . . . . .Michael W Triplett, Sr
President, Small Bus Seg. . . . . .Dennis Wilson
President, Group Ins . . . . .Gregory Wolf
Sr VP/Sales . . . . .Gary Kirkner
Sr VP/Marketing . . . . .Jay Menario
Chief Financial Officer . . . . .Peter J Vogt

814 CoreSource: North Carolina

5200 Seventy-Seven Center Drive
Suite 400
Charlotte, NC 28217
Toll-Free: 800-327-5462
Phone: 704-554-44400
www.coresource.com
Subsidiary of: Trustmark
Year Founded: 1980
Total Enrollment: 1,100,000

Healthplan and Services Defined
PLAN TYPE: Multiple
Other Type: TPA
Model Type: Network
Plan Specialty: Claims Administration, TPA
Benefits Offered: Behavioral Health, Home Care, Prescription, Transplant

Type of Coverage
Commercial

Geographic Areas Served
Nationwide

Accreditation Certification
Utilization Review, Pre-Admission Certification

Key Personnel

President	Nancy Eckrich
COO	Lloyd Sarrel
VP/Planning	Rob Corrigan
CFO	Clare Smith
VP/Healthcare Mgmt	Donna Heiser
VP/Product Development	Steve Horvath

815 Crescent Health Solutions

1200 Ridgefield Boulevard
Suite 215
Asheville, NC 28806
Phone: 828-670-9145
Fax: 828-670-9155
www.crescenths.com
Non-Profit Organization: Yes
Year Founded: 1999
Physician Owned Organization: Yes
Number of Affiliated Hospitals: 15
Number of Primary Care Physicians: 1,900
Number of Referral/Specialty Physicians: 2,400
Total Enrollment: 40,000
State Enrollment: 40,000

Healthplan and Services Defined
PLAN TYPE: PPO
Benefits Offered: Disease Management, Prescription, Wellness, Case Management, UR, TPA Services

Type of Coverage
Commercial, Individual

Geographic Areas Served
16 counties in Western North Carolina

Peer Review Type
Utilization Review: Yes
Case Management: Yes

Key Personnel

CEO	Myrna Harris
COO	Jennifer Moore
CFO	Tara Pressley
Director, Business Dev.	Desiree Greene
Chief Medical Officer	J. Paul Martin, MD
Dir., Provider Relations	Deana Gardner

816 Delta Dental of North Carolina

4208 Six Forks Road
Suite 912
Raleigh, NC 27609
Toll-Free: 800-662-8856
www.deltadentalnc.org
Mailing Address: PO Box 9085, Farmington Hills, MI 48333-9085
Non-Profit Organization: Yes
Number of Primary Care Physicians: 198,000
Total Enrollment: 54,000,000

Healthplan and Services Defined
PLAN TYPE: Dental
Other Type: Dental PPO
Plan Specialty: Dental
Benefits Offered: Dental

Type of Coverage
Commercial

Type of Payment Plans Offered
POS, DFFS, FFS

Geographic Areas Served
Statewide

Key Personnel

President & CEO	Curtis Ladig

Dir/Media & Public Affair .... Elizabeth Risberg
415-972-8423

817 eHealthInsurance Services Inc.

11919 Foundation Place
Gold River, CA 95670
Toll-Free: 800-644-3491
webmaster@healthinsurance.com
www.e.healthinsurance.com
Year Founded: 1997

Healthplan and Services Defined
PLAN TYPE: HMO/PPO
Benefits Offered: Dental, Life, STD

Type of Coverage
Commercial, Individual, Medicare

Geographic Areas Served
All 50 states in the USA and District of Columbia

Key Personnel

Chairman & CEO	Gary L. Lauer
EVP/Business & Corp. Dev.	Bruce Telkamp
EVP/Chief Technology	Dr. Sheldon X. Wang
SVP & CFO	Stuart M. Huizinga
Pres. of eHealth Gov. Sys	Samuel C. Gibbs
SVP of Sales & Operations	Robert S. Hurley
Director Public Relations	Nate Purpura
650-210-3115	

818 FirstCarolinaCare

42 Memorial Drive
Pinehurst, NC 28374
Toll-Free: 800-811-3298
www.firstcarolinacare.com
Subsidiary of: FirstHealth of the Carolinas
Total Enrollment: 13,000
State Enrollment: 13,000

Healthplan and Services Defined
PLAN TYPE: HMO
Offers Demand Management Patient Information Service: Yes
DMPI Services Offered: Nurse Helpline

Key Personnel

President	Kenneth Lewis
Executive Director	Charles Frock
Corporate Communications	Emily Sloan
910-715-5376	

819 Great-West Healthcare North Carolina

6100 Fairview Road
Suite 650
Charlotte, NC 28210
Toll-Free: 888-663-3188
Phone: 704-556-9033
eliginquiries@cigna.com
www.cignaforhealth.com
Secondary Address: 620 Green Valley Road, Suite 101, Greensboro, NC 27408
Subsidiary of: CIGNA HealthCare
Acquired by: CIGNA
For Profit Organization: Yes
Total Enrollment: 56,422
State Enrollment: 53,379

Healthplan and Services Defined
PLAN TYPE: HMO/PPO
Benefits Offered: Disease Management, Prescription, Wellness

Type of Coverage
Commercial

Type of Payment Plans Offered
POS, FFS

Geographic Areas Served
North Carolina

Accreditation Certification
URAC

Specialty Managed Care Partners
Caremark Rx

820 Humana Health Insurance of North Carolina

2000 Regency Parkway
Suite 470
Cary, NC 27518
Toll-Free: 866-653-7295
Phone: 919-465-1367
Fax: 919-468-8556
www.humana.com
For Profit Organization: Yes
Total Enrollment: 494,200
State Enrollment: 17,400

Healthplan and Services Defined
PLAN TYPE: HMO/PPO
Plan Specialty: ASO
Benefits Offered: Disease Management, Prescription, Wellness

Type of Coverage
Commercial, Individual

Geographic Areas Served
North Carolina, South Carolina, Virginia

Accreditation Certification
URAC, NCQA, CORE

Key Personnel
President . . . . Alan Guzzino

Specialty Managed Care Partners
Caremark Rx

Employer References
Tricare

821 MedCost

165 Kimel Park Drive
Winston Salem, NC 27103
Toll-Free: 800-433-9178
www.medcost.com
Subsidiary of: Carolinas HealthCare System
For Profit Organization: Yes
Year Founded: 1983
Number of Affiliated Hospitals: 191
Number of Primary Care Physicians: 12,349
Number of Referral/Specialty Physicians: 21,295
Total Enrollment: 670,000
State Enrollment: 670,000

Healthplan and Services Defined
PLAN TYPE: PPO
Model Type: Network
Plan Specialty: UR, PPO Network, Maternity Management, Case
Management, Nurse Coaching
Benefits Offered: Home Care, Inpatient SNF, Long-Term Care,
Physical Therapy, Podiatry, Psychiatric, Transplant, Vision,
Wellness, Medical, Hospice, Durable Medical Equipment

Type of Coverage
Commercial

Type of Payment Plans Offered
FFS

Geographic Areas Served
North Carolina and South Carolina

Subscriber Information
Average Subscriber Co-Payment:
Primary Care Physician: Varies
Non-Network Physician: Varies
Prescription Drugs: Varies
Hospital ER: Varies
Home Health Care: Varies
Home Health Care Max. Days/Visits Covered: Varies
Nursing Home: Varies
Nursing Home Max. Days/Visits Covered: Varies

Peer Review Type
Utilization Review: Yes
Second Surgical Opinion: Yes
Case Management: Yes

Publishes and Distributes Report Card: Yes

Accreditation Certification
URAC

822 Mid Atlantic Medical Services: North Carolina

The Atrium at 77 South
4421 Stuart Andrews Blvd, Suite 600
Charlotte, NC 28217
Toll-Free: 800-469-8471
Phone: 704-529-1211
Fax: 704-529-6078
www.mamsiunitedhealthcare.com
Secondary Address: 627 Davis Drive, Suite 100, Morrisville, NC
27560
Subsidiary of: UnitedHealthCare/UnitedHealth Group
Federally Qualified: Yes
Number of Affiliated Hospitals: 342
Number of Primary Care Physicians: 3,276
Total Enrollment: 180,000

Healthplan and Services Defined
PLAN TYPE: HMO/PPO
Benefits Offered: Behavioral Health, Dental, Disease Management,
Home Care, Prescription, Psychiatric, Vision, Wellness, AD&D,
Life, STD, Hospice, discounts on value-added services such as laser
vision correction, acupuncture, chiropractic services, massage

Accreditation Certification
NCQA

Key Personnel
President/CEO . . . . Thomas P Barbera

Specialty Managed Care Partners
HomeCall, FirstCall, HomeCall Pharmaceutical Services, HomeCall
Hospice Services

823 OptiCare Managed Vision

112 Zebulon Court
Rocky Mount, NC 27804
Toll-Free: 800-334-3937
Fax: 877-940-9243
www.opticare.com
Secondary Address: 3120 Highwoods Boulevard, Raleigh, NC 27604
For Profit Organization: Yes
Year Founded: 1955
Number of Primary Care Physicians: 20,000
Total Enrollment: 1,000,000

Healthplan and Services Defined
PLAN TYPE: Vision
Model Type: Network
Plan Specialty: Vision
Benefits Offered: Vision

Type of Coverage
Commercial, Medicare, Supplemental Medicare, Medicaid

Type of Payment Plans Offered
POS, DFFS, Capitated, FFS, Combination FFS & DFFS

Geographic Areas Served
Nationwide

Peer Review Type
Utilization Review: Yes
Case Management: Yes

Accreditation Certification
AAAHC, NCQA, State Licensure

Key Personnel
President/CEO................................David Lavely
SVP, Information Systems.......................Juan Marrero
SVP, Regulatory Affairs.........................Larry Keeley
SVP, Quality Management ....Tara Price
SVP, Finance ....George Verrastro
VP, Member/Provider Svcs..................Shaheen Chaundhry
VP, Business Development ....Michael Grover
Director, Finance ....Louis Martin
Director, Sales..............................Doug Newcom
Manager, Marketing/Comm....................Annie Mayo
Manager, Provider Affairs ....Jay Myers
National Medical Director ....Mark Ruchman

Employer References
Wilmer-Hutchins Independent School D+strict

---

824 Preferred Care Select

5901 Chapel Hill Road
Durham, NC 27707
Toll-Free: 1-800-446-8053
Phone: 919-489-7431
Fax: 919-765-4459
www.bcbsnc.com
Mailing Address: PO Box 2291, Durham, NC 27702-2291
Subsidiary of: Blue Cross Blue Shield
Acquired by: Blue Cross & Blue Shield
Non-Profit Organization: Yes
Year Founded: 1994
Number of Affiliated Hospitals: 109
Number of Primary Care Physicians: 4,425
State Enrollment: 822,170

Healthplan and Services Defined
  PLAN TYPE: PPO
  Model Type: Network
  Plan Specialty: ASO, Behavioral Health, Chiropractic, Dental,
    Disease Management, Lab, PBM, Vision, Radiology, UR
  Benefits Offered: Behavioral Health, Chiropractic, Complementary
    Medicine, Dental, Disease Management, Home Care, Inpatient
    SNF, Long-Term Care, Physical Therapy, Podiatry, Prescription,
    Psychiatric, Transplant, Vision, Wellness, AD&D, Life, LTD, STD
  Offers Demand Management Patient Information Service: Yes
  DMPI Services Offered: Health Line Blue Nurseline, VitaBlue, Optic
    Blue, Atl Med Blue, Active Blue Magazine

Type of Coverage
Commercial

Type of Payment Plans Offered
POS, DFFS, FFS, Combination FFS & DFFS

Subscriber Information
Average Monthly Fee Per Subscriber
  (Employee + Employer Contribution):
    Employee Only (Self): Varies by plan
Average Annual Deductible Per Subscriber:
    Employee Only (Self): $500.00
    Employee & 1 Family Member: $500.00
    Employee & 2 Family Members: $500.00
Average Subscriber Co-Payment:
    Primary Care Physician: $15.00
    Non-Network Physician: 30%
    Prescription Drugs: $10.00/20.00/30.00

Hospital ER: 75.00 and 20%
Home Health Care: 10%
Home Health Care Max. Days/Visits Covered: 60 days
Nursing Home: 10%
Nursing Home Max. Days/Visits Covered: 60 days

Network Qualifications
Pre-Admission Certification: Yes

Peer Review Type
Utilization Review: Yes
Second Surgical Opinion: Yes
Case Management: Yes

Key Personnel
President/CEO ....Robert J Greczyn, Jr
  bob.greczyn@bcbsnc.com
CFO ....Daniel E Glaser
  dan.glaser@bcbsnc.com
Sr VP/Strategic Develop ....Frederick Goldwater
Chief Medical Officer ....Robert T Harris, MD
Sr VP/General Counsel ....Maureen K O'Connor
Sr VP/Sales & Marketing ....John T Roos
Chief Information Officer ....John S Sternbergh
Exec VP/Chief Admin Off ....J Bradley Wilson
Sr VP/Human Resources ....Robert T Vavrina, Jr

Average Claim Compensation
Physician's Fees Charged: 43%
Hospital's Fees Charged: 35%

Specialty Managed Care Partners
Health Dialog, Merck-Medco, Ceridian Benefits Services,
  Chiropractic Network, OptiCare Eye Health, Dental Benefits
  Providers

---

825 Southeast Community Care

4600 Marriott Drive
Suite 100
Raleigh, NC 27612
Toll-Free: 877-268-3866
Phone: 919-781-8000
Fax: 919-781-8088
www.southeastcommunitycare.com
Subsidiary of: Arcadian Health Plans

Healthplan and Services Defined
  PLAN TYPE: Medicare

Type of Coverage
Medicare

---

826 United Concordia: North Carolina

10700 Sikes Blvd.
Suite 331
Charlotte, NC 28277
Phone: 704-845-8224
ucproducer@ucci.com
www.secure.ucci.com
For Profit Organization: Yes
Year Founded: 1971
Number of Primary Care Physicians: 111,000
Total Enrollment: 8,000,000

Healthplan and Services Defined
  PLAN TYPE: Dental
  Plan Specialty: Dental
  Benefits Offered: Dental

Type of Coverage
Commercial, Individual

Geographic Areas Served
Military personnel and their families, nationwide

827 UnitedHealthCare of North Carolina

1001 Winstead Drive, Suite 200
Cary, NC 27513
Toll-Free: 800-362-0655
Fax: 803-454-1340
carolinaprteam@uhc.com
www.uhc.com
Secondary Address: 6101 Carnegie Blvd, Suite 500, Charlotte, NC 28209, 800-362-0655
Subsidiary of: UnitedHealth Group
For Profit Organization: Yes
Year Founded: 1985
Number of Affiliated Hospitals: 107
Number of Primary Care Physicians: 4,364
Number of Referral/Specialty Physicians: 7,182
Total Enrollment: 75,000,000
State Enrollment: 357,768

Healthplan and Services Defined
  PLAN TYPE: HMO/PPO
  Model Type: IPA
  Benefits Offered: Disease Management, Prescription, Wellness
  Offers Demand Management Patient Information Service: Yes

Type of Coverage
  Catastrophic Illness Benefit: Maximum $2M

Type of Payment Plans Offered
  POS, DFFS, FFS, Combination FFS & DFFS

Geographic Areas Served
  All 100 counties within North Carolina, with operational provider networks in these 57 counties: Alamance, Alexander, Bladen, Brunswick, Buncombe, Burke, Cabarrus, Caldwell, Caswell, Catawba, Cleveland, Columbus, Cumberland, Davidson, Davie, Duplin,Durham, Forsyth, Franklin, Gaston, Guilford, Harnett, Haywood, Henderson, Hoke, Irepell, Jackson, Lee, Lincoln, Madison, McDowell, Mecklenburg, Moore, New Hanover, Onslow, Orange, Pender, Person, Polk, Randolph, Richmond

Subscriber Information
  Average Subscriber Co-Payment:
    Primary Care Physician: $10.00
    Non-Network Physician: 20%
    Prescription Drugs: $10.00
    Hospital ER: $35.00
    Home Health Care: $0
    Home Health Care Max. Days/Visits Covered: 30 days
    Nursing Home: 20%
    Nursing Home Max. Days/Visits Covered: 30 days

Network Qualifications
  Pre-Admission Certification: Yes

Peer Review Type
  Utilization Review: Yes
  Second Surgical Opinion: No
  Case Management: Yes

Publishes and Distributes Report Card: Yes

Accreditation Certification
  TJC Accreditation, Utilization Review, Pre-Admission Certification, State Licensure, Quality Assurance Program

Key Personnel
  President/CEO . . . . .Frank J Branchini
  COO. . . . . .Donna Lynne
  CFO . . . . .Joseph Capezza
  Claims. . . . . .Howard Greenburg
  Network Contracting . . . . .Caroline Green
  Credentialing . . . . .Caroline Green
  Dental . . . . .John Baackes
  In House Formulary. . . . . .Steve Kessler
  Marketing . . . . .David Henderson
  Materials Management . . . . .Joseph Capezza
  Medical Affairs. . . . . .Aran Ron, MD
  Member Services. . . . . .Marilyn DeQuatro

  Information Systems . . . . .Philip Berman
  Provider Services . . . . .Caroline Greene
  Sales . . . . .David Henderson
  Media Contact. . . . . .Roger Rollman
    roger_f_rollman@uhc.com

828 WellPath: A Coventry Health Care Plan

2801 Slater Road, Suite 200
Morrisville, NC 27560
Toll-Free: 800-935-7284
http://chcnorthcarolina.coventryhealthcare.com
Secondary Address: 2815 Coliseum Center Drive, Suite 550, Charlotte, NC 28217
Subsidiary of: Coventry Health Care
For Profit Organization: Yes
Year Founded: 1995
Number of Affiliated Hospitals: 65
Number of Primary Care Physicians: 24,000
Number of Referral/Specialty Physicians: 5,000
Total Enrollment: 160,000
State Enrollment: 160,000

Healthplan and Services Defined
  PLAN TYPE: HMO
  Model Type: Network
  Plan Specialty: Chiropractic, Vision
  Benefits Offered: Prescription

Type of Coverage
  Medicare
  Catastrophic Illness Benefit: Unlimited

Type of Payment Plans Offered
  POS, Capitated, FFS

Geographic Areas Served
  North Carolina: Alamance, Buncombe, Burke, Cabarrus, Carteret, Caswell, Catawba, Chatham, Cleveland, Columbus, Craven, Cumberland, Davidson, Davie, Durham, Forsyth, Franklin, Gaston, Granville, Guilford, Harnett, Iredell, Johnston, Lee, Lincoln, Mecklenburg, Moore, Nash, Orange, Person, Randolph, Robeson, Rockingham, Rowan, Scotland, Stanly, Stokes, Surry, Union, Vance, Wake, Wilson, Warren & Yadkin; South Carolina: Anderson, Cherokee, Chester, Greenville, Lancaster

Subscriber Information
  Average Monthly Fee Per Subscriber
    (Employee + Employer Contribution):
      Employee Only (Self): Varies by plan
  Average Subscriber Co-Payment:
    Primary Care Physician: $10.00
    Prescription Drugs: $15.00
    Hospital ER: $50.00
    Home Health Care: $0
    Home Health Care Max. Days/Visits Covered: Unlimited
    Nursing Home: $0
    Nursing Home Max. Days/Visits Covered: 60 days

Network Qualifications
  Pre-Admission Certification: Yes

Peer Review Type
  Utilization Review: Yes
  Second Surgical Opinion: Yes
  Case Management: Yes

Publishes and Distributes Report Card: Yes

Accreditation Certification
  URAC
  TJC Accreditation, Medicare Approved, Utilization Review, Pre-Admission Certification, State Licensure, Quality Assurance Program

Specialty Managed Care Partners
  Magellan Health, Avefif

Health Insurance Coverage Status and Type of Coverage by Age

Category	All Persons		Under 18 years		Under 65 years		65 years and over	
	Number	%	Number	%	Number	%	Number	%
Total population	708	-	160	-	612	-	96	-
Covered by some type of health insurance	635 (5)	89.6 (0.8)	148 (2)	92.1 (1.2)	539 (6)	88.0 (0.9)	96 (1)	99.8 (0.1)
Covered by private health insurance	560 (7)	79.1 (1.0)	121 (3)	75.1 (1.9)	486 (6)	79.5 (1.1)	74 (2)	76.5 (1.9)
Employment based	433 (8)	61.1 (1.2)	101 (4)	63.0 (2.3)	406 (8)	66.3 (1.3)	27 (2)	27.9 (2.3)
Direct purchase	134 (6)	18.9 (0.8)	16 (2)	10.2 (1.5)	81 (5)	13.2 (0.9)	53 (2)	54.6 (2.1)
Covered by TRICARE	29 (4)	4.0 (0.5)	8 (2)	4.7 (1.0)	24 (4)	3.8 (0.6)	5 (1)	5.3 (1.1)
Covered by government health insurance	168 (5)	23.8 (0.6)	35 (3)	21.7 (1.8)	75 (4)	12.2 (0.7)	94 (1)	97.2 (0.8)
Covered by Medicaid	72 (5)	10.2 (0.7)	34 (3)	21.5 (1.8)	61 (4)	10.0 (0.7)	11 (1)	11.5 (1.4)
Also by private insurance	21 (3)	3.0 (0.4)	7 (2)	4.6 (0.9)	15 (3)	2.4 (0.4)	6 (1)	6.6 (1.2)
Covered by Medicare	105 (2)	14.9 (0.3)	1 (Z)	0.4 (0.3)	12 (2)	1.9 (0.3)	94 (1)	97.1 (0.8)
Also by private insurance	75 (2)	10.6 (0.3)	Z (Z)	0.1 (0.1)	4 (1)	0.7 (0.2)	71 (2)	73.8 (2.0)
Also by Medicaid	17 (2)	2.4 (0.3)	1 (Z)	0.3 (0.3)	6 (1)	1.0 (0.2)	11 (1)	11.5 (1.4)
Covered by VA Care	19 (2)	2.7 (0.3)	Z (Z)	0.2 (0.1)	8 (1)	1.4 (0.2)	11 (1)	11.3 (1.0)
Not covered at any time during the year	73 (6)	10.4 (0.8)	13 (2)	7.9 (1.2)	73 (6)	12.0 (0.9)	Z (Z)	0.2 (0.1)

Note: Numbers in thousands; Figures cover 2013; Margin of error appears in parenthesis; A "Z" indicates that the value either represents or rounds to zero.
Source: U.S. Census Bureau, 2013 American Community Survey, Table HI05. Health Insurance Coverage Status and Type of Coverage by State and Age for All People: 2013

North Dakota

829 Aetna Health of North Dakota

151 Farmington Avenue
Hartford, CT 06156
Toll-Free: 800-872-3862
Phone: 860-273-0123
www.aetna.com
Partnered with: eHealthInsurance Services Inc.
For Profit Organization: Yes
Total Enrollment: 11,596,230

Healthplan and Services Defined
PLAN TYPE: PPO
Other Type: POS
Plan Specialty: EPO
Benefits Offered: Dental, Disease Management, Long-Term Care, Prescription, Wellness, Life, LTD, STD

Type of Coverage
Commercial, Individual

Type of Payment Plans Offered
POS, FFS

Geographic Areas Served
Statewide

Key Personnel
Chairman/CEO/President.....................Mark T Bertolini
EVP, General Counsel.....................William J Casazza
EVP/CFO................................Shawn M Guertin

830 CIGNA HealthCare of North Dakota

525 W Monroe Street
Suite 300
Chicago, IL 60661
Toll-Free: 866-438-2446
Phone: 312-648-2460
Fax: 312-648-3617
www.cigna.com
For Profit Organization: Yes
Year Founded: 1986

Healthplan and Services Defined
PLAN TYPE: HMO
Other Type: POS
Model Type: IPA, Network
Plan Specialty: ASO, Behavioral Health, Dental
Benefits Offered: Behavioral Health, Complementary Medicine, Dental, Disease Management, Prescription, Transplant, Vision, Wellness

Type of Coverage
Commercial, Indemnity

Type of Payment Plans Offered
POS, DFFS, FFS

Geographic Areas Served
Illinois: Bureau, Coles, Cook, DuPage, Grundy, Kane, Kankakee, Lake, LaSalle, Livingston, Madison, Massac, McHenry, Monroe, Saint Clair, Shelby, Vermilion, Will counties

Network Qualifications
Pre-Admission Certification: Yes

Peer Review Type
Utilization Review: Yes

Publishes and Distributes Report Card: Yes

Accreditation Certification
NCQA
TJC Accreditation, Medicare Approved, Utilization Review, Pre-Admission Certification, State Licensure, Quality Assurance Program

831 Delta Dental of North Dakota

3560 Delta Dental Drive
Eagan, MN 55122-3166
Toll-Free: 800-448-3815
Phone: 651-406-5900
Fax: 651-768-1357
www.deltadental.com
Mailing Address: PO Box 9304, Minneapolis, MN 55440-9304
Non-Profit Organization: Yes
Year Founded: 1969
Number of Primary Care Physicians: 1,500
Total Enrollment: 54,000,000

Healthplan and Services Defined
PLAN TYPE: Dental
Other Type: Dental PPO
Model Type: Network
Plan Specialty: ASO, Dental
Benefits Offered: Dental

Type of Coverage
Commercial, Individual, Group
Catastrophic Illness Benefit: None

Geographic Areas Served
Minnesota, North Dakota

Subscriber Information
Average Monthly Fee Per Subscriber
(Employee + Employer Contribution):
Employee Only (Self): Varies
Employee & 1 Family Member: Varies
Employee & 2 Family Members: Varies
Average Annual Deductible Per Subscriber:
Employee Only (Self): Varies
Employee & 1 Family Member: Varies
Employee & 2 Family Members: Varies
Average Subscriber Co-Payment:
Prescription Drugs: $0
Home Health Care: $0
Nursing Home: $0

Key Personnel
President..................................David B Morse
CFO.......................................Dani Fjelstad
Exec VP/Sales & Marketing..................Mark A Moksnes
Exec VP/Operations......................Norman C Storbakken
Media Contact..............................Ann Johnson
651-994-5248
ajohnson@deltadentalmn.org
Dir/Media & Public Affair..................Elizabeth Risberg
415-972-8423

832 eHealthInsurance Services Inc.

11919 Foundation Place
Gold River, CA 95670
Toll-Free: 800-644-3491
webmaster@healthinsurance.com
www.e.healthinsurance.com
Year Founded: 1997

Healthplan and Services Defined
PLAN TYPE: HMO/PPO
Benefits Offered: Dental, Life, STD

Type of Coverage
Commercial, Individual, Medicare

Geographic Areas Served
All 50 states in the USA and District of Columbia

Key Personnel
Chairman & CEO.............................Gary L. Lauer
EVP/Business & Corp. Dev....................Bruce Telkamp
EVP/Chief Technology...................Dr. Sheldon X. Wang
SVP & CFO................................Stuart M. Huizinga

Pres. of eHealth Gov. Sys . . . . Samuel C. Gibbs
SVP of Sales & Operations . . . . Robert S. Hurley
Director Public Relations. . . . . Nate Purpura
650-210-3115

833   Great-West Healthcare North Dakota

525 West Monroe Street
Suite 300
Chicago, IL 60661-3629
Toll-Free: 877-809-8211
Phone: 312-648-2460
eliginquiries@cigna.com
www.cignaforhealth.com
Subsidiary of: CIGNA HealthCare
Acquired by: CIGNA
For Profit Organization: Yes
Total Enrollment: 884
State Enrollment: 503

Healthplan and Services Defined
PLAN TYPE: HMO/PPO
Benefits Offered: Disease Management, Prescription, Wellness

Type of Coverage
Commercial

Type of Payment Plans Offered
POS, FFS

Geographic Areas Served
North Dakota

Accreditation Certification
URAC

Specialty Managed Care Partners
Caremark Rx

834   Heart of America Health Plan

210 South Main Avenue
Rugby, ND 58368
Toll-Free: 800-525-5661
Phone: 701-776-5848
hoahp@gondtc.com
www.hoahp.com
Non-Profit Organization: Yes
Year Founded: 1982
Number of Affiliated Hospitals: 1
Number of Primary Care Physicians: 15
Number of Referral/Specialty Physicians: 500
Total Enrollment: 1,000
State Enrollment: 2,049

Healthplan and Services Defined
PLAN TYPE: HMO
Model Type: Group
Benefits Offered: Behavioral Health, Disease Management,
Psychiatric, Wellness, LTD, substance abuse, maternity

Type of Coverage
Supplemental Medicare

Type of Payment Plans Offered
POS, DFFS

Geographic Areas Served
North Central North Dakota: Pierce, Rolette, Bottineau,
McHenry,ÆTowner, Ward and Renville counties in North Dakota and
portions of Benson, Wells, Sheridan, McLean, Mountrail and Burke
counties

Subscriber Information
Average Annual Deductible Per Subscriber:
Employee Only (Self): $600
Employee & 1 Family Member: $0
Employee & 2 Family Members: $0
Medicare: $0

Average Subscriber Co-Payment:
Primary Care Physician: $10.00
Non-Network Physician: 20%
Prescription Drugs: $0.00
Hospital ER: $30.00

Accreditation Certification
TJC Accreditation

Average Claim Compensation
Physician's Fees Charged: 1%
Hospital's Fees Charged: 1%

Employer References
Federal Employee Plan

835   Humana Health Insurance of North Dakota

1611 Alderson Avenue
Billings, ND 59102
Toll-Free: 800-967-2308
Phone: 406-238-7130
Fax: 406-508-3186
www.humana.com
For Profit Organization: Yes

Healthplan and Services Defined
PLAN TYPE: HMO/PPO

Type of Coverage
Commercial, Individual

Accreditation Certification
URAC, NCQA, CORE

836   Medica: North Dakota

1711 Gold Drive South
Suite 210
Fargo, ND 57104
Phone: 701-293-4700
www.medica.com
Non-Profit Organization: Yes
Year Founded: 1974
Number of Affiliated Hospitals: 158
Number of Primary Care Physicians: 24,000
Total Enrollment: 1,600,000

Healthplan and Services Defined
PLAN TYPE: HMO
Model Type: IPA
Benefits Offered: Behavioral Health, Chiropractic, Dental, Disease
Management, Prescription, Wellness, AD&D, Life, LTD, STD
Offers Demand Management Patient Information Service: Yes

Type of Coverage
Medicare
Catastrophic Illness Benefit: Covered

Type of Payment Plans Offered
Capitated, FFS, Combination FFS & DFFS

Geographic Areas Served
Aitkin, Anoka, Becker, Beltrami, Benton, Big Stone, Blue Earth,
Brown, Carlton, Carver, Cass, Chisago, Clay, Clearwater,
Cottonwood, Crow Wing, Dakota, Dodge, Douglas, Fillmore,
Goodhue, Grant, Hennepin, Hubbard, Isanti, Itaska, Kanabec,
Kandiyohi, Koochiching, Jackson, Lac Qui Parle, Lake, Le Sueur,
Lincoln, Lyon, Mahnomen, McLeod, Meeker, Mille Lacs, Morrison,
Murray, Nicollet, Norman, Olnsted, Otter Tail, Pine, Polk, Pope,
Ramsey, Renville, Rice, Rock, Scott

Subscriber Information
Average Monthly Fee Per Subscriber
(Employee + Employer Contribution):
Employee Only (Self): Varies by plan
Average Subscriber Co-Payment:
Primary Care Physician: $15.00
Non-Network Physician: Deductible + 20%

Prescription Drugs: $11.00
Hospital ER: $60.00
Home Health Care: 20%
Nursing Home: 20%

Network Qualifications
Pre-Admission Certification: Yes

Peer Review Type
Utilization Review: Yes
Second Surgical Opinion: Yes
Case Management: Yes

Publishes and Distributes Report Card: Yes

Accreditation Certification
NCQA
TJC Accreditation, Medicare Approved, Utilization Review, Pre-Admission Certification, State Licensure, Quality Assurance Program

Key Personnel
President/CEO................................David Tilford
SVP, Government Programs......................Glenn Andis
SVP/CFO ....Mark Baird
SVP/General Manager......................Dannette Coleman
SVP/General Counsel ....Jim Jacobson
SVP Health Provider Svcs. ....Jana Johnson
SVP, Human Resources ....Deb Knutson
SVP, Marketing/Comm.......................Rob Longendyke
SVP, Commercial Markets ....John Naylor
SVP/CIO ....Tim Thull
Chief Innovation Officer...................Mark Werner, MD

Average Claim Compensation
Physician's Fees Charged: 65%
Hospital's Fees Charged: 60%

Specialty Managed Care Partners
Express Scrips, Vision Service Plan, National Healthcare Resources, Cigna Behavioral Resources
Enters into Contracts with Regional Business Coalitions: Yes

Employer References
Construction Industry Laborers Welfare Fund-Jefferson City, District 9 Machinists (Missouri/Welfare Plan), Government Employees Hospital Association/GEHA, Missouri Highway & Transportation Department/Highway Patrol

837   Noridian Insurance Services
4510 13th Avenue
Fargo, ND 58103
Toll-Free: 888-838-3106
Phone: 701-297-1595
www.mynisi.com
Mailing Address: PO Box 1872, Fargo, ND 58107-1872
For Profit Organization: Yes
Total Enrollment: 434,000

Healthplan and Services Defined
PLAN TYPE: PPO
Benefits Offered: Dental, Long-Term Care, AD&D, Life, LTD, STD

Type of Coverage
Commercial, Indemnity

Geographic Areas Served
North Dakota and northwest Minnesota

Key Personnel
Worksite Benefit Consult....................Maggy Penderson
LT Care Consulting Spec......................Rhonda Peterson
NISI Agency Manager ....Peg Dickelman

838   UnitedHealthCare of North Dakota
9700 Health Care Lane
Minnetonka, MN 55343
Toll-Free: 800-842-3585
www.uhc.com
Subsidiary of: UnitedHealth Group
For Profit Organization: Yes
Year Founded: 1977
Number of Affiliated Hospitals: 4,200
Number of Primary Care Physicians: 460,000
Total Enrollment: 75,000,000

Healthplan and Services Defined
PLAN TYPE: HMO/PPO
Model Type: Network
Plan Specialty: Lab, Radiology
Benefits Offered: Behavioral Health, Dental, Disease Management, Home Care, Physical Therapy, Prescription, Psychiatric, Wellness, AD&D, Life, LTD, STD

Type of Coverage
Commercial, Individual, Indemnity, Medicare
Catastrophic Illness Benefit: Varies per case

Geographic Areas Served
Statewide

Publishes and Distributes Report Card: Yes

Accreditation Certification
TJC Accreditation, Medicare Approved

Specialty Managed Care Partners
Enters into Contracts with Regional Business Coalitions: Yes

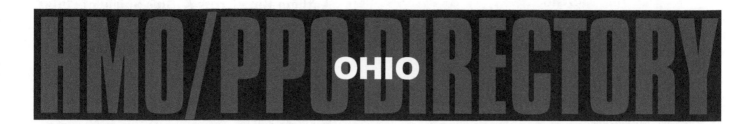
Health Insurance Coverage Status and Type of Coverage by Age

Category	All Persons		Under 18 years		Under 65 years		65 years and over	
	Number	%	Number	%	Number	%	Number	%
Total population	11,398	-	2,645	-	9,717	-	1,681	-
Covered by some type of health insurance	10,141 *(21)*	89.0 *(0.2)*	2,504 *(10)*	94.7 *(0.4)*	8,468 *(21)*	87.1 *(0.2)*	1,673 *(4)*	99.5 *(0.1)*
Covered by private health insurance	7,814 *(41)*	68.6 *(0.4)*	1,656 *(20)*	62.6 *(0.7)*	6,717 *(40)*	69.1 *(0.4)*	1,097 *(11)*	65.2 *(0.7)*
Employment based	6,806 *(42)*	59.7 *(0.4)*	1,529 *(21)*	57.8 *(0.8)*	6,112 *(42)*	62.9 *(0.4)*	695 *(11)*	41.3 *(0.6)*
Direct purchase	1,220 *(22)*	10.7 *(0.2)*	128 *(7)*	4.8 *(0.3)*	696 *(19)*	7.2 *(0.2)*	523 *(9)*	31.1 *(0.5)*
Covered by TRICARE	174 *(8)*	1.5 *(0.1)*	31 *(4)*	1.2 *(0.2)*	117 *(7)*	1.2 *(0.1)*	57 *(4)*	3.4 *(0.2)*
Covered by government health insurance	3,697 *(35)*	32.4 *(0.3)*	956 *(21)*	36.2 *(0.8)*	2,066 *(34)*	21.3 *(0.4)*	1,631 *(5)*	97.0 *(0.2)*
Covered by Medicaid	1,976 *(34)*	17.3 *(0.3)*	949 *(21)*	35.9 *(0.8)*	1,803 *(33)*	18.6 *(0.3)*	173 *(6)*	10.3 *(0.4)*
Also by private insurance	280 *(11)*	2.5 *(0.1)*	107 *(8)*	4.0 *(0.3)*	200 *(11)*	2.1 *(0.1)*	80 *(4)*	4.7 *(0.2)*
Covered by Medicare	1,921 *(10)*	16.9 *(0.1)*	15 *(3)*	0.6 *(0.1)*	292 *(9)*	3.0 *(0.1)*	1,629 *(5)*	96.9 *(0.2)*
Also by private insurance	1,134 *(12)*	10.0 *(0.1)*	2 *(1)*	0.1 *(0.1)*	79 *(4)*	0.8 *(0.1)*	1,055 *(11)*	62.7 *(0.6)*
Also by Medicaid	292 *(9)*	2.6 *(0.1)*	9 *(3)*	0.3 *(0.1)*	119 *(6)*	1.2 *(0.1)*	173 *(6)*	10.3 *(0.4)*
Covered by VA Care	248 *(7)*	2.2 *(0.1)*	1 *(1)*	0.1 *(0.1)*	115 *(6)*	1.2 *(0.1)*	133 *(4)*	7.9 *(0.3)*
Not covered at any time during the year	1,258 *(21)*	11.0 *(0.2)*	141 *(9)*	5.3 *(0.4)*	1,249 *(21)*	12.9 *(0.2)*	9 *(2)*	0.5 *(0.1)*

Note: Numbers in thousands; Figures cover 2013; Margin of error appears in parenthesis; A "Z" indicates that the value either represents or rounds to zero.
Source: U.S. Census Bureau, 2013 American Community Survey, Table HI05. Health Insurance Coverage Status and Type of Coverage by State and Age for All People: 2013

Ohio

839 Aetna Health of Ohio
1 South Wacker Drive
Mail Stop F643
Chicago, IL 60606
Toll-Free: 866-582-9629
www.aetna.com
For Profit Organization: Yes
Year Founded: 1930
Number of Affiliated Hospitals: 25
Total Enrollment: 159,375
State Enrollment: 159,375

Healthplan and Services Defined
PLAN TYPE: HMO
Other Type: POS
Model Type: IPA
Benefits Offered: Disease Management, Wellness

Type of Payment Plans Offered
POS

Geographic Areas Served
Statewide

Subscriber Information
Average Subscriber Co-Payment:
Primary Care Physician: $5.00
Prescription Drugs: $5.00
Hospital ER: $25.00
Home Health Care: $25.00
Home Health Care Max. Days/Visits Covered: Unlimited

Network Qualifications
Pre-Admission Certification: No

Peer Review Type
Utilization Review: Yes
Second Surgical Opinion: Yes
Case Management: Yes

Publishes and Distributes Report Card: Yes

Accreditation Certification
NCQA
TJC Accreditation, Utilization Review, Pre-Admission Certification, State Licensure, Quality Assurance Program

Specialty Managed Care Partners
Enters into Contracts with Regional Business Coalitions: Yes

840 Amerigroup Ohio
10123 Alliance Road
Suites 140 & 320
Blue Ash, OH 45242
Toll-Free: 800-324-8680
Phone: 513-733-2300
www.realsolutions.com
For Profit Organization: Yes
Year Founded: 2006
Total Enrollment: 1,900,000

Healthplan and Services Defined
PLAN TYPE: HMO

Type of Coverage
Medicaid, SCHIP

Key Personnel
Chairman/President . . . . James Carlson
EVP/External Affairs . . . . John Littel
Chief Medical Officer . . . . Mary McCcluskey
EVP/General Counsel . . . . Nicholas Pace

841 Anthem Blue Cross & Blue Shield of Ohio
4361 Irwin Simpson Road
Building II
Mason, OH 45040
Toll-Free: 800-442-1832
Phone: 513-872-8100
www.anthem.com
Secondary Address: 86 Columbus Road, Athens, OH 45701
For Profit Organization: Yes
Year Founded: 1944
Owned by an Integrated Delivery Network (IDN): Yes
Number of Affiliated Hospitals: 568
Number of Primary Care Physicians: 25,000
Number of Referral/Specialty Physicians: 61,728
Total Enrollment: 3,000,000
State Enrollment: 3,000,000

Healthplan and Services Defined
PLAN TYPE: PPO
Plan Specialty: ASO, Behavioral Health, Chiropractic, Dental, Disease Management, Lab, PBM, Vision, Radiology, Worker's Compensation, UR
Benefits Offered: Behavioral Health, Chiropractic, Dental, Disease Management, Home Care, Inpatient SNF, Physical Therapy, Podiatry, Prescription, Psychiatric, Transplant, Vision, Wellness, Worker's Compensation
Offers Demand Management Patient Information Service: Yes
DMPI Services Offered: Iris Program, Care Wise (24/7 Nurse Line), Dental, Vision

Type of Coverage
Commercial, Individual, Indemnity, Medicare

Type of Payment Plans Offered
POS, DFFS, Capitated, FFS

Subscriber Information
Average Monthly Fee Per Subscriber
(Employee + Employer Contribution):
Employee Only (Self): Proprietary
Employee & 1 Family Member: Proprietary
Employee & 2 Family Members: Proprierary
Medicare: Proprietary
Average Annual Deductible Per Subscriber:
Employee Only (Self): Proprietary
Employee & 1 Family Member: Proprietary
Employee & 2 Family Members: Proprietary
Medicare: Proprietary

Network Qualifications
Pre-Admission Certification: Yes

Peer Review Type
Utilization Review: Yes
Second Surgical Opinion: Yes
Case Management: Yes

Accreditation Certification
URAC, NCQA
TJC Accreditation, Medicare Approved, Utilization Review, Pre-Admission Certification, State Licensure, Quality Assurance Program

Key Personnel
President . . . . Erin Hoeflinger
Marketing Director . . . . Shelley Hahn
Medical Director . . . . Barry Malinowski, MD
Media Contact . . . . Kim Ashley
513-682-8863
kim.ashley@anthem.com

Specialty Managed Care Partners
Anthem Dental, Anthem Prescription Management LLC, Anthem Vision, Anthem Life

842   **Assurant Employee Benefits: Ohio**
312 Elm Street
Suite 1500
Cincinnati, OH 45202
Phone: 513-621-1924
Fax: 513-621-4553
benefits@assurant.com
www.assurantemployeebenefits.com
Subsidiary of: Assurant, Inc
For Profit Organization: Yes
Number of Primary Care Physicians: 112,000
Total Enrollment: 47,000

Healthplan and Services Defined
   PLAN TYPE: Multiple
   Plan Specialty: Dental, Vision, Long & Short-Term Disability
   Benefits Offered: Dental, Vision, Wellness, AD&D, Life, LTD, STD

Type of Coverage
   Commercial, Indemnity, Individual Dental Plans

Geographic Areas Served
   Statewide

Subscriber Information
   Average Monthly Fee Per Subscriber
     (Employee + Employer Contribution):
       Employee Only (Self): Varies by plan

Key Personnel
   Business Manager . . . . Maureen Seubert
   PR Specialist. . . . . Megan Hutchison
     816-556-7815
     megan.hutchison@assurant.com

843   **Aultcare Corporation**
2600 Sixth Street SW
Canton, OH 44710
Toll-Free: 800-344-8858
Phone: 330-363-6360
www.aultcare.com
Non-Profit Organization: Yes
Year Founded: 1985
Number of Affiliated Hospitals: 14
Number of Primary Care Physicians: 3,500
Number of Referral/Specialty Physicians: 6,800
Total Enrollment: 500,000
State Enrollment: 5,151

Healthplan and Services Defined
   PLAN TYPE: HMO/PPO
   Model Type: Network
   Benefits Offered: Dental, Disease Management, Vision, Worker's
     Compensation, STD, Flexible Spending Accounts

Type of Coverage
   Commercial, Individual

Geographic Areas Served
   Carroll, Holmes, Stark, Summit, Tuscarawas and Wayne counties

Network Qualifications
   Pre-Admission Certification: Yes

Peer Review Type
   Utilization Review: Yes
   Second Surgical Opinion: Yes
   Case Management: Yes

Accreditation Certification
   NCQA

Employer References
   Maytag, Timken Company

844   **CareSource**
230 N Main Street
Dayton, OH 45402
Phone: 937-224-3300
Fax: 937-425-0864
www.caresource.com
Mailing Address: PO Box 8738, Dayton, OH 45401-8738
Non-Profit Organization: Yes
Year Founded: 1989
Total Enrollment: 840,000
State Enrollment: 501,086

Healthplan and Services Defined
   PLAN TYPE: HMO
   Model Type: IPA
   Benefits Offered: Disease Management, Wellness

Type of Coverage
   Medicaid

Type of Payment Plans Offered
   Capitated

Geographic Areas Served
   Ohio and Michigan

Key Personnel
   President & CEO . . . . Pamela Morris
     937-531-2201
     pamela.morris@csmg-online.com
   Chief Financial Officer . . . . Tarlton Thomas
   Chief Operating Officer . . . . Bobby Jones
   SVP, Care Management . . . . Pam Tropiano
     937-531-2033
     pam.tropiano@csmg-online.com
   SVP, Bus Dev & Reg Affair . . . . Janet Grant
   Director, Communications. . . . . Jenny Michael
   EVP, General Counsel. . . . . Mark Chilson
   EVP, Business Development. . . . . Janet Grant
   Chief Medical Officer. . . . . Craig Thiele, MD
   Director of Communication. . . . . Jenny Michael
     937-531-2910
     jenny.michael@caresource.com

845   **CIGNA HealthCare of Ohio**
5005 Rockside Road
Independence, OH 44131
Toll-Free: 800-541-7526
Phone: 216-642-1700
Fax: 216-642-1820
www.cigna.com
Secondary Address: 440 Polaris Parkway, Suite 300, Columbus, OH
43240
For Profit Organization: Yes

Healthplan and Services Defined
   PLAN TYPE: PPO

Type of Coverage
   Commercial

846   **CoreSource: Ohio**
5200 Upper Metro Place
Suite 300
Dublin, OH 43017
Toll-Free: 800-282-3920
Phone: 614-336-9604
www.coresource.com
Subsidiary of: Trustmark
Year Founded: 1980
Total Enrollment: 1,100,000

Healthplan and Services Defined
   PLAN TYPE: Multiple

Other Type: TPA
Model Type: Network
Plan Specialty: Claims Administration, TPA
Benefits Offered: Behavioral Health, Home Care, Prescription,
Transplant

Type of Coverage
Commercial

Geographic Areas Served
Nationwide

Accreditation Certification
Utilization Review, Pre-Admission Certification

Key Personnel
President . . . . Nancy Ekrich
Chief Operating Officer . . . . Lloyd Sarrel
VP & Chief Financial Offi . . . . Clare Smith
VP, Healthcare Management. Donna Heiser
VP, Product Management & . . . . Rob Corrigan

847   Delta Dental of Michigan, Ohio and Indiana

550 Polaris Parkway
Suite 550
Westerville, OH 43082
Toll-Free: 800-537-5527
Phone: 614-890-1117
Fax: 614-890-1274
www.deltadentaloh.com
Secondary Address: 6000 Lombardo, Suite 140, Seven Hills, OH
44131
Non-Profit Organization: Yes
Year Founded: 1960
Total Enrollment: 54,000,000
State Enrollment: 952,000

Healthplan and Services Defined
PLAN TYPE: Dental
Other Type: Dental PPO
Plan Specialty: Dental
Benefits Offered: Dental

Type of Coverage
Commercial

Type of Payment Plans Offered
POS

Geographic Areas Served
Indiana, Ohio and Michigan

Network Qualifications
Pre-Admission Certification: Yes

Peer Review Type
Second Surgical Opinion: Yes
Case Management: No

Publishes and Distributes Report Card: Yes

Accreditation Certification
Utilization Review

Key Personnel
President/CEO. . . . . Laura L. Czelada, DDS
SVP/CFO . . . . Goran Jurkovic, CPA
EVP/CIO . . . . Brenda Laird
VP/Administration . . . . Judge Patrick T Cahill
VP/Operations . . . . Sherry L Crisp
VP/Corporate Affairs. . . . . Nancy E Hostetier
Dental Director . . . . Jed J Jacobson, DDS
VP/Sales . . . . Charles D Floyd, CEBS
VP/Marketing . . . . E Craig Lesley
Communications Admin . . . . Ari B Adler
517-347-5292
aadler@deltadentalmi.com
Dir/Media & Public Affair . . . . Elizabeth Risberg
415-972-8423

Specialty Managed Care Partners
Enters into Contracts with Regional Business Coalitions: Yes

848   eHealthInsurance Services Inc.

11919 Foundation Place
Gold River, CA 95670
Toll-Free: 800-644-3491
webmaster@healthinsurance.com
www.e.healthinsurance.com
Year Founded: 1997

Healthplan and Services Defined
PLAN TYPE: HMO/PPO
Benefits Offered: Dental, Life, STD

Type of Coverage
Commercial, Individual, Medicare

Geographic Areas Served
All 50 states in the USA and District of Columbia

Key Personnel
Chairman & CEO. . . . . Gary L. Lauer
EVP/Business & Corp. Dev. . . . . Bruce Telkamp
EVP/Chief Technology . . . . Dr. Sheldon X. Wang
SVP & CFO . . . . Stuart M. Huizinga
Pres. of eHealth Gov. Sys . . . . Samuel C. Gibbs
SVP of Sales & Operations . . . . Robert S. Hurley
Director Public Relations. . . . . Nate Purpura
650-210-3115

849   Emerald Health PPO

Tower At Erie View, 24th Floor
1301 East 9th Street
Cleveland, OH 44114
Toll-Free: 800-681-6912
Phone: 216-479-2030
Fax: 216-479-2039
healthsmartrx@healthsmart.com
www.healthsmart.com
Subsidiary of: Healthsmart Preferred
Acquired by: HealthSmart
For Profit Organization: Yes
Year Founded: 1983
Number of Affiliated Hospitals: 225
Number of Primary Care Physicians: 2,500
Number of Referral/Specialty Physicians: 30,000
State Enrollment: 300,000

Healthplan and Services Defined
PLAN TYPE: PPO
Model Type: No Health Insurance
Plan Specialty: ASO, Behavioral Health, Chiropractic, Dental,
Disease Management, Lab, MSO, PBM, Vision, Radiology, UR,
Nurse Coach, Case Management, Benefits Design & Solutions,
eDataWorks/Analytics
Benefits Offered: Behavioral Health, Chiropractic, Complementary
Medicine, Dental, Disease Management, Home Care, Inpatient
SNF, Long-Term Care, Physical Therapy, Podiatry, Prescription,
Psychiatric, Transplant, Vision, Wellness, Worker's Compensation

Type of Coverage
Catastrophic Illness Benefit: Maximum $2M

Type of Payment Plans Offered
DFFS

Geographic Areas Served
Ohio, Eastern Indiana, Western Pennsylvania, Northern Kentucky,
Northern West Virginia and Southern Michigan

Peer Review Type
Utilization Review: Yes
Second Surgical Opinion: Yes
Case Management: Yes

Publishes and Distributes Report Card: No

Accreditation Certification
TJC Accreditation, Utilization Review

Key Personnel
President . . . . .James M. Penington
Chairman . . . . .Daniel D. Crowley
SVP & Chief Financial Off . . . . .William Dembereckyj
Sr VP Health Economics . . . . .Deanna Weber
VP Operations . . . . .Joseph T Pernici, II
SVP, Sales & Marketing . . . . .Scott Settle
    ssettle@interplanhealth.com
Sr VP Sales . . . . .Michael Hotz

Specialty Managed Care Partners
EBRx
Enters into Contracts with Regional Business Coalitions: Yes

850   EyeMed Vision Care
4000 Luxottica Place
Mason, OH 45040
Toll-Free: 866-939-3633
http://portal.eyemedvisioncare.com
For Profit Organization: Yes
Year Founded: 1988
Total Enrollment: 159,000,000

Healthplan and Services Defined
   PLAN TYPE: Vision
   Plan Specialty: Vision
   Benefits Offered: Vision

Type of Coverage
   Commercial

Key Personnel
SVP, General Counsel . . . . .Michael Boxer
SVP, Human Resources . . . . .Mildred Curtis

851   Health Maintenance Plan
1351 William Howard Taft Road
Cincinnati, OH 45206
Toll-Free: 800-442-1832
Phone: 513-872-8100
Fax: 513-336-2425
Subsidiary of: Wellpoint
Acquired by: Anthem BlueCross & BlueShield of Ohio
For Profit Organization: Yes

Healthplan and Services Defined
   PLAN TYPE: HMO

Geographic Areas Served
   Allen, Ashland, Ashtabula, Athens, Brown, Butler, Carroll,
   Champaign, Clark, Clermont, Clinton, Columbiana, Coshocton,
   Cuyahoga, Drake, Defiance, Delaware, Erie, Fairfield, Fayette,
   Franklin, Fulton, Geauga, Greene, Hamilton, Hancock, Harrison,
   Henry, Highland, Holmes, Huron, Jefferson, Lake, Licking, Logan,
   Lorain, Lucas, Madison, Mahoning, Medina, Miami, Montgomery,
   Ottawa, Paulding, Pickaway, Portage, Preble, Putnam, Sandusky,
   Seneca, Shelby, Stark, Summit

Peer Review Type
   Case Management: Yes

Publishes and Distributes Report Card: Yes

Key Personnel
President and CEO . . . . .Larry Glasscock

852   HealthSpan
Pictoria Tower 1
225 Pictoria Drive, Suite 320
Cincinnati, OH 45246
Toll-Free: 888-914-7726
Phone: 513-551-1400
Fax: 513-551-1469
dpwoods@health-partners.org
www.healthspannetwork.com
Subsidiary of: Mercy Health Partners
For Profit Organization: Yes
Year Founded: 1991
Physician Owned Organization: Yes
Number of Affiliated Hospitals: 86
Number of Primary Care Physicians: 8,400
Total Enrollment: 108,000
State Enrollment: 81,760

Healthplan and Services Defined
   PLAN TYPE: PPO
   Benefits Offered: Disease Management, Wellness

Type of Coverage
   Commercial, Individual

Geographic Areas Served
   Indiana, Kentucky, Ohio

Peer Review Type
   Utilization Review: Yes
   Case Management: Yes

Accreditation Certification
   URAC

Key Personnel
President & CEO . . . . .Kenneth Page
Chief Operations Officer .Daniel Hounchell
Medical Director . . . . .Anthony Behler
CMO . . . . .Anthony Behler, MD
Director . . . . .Barbara Durr
Director . . . . .Jane Hawkins
Marketing Director . . . . .Dawn Woods
Member Services . . . . .Chris Crapsey
Member Services . . . . .Diane Oliver
Information Systems . . . . .Melissa Mehring
Provider Services . . . . .Barbara Durr
Media Contact . . . . .Dawn Woods, APR
   513-675-3885
   dpwoods@health-partners.org

853   HMO Health Ohio
2060 East 9th Street
Cleveland, OH 44115
Toll-Free: 800-382-5729
Phone: 216-687-7000
Fax: 216-687-6585
www.medmutual.com
Mailing Address: PO Box 94917, Cleveland, OH 44101-4917
Subsidiary of: Medical Mutual of Ohio
Year Founded: 1978
Number of Primary Care Physicians: 21
State Enrollment: 55,000

Healthplan and Services Defined
   PLAN TYPE: HMO
   Model Type: Staff
   Benefits Offered: Prescription
   Offers Demand Management Patient Information Service: Yes

Type of Payment Plans Offered
   DFFS, Capitated, FFS, Combination FFS & DFFS

Geographic Areas Served
   Ohio

Network Qualifications
Pre-Admission Certification: Yes

Publishes and Distributes Report Card: Yes

Accreditation Certification
NCQA

Key Personnel

Chairman/President/CEO	Rick Chiricosta
EVP/Chief Marketing & Com	Jared Chaney
EVP/Chief Legal Officer	Pat Dugan
EVP, Chief Managed Care	George Stadtlander
EVP, CFO	Dennis Jansey
EVP, Chief Experience Ofc	Sue Tyler
VP, Govt Relations	Joseph F Gibbons, Jr
Dir, Community Relations	Debra Green
VP, New Market Dev	Lincoln LaFayette
Chief Diversity Officer	Patricia Lattimore
Chief Medical Officer	Robert Rzewnicki
VP, Internal Audit	Kathy Golovan
Chief Information Officer	Kenneth Sidon
VP, Healthcare Finance	Kevin S Lauterjung
SVP, Business Development	Jeff Perry
Mgr, Media Relations	Ed Byers

216-687-2685

VP, Finance	Steffany Matticola

Specialty Managed Care Partners
Enters into Contracts with Regional Business Coalitions: Yes

854 Humana Health Insurance of Ohio

640 Eden Park Drive
Cincinnati, OH 45202
Phone: 502-580-1000
Fax: 513-442-7668
www.humana.com
Secondary Address: 4690 Munson Street NW, Suite D, Canton, OH
44718, 330-498-0537
For Profit Organization: Yes
Year Founded: 1979
Owned by an Integrated Delivery Network (IDN): Yes
Number of Affiliated Hospitals: 12
Number of Primary Care Physicians: 3,121
Total Enrollment: 100,000
State Enrollment: 404,052

Healthplan and Services Defined
PLAN TYPE: HMO/PPO
Model Type: Group
Plan Specialty: ASO, Dental, Vision, Radiology, Worker's
Compensation
Benefits Offered: Behavioral Health, Chiropractic, Disease
Management, Inpatient SNF, Physical Therapy, Podiatry,
Prescription, Psychiatric, Transplant, Vision, Wellness
Offers Demand Management Patient Information Service: Yes

Type of Coverage
Commercial, Individual, Medicare, Medicaid

Type of Payment Plans Offered
POS, DFFS, Capitated, FFS, Combination FFS & DFFS

Geographic Areas Served
Cincinnati, Dayton Southern Ohio, Northern Kentucky and
Southeastern Indiana

Subscriber Information
Average Subscriber Co-Payment:
Home Health Care: $0
Nursing Home: $0

Network Qualifications
Pre-Admission Certification: Yes

Peer Review Type
Utilization Review: Yes
Case Management: Yes

Publishes and Distributes Report Card: No

Accreditation Certification
URAC, NCQA, CORE
Utilization Review, Pre-Admission Certification, State Licensure,
Quality Assurance Program

Key Personnel

President/CEO	Michael B McCallister
Chief Operating Officer	James E Murray
VP/Chief Actuary	John M Bertko, FSA
Chief Financial Officer	James H Bloem
Chief Informatin Officer	Bruce J Goodman
Chief Human Resources Off	Bonita C Hathcock
General Counsel	Arthur P Hipwell
Sr VP/Corporate Devel	Thomas J Liston
Chief Innovation Officer	Jonathan T Lord, MD
Sr VP/Government Relation	Heidi S Margulis
Vice President/Controller	Steven E McCulley
Sr VP/Chief Marketing Officer	Steven O Moya

Specialty Managed Care Partners
Enters into Contracts with Regional Business Coalitions: No

855 Interplan Health Group

1301 East Ninth Street
Tower at Erieview, 24th Floor
Cleveland, OH 44114
Toll-Free: 800-683-6830
healthsmartrx@healthsmart.com
www.interplanhealth.com
Subsidiary of: A HealthSmart Network
Acquired by: HealthSmart
For Profit Organization: Yes
Year Founded: 1982
Number of Affiliated Hospitals: 300
Number of Primary Care Physicians: 32,000
Number of Referral/Specialty Physicians: 1,400
Total Enrollment: 1,000,000

Healthplan and Services Defined
PLAN TYPE: PPO
Model Type: Network
Plan Specialty: Behavioral Health, EPO, Worker's Compensation,
TPA
Benefits Offered: Behavioral Health, Prescription, Transplant,
Worker's Compensation

Type of Coverage
Commercial

Geographic Areas Served
Illinois, Indiana, eastern Iowa, Wisconsin

Network Qualifications
Pre-Admission Certification: Yes

Peer Review Type
Utilization Review: Yes
Case Management: Yes

Accreditation Certification
TJC Accreditation, Medicare Approved, Utilization Review,
Pre-Admission Certification, State Licensure, Quality Assurance
Program

Key Personnel

President	James M. Penington
Chairman	Daniel D. Crowley
SVP & Chief Financial Off	William Dembereckyj
Sr VP Sales/Marketing	Michael Mitchell

856   Kaiser Permanente Health Plan Ohio

1001 Lakeside Avenue
Suite 1200
Cleveland, OH 44114
Toll-Free: 800-493-6004
www.kaiserpermanente.org
Non-Profit Organization: Yes
Year Founded: 1964
Owned by an Integrated Delivery Network (IDN): Yes
Number of Affiliated Hospitals: 35
Number of Primary Care Physicians: 15,129
Total Enrollment: 110,000
State Enrollment: 134,949

Healthplan and Services Defined
PLAN TYPE: HMO
Model Type: Staff
Plan Specialty: Dental, Disease Management, Vision
Benefits Offered: Disease Management, Prescription, Wellness

Type of Coverage
Individual, Medicare

Type of Payment Plans Offered
POS

Geographic Areas Served
Cuyahoga, Geauga, Lake, Lorain, Medina, Portage, Stark, Summit
and Wayne counties

Subscriber Information
Average Monthly Fee Per Subscriber
(Employee + Employer Contribution):
Employee Only (Self): Varies by plan
Average Subscriber Co-Payment:
Primary Care Physician: $5.00-10.00
Non-Network Physician: Not covered
Prescription Drugs: $5.00-10.00
Hospital ER: $35.00-45.00
Home Health Care Max. Days/Visits Covered: Unlimited
Nursing Home Max. Days/Visits Covered: 100/year

Network Qualifications
Pre-Admission Certification: Yes

Peer Review Type
Utilization Review: Yes
Second Surgical Opinion: Yes
Case Management: Yes

Publishes and Distributes Report Card: Yes

Accreditation Certification
NCQA
TJC Accreditation, Medicare Approved, Utilization Review,
Pre-Admission Certification, State Licensure, Quality Assurance
Program

Key Personnel
Regional President . . . . Patricia D Kennedy-Scott
President & Med Director . . . . Ronald Louis Copeland, MD
Media Relation Specialist . . . . Renee M Deluca
216-479-5079
Media Contact . . . . Renee DeLuca
216-479-5079
renee.m.deluca@kp.org

Specialty Managed Care Partners
Federal Government, City of Cleveland, State of Ohio, Chrysler
Enters into Contracts with Regional Business Coalitions: No

857   Medical Mutual of Ohio

2060 E 9th Street
Cleveland, OH 44115
Toll-Free: 800-700-2583
Phone: 216-687-7000
www.medmutual.com

Year Founded: 1934
Number of Affiliated Hospitals: 202
Number of Primary Care Physicians: 7,728
Number of Referral/Specialty Physicians: 18,736
Total Enrollment: 1,107,000

Healthplan and Services Defined
PLAN TYPE: HMO/PPO
Model Type: Group, Network, PPO, TPA, HMO
Benefits Offered: Dental, Prescription, Vision, Wellness, Life, Health

Type of Coverage
Commercial, Individual

Geographic Areas Served
Ohio, seven other states via subsidiaries

Network Qualifications
Pre-Admission Certification: Yes

Peer Review Type
Utilization Review: Yes
Second Surgical Opinion: Yes
Case Management: Yes

Publishes and Distributes Report Card: Yes

Accreditation Certification
NCQA

Key Personnel
President/CEO . . . . Rick Chiricosta
Chief Communications Offc . . . . Jared Chaney
Chief Legal Officer . . . . Pat Dugan
EVP, Chief Managed Care . . . . George Stadtlander
EVP, CFO . . . . Dennis Janscy
EVP, Chief Experience Ofc . . . . Sue Tyler
VP, Govt Relations . . . . Joseph F Gibbons, Jr
Dir, Community Relations . . . . Debra Green
VP, New Market Dev . . . . Lincoln LaFayette
Chief Diversity Officer . . . . Patricia Lattimore
Chief Medical Officer . . . . Robert Rzewnicki
VP, Internal Audit . . . . Kathy Golovan
Chief Information Officer . . . . Kenneth Sidon
VP, Healthcare Finance . . . . Kevin S Lauterjung
SVP, Business Development . . . . Jeff Perry
Mgr, Media Relations . . . . Ed Byers
216-687-2685
VP, Finance . . . . Steffany Matticola

858   Medical Mutual of Ohio Medicare Plan

2060 East Ninth Street
Cleveland, OH 44115
Toll-Free: 800-700-2583
Phone: 216-687-7000
www.medmutual.com

Healthplan and Services Defined
PLAN TYPE: Medicare
Benefits Offered: Chiropractic, Dental, Disease Management, Home
Care, Inpatient SNF, Physical Therapy, Podiatry, Prescription,
Psychiatric, Vision, Wellness

Type of Coverage
Individual, Medicare

Geographic Areas Served
Available within Ohio only

Subscriber Information
Average Monthly Fee Per Subscriber
(Employee + Employer Contribution):
Employee Only (Self): Varies
Medicare: Varies
Average Annual Deductible Per Subscriber:
Employee Only (Self): Varies
Medicare: Varies
Average Subscriber Co-Payment:
Primary Care Physician: Varies

Non-Network Physician: Varies
Prescription Drugs: Varies
Hospital ER: Varies
Home Health Care: Varies
Home Health Care Max. Days/Visits Covered: Varies
Nursing Home: Varies
Nursing Home Max. Days/Visits Covered: Varies

Key Personnel
President/CEO . . . . Rick Chiricosta
Chief Communications Offc . . . . Jared Chaney
Chief Legal Officer. . . . . Pat Dugan
EVP, Chief Managed Care . . . . George Stadtlander
EVP, CFO. . . . . Dennis Janscy
EVP, Chief Experience Ofc . . . . Sue Tyler
VP, Govt Relations . . . . Joseph F Gibbons, Jr
Dir, Community Relations . . . . Debra Green
VP, New Market Dev. . . . . Lincoln LaFayette
Chief Diversity Officer. . . . . Patricia Lattimore
Chief Medical Officer . . . . Robert Rzewnicki
VP, Internal Audit. . . . . Kathy Golovan
Chief Information Officer. . . . . Kenneth Sidon
VP, Healthcare Finance . . . . Kevin S Lauterjung
SVP, Business Development . . . . Jeff Perry
Mgr, Media Relations. . . . . Ed Byers
216-687-2685
VP, Finance . . . . Steffany Matticola

859 Meritain Health: Ohio
24651 Center Ridge Road
2nd Floor, Ste 200, Point 6 Office Bldg
Westlake, OH 44145
Toll-Free: 800-356-6226
sales@meritain.com
www.meritain.com
For Profit Organization: Yes
Year Founded: 1983
Number of Affiliated Hospitals: 110
Number of Primary Care Physicians: 3,467
Number of Referral/Specialty Physicians: 5,720
Total Enrollment: 500,000
State Enrollment: 450,000

Healthplan and Services Defined
  PLAN TYPE: PPO
  Model Type: Network
  Plan Specialty: Dental, Disease Management, Vision, Radiology, UR
  Benefits Offered: Prescription
  Offers Demand Management Patient Information Service: Yes

Type of Coverage
  Commercial

Geographic Areas Served
  Nationwide

Subscriber Information
  Average Monthly Fee Per Subscriber
    (Employee + Employer Contribution):
      Employee Only (Self): Varies by plan

Accreditation Certification
  URAC
  TJC Accreditation, Medicare Approved, Utilization Review,
    Pre-Admission Certification, State Licensure, Quality Assurance
    Program

Key Personnel
  EVP, Chief Financial Offi. Vincent DiMura

Average Claim Compensation
  Physician's Fees Charged: 78%
  Hospital's Fees Charged: 90%

Specialty Managed Care Partners
  Express Scripts, LabOne, Interactive Health Solutions

860 Molina Healthcare: Ohio
8101 High Street
Columbus, OH 43235
Toll-Free: 800-357-0146
www.molinahealthcare.com
For Profit Organization: Yes
Year Founded: 1980
Physician Owned Organization: Yes
Number of Affiliated Hospitals: 84
Number of Primary Care Physicians: 2,167
Number of Referral/Specialty Physicians: 6,184
Total Enrollment: 1,400,000

Healthplan and Services Defined
  PLAN TYPE: HMO
  Model Type: Network
  Benefits Offered: Chiropractic, Dental, Home Care, Inpatient SNF,
    Long-Term Care, Podiatry, Vision

Type of Coverage
  Commercial, Medicare, Supplemental Medicare, Medicaid

Accreditation Certification
  URAC, NCQA

Key Personnel
  President/CEO. . . . . J. Mario Molina
  Chief Financial Officer. . . . . John C. Molina
  Chief Operating Officer . . . . Terry P. Bayer

861 Mount Carmel Health Plan Inc (MediGold)
6150 East Broad Street
Suite EE320
Columbus, OH 43213
Toll-Free: 800-964-4525
Fax: 614-546-3108
www.medigold.com
Non-Profit Organization: Yes
Year Founded: 1997
Federally Qualified: Yes
Number of Affiliated Hospitals: 23
Number of Primary Care Physicians: 1,050
Number of Referral/Specialty Physicians: 1,850
Total Enrollment: 28,125
State Enrollment: 28,125

Healthplan and Services Defined
  PLAN TYPE: Medicare
  Model Type: Network, Medicare
  Benefits Offered: Behavioral Health, Chiropractic, Dental, Disease
    Management, Home Care, Inpatient SNF, Physical Therapy,
    Podiatry, Prescription, Psychiatric, Vision, Wellness, Medical, OP
    Services, Drug Coverage

Type of Coverage
  Individual, Medicare
  Catastrophic Illness Benefit: Unlimited

Type of Payment Plans Offered
  Combination FFS & DFFS

Geographic Areas Served
  Clark, Delaware, Fairfield, Fayette, Franklin, Greene, Knox, Licking,
    Madison, Montgomery, Pickaway, Ross, Union counties

Subscriber Information
  Average Monthly Fee Per Subscriber
    (Employee + Employer Contribution):
      Employee Only (Self): Varies
      Medicare: Varies
  Average Annual Deductible Per Subscriber:
      Employee Only (Self): Varies
      Medicare: Varies
  Average Subscriber Co-Payment:
      Primary Care Physician: Varies
      Non-Network Physician: Varies

Prescription Drugs: Varies
Hospital ER: Varies
Home Health Care: Varies
Home Health Care Max. Days/Visits Covered: Varies
Nursing Home: Varies
Nursing Home Max. Days/Visits Covered: Varies

Network Qualifications
Pre-Admission Certification: Yes

Peer Review Type
Utilization Review: Yes
Case Management: Yes

Publishes and Distributes Report Card: Yes

Accreditation Certification
TJC Accreditation, Medicare Approved, Utilization Review,
Pre-Admission Certification, State Licensure, Quality Assurance
Program

Key Personnel
Chief Information Officer . . . . Cindy Sheets

Specialty Managed Care Partners
PBM-CAREMARK

Employer References
Timken, Mount Carmel Trinity

862 Nationwide Better Health

Three Nationwide Plaza
Columbus, OH 43215
Toll-Free: 866-404-6924
Phone: 614-222-0043
nbhsales@nwbetterhealth.com
www.nwbetterhealth.com
Secondary Address: 5100 Rings Road, Dublin, OH 43017
For Profit Organization: Yes
Year Founded: 1925
Number of Affiliated Hospitals: 148
Number of Primary Care Physicians: 5,800
Number of Referral/Specialty Physicians: 8,400

Healthplan and Services Defined
PLAN TYPE: HMO
Model Type: IPA
Benefits Offered: Behavioral Health, Chiropractic, Dental, Home
Care, Inpatient SNF, Long-Term Care, Physical Therapy, Podiatry,
Prescription, Psychiatric, Transplant, Vision, Wellness

Type of Coverage
Commercial, Individual
Catastrophic Illness Benefit: Varies per case

Type of Payment Plans Offered
POS, DFFS, FFS

Geographic Areas Served
Statewide

Network Qualifications
Pre-Admission Certification: Yes

Peer Review Type
Utilization Review: Yes
Second Surgical Opinion: Yes
Case Management: Yes

Publishes and Distributes Report Card: No

Accreditation Certification
URAC
TJC Accreditation, Medicare Approved, Utilization Review,
Pre-Admission Certification, State Licensure, Quality Assurance
Program

Key Personnel
President . . . . Terri Hill
Chief Financial Officer . . . . Mark Beres, CPA
Director, Operations . . . . Carol Blaine, MBA
Chief of Staff . . . . Todd Christian, MBA

Chief Medical Officer . . . . Neil Gordon, MD
VP, Specialty Health . . . . Melissa Gutierrez, CLU
Chief Information Offc . . . . Kara Kneidel, MBA
Chief Marketing Officer . . . . Eric Motter, MBA
VP, Sales . . . . Eugene Pompili
Chief Health & Prod Offc . . . . Claire Rosse, RN
Chief Operations Officer . . . . Marwan Shiblaq, MBA
AVP, Product Development . . . . David Underhill
EVP, Sales . . . . Bill Evans
nbhsales@nwbetterhealth.com
Media Relations . . . . Elizabeth Stelzer
614-249-5755
stelzee@nationwide.com

Specialty Managed Care Partners
Carwel Behavioral Health, American Chiropractic
Enters into Contracts with Regional Business Coalitions: No

Employer References
Nationwide Insurance, Abbott Labs, Merck-Medco, PPG Industrials,
Ohio Lumberman's Association

863 Ohio Health Choice

PO Box 2090
Akron, OH 44309-2090
Toll-Free: 800-554-0027
www.ohiohealthchoice.com
For Profit Organization: Yes
Year Founded: 1982
Number of Affiliated Hospitals: 198
Number of Primary Care Physicians: 7,932
Number of Referral/Specialty Physicians: 18,022
Total Enrollment: 370,000
State Enrollment: 370,000

Healthplan and Services Defined
PLAN TYPE: PPO
Model Type: Network
Plan Specialty: Chiropractic, Disease Management, EPO, UR
Benefits Offered: Behavioral Health, Chiropractic, Disease
Management, Home Care, Inpatient SNF, Long-Term Care,
Physical Therapy, Podiatry, Psychiatric, Transplant, Wellness,
Audiology, durable medical equipment, sleep disorder services,
speech therapy

Type of Coverage
Commercial, Individual, Indemnity, Medicare

Type of Payment Plans Offered
POS, FFS

Geographic Areas Served
Throughout Ohio as well as the contiguous counties of Boone, Boyd,
Campbell, Grant and Kenton in Kentucky; Dearborn in Indiana;
Mercer and Erie in Pennsylvania; and Wood, Hancock and Ohio in
West Virginia

Peer Review Type
Utilization Review: Yes
Second Surgical Opinion: Yes
Case Management: Yes

Key Personnel
Materials Management . . . . Edward Martin
Manager Medical Affairs . . . . Christy Barnes
Member Services . . . . Mona Delvalle
Information Services . . . . Adam Yanchak
Director Provider Services . . . . Leslie Colvin
Sales Director . . . . Melissa Lewis

864 Ohio State University Health Plan Inc.

700 Ackerman Road
Suite 440
Columbus, OH 43202
Toll-Free: 800-678-6269
Phone: 614-292-4700
OSUHealthPlanCS@osumc.edu
www.osuhealthplan.com
Non-Profit Organization: Yes
Year Founded: 1991
Number of Affiliated Hospitals: 95
Number of Primary Care Physicians: 3,250
Number of Referral/Specialty Physicians: 7,950
Total Enrollment: 52,000
State Enrollment: 52,000

Healthplan and Services Defined
PLAN TYPE: Multiple
Model Type: IPA
Plan Specialty: ASO, Behavioral Health, Disease Management, EPO
Benefits Offered: Behavioral Health, Chiropractic, Complementary
   Medicine, Dental, Disease Management, Home Care, Inpatient
   SNF, Physical Therapy, Podiatry, Prescription, Psychiatric,
   Transplant, Vision, Wellness
Offers Demand Management Patient Information Service: Yes
DMPI Services Offered: Faculty and Staff Assistance Program,
   University Health Connection

Type of Payment Plans Offered
DFFS, Capitated, Combination FFS & DFFS

Geographic Areas Served
Ohio State University employees and their dependents

Subscriber Information
Average Annual Deductible Per Subscriber:
   Employee Only (Self): $0
   Employee & 1 Family Member: $0
   Employee & 2 Family Members: $0
   Medicare: $0
Average Subscriber Co-Payment:
   Primary Care Physician: $15.00
   Non-Network Physician: 30%
   Prescription Drugs: 20% (generic)
   Hospital ER: $75.00
   Home Health Care: 20%
   Home Health Care Max. Days/Visits Covered: Unlimited
   Nursing Home: $0
   Nursing Home Max. Days/Visits Covered: 60 days

Network Qualifications
Pre-Admission Certification: Yes

Peer Review Type
Utilization Review: Yes
Second Surgical Opinion: No
Case Management: Yes

Publishes and Distributes Report Card: No

Accreditation Certification
NCQA
TJC Accreditation, Medicare Approved, Utilization Review,
   Pre-Admission Certification, State Licensure, Quality Assurance
   Program

Key Personnel
Chief Executive Officer . . . . Dan Vulkner
Chief Financial Officer . . . . Kelly Hamilton
Medical Director . . . . Bruce Wall
Chief Pharmacy Officer . . . . Jim Ballenger
Director, IT . . . . Tom Gessells
Dir., Medical Management. Lorena Owings
Dir., Marketing. . . . . Susan Meyer

Specialty Managed Care Partners
Enters into Contracts with Regional Business Coalitions: No

Employer References
Ohio State University

865 OhioHealth Group

155 East Broad Street
Suite 1700
Columbus, OH 43215
Toll-Free: 800-455-4460
Phone: 614-566-0056
www.ohiohealthgroup.com
For Profit Organization: Yes
Year Founded: 1985
Physician Owned Organization: Yes
Number of Affiliated Hospitals: 68
Number of Primary Care Physicians: 5,900
Number of Referral/Specialty Physicians: 10,000
Total Enrollment: 100,000
State Enrollment: 100,000

Healthplan and Services Defined
PLAN TYPE: PPO
Model Type: TPA
Benefits Offered: Disease Management, Prescription, Wellness

Type of Coverage
Commercial, Individual

Geographic Areas Served
Ohio

Peer Review Type
Utilization Review: Yes
Case Management: Yes

Key Personnel
CEO . . . . Randy Hoffman
COO . . . . Ron Kadylak
CFO. . . . . Kathy Savenko
CMO . . . . Bruce A Wall
Marketing. . . . . Ed Piela
Member Relations . . . . Lora Heddleston
Pharmacy Director. . . . . Maria Eileen Murpht

866 Paramount Elite Medicare Plan

1901 Indian Wood Circle
Maumee, OH 43537
Toll-Free: 800-462-3589
Phone: 419-887-2500
Fax: 419-887-2017
www.paramounthealthcare.com
Mailing Address: PO Box 928, Toledo, OH 43697-0928
Year Founded: 1988
Number of Affiliated Hospitals: 34
Number of Primary Care Physicians: 1,900
Total Enrollment: 187,000

Healthplan and Services Defined
PLAN TYPE: Medicare
Benefits Offered: Chiropractic, Dental, Disease Management, Home
   Care, Inpatient SNF, Physical Therapy, Podiatry, Prescription,
   Psychiatric, Vision

Type of Coverage
Individual, Medicare

Geographic Areas Served
Paramount Elite is available to persons currently enrolled in Medicare
   Parts A and B who permanently reside in Lucas or Wood counties in
   Ohio, or, within Monroe County in Michigan

Subscriber Information
Average Monthly Fee Per Subscriber
   (Employee + Employer Contribution):
      Employee Only (Self): Varies
      Medicare: Varies

Average Annual Deductible Per Subscriber:
    Employee Only (Self): Varies
    Medicare: Varies
Average Subscriber Co-Payment:
    Primary Care Physician: Varies
    Non-Network Physician: Varies
    Prescription Drugs: Varies
    Hospital ER: Varies
    Home Health Care: Varies
    Home Health Care Max. Days/Visits Covered: Varies
    Nursing Home: Varies
    Nursing Home Max. Days/Visits Covered: Varies

Key Personnel
President . . . . John C Randolph
    419-887-2500
VP, Finance . . . . Jeff Martin
Managed Care Admin . . . . Steve Gullett
Director, Marketing . . . . Jeff O'Connell
VP, Medical Services . . . . John Meier
Member Relations . . . . Karen Eichenberg

867   Paramount Health Care

1901 Indian Wood Circle
Maumee, OH 43537
Toll-Free: 800-462-3589
Phone: 419-887-2500
Fax: 419-887-2017
paramount.marketing@promedica.org
www.paramounthealthcare.com
Secondary Address: 106 Park Place, Dundee, MI 48131,
    734-529-7800
Subsidiary of: ProMedica Health System
For Profit Organization: Yes
Year Founded: 1988
Number of Affiliated Hospitals: 34
Number of Primary Care Physicians: 1,900
Number of Referral/Specialty Physicians: 900
Total Enrollment: 187,000

Healthplan and Services Defined
    PLAN TYPE: HMO/PPO
    Model Type: Network
    Benefits Offered: Prescription

Geographic Areas Served
    Northwest Ohio

Subscriber Information
Average Monthly Fee Per Subscriber
    (Employee + Employer Contribution):
        Employee Only (Self): Varies by plan
Average Annual Deductible Per Subscriber:
    Employee Only (Self): Varies
    Employee & 1 Family Member: Varies
    Employee & 2 Family Members: Varies
Average Subscriber Co-Payment:
    Primary Care Physician: Varies
    Prescription Drugs: Varies
    Hospital ER: $25.00
    Home Health Care: $0
    Home Health Care Max. Days/Visits Covered: Unlimited
    Nursing Home: $0
    Nursing Home Max. Days/Visits Covered: 100 days

Network Qualifications
    Pre-Admission Certification: Yes

Peer Review Type
    Second Surgical Opinion: Yes

Publishes and Distributes Report Card: Yes

Accreditation Certification
    URAC, NCQA

Key Personnel
President . . . . John C Randolph
    419-887-2500
VP, Finance . . . . Jeff Martin
Managed Care Admin . . . . Steve Gullett
Director, Marketing . . . . Jeff O'Connell
VP, Medical Services . . . . John Meier
Member Relations . . . . Karen Eichenberg

868   Prime Time Health Medicare Plan

214 Dartmouth Ave SW
Canton, OH 44710
Toll-Free: 800-577-5084
Phone: 330-363-7407
aultconnect@aultcare.com
www.primetimehealthplan.com
Subsidiary of: Aultcare

Healthplan and Services Defined
    PLAN TYPE: Medicare
    Benefits Offered: Chiropractic, Dental, Disease Management, Home
        Care, Inpatient SNF, Physical Therapy, Podiatry, Prescription,
        Psychiatric, Vision, Wellness

Type of Coverage
    Individual, Medicare, Medicaid

Geographic Areas Served
    Stark, Carroll, Columbiana, Holmes, Harrison, Jefferson, Mahoning,
    Tuscarawas and Wayne counties

Subscriber Information
Average Monthly Fee Per Subscriber
    (Employee + Employer Contribution):
        Employee Only (Self): Varies
        Medicare: Varies
Average Annual Deductible Per Subscriber:
    Employee Only (Self): Varies
    Medicare: Varies
Average Subscriber Co-Payment:
    Primary Care Physician: Varies
    Non-Network Physician: Varies
    Prescription Drugs: Varies
    Hospital ER: Varies
    Home Health Care: Varies
    Home Health Care Max. Days/Visits Covered: Varies
    Nursing Home: Varies
    Nursing Home Max. Days/Visits Covered: Varies

Key Personnel
President/CEO . . . . Rick Haines
Chief Financial Officer . . . . George Film
Medical Director . . . . Gregory Haban

869   S&S Healthcare Strategies

1385 Kemper Meadow Drive
Cincinnati, OH 45240
Toll-Free: 800-717-2872
Phone: 513-772-8866
Fax: 513-772-9174
info@ss-healthcare.com
www.ss-healthcare.com
Subsidiary of: International Managed Care Strategies (IMCS)
Year Founded: 1994

Healthplan and Services Defined
    PLAN TYPE: PPO
    Model Type: Network
    Benefits Offered: Dental, Prescription, Vision

Type of Payment Plans Offered
    POS, DFFS, FFS

Network Qualifications
    Pre-Admission Certification: Yes

Peer Review Type
  Second Surgical Opinion: No
  Case Management: No

Publishes and Distributes Report Card: Yes

Key Personnel
  President/CEO..............................Gale Schweitzer
  Information Services..........................Michael Ward

Specialty Managed Care Partners
  Enters into Contracts with Regional Business Coalitions: Yes

---

870   SummaCare Health Plan

10 North Main Street
Akron, OH 44308
Toll-Free: 800-996-8411
Phone: 330-996-8410
Fax: 330-996-8454
individualinfo@summacare.com
www.summacare.com
Mailing Address: PO Box 3620, Akron, OH 44309
Subsidiary of: Summa Health System
For Profit Organization: Yes
Year Founded: 1993
Physician Owned Organization: Yes
Number of Affiliated Hospitals: 50
Number of Primary Care Physicians: 6,000
Number of Referral/Specialty Physicians: 2,733
Total Enrollment: 155,000
State Enrollment: 155,000

Healthplan and Services Defined
  PLAN TYPE: HMO/PPO
  Other Type: POS
  Model Type: IPA, PPO, POS
  Plan Specialty: ASO, Behavioral Health, Chiropractic, Dental,
    Disease Management, EPO
  Benefits Offered: Behavioral Health, Chiropractic, Complementary
    Medicine, Dental, Disease Management, Home Care, Inpatient
    SNF, Physical Therapy, Podiatry, Prescription, Psychiatric,
    Transplant, Vision, Wellness, AD&D, Life
  Offers Demand Management Patient Information Service: Yes
  DMPI Services Offered: Nurses Line

Type of Coverage
  Catastrophic Illness Benefit: Covered

Type of Payment Plans Offered
  POS, DFFS, FFS

Geographic Areas Served
  Northeast Ohio: Cuyahoga, Geauga, Medina, Portage, Stark,
    Summit, Wayne, Tuscarawas, Ashtabula, Caroll, Mahoning, Trumbull
    & Lorain counties

Subscriber Information
  Average Monthly Fee Per Subscriber
    (Employee + Employer Contribution):
      Employee Only (Self): Proprietary
  Average Annual Deductible Per Subscriber:
      Employee Only (Self): $0
      Employee & 1 Family Member: $0
      Employee & 2 Family Members: $0
      Medicare: $45.00
  Average Subscriber Co-Payment:
      Primary Care Physician: $5.00/10.00
      Prescription Drugs: $5.00/10.00
      Hospital ER: $50.00
      Home Health Care: $0 if in-network
      Home Health Care Max. Days/Visits Covered: 30 days
      Nursing Home: $0 if in-network
      Nursing Home Max. Days/Visits Covered: 100 days

Network Qualifications
  Pre-Admission Certification: Yes

Peer Review Type
  Utilization Review: Yes
  Second Surgical Opinion: Yes
  Case Management: Yes

Accreditation Certification
  NCQA
  TJC Accreditation, Medicare Approved, Utilization Review,
    Pre-Admission Certification, State Licensure, Quality Assurance
    Program

Key Personnel
  President/CEO..............................Martin P Hauser
    330-996-8410
    hauserm@summacare.com
  CFO...Ernie Humbert
    330-996-8410
    humberte@summacare.com
  COO.......................................Claude Vincenti
    330-996-8410
    vincentic@summacare.com
  Director Operations ....Kevin Armbruster
    330-996-8410
    armbrusterk@summacare.com
  Contracting Coordinator.........................Anne Armao
    330-996-8410
    armaoa@summacare.com
  Manager Credentialing........................Janna Kennedy
    330-996-8410
    kennedyj@summacare.com
  QA/UR.......................................Nancy Markle
    330-996-8410
    marklen@summacare.com
  Director Pharmacy...........................Tracy Dankoff
    330-996-8410
    dankofft@summacare.com
  VP Sales and Marketing ....Kevin Cavalier
    330-996-8410
    cavalierk@summacare.com
  Manager Public Relations ....Tracie Babarick
    330-996-8410
    babarickt@summacare.com
  Chief Medical Officer.......................Tere Koenig, MD
    330-996-8410
    koenigt@summacare.com
  Director Operations ....Kevin Armbruster
    330-996-8410
    armbrusterk@summacare.com
  Information Systems ....Claude Vincenti
    vincentic@summacare.com
  Director Provider Relations ....Anne Armao
    330-996-8410
    armaoa@summacare.com
  VP Health Service Mgr........................Kevin Cavalier
    330-996-8410
    cavalierk@summacare.com
  Dir, Public Relations ....Mike Bernstein
    330-375-7930

Specialty Managed Care Partners
  Enters into Contracts with Regional Business Coalitions: Yes
  Akron Regional Development Board, Canton Regional Chamber of
    Commerce, Home Builders Association

Employer References
  Goodyear, Summa Health System, Cuyahoga County, University of
    Akron, Akron Public Schools

---

871   SummaCare Medicare Advantage Plan

10 North Main Street
Akron, OH 44308
Phone: 330-996-8410
www.summacare.com

Subsidiary of: Summa Health System
For Profit Organization: Yes
Year Founded: 1993
Physician Owned Organization: Yes
Number of Affiliated Hospitals: 50
Number of Primary Care Physicians: 6,000
Number of Referral/Specialty Physicians: 3,596
Total Enrollment: 26,000
State Enrollment: 73,724

Healthplan and Services Defined
  PLAN TYPE: Medicare
  Model Type: IPA, PPO, POS
  Benefits Offered: Behavioral Health, Chiropractic, Complementary
    Medicine, Dental, Disease Management, Home Care, Inpatient
    SNF, Physical Therapy, Podiatry, Prescription, Psychiatric,
    Transplant, Vision, Wellness, AD&D, Life
  Offers Demand Management Patient Information Service: Yes
  DMPI Services Offered: Nurses Line

Type of Coverage
  Medicare
  Catastrophic Illness Benefit: Covered

Type of Payment Plans Offered
  POS, DFFS, FFS

Geographic Areas Served
  Northeast Ohio: Cuyahoga, Geauga, Medina, Portage, Stark,
  Summit, Wayne, Tuscarawas, Ashtabula, Caroll, Mahoning, Trumbull
  & Lorain counties

Subscriber Information
  Average Monthly Fee Per Subscriber
    (Employee + Employer Contribution):
      Employee Only (Self): Proprietary
  Average Annual Deductible Per Subscriber:
      Employee Only (Self): $0
      Employee & 1 Family Member: $0
      Employee & 2 Family Members: $0
      Medicare: $45.00
  Average Subscriber Co-Payment:
      Primary Care Physician: $5.00/10.00
      Prescription Drugs: $5.00/10.00
      Hospital ER: $50.00
      Home Health Care: $0 if in-network
      Home Health Care Max. Days/Visits Covered: 30 days
      Nursing Home: $0 if in-network
      Nursing Home Max. Days/Visits Covered: 100 days

Network Qualifications
  Pre-Admission Certification: Yes

Peer Review Type
  Utilization Review: Yes
  Second Surgical Opinion: Yes
  Case Management: Yes

Accreditation Certification
  NCQA
  TJC Accreditation, Medicare Approved, Utilization Review,
    Pre-Admission Certification, State Licensure, Quality Assurance
    Program

Specialty Managed Care Partners
  Enters into Contracts with Regional Business Coalitions: Yes
  Akron Regional Development Board, Canton Regional Chamber of
    Commerce, Home Builders Association

Employer References
  Goodyear, Summa Health System, Cuyahoga County, University of
    Akron, Akron Public Schools

---

872 ## Superior Dental Care

6683 Centerville Business Parkway
Dayton, OH 45459
Toll-Free: 800-762-3159
Phone: 937-438-0283
Fax: 937-291-8695
www.superiordental.com
Year Founded: 1986
Physician Owned Organization: Yes
Number of Primary Care Physicians: 4,200
Number of Referral/Specialty Physicians: 10,000
State Enrollment: 135,000

Healthplan and Services Defined
  PLAN TYPE: Dental
  Model Type: IPA
  Plan Specialty: Dental
  Benefits Offered: Dental, Vision, Ceridian Products

Type of Payment Plans Offered
  FFS

Geographic Areas Served
  Ohio, Kentucky

Subscriber Information
  Average Monthly Fee Per Subscriber
    (Employee + Employer Contribution):
      Employee Only (Self): $18.00
      Employee & 1 Family Member: $38.00
      Employee & 2 Family Members: $56.00

Publishes and Distributes Report Card: Yes

Key Personnel
  President/Dental Director. . . . . Richard W Portune, DDS
  CEO. . . . . .Rebecca York
  Secretary. . . . . .Roger E Clark, DDS
  Treasurer . . . . .Douglas R Hoefling, DDS
  Director . . . . .Dennis A Burns, DDS
  Director. . . . . .L Don Schumaker, DDS
  Director . . . . .James L Sims, DDS
  Chief Marketing Officer . . . . .Traci Harrell
  CFO . . . . .Wendy Glover
  VP/Dental Director. . . . . Richard W Portune, DDS

---

873 ## SuperMed One

2060 E 9th Street
Cleveland, OH 44115
Toll-Free: 800-722-7331
Phone: 216-687-7000
Fax: 216-687-7274
sm1@insuredonebenefits.com
www.supermedone.com
Subsidiary of: Medical Mutual of Ohio
Non-Profit Organization: Yes
Year Founded: 1934
Number of Affiliated Hospitals: 150
Number of Primary Care Physicians: 3,977
Number of Referral/Specialty Physicians: 6,761

Healthplan and Services Defined
  PLAN TYPE: PPO
  Model Type: IPA, Group, Network
  Benefits Offered: Prescription
  Offers Demand Management Patient Information Service: Yes

Type of Coverage
  Commercial
  Catastrophic Illness Benefit: Varies per case

Type of Payment Plans Offered
  POS, Combination FFS & DFFS

Geographic Areas Served
  Statewide

Network Qualifications
Pre-Admission Certification: Yes

Peer Review Type
Utilization Review: Yes
Second Surgical Opinion: Yes
Case Management: Yes

Publishes and Distributes Report Card: Yes

Accreditation Certification
NCQA
TJC Accreditation, Medicare Approved, Utilization Review,
Pre-Admission Certification, State Licensure, Quality Assurance
Program

Key Personnel
President/CEO . . . . Rick Chiricosta
Chief Communications Offc . . . . Jared Chaney
Chief Legal Officer. . . . . Pat Dugan
EVP, Chief Managed Care . . . . George Stadtlander
EVP, CFO. . . . . Dennis Janscy
EVP, Chief Experience Ofc . . . . Sue Tyler
VP, Govt Relations . . . . Joseph F Gibbons, Jr
Dir, Community Relations . . . . Debra Green
VP, New Market Dev. . . . . Lincoln LaFayette
Chief Diversity Officer. Patricia Lattimore
Chief Medical Officer . . . . Robert Rzewnicki
VP, Internal Audit. . . . . Kathy Golovan
Chief Information Officer . . . . Kenneth Sidon
VP, Healthcare Finance . . . . Kevin S Lauterjung
SVP, Business Development . . . . Jeff Perry
Mgr, Media Relations. . . . . Ed Byers
216-687-2685
VP, Finance . . . . Steffany Matticola

Specialty Managed Care Partners
Enters into Contracts with Regional Business Coalitions: Yes

874   The Dental Care Plus Group
100 Crowne Point Place
Cincinnati, OH 45241
Toll-Free: 800-367-9466
Phone: 513-554-1100
Fax: 513-554-3187
info@dentalcareplus.com
www.dentalcareplus.com
For Profit Organization: Yes
Year Founded: 1988
Physician Owned Organization: Yes
Number of Primary Care Physicians: 4,179
Number of Referral/Specialty Physicians: 850
Total Enrollment: 269,392

Healthplan and Services Defined
PLAN TYPE: Dental
Model Type: IPA
Plan Specialty: Dental
Benefits Offered: Dental, Vision

Type of Coverage
Dental & Vision Insurance

Type of Payment Plans Offered
POS

Geographic Areas Served
Ohio, Kentucky, Indiana

Subscriber Information
Average Monthly Fee Per Subscriber
(Employee + Employer Contribution):
Employee Only (Self): $23.50
Employee & 1 Family Member: $45.85
Employee & 2 Family Members: $82.28
Average Annual Deductible Per Subscriber:
Employee Only (Self): $50.00

Employee & 1 Family Member: $50.00
Employee & 2 Family Members: $50.00

Peer Review Type
Utilization Review: Yes

Key Personnel
President and CEO. . . . . Anthony A Cook
513-554-1100
CFO. . . . . Robert C Hodgkins, Jr
Chief Sales/Marketing . . . . Ann Young
Dir, Corp Communications . . . . Allison Dubbs
513-554-1100

875   The Health Plan of the Ohio Valley/Mountaineer Region

, OH
Toll-Free: 888-847-7902
Phone: 740-695-7902
Fax: 740-699-6163
information@healthplan.org
www.healthplan.org
Non-Profit Organization: Yes
Year Founded: 1979
Federally Qualified: Yes
Number of Affiliated Hospitals: 63
Number of Primary Care Physicians: 4,000
Number of Referral/Specialty Physicians: 1,000
Total Enrollment: 380,000
State Enrollment: 380,000

Healthplan and Services Defined
PLAN TYPE: HMO/PPO
Other Type: POS
Model Type: IPA
Plan Specialty: ASO, Disease Management, Worker's Compensation,
UR, TPA
Benefits Offered: Behavioral Health, Chiropractic, Disease
Management, Home Care, Inpatient SNF, Physical Therapy,
Podiatry, Prescription, Psychiatric, Transplant, Vision, Worker's
Compensation, AD&D, Life, LTD, STD
Offers Demand Management Patient Information Service: No

Type of Coverage
Individual, Medicare, Medicaid
Catastrophic Illness Benefit: Unlimited

Type of Payment Plans Offered
POS, DFFS

Geographic Areas Served
Eastern Ohio, Northern & Central West Virginia

Subscriber Information
Average Monthly Fee Per Subscriber
(Employee + Employer Contribution):
Employee Only (Self): Varies
Medicare: Varies
Average Annual Deductible Per Subscriber:
Employee Only (Self): Varies
Medicare: Varies
Average Subscriber Co-Payment:
Primary Care Physician: Varies
Non-Network Physician: Varies
Prescription Drugs: Varies
Hospital ER: Varies
Home Health Care: Varies
Home Health Care Max. Days/Visits Covered: Varies
Nursing Home: Varies
Nursing Home Max. Days/Visits Covered: Varies

Network Qualifications
Pre-Admission Certification: Yes

Peer Review Type
Utilization Review: Yes
Second Surgical Opinion: Yes
Case Management: Yes

Publishes and Distributes Report Card: Yes

Accreditation Certification
NCQA
TJC Accreditation, Medicare Approved, Utilization Review,
Pre-Admission Certification, State Licensure, Quality Assurance
Program

876   Unison Health Plan of Ohio

2800 Corporate Exchange Drive
Suite 200
Columbus, OH 43231
Toll-Free: 877-886-4733
Phone: 614-890-6850
Fax: 877-877-7697
www.unisonhealthplan.com
Subsidiary of: AmeriChoice, A UnitedHealth Group Company
Total Enrollment: 103,000

Healthplan and Services Defined
PLAN TYPE: HMO

Key Personnel
Chief Executive Officer...........................Jeff Corzine
Finance Director ....Tim Brinkley
Marketing Director.............................Jackie Lewis
Chief Medical Officer ....Linda Post, MD
Provider Services ....Suzanne Pierce
Media Contact.................................Jeff Smith
    952-931-5685
    jeff.smith@uhc.com

877   UnitedHealthCare of Ohio: Columbus

9200 Worthington Road
Westerville, OH 43082
Toll-Free: 800-328-8835
Phone: 614-410-7000
www.uhc.com
Subsidiary of: UnitedHealth Group
For Profit Organization: Yes
Year Founded: 1980
Number of Affiliated Hospitals: 34
Number of Primary Care Physicians: 2,442
Number of Referral/Specialty Physicians: 3,304
Total Enrollment: 75,000,000
State Enrollment: 82,000

Healthplan and Services Defined
PLAN TYPE: HMO/PPO
Model Type: IPA
Plan Specialty: Dental, Vision
Benefits Offered: Disease Management, Prescription, Wellness

Geographic Areas Served
Statewide

Subscriber Information
Average Subscriber Co-Payment:
    Primary Care Physician: $15.00
    Prescription Drugs: $15.00

Accreditation Certification
NCQA

Key Personnel
CEO..Tom Brady
    614-410-7102
CFO..Ralph O'Brien
Regional Dir/Operations.......................Leslie Worley
Medical Affairs.......................Steve Richardson, MD

Provider Services............................Lyn Flanagan
Sales..Christine Kyle
Media Contact ....Debora Spano
    debora_m_spano@uhc.com

878   UnitedHealthCare of Ohio: Dayton & Cincinnati

9050 Centre Point Drive
Suite 400
West Chester, OH 45069
Toll-Free: 800-861-4037
Phone: 513-603-6200
Fax: 3
www.uhc.com
Subsidiary of: UnitedHealth Group
For Profit Organization: Yes
Year Founded: 1980
Number of Affiliated Hospitals: 34
Number of Primary Care Physicians: 2,442
Number of Referral/Specialty Physicians: 3,304
Total Enrollment: 75,000,000
State Enrollment: 82,000

Healthplan and Services Defined
PLAN TYPE: HMO/PPO
Model Type: IPA
Plan Specialty: Dental, Vision
Benefits Offered: Disease Management, Prescription, Wellness

Geographic Areas Served
Statewide

Subscriber Information
Average Subscriber Co-Payment:
    Primary Care Physician: $15.00
    Prescription Drugs: $15.00

Accreditation Certification
NCQA

Key Personnel
CEO..Tom Brady
    614-410-7000
CFO..Ralph O'Brien
Regional Dir/Operations........................Leslie Worley
VP Network Management........................Lyn Flanagan
Medical Affairs.......................Steve Richardson, MD
VP Network Management & P ....Lyn Flanagan
Sales..Christine Kyle
Media Contact ....Debora Spano
    debora_m_spano@uhc.com

879   VSP: Vision Service Plan of Ohio

4450 Belden Village Street NW
#808
Canton, OH 44718-2552
Phone: 330-759-4877
webmaster@vsp.com
www.vsp.com
Year Founded: 1955
Number of Primary Care Physicians: 26,000
Total Enrollment: 55,000,000

Healthplan and Services Defined
PLAN TYPE: Vision
Plan Specialty: Vision
Benefits Offered: Vision

Type of Payment Plans Offered
Capitated

Geographic Areas Served
Statewide

Network Qualifications
Pre-Admission Certification: Yes

Peer Review Type
Utilization Review: Yes

Accreditation Certification
Utilization Review, Quality Assurance Program

Key Personnel
President . . . . Rob Lynch

Health Insurance Coverage Status and Type of Coverage by Age

Category	All Persons		Under 18 years		Under 65 years		65 years and over	
	Number	%	Number	%	Number	%	Number	%
Total population	3,770	-	946	-	3,242	-	528	-
Covered by some type of health insurance	3,104 *(13)*	82.3 *(0.3)*	851 *(5)*	90.0 *(0.5)*	2,580 *(13)*	79.6 *(0.4)*	525 *(2)*	99.3 *(0.1)*
Covered by private health insurance	2,300 *(20)*	61.0 *(0.5)*	480 *(9)*	50.8 *(1.0)*	1,963 *(19)*	60.6 *(0.6)*	337 *(5)*	63.8 *(0.8)*
Employment based	1,850 *(18)*	49.1 *(0.5)*	401 *(10)*	42.3 *(1.0)*	1,680 *(18)*	51.8 *(0.5)*	170 *(4)*	32.1 *(0.8)*
Direct purchase	445 *(12)*	11.8 *(0.3)*	63 *(5)*	6.6 *(0.5)*	267 *(10)*	8.2 *(0.3)*	178 *(5)*	33.7 *(0.9)*
Covered by TRICARE	147 *(7)*	3.9 *(0.2)*	31 *(3)*	3.3 *(0.3)*	101 *(5)*	3.1 *(0.2)*	47 *(3)*	8.8 *(0.6)*
Covered by government health insurance	1,252 *(15)*	33.2 *(0.4)*	410 *(9)*	43.4 *(1.0)*	737 *(14)*	22.7 *(0.4)*	515 *(2)*	97.5 *(0.3)*
Covered by Medicaid	666 *(14)*	17.7 *(0.4)*	402 *(9)*	42.5 *(1.0)*	609 *(13)*	18.8 *(0.4)*	58 *(3)*	10.9 *(0.6)*
Also by private insurance	89 *(6)*	2.4 *(0.1)*	37 *(3)*	4.0 *(0.4)*	66 *(5)*	2.0 *(0.2)*	23 *(2)*	4.4 *(0.4)*
Covered by Medicare	632 *(6)*	16.8 *(0.1)*	9 *(2)*	1.0 *(0.2)*	118 *(5)*	3.7 *(0.2)*	514 *(2)*	97.2 *(0.3)*
Also by private insurance	357 *(6)*	9.5 *(0.1)*	2 *(1)*	0.2 *(0.1)*	30 *(3)*	0.9 *(0.1)*	327 *(4)*	61.9 *(0.8)*
Also by Medicaid	100 *(5)*	2.7 *(0.1)*	3 *(1)*	0.3 *(0.1)*	42 *(3)*	1.3 *(0.1)*	58 *(3)*	10.9 *(0.6)*
Covered by VA Care	123 *(4)*	3.3 *(0.1)*	2 *(1)*	0.3 *(0.1)*	62 *(4)*	1.9 *(0.1)*	61 *(3)*	11.5 *(0.5)*
Not covered at any time during the year	666 *(13)*	17.7 *(0.3)*	95 *(5)*	10.0 *(0.5)*	662 *(13)*	20.4 *(0.4)*	4 *(1)*	0.7 *(0.1)*

Note: Numbers in thousands; Figures cover 2013; Margin of error appears in parenthesis; A "Z" indicates that the value either represents or rounds to zero.
Source: U.S. Census Bureau, 2013 American Community Survey, Table HI05. Health Insurance Coverage Status and Type of Coverage by State and Age for All People: 2013

Oklahoma

880   Aetna Health of Oklahoma

2777 Stemmons Freeway
Suite 300
Dallas, TX 75207
Toll-Free: 866-582-9629
www.aetna.com
For Profit Organization: Yes
Year Founded: 1998
Number of Affiliated Hospitals: 5,300
Number of Primary Care Physicians: 597,000
Number of Referral/Specialty Physicians: 300,000
Total Enrollment: 22,000,000
State Enrollment: 31,363

Healthplan and Services Defined
 PLAN TYPE: HMO
 Other Type: POS
 Model Type: IPA
 Benefits Offered: Behavioral Health, Chiropractic, Dental, Disease
  Management, Home Care, Inpatient SNF, Long-Term Care,
  Physical Therapy, Podiatry, Prescription, Psychiatric, Transplant,
  Vision, Wellness, AD&D, Life, LTD, STD, Alternative Heatlh
  Care programs, Informed H

Type of Coverage
 Commercial

Type of Payment Plans Offered
 DFFS, Capitated, FFS

Geographic Areas Served
 Statewide

Subscriber Information
 Average Subscriber Co-Payment:
  Primary Care Physician: $20.00
  Non-Network Physician: $30.00
  Prescription Drugs: $15/30/60
  Hospital ER: $150.00

Peer Review Type
 Second Surgical Opinion: Yes
 Case Management: Yes

Accreditation Certification
 URAC, NCQA

Key Personnel
 General Manager . . . . Melissa Heim-lawrence
 Sr Vice President . . . . Bill Roth
 Business Development . . . . Brian Forbes
 Medical Director . . . . David Valdez, MD
 Sales Manager . . . . Jeff Miller

881   Assurant Employee Benefits: Oklahoma

22323 E 62nd Street South
Broken Arrow, OK 74014-2006
Phone: 918-355-4150
benefits@assurant.com
www.assurantemployeebenefits.com
Subsidiary of: Assurant, Inc
For Profit Organization: Yes
Number of Primary Care Physicians: 112,000
Total Enrollment: 47,000

Healthplan and Services Defined
 PLAN TYPE: Multiple
 Plan Specialty: Dental, Vision, Long & Short-Term Disability
 Benefits Offered: Dental, Vision, Wellness, AD&D, Life, LTD, STD

Type of Coverage
 Commercial, Indemnity, Individual Dental Plans

Geographic Areas Served
 Statewide

Subscriber Information
 Average Monthly Fee Per Subscriber
  (Employee + Employer Contribution):
   Employee Only (Self): Varies by plan

Key Personnel
 Branch Manager . . . . Robert Burkeen
 PR Specialist . . . . Megan Hutchison
  816-556-7815
  megan.hutchison@assurant.com

882   Blue Cross & Blue Shield of Oklahoma

3401 NW 63rd
Oklahoma City, OK 74102
Phone: 918-560-3500
Okmarketingoperations@bcbsok.com
www.bcbsok.com
Mailing Address: PO Box 60545, Oklahoma City, OK 73146-0545
Non-Profit Organization: Yes
Year Founded: 1940
Number of Affiliated Hospitals: 88
Number of Primary Care Physicians: 1,551
Number of Referral/Specialty Physicians: 6,000
Total Enrollment: 600,000
State Enrollment: 600,000

Healthplan and Services Defined
 PLAN TYPE: HMO/PPO
 Model Type: IPA
 Plan Specialty: ASO, Behavioral Health, Chiropractic, Dental,
  Disease Management, Lab, MSO, PBM, Vision, Radiology, UR
 Benefits Offered: Behavioral Health, Chiropractic, Dental, Disease
  Management, Home Care, Inpatient SNF, Long-Term Care,
  Physical Therapy, Podiatry, Prescription, Psychiatric, Transplant,
  Vision, Worker's Compensation, Life, LTD, STD

Type of Coverage
 Commercial, Individual, Indemnity, Supplemental Medicare

Type of Payment Plans Offered
 POS, FFS

Geographic Areas Served
 State wide

Subscriber Information
 Average Annual Deductible Per Subscriber:
  Employee Only (Self): $500.00
 Average Subscriber Co-Payment:
  Primary Care Physician: $10.00
  Prescription Drugs: 10/20/30%

Network Qualifications
 Pre-Admission Certification: Yes

Peer Review Type
 Utilization Review: Yes
 Second Surgical Opinion: Yes
 Case Management: Yes

Accreditation Certification
 URAC

Key Personnel
 President . . . . Bert Marshall
 EVP Subsidiary . . . . Michael Rhoads
 Executive VP/Internal Ops . . . . Jerry L Hudson
 General Counsel . . . . Jacqueline Haglund
 VP/Benefits Admin . . . . Nequita K Hanna
 Chief Information Officer . . . . Jerry D Scherer
 VP Marketing . . . . Lisa Putt
 Chief Medical Officer . . . . Joseph Nicholson
 Chief Medical Director . . . . Charles Knife

Media Contact .... Nicole Amend
918-551-3339
namend@bcbsok.com

Specialty Managed Care Partners
Enters into Contracts with Regional Business Coalitions: Yes

Employer References
Federal Employee Program, The Williams Companies, OneOK, Helmerich & Payne, Bank of Oklahoma

883   BlueLincs HMO
1400 S Boston Avenue
Tulsa, OK 74119
Phone: 918-551-3500
Fax: 918-561-9980
Okmarketingoperations@bcbsok.com
www.bcbsok.com
Mailing Address: PO Box 3283, Tulsa, OK 74102-3282
Subsidiary of: Blue Cross Blue Shield of Oklahoma
Acquired by: BlueCross BlueShield of Oklahoma
For Profit Organization: Yes
Year Founded: 1984
Owned by an Integrated Delivery Network (IDN): Yes
Number of Affiliated Hospitals: 6,000
Number of Primary Care Physicians: 438
Number of Referral/Specialty Physicians: 1,213
Total Enrollment: 522,248
State Enrollment: 15,248

Healthplan and Services Defined
PLAN TYPE: HMO
Model Type: IPA
Plan Specialty: Disease Management, PBM, Vision, UR
Benefits Offered: Behavioral Health, Chiropractic, Disease Management, Home Care, Inpatient SNF, Long-Term Care, Physical Therapy, Podiatry, Prescription, Psychiatric, Transplant, Vision, Worker's Compensation, Life, LTD, STD

Type of Coverage
Commercial
Catastrophic Illness Benefit: Unlimited

Type of Payment Plans Offered
Capitated, FFS

Geographic Areas Served
80% of Oklahoma

Subscriber Information
Average Annual Deductible Per Subscriber:
Employee Only (Self): $0
Employee & 2 Family Members: $0
Average Subscriber Co-Payment:
Primary Care Physician: $10.00
Prescription Drugs: $5/20/30
Hospital ER: $75.00
Nursing Home: $0

Network Qualifications
Pre-Admission Certification: Yes

Peer Review Type
Utilization Review: Yes
Second Surgical Opinion: Yes
Case Management: Yes

Key Personnel
President.................................... Wyndham Kidd
EVP Subsidiary .... Michael Rhoads
GVP Bluelincs HMO........................... Lyndle Ellis
VP BlueLincs Operations .... Mike Edmondson
VP Health Industry .... C Wayne Wallace
Medical Affairs .... Elaine Olzawski, RN
Pharmacy Manager .... Thomas Kaye, RPH
GVP Marketing .... James Roberts
Manager of Facilities .... Steven Berry

HMO Medical Director...................... Paula Root, MD
Information Services .... Dennis Timms
Sales .... James Roberts

Specialty Managed Care Partners
Behavioral Health Center, Saint John Behavioral Health, Magellan Behavioral Health, Prime Therapeutics
Enters into Contracts with Regional Business Coalitions: Yes

Employer References
Local Oklahoma Bank, Hillcrest Health Systems, National Steak and Poultry

884   CIGNA HealthCare of Oklahoma
1640 Dallas Parkway
4th Floor
Plano, TX 75093
Toll-Free: 866-438-2446
Phone: 972-863-4300
www.cigna.com
For Profit Organization: Yes
Year Founded: 1992
Number of Primary Care Physicians: 1,000
Total Enrollment: 75,000,000
State Enrollment: 22,300

Healthplan and Services Defined
PLAN TYPE: HMO/PPO
Model Type: IPA
Benefits Offered: Disease Management, Prescription, Transplant, Wellness, Womens and Mens Health Programs
Offers Demand Management Patient Information Service: Yes
DMPI Services Offered: Language Links Service, 24 hour health information line, Health Information Library, Automated ReferralLine

Type of Coverage
Commercial

Type of Payment Plans Offered
POS

Geographic Areas Served
Creek, Lincoln, Mayes, Muskogee, Okmulgee, Osage, Rogers, Tulsa and Washington counties

Accreditation Certification
URAC, NCQA

885   CommunityCare Managed Healthcare Plans of Oklahoma
218 West Sixth Street
Tulsa, OK 74119
Toll-Free: 800-278-7563
Phone: 918-594-5200
Fax: 918-594-5210
ccare@ccok.com
www.ccok.com
For Profit Organization: Yes
Number of Affiliated Hospitals: 30
Number of Primary Care Physicians: 3,000
Number of Referral/Specialty Physicians: 1,300
Total Enrollment: 250,000
State Enrollment: 250,000

Healthplan and Services Defined
PLAN TYPE: HMO/PPO
Other Type: POS
Benefits Offered: Disease Management, Prescription, Vision, Wellness, Womens health, EAP
Offers Demand Management Patient Information Service: Yes
DMPI Services Offered: 24 hour nurse line

Type of Coverage
Commercial, Medicare, Supplemental Medicare

Type of Payment Plans Offered
POS

Geographic Areas Served
Arkansas, Kansas, Missouri, Oklahoma

Key Personnel

CEO	Richard Todd
COO	Nancy Horstmann
VP, CFO	John Thomas
CMO	Jack Sommers, MD
General Counsel	Rem Beitel
Provider Relations	Kelly Ross
Marketing	Cindy Giddings
Member Relations	Pat Hall
Pharmacy Director	Melanie Maxwell
Public Relations	Betsy Panturf
VP	William Hancock

Specialty Managed Care Partners
PrecisionRX

---

886   CommunityCare Medicare Plan

218 W 6th Street
Tulsa, OK 74119
Toll-Free: 800-278-7563
Phone: 918-594-5200
Fax: 918-594-5209
ccare@ccok.com
www.ccok.com/CommunityCare%20Medicare/

Healthplan and Services Defined
PLAN TYPE: Medicare
Benefits Offered: Chiropractic, Dental, Disease Management, Home
Care, Inpatient SNF, Physical Therapy, Podiatry, Prescription,
Psychiatric, Vision, Wellness

Type of Coverage
Individual, Medicare

Geographic Areas Served
Available within Oklahoma only

Subscriber Information
Average Monthly Fee Per Subscriber
(Employee + Employer Contribution):
Employee Only (Self): Varies
Medicare: Varies
Average Annual Deductible Per Subscriber:
Employee Only (Self): Varies
Medicare: Varies
Average Subscriber Co-Payment:
Primary Care Physician: Varies
Non-Network Physician: Varies
Prescription Drugs: Varies
Hospital ER: Varies
Home Health Care: Varies
Home Health Care Max. Days/Visits Covered: Varies
Nursing Home: Varies
Nursing Home Max. Days/Visits Covered: Varies

Key Personnel

President	Richard W Todd
Vice President	William H Hancock
VP/CFO	John Thomas
Human Resources Director	Candia Fields

---

887   Delta Dental of Oklahoma

16 NW 63rd Street
Suite 201
Oklahoma City, OK 73116
Toll-Free: 800-522-0188
Phone: 405-607-2100
customerservice@deltadentalok.org
www.deltadentalok.org

Mailing Address: PO Box 54709, Oklahoma City, OK 73154-1709
Non-Profit Organization: Yes
Year Founded: 1973
Total Enrollment: 54,000,000
State Enrollment: 700,000

Healthplan and Services Defined
PLAN TYPE: Dental
Other Type: Dental PPO
Model Type: Network
Plan Specialty: ASO, Dental
Benefits Offered: Dental

Type of Coverage
Commercial, Individual, Group
Catastrophic Illness Benefit: None

Geographic Areas Served
Statewide

Subscriber Information
Average Monthly Fee Per Subscriber
(Employee + Employer Contribution):
Employee Only (Self): Varies
Employee & 1 Family Member: Varies
Employee & 2 Family Members: Varies
Average Annual Deductible Per Subscriber:
Employee Only (Self): Varies
Employee & 1 Family Member: Varies
Employee & 2 Family Members: Varies
Average Subscriber Co-Payment:
Prescription Drugs: $0
Home Health Care: $0
Nursing Home: $0

Key Personnel

Chief Executive Officer	John Gladden
Dir, Corporate Comm	Thomas J Searls

405-607-2100
corpcomm@deltadentalok.org

Dir/Media & Public Affair	Elizabeth Risberg

415-972-8423

---

888   eHealthInsurance Services Inc.

11919 Foundation Place
Gold River, CA 95670
Toll-Free: 800-644-3491
webmaster@healthinsurance.com
www.e.healthinsurance.com
Year Founded: 1997

Healthplan and Services Defined
PLAN TYPE: HMO/PPO
Benefits Offered: Dental, Life, STD

Type of Coverage
Commercial, Individual, Medicare

Geographic Areas Served
All 50 states in the USA and District of Columbia

Key Personnel

Chairman & CEO	Gary L. Lauer
EVP/Business & Corp. Dev.	Bruce Telkamp
EVP/Chief Technology	Dr. Sheldon X. Wang
SVP & CFO	Stuart M. Huizinga
Pres. of eHealth Gov. Sys	Samuel C. Gibbs
SVP of Sales & Operations	Robert S. Hurley
Director Public Relations	Nate Purpura

650-210-3115

889   Great-West Healthcare Oklahoma

8350 North Central Expressway
Suite M1000
Dallas, TX 75206
Toll-Free: 800-284-2138
Phone: 972-813-6630
eliginquiries@cigna.com
www.cigna.com
Subsidiary of: CIGNA HealthCare
Acquired by: CIGNA
For Profit Organization: Yes
Total Enrollment: 18,335
State Enrollment: 16,882

Healthplan and Services Defined
    PLAN TYPE: HMO/PPO
    Benefits Offered: Disease Management, Prescription, Wellness

Type of Coverage
    Commercial

Type of Payment Plans Offered
    POS, FFS

Geographic Areas Served
    Oklahoma

Accreditation Certification
    URAC

Key Personnel
    President & CEO......................Raymond L. McFeetors
    Executive Vice President ....Richard F. Rivers
    Chief Medical Officer.........................Dr. Terry Fouts

Specialty Managed Care Partners
    Caremark Rx

890   Humana Health Insurance of Oklahoma

7104 S Sheridan
Suite 10A
Tulsa, OK 74133
Toll-Free: 800-681-0637
Phone: 918-477-9357
Fax: 918-499-2297
www.humana.com
For Profit Organization: Yes

Healthplan and Services Defined
    PLAN TYPE: HMO/PPO

Type of Coverage
    Commercial, Individual

Accreditation Certification
    URAC, NCQA, CORE

891   Mercy Health Plans: Oklahoma

14528 South Outer 40
Suite 300
Chesterfield, MO 63017-5743
Toll-Free: 800-830-1918
Phone: 314-214-8100
Fax: 314-810-8101
www.mercyhealthplans.com
Non-Profit Organization: Yes
Total Enrollment: 73,000

Healthplan and Services Defined
    PLAN TYPE: HMO

Type of Coverage
    Commercial, Individual

Key Personnel
    Interim CEO ....Chris Knackstedt
    EVP, COO....................................Mike Treash

    Executive Vice President ....Janet Pursley
    CFO, Treasurer.............................George Schneider
    VP, General Counsel ....Charles Gilham
    Chief Medical Officer..................Stephen Spurgeon, MD
    VP, Human Resources.......................Donna McDaniel
    VP, Mission & Ethics ....Michael Doyle
    VP, Sales & Service...........................Carl Schultz

892   PacifiCare of Oklahoma

7666 E 61st Street
Suite 500
Tulsa, OK 74133
Phone: 918-459-1100
Fax: 918-459-1450
www.pacificare.com
Subsidiary of: UnitedHealthCare
For Profit Organization: Yes
Year Founded: 1985
Owned by an Integrated Delivery Network (IDN): Yes
Number of Affiliated Hospitals: 15
Number of Primary Care Physicians: 474
Total Enrollment: 43,000
State Enrollment: 78,785

Healthplan and Services Defined
    PLAN TYPE: HMO
    Model Type: Network
    Plan Specialty: ASO, Behavioral Health, Chiropractic, Dental,
        Disease Management, EPO, Lab, MSO, PBM, Vision, Radiology,
        Worker's Compensation
    Benefits Offered: Prescription
    Offers Demand Management Patient Information Service: Yes

Type of Coverage
    Commercial, Individual, Indemnity, Medicare, Supplemental
        Medicare
    Catastrophic Illness Benefit: Covered

Type of Payment Plans Offered
    POS, Combination FFS & DFFS

Geographic Areas Served
    Tulsa, Canadian, Cleveland, Creek, Grady, Kingfisher, Lincoln,
    Logan, Mayes, McClain, Muskogee, Okfuskee, Oklahoma, Okmulgee,
    Osage, Pawnee, Payne, Pottawatomie, Rogers, Seminole, Wagoner, &
    Washington counties

Subscriber Information
    Average Monthly Fee Per Subscriber
        (Employee + Employer Contribution):
            Employee Only (Self): Varies by plan
    Average Subscriber Co-Payment:
        Primary Care Physician: $10.00
        Hospital ER: $50.00
        Home Health Care: $10.00
        Home Health Care Max. Days/Visits Covered: Unlimited

Network Qualifications
    Pre-Admission Certification: Yes

Peer Review Type
    Utilization Review: Yes
    Second Surgical Opinion: No
    Case Management: Yes

Publishes and Distributes Report Card: Yes

Accreditation Certification
    NCQA
    TJC Accreditation, Medicare Approved, Pre-Admission Certification,
        State Licensure, Quality Assurance Program

Key Personnel
    President/CEO ....George H Becker, Jr
    CFO.......................................Daniel J Comrie
    Marketing ....Victor J Pluto
    Medical Affairs.........................Steve Sanders, DO

893   UnitedHealthCare of Oklahoma
5800 Granite Parkway
Suite 700
Plano, TX 75024
Toll-Free: 800-842-2481
Fax: 469-633-8856
www.uhc.com
Secondary Address: 7440 Woodland Drive, Indianapolis, IN 46278,
   888-545-5205
For Profit Organization: Yes
Year Founded: 1986
Number of Affiliated Hospitals: 5,609
Number of Primary Care Physicians: 726,537
Total Enrollment: 70,000,000
State Enrollment: 177,243

Healthplan and Services Defined
   PLAN TYPE: HMO/PPO
   Model Type: IPA
   Benefits Offered: Dental, Disease Management, Prescription,
      Wellness, AD&D, Life, LTD, STD

Type of Coverage
   Commercial, Individual, Medicare

Geographic Areas Served
   Statewide

Network Qualifications
   Pre-Admission Certification: Yes

Publishes and Distributes Report Card: Yes

Accreditation Certification
   AAPI, NCQA

Specialty Managed Care Partners
   Enters into Contracts with Regional Business Coalitions: Yes

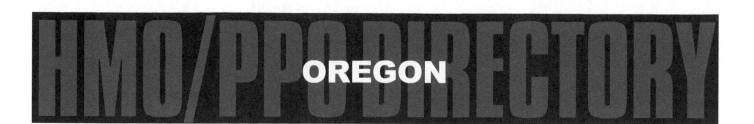
Health Insurance Coverage Status and Type of Coverage by Age

Category	All Persons		Under 18 years		Under 65 years		65 years and over	
	Number	%	Number	%	Number	%	Number	%
Total population	3,893	-	858	-	3,299	-	594	-
Covered by some type of health insurance	3,322 (15)	85.3 (0.4)	808 (5)	94.2 (0.6)	2,731 (16)	82.8 (0.5)	592 (2)	99.6 (0.1)
Covered by private health insurance	2,558 (25)	65.7 (0.6)	518 (12)	60.3 (1.4)	2,164 (23)	65.6 (0.7)	394 (6)	66.2 (1.0)
Employment based	2,054 (26)	52.8 (0.7)	454 (11)	52.9 (1.3)	1,874 (24)	56.8 (0.7)	180 (6)	30.4 (1.0)
Direct purchase	564 (15)	14.5 (0.4)	68 (6)	8.0 (0.7)	324 (14)	9.8 (0.4)	240 (7)	40.4 (1.2)
Covered by TRICARE	72 (5)	1.8 (0.1)	8 (2)	0.9 (0.2)	38 (4)	1.1 (0.1)	34 (3)	5.7 (0.5)
Covered by government health insurance	1,264 (19)	32.5 (0.5)	323 (11)	37.6 (1.3)	684 (18)	20.7 (0.6)	580 (3)	97.6 (0.3)
Covered by Medicaid	662 (18)	17.0 (0.5)	320 (11)	37.2 (1.3)	587 (17)	17.8 (0.5)	75 (4)	12.6 (0.7)
Also by private insurance	111 (7)	2.9 (0.2)	32 (4)	3.7 (0.5)	75 (6)	2.3 (0.2)	36 (2)	6.1 (0.4)
Covered by Medicare	677 (7)	17.4 (0.2)	4 (2)	0.4 (0.2)	98 (6)	3.0 (0.2)	579 (3)	97.4 (0.3)
Also by private insurance	412 (7)	10.6 (0.2)	Z (Z)	0.0 (0.1)	31 (3)	0.9 (0.1)	381 (6)	64.2 (1.1)
Also by Medicaid	119 (5)	3.1 (0.1)	1 (1)	0.2 (0.1)	44 (4)	1.3 (0.1)	75 (4)	12.6 (0.7)
Covered by VA Care	112 (4)	2.9 (0.1)	1 (1)	0.1 (0.1)	54 (4)	1.6 (0.1)	58 (3)	9.8 (0.5)
Not covered at any time during the year	571 (15)	14.7 (0.4)	50 (5)	5.8 (0.6)	568 (15)	17.2 (0.5)	3 (1)	0.4 (0.1)

Note: Numbers in thousands; Figures cover 2013; Margin of error appears in parenthesis; A "Z" indicates that the value either represents or rounds to zero.
Source: U.S. Census Bureau, 2013 American Community Survey, Table HI05. Health Insurance Coverage Status and Type of Coverage by State and Age for All People: 2013

Oregon

894 Aetna Health of Oregon
151 Farmington Avenue
Hartford, CT 06156
Toll-Free: 800-872-3862
Phone: 860-273-0123
www.aetna.com
Partnered with: eHealthInsurance Services Inc.
For Profit Organization: Yes
Total Enrollment: 11,596,230

Healthplan and Services Defined
PLAN TYPE: PPO
Other Type: POS
Plan Specialty: EPO
Benefits Offered: Dental, Disease Management, Long-Term Care, Prescription, Wellness, Life, LTD, STD

Type of Coverage
Commercial, Individual

Type of Payment Plans Offered
POS, FFS

Geographic Areas Served
Statewide

Key Personnel
Chairman/CEO/President . . . . Mark T Bertolini
EVP, General Counsel . . . . William J Casazza
EVP/CFO . . . . Shawn M Guertin

895 Assurant Employee Benefits: Oregon
1515 SW 5th Avenue
Suite 645
Portland, OR 97201
Phone: 503-228-4511
Fax: 503-228-4286
benefits@assurant.com
www.assurantemployeebenefits.com
Subsidiary of: Assurant, Inc
For Profit Organization: Yes
Number of Primary Care Physicians: 112,000
Total Enrollment: 47,000

Healthplan and Services Defined
PLAN TYPE: Multiple
Plan Specialty: Dental, Vision, Long & Short-Term Disability
Benefits Offered: Dental, Vision, Wellness, AD&D, Life, LTD, STD

Type of Coverage
Commercial, Indemnity, Individual Dental Plans

Geographic Areas Served
Statewide

Subscriber Information
Average Monthly Fee Per Subscriber
(Employee + Employer Contribution):
Employee Only (Self): Varies by plan

Key Personnel
Account Manager . . . . Sarah Trinh
PR Specialist . . . . Megan Hutchison
816-556-7815
megan.hutchison@assurant.com

896 Atrio Health Plans
2270 NW Aviation Drive
Suite 3
Roseburg, OR 97470
Toll-Free: 877-672-8620
Phone: 541-672-8620
Fax: 541-672-8670
www.atriohp.com

Healthplan and Services Defined
PLAN TYPE: Medicare
Other Type: HMO, PPO
Benefits Offered: Chiropractic, Dental, Disease Management, Home Care, Inpatient SNF, Physical Therapy, Podiatry, Prescription, Psychiatric, Vision, Wellness

Type of Coverage
Individual, Medicare

Geographic Areas Served
Douglas, Klamath & Washington counties in Oregon

Subscriber Information
Average Monthly Fee Per Subscriber
(Employee + Employer Contribution):
Employee Only (Self): Varies
Medicare: Varies
Average Annual Deductible Per Subscriber:
Employee Only (Self): Varies
Medicare: Varies
Average Subscriber Co-Payment:
Primary Care Physician: Varies
Non-Network Physician: Varies
Prescription Drugs: Varies
Hospital ER: Varies
Home Health Care: Varies
Home Health Care Max. Days/Visits Covered: Varies
Nursing Home: Varies
Nursing Home Max. Days/Visits Covered: Varies

897 CareOregon Health Plan
315 SW Fifth Avenue
Suite 900
Portland, OR 97204
Toll-Free: 800-224-4840
Phone: 503-416-4100
www.careoregon.org
Non-Profit Organization: Yes
Year Founded: 1993
Number of Affiliated Hospitals: 33
Number of Primary Care Physicians: 950
Number of Referral/Specialty Physicians: 3,000
Total Enrollment: 131,096
State Enrollment: 131,096

Healthplan and Services Defined
PLAN TYPE: Medicare

Type of Coverage
Medicare

Geographic Areas Served
20 counties in Oregon

Key Personnel
CEO . . . . Patrick Curran

898　CareSource Mid Rogue Health Plan

740 SE 7th Street
Grants Pass, OR 97526
Toll-Free: 888-460-0185
Phone: 541-471-4106
Fax: 541-471-1524
info@caresourcehealthplan.com
www.caresourcehp.com
Secondary Address: 1390 Biddle Road, Suite 105, Medford, OR 97504
Year Founded: 1995

Healthplan and Services Defined
　PLAN TYPE: Medicare
　Benefits Offered: Chiropractic, Dental, Disease Management, Home Care, Inpatient SNF, Physical Therapy, Podiatry, Prescription, Psychiatric, Vision, Wellness

Type of Coverage
　Individual, Medicare

Geographic Areas Served
　Available within Oregon only

Subscriber Information
　Average Monthly Fee Per Subscriber
　　(Employee + Employer Contribution):
　　　Employee Only (Self): Varies
　　　Medicare: Varies
　Average Annual Deductible Per Subscriber:
　　　Employee Only (Self): Varies
　　　Medicare: Varies
　Average Subscriber Co-Payment:
　　　Primary Care Physician: Varies
　　　Non-Network Physician: Varies
　　　Prescription Drugs: Varies
　　　Hospital ER: Varies
　　　Home Health Care: Varies
　　　Home Health Care Max. Days/Visits Covered: Varies
　　　Nursing Home: Varies
　　　Nursing Home Max. Days/Visits Covered: Varies

Key Personnel
　Director . . . . Cynthia Ackerman
　Chief Executive Officer . . . . Doug Flow
　Chief Executive Officer. . . . . Jan Buffa
　Medical Director . . . . Chris Kirk
　Marketing Director. . . . . Freddy Senhauser
　Medicare Advantage Spec . . . . Grace Ely

899　CIGNA HealthCare of Oregon

121 SW Morrison
Suite 525
Portland, OR 97204
Toll-Free: 800-274-0143
Phone: 503-224-0143
Fax: 505-262-3867
www.cigna.com
For Profit Organization: Yes
Total Enrollment: 126,000

Healthplan and Services Defined
　PLAN TYPE: PPO
　Model Type: Gatekeeper/ConsumerDriven
　Benefits Offered: Behavioral Health, Dental, Prescription, Medical

Type of Coverage
　Commercial

Type of Payment Plans Offered
　POS, FFS

Geographic Areas Served
　Oregon & Southwest Washington

Key Personnel
　President & General Mgr . . . . Chris Blanton

900　Clear One Health Plans

2965 NE Conners Avenue
Bend, OR 97701
Toll-Free: 800-624-6052
Phone: 541-385-5315
Fax: 541-382-4217
marketing&sales@clearonehp.com
www.clearonehp.com
Mailing Address: PO Box 7469, Bend, OR 97708
Subsidiary of: PacificSource Health Plans
Acquired by: PacificSource Health Plans
Year Founded: 1995
Physician Owned Organization: Yes
Federally Qualified: Yes
Number of Primary Care Physicians: 525
Total Enrollment: 35,000
State Enrollment: 35,000

Healthplan and Services Defined
　PLAN TYPE: Multiple
　Model Type: Network
　Plan Specialty: Behavioral Health, Chiropractic, Dental, Disease Management, Lab, Vision, Radiology
　Benefits Offered: Behavioral Health, Chiropractic, Complementary Medicine, Dental, Disease Management, Home Care, Inpatient SNF, Physical Therapy, Podiatry, Prescription, Psychiatric, Transplant, Vision, Wellness

Type of Coverage
　Commercial, Medicare, Supplemental Medicare

Geographic Areas Served
　Available within Oregon only

Subscriber Information
　Average Monthly Fee Per Subscriber
　　(Employee + Employer Contribution):
　　　Employee Only (Self): Varies
　　　Employee & 1 Family Member: Varies
　　　Employee & 2 Family Members: Varies
　　　Medicare: Varies
　Average Annual Deductible Per Subscriber:
　　　Employee Only (Self): Varies
　　　Employee & 1 Family Member: Varies
　　　Employee & 2 Family Members: Varies
　　　Medicare: Varies
　Average Subscriber Co-Payment:
　　　Primary Care Physician: Varies
　　　Non-Network Physician: Varies
　　　Prescription Drugs: Varies
　　　Hospital ER: Varies
　　　Home Health Care: Varies
　　　Home Health Care Max. Days/Visits Covered: Varies
　　　Nursing Home: Varies
　　　Nursing Home Max. Days/Visits Covered: Varies

Publishes and Distributes Report Card: Yes

Key Personnel
　President/CEO . . . . Patricia J Gibford
　VP/Medical Director. . . . . Michael Patmas, MD
　Manager, Customer Service . . . . Robert Brown
　Chief Financial Officer . . . . P Gunnar Hansen, Jr
　Chief Information Officer . . . . Sandra Loder
　SVP, Government Programs . . . . Peter Mggarry
　Media/PacificSource. . . . . Colleen Thompson
　　541-684-5453
　　cthompson@pacificsource.com

901 Dental Health Services of Oregon

205 SE Spokane Street
Suite 334
Portland, OR 97202
Toll-Free: 800-637-6453
www.dentalhealthservices.com
Secondary Address: 100 West Harrison Street, Suite S-440, South
    Tower, Seattle, WA 98119
For Profit Organization: Yes
Year Founded: 1974

Healthplan and Services Defined
    PLAN TYPE: Dental

Geographic Areas Served
    Washington State

Accreditation Certification
    URAC, NCQA

902 eHealthInsurance Services Inc.

11919 Foundation Place
Gold River, CA 95670
Toll-Free: 800-644-3491
webmaster@healthinsurance.com
www.e.healthinsurance.com
Year Founded: 1997

Healthplan and Services Defined
    PLAN TYPE: HMO/PPO
    Benefits Offered: Dental, Life, STD

Type of Coverage
    Commercial, Individual, Medicare

Geographic Areas Served
    All 50 states in the USA and District of Columbia

Key Personnel
    Chairman & CEO . . . . Gary L. Lauer
    EVP/Business & Corp. Dev. . . . . Bruce Telkamp
    EVP/Chief Technology . . . . Dr. Sheldon X. Wang
    SVP & CFO . . . . Stuart M. Huizinga
    Pres. of eHealth Gov. Sys . . . . Samuel C. Gibbs
    SVP of Sales & Operations . . . . Robert S. Hurley
    Director Public Relations . . . . Nate Purpura
        650-210-3115

903 FamilyCare Health Medicare Plan

825 NE Multnomah
Suite 300
Portland, OR 97232
Toll-Free: 800-458-9518
Phone: 503-222-2880
Fax: 503-222-2392
www.familycareinc.org
For Profit Organization: Yes
Year Founded: 1984
Total Enrollment: 2,000

Healthplan and Services Defined
    PLAN TYPE: Medicare
    Benefits Offered: Chiropractic, Dental, Disease Management, Home
        Care, Inpatient SNF, Physical Therapy, Podiatry, Prescription,
        Psychiatric, Vision, Wellness

Type of Coverage
    Individual, Medicare, Medicaid

Geographic Areas Served
    Clackamas, Clatsop, Morrow, Multnomah, Umatilla and Washington
        counties

Subscriber Information
    Average Monthly Fee Per Subscriber
        (Employee + Employer Contribution):

Employee Only (Self): Varies
    Medicare: Varies
Average Annual Deductible Per Subscriber:
    Employee Only (Self): Varies
    Medicare: Varies
Average Subscriber Co-Payment:
    Primary Care Physician: Varies
    Non-Network Physician: Varies
    Prescription Drugs: Varies
    Hospital ER: Varies
    Home Health Care: Varies
    Home Health Care Max. Days/Visits Covered: Varies
    Nursing Home: Varies
    Nursing Home Max. Days/Visits Covered: Varies

Key Personnel
    President/CEO . . . . Jeff S. Heatherington

904 Great-West Healthcare Oregon

121 SW Morrison
Suite 525
Portland, OR 97204-3247
Toll-Free: 800-274-0143
Phone: 503-224-0143
eliginquiries@cigna.com
www.cignaforhealth.com
Subsidiary of: CIGNA HealthCare
Acquired by: CIGNA
For Profit Organization: Yes
Total Enrollment: 39,334
State Enrollment: 3,487

Healthplan and Services Defined
    PLAN TYPE: HMO/PPO
    Benefits Offered: Disease Management, Prescription, Wellness

Type of Coverage
    Commercial

Type of Payment Plans Offered
    POS, FFS

Geographic Areas Served
    Oregon

Key Personnel
    General Manager . . . . John Casper

Specialty Managed Care Partners
    Caremark Rx

905 Health Net Health Plan of Oregon

13221 SW 68th Parkway
Suite 200
Portland, OR 97223
Toll-Free: 888-802-7001
Phone: 503-213-5000
service@healthnet.com
www.healthnet.com
Subsidiary of: Health Net
For Profit Organization: Yes
Number of Affiliated Hospitals: 39
Number of Primary Care Physicians: 4,400
Number of Referral/Specialty Physicians: 6,000
Total Enrollment: 123,000
State Enrollment: 17,100

Healthplan and Services Defined
    PLAN TYPE: HMO/PPO
    Model Type: IPA
    Benefits Offered: Behavioral Health, Chiropractic, Complementary
        Medicine, Dental, Disease Management, Home Care, Inpatient
        SNF, Physical Therapy, Podiatry, Prescription, Psychiatric,
        Transplant, Vision, Wellness

Type of Coverage
Commercial, Individual, Indemnity, Supplemental Medicare

Type of Payment Plans Offered
POS, DFFS, Capitated, FFS, Combination FFS & DFFS

Geographic Areas Served
18 Oregon counties

Subscriber Information
Average Subscriber Co-Payment:
Primary Care Physician: $25.00
Non-Network Physician: 50%
Hospital ER: $100.00

Key Personnel
President . . . . .Chris Ellertson
Claims . . . . .Kitty Oreskovich
Network Contracting . . . . .Gerry Weiner
Credentialing . . . . .Renee Claborn
Dental . . . . .Kitty Oreskovich
In-House Formulary . . . . .Renee Claborn
Marketing . . . . .Richard Skayhan
Materials Management . . . . .Richard Skayhan
Provider Services . . . . .Gerry Weiner
Sales . . . . .Greg O'Hanlon
Director, Communications . . . . .Amy Sheyer
818-676-8304
amy.l.sheyer@healthnet.com

Average Claim Compensation
Physician's Fees Charged: 30%
Hospital's Fees Charged: 35%

Specialty Managed Care Partners
Mhn, Vsp, Chp

Employer References
COSTCO, Willamette ESD

---

906 Humana Health Insurance of Oregon
1498 SE Tech Center Place
Suite 300
Vancouver, WA 98683
Toll-Free: 800-781-4203
Phone: 360-253-7523
Fax: 360-253-7524
www.humana.com
For Profit Organization: Yes

Healthplan and Services Defined
PLAN TYPE: HMO/PPO

Type of Coverage
Commercial, Individual

Accreditation Certification
URAC, NCQA, CORE

Key Personnel
President/CEO . . . . .Michael McCallister

---

907 Kaiser Permanente Health Plan of the Northwest
500 NE Multnomah Street
Suite 100
Portland, OR 97232
Toll-Free: 877-221-8221
www.kaiserpermanente.org
Subsidiary of: Kaiser Foundation Health Plan
Non-Profit Organization: Yes
Year Founded: 1945
Owned by an Integrated Delivery Network (IDN): Yes
Number of Affiliated Hospitals: 35
Number of Primary Care Physicians: 15,129
Number of Referral/Specialty Physicians: 11,000

Total Enrollment: 471,000
State Enrollment: 471,000

Healthplan and Services Defined
PLAN TYPE: HMO
Model Type: Group
Plan Specialty: Behavioral Health, Disease Management, Lab, Vision, Radiology, Worker's Compensation
Benefits Offered: Behavioral Health, Chiropractic, Complementary Medicine, Dental, Disease Management, Home Care, Inpatient SNF, Physical Therapy, Prescription, Psychiatric, Transplant, Vision, Wellness, Worker's Compensation

Type of Coverage
Commercial, Individual, Medicare, Medicaid

Type of Payment Plans Offered
POS, Capitated

Geographic Areas Served
Northwestern Oregon & Southwestern Washington

Subscriber Information
Average Monthly Fee Per Subscriber
(Employee + Employer Contribution):
Employee Only (Self): Varies
Employee & 1 Family Member: Varies
Employee & 2 Family Members: Varies
Medicare: Varies
Average Subscriber Co-Payment:
Primary Care Physician: Varies
Non-Network Physician: Varies
Prescription Drugs: Varies
Hospital ER: Varies
Home Health Care: Varies
Home Health Care Max. Days/Visits Covered: Varies
Nursing Home: Varies
Nursing Home Max. Days/Visits Covered: Varies

Network Qualifications
Pre-Admission Certification: Yes

Peer Review Type
Utilization Review: Yes

Publishes and Distributes Report Card: Yes

Accreditation Certification
TJC, NCQA

Key Personnel
Regional President . . . . .Andrew R McCulloch
Exec Medical Director . . . . .Sharon M Higgins, MD
Dental Director & CEO . . . . .John J Snyder, DMD
Media Contact . . . . .David Northfield
503-813-4235
david.t.northfield@kp.org

Specialty Managed Care Partners
Complementary Health Plan

Employer References
Federal Employees, State of Oregon, Oregon PERS, State of Washington

---

908 Liberty Health Plan: Corporate Office
100 Liberty Way
Dover, OR 03820
Toll-Free: 888-398-8924
Phone: 503-239-5800
Fax: 503-736-7303
customerservice.center@libertynorthwest.com
www.libertynorthwest.com
For Profit Organization: Yes
Year Founded: 1983

Healthplan and Services Defined
PLAN TYPE: PPO
Model Type: Group
Plan Specialty: Worker's Compensation

Benefits Offered: Prescription

Type of Payment Plans Offered
POS, DFFS, FFS, Combination FFS & DFFS

Geographic Areas Served
Baker, Benton, Clackamas, Columbia, Coos, Crook, Curry, Deschutes, Douglas, Gilliam, Grant, Harney, Hood River, Jackson, Jefferson, Josephine, Klamath, Lake, Lane, Lincoln counties

Network Qualifications
Pre-Admission Certification: Yes

Peer Review Type
Case Management: Yes

Publishes and Distributes Report Card: No

Key Personnel
President/CEO . . . . Matt Nickerson
CFO . . . . Jim McKittrick
Controller . . . . Mary Augustyn
Vice Presdient, Claims . . . . Margie Cooper
Vp/Corporate Marketing . . . . Beth Shia
  503-736-7003
  beth.shia@libertynorthwest.com
VP/Public Affairs . . . . Brian Boe
  503-736-7027
  brian.boe@libertynorthwest.com
Medical Affairs . . . . Chris Fassenfelt
Member Services . . . . Phil Wentz
Information Systems . . . . Jim Scott
Media Contact . . . . Christopher Goetcheus
  774-279-5923
  christopher.goetcheus@libertynorthwest.c

Specialty Managed Care Partners
Enters into Contracts with Regional Business Coalitions: No

---

909   Lifewise Health Plan of Oregon

2020 SW Fourth Street
Suite 1000
Portland, OR 97201
Toll-Free: 800-596-3440
Phone: 503-295-6707
Fax: 503-279-5295
www.lifewiseor.com
Mailing Address: PO Box 7709, Bend, OR 97702-7709
For Profit Organization: Yes
Number of Primary Care Physicians: 9,000
Total Enrollment: 1,500,000
State Enrollment: 82,000

Healthplan and Services Defined
  PLAN TYPE: PPO

Key Personnel
President/CEO . . . . Majd El-Azma
VP, Sales & Marketing . . . . David Lechner
VP, Underwriting . . . . Sharon Howe
VP, Underwriting . . . . Sharon Howe
VP, Sales & Marketing . . . . David Lechner
Communications Team Lead . . . . Deanna Strunk
  541-318-2071
  deana.strunk@lifewisehealth.com

---

910   Managed HealthCare Northwest

422 East Burnside Street
#215, PO Box 4629
Portland, OR 97208-4629
Toll-Free: 800-648-6356
Phone: 503-413-5800
Fax: 503-413-5801
www.mhninc.com
Subsidiary of: Legacy Health & Adventist Medical Center

For Profit Organization: Yes
Year Founded: 1988
Number of Affiliated Hospitals: 22
Number of Primary Care Physicians: 1,435
Number of Referral/Specialty Physicians: 4,236
Total Enrollment: 129,120
State Enrollment: 129,120

Healthplan and Services Defined
  PLAN TYPE: PPO
  Model Type: Network
  Plan Specialty: Worker's Compensation, MCO, Precertification, Utilization Review, Case Management
  Benefits Offered: Worker's Compensation, MCO, Precertification, Utilization Review, Case Management

Type of Coverage
  Commercial, Individual, Group Workers' Comp, MCO

Geographic Areas Served
  Oregon: Clackamas, Columbia, Coos, Hood River, Lane, Marion, Multnomah, Polk, Wasco, Washington & Yamhill counties; Washington: Clark, Klickitat & Skamania counties

Network Qualifications
  Pre-Admission Certification: Yes

Peer Review Type
  Utilization Review: Yes
  Second Surgical Opinion: Yes
  Case Management: Yes

Publishes and Distributes Report Card: No

Key Personnel
President and CEO . . . . Dolores Russell
Marketing Manager . . . . Jody Ordway
Commercial Care Mgmt . . . . Jan Munro
Workers' Comp MCO . . . . Rhea Schnitzer
IS Director, Finance Dir . . . . David Pyle
Provider Relations Dir . . . . Jennifer Kirk

Specialty Managed Care Partners
  Enters into Contracts with Regional Business Coalitions: Yes

Employer References
  City of Portland, SAIF Corporation, Adventist Medical Center, Legacy Health System

---

911   ODS Health Plan

601 Southwest Second Avenue
Portland, OR 97204
Toll-Free: 877-299-9062
Phone: 503-228-6554
www.odscompanies.com
Mailing Address: PO Box 40384, Portland, OR 97240-0384
Year Founded: 1955
Total Enrollment: 1,500,000
State Enrollment: 1,500,000

Healthplan and Services Defined
  PLAN TYPE: Multiple
  Other Type: PPO, POS, Dental
  Benefits Offered: Chiropractic, Dental, Disease Management, Home Care, Inpatient SNF, Physical Therapy, Podiatry, Prescription, Psychiatric, Vision, Wellness

Type of Coverage
  Commercial, Individual, Medicare

Geographic Areas Served
  Available within Oregon only

Subscriber Information
  Average Monthly Fee Per Subscriber
    (Employee + Employer Contribution):
      Employee Only (Self): Varies
      Medicare: Varies
  Average Annual Deductible Per Subscriber:
      Employee Only (Self): Varies

Medicare: Varies
Average Subscriber Co-Payment:
  Primary Care Physician: Varies
  Non-Network Physician: Varies
  Prescription Drugs: Varies
  Hospital ER: Varies
  Home Health Care: Varies
  Home Health Care Max. Days/Visits Covered: Varies
  Nursing Home: Varies
  Nursing Home Max. Days/Visits Covered: Varies

Key Personnel
President....................................William Johnson
Chief Executive Officer.......................Robert Gootee
Senior Vice President.......................Robin Richardson
Executive Vice President........................Steve Wynne
SVP, Dental Services............................Bill Ten Pas
VP, Corp Communications ....Jonathan Nicholas
  503-219-3673

912 PacifiCare of Oregon
5 Centerpointe Drive
Suite 600
Lake Oswego, OR 97035
Toll-Free: 800-922-1444
Phone: 503-603-7355
Fax: 503-624-5162
www.pacificare.com
Mailing Address: PO Box 6090, Cypress, CA 90630-0092
Subsidiary of: UnitedHealthCare
For Profit Organization: Yes
Year Founded: 1985
Number of Affiliated Hospitals: 25
Number of Primary Care Physicians: 4,200
Total Enrollment: 29,000
State Enrollment: 49,455

Healthplan and Services Defined
PLAN TYPE: HMO
Model Type: Mixed
Benefits Offered: Behavioral Health, Chiropractic, Complementary Medicine, Dental, Disease Management, Home Care, Inpatient SNF, Physical Therapy, Podiatry, Prescription, Psychiatric, Transplant, Vision, Wellness, Life, LTD, STD

Type of Coverage
Commercial, Individual, Indemnity, Medicare

Accreditation Certification
NCQA

Key Personnel
CEO.......................................Randy Wardlow
Medical Director ....Bill Hopper, MD

913 PacificSource Health Plans: Corporate Headquarters
110 International Way
Springfield, OR 97477
Toll-Free: 800-624-6052
Phone: 541-686-1242
Fax: 541-485-0915
www.pacificsource.com
Secondary Address: 2965 NE Conners Avenue, Bend, OR 97701
Non-Profit Organization: Yes
Year Founded: 1933
Number of Primary Care Physicians: 34,000
Total Enrollment: 280,000

Healthplan and Services Defined
PLAN TYPE: HMO/PPO

Benefits Offered: Dental, Disease Management, Prescription, Vision, Wellness

Type of Coverage
Commercial, Individual

Type of Payment Plans Offered
POS, Combination FFS & DFFS

Geographic Areas Served
Oregon and Idaho

Key Personnel
President & CEO............................Ken Provencher
EVP, COO ....Sujata Sanghvi
EVP, CFO ....Peter Davidson
SVP, Director ID & WA ....Dave Self
VP, Large Group & ASO ....Steve Schmidt
VP, Administration ....Paul Wynkoop
VP, Finance & Controller......................Kari Patterson
VP, Business Development ....Lisz Zenev
Reg VP, Marketing Officer ....Troy Kirk
SVP, Chief Medical Offc ....Steven D Marks, MD
SVP, Chief Info Officer.........................Erick Doolen
VP, Provider Network ....Peter McGarry
VP, Actuarial ....Victor Paguia
Media Contact...........................Colleen Thompson
  541-684-5453
  cthompson@pacificsource.com

Specialty Managed Care Partners
Caremark Rx

914 Providence Health Plans
3601 SW Murray Boulevard
Suite 109
Beaverton, OR 97005
Toll-Free: 877-245-4077
Phone: 503-574-7440
Fax: 503-215-7543
www.providence.org/healthplans
Mailing Address: PO Box 4327, Portland, OR 97208-4327
Subsidiary of: Providence Health Systems
Non-Profit Organization: Yes
Year Founded: 1985
Number of Affiliated Hospitals: 31
Number of Primary Care Physicians: 1,366
Number of Referral/Specialty Physicians: 3,042
Total Enrollment: 350,000
State Enrollment: 350,000

Healthplan and Services Defined
PLAN TYPE: HMO/PPO
Model Type: IPA, Group, PHO
Plan Specialty: Disease Management, EPO, Vision, UR
Benefits Offered: Behavioral Health, Chiropractic, Complementary Medicine, Disease Management, Home Care, Inpatient SNF, Physical Therapy, Podiatry, Prescription, Psychiatric, Transplant, Vision, Wellness
Offers Demand Management Patient Information Service: Yes
DMPI Services Offered: 24 Hour Telephone Advice Nurse, Website, Fitness Wellness Classes, Resource Telephone Service, Discounted Vision Service

Type of Coverage
Commercial, Medicare, Medicaid

Type of Payment Plans Offered
POS, FFS

Geographic Areas Served
Oregon: Benton, Clackamas, Crook, Deschules, Grant, Harney, Jefferson, Josephine, Lake, Marion, Multnomah, Tillamook, Washington, Wheeler, and Yamhill; WA: Clark and Skamania

Subscriber Information
Average Monthly Fee Per Subscriber
(Employee + Employer Contribution):
Employee Only (Self): Varies by plan
Average Subscriber Co-Payment:
Home Health Care Max. Days/Visits Covered: 30 days
Nursing Home Max. Days/Visits Covered: 60 days

Network Qualifications
Pre-Admission Certification: Yes

Peer Review Type
Utilization Review: Yes
Second Surgical Opinion: Yes
Case Management: Yes

Publishes and Distributes Report Card: Yes

Accreditation Certification
NCQA
Medicare Approved, Utilization Review, Pre-Admission
Certification, State Licensure, Quality Assurance Program

Key Personnel
Chairman .... Sister Lucille Dean
Chief Operating Officer .... Michael White
Chief Service Officer .... Alison Schrupp
Dir, Mission Integration .... Margaret Pastro, SP
Dir, Regulatory Compl .... Carrie Smith
Chief Sales & Mktg Offc .... Barbara Christensen

Average Claim Compensation
Physician's Fees Charged: 55%
Hospital's Fees Charged: 48%

Specialty Managed Care Partners
PBH Behavioral Health, ARGUS (PBM), Complementary Health
Care, Well Partner
Enters into Contracts with Regional Business Coalitions: No

Employer References
Providence Health System, PeaceHealth, Portland Public School
District, Oregon PERS, Tektonix

---

915 Regence Blue Cross & Blue Shield of Oregon
100 SW Market Street
Portland, OR 97201
Toll-Free: 888-675-6570
Phone: 503-225-5221
Fax: 503-225-5274
dmglass@regence.com
www.or.regence.com
Mailing Address: PO Box 1071, Portland, OR 97207
Subsidiary of: The Regence Group
Non-Profit Organization: Yes
Year Founded: 1941
Owned by an Integrated Delivery Network (IDN): Yes
Number of Affiliated Hospitals: 48
Number of Primary Care Physicians: 10,425
Total Enrollment: 2,500,000
State Enrollment: 800,000

Healthplan and Services Defined
PLAN TYPE: PPO
Model Type: IPA
Benefits Offered: Behavioral Health, Dental, Disease Management,
Prescription, Vision, Wellness, Hearing Care, Local Gym
Memberships, Weight Loss Programs, Child Health & Safety
Products

Type of Coverage
Commercial, Individual, Indemnity, Medicare, Supplemental
Medicare
Catastrophic Illness Benefit: Maximum $2M

Type of Payment Plans Offered
POS, DFFS, Capitated, FFS, Combination FFS & DFFS

Geographic Areas Served
All Oregon and Clark County, WA

Subscriber Information
Average Annual Deductible Per Subscriber:
Employee Only (Self): $250.00
Average Subscriber Co-Payment:
Primary Care Physician: $15.00/100.00
Prescription Drugs: $10/30/50
Hospital ER: $100.00
Home Health Care: $180 days

Network Qualifications
Pre-Admission Certification: Yes

Peer Review Type
Utilization Review: Yes
Second Surgical Opinion: Yes
Case Management: Yes

Publishes and Distributes Report Card: Yes

Accreditation Certification
NCQA
TJC Accreditation, Medicare Approved, Pre-Admission Certification,
State Licensure

Key Personnel
President .... Don Antonucci
EVP, Healthcare Services/................... Dr. Richard Popiel
SVP, Govt. Programs .... Lisa Brubaker
Chief Marketing Executive .... Mohan Nair
EVP, Chief Legal Officer .... Kerry Barnett
Chief Financial Officer......................... Vince Price
Sr VP/Human Resources .... Tom Kennedy
EVP, Chief Marketing Exec...................... Mohan Nair
SVP, Enterprise Mgmt .... Jo Ann Long
President, Regence WA .... Johathan Hensley
President, Regence UT......................... Robert A Hatch
President, Regence ID .... Scott Kreiling
President, Regence OR .... Jared L Short
Oregon Media Inquiries....................... Samantha Meese
503-225-5332
sxmeese@regence.com
Vice President.............................. Peggy Maguire

Specialty Managed Care Partners
Magellan, Ceres Behavioral, Advance Masters, Northwest Mental
Health, Alternare, Heart Masters

---

916 Samaritan Health Plan
815 Northwest 9th Street
Corvallis, OR 97330
Toll-Free: 800-832-4580
Phone: 541-768-4550
Fax: 541-768-4482
advantage@samhealth.org
www.samhealth.org/shplans
Mailing Address: PO Box 1510, Corvallis, OR 97339
Year Founded: 1993
Total Enrollment: 30,000
State Enrollment: 30,000

Healthplan and Services Defined
PLAN TYPE: Multiple
Benefits Offered: Chiropractic, Dental, Disease Management, Home
Care, Inpatient SNF, Physical Therapy, Podiatry, Prescription,
Psychiatric, Vision, Wellness

Type of Coverage
Individual, Medicare

Geographic Areas Served
Available within Oregon only

Subscriber Information
Average Monthly Fee Per Subscriber
(Employee + Employer Contribution):

Employee Only (Self): Varies
Medicare: Varies
Average Annual Deductible Per Subscriber:
Employee Only (Self): Varies
Medicare: Varies
Average Subscriber Co-Payment:
Primary Care Physician: Varies
Non-Network Physician: Varies
Prescription Drugs: Varies
Hospital ER: Varies
Home Health Care: Varies
Home Health Care Max. Days/Visits Covered: Varies
Nursing Home: Varies
Nursing Home Max. Days/Visits Covered: Varies

Key Personnel
President & CEO . . . . Larry A Mullins, DHA
Chief Executive Officer . . . . Kelley C Kaiser, MPH
Chief Operations Officer . . . . Kim R Whitley, MPA
CFO . . . . Ronald S Stevens, MBA
Medical Director . . . . Rick Wopat, MD

917   Trillium Community Health Plan

UO Riverfront Research Park
1800 Millrace Drive
Eugene, OR 97403
Toll-Free: 800-910-3906
Phone: 541-431-1950
Fax: 541-984-5685
customerservice@trilliumchp.com
www.trilliumchp.com
Mailing Address: PO Box 11756, Eugene, OR 97440-3956
Subsidiary of: Lane Individual Practice Association (LIPA)

Healthplan and Services Defined
PLAN TYPE: Medicare
Benefits Offered: Chiropractic, Dental, Disease Management, Home
Care, Inpatient SNF, Physical Therapy, Podiatry, Prescription,
Psychiatric, Vision, Wellness

Type of Coverage
Individual, Medicare, Sprout Healthy KidsConnect

Geographic Areas Served
Available within Oregon only

Subscriber Information
Average Monthly Fee Per Subscriber
(Employee + Employer Contribution):
Employee Only (Self): Varies
Medicare: Varies
Average Annual Deductible Per Subscriber:
Employee Only (Self): Varies
Medicare: Varies
Average Subscriber Co-Payment:
Primary Care Physician: Varies
Non-Network Physician: Varies
Prescription Drugs: Varies
Hospital ER: Varies
Home Health Care: Varies
Home Health Care Max. Days/Visits Covered: Varies
Nursing Home: Varies
Nursing Home Max. Days/Visits Covered: Varies

Key Personnel
President . . . . Thomas K Wuest, MD
Chief Financial Officer . . . . David L Cole
Chief Medical Officer . . . . Robert R Wheeler
Chief Admin Officer . . . . Kent M Noah
Governmental Affairs . . . . Rhonda J Busek
Secretary . . . . Terry W Coplin
Board of Directors/CEO . . . . Peter Fletcher Davidson
Board of Directors . . . . Dean Raymond Kortge
Board of Directors . . . . Mary Frances Theresa Spilde

Medicare Director . . . . Shannon Conley
Medical Directori . . . . John Sattenspiel
Medicare Compliance Dir . . . . Cheryl Lund
Enrollment Specialist . . . . Billie Stoltz
Claims Analyst . . . . Terri Maack

918   United Concordia: Oregon

121 Southwest Salmon Street
Suite 1132
Portland, OR 97024-2908
Toll-Free: 888-815-8224
Phone: 503-471-1449
Fax: 503-471-1442
ucproducer@ucci.com
www.secure.ucci.com
For Profit Organization: Yes
Year Founded: 1971
Number of Primary Care Physicians: 111,000
Total Enrollment: 8,000,000

Healthplan and Services Defined
PLAN TYPE: Dental
Plan Specialty: Dental
Benefits Offered: Dental

Type of Coverage
Commercial, Individual

Geographic Areas Served
Military personnel and their families, nationwide

919   UnitedHealthCare of Oregon

5 Centerpointe Drive
Suite 600
Lake Oswego, OR 97035
Toll-Free: 800-922-1444
www.uhc.com
Subsidiary of: UnitedHealth Group
For Profit Organization: Yes
Total Enrollment: 75,000,000
State Enrollment: 231,125

Healthplan and Services Defined
PLAN TYPE: HMO/PPO

Geographic Areas Served
Statewide

Key Personnel
Chief Executive Officer . . . . David Hansen
Marketing . . . . Lya Selby
Medical Director . . . . Roger Muller, MD
Media Contact . . . . Will Shanley
will.shanley@uhc.com

920   VSP: Vision Service Plan of Oregon

121 SW Morrison Street
Suite 1050
Portland, OR 97024
Toll-Free: 800-852-7600
Phone: 503-232-8187
webmaster@vsp.com
www.vsp.com
Year Founded: 1955
Number of Primary Care Physicians: 26,000
Total Enrollment: 55,000,000

Healthplan and Services Defined
PLAN TYPE: Vision
Plan Specialty: Vision
Benefits Offered: Vision

Type of Payment Plans Offered
Capitated

Geographic Areas Served
Statewide

Network Qualifications
Pre-Admission Certification: Yes

Peer Review Type
Utilization Review: Yes

Accreditation Certification
Utilization Review, Quality Assurance Program

Key Personnel
Manager.......................................Steve Hanks
Mgr Information Security ....Douglas Ljung
Manager....................................Jennifer Aberg

---

921 Willamette Dental Insurance

6950 NE Campus Way
Hillsboro, OR 97124
Toll-Free: 800-460-7644
Phone: 503-952-2000
Fax: 503-952-2200
info@willamettedental.com
www.willamettedental.com
Subsidiary of: Willamette Dental Group
For Profit Organization: Yes
Year Founded: 1970
Number of Primary Care Physicians: 245

Healthplan and Services Defined
PLAN TYPE: Dental
Model Type: Staff
Plan Specialty: Dental
Benefits Offered: Dental

Type of Payment Plans Offered
POS, FFS

Geographic Areas Served
Oregon: Washington: Idaho: Nevada

Network Qualifications
Pre-Admission Certification: Yes

Peer Review Type
Case Management: Yes

Publishes and Distributes Report Card: No

Key Personnel
President/CEO ....Steve Petruzelli
COO ....Yuen Chin
CFO ....Wee Chin
Marketing..................................Doug Wohlman
VP, Human Resources.......................Chris Holgerson
VP Marketing..............................Doug Wohlman
Information Services ....Don Mason
VP, Operations ....April Kniess

Specialty Managed Care Partners
Enters into Contracts with Regional Business Coalitions: No

Health Insurance Coverage Status and Type of Coverage by Age

Category	All Persons		Under 18 years		Under 65 years		65 years and over	
	Number	%	Number	%	Number	%	Number	%
Total population	12,569	-	2,709	-	10,558	-	2,011	-
Covered by some type of health insurance	11,347 (22)	90.3 (0.2)	2,562 (8)	94.6 (0.3)	9,348 (22)	88.5 (0.2)	1,999 (3)	99.4 (0.1)
Covered by private health insurance	9,075 (39)	72.2 (0.3)	1,742 (19)	64.3 (0.7)	7,654 (38)	72.5 (0.4)	1,422 (8)	70.7 (0.4)
Employment based	7,550 (36)	60.1 (0.3)	1,581 (18)	58.4 (0.7)	6,844 (35)	64.8 (0.3)	706 (10)	35.1 (0.5)
Direct purchase	1,800 (19)	14.3 (0.2)	173 (7)	6.4 (0.3)	946 (17)	9.0 (0.2)	854 (10)	42.5 (0.5)
Covered by TRICARE	167 (8)	1.3 (0.1)	25 (3)	0.9 (0.1)	102 (7)	1.0 (0.1)	65 (4)	3.2 (0.2)
Covered by government health insurance	4,057 (29)	32.3 (0.2)	962 (18)	35.5 (0.7)	2,108 (29)	20.0 (0.3)	1,949 (5)	96.9 (0.2)
Covered by Medicaid	2,086 (29)	16.6 (0.2)	956 (18)	35.3 (0.7)	1,854 (29)	17.6 (0.3)	232 (6)	11.5 (0.3)
Also by private insurance	408 (11)	3.2 (0.1)	141 (7)	5.2 (0.3)	286 (9)	2.7 (0.1)	122 (5)	6.1 (0.2)
Covered by Medicare	2,277 (9)	18.1 (0.1)	12 (2)	0.4 (0.1)	330 (9)	3.1 (0.1)	1,947 (5)	96.8 (0.2)
Also by private insurance	1,478 (10)	11.8 (0.1)	2 (1)	0.1 (0.1)	108 (5)	1.0 (0.1)	1,370 (8)	68.1 (0.4)
Also by Medicaid	392 (8)	3.1 (0.1)	7 (2)	0.2 (0.1)	160 (7)	1.5 (0.1)	232 (6)	11.5 (0.3)
Covered by VA Care	262 (6)	2.1 (0.1)	1 (1)	0.0 (0.1)	110 (5)	1.0 (0.1)	152 (4)	7.6 (0.2)
Not covered at any time during the year	1,222 (22)	9.7 (0.2)	147 (8)	5.4 (0.3)	1,211 (22)	11.5 (0.2)	12 (2)	0.6 (0.1)

Note: Numbers in thousands; Figures cover 2013; Margin of error appears in parenthesis; A "Z" indicates that the value either represents or rounds to zero.
Source: U.S. Census Bureau, 2013 American Community Survey, Table HI05. Health Insurance Coverage Status and Type of Coverage by State and Age for All People: 2013

Pennsylvania

922 Aetna Health of Pennsylvania

151 Farmington Avenue
Hartford, CT 06156
Toll-Free: 800-872-3862
Phone: 860-273-0123
www.aetna.com
For Profit Organization: Yes
Year Founded: 1987
Number of Affiliated Hospitals: 52
Number of Primary Care Physicians: 1,524
Number of Referral/Specialty Physicians: 3,928
Total Enrollment: 409,265
State Enrollment: 409,265

Healthplan and Services Defined
PLAN TYPE: HMO
Other Type: POS
Model Type: IPA
Benefits Offered: Disease Management, Prescription, Wellness
Offers Demand Management Patient Information Service: Yes

Geographic Areas Served
Statewide

Network Qualifications
Pre-Admission Certification: Yes

Peer Review Type
Utilization Review: Yes
Second Surgical Opinion: Yes
Case Management: Yes

Publishes and Distributes Report Card: Yes

Accreditation Certification
URAC, NCQA

Key Personnel
Chairman/CEO/President.....................Mark T Bertolini
EVP/General Counsel ....William J Casazza
EVP/CFO ....Shawn M Guertin

Specialty Managed Care Partners
Enters into Contracts with Regional Business Coalitions: Yes

923 American Health Care Group

1910 Cochran Road
Manor Oak One, Suite 405
Pittsburgh, PA 15220
Phone: 412-563-8800
Fax: 412-563-8319
info@american-healthcare.net
www.american-healthcare.net
For Profit Organization: Yes
Year Founded: 1996
Number of Affiliated Hospitals: 30
Total Enrollment: 60,000

Healthplan and Services Defined
PLAN TYPE: HMO/PPO
Model Type: Network
Plan Specialty: ASO, Chiropractic, Dental, MSO, Worker's
Compensation
Benefits Offered: Behavioral Health, Chiropractic, Complementary
Medicine, Dental, Disease Management, Home Care, Inpatient
SNF, Long-Term Care, Physical Therapy, Podiatry, Prescription,
Psychiatric, Transplant, Vision, Wellness, Worker's Compensation,
Offers a variety of
Offers Demand Management Patient Information Service: Yes
DMPI Services Offered: PPO Network, Workers Complaint,
Customize Network Development, Information Systems

Type of Payment Plans Offered
FFS

Geographic Areas Served
Pennsylvania, Eastern Ohio, Northwestern Virgina

Peer Review Type
Utilization Review: Yes
Second Surgical Opinion: Yes
Case Management: Yes

Accreditation Certification
State Licensure

Key Personnel
President/CEO ....Robert E Hagan Jr.
bhagan@american-healthcare.net
Chief medical Officer ....Joseph C. Maroon
Marketing Manager..........................Mary Double
mdouble@american-healthcare.net
Financial Operations ....Lynn Hagan
lhagan@american-healthcare.net
Chief Medical Officer ....Joseph C Maroon, MD
Medical Management Svcs ....Sarah Doyle Steranka
ssteranka@american-healthcare.net
Wellness Program Manager ....Liz Kanche
lhkanche@american-healthcare.net
Health Benefit Services ....Erin E Hart
ehart@american-healthcare.net

924 American WholeHealth Network

21251 Ridgetop Circle
Suite 150
Sterling, PA 20166
Toll-Free: 800-274-7526
Phone: 703-547-5100
Fax: 703-547-5573
ContactUs1@awhinc.com
www.americanwholehealth.com
Secondary Address: Healthways, Inc., 701 Cool Springs Blvd,
Franklin, TN 37067
Subsidiary of: Healthways, Inc.
For Profit Organization: Yes
Year Founded: 1975
Owned by an Integrated Delivery Network (IDN): Yes
Number of Referral/Specialty Physicians: 4,000
Total Enrollment: 3,100,000

Healthplan and Services Defined
PLAN TYPE: PPO
Model Type: IPA, Network
Plan Specialty: Chiropractic, MSO, Physical Therapy
Benefits Offered: Chiropractic, Complementary Medicine, Disease
Management, Physical Therapy, Wellness

Type of Payment Plans Offered
POS, DFFS, FFS

Geographic Areas Served
Arizona, California, Connecticut, Delaware, Florida, Georgia,
Massachusetts, Maryland, Minnesota, North Carolina, New Jersey,
Nevada, New York, Pennsylvania, Rhode Island, South Carolina,
Tennessee and Washington, DC

Subscriber Information
Average Monthly Fee Per Subscriber
(Employee + Employer Contribution):
Employee Only (Self): Varies
Employee & 1 Family Member: Varies
Employee & 2 Family Members: Varies
Medicare: Varies
Average Annual Deductible Per Subscriber:
Employee Only (Self): Varies
Employee & 1 Family Member: Varies
Employee & 2 Family Members: Varies
Medicare: Varies

Network Qualifications
Pre-Admission Certification: Yes

Peer Review Type
　Utilization Review: Yes
　Case Management: Yes

Accreditation Certification
　URAC
　Utilization Review, Pre-Admission Certification, Quality Assurance
　　Program

Key Personnel
　President and CEO . . . . William P Dorney, Dr
　VP/Operations . . . . Vincent J Love
　Controller . . . . Lori Piccioni
　Director . . . . Walter Channing, Jr
　Director . . . . H Tomkins O'Connor
　Director . . . . Sam Havens
　Information Technology . . . . Billie York
　Sales . . . . William Dorney, MD
　Media Contact . . . . Melissa Wyllie
　　615-614-4466
　　melissa.wyllie@healthways.com

Specialty Managed Care Partners
　Enters into Contracts with Regional Business Coalitions: Yes

---

925　Americhoice of Pennsylvania

The Wanamaker Building
100 Penn Square E, Suite 900
Philadelphia, PA 19107
Phone: 215-832-4500
Fax: 215-832-4644
www.americhoice.com
Subsidiary of: UnitedHealth Group
For Profit Organization: Yes
Year Founded: 1988
Number of Affiliated Hospitals: 42
Number of Primary Care Physicians: 1,100
Number of Referral/Specialty Physicians: 3,400
Total Enrollment: 71,000
State Enrollment: 110,736

Healthplan and Services Defined
　PLAN TYPE: Multiple
　Model Type: IPA
　Benefits Offered: Disease Management, Prescription, Wellness

Type of Coverage
　Medicare, Supplemental Medicare, Medicaid

Type of Payment Plans Offered
　DFFS, Capitated, Combination FFS & DFFS

Geographic Areas Served
　Bucks, Chester, Delaware, Montgomery & Philadelphia counties

Accreditation Certification
　NCQA
　TJC Accreditation, Medicare Approved, Utilization Review,
　　Pre-Admission Certification, State Licensure, Quality Assurance
　　Program

Key Personnel
　CEO . . . . Ernest Montiletto
　President . . . . Rick Jelinek
　Acting CFO . . . . Andy Bhugra

926　AmeriHealth Medicare Plan

1901 Market Street
Philadelphia, PA 19103-1480
Toll-Free: 866-681-7373
www.amerihealth.com/amerihealth65/index.html
Secondary Address: 580 Swedesford Road, Wayne, PA 19087

Healthplan and Services Defined
　PLAN TYPE: Medicare
　Other Type: POS

Benefits Offered: Chiropractic, Dental, Disease Management, Home
　Care, Inpatient SNF, Physical Therapy, Podiatry, Prescription,
　Psychiatric, Vision, Wellness

Type of Coverage
　Individual, Medicare

Geographic Areas Served
　Available within mutliple states

Subscriber Information
　Average Monthly Fee Per Subscriber
　　(Employee + Employer Contribution):
　　　Employee Only (Self): Varies
　　　Medicare: Varies
　Average Annual Deductible Per Subscriber:
　　　Employee Only (Self): Varies
　　　Medicare: Varies
　Average Subscriber Co-Payment:
　　　Primary Care Physician: Varies
　　　Non-Network Physician: Varies
　　　Prescription Drugs: Varies
　　　Hospital ER: Varies
　　　Home Health Care: Varies
　　　Home Health Care Max. Days/Visits Covered: Varies
　　　Nursing Home: Varies
　　　Nursing Home Max. Days/Visits Covered: Varies

Key Personnel
　President . . . . Judith Roman
　VP Provider Relations . . . . Paul E Portsmore, Jr
　CEO . . . . Joseph A Frick
　VP Deputy General Counsel . . . . Lilton R Taliaferro, Jr
　VP Marketing . . . . Susan L Sendlewski
　VP Medical Director . . . . Allan B Goldstein
　Media Contact . . . . Kate Wilhelmi
　　856-778-6552

927　Assurant Employee Benefits: Pennsylvania

676 Swedesford Road
Tredyffrin, PA 19312
Toll-Free: 800-373-1021
Phone: 484-254-9000
Fax: 412-921-7343
pittsburgh.rfp@assurant.com
www.assurantemployeebenefits.com
Subsidiary of: Assurant, Inc
For Profit Organization: Yes
Number of Primary Care Physicians: 112,000
Total Enrollment: 47,000

Healthplan and Services Defined
　PLAN TYPE: Multiple
　Plan Specialty: Dental, Vision, Long & Short-Term Disability
　Benefits Offered: Dental, Vision, Wellness, AD&D, Life, LTD, STD

Type of Coverage
　Commercial, Indemnity, Individual Dental Plans

Geographic Areas Served
　Statewide

Subscriber Information
　Average Monthly Fee Per Subscriber
　　(Employee + Employer Contribution):
　　　Employee Only (Self): Varies by plan

Key Personnel
　Manager . . . . Ray Brady
　PR Specialist . . . . Megan Hutchison
　　816-556-7815
　　megan.hutchison@assurant.com

928 Berkshire Health Partners

50 Commerce Drive
Wyomissing, PA 19610
Toll-Free: 800-647-2500
Phone: 610-372-8417
Fax: 484-334-7027
glounert@bhp.org
www.bhp.org
Non-Profit Organization: Yes
Year Founded: 1986
Physician Owned Organization: Yes
Number of Affiliated Hospitals: 16
Number of Primary Care Physicians: 825
Number of Referral/Specialty Physicians: 3,120
Total Enrollment: 60,353
State Enrollment: 60,353

Healthplan and Services Defined
 PLAN TYPE: PPO
 Model Type: Preferred Provider
 Plan Specialty: PPO
 Benefits Offered: Large provider network, claims repricing, case
  mgmt, wellness and disease mgmt and short term disability case
  mgmt

Type of Coverage
 Commercial, Individual, Indemnity, Catastrophic, Self-Funded -ASO,
  Fully-Insured
 Catastrophic Illness Benefit: Varies per case

Type of Payment Plans Offered
 FFS

Geographic Areas Served
 Berks, Upper Bucks, Lancaster, Lehigh, Montgomery, Northampton,
 Schuylkill counties in PA

Subscriber Information
 Average Monthly Fee Per Subscriber
  (Employee + Employer Contribution):
   Employee Only (Self): Varies
 Average Annual Deductible Per Subscriber:
   Employee Only (Self): Varies
   Employee & 2 Family Members: Varies
 Average Subscriber Co-Payment:
   Primary Care Physician: Varies
   Prescription Drugs: Varies
   Hospital ER: Varies
   Nursing Home Max. Days/Visits Covered: Varies

Peer Review Type
 Utilization Review: Yes
 Second Surgical Opinion: Yes
 Case Management: Yes

Accreditation Certification
 URAC, NCQA

Key Personnel
 President & CEO . . . . .Charles Wills
  610-372-8044
 Director Operations. . . . . .Tanya Glouner
 Claims Manager . . . . .Lori Calpino
 Marketing/Sales . . . . .Natalie Zimmerman
 Dir, Medical Management. . . . . .Dawn Dreibelbis
 Mgr, Medical Management .Robin Riegner
 Provider Services. . . . . .Tanya Glouner
 Dir, Business Development. . . . . .Natalie Zimmerman
  610-372-8044
  zimmermann@bhp.org

Specialty Managed Care Partners
 Enters into Contracts with Regional Business Coalitions: Yes
 PPHN, Unity

929 Blue Cross of Northeastern Pennsylvania

19 N Main Street
Wilkes Barre, PA 18711-0302
Toll-Free: 800-822-8753
Phone: 570-200-4300
Fax: 570-200-6888
www.bcnepa.com
Non-Profit Organization: Yes
Year Founded: 1938
Number of Affiliated Hospitals: 30
Total Enrollment: 550,000
State Enrollment: 550,000

Healthplan and Services Defined
 PLAN TYPE: HMO/PPO
 Other Type: EPO
 Model Type: IPA
 Plan Specialty: Dental, Vision
 Benefits Offered: Dental, Disease Management, Prescription, Vision,
  Wellness

Type of Coverage
 Commercial, Individual

Geographic Areas Served
 Northeast Pennsylvania

Network Qualifications
 Pre-Admission Certification: Yes

Peer Review Type
 Second Surgical Opinion: Yes

Publishes and Distributes Report Card: Yes

Accreditation Certification
 URAC, NCQA

Key Personnel
 CEO . . . . .Denise Cesare
 CFO. . . . . .Michael Gallagher
 COO . . . . .Cathy Stitzer
 VP of Customer Service . . . . .Edward Fennel
 Officer . . . . .Trish Savitsky
 Manager . . . . .Alan Pawlenok
 Information Technology. . . . . .Paul Fort
 Medical Affairs .Carmella Sabastian, MD
 Project Manager . . . . .Linda Moharsky

Specialty Managed Care Partners
 Enters into Contracts with Regional Business Coalitions: Yes

930 Blue Ridge Health Network

1500 W End Ave
Pottsville, PA 17901
Toll-Free: 800-730-0134
Phone: 570-628-1880
Fax: 570-628-1880
contact_us@blueridgehealthnetwork.com
www.blueridgehealthnetwork.com
Mailing Address: PO Box 674, Sch. Haven, PA 17972
Year Founded: 1995
Number of Affiliated Hospitals: 15
Number of Primary Care Physicians: 1,395
Number of Referral/Specialty Physicians: 5,125
Total Enrollment: 50,000
State Enrollment: 50,000

Healthplan and Services Defined
 PLAN TYPE: PPO
 Model Type: Network
 Plan Specialty: Advantage Plus
 Benefits Offered: Chiropractic, Prescription
 Offers Demand Management Patient Information Service: Yes

Type of Coverage
 Catastrophic Illness Benefit: Maximum $1M

Geographic Areas Served
Carbon, Lebanon, Monroe, Schuylkill, Luzerne, Columbia, Northumberland, Montour

Subscriber Information
Average Annual Deductible Per Subscriber:
Employee Only (Self): $500.00
Employee & 1 Family Member: $1000.00
Employee & 2 Family Members: $1000.00
Average Subscriber Co-Payment:
Primary Care Physician: $20.00-25.00
Non-Network Physician: 30%
Prescription Drugs: $15.00-40.00
Hospital ER: $50.00
Home Health Care: Yes
Home Health Care Max. Days/Visits Covered: 90 visits
Nursing Home: Yes
Nursing Home Max. Days/Visits Covered: 90 days

Network Qualifications
Pre-Admission Certification: Yes

Peer Review Type
Utilization Review: Yes
Second Surgical Opinion: No
Case Management: Yes

Accreditation Certification
TJC Accreditation, Medicare Approved, Utilization Review, Pre-Admission Certification, State Licensure, Quality Assurance Program

Key Personnel
President/CEO . . . . Robert Jones
CFO. . . . . Lisa A Laudeman

Average Claim Compensation
Physician's Fees Charged: 51%
Hospital's Fees Charged: 34%

Specialty Managed Care Partners
Enters into Contracts with Regional Business Coalitions: Yes

---

931 Bravo Health: Pennsylvania
1500 Spring Garden Street
Suite 800
Philadelphia, PA 19130
Toll-Free: 800-291-0396
www.bravohealth.com
Secondary Address: Foster Plaza - 5, 651 Holiday Drive, 4th Floor, Pittsburgh, PA 15220, 412-250-2424
Subsidiary of: Health Spring Co.
Year Founded: 1996
Number of Primary Care Physicians: 30,000
Total Enrollment: 360,000

Healthplan and Services Defined
PLAN TYPE: Medicare

Type of Coverage
Medicare, Supplemental Medicare

Geographic Areas Served
Delaware, Maryland, Pennslyvania, Texas, Washington DC, New Jersey

Key Personnel
SVP, Executive Director . . . . Jason Feuerman

---

932 Capital Blue Cross
2500 Elmerton Avenue
Harrisburg, PA 17177
Toll-Free: 800-962-2242
Phone: 717-541-7000
Fax: 717-541-6915
www.capbluecross.com
Secondary Address: 1221 West Hamilton Street, Allentown, PA 18101

Non-Profit Organization: Yes
Year Founded: 1938
Number of Affiliated Hospitals: 37
Number of Primary Care Physicians: 11,000
Total Enrollment: 121,000
State Enrollment: 116,465

Healthplan and Services Defined
PLAN TYPE: HMO/PPO
Benefits Offered: Home Care, Inpatient SNF, Physical Therapy, Prescription, Psychiatric, Transplant, Wellness

Type of Coverage
Commercial

Type of Payment Plans Offered
FFS

Geographic Areas Served
A 21-county area in central Pennsylvania and the Lehigh Valley

Peer Review Type
Second Surgical Opinion: Yes
Case Management: Yes

Accreditation Certification
TJC Accreditation, Medicare Approved, Utilization Review, Pre-Admission Certification, State Licensure, Quality Assurance Program

Key Personnel
Chief Executive Officer . . . . William Lehr, Jr
Sr Exec Vice President . . . . Ronald Drnevich
Pres, Capital BlueCross. . . . . Gary St. Hilaire
SVP, Sales & Marketing . . . . Marc Backon
Media Relations Spec. . . . . Joe Butera
717-541-6139
joe.butera@capbluecross.com

---

933 Central Susquehanna Healthcare Providers
1 Hospital Drive
Lewisburg, PA 17837
Toll-Free: 866-890-2747
Phone: 570-522-4034
Fax: 570-768-3911
kwagner2@evanhospital.com
www.cshpnetwork.com
Subsidiary of: Evangelical Community Hosptial
Non-Profit Organization: Yes
Year Founded: 1987
Number of Affiliated Hospitals: 8
Number of Primary Care Physicians: 274
Number of Referral/Specialty Physicians: 825
Total Enrollment: 12,700
State Enrollment: 12,700

Healthplan and Services Defined
PLAN TYPE: PPO
Model Type: Network
Benefits Offered: Behavioral Health, Home Care, Inpatient SNF, Long-Term Care, Physical Therapy, Podiatry, Prescription, Psychiatric, Transplant, Vision, Wellness

Type of Coverage
Commercial, Individual, Indemnity, Medicaid
Catastrophic Illness Benefit: Maximum $2M

Type of Payment Plans Offered
DFFS, Combination FFS & DFFS

Geographic Areas Served
Central Pennsylvania

Network Qualifications
Pre-Admission Certification: No

Key Personnel
Director. . . . . Kelly Geise

Director. . . . . .Kelly Geise
   570-522-4035
   kgeise@evanhospital.com
Contract Analyst . . . . .Rahmaire Brooks
   570-522-4073
   rbrooks@evanhospital.com
Credentialing . . . . .Lisa Featherman
   570-522-2798
   lfeatherman@evanhospital.com
Managed Care Coordinator . . . . .Renee Ferry
   570-522-4034
   rferry@evanhospital.com
Media Contact . . . . .Liz Hendricks
   570-522-4160
   lhendricks@evanhospital.com

Average Claim Compensation
   Physician's Fees Charged: 25%
   Hospital's Fees Charged: 16%

934   CIGNA HealthCare of Pennsylvania

1 Beaver Valley Road
Wilmington, PA 19803-1115
Toll-Free: 800-345-9458
Phone: 215-283-3300
Fax: 215-283-3920
www.cigna.com
Secondary Address: 3101 Park Lane Drive, Pittsburgh, PA 15272,
   412-747-4410
For Profit Organization: Yes
Federally Qualified: Yes
Total Enrollment: 143,488
State Enrollment: 13

Healthplan and Services Defined
   PLAN TYPE: HMO
   Model Type: IPA, Group, Network
   Benefits Offered: Disease Management, Prescription, Transplant,
     Wellness

Type of Coverage
   Commercial

Publishes and Distributes Report Card: Yes

Accreditation Certification
   NCQA
   TJC Accreditation, Medicare Approved, Utilization Review,
     Pre-Admission Certification, State Licensure, Quality Assurance
     Program

Key Personnel
   President/CEO. . . . . .Mitchell T.G. Graye
   In House Formulary . . . . .David Burton
   Materials Management . . . . .Jim Hicks
   Medical Affairs. . . . . .John Tudor, MD
   Member Services. . . . . .Martha Spoor
   Provider Services. . . . . .Josh Nelson
   Sales . . . . .Robert Immitt

935   CIGNA: Corporate Headquarters

1601 Chestnut Street
Philadelphia, PA 19192
Toll-Free: 866-438-2446
Phone: 610-250-1600
www.cigna.com
For Profit Organization: Yes
Year Founded: 1982
Number of Affiliated Hospitals: 5,400
Number of Primary Care Physicians: 612,000
Total Enrollment: 11,000,000
State Enrollment: 11,969

Healthplan and Services Defined
   PLAN TYPE: HMO
   Other Type: POS
   Benefits Offered: Disease Management, Transplant, Wellness

Type of Coverage
   Commercial

Type of Payment Plans Offered
   POS

Geographic Areas Served
   Nationwide and international

Publishes and Distributes Report Card: Yes

Key Personnel
   President & CEO. . . . . .David M Cordani
   President, CIGNA Intl. . . . . .William L Atwell
   President, US Service. . . . . .Matthew G Manders
   Acting CFO . . . . .Thomas A McCarthy
   EVP, Human Resources . . . . .John M Murabito
   EVP, General Counsel. . . . . .Carol Ann Petren
   President, US Commercial .Bertram Scott
   EVP, Chief Information Of. . . . . .Michael D Woeller
   VP, Chief Accounting Offc . . . . .Marty T Hoeltzel

936   CoreSource: Pennsylvania

1280 North Plum Street
Lancaster, PA 17601
Toll-Free: 800-223-3943
Phone: 717-295-9201
www.coresource.com
Subsidary of: Trustmark
Year Founded: 1980
Total Enrollment: 1,100,000

Healthplan and Services Defined
   PLAN TYPE: Multiple
   Other Type: TPA
   Model Type: Network
   Plan Specialty: Claims Administration, TPA
   Benefits Offered: Behavioral Health, Home Care, Prescription,
     Transplant

Type of Coverage
   Commercial

Geographic Areas Served
   Nationwide

Accreditation Certification
   Utilization Review, Pre-Admission Certification

Key Personnel
   President . . . . .Nancy Ekrich
   Chief Operating Officer . . . . .Lloyd Sarrel
   VP, Chief Financial Offic. . . . . .Clare Smith
   VP, Healthcare Management. . . . . .Donna Heiser
   VP, Product Management & . . . . .Rob Corrigan
   VP, Product Development & . . . . .Steve Horvath

937   Delta Dental of the Mid-Atlantic

One Delta Drive
Mechanicsburg, PA 17055-6999
Toll-Free: 800-932-0783
Fax: 717-766-8719
www.deltadentalins.com
Non-Profit Organization: Yes
Total Enrollment: 54,000,000

Healthplan and Services Defined
   PLAN TYPE: Dental
   Other Type: Dental PPO

Type of Coverage
   Commercial

Geographic Areas Served
Statewide

Key Personnel
President/CEO...............................Gary D Radine
VP, Public & Govt Affairs ....Jeff Album
   415-972-8418
Dir/Media & Public Affair...................Elizabeth Risberg
   415-972-8423

938   Devon Health Services

1100 First Avenue
Suite 100
King of Prussia, PA 19406
Toll-Free: 800-431-2273
Fax: 800-221-0002
dbehuniak@devonhealth.com
www.devonhealth.com
For Profit Organization: Yes
Year Founded: 1991
Physician Owned Organization: Yes
Number of Affiliated Hospitals: 675
Number of Primary Care Physicians: 20,000
Number of Referral/Specialty Physicians: 325,000
Total Enrollment: 3,000,000
State Enrollment: 3,000,000

Healthplan and Services Defined
  PLAN TYPE: PPO
  Model Type: Network
  Plan Specialty: Chiropractic, Dental, Lab, Vision, Radiology,
    Worker's Compensation, Group Health & Pharmacy Plans
  Benefits Offered: Dental, Inpatient SNF, Physical Therapy, Vision,
    Worker's Compensation, Group Health & Pharmacy Plans

Type of Coverage
Commercial

Type of Payment Plans Offered
DFFS, FFS, Combination FFS & DFFS

Geographic Areas Served
Pennsylvania, New Jersey, New York, Ohio, Delaware and Maryland

Subscriber Information
Average Subscriber Co-Payment:
    Primary Care Physician: $10.00-20.00
    Hospital ER: $25-50.00
    Home Health Care: Varies
    Nursing Home: Varies

Network Qualifications
Pre-Admission Certification: Yes

Publishes and Distributes Report Card: No

Key Personnel
President ....Charles Falcone
   800-431-2273
CEO ....John A Bennett, MD
   800-431-2273
Chief Legal Counsel ....Galen Hawk
VP Operations................................Andrea Fisher
   800-431-2273
VP, Network Development........................Bill Bruce
   800-431-2273
VP, Client Services ....Mike Tosti
   800-431-2273
Chief Financial Officer.........................Francis Lutz
VP, Sales.......................................Jeff Penn
   800-431-2273
Dir, Marketing & Comm ....Darren Behuniak
   800-431-2273
   dbehuniak@devonhealth.com

Average Claim Compensation
Physician's Fees Charged: 55%

Hospital's Fees Charged: 58%

Specialty Managed Care Partners
Medimpact
Enters into Contracts with Regional Business Coalitions: Yes

Employer References
Mid-Jersey trucking Industry & Local 701 Welfare Fund,
   Pennsylvania Public School Health Care Trust, International
   Brotherhood of Teamsters

939   eHealthInsurance Services Inc.

11919 Foundation Place
Gold River, CA 95670
Toll-Free: 800-644-3491
webmaster@healthinsurance.com
www.e.healthinsurance.com
Year Founded: 1997

Healthplan and Services Defined
  PLAN TYPE: HMO/PPO
  Benefits Offered: Dental, Life, STD

Type of Coverage
Commercial, Individual, Medicare

Geographic Areas Served
All 50 states in the USA and District of Columbia

Key Personnel
Chairman & CEO ....Gary L. Lauer
EVP/Business & Corp. Dev.....................Bruce Telkamp
EVP/Chief Technology...................Dr. Sheldon X. Wang
SVP & CFO ....Stuart M. Huizinga
Pres. of eHealth Gov. Sys ....Samuel C. Gibbs
SVP of Sales & Operations ....Robert S. Hurley
Director Public Relations.......................Nate Purpura
   650-210-3115

940   EHP

PO Box 7777
Lancaster, PA 17604-7777
Toll-Free: 888-498-9648
Phone: 717-735-7760
Fax: 717-399-1693
kwilliams@significabenefits.com
www.ehpservices.com
Subsidiary of: Significa Insurance Group
Non-Profit Organization: Yes
Year Founded: 1996
Number of Affiliated Hospitals: 179
Number of Primary Care Physicians: 49,000

Healthplan and Services Defined
  PLAN TYPE: PPO
  Plan Specialty: Offers EHP Healthy Benefits including discounts for
    members to health clubs.
  Benefits Offered: Disease Management, Wellness

Geographic Areas Served
Berks, Lancaster & York counties

Subscriber Information
Average Monthly Fee Per Subscriber
   (Employee + Employer Contribution):
    Employee Only (Self): $3.00

Key Personnel
President/CEO ....Larry W Rodabaugh
Provider Services ....Kris Danz

941 EHP Signifia

PO Box 7777
Lancaster, PA 17604-7777
Toll-Free: 800-433-3746
Phone: 717-581-1300
info@significa-ins.com
www.ehpsignifica.com
Subsidiary of: Significa Insurance Group
Non-Profit Organization: Yes
Number of Affiliated Hospitals: 179
Number of Primary Care Physicians: 49,000

Healthplan and Services Defined
  PLAN TYPE: PPO

Type of Coverage
  Commercial

942 First Priority Health

19 N Main Street
Wilkes Barre, PA 18711-0302
Toll-Free: 800-822-8753
www.bcnepa.com
Subsidiary of: Blue Cross of Northeastern Pennsylvania
Acquired by: Blue Cross of NE Pennsylvania
Non-Profit Organization: Yes
Year Founded: 1986
Number of Affiliated Hospitals: 36
Number of Primary Care Physicians: 637
Total Enrollment: 115,400

Healthplan and Services Defined
  PLAN TYPE: HMO
  Model Type: IPA
  Benefits Offered: Disease Management, Prescription, Wellness, Case
    Management

Type of Coverage
  Catastrophic Illness Benefit: Unlimited

Geographic Areas Served
  Bradford, Clinton, Lackawanna, Luzerne, Lycoming, Monroe, Pike,
    Sullivan, Susquehanna, Carbon, Tioga, Wayne & Wyoming counties

Publishes and Distributes Report Card: Yes

Accreditation Certification
  URAC, NCQA

Key Personnel
  President/CEO . . . . .Thomas Ward
  VP/Marketing and Sales. . . . . .William Phelps
  VP/COO. . . . . .Denise Cesare
  Senior VP/Treasurer. . . . . .Michael Gallagher, Sr
  VP/Medical Affairs . . . . .Edward Rolde, MD

Specialty Managed Care Partners
  Express Scripts, Inc, Community Behavioral Healthcare of
    Northeastern Pennsylvania
  Enters into Contracts with Regional Business Coalitions: Yes

943 Gateway Health Plan

Four Gateway Center
444 Liberty Ave, Suite 2100
Pittsburgh, PA 15222-1222
Toll-Free: 877-428-3929
Phone: 412-255-4640
Fax: 412-255-4670
www.gatewayhealthplan.com
For Profit Organization: Yes
Year Founded: 1992
Number of Affiliated Hospitals: 135
Number of Primary Care Physicians: 8,000
Number of Referral/Specialty Physicians: 4,650

Total Enrollment: 244,000
State Enrollment: 244,000

Healthplan and Services Defined
  PLAN TYPE: HMO
  Other Type: Medicaid
  Model Type: Network
  Plan Specialty: Dental, Disease Management, Vision, UR, Prospective
    Care Managment
  Benefits Offered: Chiropractic, Dental, Disease Management, Home
    Care, Inpatient SNF, Physical Therapy, Podiatry, Prescription,
    Transplant, Vision, Wellness

Type of Coverage
  Medicare, Medicaid

Type of Payment Plans Offered
  DFFS, Capitated, FFS

Geographic Areas Served
  Allegheny, Armstrong, Beaver, Berks, Blair, Butler, Cambria, Clarion,
    Cumberland, Dauphin, Erie, Fayette, Greene, Indiana, Jefferson,
    Lawrence, Lehigh, Mercer, Montour, Northumberland, Schulkill,
    Somerset, Washington and Westmoreland counties

Peer Review Type
  Utilization Review: Yes
  Second Surgical Opinion: Yes
  Case Management: Yes

Accreditation Certification
  NCQA
  Utilization Review, State Licensure, Quality Assurance Program

Key Personnel
  President/CEO . . . . .Michael Blackwood
  Physician Advisor. . . . . .Ronald Mohan, MD
  Medical Director . . . . .Maria E Moutinho, MD
  Pediatric Physician Adv . . . . .Barbara Negrini, MD
  Chief Medical Officer . . . . .Michael Madden, MD
  Medical Director . . . . .Caesar A DeLeo, MD
  Physician Advisor . . . . .Shawn C Files, MD
  Medical Director. . . . . .Edwin J Kairis, MD
  Medical Director . . . . .Renee Miskimmin, MD

Specialty Managed Care Partners
  Clarity Vision, Dental Benefit Providers, National Imaging
    Association, Merck-Medco

944 Geisinger Health Plan

100 North Academy Avenue
Danville, PA 17822-3040
Toll-Free: 800-498-9731
Phone: 570-271-8771
Fax: 570-271-7218
media@thehealthplan.com
www.thehealthplan.com
Mailing Address: PO Box 8200, Danville, PA 17821-8200
Non-Profit Organization: Yes
Year Founded: 1985
Number of Affiliated Hospitals: 104
Number of Primary Care Physicians: 4,426
Number of Referral/Specialty Physicians: 39,423
Total Enrollment: 290,000

Healthplan and Services Defined
  PLAN TYPE: HMO/PPO
  Benefits Offered: Chiropractic, Dental, Disease Management, Home
    Care, Inpatient SNF, Physical Therapy, Podiatry, Prescription,
    Psychiatric, Vision, Wellness

Type of Coverage
  Commercial, Individual, Medicare, Supplemental Medicare, CHIP

Geographic Areas Served
  Adams, Bedford, Berks, Blair, Bradford, Cambria, Cameron, Carbon,
    Centre, Clearfield, Clinton, Columbia, Cumberland, Dauphin, Elk,
    Fulton, Huntingdon, Jefferson, Juanita, Lackawanna, Lancaster,

Lebanon, Lehigh, Luzerne, Lycoming, Miffin, Monroe, Montour, Northumberland, Northampton, Perry, Pike, Potter, Schuyikill, Somerset, Snyder, Sullivan, Susquehana, Tioga, Union, Wayne, York counties

Subscriber Information
Average Monthly Fee Per Subscriber
(Employee + Employer Contribution):
Employee Only (Self): Varies
Medicare: Varies
Average Annual Deductible Per Subscriber:
Employee Only (Self): Varies
Medicare: Varies
Average Subscriber Co-Payment:
Primary Care Physician: Varies
Non-Network Physician: Varies
Prescription Drugs: Varies
Hospital ER: Varies
Home Health Care: Varies
Home Health Care Max. Days/Visits Covered: Varies
Nursing Home: Varies
Nursing Home Max. Days/Visits Covered: Varies

Accreditation Certification
NCQA

Key Personnel
CEO ....Jean Haynes, RN
COO ....Richard Kwei
CFO................................George Schneider, CPA
VP, Chief Medical Offc ....Duane E Davis, MD
Assoc Chief Legal Officer.................David J Weader, JD
Chief Sales Officer ....Joseph Haddock, MHA
Dir, Group & Brand Mktg.....................Lisa D Hartman
570-271-8135

945 Great-West Healthcare Pennsylvania
1023 E Baltimore Pike
#200
Media, NJ 19063-5126
Toll-Free: 866-494-2111
Phone: 610-566-1316
eliginquiries@cigna.com
www.cignaforhealth.com
Subsidiary of: CIGNA HealthCare
Acquired by: CIGNA
For Profit Organization: Yes
Total Enrollment: 26,411
State Enrollment: 21,997

Healthplan and Services Defined
PLAN TYPE: HMO/PPO
Benefits Offered: Disease Management, Prescription, Wellness

Type of Coverage
Commercial

Type of Payment Plans Offered
POS, FFS

Geographic Areas Served
Pennsylvania

Accreditation Certification
URAC

Specialty Managed Care Partners
Caremark Rx

946 Health Partners Medicare Plan
901 Market Street
Suite 500
Philadelphia, PA 19107
Toll-Free: 800-883-2177
Phone: 952-883-5000
contact@healthpart.com
www.healthpart.com
Non-Profit Organization: Yes
Physician Owned Organization: Yes
Total Enrollment: 170,000
State Enrollment: 170,000

Healthplan and Services Defined
PLAN TYPE: Medicare
Benefits Offered: Chiropractic, Dental, Disease Management, Home Care, Inpatient SNF, Physical Therapy, Podiatry, Prescription, Psychiatric, Vision, Wellness

Type of Coverage
Medicare, Medicaid

Geographic Areas Served
Available within Pennsylvania only

Subscriber Information
Average Monthly Fee Per Subscriber
(Employee + Employer Contribution):
Employee Only (Self): Varies
Medicare: Varies
Average Annual Deductible Per Subscriber:
Employee Only (Self): Varies
Medicare: Varies
Average Subscriber Co-Payment:
Primary Care Physician: Varies
Non-Network Physician: Varies
Prescription Drugs: Varies
Hospital ER: Varies
Home Health Care: Varies
Home Health Care Max. Days/Visits Covered: Varies
Nursing Home: Varies
Nursing Home Max. Days/Visits Covered: Varies

Key Personnel
President/CEO ....William George
SVP/COO ....Elaine Markezin
SVP Business Development ....Judy B Harrington
SVP/Compliance/Resources ....Vicki Sessoms
SVP/Pharmacy Business ....Don Daddario
SVP/Operations ....Debra A Kircher
SVP/Chief Medical Officer ....Mary K Stom, MD
SVP, CFO....................................Martin J Brill
Senior Communications Spc.................Felicia R Phillips
215-991-4580
fphillips@healthpart.com

947 HealthAmerica
100 State St
Erie, PA 16501
Toll-Free: 800-255-4281
Phone: 814-878-1700
Fax: 814-878-1820
www.healthamerica.cvty.com
Secondary Address: 3721 TecPort Drive, PO Box 67103, Harrisburg, PA 17106-6445
Subsidiary of: A Coventry Health Care Plan
For Profit Organization: Yes
Year Founded: 1994
Number of Affiliated Hospitals: 36
Number of Primary Care Physicians: 370
Number of Referral/Specialty Physicians: 605
Total Enrollment: 500,000
State Enrollment: 395,000

Healthplan and Services Defined
  PLAN TYPE: Multiple
  Other Type: HMO, POS, Medicare
  Model Type: IPA, Network
  Plan Specialty: ASO, Behavioral Health, Disease Management
  Benefits Offered: Chiropractic, Dental, Disease Management, Home
    Care, Inpatient SNF, Physical Therapy, Podiatry, Prescription,
    Psychiatric, Transplant, Vision, Wellness

Type of Coverage
  Commercial, Indemnity
  Catastrophic Illness Benefit: Maximum $1M

Type of Payment Plans Offered
  POS, DFFS, Capitated, Combination FFS & DFFS

Geographic Areas Served
  Pennsylvania and Ohio

Subscriber Information
  Average Monthly Fee Per Subscriber
    (Employee + Employer Contribution):
      Employee Only (Self): $170.42
      Employee & 1 Family Member: $525.00
      Employee & 2 Family Members: $525.00
  Average Subscriber Co-Payment:
      Primary Care Physician: $10.00
      Prescription Drugs: $10.00/25.00
      Hospital ER: $35.00
      Nursing Home: $0

Network Qualifications
  Minimum Years of Practice: 3
  Pre-Admission Certification: Yes

Peer Review Type
  Utilization Review: Yes
  Second Surgical Opinion: Yes
  Case Management: Yes

Accreditation Certification
  NCQA, 3yr excellent

Key Personnel
  President...........................Thomas P McDonough
  Executive VP ....Harvey C DeMovick, Jr
  CEO...................................Dale B Wolf
  Executive VP/CFO.......................Shawn M Guertin
  Marketing ....Alfred Dore, Jr
  Medical Affairs...........................John Bauers, MD
  Director Health Plan Operations ....Patricia Carns
  Information Systems.........................Patricia Carns
  Provider Services ....Patricia Carns

Specialty Managed Care Partners
  Enters into Contracts with Regional Business Coalitions: Yes

---

948 HealthAmerica Pennsylvania

3721 TecPort Drive
PO Box 67103
Harrisburg, PA 17106-7103
Toll-Free: 800-788-7895
Phone: 717-540-4260
http://healthamerica.coventryhealthcare.com
Secondary Address: 11 Stanwix Street, Suite 2300, Pittsburgh, PA
  15222
Subsidiary of: Coventry Health Care
For Profit Organization: Yes
Year Founded: 1974
Owned by an Integrated Delivery Network (IDN): Yes
Number of Affiliated Hospitals: 127
Number of Primary Care Physicians: 3,915
Number of Referral/Specialty Physicians: 8,358
Total Enrollment: 500,000
State Enrollment: 395,000

Healthplan and Services Defined
  PLAN TYPE: Multiple
  Model Type: Network
  Plan Specialty: ASO, Behavioral Health, Chiropractic, Dental,
    Disease Management, Lab, Vision, Radiology
  Benefits Offered: Behavioral Health, Chiropractic, Complementary
    Medicine, Dental, Disease Management, Home Care, Inpatient
    SNF, Physical Therapy, Podiatry, Prescription, Psychiatric,
    Transplant, Vision, Wellness
  Offers Demand Management Patient Information Service: Yes

Type of Coverage
  Commercial, Medicare, Medicaid

Type of Payment Plans Offered
  Capitated, FFS

Geographic Areas Served
  Central Pennsylvania-Clinton, Lycomuing, Centre, Blair, Huntington,
    Franklin, Adams, Cumberland, Perry, Juniata, Mifflin, Union, Snyder,
    Dauphin, York, Northumberland, Erie, Crawford, Warren, Venangom,
    Forest; Ohio-Thumbull, Mahoning, Columbiana, Jefferson, Harrison,
    Belmont

Subscriber Information
  Average Monthly Fee Per Subscriber
    (Employee + Employer Contribution):
      Employee Only (Self): Proprietary
      Employee & 1 Family Member: Proprietary
      Employee & 2 Family Members: Proprietary
      Medicare: Proprietary
  Average Annual Deductible Per Subscriber:
      Employee Only (Self): Proprietary
      Employee & 1 Family Member: Proprietary
      Employee & 2 Family Members: Proprietary
      Medicare: Proprietary
  Average Subscriber Co-Payment:
      Primary Care Physician: $10.00
      Non-Network Physician: $20.00
      Prescription Drugs: $10.00/20.00
      Hospital ER: Varies
      Home Health Care Max. Days/Visits Covered: 120
      Nursing Home Max. Days/Visits Covered: 100

Network Qualifications
  Pre-Admission Certification: Yes

Peer Review Type
  Utilization Review: Yes
  Case Management: Yes

Accreditation Certification
  TJC, NCQA
  Medicare Approved, Utilization Review, Pre-Admission Certification,
    State Licensure, Quality Assurance Program

Key Personnel
  CEO.....................................Timothy E Nolan
  Executive VP ....Mary Lou Osborne
  CFO......................................Stephen Dengler
  VP/Sales ....Darin Hayes
  VP/Health Services ....Angel Oddo
  VP/Quality and Cost Mgmt ....Joshua Bennett, MD
  Regional Director NWPA ....Eric Hays
  VP/Medical Affairs ....Eugene Sun, MD
  VP/Medicare Operations ....Pauline Degenfelder
  VP Business Development ....Jayne Olshanski

Specialty Managed Care Partners
  ValueOptions, CareMark, Dominion Dental (WPA) Delta Dental
    (EPA), Quest Diagnostics (EPA) LabCorp (WPA), National Vision
    Administrators (NVA)

Employer References
  Federal Government, Penn State University, US Airways, City of
    Pittsburgh, General Motors

949   Highmark Blue Cross & Blue Shield

501 Penn Avenue Place
Pittsburgh, PA 15222-3099
Toll-Free: 800-294-9568
Phone: 412-544-7000
Fax: 412-544-8368
cynthia.dellecker@highmark.com
www.highmarkbcbs.com
Mailing Address: PO Box 226, Pittsburgh, PA 15222
For Profit Organization: Yes
Year Founded: 1996
Owned by an Integrated Delivery Network (IDN): Yes
Number of Affiliated Hospitals: 50
Number of Primary Care Physicians: 1,200
Number of Referral/Specialty Physicians: 4,552
Total Enrollment: 4,900,000
State Enrollment: 4,900,000

Healthplan and Services Defined
  PLAN TYPE: HMO/PPO
  Model Type: IPA
  Benefits Offered: Dental, Disease Management, Prescription, Vision,
    Wellness
  Offers Demand Management Patient Information Service: Yes

Type of Coverage
  Commercial, Individual
  Catastrophic Illness Benefit: Unlimited

Type of Payment Plans Offered
  POS, DFFS, Capitated, FFS, Combination FFS & DFFS

Geographic Areas Served
  Allegheny, Armstrong, Beaver, Bedford, Blair, Butler, Cambria,
  Clarion, Clearfield, Crawford, Erie, Fayette, Forest, Greene,
  Huntingdon, Indiana, Jefferson, Lawrence, McKean, Mercer,
  Somerset, Venango, Washington, Cameron, Elk, Potter, Warren and
  Westmoreland counties

Subscriber Information
  Average Monthly Fee Per Subscriber
    (Employee + Employer Contribution):
      Employee Only (Self): $205.00
      Employee & 1 Family Member: $620.00
      Employee & 2 Family Members: $470.00
      Medicare: $39.50
  Average Annual Deductible Per Subscriber:
      Employee Only (Self): $0
      Employee & 1 Family Member: $0
      Employee & 2 Family Members: $0
      Medicare: $0
  Average Subscriber Co-Payment:
      Primary Care Physician: $5.00
      Non-Network Physician: $0
      Prescription Drugs: $2.00/8.00
      Hospital ER: $25.00
      Home Health Care: $0
      Home Health Care Max. Days/Visits Covered: Varies
      Nursing Home: $0
      Nursing Home Max. Days/Visits Covered: 100 days

Network Qualifications
  Pre-Admission Certification: Yes

Peer Review Type
  Utilization Review: Yes
  Second Surgical Opinion: No
  Case Management: Yes

Publishes and Distributes Report Card: No

Accreditation Certification
  URAC, NCQA
  Medicare Approved, Pre-Admission Certification, State Licensure

Key Personnel
  Chairman of the Board.....................J Robert Baum, PhD
  President/CEO.........................Kenneth R Melani, MD

  EVP, Chief Financial Offc ....Nanette P DeTurk
  EVP, Chief Legal Officer......................Maureen Hogel
  EVP, Vision Services ....David L Holmberg
  EVP, Government Services...................David M O'Brien
  SVP, Chief Audit Exec...................Elizabeth A Farbacher
  EVP, Comm & Strategy ....Thomas Kerr
  EVP, Subsidiary Business ....Daniel J Lebish
  EVP, Health Services......................Deborah L Rice
  Client Svcs, Enrollment ....Nadina Bowman
  Provider Relations ....Bill Jarrett
  Public Relations ....Aaron Billger
    412-544-7826
    aaron.billger@highmark.com

Average Claim Compensation
  Physician's Fees Charged: 50%
  Hospital's Fees Charged: 61%

Specialty Managed Care Partners
  Enters into Contracts with Regional Business Coalitions: No

950   Highmark Blue Shield

1800 Center Street
Camp Hill, PA 17011
Toll-Free: 866-856-6166
Phone: 412-544-7000
webmaster@highmark.com
www.highmarkblueshield.com
Mailing Address: PO Box 890173, Camp Hill, PA 17089-0173
Non-Profit Organization: Yes
Year Founded: 1932
Total Enrollment: 600,000
State Enrollment: 375,300

Healthplan and Services Defined
  PLAN TYPE: PPO
  Model Type: Network
  Benefits Offered: Disease Management, Prescription, Wellness
  Offers Demand Management Patient Information Service: Yes

Type of Payment Plans Offered
  POS, DFFS, Combination FFS & DFFS

Geographic Areas Served
  Statewide

Network Qualifications
  Pre-Admission Certification: Yes

Peer Review Type
  Second Surgical Opinion: Yes

Publishes and Distributes Report Card: Yes

Accreditation Certification
  URAC, NCQA

Key Personnel
  President ....Deborah L. Rice-Johnson, MD
  Treasurer ....Nanette P. DeTurk
  Secretary ....Thomas L. VanKirk
  EVP, Chief Financial Offc ....Nanette P DeTurk
  EVP, Vision Services ....David L Holmberg
  EVP/Government Services...................David M O'Brien
  SVP/Chief Auditor ....Elizabeth A Farbacher
  EVP/Chief Strategy Offc ....Thomas Kerr
  EVP/Subsidiary Business......................Daniel J Lebish
  EVP/Health Services.........................Deborah L Rice
  Public Relations ....Aaron Billger
    412-544-7826
    aaron.billger@highmark.com
  Corp Media Relations......................Michael Weinstein
    412-544-7903
    michael.weinstein@highmark.com

Specialty Managed Care Partners
  Enters into Contracts with Regional Business Coalitions: Yes

951 Humana Health Insurance of Pennsylvania
5000 Ritter Road
Suite 101
Mechanicsburg, PA 17055
Phone: 717-766-6040
Fax: 717-795-1951
www.humana.com
For Profit Organization: Yes

Healthplan and Services Defined
PLAN TYPE: HMO/PPO

Type of Coverage
Commercial, Individual

Accreditation Certification
URAC, NCQA, CORE

952 Independence Blue Cross
1901 Market Street
Philadelphia, PA 19103
Toll-Free: 800-275-2583
Phone: 215-241-2920
www.ibx.com
Non-Profit Organization: Yes
Year Founded: 1938
Number of Affiliated Hospitals: 159
Number of Primary Care Physicians: 38,053
Total Enrollment: 3,300,000
State Enrollment: 3,300,000

Healthplan and Services Defined
PLAN TYPE: HMO/PPO
Other Type: POS
Benefits Offered: Dental, Disease Management, Prescription, Vision, Wellness, Life

Type of Coverage
Commercial, Individual, Medicare, Supplemental Medicare

Type of Payment Plans Offered
POS, FFS

Geographic Areas Served
Philadelphia and southeastern Pennsylvania

Key Personnel
Chairman of the Board . . . . M Walter D'Alessio
President & CEO. . . . . Joseph A Frick
Executive Vice President. Christopher Butler
EVP, Health Markets . . . . Daniel J Hilferty
SVP, Chief Admin Officer. Yvette D Bright
SVP, Corp & Public Affair. . . . . Christopher Cashman
SVP, Provider Networks . . . . Douglas L Chaet
SVP, Underwriting. . . . . Kathryn A Galareau, FSA
SVP, Marketing Services. . . . . John R Janney, Jr
SVP, Chief Financial Offc. . . . . Alan Krigstein
EVP Health Services . . . . I Steven Udvarhelyi, MD
SVP, Internal Audit . . . . Karen Lessin
SVP, Chief Info Officer . . . . Carolyn W Luther
Senior Vice President . . . . Richard J Neeson
SVP, Operations . . . . Stephen R Roker
SPV, Chief Marketing . . . . Linda M Taylor
SVP, General Counsel . . . . Paul A Tufano, Esq

Specialty Managed Care Partners
Caremark Rx

953 InterGroup Services Corporation
Valleybrooke III, 101 Lindenwood Drive
Suite 150
Malvern, PA 19355
Toll-Free: 800-537-9389
Phone: 610-647-5383
Fax: 610-647-5383
www.igs-ppo.com
Secondary Address: 401 Shady Avenue, Suite B108, Pittsburgh, PA 15206, 800-496-8098
For Profit Organization: Yes
Year Founded: 1985
Number of Affiliated Hospitals: 330
Number of Primary Care Physicians: 89,000
Total Enrollment: 700,000

Healthplan and Services Defined
PLAN TYPE: PPO
Model Type: Network
Plan Specialty: ASO, Behavioral Health, Chiropractic, EPO, Lab, MSO, PBM, Vision, Radiology, Worker's Compensation
Benefits Offered: Behavioral Health, Disease Management, Prescription, Wellness, Worker's Compensation

Type of Coverage
Commercial

Geographic Areas Served
Delaware, New Jersey, Pennsylvania, West Virginia

Network Qualifications
Pre-Admission Certification: Yes

Key Personnel
President . . . . John George
800-537-9389
CFO . . . . Caren Ryan
800-537-9389
CEO/COO . . . . G Martin Dudley
800-537-9389
mdudley@igs-ppo.com
Manager Claims Repricing . . . . Jennifer McNatt
800-537-9389
jmcnatt@igs-ppo.com
Network Contracting. . . . . Gregory Dudley
800-537-9389
gdudley@igs-ppo.com
Marketing . . . . Joe McLaughlin
800-537-9389
jmclaughlin@igs-ppo.com
Member Services. . . . . Joe McLaughlin
800-537-9389
jmclaughlin@igs-ppo.com
Dir Information Systems. . . . . Gregory Dudley
800-537-9389
gdudley@igs-ppo.com
VP Provider Relations. Gregory Dudley
800-537-9389
gdudley@igs-ppo.com

Specialty Managed Care Partners
Chiropractic Network

954 Keystone Health Plan Central
2500 Elmerton Avenue
PO Box 779519
Harrisburg, PA 17177-9519
Toll-Free: 800-962-2242
Phone: 717-541-6915
Fax: 717-541-6915
info@pahealthcoverage.com
www.capbluecross.com
Secondary Address: 1221 West Hamilton Street, Allentown, PA

Subsidiary of: Capital Blue Cross
Acquired by: Capital Blue Cross
For Profit Organization: Yes
Year Founded: 1982
Number of Affiliated Hospitals: 51
Total Enrollment: 93,000

Healthplan and Services Defined
   PLAN TYPE: HMO
   Model Type: IPA
   Plan Specialty: ASO
   Benefits Offered: Behavioral Health, Chiropractic, Disease
      Management, Home Care, Inpatient SNF, Long-Term Care,
      Physical Therapy, Prescription, Psychiatric, Transplant, Wellness

Type of Coverage
   Commercial, Medicare
   Catastrophic Illness Benefit: None

Type of Payment Plans Offered
   Capitated, Combination FFS & DFFS

Geographic Areas Served
   Adams, Berks, Centre, Columbia, Cumberland, Dauphin, Juniata,
      Lancaster, Lebanon, Lehigh, Mifflin, Montour, Northampton,
      Northumberland, Perry, Schuylkill, Snyder, Union & York counties

Subscriber Information
   Average Monthly Fee Per Subscriber
      (Employee + Employer Contribution):
         Employee Only (Self): $202.46
         Employee & 1 Family Member: $414.91
         Employee & 2 Family Members: $534.07
   Average Subscriber Co-Payment:
      Primary Care Physician: $10.00
      Prescription Drugs: 50%
      Hospital ER: $25.00
      Home Health Care: 100%
      Home Health Care Max. Days/Visits Covered: 100/yr.
      Nursing Home: $0

Network Qualifications
   Pre-Admission Certification: Yes

Peer Review Type
   Utilization Review: Yes
   Second Surgical Opinion: Yes
   Case Management: Yes

Publishes and Distributes Report Card: Yes

Accreditation Certification
   NCQA

Key Personnel
   President . . . . .Joseph Pfister
   CFO . . . . .Brian Britt
   Sales . . . . .Tona Shaver
   Media Relations Spec. . . . . .Joe Butera
      717-541-6139
      joe.butera@capbluecross.com

Specialty Managed Care Partners
   PacifiCare

Employer References
   Pennsylvania Employees Benefit Trust Fund, Air Products &
      Chemicals, East Penn Manufacturing, Dentsply, Dayphin County

---

955 Keystone Health Plan East
1901 Market Street
PO Box 8489
Philadelphia, PA 19103-1480
Toll-Free: 800-555-1514
Phone: 215-636-9559
Fax: 215-241-0403
www.ibx.com
Subsidiary of: Independence Blue Cross (IBC)
Acquired by: Independence Blue Cross

Non-Profit Organization: Yes
Year Founded: 1986
Number of Affiliated Hospitals: 109
Number of Primary Care Physicians: 10,000
Number of Referral/Specialty Physicians: 24,866
Total Enrollment: 3,400,000
State Enrollment: 2,600,000

Healthplan and Services Defined
   PLAN TYPE: HMO/PPO
   Benefits Offered: Dental, Prescription, Vision, Worker's
      Compensation, AD&D, Life, LTD, STD
   Offers Demand Management Patient Information Service: Yes

Type of Coverage
   Individual, Indemnity, Medicaid

Type of Payment Plans Offered
   DFFS, FFS, Combination FFS & DFFS

Geographic Areas Served
   Berks, Bucks, Chester, Delaware, Lancaster, Lehigh, Mongomery,
      Northhampton, Philadelphia

Network Qualifications
   Pre-Admission Certification: Yes

Peer Review Type
   Utilization Review: Yes
   Second Surgical Opinion: No
   Case Management: Yes

Publishes and Distributes Report Card: Yes

Accreditation Certification
   NCQA
   TJC Accreditation, Medicare Approved, Utilization Review,
      Pre-Admission Certification, State Licensure, Quality Assurance
      Program

Key Personnel
   President/CEO. . . . . .Joseph A Frick
   CFO. . . . . .John G Foos
   Chairman. . . . . .Robert H Young
   Public Relations . . . . .Liz Williams
      215-241-2220

Specialty Managed Care Partners
   Magellan Behavioral Health, United Concorida, Medco Health
      Solutions
   Enters into Contracts with Regional Business Coalitions: Yes

---

956 Mid Atlantic Medical Services: Pennsylvania
2 West Rolling Crossroads
Suite 11
Baltimore, MD 21228
Toll-Free: 800-782-1966
Phone: 410-869-7400
Fax: 410-869-7583
masales99@uhc.com
www.mamsiunitedhealthcare.com
Subsidiary of: United Healthcare/United Health Group
Year Founded: 1986
Number of Affiliated Hospitals: 342
Number of Primary Care Physicians: 3,276
Total Enrollment: 180,000

Healthplan and Services Defined
   PLAN TYPE: HMO/PPO
   Model Type: IPA, Network
   Benefits Offered: Disease Management, Prescription, Wellness

Type of Payment Plans Offered
   Combination FFS & DFFS

Geographic Areas Served
   Delaware, Maryland, North Carolina, Pennsylvania, Virginia,
      Washington DC, West Virginia

Network Qualifications
Pre-Admission Certification: Yes

Peer Review Type
Utilization Review: Yes
Second Surgical Opinion: Yes
Case Management: Yes

Publishes and Distributes Report Card: No

Accreditation Certification
TJC, NCQA

Specialty Managed Care Partners
Enters into Contracts with Regional Business Coalitions: Yes

957 Penn Highlands Health Plan
1086 Franklin Street
Johnstown, PA 15905
Toll-Free: 888-722-0805
Phone: 814-536-7525
Fax: 814-534-1544
mgbarret@conemaugh.org
www.pennhighlands.com
Subsidiary of: Conemaugh Health Plan, Highlands Preferred
Physicians
Non-Profit Organization: Yes
Year Founded: 1985
Number of Affiliated Hospitals: 7
Number of Primary Care Physicians: 425
Number of Referral/Specialty Physicians: 4,100
Total Enrollment: 18,500
State Enrollment: 18,500

Healthplan and Services Defined
PLAN TYPE: PPO
Model Type: IPA
Plan Specialty: ASO, Behavioral Health, Disease Management, EPO,
Lab, MSO, Radiology, Worker's Compensation, UR
Benefits Offered: Behavioral Health, Chiropractic, Disease
Management, Home Care, Inpatient SNF, Long-Term Care,
Physical Therapy, Podiatry, Psychiatric, Transplant, Wellness,
Worker's Compensation
Offers Demand Management Patient Information Service: Yes

Type of Coverage
Commercial

Type of Payment Plans Offered
POS, DFFS, Combination FFS & DFFS

Geographic Areas Served
Bedford, Blair, Cambria and Somerset counties

Subscriber Information
Average Annual Deductible Per Subscriber:
Employee & 2 Family Members: $200.00
Average Subscriber Co-Payment:
Primary Care Physician: $10.00
Non-Network Physician: 50%
Hospital ER: $50.00

Network Qualifications
Pre-Admission Certification: Yes

Peer Review Type
Utilization Review: Yes
Second Surgical Opinion: No
Case Management: Yes

Publishes and Distributes Report Card: Yes

Accreditation Certification
AAAHC, URAC
TJC Accreditation, Medicare Approved, Pre-Admission Certification,
State Licensure

Key Personnel
President . . . . Renee A Staib
CFO . . . . Ed De Pasquale

Medical Director . . . . Richard S Wozniak, MD
Provider Services . . . . Robert Schalles

Average Claim Compensation
Physician's Fees Charged: 1%
Hospital's Fees Charged: 1%

Specialty Managed Care Partners
Enters into Contracts with Regional Business Coalitions: No

958 Preferred Care
1300 Virginia Drive
Suite 315
Fort Washington, PA 19034
Toll-Free: 800-222-3085
Phone: 215-639-6208
Fax: 215-639-2674
info@preferredcareinc.net
www.preferredcareinc.net
For Profit Organization: Yes
Year Founded: 1985
Number of Affiliated Hospitals: 1,200
Number of Primary Care Physicians: 300,000
Number of Referral/Specialty Physicians: 300,000
Total Enrollment: 186,425
State Enrollment: 146,000

Healthplan and Services Defined
PLAN TYPE: PPO
Other Type: TPA
Model Type: Group, Network
Plan Specialty: Chiropractic, PBM
Benefits Offered: Behavioral Health, Chiropractic, Dental, Physical
Therapy, Podiatry, Vision, Life

Type of Payment Plans Offered
DFFS, Capitated, FFS

Geographic Areas Served
Delaware, New Jersey, New York, Pennsylvania: (Bucks, Chester,
Delaware, Lehigh, Montgomery, Philadelphia & Northhampton
counties)

Network Qualifications
Pre-Admission Certification: Yes

Peer Review Type
Utilization Review: Yes
Second Surgical Opinion: Yes
Case Management: Yes

Publishes and Distributes Report Card: No

Accreditation Certification
TJC Accreditation, Medicare Approved, Utilization Review,
Pre-Admission Certification, State Licensure, Quality Assurance
Program

Key Personnel
President . . . . Richard Wehr
PPO President . . . . Richard Matthew
Manager Claims . . . . Maureen Rensom
Contracting . . . . Carole Chapman
Credentialing . . . . Carol Chapman
Marketing . . . . Patricia McGovern
Medical Affairs . . . . H Newton Spencer
QA/UR . . . . Carol Chapman

Specialty Managed Care Partners
Mental Health Consultants, Foot Care Network
Enters into Contracts with Regional Business Coalitions: No

959   Preferred Health Care

Urban Place 480 New Holland Ave
Suite #7203
Lancaster, PA 17602
Phone: 717-560-9290
Fax: 717-560-2312
info@phcunity.com
www.phcunity.com
Non-Profit Organization: Yes
Year Founded: 1984
Number of Affiliated Hospitals: 19
Number of Primary Care Physicians: 1,900
Total Enrollment: 80,316

Healthplan and Services Defined
  PLAN TYPE: PPO
  Model Type: Network
  Offers Demand Management Patient Information Service: Yes

Type of Payment Plans Offered
  FFS

Geographic Areas Served
  Lancaster, Chester, York, Tioga, Bradford and Potter counties

Subscriber Information
  Average Subscriber Co-Payment:
    Primary Care Physician: 20%
    Non-Network Physician: 30%-40%
    Home Health Care: 20%

Peer Review Type
  Utilization Review: Yes
  Case Management: Yes

Accreditation Certification
  TJC Accreditation, Medicare Approved, Utilization Review,
    Pre-Admission Certification, State Licensure, Quality Assurance
    Program

Key Personnel
  President/CEO . . . . Eric E Buck
    717-560-9290
    ebuck@phcunity.com
  VP, Operations . . . . Sherry Wolgemuth
  Medical Director . . . . Dr. C David Noll
    swolgemuth@phcunity.com
  Medical Director . . . . David Bowers, MD
    dbowers@phcunity.com
  Network Affairs Rep . . . . Roger Milner
    rmilner@phcuinity.com
  Media Contact . . . . Roger Milner
    717-560-9290
    rmilner@phcunity.com

960   Preferred Healthcare System

3223 Route 764
Duncansville, PA 16635
Toll-Free: 800-238-9900
Phone: 814-317-5063
Fax: 814-317-5139
mfrucella.preferred@altanticbbn.net
www.phsppo.com
For Profit Organization: Yes
Year Founded: 1985
Physician Owned Organization: Yes
Number of Affiliated Hospitals: 14
Number of Primary Care Physicians: 150
Number of Referral/Specialty Physicians: 448
Total Enrollment: 20,000

Healthplan and Services Defined
  PLAN TYPE: PPO
  Model Type: Network

Plan Specialty: ASO, Behavioral Health, Chiropractic, Dental,
  Disease Management, EPO, PBM, Vision, Worker's Compensation,
  Health
Benefits Offered: Behavioral Health, Chiropractic, Complementary
  Medicine, Dental, Disease Management, Home Care, Inpatient
  SNF, Long-Term Care, Physical Therapy, Podiatry, Prescription,
  Psychiatric, Transplant, Vision, Wellness, AD&D, Life, STD,
  Durable Medical Equipment

Type of Coverage
  Commercial, Individual, Indemnity
  Catastrophic Illness Benefit: Maximum $1M

Type of Payment Plans Offered
  Combination FFS & DFFS

Geographic Areas Served
  Clearfield, Centre, Cambria, Blair, Huntingdon, Mifflin, Bedford,
  Fulton, Sommerset and Juniata counties

Subscriber Information
  Average Monthly Fee Per Subscriber
    (Employee + Employer Contribution):
      Employee Only (Self): Varies
      Employee & 1 Family Member: Varies
      Employee & 2 Family Members: Varies
      Medicare: Varies
  Average Annual Deductible Per Subscriber:
      Employee Only (Self): Varies
      Employee & 1 Family Member: Varies
      Employee & 2 Family Members: Varies
      Medicare: Varies
  Average Subscriber Co-Payment:
    Prescription Drugs: Varies
    Hospital ER: Varies
    Home Health Care: Varies
    Home Health Care Max. Days/Visits Covered: Varies
    Nursing Home: Varies
    Nursing Home Max. Days/Visits Covered: Varies

Network Qualifications
  Pre-Admission Certification: Yes

Peer Review Type
  Utilization Review: Yes
  Second Surgical Opinion: Yes

Publishes and Distributes Report Card: No

Accreditation Certification
  TJC Accreditation, Utilization Review, Pre-Admission Certification,
    State Licensure, Quality Assurance Program

Key Personnel
  President . . . . Maureen Frucella
  Chief Executive Officer . . . . Brian Brumbaugh
  Utilization Review . . . . Jessie E Bradfield

Average Claim Compensation
  Physician's Fees Charged: 70%
  Hospital's Fees Charged: 70%

Specialty Managed Care Partners
  Enters into Contracts with Regional Business Coalitions: Yes

961   Prime Source Health Network

3421 Concord Road
York, PA 17402
Toll-Free: 800-842-1768
Phone: 717-851-6800
www.primesourcehealthnetwork.com
Subsidiary of: South Central Preferred Health Network
Non-Profit Organization: Yes
Year Founded: 1992
Number of Affiliated Hospitals: 16
Number of Primary Care Physicians: 6,150
Number of Referral/Specialty Physicians: 1,275
Total Enrollment: 33,000

State Enrollment: 33,000

Healthplan and Services Defined
  PLAN TYPE: PPO
  Model Type: PHO
  Plan Specialty: Behavioral Health, Chiropractic, Radiology
  Benefits Offered: Behavioral Health, Chiropractic, Home Care,
    Inpatient SNF, Long-Term Care, Physical Therapy, Podiatry,
    Psychiatric, Transplant

Type of Coverage
  Catastrophic Illness Benefit: None

Type of Payment Plans Offered
  Capitated

Geographic Areas Served
  Cumberland, Dauphin, Lebanon, Perry and Northern York counties

Subscriber Information
  Average Monthly Fee Per Subscriber
    (Employee + Employer Contribution):
      Employee Only (Self): $6.75 per employee

Network Qualifications
  Pre-Admission Certification: No

Peer Review Type
  Utilization Review: Yes

Average Claim Compensation
  Physician's Fees Charged: 64%
  Hospital's Fees Charged: 70%

962 SelectCare Access Corporation
Manor Oak Township, Suite 605
1910 Cochran Road
Pittsburgh, PA 15220
Toll-Free: 800-922-4966
Phone: 412-922-2803
Fax: 412-922-3071
www.mcoa.com
Subsidiary of: Managed Care of America, Inc.
For Profit Organization: Yes
Year Founded: 1991
Number of Affiliated Hospitals: 55
Number of Primary Care Physicians: 1,375
Number of Referral/Specialty Physicians: 3,609
Total Enrollment: 15,700

Healthplan and Services Defined
  PLAN TYPE: PPO
  Model Type: Network
  Benefits Offered: Prescription

Type of Payment Plans Offered
  POS, DFFS, FFS, Combination FFS & DFFS

Geographic Areas Served
  Statewide

Network Qualifications
  Pre-Admission Certification: No

Peer Review Type
  Utilization Review: Yes
  Second Surgical Opinion: No
  Case Management: Yes

Accreditation Certification
  TJC Accreditation, Utilization Review, State Licensure

Key Personnel
  President/CFO.............................Phyllis Shehab
    412-922-0780
  COO......................................Richard Adams
    412-922-0780
    rladams@mcoa.com
  Legal Counsel..........................Charles E Davidson
    412-922-0780
    cedavidson@mcoa.com

  Credentialing.............................Jane Kwiecinski
    412-922-0780
    ljkwiecinski@mcoa.com
  VP Marketing ....Dennis Casey
    412-922-0780
  Dir. Provider Services.....................Tracey M Shank
    412-922-0780
    tmshank@mcoa.com

963 South Central Preferred
1803 Mount Rose Avenue
B-5
York, PA 17403
Toll-Free: 800-842-1768
Phone: 717-851-6800
Fax: 717-851-6775
www.scphealth.com
Subsidiary of: WellSpan
Non-Profit Organization: Yes
Year Founded: 1992
Number of Affiliated Hospitals: 16
Number of Primary Care Physicians: 6,150
Total Enrollment: 56,000
State Enrollment: 56,000

Healthplan and Services Defined
  PLAN TYPE: PPO
  Benefits Offered: Wellness, Self-funded Administration & PPO
    Network, EAP

Type of Coverage
  Commercial, Individual

Geographic Areas Served
  South Central Pennsylvania

Peer Review Type
  Utilization Review: Yes
  Case Management: Yes

Key Personnel
  COO ....Jim Cochran
  Finance ....Bill Smith
  CMO ....Neal Friedman
  Provider Relations.........................Jane Grove
  Marketing................................Andy Seebold
    aseebold@wellspan.org
  Claims....................................Deb Kehres
  Customer Service....................Rebecca Timmermans

Specialty Managed Care Partners
  Express Scripts

964 Susquehanna EHP Significa
1871 Santa Barbara Road
Lancaster, PA 17601
Toll-Free: 800-432-8877
Phone: 717-581-1245
www.sh-ehpsig.com
Subsidiary of: Significa Insurance Group
Non-Profit Organization: Yes
Number of Affiliated Hospitals: 179
Number of Primary Care Physicians: 49,000

Healthplan and Services Defined
  PLAN TYPE: PPO

Type of Coverage
  Commercial

Geographic Areas Served
  Bradford, Centre, Clinton, Columbia, Lycoming, Montour,
  Northumberland, Snyder, Tioga and Union counties in Pennsylvania

965 Susquehanna Health Care

109 North Mulberry Street
Berwick, PA 18603
Phone: 570-759-1702
Fax: 570-759-2559
no website
For Profit Organization: Yes
Year Founded: 1985
Physician Owned Organization: Yes
Number of Affiliated Hospitals: 33
Number of Primary Care Physicians: 1,090
Total Enrollment: 45,000
State Enrollment: 45,000

Healthplan and Services Defined
PLAN TYPE: PPO
Model Type: Network
Benefits Offered: Prescription

Type of Coverage
Catastrophic Illness Benefit: Maximum $2M

Geographic Areas Served
Central & Northeastern Pennsylvania, 17 counties

Subscriber Information
Average Monthly Fee Per Subscriber
(Employee + Employer Contribution):
Employee Only (Self): $140
Employee & 1 Family Member: $275
Employee & 2 Family Members: $410
Average Annual Deductible Per Subscriber:
Employee Only (Self): $500
Average Subscriber Co-Payment:
Primary Care Physician: $30.00
Non-Network Physician: $52.00
Hospital ER: $75.00
Home Health Care: 15%
Home Health Care Max. Days/Visits Covered: 100 days
Nursing Home Max. Days/Visits Covered: 30/confinement

Network Qualifications
Pre-Admission Certification: Yes

Peer Review Type
Utilization Review: Yes
Second Surgical Opinion: Yes

Publishes and Distributes Report Card: No

Accreditation Certification
Medicare Approved, Utilization Review, Pre-Admission
Certification, State Licensure, Quality Assurance Program

Key Personnel
President/CEO . . . . Steven P. Johnson, Jr
Communications Director . . . . Kendall Marcocci

Specialty Managed Care Partners
Enters into Contracts with Regional Business Coalitions: Yes

966 Unison Health Plan of Pennsylvania

1001 Brinton Road
Unison Plaza
Pittsburgh, PA 15221
Toll-Free: 800-600-9007
Phone: 412-858-4000
www.uhccommunityplan.com
Subsidiary of: AmeriChoice, A UnitedHealth Group Company
Total Enrollment: 160,000

Healthplan and Services Defined
PLAN TYPE: Multiple
Benefits Offered: Chiropractic, Dental, Disease Management, Home
Care, Inpatient SNF, Physical Therapy, Podiatry, Prescription,
Psychiatric, Vision, Wellness

Type of Coverage
Individual, Medicare

Geographic Areas Served
Available within Pennsylvania, South Carolina, Ohio, and Tennesse

Subscriber Information
Average Monthly Fee Per Subscriber
(Employee + Employer Contribution):
Employee Only (Self): Varies
Medicare: Varies
Average Annual Deductible Per Subscriber:
Employee Only (Self): Varies
Medicare: Varies
Average Subscriber Co-Payment:
Primary Care Physician: Varies
Non-Network Physician: Varies
Prescription Drugs: Varies
Hospital ER: Varies
Home Health Care: Varies
Home Health Care Max. Days/Visits Covered: Varies
Nursing Home: Varies
Nursing Home Max. Days/Visits Covered: Varies

Accreditation Certification
URAC, NCQA

Key Personnel
President/Pennsylvania . . . . Jennifer Kessler
SVP/Medical Operations . . . . Shirley Blevins
Chief Operating Officer . . . . Fred Madill
SVP/General Counsel . . . . David Thomas
Compliance Officer . . . . John G Beck
President/South Carolina . . . . Dan Gallagher
President/Ohio . . . . Scott A Bowers
President/Tennessee . . . . Matthew Moore
VP/Medicare Products . . . . Keith Volberg
VP/Network Administration. . . . . Healther Cianfrocco
Contact . . . . Tyler Mason
714-229-5730
brandon.moser@unisonhealthplan.com

967 United Concordia

4401 Deer Path Road
Harrisburg, PA 17110
Toll-Free: 800-345-3837
Phone: 877-438-8224
Fax: 717-433-9871
ucproducer@ucci.com
www.secure.ucci.com/ducdws/home.xhtml
Secondary Address: Claim Submission, PO Box 69421, Harrisburg, PA
17106-9421
For Profit Organization: Yes
Year Founded: 1971
Number of Primary Care Physicians: 111,000
Total Enrollment: 6,000,000

Healthplan and Services Defined
PLAN TYPE: Dental
Plan Specialty: Dental
Benefits Offered: Dental

Type of Coverage
Commercial, Individual

Geographic Areas Served
Military personnel and their families, nationwide

Accreditation Certification
URAC

Key Personnel
Chairman & CEO . . . . Daniel Lebish
SVP, Finance . . . . Daniel Wright
SVP, Sales & Marketing . . . . Sharon Muscarella

968 UPMC Health Plan

1 Chatham Center
112 Washington Place
Pittsburgh, PA 15219
Toll-Free: 866-778-6073
Phone: 412-434-1200
Fax: 412-454-7711
hponeline@upmc.edu
www.upmchealthplan.com
Secondary Address: U.S. Steel Tower, 600 Grant Street, Pittsburgh, PA
  15219
Subsidiary of: University of Pittsburgh Medical Center
For Profit Organization: Yes
Year Founded: 1996
Physician Owned Organization: Yes
Number of Affiliated Hospitals: 80
Number of Primary Care Physicians: 7,600
Total Enrollment: 101,000
State Enrollment: 209,211

Healthplan and Services Defined
  PLAN TYPE: Multiple
  Benefits Offered: Behavioral Health, Chiropractic, Complementary
    Medicine, Dental, Disease Management, Home Care, Inpatient
    SNF, Physical Therapy, Podiatry, Prescription, Psychiatric,
    Transplant, Vision, Wellness

Type of Coverage
  Commercial, Individual, Medicare, Medicaid

Type of Payment Plans Offered
  POS

Geographic Areas Served
  26 counties in western Pennsylvania

Subscriber Information
  Average Monthly Fee Per Subscriber
    (Employee + Employer Contribution):
      Employee Only (Self): Varies
      Employee & 1 Family Member: Varies
      Employee & 2 Family Members: Varies
      Medicare: Varies
  Average Annual Deductible Per Subscriber:
      Employee Only (Self): Varies
      Employee & 1 Family Member: Varies
      Employee & 2 Family Members: Varies
      Medicare: Varies
  Average Subscriber Co-Payment:
      Primary Care Physician: Varies
      Non-Network Physician: Varies
      Prescription Drugs: Varies
      Hospital ER: Varies
      Home Health Care: Varies
      Home Health Care Max. Days/Visits Covered: Varies
      Nursing Home: Varies
      Nursing Home Max. Days/Visits Covered: Varies

Accreditation Certification
  NCQA

Key Personnel
  President and CEO . . . . Diane P Holder
  CFO. . . . . Scott Lammie
  Senior Vice President and. . . . . Mary Beth Jenkins
  VP, Medicare. . . . . Cathy Batteer
  VP, Network/Provider Rel. . . . . Sandra E McAnallen
  VP, Quality, Audit, Fraud. . . . . William Gedmen, CPA
  CEO, Askesis Dev Group . . . . Sharon Hicks
  VP, Marketing & Comm . . . . Jeffrey Nelson
  VP Business Development . . . . Anthony Benevento
  VP, Medical Affairs. . . . . Michael Culyba, MD
  VP, Human Resources. Sharon Czyzewski
  Chief Medical Officer . . . . Anne Boland Docimo, MD
  President, UPMC For You. John Lovelace

VP, Sales & Marketing . . . . Anthony Benevento
Dir, Public Relations . . . . Gina Pferdehirt
  412-454-4953
  pferdehirtgm@upmc.edu
VP, Pharmacy . . . . Chronis Manolis, RPh

969 Val-U-Health

520 Pleasant Valley Road
Trafford, PA 15085
Toll-Free: 877-688-5977
Fax: 855-439-2443
vbhpawebmaster@valueoptions.com
www.vbh-pa.com
Acquired by: Value Behavioral Health of PA
Non-Profit Organization: Yes
Year Founded: 1995
Number of Primary Care Physicians: 140
Total Enrollment: 2,375

Healthplan and Services Defined
  PLAN TYPE: PPO
  Model Type: Network
  Benefits Offered: Prescription

Type of Coverage
  Catastrophic Illness Benefit: Covered

Geographic Areas Served
  Southern Allegheny, Fayette, Greene, Washington & Central
  Westmoreland counties

Subscriber Information
  Average Annual Deductible Per Subscriber:
      Employee Only (Self): $200.00
      Employee & 1 Family Member: $400.00
      Employee & 2 Family Members: $400.00

Peer Review Type
  Case Management: Yes

Accreditation Certification
  TJC, CARF, COA and AOA

Key Personnel
  President and Chairman . . . . Dr Ronald Dozoretz
    724-379-4011
    smf@vuhealth.com
  Director Quality Mgmt. . . . . Trina L Curcio
    tlc@vuhealth.com
  Director Operations. . . . . Lois Weaver
    ljw@vuhealth.com

970 Valley Preferred

1605 N Cedar Crest Blvd
Suite 411
Allentown, PA 18104-2351
Toll-Free: 800-955-6620
Phone: 610-969-0480
Fax: 610-969-0439
selicia.chronister@valleypreferred.com
www.valleypreferred.com
Non-Profit Organization: Yes
Year Founded: 1994
Physician Owned Organization: Yes
Federally Qualified: Yes
Number of Affiliated Hospitals: 18
Number of Primary Care Physicians: 778
Number of Referral/Specialty Physicians: 2,977
Total Enrollment: 174,309
State Enrollment: 174,209

Healthplan and Services Defined
  PLAN TYPE: Multiple
  Model Type: PHO

Geographic Areas Served
Lehigh, Northampton, Berks, Bucks, Montgomery, Dauphin, Schuylkill, Columbia, Luzerne, Carbon and Lackawanna counties

Accreditation Certification
TJC, NCQA

Key Personnel

Executive Director and CE . . . . Gregory Kile
Interim Exec Director . . . . Jack A Lenhart
General Manager. . . . . Laura J Mertz
Dir, Info Technology . . . . Louis W Bottitta
GLVIPA Coordinator . . . . Maryann Curcio
Admin, Health Services . . . . Christina Lewisr
Provider Relations . . . . Patricia A Sank
Medical Director. . . . . Jack A Lenhart
Sales and Marketing Assis . . . . Kaye Long

Specialty Managed Care Partners
Enters into Contracts with Regional Business Coalitions: No
NPRHCC

---

971   **Value Behavioral Health of Pennsylvania**

520 Pleasant Valley Road
Trafford, PA 15085
Toll-Free: 877-615-8503
Phone: 724-744-6361
Fax: 724-744-6379
vbhpawebmaster@valueoptions.com
www.vbh-pa.com
Subsidiary of: A ValueOptions Company
For Profit Organization: Yes
Year Founded: 1983
Physician Owned Organization: Yes
Number of Affiliated Hospitals: 1,225
Number of Referral/Specialty Physicians: 6,000
Total Enrollment: 22,000,000

Healthplan and Services Defined
PLAN TYPE: PPO
Model Type: Network
Plan Specialty: ASO, Behavioral Health, UR
Benefits Offered: Behavioral Health, Psychiatric, EAP

Type of Coverage
Commercial, Indemnity, Medicaid

Type of Payment Plans Offered
POS, DFFS, Combination FFS & DFFS

Geographic Areas Served
Armstrong, Beaver, Butler, Cambria, Crawford, Erie, Fayette, Greene, Indiana, Lawrence, Mercer, Venango, Washington and Westmoreland counties

Peer Review Type
Case Management: Yes

Publishes and Distributes Report Card: Yes

Accreditation Certification
TJC, URAC, NCQA, CARF, COA and AOA

Key Personnel

President and Chairman . . . . Dr Ronald Dozoretz
COO . . . . John Hill
CFO. . . . . Ed Hackett
Director, Marketing/Sales . . . . Lisa Todd

Health Insurance Coverage Status and Type of Coverage by Age

Category	All Persons		Under 18 years		Under 65 years		65 years and over	
	Number	%	Number	%	Number	%	Number	%
Total population	na	na	na	na	na	na	na	na
Covered by some type of health insurance	na	na	na	na	na	na	na	na
Covered by private health insurance	na	na	na	na	na	na	na	na
Employment based	na	na	na	na	na	na	na	na
Own employment based	na	na	na	na	na	na	na	na
Direct purchase	na	na	na	na	na	na	na	na
Covered by government health insurance	na	na	na	na	na	na	na	na
Covered by Medicaid	na	na	na	na	na	na	na	na
Also by private insurance	na	na	na	na	na	na	na	na
Covered by Medicare	na	na	na	na	na	na	na	na
Also by private insurance	na	na	na	na	na	na	na	na
Also by Medicaid	na	na	na	na	na	na	na	na
Covered by military health care	na	na	na	na	na	na	na	na
Not covered at any time during the year	na	na	na	na	na	na	na	na

Note: Data was not available for Puerto Rico

Puerto Rico

972 CIGNA HealthCare of Puerto Rico
Hato Rey Tower
268 Munoz Rivera Avenue, Suite 700
San Juan, PR 00918
Toll-Free: 866-438-2446
www.cigna.com
For Profit Organization: Yes
Total Enrollment: 75,000,000

Healthplan and Services Defined
PLAN TYPE: PPO

Type of Coverage
Commercial

Accreditation Certification
URAC, NCQA

973 First Medical Health Plan
Ext Villa Caparra Mar Buch 530
Guaynabo, PR 00968
Toll-Free: 888-318-0274
www.firstmedicalpr.com
For Profit Organization: Yes
Year Founded: 1977
Number of Affiliated Hospitals: 12
Total Enrollment: 180,000
State Enrollment: 180,000

Healthplan and Services Defined
PLAN TYPE: Multiple

Key Personnel
President . . . . Francisco Javier Artau Feliciano

974 Humana Health Insurance of Puerto Rico
383 Franklin Delano Roosevelt Ave
San Juan, PR 00918
Toll-Free: 866-836-6162
Phone: 502-301-1903
Fax: 888-899-8319
www.humana.com
Subsidiary of: LifeSynch
For Profit Organization: Yes
Total Enrollment: 370,000

Healthplan and Services Defined
PLAN TYPE: HMO/PPO

Type of Coverage
Commercial, Individual

Accreditation Certification
URAC, NCQA, CORE

975 Medical Card System (MCS)
Bird Ponce De Leon #255
Suite 1600, Floor 9
San Juan, PR 00917
Toll-Free: 888-758-1616
Phone: 787-758-2500
Fax: 787-250-0380
www.mcs.com.pr
For Profit Organization: Yes
Year Founded: 1983
Number of Affiliated Hospitals: 57
Number of Primary Care Physicians: 11
Total Enrollment: 300,000

Healthplan and Services Defined
PLAN TYPE: Multiple
Model Type: Group, Network
Plan Specialty: ASO, Behavioral Health, Chiropractic, Dental, Disease Management, EPO, Lab, MSO, PBM, Vision, Radiology
Benefits Offered: Behavioral Health, Chiropractic, Complementary Medicine, Dental, Disease Management, Home Care, Inpatient SNF, Physical Therapy, Podiatry, Prescription, Psychiatric, Transplant, Vision, Wellness, Life, LTD

Type of Coverage
Commercial, Individual, Indemnity, Medicare, Supplemental Medicare, Medicaid, Catastrophic

Type of Payment Plans Offered
POS, Capitated

Geographic Areas Served
Puerto Rico

Subscriber Information
Average Monthly Fee Per Subscriber
    (Employee + Employer Contribution):
        Employee Only (Self): Varies
        Employee & 1 Family Member: Varies
        Employee & 2 Family Members: Varies
        Medicare: Varies
Average Annual Deductible Per Subscriber:
        Employee Only (Self): Varies
        Employee & 1 Family Member: Varies
        Employee & 2 Family Members: Varies
        Medicare: Varies
Average Subscriber Co-Payment:
        Primary Care Physician: Varies
        Non-Network Physician: Varies
        Prescription Drugs: Varies
        Hospital ER: Varies
        Home Health Care: Varies
        Home Health Care Max. Days/Visits Covered: Varies
        Nursing Home: Varies
        Nursing Home Max. Days/Visits Covered: Varies

Network Qualifications
Pre-Admission Certification: Yes

Peer Review Type
Utilization Review: Yes
Second Surgical Opinion: Yes
Case Management: Yes

Accreditation Certification
Medicare Approved, Pre-Admission Certification, State Licensure

Key Personnel
President . . . . Dr. David Scanavino
President MCS Life Insura . . . . Jos, Dur n
Chief Executive Officer . . . . Jim O 'Drobinak
Chief Legal Officer . . . . Maritza I Munich
VP, Chief Audit Executive . . . . A Tian See
MCS HMO President . . . . Jose Mirabal
MCS HMO Vice President . . . . Lilia Sabater
Controller . . . . Brendan Shanahan
VP, Finance . . . . David Schaffer
VP, Underwriting . . . . Eduardo Zetina
Chief Medical Officer . . . . Ines Hernandez, MD
Vice President Membership . . . . Richard Moon
Chief Information Officer . . . . Ivars Blums
VP, Service & Renewals . . . . Carmen Molina
VP, Individual Sales . . . . Richard Luna

Employer References
Sensormatic, El Nuevo Dia, Pan Pepin, Nypro Puerto Rico, Cardinal Health

976 MMM Healthcare

350 Chardon Ave
Suite 500, Torre Chardon
San Juan, PR 00918-2137
Toll-Free: 866-333-5469
Phone: 787-620-2397
Fax: 787-629-2399
www.mmm-pr.com
Year Founded: 2001
Total Enrollment: 126,000

Healthplan and Services Defined
  PLAN TYPE: Multiple

Type of Coverage
  Individual, Medicare

Geographic Areas Served
  Puerto Rico

Accreditation Certification
  NCQA

Key Personnel
  President..................................Orlando Gonzalez
  CEO.......................................Richard Shinto

977 PMC Medicare Choice

350 Avenida Chardon
Suite 500, Torre Chardon
San Juan, PR 00918-2101
Toll-Free: 877-568-0808
Phone: 787-622-3000
Fax: 787-999-1762
www.pmcpr.org
Secondary Address: Edif. Gatsby Plaza, Piso 3, Avenida Jos,
  Mercado, Caguas, PR 00725, 787-622-3000
For Profit Organization: Yes
Year Founded: 2004
Number of Primary Care Physicians: 7
Total Enrollment: 53,000

Healthplan and Services Defined
  PLAN TYPE: Medicare

Type of Coverage
  Medicare

Geographic Areas Served
  Puerto Rico

Accreditation Certification
  NCQA

Key Personnel
  President ....Orlando Gonzalez, MD
  Chief Executive Officer ....Richard Shinto, Esq

978 Triple-S Salud Blue Cross Blue Shield of Puerto Rico

PO Box 363628
San Juan, PR 00920
Toll-Free: 800-981-3241
Phone: 787-774-6060
Fax: 787-706-2833
www.ssspr.com
Year Founded: 1959
Total Enrollment: 100,000
State Enrollment: 100,000

Healthplan and Services Defined
  PLAN TYPE: Multiple
  Benefits Offered: Chiropractic, Dental, Disease Management, Home
    Care, Inpatient SNF, Physical Therapy, Podiatry, Prescription,
    Psychiatric, Vision, Wellness

Type of Coverage
  Individual, Medicare, Supplemental Medicare

Geographic Areas Served
  Puerto Rico

Subscriber Information
  Average Monthly Fee Per Subscriber
    (Employee + Employer Contribution):
      Employee Only (Self): Varies
      Employee & 1 Family Member: Varies
      Employee & 2 Family Members: Varies
      Medicare: Varies
  Average Annual Deductible Per Subscriber:
      Employee Only (Self): Varies
      Employee & 1 Family Member: Varies
      Employee & 2 Family Members: Varies
      Medicare: Varies
  Average Subscriber Co-Payment:
      Primary Care Physician: Varies
      Non-Network Physician: Varies
      Prescription Drugs: Varies
      Hospital ER: Varies
      Home Health Care: Varies
      Home Health Care Max. Days/Visits Covered: Varies
      Nursing Home: Varies
      Nursing Home Max. Days/Visits Covered: Varies

Accreditation Certification
  TJC, URAC, NCQA

Key Personnel
  President............................Jesus R Sanchez Colon
  Vice President.......................Jose Hawayek Alemany
  Secretary.........................Ing. Jorge Fuentes Benejam
  Media Contact.............................Vivian Lopez
    787-749-4112
    vivian.lopez@ssspr.com

979 UnitedHealthCare of Puerto Rico

9700 Health Care Lane
Minnetonka, MN 55343
Toll-Free: 800-842-3585
www.uhc.com
Subsidiary of: UnitedHealth Group
Year Founded: 1977
Number of Affiliated Hospitals: 4,200
Number of Primary Care Physicians: 460,000
Total Enrollment: 75,000,000

Healthplan and Services Defined
  PLAN TYPE: HMO/PPO
  Model Type: IPA, Group, Network
  Plan Specialty: Lab, Radiology
  Benefits Offered: Chiropractic, Dental, Physical Therapy,
    Prescription, Wellness, AD&D, Life, LTD, STD
  Offers Demand Management Patient Information Service: Yes

Type of Coverage
  Commercial, Individual, Indemnity, Medicare

Geographic Areas Served
  Statewide

Network Qualifications
  Pre-Admission Certification: Yes

Peer Review Type
  Utilization Review: Yes
  Second Surgical Opinion: Yes
  Case Management: Yes

Publishes and Distributes Report Card: Yes

Accreditation Certification
  TJC, NCQA

Specialty Managed Care Partners
  Enters into Contracts with Regional Business Coalitions: Yes

Health Insurance Coverage Status and Type of Coverage by Age

Category	All Persons		Under 18 years		Under 65 years		65 years and over	
	Number	%	Number	%	Number	%	Number	%
Total population	1,036	-	212	-	881	-	155	-
Covered by some type of health insurance	916 *(7)*	88.4 *(0.7)*	201 *(2)*	94.6 *(1.1)*	761 *(7)*	86.4 *(0.8)*	155 *(1)*	99.7 *(0.2)*
Covered by private health insurance	714 *(11)*	68.9 *(1.1)*	134 *(4)*	63.2 *(2.1)*	616 *(11)*	69.9 *(1.2)*	98 *(3)*	63.2 *(2.2)*
Employment based	596 *(11)*	57.6 *(1.0)*	120 *(4)*	56.6 *(2.1)*	546 *(10)*	62.0 *(1.1)*	50 *(3)*	32.5 *(1.9)*
Direct purchase	130 *(6)*	12.5 *(0.6)*	12 *(2)*	5.8 *(1.1)*	76 *(5)*	8.6 *(0.6)*	54 *(3)*	34.7 *(2.0)*
Covered by TRICARE	22 *(4)*	2.1 *(0.4)*	5 *(2)*	2.4 *(0.7)*	14 *(3)*	1.6 *(0.4)*	8 *(1)*	5.0 *(0.9)*
Covered by government health insurance	329 *(9)*	31.8 *(0.8)*	78 *(5)*	36.8 *(2.2)*	179 *(8)*	20.4 *(1.0)*	150 *(1)*	96.6 *(0.7)*
Covered by Medicaid	184 *(9)*	17.8 *(0.8)*	78 *(5)*	36.8 *(2.2)*	161 *(8)*	18.3 *(1.0)*	23 *(3)*	14.5 *(1.6)*
Also by private insurance	34 *(4)*	3.3 *(0.4)*	12 *(3)*	5.4 *(1.2)*	26 *(4)*	2.9 *(0.4)*	8 *(1)*	5.3 *(0.8)*
Covered by Medicare	179 *(3)*	17.3 *(0.3)*	1 *(1)*	0.3 *(0.3)*	30 *(3)*	3.4 *(0.3)*	150 *(1)*	96.4 *(0.7)*
Also by private insurance	102 *(3)*	9.8 *(0.3)*	Z *(Z)*	0.0 *(0.1)*	8 *(1)*	1.0 *(0.2)*	93 *(3)*	60.1 *(2.0)*
Also by Medicaid	40 *(4)*	3.8 *(0.3)*	1 *(1)*	0.3 *(0.3)*	17 *(2)*	1.9 *(0.3)*	23 *(3)*	14.5 *(1.6)*
Covered by VA Care	20 *(2)*	1.9 *(0.2)*	Z *(Z)*	0.0 *(0.1)*	7 *(2)*	0.8 *(0.2)*	13 *(2)*	8.5 *(1.0)*
Not covered at any time during the year	120 *(7)*	11.6 *(0.7)*	12 *(2)*	5.4 *(1.1)*	120 *(7)*	13.6 *(0.8)*	1 *(Z)*	0.3 *(0.2)*

Note: Numbers in thousands; Figures cover 2013; Margin of error appears in parenthesis; A "Z" indicates that the value either represents or rounds to zero.
Source: U.S. Census Bureau, 2013 American Community Survey, Table HI05. Health Insurance Coverage Status and Type of Coverage by State and Age for All People: 2013

Rhode Island

980 Aetna Health of Rhode Island

151 Farmington Avenue
Hartford, CT 06156
Toll-Free: 800-872-3862
Phone: 860-273-0123
www.aetna.com
Partnered with: eHealthInsurance Services Inc.
For Profit Organization: Yes
Total Enrollment: 11,596,230

Healthplan and Services Defined
PLAN TYPE: PPO
Other Type: POS
Plan Specialty: EPO
Benefits Offered: Dental, Disease Management, Long-Term Care,
Prescription, Wellness, Life, LTD, STD

Type of Coverage
Commercial, Individual

Type of Payment Plans Offered
POS, FFS

Geographic Areas Served
Statewide

Key Personnel
Chairman/CEO/President. . . . . Mark T Bertolini
SVP/General Counsel . . . . William J Casazza
EVP/CFO . . . . Shawn M Guertin

981 Blue Cross & Blue Shield of Rhode Island

500 Exchange Street
Providence, RI 02903
Toll-Free: 800-637-3718
Phone: 401-459-1000
www.bcbsri.com
Subsidiary of: Health and Wellness Institute
Non-Profit Organization: Yes
Year Founded: 1939
Number of Primary Care Physicians: 100,000
Total Enrollment: 600,000

Healthplan and Services Defined
PLAN TYPE: HMO
Model Type: Staff
Benefits Offered: Disease Management, Wellness

Type of Payment Plans Offered
DFFS

Peer Review Type
Case Management: Yes

Publishes and Distributes Report Card: Yes

Accreditation Certification
URAC, NCQA

Key Personnel
President & CEO . . . . Peter Andruszkiewicz
401-459-1200
COO . . . . William K Wray
401-459-1232
Executive Vice President . . . . Michael Hudson
401-459-2519
Executive Vice President . . . . Michele B Lederberg
401-459-1202
Senior Vice President, Ne . . . . Mark Waggoner
401-459-1400
VP, Human Resources . . . . Eric Gasbaro
Senior Vice President and . . . . Shanna Marzilli
401-459-1633

SVP/Chief Medical Officer . . . . Gus Manocchia, MD
401-459-5621
Vice President, Informati . . . . Paul Hanlon
401-459-5054
Vice President and Chief . . . . Bob Wolfkiel
401-459-5470
Dir, Media Relations . . . . Kimberly Reingold
401-459-5611
kimberly.reingold@bcbsri.org

982 CIGNA HealthCare of Rhode Island

Three Newton Executive Park
2223 Washington Street
Newton, MA 02462
Toll-Free: 866-438-2446
Phone: 617-630-4300
Fax: 617-630-4380
www.cigna.com
For Profit Organization: Yes

Healthplan and Services Defined
PLAN TYPE: PPO

Type of Coverage
Commercial

983 CVS CareMark

One CVS Drive
Woonsocket, RI 02895
Toll-Free: 800-552-8159
Phone: 401-765-1500
CommunityMailbox@cvscaremark.com
www.cvscaremark.com
For Profit Organization: Yes
Year Founded: 1963
Owned by an Integrated Delivery Network (IDN): Yes
Number of Affiliated Hospitals: 650
Number of Primary Care Physicians: 60,000
Total Enrollment: 70,000,000

Healthplan and Services Defined
PLAN TYPE: Other
Other Type: PBM
Model Type: Staff
Plan Specialty: Disease Management, PBM
Benefits Offered: Disease Management, Prescription

Type of Payment Plans Offered
POS, DFFS, FFS

Geographic Areas Served
Nationwide

Peer Review Type
Second Surgical Opinion: Yes
Case Management: Yes

Publishes and Distributes Report Card: Yes

Accreditation Certification
TJC, URAC

Key Personnel
President & CEO. . . . . Larry J Merlo
Executive Vice President. . . . . Mark Cosby
EVP, Chief Financial Offc . . . . David M Denton
Executive Vice President . . . . Thomas M Moriarty
President, Pharmacy Svcs . . . . Per Lofberg
Executive Vice President . . . . Helena B Foulkes
PBM Chief Operating Offc. . . . . Jonathan C. Roberts
EVP & Chief Medical Off. . . . . Troyen A. Brennan, MD
SVP, Chief Human Resource . . . . Lisa Bisaccia
SVP, Chief Info Officer . . . . Stephen J Gold
Executive Vice President . . . . J David Joyner

Dir, Public Relations . . . . Christine Cramer
401-770-3317
ckcramer@cvs.com
EVP, Chief Legal Officer . . . . Douglas A. Sgarro

Specialty Managed Care Partners
Enters into Contracts with Regional Business Coalitions: Yes

984 Delta Dental of Rhode Island

10 Charles Street
Providence, RI 02904-2208
Toll-Free: 800-598-6684
Phone: 401-752-6000
Fax: 401-752-6060
email@deltadentalri.com
www.deltadentalri.com
Mailing Address: PO Box 1517, Providence, RI 02901-1517
Non-Profit Organization: Yes
Year Founded: 1959
Total Enrollment: 59,500,000
State Enrollment: 587,000

Healthplan and Services Defined
PLAN TYPE: Dental
Other Type: Dental PPO
Plan Specialty: Dental
Benefits Offered: Dental

Type of Coverage
Commercial

Geographic Areas Served
Statewide

Peer Review Type
Case Management: Yes

Publishes and Distributes Report Card: Yes

Key Personnel
President & CEO . . . . Joseph A Nagle
VP, Chief Financial Offc . . . . Richard A Fritz
VP, Chief Actuary . . . . Craig W Lewis
VP, Sales, Altus Dental . . . . Joseph Perroni
VP, External Affairs . . . . Kathryn M Shanley
VP, Operations . . . . Stephen J Sperandio
VP, Chief Info Officer . . . . Thomas D Chase
VP, Sales, Delta Dental . . . . Angelo Pezzullo
Corporate Communications . . . . Mary Sommer
401-752-6265
msommer@deltadentalri.com
Dir/Media & Public Affair . . . . Elizabeth Risberg
415-972-8423

985 eHealthInsurance Services Inc.

11919 Foundation Place
Gold River, CA 95670
Toll-Free: 800-644-3491
webmaster@healthinsurance.com
www.e.healthinsurance.com
Year Founded: 1997

Healthplan and Services Defined
PLAN TYPE: HMO/PPO
Benefits Offered: Dental, Life, STD

Type of Coverage
Commercial, Individual, Medicare

Geographic Areas Served
All 50 states in the USA and District of Columbia

Key Personnel
Chairman & CEO . . . . Gary L. Lauer
EVP/Business & Corp. Dev. Bruce Telkamp
EVP/Chief Technology . . . . Dr. Sheldon X. Wang
SVP & CFO . . . . Stuart M. Huizinga

Pres. of eHealth Gov. Sys . . . . Samuel C. Gibbs
SVP of Sales & Operations . . . . Robert S. Hurley
Director Public Relations . . . . Nate Purpura
650-210-3115

986 Humana Health Insurance of Rhode Island

One International Boulevard
Suite 904
Mahwah, NJ 07495
Toll-Free: 800-967-2370
www.humana.com
For Profit Organization: Yes

Healthplan and Services Defined
PLAN TYPE: HMO/PPO

Type of Coverage
Commercial, Individual

Accreditation Certification
URAC, NCQA, CORE

987 Neighborhood Health Plan of Rhode Island

299 Promenade Street
Providence, RI 02908
Toll-Free: 800-963-1001
Phone: 401-459-6000
Fax: 401-459-6175
www.nhpri.org
Non-Profit Organization: Yes
Year Founded: 1993
Number of Primary Care Physicians: 900
Number of Referral/Specialty Physicians: 2,700
Total Enrollment: 90,000
State Enrollment: 90,000

Healthplan and Services Defined
PLAN TYPE: HMO
Model Type: Network
Benefits Offered: Disease Management, Wellness

Type of Coverage
Medicaid

Peer Review Type
Case Management: Yes

Publishes and Distributes Report Card: Yes

Accreditation Certification
NCQA

Key Personnel
Chairman . . . . Merrill Thomas
Vice-Chairwoman . . . . Jane Hayward
Treasurer . . . . Peter Walsh
Secretary . . . . Brenda Dowlatshahi
President/CEO . . . . James A. Hooley
MD . . . . Francisco Paco"", Trilla
Chief Medica
Media . . . . Y

988 Tufts Health Plan: Rhode Island

1 West Exchange Place
Providence, RI 02903
Toll-Free: 800-682-8059
Phone: 401-272-3499
www.tuftshealthplan.com
Non-Profit Organization: Yes
Year Founded: 1979
Number of Affiliated Hospitals: 90
Number of Primary Care Physicians: 25,000
Number of Referral/Specialty Physicians: 12,500
Total Enrollment: 1,018,589

Healthplan and Services Defined
 PLAN TYPE: HMO/PPO
 Model Type: IPA
 Plan Specialty: ASO, Behavioral Health, Chiropractic, Disease
  Management, EPO, Lab, PBM, Vision, Radiology, UR, Pharmacy
 Benefits Offered: Behavioral Health, Chiropractic, Complementary
  Medicine, Disease Management, Home Care, Inpatient SNF,
  Physical Therapy, Podiatry, Prescription, Psychiatric, Transplant,
  Vision, Wellness

Type of Coverage
 Commercial, Individual, Medicare, Supplemental Medicare

Type of Payment Plans Offered
 POS, DFFS, FFS, Combination FFS & DFFS

Geographic Areas Served
 Massachusetts, New Hampshire and Rhode Island

Subscriber Information
 Average Monthly Fee Per Subscriber
  (Employee + Employer Contribution):
   Employee Only (Self): $190.00-220.00
   Employee & 2 Family Members: $800.00-950.00
   Medicare: $150.00
 Average Annual Deductible Per Subscriber:
   Employee Only (Self): $1000.00
   Employee & 1 Family Member: $500.00
   Employee & 2 Family Members: $3000.00
 Average Subscriber Co-Payment:
   Primary Care Physician: $10.00
   Non-Network Physician: 20%
   Prescription Drugs: $10/20/35
   Hospital ER: $50.00
   Home Health Care: $0
   Home Health Care Max. Days/Visits Covered: 120 days
   Nursing Home: $0
   Nursing Home Max. Days/Visits Covered: 120 days

Network Qualifications
 Pre-Admission Certification: No

Peer Review Type
 Utilization Review: Yes
 Case Management: Yes

Publishes and Distributes Report Card: Yes

Accreditation Certification
 TJC, AAPI, NCQA

Key Personnel
 Principal . . . . .Mark Cenachetti
 Account Executive . . . . .Sarah Nowicki

Average Claim Compensation
 Physician's Fees Charged: 75%
 Hospital's Fees Charged: 70%

Specialty Managed Care Partners
 Advance PCS, Private Healthe Care Systems

Employer References
 Commonwealth of Massachuestts, Fleet Boston, Roman Catholic
  Archdiocese of Boston, City of Boston, State Street Corporation

---

989   UnitedHealthCare of Rhode Island
475 Kilvert Street
Warwick, RI 02886
Toll-Free: 800-447-1245
Phone: 401-737-6900
RhodeIsland_PR_Team@uhc.com
www.uhc.com
For Profit Organization: Yes
Year Founded: 1983
Owned by an Integrated Delivery Network (IDN): Yes
Number of Affiliated Hospitals: 5,609
Number of Primary Care Physicians: 726,537
Total Enrollment: 70,000,000

State Enrollment: 92,000

Healthplan and Services Defined
 PLAN TYPE: HMO/PPO
 Model Type: IPA
 Plan Specialty: Behavioral Health, Chiropractic, Dental, Disease
  Management, Lab, PBM, Vision, Radiology
 Benefits Offered: Prescription
 Offers Demand Management Patient Information Service: Yes

Type of Coverage
 Commercial

Type of Payment Plans Offered
 Combination FFS & DFFS

Geographic Areas Served
 Rhode Island & Southeastern Massachusetts

Publishes and Distributes Report Card: Yes

Accreditation Certification
 AAPI, NCQA

Key Personnel
 CFO. . . . . .Donald H Powers
 In House Formulary. . . . . .Scott E Enos, RPh
 Marketing . . . . .James Moniz, Jr
 Materials Management . . . . .Diane McDole
 Medical Affairs . . . . .William Corrao, MD
 Media Contact . . . . .Debora Spano
  debora_m_spano@uhc.com

Specialty Managed Care Partners
 G Tec, State of RI

Health Insurance Coverage Status and Type of Coverage by Age

Category	All Persons		Under 18 years		Under 65 years		65 years and over	
	Number	%	Number	%	Number	%	Number	%
Total population	4,678	-	1,077	-	3,970	-	708	-
Covered by some type of health insurance	3,939 *(18)*	84.2 *(0.4)*	1,004 *(7)*	93.3 *(0.6)*	3,236 *(18)*	81.5 *(0.5)*	704 *(2)*	99.4 *(0.1)*
Covered by private health insurance	2,912 *(28)*	62.3 *(0.6)*	570 *(11)*	53.0 *(1.1)*	2,465 *(27)*	62.1 *(0.7)*	447 *(7)*	63.2 *(1.0)*
Employment based	2,370 *(27)*	50.7 *(0.6)*	489 *(11)*	45.4 *(1.0)*	2,135 *(25)*	53.8 *(0.6)*	235 *(7)*	33.3 *(1.0)*
Direct purchase	537 *(16)*	11.5 *(0.3)*	60 *(6)*	5.6 *(0.6)*	307 *(13)*	7.7 *(0.3)*	230 *(7)*	32.6 *(1.0)*
Covered by TRICARE	220 *(10)*	4.7 *(0.2)*	41 *(4)*	3.8 *(0.4)*	146 *(9)*	3.7 *(0.2)*	74 *(4)*	10.5 *(0.6)*
Covered by government health insurance	1,615 *(19)*	34.5 *(0.4)*	471 *(11)*	43.7 *(1.1)*	923 *(19)*	23.2 *(0.5)*	692 *(3)*	97.9 *(0.3)*
Covered by Medicaid	869 *(20)*	18.6 *(0.4)*	465 *(12)*	43.2 *(1.1)*	777 *(19)*	19.6 *(0.5)*	92 *(5)*	13.0 *(0.7)*
Also by private insurance	122 *(6)*	2.6 *(0.1)*	35 *(4)*	3.3 *(0.3)*	84 *(5)*	2.1 *(0.1)*	38 *(4)*	5.4 *(0.5)*
Covered by Medicare	845 *(8)*	18.1 *(0.2)*	8 *(2)*	0.7 *(0.2)*	153 *(8)*	3.9 *(0.2)*	692 *(3)*	97.7 *(0.3)*
Also by private insurance	482 *(8)*	10.3 *(0.2)*	2 *(1)*	0.2 *(0.1)*	46 *(4)*	1.2 *(0.1)*	435 *(7)*	61.5 *(1.0)*
Also by Medicaid	157 *(8)*	3.3 *(0.2)*	4 *(1)*	0.3 *(0.1)*	65 *(5)*	1.6 *(0.1)*	92 *(5)*	13.0 *(0.7)*
Covered by VA Care	142 *(5)*	3.0 *(0.1)*	2 *(1)*	0.2 *(0.1)*	75 *(5)*	1.9 *(0.1)*	67 *(3)*	9.5 *(0.4)*
Not covered at any time during the year	739 *(18)*	15.8 *(0.4)*	73 *(7)*	6.7 *(0.6)*	735 *(18)*	18.5 *(0.5)*	4 *(1)*	0.6 *(0.1)*

Note: Numbers in thousands; Figures cover 2013; Margin of error appears in parenthesis; A "Z" indicates that the value either represents or rounds to zero.
Source: U.S. Census Bureau, 2013 American Community Survey, Table HI05. Health Insurance Coverage Status and Type of Coverage by State and Age for All People: 2013

South Carolina

990　Aetna Health of the Carolinas
11675 Great Oaks Way
Suite 330
Alpharetta, GA 30022
Toll-Free: 866-582-9629
www.aetna.com
For Profit Organization: Yes
Total Enrollment: 18,960

Healthplan and Services Defined
　PLAN TYPE: HMO
　Other Type: POS
　Plan Specialty: EPO
　Benefits Offered: Dental, Disease Management, Long-Term Care,
　　Prescription, Wellness, Life, LTD, STD

Type of Coverage
　Commercial, Individual

Type of Payment Plans Offered
　POS, FFS

Geographic Areas Served
　Statewide

991　Assurant Employee Benefits: South Carolina
5 Foot Point Road
Columbia, SC 29209-0846
Phone: 803-782-2132
benefits@assurant.com
www.assurantemployeebenefits.com
For Profit Organization: Yes
Number of Primary Care Physicians: 112,000
Total Enrollment: 47,000

Healthplan and Services Defined
　PLAN TYPE: Multiple
　Plan Specialty: Dental, Vision, Long & Short-Term Disability
　Benefits Offered: Dental, Vision, Wellness, AD&D, Life, LTD, STD

Type of Coverage
　Commercial, Indemnity, Individual Dental Plans

Geographic Areas Served
　Statewide

Subscriber Information
　Average Monthly Fee Per Subscriber
　　(Employee + Employer Contribution):
　　　Employee Only (Self): Varies by plan

Accreditation Certification
　TJC

Key Personnel
　Manager ....Dan Pruitt
　PR Specialist............................Megan Hutchison
　　816-556-7815
　　megan.hutchison@assurant.com

992　Blue Cross & Blue Shield of South Carolina
I-20 Alpine Road
Columbia, SC 29219
Toll-Free: 800-288-2227
Phone: 803-264-7258
Fax: 803-264-7257
www.bcbssc.com
Subsidiary of: Blue Choice Health Plan of South Carolina
For Profit Organization: Yes
Year Founded: 1946
Number of Affiliated Hospitals: 64
Number of Primary Care Physicians: 3,434

Number of Referral/Specialty Physicians: 5,473
Total Enrollment: 950,000
State Enrollment: 950,000

Healthplan and Services Defined
　PLAN TYPE: HMO/PPO
　Model Type: Network
　Plan Specialty: ASO, Behavioral Health, Chiropractic, Dental,
　　Disease Management, EPO, Lab, PBM, Vision, Radiology, UR
　Benefits Offered: Behavioral Health, Chiropractic, Complementary
　　Medicine, Dental, Disease Management, Physical Therapy,
　　Podiatry, Prescription, Psychiatric, Transplant, Vision, Wellness
　Offers Demand Management Patient Information Service: Yes

Type of Coverage
　Commercial, Individual, Medicare

Type of Payment Plans Offered
　POS, DFFS, Capitated, FFS, Combination FFS & DFFS

Geographic Areas Served
　Statewide

Network Qualifications
　Pre-Admission Certification: Yes

Peer Review Type
　Utilization Review: Yes
　Second Surgical Opinion: Yes

Publishes and Distributes Report Card: Yes

Accreditation Certification
　URAC, NCQA
　TJC Accreditation, Utilization Review, Pre-Admission Certification,
　　State Licensure, Quality Assurance Program

Key Personnel
　Chairman.......................................Ed Sellers
　President ....David Pankau
　EVP/COO.................................Thomas Faulds
　VP/Managed Care Services ....Robert Leichtle
　SVP/Actuarial Services....................William R Schrader
　Media/Press Relations...........................Dale Rish
　Small Group & Indiv Oper.........................Terry Peace
　Marketing ....Mike Griggs
　Medical Affairs ....John Little
　Information Systems ....Stephen Wiggins
　Sales ....Mike Griggs
　Media Contact ....Elizabeth Hammond
　　803-264-4626

Specialty Managed Care Partners
　Enters into Contracts with Regional Business Coalitions: Yes

993　BlueChoice Health Plan of South Carolina
PO Box 6170
Columbia, SC 29223
Toll-Free: 800-327-3183
Phone: 803-786-8466
Fax: 803-754-6386
ann.weldon@bluechoicesc.com
www.bluechoicesc.com
Secondary Address: 4101 Percival Road, Columbia, SC 29229
For Profit Organization: Yes
Year Founded: 1984
Owned by an Integrated Delivery Network (IDN): Yes
Federally Qualified: Yes
Number of Affiliated Hospitals: 68
Number of Primary Care Physicians: 7,700
Number of Referral/Specialty Physicians: 4,199
Total Enrollment: 205,000
State Enrollment: 205,000

Healthplan and Services Defined
　PLAN TYPE: Multiple
　Model Type: IPA
　Plan Specialty: ASO, Disease Management, EPO, PBM, Vision, UR

Benefits Offered: Behavioral Health, Chiropractic, Complementary Medicine, Dental, Disease Management, Home Care, Inpatient SNF, Physical Therapy, Podiatry, Prescription, Psychiatric, Transplant, Vision, Wellness, AD&D, Life, LTD, STD, EAP
Offers Demand Management Patient Information Service: Yes

Type of Coverage
Commercial, Individual, Medicare, Medicaid, Medicare Advantage
Catastrophic Illness Benefit: Maximum $2M

Type of Payment Plans Offered
POS, DFFS, Combination FFS & DFFS

Geographic Areas Served
South Carolina

Subscriber Information
Average Annual Deductible Per Subscriber:
  Employee Only (Self): $0
  Employee & 1 Family Member: $0
  Employee & 2 Family Members: $0
Average Subscriber Co-Payment:
  Primary Care Physician: $15.00
  Non-Network Physician: $25.00
  Prescription Drugs: $3 tier
  Hospital ER: 10%
  Home Health Care: 10%
  Home Health Care Max. Days/Visits Covered: Unlimited
  Nursing Home Max. Days/Visits Covered: 120 days

Network Qualifications
Pre-Admission Certification: Yes

Peer Review Type
Utilization Review: Yes
Second Surgical Opinion: Yes
Case Management: Yes

Publishes and Distributes Report Card: Yes

Accreditation Certification
NCQA
Quality Assurance Program

Key Personnel
President/COO . . . . Mary P Mazzola-Spivey
  803-786-8466
Finance Director . . . . Timothy L Vaughn
  803-786-8466
VP Operations . . . . Toni Hankins
Assistant VP Operations . . . . Toni J Hankins
  803-786-8466
VP Health Care Network . . . . Ann T Burnett
  803-786-8466
Chief Medical Officer . . . . Laura B Long, MD
  803-786-8466
In House Formulary . . . . Laura B Long, MD
VP Marketing . . . . Bill Ferguson
  803-786-8466
QA/UR . . . . Laura B Long, MD
Medical Affairs. . . . . Laura B Long, MD
Manager Info. Services . . . . Mark Rush
  803-786-8466
VP Health Network . . . . Ann T Burnett
  803-786-8466
VP Sales. . . . . Bill Ferguson
  803-786-8466

Average Claim Compensation
Physician's Fees Charged: 65%
Hospital's Fees Charged: 65%

Specialty Managed Care Partners
Companion Benefit Alternatives (CBA)

Employer References
Alltel Corporation, Bank of America, Kimberley Clark, BellSouth, United Parcel Service

994 Carolina Care Plan

201 Executive Center Drive
Suite 300
Columbia, SC 29210
Toll-Free: 800-868-6734
Phone: 803-750-7400
Fax: 803-750-7474
www.carolinacareplan.com
Secondary Address: 3535 Pelham Road, Suite 102, Greenville, SC 29615
Subsidiary of: A Medical Mutual of Ohio Company
For Profit Organization: Yes
Year Founded: 1984
Number of Affiliated Hospitals: 61
Number of Primary Care Physicians: 7,332
Total Enrollment: 123,000
State Enrollment: 123,000

Healthplan and Services Defined
  PLAN TYPE: HMO
  Other Type: POS
  Benefits Offered: Chiropractic, Dental, Disease Management, Home Care, Inpatient SNF, Physical Therapy, Podiatry, Prescription, Psychiatric, Vision, Wellness

Type of Coverage
Commercial, Individual, Medicare

Geographic Areas Served
South Carolina

Subscriber Information
Average Monthly Fee Per Subscriber
  (Employee + Employer Contribution):
    Employee Only (Self): Varies
    Employee & 1 Family Member: Varies
    Employee & 2 Family Members: Varies
    Medicare: Varies
Average Annual Deductible Per Subscriber:
    Employee Only (Self): Varies
    Employee & 1 Family Member: Varies
    Employee & 2 Family Members: Varies
    Medicare: Varies
Average Subscriber Co-Payment:
    Primary Care Physician: Varies
    Non-Network Physician: Varies
    Prescription Drugs: Varies
    Hospital ER: Varies
    Home Health Care: Varies
    Home Health Care Max. Days/Visits Covered: Varies
    Nursing Home: Varies
    Nursing Home Max. Days/Visits Covered: Varies

Accreditation Certification
URAC

Key Personnel
President. . . . . Carson Meehan
VP/COO/Medical Affairs . . . . Belinda Cox, RN/CPHQ
VP/CFO. . . . . Mark T Corcoran
Medical Director . . . . Edward D Hutt, MD
VP Network Management . . . . Donald Pifer
Marketing. . . . . Robert M Dickes
Pharmacy Director. . . . . Jim Shelley, PhD
Compliance Officer . . . . Pat Mack
Manager, Media Relations . . . . Ed Byers
  216-687-2685
Sr Communications Spec. Kasey Stround
  803-561-7707

Specialty Managed Care Partners
Express Scripts

Employer References
South Carolina Bar, South Carolina Home Builders Association, Low County Manufactures Council, South Carolina Federal Employees

995 CIGNA HealthCare of South Carolina

250 Commonwealth Drive
Suite 110
Greenville, SC 29615
Toll-Free: 800-962-8811
Phone: 864-987-1350
Fax: 864-987-1389
www.cigna.com
For Profit Organization: Yes
Year Founded: 1987
Number of Primary Care Physicians: 8,100
Total Enrollment: 75,000,000
State Enrollment: 14,341

Healthplan and Services Defined
　PLAN TYPE: HMO
　Model Type: IPA
　Benefits Offered: Chiropractic, Complementary Medicine, Dental,
　　Disease Management, Home Care, Inpatient SNF, Long-Term
　　Care, Podiatry, Prescription, Psychiatric, Transplant, Vision,
　　Wellness

Type of Coverage
　Commercial

Type of Payment Plans Offered
　POS

Accreditation Certification
　URAC, NCQA

Key Personnel
　President/CEO . . . . H Edward Hanaway
　Executive VP/CFO . . . . Michael W Bell
　Ex VP Operations/Tech . . . . Scott A Storrer
　Chairman Audit Committee . . . . Robert H Campbell
　Corporate Governance . . . . Marilyn Ware
　Finance Committee . . . . Peter N Larson

996 Delta Dental of South Carolina

1320 Main Street
Suite 650
Columbia, SC 29201
Toll-Free: 800-529-3268
Phone: 803-731-2495
Fax: 803-731-0273
service@ddpmo.org
www.deltadentalsc.com
Secondary Address: 12399 Gravois Road, Saint Louis, MO
　63127-1702, 314-656-3000
Non-Profit Organization: Yes
Year Founded: 1969
Number of Primary Care Physicians: 180,000
Total Enrollment: 1,400,000

Healthplan and Services Defined
　PLAN TYPE: Dental
　Other Type: Dental PPO
　Model Type: Network
　Plan Specialty: ASO, Dental
　Benefits Offered: Dental

Type of Coverage
　Commercial, Individual, Group
　Catastrophic Illness Benefit: None

Geographic Areas Served
　Statewide

Subscriber Information
　Average Monthly Fee Per Subscriber
　　(Employee + Employer Contribution):
　　　Employee Only (Self): Varies
　　　Employee & 1 Family Member: Varies
　　　Employee & 2 Family Members: Varies

Average Annual Deductible Per Subscriber:
　Employee Only (Self): Varies
　Employee & 1 Family Member: Varies
　Employee & 2 Family Members: Varies
Average Subscriber Co-Payment:
　Prescription Drugs: $0
　Home Health Care: $0
　Nursing Home: $0

997 eHealthInsurance Services Inc.

11919 Foundation Place
Gold River, CA 95670
Toll-Free: 800-644-3491
webmaster@healthinsurance.com
www.e.healthinsurance.com
Year Founded: 1997

Healthplan and Services Defined
　PLAN TYPE: HMO/PPO
　Benefits Offered: Dental, Life, STD

Type of Coverage
　Commercial, Individual, Medicare

Geographic Areas Served
　All 50 states in the USA and District of Columbia

Key Personnel
　Chairman & CEO . . . . Gary L. Lauer
　EVP/Business & Corp. Dev. Bruce Telkamp
　EVP/Chief Technology . . . . Dr. Sheldon X. Wang
　SVP & CFO . . . . Stuart M. Huizinga
　Pres. of eHealth Gov. Sys . . . . Samuel C. Gibbs
　SVP of Sales & Operations . . . . Robert S. Hurley
　Director Public Relations . . . . Nate Purpura
　650-210-3115

998 Great-West Healthcare South Carolina

250 Commonwealth Drive
Suite 110
Greenville, NC 29615
Toll-Free: 866-494-2111
Phone: 864-987-1350
eliginquiries@cigna.com
www.cignaforhealth.com
Subsidiary of: CIGNA HealthCare
Acquired by: CIGNA
For Profit Organization: Yes
Total Enrollment: 16,852
State Enrollment: 15,452

Healthplan and Services Defined
　PLAN TYPE: HMO/PPO
　Benefits Offered: Disease Management, Prescription, Wellness

Type of Coverage
　Commercial

Type of Payment Plans Offered
　POS, FFS

Geographic Areas Served
　South Carolina

Accreditation Certification
　URAC

Specialty Managed Care Partners
　Caremark Rx

999   Humana Health Insurance of South Carolina

240 Harbison Boulevard
Suite H
Columbia, SC 29212
Toll-Free: 877-486-2622
Phone: 803-865-7663
Fax: 803-865-1760
www.humana.com
Secondary Address: 430 Roper Mountain Road, Suite G, Greenville,
   SC 29615, 803-865-7663
Subsidiary of: LifeSynch
For Profit Organization: Yes

Healthplan and Services Defined
   PLAN TYPE: HMO/PPO

Type of Coverage
   Commercial, Individual

Accreditation Certification
   URAC, NCQA, CORE

Geographic Areas Served
   North and South Carolina

Peer Review Type
   Utilization Review: Yes
   Second Surgical Opinion: Yes
   Case Management: Yes

Accreditation Certification
   AAAHC, URAC
   Utilization Review

Key Personnel
   President and CEO . . . . .Kenneth U. Kuk
   VP/Operations . . . . .Russell J Prepenbring
   Claims . . . . .B Shelton Rice
   Network Contracting . . . . .Patricia England
   Marketing. . . . . .Scott McEwen
   Provider Services . . . . .Pat England

Specialty Managed Care Partners
   Enters into Contracts with Regional Business Coalitions: Yes

1000   InStil Health

P.O. Box 100295
Mail Code AG-795
Columbia, SC 29202-3294
Toll-Free: 877-446-7845
Phone: 803-763-6620
Fax: 803-666-3705
sandy.collins@myinstil.com
www.myinstil.com
Total Enrollment: 30,000

Healthplan and Services Defined
   PLAN TYPE: Medicare

Type of Coverage
   Medicare, Supplemental Medicare

Accreditation Certification
   URAC

Key Personnel
   Network Manager. . . . . .Sandy Collins
   Assistant VP . . . . .Jennifer N. Pendleton
   Director, TRICARE SC . . . . .Vivian B. Mills

1001   Kanawha Healthcare Solutions

PO Box 7000
210 South White Street
Lancaster, SC 29721
Toll-Free: 888-313-4534
Phone: 803-283-5300
Fax: 803-416-5925
salessupport@kmgamerica.com
www.kmgamerica.com
Subsidiary of: KMG America
Acquired by: Humana, Inc.
For Profit Organization: Yes
Year Founded: 1992
Number of Affiliated Hospitals: 84
Number of Primary Care Physicians: 455
Number of Referral/Specialty Physicians: 1,427
Total Enrollment: 19,468
State Enrollment: 19,468

Healthplan and Services Defined
   PLAN TYPE: PPO
   Model Type: Network
   Benefits Offered: Long-Term Care, Life, LTD

Type of Coverage
   Self-funded plans only
   Catastrophic Illness Benefit: Unlimited

1002   Medical Mutual Services

PO Box 1640
Columbia, SC 29202-1640
Toll-Free: 800-773-1445
Phone: 803-214-3384
Fax: 803-214-3388
www.supermednetwork.com
Subsidiary of: SuperMed Network
Total Enrollment: 144,000

Healthplan and Services Defined
   PLAN TYPE: PPO

Type of Coverage
   Commercial, Self Funded, Insurance Companies

Geographic Areas Served
   South Carolina, Georgia, Ohio

Accreditation Certification
   TJC, NCQA

Key Personnel
   Director Sales/Marketing. . . . . .Dee Nash
   dee.nash@medmutual.com

1003   Select Health of South Carolina

PO Box 40849
Charleston, SC 29423
Toll-Free: 800-741-6605
Phone: 843-569-1759
www.selecthealthofsc.com
Secondary Address: 3315 Broad River Road, Columbia, SC 29210
Subsidiary of: AmeriHealth Mercy
For Profit Organization: Yes
Number of Affiliated Hospitals: 67
Number of Primary Care Physicians: 2,030
Number of Referral/Specialty Physicians: 4,490
Total Enrollment: 234,000
State Enrollment: 234,000

Healthplan and Services Defined
   PLAN TYPE: HMO
   Model Type: Medicaid
   Plan Specialty: Medicaid
   Benefits Offered: Medicaid

Type of Coverage
   Medicaid

Peer Review Type
   Case Management: Yes

Publishes and Distributes Report Card: Yes

Accreditation Certification
TJC, URAC, NCQA

Key Personnel

President/CEO	J Michael Jernigan
Executive Director	Cindy Helling
CFO	Rob Church
Dir, Data & Tech Services	John McFadden
Dir, Network Management	Peggy Vickery
Dir, Provider Relations	Philip Fairchild
Dir, Quaility Improvement	Rebecca Engelman, RN
Regional Dir Marketing	Tina Davis
Community Liason Director	Terry J Davenport
Chief Medical Officer	Fred Volkman, MD
Director of Member Services	Kevin Vaughan, MD
Medical Director	William Burnham, MD
Reg Dir, Marketing	Lillian Suarez
Dir, Communications	Tracy Pou
Dir, Member Services	Kevin Vaughn

1004 Southeast Community Care

7301 Rivers Avenue
Suite 100
North Charleston, SC 29406-4650
Toll-Free: 888-998-3055
Phone: 843-553-9996
Fax: 843-553-9838
www.southeastcommunitycare.com
Subsidiary of: Arcadian Health Plans

Healthplan and Services Defined
PLAN TYPE: Medicare

Type of Coverage
Medicare

1005 Unison Health Plan of South Carolina

, SC
Toll-Free: 800-414-9025
www.uhccommunityplan.com

Healthplan and Services Defined
PLAN TYPE: HMO

Geographic Areas Served
Abbeville, Aiken, Allendale, Anderson, Bamberg, Barnwell, Beaufort, Berkeley, Calhoun, Chester, Clarendon, Colleton, Darlington, Dillon, Dorchester, Edgefield, Florence, Georgetown, Greenville, Hampton, Horry, Jasper, Lancaster, Laurens, Lee, Lexington, Marion, Marlboro, Newberry, Oconee, Orangeburg, Pickens, Richland, Saluda, Sumter, Union, Williamsburg, York

Accreditation Certification
NCQA

Key Personnel

Chief Executive Officer	Dan Gallagher
Finance Director	Jeff Skobel
Operations Director	Mary Ann Kelleher
Chief Medical Officer	Brenna DeLaine, MD
Media Contact	Jeff Smith

952-931-5685
jeff.smith@uhc.com

1006 UnitedHealthCare of South Carolina

107 Westpark Blvd
Suite 110
Columbia, SC 29210
Toll-Free: 800-660-5378
Phone: 803-551-1170
Fax: 803-454-1340
CarolinasPRTeam@uhc.com
www.uhc.com
Secondary Address: Golden Rule Insurance, 7440 Woodland Drive, Indianapolis, IN 46278, 888-545-5205
For Profit Organization: Yes
Number of Affiliated Hospitals: 5,609
Number of Primary Care Physicians: 726,537
Total Enrollment: 70,000,000
State Enrollment: 148,404

Healthplan and Services Defined
PLAN TYPE: HMO/PPO

Geographic Areas Served
Statewide

Accreditation Certification
AAPI, NCQA

Key Personnel

Media Contact	Roger Rollman

roger_f_rollman@uhc.com

1007 VSP: Vision Service Plan of South Carolina

11 Brendan Way
Suite B33
Greenville, SC 26915-3612
Toll-Free: 800-877-7195
Phone: 864-421-0707
webmaster@vsp.com
www.vsp.com
Year Founded: 1955
Number of Primary Care Physicians: 26,000
Total Enrollment: 55,000,000

Healthplan and Services Defined
PLAN TYPE: Vision
Plan Specialty: Vision
Benefits Offered: Vision

Type of Payment Plans Offered
Capitated

Geographic Areas Served
Statewide

Network Qualifications
Pre-Admission Certification: Yes

Peer Review Type
Utilization Review: Yes

Accreditation Certification
NCQA
Utilization Review, Quality Assurance Program

Key Personnel

Manager	Warren Laird

Health Insurance Coverage Status and Type of Coverage by Age

Category	All Persons		Under 18 years		Under 65 years		65 years and over	
	Number	%	Number	%	Number	%	Number	%
Total population	827	-	207	-	709	-	118	-
Covered by some type of health insurance	734 (6)	88.7 (0.7)	194 (2)	93.7 (1.1)	616 (6)	86.9 (0.8)	117 (1)	99.5 (0.4)
Covered by private health insurance	593 (7)	71.7 (0.9)	134 (4)	64.5 (1.9)	514 (7)	72.6 (1.0)	78 (2)	66.2 (1.7)
Employment based	442 (9)	53.4 (1.0)	110 (4)	53.1 (2.0)	419 (8)	59.1 (1.1)	23 (2)	19.7 (1.7)
Direct purchase	156 (6)	18.8 (0.7)	22 (2)	10.5 (1.0)	99 (5)	13.9 (0.7)	57 (2)	48.6 (2.1)
Covered by TRICARE	33 (4)	4.0 (0.4)	8 (2)	3.8 (0.8)	26 (3)	3.6 (0.5)	8 (1)	6.4 (1.1)
Covered by government health insurance	250 (6)	30.3 (0.7)	71 (4)	34.4 (1.8)	135 (6)	19.0 (0.8)	115 (1)	97.8 (0.6)
Covered by Medicaid	125 (6)	15.1 (0.7)	71 (4)	34.1 (1.8)	112 (6)	15.8 (0.8)	13 (2)	11.1 (1.3)
Also by private insurance	26 (3)	3.2 (0.3)	11 (2)	5.1 (0.8)	19 (3)	2.7 (0.4)	7 (1)	6.2 (1.0)
Covered by Medicare	134 (2)	16.3 (0.3)	1 (Z)	0.4 (0.2)	19 (2)	2.7 (0.3)	115 (1)	97.7 (0.7)
Also by private insurance	82 (3)	9.9 (0.3)	Z (Z)	0.2 (0.2)	6 (1)	0.8 (0.1)	76 (2)	64.4 (1.8)
Also by Medicaid	23 (2)	2.7 (0.3)	Z (Z)	0.2 (0.1)	10 (2)	1.3 (0.2)	13 (2)	11.1 (1.3)
Covered by VA Care	30 (2)	3.6 (0.3)	Z (Z)	0.1 (0.1)	15 (2)	2.1 (0.3)	15 (1)	12.7 (1.1)
Not covered at any time during the year	93 (5)	11.3 (0.7)	13 (2)	6.3 (1.1)	93 (5)	13.1 (0.8)	1 (Z)	0.5 (0.4)

Note: Numbers in thousands; Figures cover 2013; Margin of error appears in parenthesis; A "Z" indicates that the value either represents or rounds to zero.
Source: U.S. Census Bureau, 2013 American Community Survey, Table HI05. Health Insurance Coverage Status and Type of Coverage by State and Age for All People: 2013

South Dakota

1008 Aetna Health of South Dakota

151 Farmington Avenue
Hartford, CT 06156
Toll-Free: 800-872-3862
Phone: 860-273-0123
www.aetna.com
Partnered with: eHealthInsurance Services Inc.
For Profit Organization: Yes
Total Enrollment: 11,596,230

Healthplan and Services Defined
PLAN TYPE: PPO
Other Type: POS
Plan Specialty: EPO
Benefits Offered: Dental, Disease Management, Long-Term Care,
Prescription, Wellness, Life, LTD, STD

Type of Coverage
Commercial, Individual

Type of Payment Plans Offered
POS, FFS

Geographic Areas Served
Statewide

Key Personnel
Chairman/CEO/President . . . . Mark T Bertolini
EVP/General Counsel . . . . William J Casazza
EVP/CFO . . . . Shawn M Guertin

1009 Americas PPO

7201 West 78th Street
Suite 100
Bloomington, MN 55439
Toll-Free: 800-948-9451
Phone: 952-896-1201
www.americasppo.com
Subsidiary of: Araz Group Inc
For Profit Organization: Yes
Year Founded: 1982
Physician Owned Organization: No
Number of Affiliated Hospitals: 260
Number of Primary Care Physicians: 18,000
Number of Referral/Specialty Physicians: 71,000
State Enrollment: 245,000

Healthplan and Services Defined
PLAN TYPE: PPO
Model Type: Staff, Group
Benefits Offered: Behavioral Health, Wellness, Worker's
Compensation, Maternity
Offers Demand Management Patient Information Service: No

Type of Coverage
Commercial, Individual, Medicaid
Catastrophic Illness Benefit: Maximum $1M

Type of Payment Plans Offered
DFFS, Capitated

Geographic Areas Served
Minnesota, South Dakota, North Dakota, Western Wisconsin

Subscriber Information
Average Monthly Fee Per Subscriber
(Employee + Employer Contribution):
Employee Only (Self): Varies by plan
Average Annual Deductible Per Subscriber:
Employee Only (Self): $500.00
Employee & 1 Family Member: $500.00
Employee & 2 Family Members: $750.00
Average Subscriber Co-Payment:
Primary Care Physician: $15.00

Non-Network Physician: $500.00-1000.00
Prescription Drugs: $10.00/15.00
Hospital ER: $150.00
Nursing Home: Varies

Network Qualifications
Pre-Admission Certification: Yes

Peer Review Type
Utilization Review: Yes
Case Management: Yes

Publishes and Distributes Report Card: No

Accreditation Certification
URAC
TJC Accreditation, Utilization Review, Pre-Admission Certification,
State Licensure, Quality Assurance Program

Key Personnel
President . . . . Amir Eftekhari
Founder and CEO . . . . Nazie Eftekhari
Executive Vice President. Elizabeth Vetter
Marketing . . . . Tim Bode
Sales. . . . . Wendy Olson

Specialty Managed Care Partners
Enters into Contracts with Regional Business Coalitions: Yes

1010 Avera Health Plans

3816 South Elmwood Ave
Sioux Falls, SD 57105-6583
Toll-Free: 888-605-3229
Phone: 605-322-4500
www.averahealthplans.com
Subsidiary of: Avera Health
Total Enrollment: 63,000
State Enrollment: 63,000

Healthplan and Services Defined
PLAN TYPE: HMO
Benefits Offered: Disease Management, Prescription, Wellness,
Health Education, EAP

Type of Coverage
Commercial, Individual

Type of Payment Plans Offered
POS

Geographic Areas Served
South Dakota and areas of North Dakota, Minnesota, Iowa and
Nebraska

Accreditation Certification
URAC

Key Personnel
Chairman . . . . Rodney Fouberg
President & CEO. . . . . John Porter
SVP, Hospital Operations . . . . Judy Blauwet

1011 CIGNA HealthCare of South Dakota

525 West Monroe Street
Suite 300
Chicago, IL 60661-3629
Toll-Free: 866-438-2446
Phone: 312-648-2460
Fax: 312-648-3617
www.cigna.com
For Profit Organization: Yes
Total Enrollment: 8,135
State Enrollment: 6,570

Healthplan and Services Defined
PLAN TYPE: PPO
Benefits Offered: Disease Management, Prescription, Transplant,
Wellness

Type of Coverage
Commercial

Type of Payment Plans Offered
POS, FFS

Geographic Areas Served
South Dakota

1012 DakotaCare

2600 W. 49th Street
P.O. Box 7406
Sioux Falls, SD 57117-7406
Toll-Free: 800-325-5598
Phone: 605-334-4000
customer-service@dakotacare.com
www.dakotacare.com
Subsidiary of: Dakotacare Administrative Services
For Profit Organization: Yes
Year Founded: 1986
Physician Owned Organization: Yes
Number of Affiliated Hospitals: 74
Number of Primary Care Physicians: 825
Number of Referral/Specialty Physicians: 950
Total Enrollment: 118,600
State Enrollment: 24,310

Healthplan and Services Defined
PLAN TYPE: HMO
Model Type: IPA
Plan Specialty: ASO, Behavioral Health, Chiropractic, Dental, Disease Management, Lab, PBM, Vision, Radiology, UR
Benefits Offered: Behavioral Health, Chiropractic, Complementary Medicine, Dental, Disease Management, Home Care, Inpatient SNF, Physical Therapy, Podiatry, Prescription, Psychiatric, Transplant, Vision, Wellness, AD&D, Life, LTD, STD
Offers Demand Management Patient Information Service: No

Type of Payment Plans Offered
POS, FFS

Geographic Areas Served
HMO: all counties in South Dakota; TPA: Nationwide

Subscriber Information
Average Monthly Fee Per Subscriber
(Employee + Employer Contribution):
Employee Only (Self): Varies by plan
Average Annual Deductible Per Subscriber:
Employee & 1 Family Member: $1500
Average Subscriber Co-Payment:
Primary Care Physician: $25.00
Non-Network Physician: $25.00
Hospital ER: $150.00

Network Qualifications
Pre-Admission Certification: Yes

Peer Review Type
Utilization Review: Yes
Case Management: Yes

Publishes and Distributes Report Card: No

Accreditation Certification
URAC
Utilization Review, Pre-Admission Certification, State Licensure, Quality Assurance Program

Key Personnel
CEO . . . . .Kirk Zimmer
605-334-4000
kzimmer@dakotacare.com
Chief Operating Officer. .Rhonda K. Mack
dkrogman@dakotacare.com
Chief Financial Officer. . . . . .John D. Graham
Asst VP, Process Improv. . . . . .Trish Zimmer
tzimmer@dakotacare.com

Enrollment . . . . .Melissa Powell
mpowell@dakotacare.com
COBRA . . . . .Joanne Curry
jcurry@dakotacare.com
Director, TPA Services. . . . . .Marti Thompson
mthompso@dakotacare.com
Chief Marketing Officer . . . . .Greg Jasmer
tnichols@dakotacare.com
Compliance/Quality. . . . . .Jacqueline Cole
jcole@dakotacare.com
Chief Medical Officer. .Paul Amundson, MD
pamundso@dakotacare.com
Dir, Customer Service. . . . . .Jill Jaacks
jjaacks@dakotacare.com
VP, Provider Services . . . . .Scott Jamison
sjamison@dakotacare.com
Director, Marketing. . . . . .Greg Jasmer
gjasmer@dakotacare.com

Specialty Managed Care Partners
Prescription benefits - CVS Caremark, Chiropractic - CASD, Transplant - Optum, Dental Benefits - Companion Life, Life Insurance Benefits - Companion Life, Sun Life Standard, STD/LTD - Companion Life
Enters into Contracts with Regional Business Coalitions: No

1013 Delta Dental of South Dakota

PO Box 1157
Pierre, SD 57501
Toll-Free: 800-627-3961
Fax: 605-224-0909
sales@deltadentalsd.com
www.deltadentalsd.com
Non-Profit Organization: Yes
Year Founded: 1963
Total Enrollment: 60,000,000
State Enrollment: 204,000

Healthplan and Services Defined
PLAN TYPE: Dental
Other Type: Dental PPO
Model Type: Network
Plan Specialty: ASO, Dental
Benefits Offered: Dental

Type of Coverage
Commercial, Individual, Group
Catastrophic Illness Benefit: None

Geographic Areas Served
Statewide

Subscriber Information
Average Monthly Fee Per Subscriber
(Employee + Employer Contribution):
Employee Only (Self): Varies
Employee & 1 Family Member: Varies
Employee & 2 Family Members: Varies
Average Annual Deductible Per Subscriber:
Employee Only (Self): Varies
Employee & 1 Family Member: Varies
Employee & 2 Family Members: Varies
Average Subscriber Co-Payment:
Prescription Drugs: $0
Home Health Care: $0
Nursing Home: $0

Key Personnel
President & CEO. . . . . .Scott Jones
VP, Operations . . . . .Mick Heckenlaible
VP, Finance . . . . .Kirby Scott
VP, Underwriting . . . . .Jeff Miller
VP, Professional Services. . . . . .Nance Orsbon
VP, Information Tech. . . . . .Gene Tetzlaff

Dir/Media & Public Affair . . . . Elizabeth Risberg
415-972-8423

Specialty Managed Care Partners
Enters into Contracts with Regional Business Coalitions: Yes

1014 eHealthInsurance Services Inc.

11919 Foundation Place
Gold River, CA 95670
Toll-Free: 800-644-3491
webmaster@healthinsurance.com
www.e.healthinsurance.com
Year Founded: 1997
Total Enrollment: 3,000,000

Healthplan and Services Defined
PLAN TYPE: HMO/PPO
Benefits Offered: Dental, Life, STD

Type of Coverage
Commercial, Individual, Medicare

Geographic Areas Served
All 50 states in the USA and District of Columbia

Key Personnel
Chairman & CEO . . . . Gary L. Lauer
EVP/Business & Corp. Dev. Bruce Telkamp
EVP/Chief Technology . . . . Dr. Sheldon X. Wang
SVP & CFO . . . . Stuart M. Huizinga
Pres. of eHealth Gov. Sys . . . . Samuel C. Gibbs
SVP of Sales & Operations . . . . Robert S. Hurley
Director Public Relations . . . . Nate Purpura
650-210-3115

1015 First Choice of the Midwest

100 S Spring Avenue
Suite 220
Sioux Falls, SD 57104-3660
Toll-Free: 888-246-9949
Phone: 605-332-5955
Fax: 605-332-5953
info@1choicem.com
www.1choicem.com
Mailing Address: PO Box 5078, Sioux Falls, SD 57117
For Profit Organization: Yes
Year Founded: 1997
Owned by an Integrated Delivery Network (IDN): Yes
Number of Referral/Specialty Physicians: 6,924
Total Enrollment: 87,000
State Enrollment: 25,000

Healthplan and Services Defined
PLAN TYPE: PPO
Model Type: Network, Open Staff
Plan Specialty: ASO, Behavioral Health, Chiropractic, Disease
Management, EPO, Lab, Radiology, Worker's Compensation
Benefits Offered: Behavioral Health, Chiropractic, Complementary
Medicine, Home Care, Inpatient SNF, Long-Term Care, Physical
Therapy, Podiatry, Prescription, Psychiatric, Transplant, Vision,
Wellness, Worker's Compensation, Durable Medical Equipment

Type of Payment Plans Offered
DFFS

Geographic Areas Served
Colorado, Iowa, North Dakota, Nebraska, Utah, South Dakota,
Minnesota, Montana, Wyoming, and Idaho

Network Qualifications
Pre-Admission Certification: No

Accreditation Certification
TJC, NCQA

Average Claim Compensation
Physician's Fees Charged: 85%
Hospital's Fees Charged: 90%

1016 Great-West Healthcare South Dakota

525 West Monroe Street
Suite 300
Chicago, IL 60661-3629
Toll-Free: 800-678-8287
Phone: 312-648-2460
eliginquiries@cigna.com
www.cignaforhealth.com
Subsidiary of: CIGNA HealthCare
Acquired by: CIGNA
For Profit Organization: Yes
Total Enrollment: 1,685
State Enrollment: 1,430

Healthplan and Services Defined
PLAN TYPE: HMO/PPO
Benefits Offered: Disease Management, Prescription, Wellness

Type of Coverage
Commercial

Type of Payment Plans Offered
POS, FFS

Geographic Areas Served
South Dakota

Accreditation Certification
URAC

Key Personnel
Executive Vice President . . . . Richard F. Rivers
Chief Medical Officer . . . . Terry Fouts, MD

Specialty Managed Care Partners
Caremark Rx

1017 Humana Health Insurance of South Dakota

1611 Alderson Avenue
Billings, SD 59102
Toll-Free: 800-967-2308
Phone: 406-238-7130
Fax: 502-508-3186
www.humana.com
Subsidiary of: LifeSynch
For Profit Organization: Yes

Healthplan and Services Defined
PLAN TYPE: HMO/PPO

Type of Coverage
Commercial, Individual

Accreditation Certification
URAC, NCQA, CORE

1018 Medica: South Dakota

110 South Phillips Ave
Suite 200
Sioux Falls, SD 57104
Toll-Free: 800-841-6753
neducafb@medica.com
www.medica.com
Non-Profit Organization: Yes
Year Founded: 1991
Number of Affiliated Hospitals: 4,000
Number of Primary Care Physicians: 27,000
Total Enrollment: 1,600,000

Healthplan and Services Defined
PLAN TYPE: HMO
Model Type: IPA

Benefits Offered: Behavioral Health, Chiropractic, Complementary Medicine, Dental, Disease Management, Home Care, Inpatient SNF, Physical Therapy, Podiatry, Prescription, Psychiatric, Transplant, Vision, Wellness, Worker's Compensation, Nurse line chat, visiting nurse, wo

Type of Coverage
Commercial, Individual, Medicare, Medicaid

Type of Payment Plans Offered
POS

Geographic Areas Served
Minnesota, Wisconsin, North Dakota, South Dakota

Accreditation Certification
NCQA

Key Personnel
President/CEO.................................David Tilford
Sr VP/Government Programs......................Glenn Andis
Sr VP/Finance..................................Mark Baird
Sr VP/Chief Info Officer ....Scott Booher
Sr VP/Chief Medical Off ....Charles Fazio, MD
Sr VP/Commercial Markets.......................Tom Henke
Sr VP/General Counsel ....Jim Jacobson
Sr VP/Operations ....Jana L Johnson
Sr VP/Human Resources ....Deb Knutson
Sr VP/Marketing ....Rob Longendyke
Exec VP/CFO ....Aaron Reynolds

1019   UnitedHealthCare of South Dakota

9700 Health Care Lane
Minnetonka, MN 55343
Toll-Free: 800-842-3585
www.uhc.com
Subsidiary of: UnitedHealth Group
Year Founded: 1977
Number of Affiliated Hospitals: 4,200
Number of Primary Care Physicians: 460,000
Total Enrollment: 75,000,000

Healthplan and Services Defined
PLAN TYPE: HMO/PPO
Model Type: IPA, Group, Network
Plan Specialty: Lab, Radiology
Benefits Offered: Chiropractic, Dental, Physical Therapy, Prescription, Wellness, AD&D, Life, LTD, STD
Offers Demand Management Patient Information Service: Yes

Type of Coverage
Commercial, Individual, Indemnity, Medicare

Geographic Areas Served
Statewide

Network Qualifications
Pre-Admission Certification: Yes

Peer Review Type
Utilization Review: Yes
Second Surgical Opinion: Yes
Case Management: Yes

Publishes and Distributes Report Card: Yes

Accreditation Certification
TJC, NCQA

Specialty Managed Care Partners
Enters into Contracts with Regional Business Coalitions: Yes

1020   Wellmark Blue Cross & Blue Shield of South Dakota

1601 W Madison Street
Sioux Falls, SD 57104
Toll-Free: 800-831-4818
Phone: 605-373-7200
www.wellmark.com
For Profit Organization: Yes
Owned by an Integrated Delivery Network (IDN): Yes
Number of Affiliated Hospitals: 6,000
Number of Primary Care Physicians: 600,000
Total Enrollment: 1,800,000
State Enrollment: 300,000

Healthplan and Services Defined
PLAN TYPE: PPO
Model Type: Network
Plan Specialty: ASO, Behavioral Health, Chiropractic, Dental, Disease Management, EPO, Lab, PBM, Vision, Radiology, UR
Benefits Offered: Behavioral Health, Chiropractic, Complementary Medicine, Dental, Disease Management, Home Care, Inpatient SNF, Physical Therapy, Podiatry, Prescription, Psychiatric, Transplant, Vision, Wellness, AD&D, Life, LTD, STD

Type of Coverage
Commercial, Individual, Indemnity, Medicare, Supplemental Medicare, Medicaid, Catastrophic
Catastrophic Illness Benefit: Maximum $1M

Geographic Areas Served
South Dakota, Iowa

Publishes and Distributes Report Card: Yes

Accreditation Certification
AAAHC, TJC, URAC, NCQA

Key Personnel
Chairman/CEO...............................John D Forsyth
President/COO Wellmark SD...................Philip M Davis
Media Contact ....Rob Schweers
515-248-5683
schweers@wellmark.com

Specialty Managed Care Partners
American Health Ways

Health Insurance Coverage Status and Type of Coverage by Age

Category	All Persons		Under 18 years		Under 65 years		65 years and over	
	Number	%	Number	%	Number	%	Number	%
Total population	6,395	-	1,490	-	5,473	-	922	-
Covered by some type of health insurance	5,508 *(19)*	86.1 *(0.3)*	1,404 *(8)*	94.3 *(0.5)*	4,591 *(19)*	83.9 *(0.3)*	917 *(3)*	99.5 *(0.1)*
Covered by private health insurance	4,079 *(32)*	63.8 *(0.5)*	831 *(13)*	55.8 *(0.9)*	3,501 *(30)*	64.0 *(0.5)*	578 *(8)*	62.7 *(0.8)*
Employment based	3,281 *(31)*	51.3 *(0.5)*	706 *(14)*	47.4 *(0.9)*	3,002 *(29)*	54.8 *(0.5)*	280 *(7)*	30.4 *(0.7)*
Direct purchase	804 *(18)*	12.6 *(0.3)*	99 *(6)*	6.6 *(0.4)*	481 *(16)*	8.8 *(0.3)*	324 *(8)*	35.1 *(0.9)*
Covered by TRICARE	226 *(12)*	3.5 *(0.2)*	48 *(5)*	3.2 *(0.3)*	156 *(11)*	2.9 *(0.2)*	70 *(5)*	7.6 *(0.6)*
Covered by government health insurance	2,197 *(22)*	34.4 *(0.3)*	631 *(14)*	42.4 *(0.9)*	1,297 *(22)*	23.7 *(0.4)*	900 *(4)*	97.7 *(0.3)*
Covered by Medicaid	1,243 *(22)*	19.4 *(0.3)*	626 *(13)*	42.0 *(0.9)*	1,116 *(21)*	20.4 *(0.4)*	127 *(6)*	13.7 *(0.6)*
Also by private insurance	181 *(9)*	2.8 *(0.1)*	57 *(6)*	3.8 *(0.4)*	127 *(9)*	2.3 *(0.2)*	54 *(4)*	5.8 *(0.4)*
Covered by Medicare	1,111 *(10)*	17.4 *(0.1)*	8 *(2)*	0.6 *(0.2)*	212 *(9)*	3.9 *(0.2)*	899 *(4)*	97.6 *(0.3)*
Also by private insurance	616 *(9)*	9.6 *(0.1)*	1 *(1)*	0.1 *(0.1)*	56 *(4)*	1.0 *(0.1)*	561 *(8)*	60.9 *(0.8)*
Also by Medicaid	219 *(8)*	3.4 *(0.1)*	5 *(2)*	0.3 *(0.1)*	93 *(6)*	1.7 *(0.1)*	127 *(6)*	13.7 *(0.6)*
Covered by VA Care	155 *(6)*	2.4 *(0.1)*	2 *(1)*	0.1 *(0.1)*	78 *(5)*	1.4 *(0.1)*	76 *(4)*	8.3 *(0.4)*
Not covered at any time during the year	887 *(20)*	13.9 *(0.3)*	85 *(8)*	5.7 *(0.5)*	882 *(19)*	16.1 *(0.3)*	5 *(1)*	0.5 *(0.1)*

Note: Numbers in thousands; Figures cover 2013; Margin of error appears in parenthesis; A "Z" indicates that the value either represents or rounds to zero.
Source: U.S. Census Bureau, 2013 American Community Survey, Table HI05. Health Insurance Coverage Status and Type of Coverage by State and Age for All People: 2013

Tennessee

1021 Aetna Health of Tennessee

11675 Great Oaks Way
Suite 500
Alpharetta, GA 30022
Toll-Free: 866-582-9629
www.aetna.com
For Profit Organization: Yes
Year Founded: 1982
Number of Affiliated Hospitals: 11
Number of Primary Care Physicians: 355
Total Enrollment: 24,054
State Enrollment: 24,054

Healthplan and Services Defined
PLAN TYPE: HMO
Other Type: POS
Model Type: Group
Benefits Offered: Behavioral Health, Disease Management, Prescription, Wellness
Offers Demand Management Patient Information Service: Yes

Type of Coverage
Commercial

Geographic Areas Served
Statewide

Subscriber Information
Average Monthly Fee Per Subscriber
(Employee + Employer Contribution):
Employee Only (Self): $56.09
Employee & 2 Family Members: $199.61
Medicare: $56.09
Average Annual Deductible Per Subscriber:
Employee Only (Self): None
Employee & 1 Family Member: None
Employee & 2 Family Members: None
Medicare: None
Average Subscriber Co-Payment:
Primary Care Physician: $20.00
Prescription Drugs: $10/20
Hospital ER: $50.00
Home Health Care: $0
Home Health Care Max. Days/Visits Covered: Unlimited
Nursing Home: $0
Nursing Home Max. Days/Visits Covered: Unlimited

Publishes and Distributes Report Card: Yes

Accreditation Certification
NCQA
TJC Accreditation, Medicare Approved, Utilization Review, Pre-Admission Certification, State Licensure, Quality Assurance Program

Key Personnel
President/CEO . . . . .Robert Wolfkiel
CFO . . . . .Chris Sluder
Network Manager . . . . .Barbara Robinson
Account Executive . . . . .Mike Watson

Employer References
Federal Employees Health Plan

1022 Amerigroup Tennessee

22 Century Blvd
Suite 310
Nashville, TN 37214
Toll-Free: 800-600-4441
Phone: 757-490-6900
MPSWeb@amerigroup.com
www.amerigroup.com/

For Profit Organization: Yes
Year Founded: 2007
Total Enrollment: 2,700,000

Healthplan and Services Defined
PLAN TYPE: HMO

Type of Coverage
TennCare

Geographic Areas Served
Middle Tennessee

Accreditation Certification
NCQA

1023 Assurant Employee Benefits: Tennessee

6055 Primacy Parkway
Suite 330
Memphis, TN 38119
Toll-Free: 800-891-8945
Phone: 901-685-3111
Fax: 901-685-1175
Memphis.rfp@assurant.com
www.assurantemployeebenefits.com
For Profit Organization: Yes
Number of Primary Care Physicians: 112,000
Total Enrollment: 47,000

Healthplan and Services Defined
PLAN TYPE: Multiple
Plan Specialty: Dental, Vision, Long & Short-Term Disability
Benefits Offered: Dental, Vision, Wellness, AD&D, Life, LTD, STD

Type of Coverage
Commercial, Indemnity, Individual Dental Plans

Geographic Areas Served
Statewide

Subscriber Information
Average Monthly Fee Per Subscriber
(Employee + Employer Contribution):
Employee Only (Self): Varies by plan

Accreditation Certification
TJC

Key Personnel
Manager . . . . .Craig Wright
PR Specialist . . . . .Megan Hutchison
816-556-7815
megan.hutchison@assurant.com

1024 Baptist Health Services Group

350 N Humphreys Boulevard
4th Floor
Memphis, TN 38120
Toll-Free: 800-522-2474
Phone: 901-227-2474
bhsginfo@bmhcc.org
www.bhsgonline.org
Subsidiary of: Baptist Memorial Health Care Corporation
Non-Profit Organization: Yes
Year Founded: 1984
Number of Affiliated Hospitals: 52
Number of Primary Care Physicians: 4,000
Number of Referral/Specialty Physicians: 2,073
Total Enrollment: 423,244

Healthplan and Services Defined
PLAN TYPE: Other
Model Type: Network, Provider Spons. Network
Plan Specialty: Worker's Compensation
Offers Demand Management Patient Information Service: No

Geographic Areas Served
E Arkansas, SW Kentucky, N Mississipi, SE Missouri, and W Tennessee

Subscriber Information
Average Monthly Fee Per Subscriber
(Employee + Employer Contribution):
Employee Only (Self): n/a
Average Annual Deductible Per Subscriber:
Employee Only (Self): n/a
Average Subscriber Co-Payment:
Primary Care Physician: n/a

Publishes and Distributes Report Card: No

Key Personnel
CEO..David R Elliott
System Director, Sales ....Kim Manning

Average Claim Compensation
Physician's Fees Charged: 1%
Hospital's Fees Charged: 1%

Specialty Managed Care Partners
Enters into Contracts with Regional Business Coalitions: Yes

1025 Blue Cross & Blue Shield of Tennessee

1 Cameron Hill Circle
Chattanooga, TN 37402
Toll-Free: 800-565-9140
Phone: 423-535-5600
www.bcbst.com
Secondary Address: 85 North Danny Thomas Blvd, Memphis, TN 38103-2398
Non-Profit Organization: Yes
Year Founded: 1945
Number of Affiliated Hospitals: 130
Number of Primary Care Physicians: 2,490
Number of Referral/Specialty Physicians: 15,000
Total Enrollment: 3,000,000
State Enrollment: 3,000,000

Healthplan and Services Defined
PLAN TYPE: HMO/PPO
Benefits Offered: Dental, Disease Management, Vision, Wellness

Type of Coverage
Medicaid

Key Personnel
President & CEO ....Vicky Gregg
EVP, CFO ....John Giblin
EVP, President Govt Bus ....Steve Coulter, MD
EVP, Pres Commercial Bus.......................Joan Harp
SVP, Chief Info Officer.....................Nick Coussoule
SVP, People Services ....Ron Harr
SVP, Treasurer ....Chris Hunter
SVP, Chief Strategy Offc ....Bob Worthington
SVP, Chief Compliance...........................Bill Young

Specialty Managed Care Partners
Magellen Health Services

Employer References
State, local and government employees

1026 Cariten Healthcare

1420 Centerpoint Boulevard
Knoxville, TN 37932
Toll-Free: 800-793-1495
Phone: 865-470-7470
Fax: 865-670-7255
www.cariten.com
Secondary Address: 101 Medtech Parkway, Suite 404, Johnson City, TN 37604
Subsidiary of: A Humana Affiliate

For Profit Organization: Yes
Year Founded: 1985
Number of Affiliated Hospitals: 60
Number of Primary Care Physicians: 1,500
Number of Referral/Specialty Physicians: 6,000
Total Enrollment: 73,000
State Enrollment: 14,477

Healthplan and Services Defined
PLAN TYPE: Multiple
Other Type: HMO/POS
Plan Specialty: Behavioral Health, Chiropractic, Disease Management, Vision, Radiology, Worker's Compensation, UR
Benefits Offered: Behavioral Health, Chiropractic, Disease Management, Home Care, Inpatient SNF, Long-Term Care, Physical Therapy, Podiatry, Prescription, Psychiatric, Transplant, Vision, Wellness, Worker's Compensation, EAP, Voc Rehab

Type of Coverage
Commercial, Medicare, Medicaid, Catastrophic
Catastrophic Illness Benefit: Covered

Type of Payment Plans Offered
POS, DFFS, Capitated, FFS, Combination FFS & DFFS

Geographic Areas Served
28 counties in East Tennessee

Subscriber Information
Average Monthly Fee Per Subscriber
(Employee + Employer Contribution):
Medicare: Varies
Average Annual Deductible Per Subscriber:
Medicare: Varies
Average Subscriber Co-Payment:
Primary Care Physician: $20.00
Prescription Drugs: $10/20/35
Hospital ER: $100.00
Home Health Care Max. Days/Visits Covered: 100 days
Nursing Home Max. Days/Visits Covered: 100 days

Network Qualifications
Pre-Admission Certification: Yes

Peer Review Type
Utilization Review: Yes
Case Management: Yes

Publishes and Distributes Report Card: Yes

Accreditation Certification
URAC, NCQA

Key Personnel
President and CEO..........................Anthony L Spezia
CFO ....Jeff Collake
Director Operations ....Linda Lyle
COO ....Douglas E Haaland
Network Contracting Mgr ....Pat Gillespie
Dir, Provider Relations........................Pat Gillespie
Director, Pharmacy..........................John Cuifo, DPh
Chairman.....................................Larry Martin
Vice Chairman ....Francis H Olmstead, Jr
Materials Management ....Mary Cogar
Medical Director ....George Andrews, MD
Member Services Manager..............Theresa Christian-Wills
VP/MIS ....Barry Robbins
Marketing Director..........................Christy Newman
Sales Manager ....Lisa Johnson

Average Claim Compensation
Physician's Fees Charged: 25%
Hospital's Fees Charged: 30%

Specialty Managed Care Partners
Express Scripts
Enters into Contracts with Regional Business Coalitions: Yes
Healthcare 21 Business Coalition

1027 Cariten Preferred

1420 Centerpoint Boulevard
Knoxville, TN 37932
Toll-Free: 800-793-1495
Phone: 865-470-7470
Fax: 865-670-7255
www.cariten.com
Secondary Address: 6101 Enterprise Park Drive, Suite 600,
Chattanooga, TN 37416
Subsidiary of: A Humana Affiliate
For Profit Organization: Yes
Year Founded: 1985
Number of Affiliated Hospitals: 69
Number of Primary Care Physicians: 20,016
Total Enrollment: 50,919
State Enrollment: 50,919

Healthplan and Services Defined
  PLAN TYPE: PPO
  Plan Specialty: Behavioral Health, Chiropractic, Disease
    Management, Vision, Radiology, Worker's Compensation, UR
  Benefits Offered: Behavioral Health, Chiropractic, Disease
    Management, Home Care, Inpatient SNF, Long-Term Care,
    Physical Therapy, Podiatry, Prescription, Psychiatric, Transplant,
    Vision, Wellness, Worker's Compensation, AD&D, Life, LTD,
    STD, EAP, Voc Rehab

Type of Coverage
  Commercial, Medicare, Medicaid

Type of Payment Plans Offered
  POS, DFFS, Capitated, Combination FFS & DFFS

Geographic Areas Served
  35 counties in East Tennessee

Peer Review Type
  Utilization Review: Yes
  Case Management: Yes

Accreditation Certification
  URAC, NCQA

Key Personnel
  President/CEO . . . . Lance Hunsinger
  CFO . . . . Jeff Collake
  Director Operations . . . . Linda Lyle
  COO . . . . Douglas E Haaland
  Dir, Provider Relations . . . . Pat Gillespie
  Network Contracting Mgr . . . . Pat Gillespie
  Director, Pharmacy . . . . John Cuifo, DPh
  Marketing Director . . . . Christy Newman
  Materials Management . . . . Mary Cogar
  Medical Director . . . . George Andrews, MD
  Member Services Manager . . . . Theresa Christian-Wills
  Information Systems . . . . Barry Robbins, VPMIS
  Sales Manager . . . . Lisa Johnson

Specialty Managed Care Partners
  ProCare Rx

1028 CIGNA HealthCare of Tennessee

1111 Market Street, BR6A
Chattanooga, TN 37402
Toll-Free: 800-832-2211
Phone: 423-321-4400
Fax: 423-321-4861
www.cigna.com
Secondary Address: 3400 Players Club Parkway, Suite 140, Memphis,
TN 38125, 901-748-4100
For Profit Organization: Yes
Year Founded: 1988
Owned by an Integrated Delivery Network (IDN): Yes
Number of Affiliated Hospitals: 300
Number of Primary Care Physicians: 15,200

Total Enrollment: 75,000,000
State Enrollment: 229,356

Healthplan and Services Defined
  PLAN TYPE: HMO
  Other Type: POS
  Model Type: Network
  Plan Specialty: ASO, Behavioral Health, Chiropractic, Dental,
    Disease Management, EPO, Lab, MSO, PBM, Vision, Radiology,
    UR
  Benefits Offered: Behavioral Health, Chiropractic, Complementary
    Medicine, Dental, Disease Management, Home Care, Long-Term
    Care, Physical Therapy, Podiatry, Prescription, Psychiatric,
    Transplant, Vision, Wellness, AD&D, Life, LTD, STD, Women's
    and Men's Health Programs
  Offers Demand Management Patient Information Service: Yes
  DMPI Services Offered: Language Links Service, 24 hour Health
    Information Line, Health Information Library, Automated
    ReferralLine

Type of Coverage
  Commercial, Indemnity, Medicare, Supplemental Medicare, Medicaid,
    Catastrophic
  Catastrophic Illness Benefit: Varies per case

Type of Payment Plans Offered
  DFFS

Geographic Areas Served
  Fayette, Shelby, Tipton, Benton, Carroll, Chester, Crockett, Decatur,
    Dyer, Gibson, Hardin, Haywood, Henderson, Henry, Lake,
    Lauderdale, Madison, McNairy, Obion and Tipton counties of
    Tennessee

Network Qualifications
  Pre-Admission Certification: Yes

Peer Review Type
  Second Surgical Opinion: Yes

Publishes and Distributes Report Card: Yes

Accreditation Certification
  AAAHC, TJC, URAC, AAPI, NCQA

Key Personnel
  CEO . . . . Ed Hanaway
  Sr Contract Negotiator . . . . Chuck Utterback
  Marketing . . . . Patrick Hoffman

Specialty Managed Care Partners
  Enters into Contracts with Regional Business Coalitions: No

1029 Delta Dental of Tennessee

240 Venture Circle
Nashville, TN 37228
Toll-Free: 800-233-3104
Fax: 615-244-8108
www.deltadentaltn.com
Non-Profit Organization: Yes
Year Founded: 1965
Total Enrollment: 1,200,000

Healthplan and Services Defined
  PLAN TYPE: Dental
  Other Type: Dental PPO
  Model Type: Network
  Plan Specialty: ASO, Dental, Fully-Insured
  Benefits Offered: Dental

Type of Coverage
  Commercial, Individual, Group
  Catastrophic Illness Benefit: None

Geographic Areas Served
  Statewide

Subscriber Information
  Average Monthly Fee Per Subscriber
    (Employee + Employer Contribution):

Employee Only (Self): Varies
Employee & 1 Family Member: Varies
Employee & 2 Family Members: Varies
Average Annual Deductible Per Subscriber:
Employee Only (Self): Varies
Employee & 1 Family Member: Varies
Employee & 2 Family Members: Varies
Average Subscriber Co-Payment:
Prescription Drugs: $0
Home Health Care: $0
Nursing Home: $0

Accreditation Certification
Website Annual Report

Key Personnel
President & CEO . . . . Dr Philip A Wenk, DDS
SVP, Operations . . . . Kaye Martin
SVP, Employee Relations . . . . Pam Dishman
SVP, CFO . . . . J. Thomas Perry

1030 eHealthInsurance Services Inc.
11919 Foundation Place
Gold River, CA 95670
Toll-Free: 800-644-3491
webmaster@healthinsurance.com
www.e.healthinsurance.com
Year Founded: 1997

Healthplan and Services Defined
PLAN TYPE: HMO/PPO
Benefits Offered: Dental, Life, STD

Type of Coverage
Commercial, Individual, Medicare

Geographic Areas Served
All 50 states in the USA and District of Columbia

Key Personnel
Chairman & CEO . . . . Gary L. Lauer
EVP/Business & Corp. Dev. . . . . Bruce Telkamp
EVP/Chief Technology . . . . Dr. Sheldon X. Wang
SVP & CFO . . . . Stuart M. Huizinga
Pres. of eHealth Gov. Sys . . . . Samuel C. Gibbs
SVP of Sales & Operations . . . . Robert S. Hurley
Director Public Relations . . . . Nate Purpura
650-210-3115

1031 Health Choice LLC
1661 International Place
Suite 150
Memphis, TN 38120
Toll-Free: 888-821-5625
Phone: 901-821-6700
Fax: 901-821-4900
info@myhealthchoice.com
www.myhealthchoice.com
Year Founded: 1985
Number of Affiliated Hospitals: 24
Number of Primary Care Physicians: 1,400
Total Enrollment: 518,000
State Enrollment: 518,000

Healthplan and Services Defined
PLAN TYPE: PPO
Model Type: PHO
Plan Specialty: ASO, Behavioral Health, Chiropractic, Disease
Management, EPO, Lab, MSO, PBM, Radiology, Worker's
Compensation, UR

Type of Payment Plans Offered
DFFS, FFS, Combination FFS & DFFS

Geographic Areas Served
Tennessee: Shelby, Tipton, Fayette; Arkansas: Crittenden, Cross;
Mississippi: Tunica, Desoto; Missouri: Pemiscott

Network Qualifications
Pre-Admission Certification: Yes

Peer Review Type
Utilization Review: Yes
Second Surgical Opinion: Yes
Case Management: Yes

Accreditation Certification
AAAHC
TJC Accreditation, Medicare Approved, Utilization Review,
Pre-Admission Certification, State Licensure, Quality Assurance
Program

Key Personnel
President/CEO . . . . Bill Breen
901-821-6700
breenb@myhealthchoice.com
COO . . . . Jan Dickson
901-821-6700
dicksonj@myhealthchoice.com
Manager Contracting . . . . Pat Abernathy
801-821-6720
abernathyp@myhealthchoice.com
CEO MetroCare . . . . Jonna Elzen
901-360-1360
VP Customer Development . . . . Wayne Lohman
901-821-6712
lohmanw@myhealthchoice.com
Chief Medical Officer . . . . Gail Thurmond, MD
901-821-6733
thurmondg@myhealthchoice.com
Director Member Services . . . . Diana Hampton
901-821-6742
hamptond@myhealthchoice.com
VP Info Systems . . . . Marty Robbins
901-821-6734
robbinsm@myhealthchoice.com
Director Provider Services . . . . Carole Caylor
901-255-9810
caylorc@myhealthchoice.com

Specialty Managed Care Partners
Lakeside Behavioral Health, Med Impact PEM
Memphis Business Group On Health

Employer References
City of Memphis Employees, Shelby County Government, Memphis
Light Gas and Water, Methodist HealthCare Associates, St. Jude
Children's Hospital

1032 HealthPartners
1804 Highway 45 Bypass
Suite 400
Jackson, TN 38305
Toll-Free: 800-694-7888
Phone: 731-512-1500
Fax: 731-661-0176
www.wth.org/body_hpartners-id=2279.cfm.html
Subsidiary of: West Tennessee Healthcare
Non-Profit Organization: Yes
Number of Affiliated Hospitals: 127
Number of Primary Care Physicians: 3,357
Total Enrollment: 48,477
State Enrollment: 48,477

Healthplan and Services Defined
PLAN TYPE: PPO
Other Type: TPA
Plan Specialty: Worker's Compensation

Benefits Offered: Dental, Disease Management, Prescription, Wellness
Offers Demand Management Patient Information Service: Yes
DMPI Services Offered: Classes and Events

Type of Coverage
Commercial, Individual

Geographic Areas Served
18 counties in West Tennessee

Peer Review Type
Utilization Review: Yes
Case Management: Yes

Key Personnel
CEO..Jim Dockins
President ....Bill Jones
COO ....Jeff Coley
CFO ....Norma Shipp
CMO.......................................Dr Paul Caudill
Provider Relations.............................Dan Rainer
Marketing..................................Sherri Kilburn
Member Relations ....Candace Yates

Specialty Managed Care Partners
Express Scripts

1033 HealthSpring Prescription Drug Plan
530 Great Circle Rd
Nashville, TN 37228
Toll-Free: 800-331-6293
Phone: 615-291-7000
www.healthspring.com

Healthplan and Services Defined
PLAN TYPE: Medicare
Benefits Offered: Prescription

Type of Coverage
Individual, Medicare

Geographic Areas Served
Available within multiple states

Subscriber Information
Average Monthly Fee Per Subscriber
(Employee + Employer Contribution):
Employee Only (Self): Varies
Medicare: Varies
Average Annual Deductible Per Subscriber:
Employee Only (Self): Varies
Medicare: Varies
Average Subscriber Co-Payment:
Primary Care Physician: Varies
Non-Network Physician: Varies
Prescription Drugs: Varies
Hospital ER: Varies
Home Health Care: Varies
Home Health Care Max. Days/Visits Covered: Varies
Nursing Home: Varies
Nursing Home Max. Days/Visits Covered: Varies

Accreditation Certification
NCQA

Key Personnel
President..................................M Shawn Morris

1034 HealthSpring: Corporate Offices
530 Great Circle Road
Nashville, TN 37228
Toll-Free: 800-668-3813
info@myhealthspring.com
www.healthspring.com
Secondary Address: 500 Great Circle Rd, Nashville, TN 37228
For Profit Organization: Yes

Year Founded: 1995
Number of Affiliated Hospitals: 42
Number of Primary Care Physicians: 4,300
Total Enrollment: 345,000
State Enrollment: 17,844

Healthplan and Services Defined
PLAN TYPE: Medicare
Model Type: Network
Plan Specialty: ASO, EPO
Benefits Offered: Behavioral Health, Chiropractic, Disease Management, Home Care, Inpatient SNF, Physical Therapy, Podiatry, Prescription, Psychiatric, Transplant, Vision

Type of Coverage
Commercial, Medicare, Supplemental Medicare, Catastrophic, Medicare PPO
Catastrophic Illness Benefit: Covered

Type of Payment Plans Offered
POS, DFFS, Capitated, Combination FFS & DFFS

Geographic Areas Served
Tennessee, Northern Mississippi, Northern Georgia

Subscriber Information
Average Monthly Fee Per Subscriber
(Employee + Employer Contribution):
Employee Only (Self): Varies by plan
Medicare: $0
Average Subscriber Co-Payment:
Primary Care Physician: Varies by plan

Network Qualifications
Minimum Years of Practice: 3
Pre-Admission Certification: Yes

Peer Review Type
Utilization Review: Yes
Case Management: Yes

Accreditation Certification
AAAHC, URAC

Key Personnel
Chairman/CEO.............................Herbert Fritch
President..................................Michael Mirt
EVP/CFO..................................Karey Witty
SVP/General Counsel.......................J Gentry Barden
SVP/Chief Actuary ....David L Terry, Jr
EVP/COO ....Mark Tullock
Chief Strategy Officer...................Sharad Mansukani, MD
SVP/Chief Medical Officer ....Dirk O Wales, MD
Corp Mgr, Media Relations ....Jolene Sharp
615-234-6710
jolene.sharp@healthspring.com

Average Claim Compensation
Physician's Fees Charged: 65%
Hospital's Fees Charged: 80%

Specialty Managed Care Partners
Magellaw, Black Vision, MedImpact

Employer References
Lifeway, Ingram Industries, AmSouth Banks

1035 Humana Health Insurance of Tennessee
6075 Poplar Avenue
Suite 221
Memphis, TN 38119
Phone: 901-685-3851
Fax: 901-685-0194
www.humana.com
Secondary Address: 320 Seven Springs Way, Suite 200, Brentwood, TN 37027, 615-370-4021
Subsidiary of: LifeSynch
For Profit Organization: Yes
Total Enrollment: 172,000

State Enrollment: 35,800

Healthplan and Services Defined
  PLAN TYPE: HMO/PPO
  Plan Specialty: ASO
  Benefits Offered: Disease Management, Prescription, Wellness

Type of Coverage
  Commercial, Individual

Geographic Areas Served
  Tennessee

Accreditation Certification
  URAC, NCQA, CORE

Key Personnel
  CEO . . . . Rick Remmers

Specialty Managed Care Partners
  Caremark Rx

Employer References
  Tricare

1036 Initial Group

6556 Jocelyn Hollow Road
Nashville, TN 37205
Toll-Free: 866-295-6586
Phone: 865-546-1893
Fax: 615-352-8782
information@initialgroup.com
www.initialgroup.com
Mailing Address: PO Box 58735, Nashville, TN 37205-8735
Subsidiary of: Baptist Health System of East Tennessee
For Profit Organization: Yes
Year Founded: 1994
Number of Affiliated Hospitals: 75
Number of Primary Care Physicians: 5,000
Number of Referral/Specialty Physicians: 4,000
Total Enrollment: 200,000
State Enrollment: 106,364

Healthplan and Services Defined
  PLAN TYPE: PPO
  Model Type: Network
  Plan Specialty: Behavioral Health, Lab, Radiology, Worker's
    Compensation
  Benefits Offered: Behavioral Health, Home Care, Inpatient SNF,
    Physical Therapy, Podiatry, Psychiatric, Transplant, Wellness,
    Worker's Compensation, Life, LTD

Type of Coverage
  Commercial, Medicare
  Catastrophic Illness Benefit: Covered

Type of Payment Plans Offered
  POS

Geographic Areas Served
  Eastern Tennessee

Subscriber Information
  Average Monthly Fee Per Subscriber
    (Employee + Employer Contribution):
      Employee Only (Self): Varies by plan
  Average Annual Deductible Per Subscriber:
      Employee Only (Self): $250.00
      Employee & 2 Family Members: $500.00
  Average Subscriber Co-Payment:
      Primary Care Physician: $15.00
      Prescription Drugs: $5.00/10.00
      Hospital ER: $30.00
      Home Health Care: $30.00

Network Qualifications
  Pre-Admission Certification: Yes

Peer Review Type
  Utilization Review: Yes

Second Surgical Opinion: Yes
Case Management: Yes

Accreditation Certification
  URAC
  TJC Accreditation, Medicare Approved, Utilization Review,
    Pre-Admission Certification, State Licensure, Quality Assurance
    Program

Key Personnel
  President/CEO . . . . Lisa J Wear
    865-546-1893
  Chief Financial Officer . . . . Cheryl Wilburn
  Executive Director . . . . Cheryl Wilburn
    865-546-1893
  Marketing . . . . Mark Field
    865-546-1893
  Information Services . . . . Julles Tarkett
    865-546-1893
  Provider Services . . . . Meredith Leeger
    865-546-1893
  Sales/Marketing. . . . . Mark Field
    865-546-1893

Specialty Managed Care Partners
  Health System

1037 John Deere Health

2033 Madowview Lane
Suite 300
Kingsport, TN 37660
Toll-Free: 888-432-3373
Phone: 423-378-5122
Fax: 865-690-2741
u.s.employeebenefits@johndeere.com
www.deere.com/healthydirections/
Subsidiary of: Healthy Directions
For Profit Organization: Yes
Year Founded: 1985
Number of Affiliated Hospitals: 26
Number of Primary Care Physicians: 1,126
Number of Referral/Specialty Physicians: 1,581
Total Enrollment: 551,309
State Enrollment: 251,418

Healthplan and Services Defined
  PLAN TYPE: HMO/PPO
  Other Type: HSA
  Model Type: IPA
  Benefits Offered: Disease Management, Prescription, Wellness
  Offers Demand Management Patient Information Service: Yes

Type of Coverage
  Commercial, Medicare, Medicaid

Type of Payment Plans Offered
  POS, DFFS

Geographic Areas Served
  Tennessee and Virginia

Network Qualifications
  Pre-Admission Certification: Yes

Peer Review Type
  Utilization Review: Yes

Publishes and Distributes Report Card: Yes

Accreditation Certification
  NCQA
  TJC Accreditation, Medicare Approved, Utilization Review,
    Pre-Admission Certification, State Licensure, Quality Assurance
    Program

Key Personnel
  President/CEO. . . . . Lowell Crawford
  Manager. . . . . Garland Scott

Specialty Managed Care Partners
Enters into Contracts with Regional Business Coalitions: Yes

1038 Signature Health Alliance

2630 Elm Hill Pike, Suite 117
Nashville, TN 37214
Toll-Free: 866-471-8770
Phone: 615-872-8770
Fax: 615-872-8938
ASOdivision@bgfh.com
www.signaturehealth.com
Mailing Address: PO Box 22419, Nashville, TN 37202-2419
Subsidiary of: Bluegrass Family Health
For Profit Organization: Yes
Year Founded: 1984
Number of Affiliated Hospitals: 191
Number of Primary Care Physicians: 20,000
Number of Referral/Specialty Physicians: 13,192
Total Enrollment: 80,000
State Enrollment: 379,224

Healthplan and Services Defined
PLAN TYPE: PPO
Model Type: Network

Geographic Areas Served
Statewide

Accreditation Certification
State Licensure

Key Personnel
Principal.....................................Susan Aldreridge
Vice President................................Mindy Brown
Director ....Deona Mitchel
Marketing ....Victoria Prendergast
vprendergast@signaturehealth.com

Specialty Managed Care Partners
Enters into Contracts with Regional Business Coalitions: Yes

1039 UnitedHealthCare of Tennessee

10 Cadillac Drive, Suite 200
Brentwood, TN 37027
Toll-Free: 800-695-1273
Phone: 615-372-3622
UHC_TN_outreach@uhc.com
www.uhc.com
Secondary Address: 1208 Pointe Centre Dr, Suite 230, Chattanooga,
TN 37421, 423-954-3400
For Profit Organization: Yes
Year Founded: 1992
Number of Affiliated Hospitals: 5,609
Number of Primary Care Physicians: 726,537
Number of Referral/Specialty Physicians: 3,369
Total Enrollment: 70,000,000
State Enrollment: 270,665

Healthplan and Services Defined
PLAN TYPE: HMO/PPO
Model Type: Fully Integrated
Plan Specialty: ASO, Behavioral Health, Chiropractic, Dental,
Disease Management, EPO, Lab, MSO, PBM, Vision, Radiology,
UR
Benefits Offered: Dental, Prescription, Vision, AD&D, Life, LTD,
STD
Offers Demand Management Patient Information Service: Yes

Type of Coverage
Commercial, Individual, Indemnity, Medicare
Catastrophic Illness Benefit: Covered

Geographic Areas Served
Statewide

Network Qualifications
Pre-Admission Certification: Yes

Accreditation Certification
AAPI, NCQA

Key Personnel
Media Contact................................Roger Rollman
roger_f_rollman@uhc.com

Specialty Managed Care Partners
United Health Group, Spectra, United Behavioral Health
Enters into Contracts with Regional Business Coalitions: Yes

1040 Windsor Medicare Extra

7100 Commerce Way, Suite 285
Brentwood, TN 37027
Toll-Free: 800-316-2273
Phone: 615-782-7800
Fax: 615-782-7828
www.windsorhealthplan.com
Total Enrollment: 75,000

Healthplan and Services Defined
PLAN TYPE: Medicare
Benefits Offered: Chiropractic, Dental, Disease Management, Home
Care, Inpatient SNF, Physical Therapy, Podiatry, Prescription,
Psychiatric, Vision, Wellness

Type of Coverage
Individual, Medicare

Geographic Areas Served
Available only within Tennessee

Subscriber Information
Average Monthly Fee Per Subscriber
(Employee + Employer Contribution):
Employee Only (Self): Varies
Medicare: Varies
Average Annual Deductible Per Subscriber:
Employee Only (Self): Varies
Medicare: Varies
Average Subscriber Co-Payment:
Primary Care Physician: Varies
Non-Network Physician: Varies
Prescription Drugs: Varies
Hospital ER: Varies
Home Health Care: Varies
Home Health Care Max. Days/Visits Covered: Varies
Nursing Home: Varies
Nursing Home Max. Days/Visits Covered: Varies

Accreditation Certification
NCQA

Key Personnel
President ....Michael Bailey
Chairman/CEO ....Philip Hertik
EVP/CFO ....Willis E Jones, III
VP, Admin & Claims..........................Robin Bradley
VP, Network Services...............Jenifer L Mariencheckr, RN
CEO, Windsor HomeCare Net ....Bart Cunningham
VP, Marketing ....John Sowell
615-782-7938
jsowell@windsorhealthgroup.com
Chief Medical Officer ....James Bracikowski, MD
VP, Customer Service..........................Pat Sheridan
Chief Infomation Officer ....Steve Yates
VP, Information Tech..........................Barry Shermer
VP, Sales....................................Gary W Adkins
Media Contact ....John Sowell
615-782-7938
jsowell@windsorhealthgroup.com

Health Insurance Coverage Status and Type of Coverage by Age

Category	All Persons		Under 18 years		Under 65 years		65 years and over	
	Number	%	Number	%	Number	%	Number	%
Total population	25,977	-	7,029	-	23,094	-	2,882	-
Covered by some type of health insurance	20,228 *(54)*	77.9 *(0.2)*	6,140 *(23)*	87.4 *(0.3)*	17,404 *(53)*	75.4 *(0.2)*	2,824 *(7)*	98.0 *(0.2)*
Covered by private health insurance	15,033 *(64)*	57.9 *(0.2)*	3,452 *(30)*	49.1 *(0.4)*	13,388 *(58)*	58.0 *(0.3)*	1,645 *(14)*	57.1 *(0.5)*
Employment based	12,664 *(65)*	48.8 *(0.3)*	2,989 *(31)*	42.5 *(0.4)*	11,712 *(61)*	50.7 *(0.3)*	952 *(12)*	33.0 *(0.4)*
Direct purchase	2,456 *(32)*	9.5 *(0.1)*	394 *(14)*	5.6 *(0.2)*	1,688 *(30)*	7.3 *(0.1)*	769 *(13)*	26.7 *(0.5)*
Covered by TRICARE	774 *(26)*	3.0 *(0.1)*	179 *(11)*	2.5 *(0.2)*	548 *(21)*	2.4 *(0.1)*	225 *(9)*	7.8 *(0.3)*
Covered by government health insurance	7,364 *(43)*	28.3 *(0.2)*	2,860 *(32)*	40.7 *(0.5)*	4,623 *(42)*	20.0 *(0.2)*	2,741 *(8)*	95.1 *(0.2)*
Covered by Medicaid	4,514 *(44)*	17.4 *(0.2)*	2,831 *(33)*	40.3 *(0.5)*	4,074 *(41)*	17.6 *(0.2)*	440 *(11)*	15.3 *(0.4)*
Also by private insurance	490 *(15)*	1.9 *(0.1)*	167 *(10)*	2.4 *(0.1)*	353 *(14)*	1.5 *(0.1)*	136 *(6)*	4.7 *(0.2)*
Covered by Medicare	3,275 *(18)*	12.6 *(0.1)*	40 *(5)*	0.6 *(0.1)*	539 *(14)*	2.3 *(0.1)*	2,736 *(8)*	94.9 *(0.2)*
Also by private insurance	1,696 *(16)*	6.5 *(0.1)*	5 *(1)*	0.1 *(0.1)*	136 *(6)*	0.6 *(0.1)*	1,560 *(15)*	54.1 *(0.5)*
Also by Medicaid	683 *(14)*	2.6 *(0.1)*	17 *(3)*	0.2 *(0.1)*	243 *(9)*	1.1 *(0.1)*	440 *(11)*	15.3 *(0.4)*
Covered by VA Care	544 *(14)*	2.1 *(0.1)*	10 *(3)*	0.1 *(0.1)*	296 *(11)*	1.3 *(0.1)*	248 *(7)*	8.6 *(0.3)*
Not covered at any time during the year	5,748 *(55)*	22.1 *(0.2)*	888 *(24)*	12.6 *(0.3)*	5,690 *(54)*	24.6 *(0.2)*	58 *(5)*	2.0 *(0.2)*

Note: Numbers in thousands; Figures cover 2013; Margin of error appears in parenthesis; A "Z" indicates that the value either represents or rounds to zero.
Source: U.S. Census Bureau, 2013 American Community Survey, Table HI05. Health Insurance Coverage Status and Type of Coverage by State and Age for All People: 2013

Texas

1041 Aetna Health of Texas

2777 Stemmons Freeway
Suite 300
Dallas, TX 75207
Toll-Free: 866-582-9629
Phone: 214-200-8000
www.aetna.com
Year Founded: 1997
Number of Affiliated Hospitals: 5,300
Number of Primary Care Physicians: 597,000
Total Enrollment: 22,000,000
State Enrollment: 294,566

Healthplan and Services Defined
PLAN TYPE: HMO
Other Type: POS
Model Type: IPA
Benefits Offered: Dental, Disease Management, Prescription,
   Transplant, Vision, Wellness, AD&D, Life, LTD, STD, Alternative
   Health Care Program, Informed Health Line, Women's Health
   Programs, National Medical Excellence Program

Type of Payment Plans Offered
POS, FFS

Geographic Areas Served
Statewide

Subscriber Information
Average Subscriber Co-Payment:
   Primary Care Physician: $15.00
   Non-Network Physician: $25.00
   Prescription Drugs: $15/25/40
   Hospital ER: $100.00

Peer Review Type
Second Surgical Opinion: Yes
Case Management: Yes

Publishes and Distributes Report Card: Yes

Accreditation Certification
URAC, NCQA
TJC Accreditation, Medicare Approved, Utilization Review,
   Pre-Admission Certification, State Licensure, Quality Assurance
   Program

Key Personnel
Chair/CEO/President.........................Mark T. Bertolini
EVP/General Counsel.......................William J. Casazza
EVP/Aetna International...................Richard di Benedetto
EVP/Human Resources ....Deanna Fidler
EVP/CFO..............................Shawn M. Guertin
EVP/Corporate Affairs ....Steven B. Kelmar
EVP/Consumer Products.......................Dijuana Lewis
EVP/Operations&Technology ....Meg McCarthy
Medical Affairs...........................Jay Lawrence, MD
Director/Sales..............................Alex Herrera
   210-515-2671
   HerraA@aetna.com

1042 Alliance Regional Health Network

1501 S. Coulter
Amarillo, TX 79106
Toll-Free: 800-887-1114
Phone: 806-354-1000
Fax: 806-354-1122
www.nwtexashealthcare.com
Subsidiary of: Northwest Texas Healthcare System
For Profit Organization: Yes
Year Founded: 1986
Number of Affiliated Hospitals: 25

Number of Primary Care Physicians: 1,000
Number of Referral/Specialty Physicians: 900
Total Enrollment: 80,000
State Enrollment: 79,500

Healthplan and Services Defined
PLAN TYPE: PPO
Model Type: Network
Plan Specialty: Behavioral Health, Radiology
Benefits Offered: Disease Management, Wellness, Worker's
   Compensation, Occupational therapy

Geographic Areas Served
Amraillo, Lubbock and the Panhandle region

Network Qualifications
Pre-Admission Certification: Yes

Accreditation Certification
Medicare Approved, Utilization Review, State Licensure, Quality
   Assurance Program

Key Personnel
CEO...Frank Lopez
   806-354-1000
Network Contracting ....Diana Avila
   806-351-5151
Credentialing Coordinator ....Patsy Smith
   806-351-5153
   PSmith@nwths.com
Director of Sales ....Scott Carlisle
   806-351-5155
   SCarlise@nwths.com
Medical Affairs ....Pablo Diaz-Esquivel, MD
Member Services ....Chris Grigo
   806-351-5152
Provider Services ....Diana Avila
Sales...Scott Carlisle

Employer References
City of Amarillo, Affilate Foods, Potter County, TPMHMR/State
   Center, Boys Ranch

1043 American PPO

391 East Las Colinas Boulevard
Suite 130
Irving, TX 75039
Phone: 972-533-0081
Fax: 214-269-8401
www.americanppo.com
For Profit Organization: Yes
Year Founded: 2000
Number of Affiliated Hospitals: 305
Number of Primary Care Physicians: 10,000
Number of Referral/Specialty Physicians: 13,000

Healthplan and Services Defined
PLAN TYPE: PPO
Model Type: Network
Benefits Offered: Behavioral Health, Chiropractic, Dental, Disease
   Management, Home Care, Inpatient SNF, Long-Term Care,
   Physical Therapy, Prescription, Vision
Offers Demand Management Patient Information Service: Yes

Type of Coverage
Commercial

Type of Payment Plans Offered
Combination FFS & DFFS

Geographic Areas Served
Arkansas, Louisiana, Mississippi, Missouri, Oklahoma, Tennessee and
Texas

Key Personnel
Sales/Marketing Director.......................Shelly Dowdy
   877-223-3372
   americanppo@aol.com

Plan/Business Dev Dir . . . . Carmen Khorram
877-223-3372
americanppo@aol.com
Network Development Dir . . . . Heather Brumley
877-223-3372
americanppo@aol.com

Specialty Managed Care Partners
Enters into Contracts with Regional Business Coalitions: Yes

1044 Amerigroup Texas
3800 Buffalo Speedway
Suite 400
Houston, TX 77098
Toll-Free: 800-600-4441
Phone: 757-490-6900
www.amerigroup.com
Secondary Address: 823 Congress Avenue, Suite 400, Austin, TX
78701
For Profit Organization: Yes
Total Enrollment: 1,900,000

Healthplan and Services Defined
PLAN TYPE: HMO

Type of Coverage
Medicare, Medicaid, SCHIP, SSI

Geographic Areas Served
Austin, Corpus Christi, Dallas, Fort Worth, San Antonio, Houston
and surrounding counties

Accreditation Certification
URAC, NCQA

Key Personnel
EVP/Pres. Gov. Business . . . . Peter D. Haytaian
CFO. . . . . Scott Anglin
VP/Customer Service Op. . . . . Ken Aversa, MBA
Medicaid Compliance Off. . . . . Georgia Dodds Foley, Esq.
SVP/Chief Medical Off. . . . . Mary T. McCluskey, MD
Manager, Procurement Serv. . . . . Anne Page
Vice President, External . . . . Maureen C. McDonnell

1045 Assurant Employee Benefits: Texas
2745 Dallas Parkway
Suite 500
Plano, TX 75093-8900
Toll-Free: 800-442-0911
Phone: 214-258-1020
Fax: 214-258-1100
dallas.rfp@assurant.com
www.assurantemployeebenefits.com
For Profit Organization: Yes
Number of Primary Care Physicians: 112,000
Total Enrollment: 47,000

Healthplan and Services Defined
PLAN TYPE: Multiple
Plan Specialty: Dental, Vision, Long & Short-Term Disability
Benefits Offered: Dental, Vision, Wellness, AD&D, Life, LTD, STD

Type of Coverage
Commercial, Indemnity, Individual Dental Plans

Geographic Areas Served
Statewide

Subscriber Information
Average Monthly Fee Per Subscriber
(Employee + Employer Contribution):
Employee Only (Self): Varies by plan

Accreditation Certification
TJC

Key Personnel
President/CEO . . . . John S. Roberts
President Of Disability . . . . Matt Gilligan
SVP/Sales. . . . . J. Marc Warrington
SVP/Marketing. . . . . Joe Sevcik
SVP/CFO. . . . . Miles Yakre
VP/Dental . . . . Stacia Almquist
PR Specialist. . . . . Megan Hutchison
816-556-7815
megan.hutchison@assurant.com

1046 Avesis: Texas
8000 IH 10 West
Suite 715
San Antonio, TX 78230
Phone: 210-384-8103
www.avesis.com
Year Founded: 1978
Number of Primary Care Physicians: 18,000
Total Enrollment: 2,000,000

Healthplan and Services Defined
PLAN TYPE: PPO
Other Type: Vision, Dental
Model Type: Network
Plan Specialty: Dental, Vision, Hearing
Benefits Offered: Dental, Vision

Type of Coverage
Commercial

Type of Payment Plans Offered
POS, Capitated, Combination FFS & DFFS

Geographic Areas Served
Nationwide and Puerto Rico

Publishes and Distributes Report Card: Yes

Accreditation Certification
AAAHC, NCQA
TJC Accreditation

Key Personnel
Chief Executive Officer. . . . . Alan Cohn
Chief Financial Officer . . . . Joel Alperstein
Chief Operation Officer . . . . Linda Chirichella
Chief Marketing Officer. Michael Reamer
Chief Information Officer. . . . . Laura Gill
Insurance Broker. . . . . Rebecca Jolly

1047 Block Vision of Texas
4100 Alpha Road
Suite 910
Dallas, TX 75244
Toll-Free: 800-914-9795
www.blockvision.com
Secondary Address: 11757 Katy Freeway, Suite 1300, Houston, TX
77079, 800-475-6810
Year Founded: 1996
State Enrollment: 4,000,000

Healthplan and Services Defined
PLAN TYPE: Vision
Model Type: Staff
Plan Specialty: Vision
Benefits Offered: Vision, Wellness

Type of Coverage
Commercial, Medicare, Medicaid, CHIP

Type of Payment Plans Offered
Combination FFS & DFFS

Geographic Areas Served
All Texas counties

Publishes and Distributes Report Card: No

Accreditation Certification
NCQA
State Licensure

Key Personnel
VP/COO . . . . .Joy Schreiber
jschreiber@blockvision.com
Medical Affairs . . . . .Barry Davis
Account Executive . . . . .Stuart Bowie
800-914-9795
sbowie@blockvision.com
Account Exec, Texas . . . . .April Sanchez
512-699-2049
asanchez@blockvision.com

Specialty Managed Care Partners
Parkland Community Health Plan, Seton Health Plan, Aetna,
Amerigroup, Community Health Plan, Texas Childrens Hospital &
Health Plan

1048 Blue Cross & Blue Shield of Texas

1001 E Lookout Drive
Richardson, TX 75082
Toll-Free: 800-521-2227
Phone: 972-766-6900
Fax: 972-766-8253
www.bcbstx.com
Mailing Address: P.O. Box 660044, Dallas, TX 75226-0044
Non-Profit Organization: Yes
Year Founded: 1929
Number of Affiliated Hospitals: 451
Number of Primary Care Physicians: 38,000
Total Enrollment: 3,645,891
State Enrollment: 310,853

Healthplan and Services Defined
PLAN TYPE: HMO/PPO
Other Type: POS
Benefits Offered: Disease Management, Wellness
Offers Demand Management Patient Information Service: Yes

Type of Coverage
Commercial, Individual, Medicare, Medicaid

Type of Payment Plans Offered
POS

Geographic Areas Served
Southwest Texas

Publishes and Distributes Report Card: Yes

Accreditation Certification
TJC, NCQA

Key Personnel
Sales & Marketing Dir. . . . . .Jack Smith
Media Contact . . . . .Margaret Jarvis
972-766-7165
margaret_jarvis@bcbstx.com

Specialty Managed Care Partners
Magellen Behavioral Health

1049 Blue Cross & Blue Shield of Texas: Houston

1800 West Loop Freeway South
Suite 600
Houston, TX 77027
Toll-Free: 800-235-0796
Phone: 713-354-7000
Fax: 713-663-1297
www.bcbstx.com
For Profit Organization: Yes
Year Founded: 1984
Number of Affiliated Hospitals: 451

Number of Primary Care Physicians: 3,800
Total Enrollment: 4,000,000
State Enrollment: 2,720,162

Healthplan and Services Defined
PLAN TYPE: HMO/PPO
Model Type: Staff, IPA
Benefits Offered: Behavioral Health, Disease Management, Physical
Therapy, Prescription, Psychiatric, Wellness, Care van

Type of Coverage
Commercial
Catastrophic Illness Benefit: Unlimited

Type of Payment Plans Offered
POS, DFFS, Capitated, FFS, Combination FFS & DFFS

Geographic Areas Served
All 254 Texas counties

Subscriber Information
Average Monthly Fee Per Subscriber
(Employee + Employer Contribution):
Employee Only (Self): Varies by plan
Average Subscriber Co-Payment:
Home Health Care Max. Days/Visits Covered: 60 days
Nursing Home Max. Days/Visits Covered: 60 days

Network Qualifications
Pre-Admission Certification: Yes

Peer Review Type
Utilization Review: Yes
Second Surgical Opinion: Yes
Case Management: Yes

Publishes and Distributes Report Card: Yes

Accreditation Certification
NCQA
TJC Accreditation, Medicare Approved, Utilization Review,
Pre-Admission Certification, State Licensure, Quality Assurance
Program

Key Personnel
Director . . . . .Art Chitty
Manager. . . . . .Betty Bialaszewsky
Administrator. . . . . .Eric Bing
Media Contact . . . . .Margaret Jarvis
972-766-7165
margaret_jarvis@bcbstx.com

Average Claim Compensation
Physician's Fees Charged: 1%
Hospital's Fees Charged: 1%

Specialty Managed Care Partners
Magellen Behavioral Health
Enters into Contracts with Regional Business Coalitions: Yes

Employer References
Brinker International, Brookshire Grocery, City of Houston,
Continental Airlines, Pilgrim's Pride

1050 Bravo Health: Texas

7551 Callaghan Road
Suite 310
San Antonio, TX 78229
Toll-Free: 888-454-0061
cignahealthspring.net
Secondary Address: 10705 Gateway Dr, Suite 10705, El Paso, TX
79935, 915-599-0927
Acquired by: Cigna
Year Founded: 1996
Number of Primary Care Physicians: 30,000
Total Enrollment: 360,000

Healthplan and Services Defined
PLAN TYPE: Medicare

Type of Coverage
  Medicare, Supplemental Medicare

Geographic Areas Served
  Delaware, Maryland, Pennslyvania, Texas, Washington DC, New Jersey

Accreditation Certification
  URAC, NCQA

Key Personnel
  President and CEO...............................Jeff Folick
  SVP, Executive Director ....Patrick Feyen

1051 Brazos Valley Health Network

4547 Lake Shore Dr
Suite 10
Waco, TX 76710
Phone: 254-202-5320
Fax: 254-202-5310
Non-Profit Organization: Yes
Year Founded: 1992
Number of Affiliated Hospitals: 10
Number of Primary Care Physicians: 305
Number of Referral/Specialty Physicians: 174
Total Enrollment: 65,300
State Enrollment: 78,139

Healthplan and Services Defined
  PLAN TYPE: PPO
  Other Type: PHO
  Model Type: Network
  Benefits Offered: Dental

Type of Payment Plans Offered
  DFFS, Combination FFS & DFFS

Geographic Areas Served
  Texas: Bell, Bosque, Brazos, Coryell, Falls, Hamilton, Hill, Limestone, McLennan, Milam, Robertson & Washington

Network Qualifications
  Pre-Admission Certification: Yes

Peer Review Type
  Utilization Review: Yes

Publishes and Distributes Report Card: No

Key Personnel
  Executive Director ....Donald K Reeves
  Medical Director ....Dr James E Grey
  Assoc Medical Director................Dr Gerard A Marrorquin
  Nurse Manager ....Judy Johnson

Specialty Managed Care Partners
  Enters into Contracts with Regional Business Coalitions: No

1052 CIGNA HealthCare of North Texas

1640 Dallas Parkway
4th Floor
Plano, TX 75093
Toll-Free: 866-438-2446
Phone: 972-863-4300
Fax: 866-530-3585
www.cigna.com
For Profit Organization: Yes
Year Founded: 1980
Number of Affiliated Hospitals: 59
Number of Primary Care Physicians: 1,454
Number of Referral/Specialty Physicians: 3,279
Total Enrollment: 75,000,000
State Enrollment: 111,877

Healthplan and Services Defined
  PLAN TYPE: HMO/PPO
  Model Type: Staff, IPA

Benefits Offered: Behavioral Health, Dental, Disease Management, Physical Therapy, Prescription, Psychiatric, Transplant, Vision, Wellness, Language Line Service, 24 hour Health Information LIne, automated ReferralLine, Women's Health
  Offers Demand Management Patient Information Service: Yes
  DMPI Services Offered: Health Information Library

Type of Coverage
  Commercial

Type of Payment Plans Offered
  POS, DFFS, Capitated, FFS, Combination FFS & DFFS

Geographic Areas Served
  All of Northern Texas including Dallas, Tyler, El Paso and Waco

Network Qualifications
  Pre-Admission Certification: Yes

Peer Review Type
  Utilization Review: Yes
  Second Surgical Opinion: Yes
  Case Management: Yes

Publishes and Distributes Report Card: Yes

Accreditation Certification
  URAC, NCQA
  Medicare Approved, Utilization Review, Pre-Admission Certification, State Licensure, Quality Assurance Program

Key Personnel
  President ....David Cordani

Specialty Managed Care Partners
  Quest
  Enters into Contracts with Regional Business Coalitions: Yes

1053 CIGNA HealthCare of South Texas

2700 Post Oak
Suite 700
Houston, TX 77056
Toll-Free: 866-438-2446
Phone: 713-576-4300
Fax: 866-530-3585
www.cigna.com
Secondary Address: 7600 North Capital of Texas Highway, Suite 335, Austin, TX 78731, 512-338-7100
For Profit Organization: Yes
Year Founded: 1982
Number of Affiliated Hospitals: 92
Number of Primary Care Physicians: 2,517
Number of Referral/Specialty Physicians: 7,947
Total Enrollment: 75,000,000
State Enrollment: 111,877

Healthplan and Services Defined
  PLAN TYPE: HMO
  Other Type: POS
  Model Type: Staff, IPA, Group
  Plan Specialty: ASO, Behavioral Health, Chiropractic, Dental, Disease Management, Lab, Vision, Radiology, UR
  Benefits Offered: Behavioral Health, Chiropractic, Complementary Medicine, Dental, Disease Management, Home Care, Long-Term Care, Physical Therapy, Prescription, Psychiatric, Transplant, Vision, Wellness, Worker's Compensation, AD&D, Life, LTD, STD, Women's and Men's Heal
  Offers Demand Management Patient Information Service: Yes
  DMPI Services Offered: Language Line Service, 24 hour Health Information Line, Health Information Library, Automated ReferralLine

Type of Coverage
  Commercial, Individual, Indemnity

Type of Payment Plans Offered
  POS, DFFS, Capitated, FFS, Combination FFS & DFFS

Geographic Areas Served

All of Southern Texas including Houston, Austin, Beaumont/Port Arthur, Corpus Christi, San Antonio and Lufkin

Subscriber Information

Average Monthly Fee Per Subscriber
(Employee + Employer Contribution):
Employee Only (Self): Varies
Employee & 1 Family Member: Varies
Employee & 2 Family Members: Varies
Medicare: Varies
Average Annual Deductible Per Subscriber:
Employee Only (Self): Varies
Employee & 1 Family Member: Varies
Employee & 2 Family Members: Varies
Medicare: Varies
Average Subscriber Co-Payment:
Hospital ER: $75.00
Home Health Care Max. Days/Visits Covered: Unlimited
Nursing Home Max. Days/Visits Covered: Unlimited

Network Qualifications

Pre-Admission Certification: Yes

Peer Review Type

Utilization Review: Yes
Second Surgical Opinion: Yes
Case Management: Yes

Publishes and Distributes Report Card: Yes

Accreditation Certification

URAC, NCQA
Utilization Review, Pre-Admission Certification, State Licensure, Quality Assurance Program

Average Claim Compensation

Physician's Fees Charged: 1%
Hospital's Fees Charged: 1%

Specialty Managed Care Partners

Quest
Enters into Contracts with Regional Business Coalitions: Yes

1054 Community First Health Plans

12238 Silicon Drive
Suite 100
San Antonio, TX 78249
Toll-Free: 800-434-2347
Phone: 210-227-2347
Fax: 210-358-6170
www.cfhp.com
Secondary Address: Avenida Guadalupe, 1410 Guadalupe Street, Suite 222, San Antonio, TX 78207
Subsidiary of: University Health System
Non-Profit Organization: Yes
Year Founded: 1995
Total Enrollment: 110,000
State Enrollment: 110,000

Healthplan and Services Defined
PLAN TYPE: HMO/PPO
Benefits Offered: Disease Management, Wellness

Type of Coverage
Commercial, Medicaid, CHIP

Geographic Areas Served
Bexar and surrounding seven counties

Key Personnel
Admin Dir, Member Rel . . . . Mary Helen Gonzalez
Claims Manager . . . . Norma Doria
Dir, Network Management . . . . Martin Jiminez
Mgr, Clinical Pharmacy . . . . Ramie Ramirez
Credentialing Manager . . . . Paul Maldonado
Underwriting Manager . . . . Eric Ashihundu

Communications Director . . . . Catherine Zambrano-Chavez
210-358-6173
czambrano-chavez@cfhp.com

1055 Concentra: Corporate Office

5080 Spectrum Drive
Suite 1200 West
Addison, TX 75001
Toll-Free: 866-944-6046
Phone: 972-364-8000
Fax: 972-387-0019
www.concentra.com
Secondary Address: Concentra Privacy Office, PO Box 1438, Louisville, KY 40202-1438, 800-819-5571
For Profit Organization: Yes
Number of Affiliated Hospitals: 320
Total Enrollment: 30,000

Healthplan and Services Defined
PLAN TYPE: HMO/PPO

Key Personnel
President . . . . Ted Bucknam
Chief of Finance, Senior . . . . Su Zan Nelson
Executive VP, COO . . . . Thomas E. Kiraly
SVP, Reimbursement and Go . . . . Greg Gilbert
EVP, General Counsel . . . . Mark A Solls
Pres, Medical Centers . . . . Ted Bucknam
Pres, Health Solutions . . . . A Michael McCollum
SVP, Therapy Director . . . . Gary C Zigenfus, PT
Chief Marketing and Sales . . . . John deLorimier
SVP, Human Resources . . . . Tammy S Steele
EVP/Chief Medical Officer . . . . W Tom Fogarty, MD
SVP, Accounting . . . . Su Zan Nelson
Senior VP, CIO . . . . Suzanne C. Kosub
SVP, Medical Operations . . . . John R Anderson, DO
Senior VP, Sales . . . . Jay B. Blakey
SVP, Medical Operations . . . . William R Lewis, MD

1056 Delta Dental of Texas

317 RR 620 South
Suite 301
Austin, TX 78734
Toll-Free: 800-852-8952
Phone: 512-306-9570
Fax: 512-306-9573
aus-txsales@delta.org
www.deltadentalins.com
Mailing Address: PO Box 1809, Alpharetta, GA 30023-1809
Non-Profit Organization: Yes
Total Enrollment: 59,000,000

Healthplan and Services Defined
PLAN TYPE: Dental
Other Type: Dental PPO

Type of Coverage
Commercial

Geographic Areas Served
Statewide

Key Personnel
President . . . . Gary D. Radine
Director, Sales . . . . Jill Balboni
972-966-3345
VP, Public & Govt Affairs . . . . Jeff Album
415-972-8418
Dir/Media & Public Affair . . . . Elizabeth Risberg
415-972-8423

1057 Dental Source: Dental Health Care Plans

101 Parklane Boulevard
Suite 301
Sugar Land, TX 77478
Toll-Free: 877-493-6282
Phone: 866-481-9473
Fax: 281-313-7155
www.densource.com
For Profit Organization: Yes
Number of Primary Care Physicians: 149
State Enrollment: 1,500

Healthplan and Services Defined
PLAN TYPE: Dental
Model Type: Network
Plan Specialty: Dental, Vision
Benefits Offered: Dental, Vision

Type of Coverage
Commercial, Individual, Indemnity

Geographic Areas Served
Kansas and Missouri

Key Personnel
President/CEO . . . . .James A Taylor
CFO . . . . .Patrick Stoner
COO. . . . . .Rick Barrett
Director Sales/Marketing. . . . . .Mark Groves

1058 eHealthInsurance Services Inc.

11919 Foundation Place
Gold River, CA 95670
Toll-Free: 800-644-3491
Phone: 877-456-6670
info@ehealthinsurance.com
www.ehealthinsurance.com
Year Founded: 1997

Healthplan and Services Defined
PLAN TYPE: HMO/PPO
Benefits Offered: Dental, Life, STD

Type of Coverage
Commercial, Individual, Medicare

Geographic Areas Served
All 50 states in the USA and District of Columbia

Key Personnel
Chairman & CEO. . . . . .Gary L. Lauer
President/COO . . . . .Bill Shaughnessy
SVP/Marketing. . . . . .Jeff Bernstein
SVP & CFO . . . . .Stuart M. Huizinga
SVP/President Of Sales . . . . .Samuel C. Gibbs, III
SVP/Sales And Operations . . . . .Robert S. Hurley
SVP/Product Management . . . . .Tom Tsao
SVP/Engineering. . . . . .Dr.Jiang Wu
SVP of Sales & Operations . . . . .Robert S. Hurley
Director Public Relations. .Nate Purpura
650-210-3115

1059 FCL Dental

101 Parklane Boulevard
Suite 301
Sugar Land, TX 77478
Toll-Free: 866-912-7131
Phone: 713-313-7155
Fax: 281-313-7155
info@dentalsolutionsplus.com
www.fcldental.com
Subsidiary of: First Continental Life & Accident Insurance
For Profit Organization: Yes

Year Founded: 1986

Healthplan and Services Defined
PLAN TYPE: Dental
Plan Specialty: Dental
Benefits Offered: Dental

Subscriber Information
Average Annual Deductible Per Subscriber:
Employee Only (Self): $0
Employee & 1 Family Member: $0
Employee & 2 Family Members: $0
Medicare: $0
Average Subscriber Co-Payment:
Primary Care Physician: $9.00

Key Personnel
President/CEO . . . . .James Taylor

1060 First Care Health Plans

12940 N Highway 183
Corporate Offices
Austin, TX 78750
Toll-Free: 800-431-7737
Phone: 806-784-4300
Fax: 512-257-6037
questions@firstcare.com
www.firstcare.com
Secondary Address: 1901 West Loop 289, Suite 9, Lubbock, TX 79407
For Profit Organization: Yes
Year Founded: 1985
Owned by an Integrated Delivery Network (IDN): Yes
Number of Affiliated Hospitals: 82
Number of Primary Care Physicians: 1,100
Number of Referral/Specialty Physicians: 2,005
Total Enrollment: 130,000
State Enrollment: 130,000

Healthplan and Services Defined
PLAN TYPE: Multiple
Model Type: IPA
Plan Specialty: ASO, Behavioral Health, Chiropractic, Dental,
Disease Management, EPO, Lab, PBM, Vision, Radiology, UR
Benefits Offered: Behavioral Health, Chiropractic, Complementary
Medicine, Dental, Disease Management, Home Care, Inpatient
SNF, Physical Therapy, Podiatry, Prescription, Psychiatric,
Transplant, Vision, Wellness, Life, HSC

Type of Coverage
Commercial, Individual, Indemnity, Medicare, Medicaid, Catastrophic
Catastrophic Illness Benefit: Unlimited

Type of Payment Plans Offered
Combination FFS & DFFS

Geographic Areas Served
108 counties in North, Central and West Texas

Subscriber Information
Average Monthly Fee Per Subscriber
(Employee + Employer Contribution):
Employee Only (Self): Varies by plan
Medicare: Varies
Average Annual Deductible Per Subscriber:
Employee Only (Self): $0
Employee & 1 Family Member: $0
Employee & 2 Family Members: $0
Medicare: Varies
Average Subscriber Co-Payment:
Primary Care Physician: $10.00
Non-Network Physician: $10.00
Prescription Drugs: $10/20/35
Hospital ER: $50.00
Home Health Care: $0
Home Health Care Max. Days/Visits Covered: Unlimited
Nursing Home: $0

Nursing Home Max. Days/Visits Covered: 100 days

Network Qualifications
Pre-Admission Certification: Yes

Peer Review Type
Utilization Review: Yes
Second Surgical Opinion: No
Case Management: Yes

Publishes and Distributes Report Card: Yes

Accreditation Certification
TJC Accreditation, Medicare Approved, Utilization Review,
Pre-Admission Certification, State Licensure, Quality Assurance
Program

Key Personnel
President/CEO . . . . .Darnell Dent
VP, Sales. . . . . .Steven Abalos
Manager TPA Services . . . . .Ken Cook
Abilene Region Sales. . . . . .Becky West
    bwest@firstcare.com
Amarillo Region Sales. . . . . .Dana Nicklaus
    amamarketing@firstcare.com
Lubbock Region Sales . . . . .Cannon Allen
    806-783-9654
    khamsmith@daains.com
Waco Region Sales . . . . .Dan Mayfield
    254-761-5802
    dmayfield@firstcare.com

Specialty Managed Care Partners
PBM, Comp Care, MH Net
Enters into Contracts with Regional Business Coalitions: No

1061 Galaxy Health Network
631 106th Street
Arlington, TX 76011
Toll-Free: 800-975-3322
Phone: 817-633-5822
Fax: 817-633-5729
contracting@ghn-mci.com
www.galaxyhealth.net
Mailing Address: PO Box 201425, Arlington, TX 76006
For Profit Organization: Yes
Year Founded: 1993
Number of Affiliated Hospitals: 2,700
Number of Primary Care Physicians: 400,000
Number of Referral/Specialty Physicians: 47,000
Total Enrollment: 3,500,000
State Enrollment: 3,200,000

Healthplan and Services Defined
    PLAN TYPE: PPO
    Model Type: Network
    Benefits Offered: Prescription
    Offers Demand Management Patient Information Service: Yes

Type of Coverage
    Catastrophic Illness Benefit: Varies per case

Type of Payment Plans Offered
    POS, DFFS, FFS, Combination FFS & DFFS

Geographic Areas Served
    National

Subscriber Information
    Average Monthly Fee Per Subscriber
        (Employee + Employer Contribution):
            Employee Only (Self): Varies by plan
    Average Annual Deductible Per Subscriber:
        Employee Only (Self): $500.00
        Employee & 1 Family Member: $1000.00
        Employee & 2 Family Members: $1000.00
    Average Subscriber Co-Payment:
        Primary Care Physician: $10.00

Network Qualifications
Pre-Admission Certification: Yes

Peer Review Type
Utilization Review: Yes
Second Surgical Opinion: Yes
Case Management: Yes

Publishes and Distributes Report Card: Yes

Accreditation Certification
URAC
Utilization Review, Pre-Admission Certification, State Licensure,
Quality Assurance Program

Key Personnel
President . . . . .P.J. Shane, Jr, Jr
    pjshaneyjr@ghn.mci.com
Executive Vice President . . . . .Dan Shadle
    dshadle@ghn-mci.com
Administrative Manager. . . . . .Venus Warner
    vmathews@ghn-mci.com
Director of Network Operations. . . . . .Susdey Sud
    susdeys@ghn-mci.com
Chief Technology Offier . . . . .Stephen Ferraro
    sferraro@ghn-mci.com
Manager, Info Services . . . . .Brandie Santillan
    bsantillan@ghn-mci.com
Vice President, Sales . . . . .Stacey Hollinger
    shollinger@ghn-mci.com

Specialty Managed Care Partners
Enters into Contracts with Regional Business Coalitions: Yes

1062 Great-West Healthcare Texas
8350 North Central Expressway
Suite M1000
Dallas, TX 75206
Toll-Free: 866-494-2111
Phone: 972-813-6630
eliginquiries@cigna.com
www.cigna.com
Subsidiary of: CIGNA HealthCare
Acquired by: CIGNA
For Profit Organization: Yes
Total Enrollment: 203,856
State Enrollment: 12,334

Healthplan and Services Defined
    PLAN TYPE: HMO/PPO
    Benefits Offered: Disease Management, Prescription, Wellness

Type of Coverage
    Commercial

Type of Payment Plans Offered
    POS, FFS

Geographic Areas Served
    Texas

Accreditation Certification
    URAC

Key Personnel
    President/CEO . . . . .Donald T. Benson

Specialty Managed Care Partners
    Caremark Rx

1063 HAS-Premier Providers
5080 Spectrum Drive
Suite 650W
Addison, TX 75001
Toll-Free: 800-683-4856
Phone: 214-267-3300
slc_call_center@viant.com
www.texastruechoice.com

Subsidiary of: Acquired by Texas True Choice
Acquired by: Texas True Choice
Non-Profit Organization: Yes
Year Founded: 1984
Number of Affiliated Hospitals: 380
Number of Primary Care Physicians: 45,000
Total Enrollment: 1,080,000
State Enrollment: 1,080,000

Healthplan and Services Defined
  PLAN TYPE: PPO
  Model Type: Network
  Plan Specialty: UR
  Benefits Offered: Behavioral Health, Prescription, Psychiatric,
    Claims Administration
  Offers Demand Management Patient Information Service: Yes

Type of Coverage
  Catastrophic Illness Benefit: Varies per case

Type of Payment Plans Offered
  DFFS, Capitated, FFS, Combination FFS & DFFS

Geographic Areas Served
  Houston

Subscriber Information
  Average Monthly Fee Per Subscriber
    (Employee + Employer Contribution):
      Employee Only (Self): Varies
      Employee & 1 Family Member: Varies
      Employee & 2 Family Members: Varies
  Average Annual Deductible Per Subscriber:
      Employee Only (Self): Varies
      Employee & 1 Family Member: Varies
      Employee & 2 Family Members: Varies
  Average Subscriber Co-Payment:
      Primary Care Physician: 15%
      Non-Network Physician: 35%
      Prescription Drugs: 15%
      Hospital ER: $25.00
      Home Health Care: $0
      Home Health Care Max. Days/Visits Covered: Varies
      Nursing Home: $0
      Nursing Home Max. Days/Visits Covered: Varies

Network Qualifications
  Pre-Admission Certification: Yes

Peer Review Type
  Utilization Review: Yes
  Second Surgical Opinion: No
  Case Management: Yes

Publishes and Distributes Report Card: No

Accreditation Certification
  TJC Accreditation, Medicare Approved, Utilization Review,
    Pre-Admission Certification, State Licensure, Quality Assurance
    Program

Key Personnel
  Chairman.....................................Steve Gauen
  Claims Director..............................Karen Odom
  VP of Operations............................Ernest Mendez
  Marketing ....William B Loweth
  Medical Affairs..............................Cheryl DeBold
  Manager of Information Services..................Jeff Haillyer
  Manager of Provider Services..................Stacy Martinez

Average Claim Compensation
  Physician's Fees Charged: 60%
  Hospital's Fees Charged: 70%

Specialty Managed Care Partners
  Enters into Contracts with Regional Business Coalitions: No

---

1064 Healthcare Partners of East Texas
410 West Grand
Marshall, TX 75670
Toll-Free: 800-362-3041
Phone: 903-935-2099
Fax: 903-935-2090
Subsidiary of: A Viant Company
Acquired by: Viant
Non-Profit Organization: Yes
Year Founded: 1994
Number of Affiliated Hospitals: 39
Number of Primary Care Physicians: 2,200
Number of Referral/Specialty Physicians: 1,913
Total Enrollment: 107,539
State Enrollment: 177,539

Healthplan and Services Defined
  PLAN TYPE: PPO
  Model Type: Group, Network, PHO, messenger
  Plan Specialty: Group

Geographic Areas Served
  East Texas, 49 counties

Network Qualifications
  Pre-Admission Certification: Yes

Key Personnel
  Executive Director ....Mark Hobgood
    mhobgood@hpet.org
  CAA ....Monika Stade
    mstade@hpet.org
  Director of Operations ....Kathy Hale
    khale@hpet.org
  Director Business Devel.....................Steve Johnston, JD
    sjohnston@hpet.org
  Credential Specialist ....Melanie Perkins
    mperkins@hpet.org
  Director Marketing...........................Mark Hobgood
    mhobgood@hpet.org
  Member Services.............................Monika Stade
    mstade@hpet.org
  Data Integration ....Glenda Fort
    gfort@hpet.org
  Provider Relations ....Llaura McLelland
    lmclelland@hpet.org
  Sales.....................................Mark Hologood

Average Claim Compensation
  Physician's Fees Charged: 80%
  Hospital's Fees Charged: 72%

Employer References
  Longview ISD, County of Greggs, Southside Bank, County of Upshur

---

1065 HealthSmart Preferred Care
222 West Las Colinas Boulevard
Suite 600N
Irving, TX 75039
Toll-Free: 888-744-6638
Phone: 214-574-3546
Fax: 214-574-3911
info.his@healthsmart.com
www.healthsmart.com
Non-Profit Organization: Yes
Year Founded: 1983
Number of Affiliated Hospitals: 63
Number of Primary Care Physicians: 400,000
Total Enrollment: 470,623
State Enrollment: 394,011

Healthplan and Services Defined
  PLAN TYPE: PPO
  Model Type: Network

Plan Specialty: ASO, EPO, UR
Benefits Offered: Behavioral Health, Disease Management, Physical
 Therapy, Wellness
Offers Demand Management Patient Information Service: Yes
DMPI Services Offered: Nurse Triage

Type of Coverage
Catastrophic Illness Benefit: Varies per case

Type of Payment Plans Offered
POS, DFFS, FFS, Combination FFS & DFFS

Geographic Areas Served
36 counties in North Central Texas, including Greater Dallas/ Fort
 Worth area. National coverage available

Subscriber Information
Average Monthly Fee Per Subscriber
 (Employee + Employer Contribution):
  Employee Only (Self): Varies
  Employee & 1 Family Member: Varies
  Employee & 2 Family Members: Varies
  Medicare: Varies
Average Annual Deductible Per Subscriber:
  Employee Only (Self): Varies
  Employee & 1 Family Member: Varies
  Employee & 2 Family Members: Varies
  Medicare: Varies
Average Subscriber Co-Payment:
  Primary Care Physician: Varies
  Non-Network Physician: Varies
  Hospital ER: Varies
  Home Health Care: Varies
  Home Health Care Max. Days/Visits Covered: Varies
  Nursing Home: Varies
  Nursing Home Max. Days/Visits Covered: Varies

Network Qualifications
Minimum Years of Practice: 1
Pre-Admission Certification: Yes

Peer Review Type
Utilization Review: Yes
Second Surgical Opinion: Yes
Case Management: Yes

Publishes and Distributes Report Card: Yes

Accreditation Certification
URAC
Medicare Approved, Utilization Review, Pre-Admission
 Certification, State Licensure, Quality Assurance Program

Key Personnel
Chairman/President . . . . Daniel D Crowley
EVP Of Business Developme. . . . . Todd E. Archer
COO/Chief Financial Offic . . . . William Dembereckyj
EVP/Casualty Claims . . . . David Cook
Chief Marketing Officer. . . . . Mark Stadler
COO/Benefit Solutions. Loren W. Claypool
SVP/Account Management . . . . Lovie Pollinger
Senior Vice President of. . . . . Mark Stadler
SVP/Care Mgmt Solutions . . . . Pamela Coffey
SVP/Information Systems. . . . . Jason Bielss
VP/General Counsel . . . . James Kelly
Senior Vice President of . . . . Jason Bielss
Senior Vice President, Sp. Charles E Busch

Specialty Managed Care Partners
Enters into Contracts with Regional Business Coalitions: Yes

Employer References
Garland ISD, Richardson ISD, Nokia, Tenet Health System, Gulf
 Stream Aerospace

1066 HealthSpring of Texas

2900 North Loop West
Suite 1300
Houston, TX 77092
Toll-Free: 800-668-3813
Phone: 832-553-3300
customerservicehelp@healthspring.com
www.cignahealthspring.com
Secondary Address: 105 Decker Court, Suite 1000, Irving, TX 75062
Subsidiary of: Health Spring Life and Health
Acquired by: Cigna
For Profit Organization: Yes
Year Founded: 2000
Total Enrollment: 1,000,000

Healthplan and Services Defined
  PLAN TYPE: Medicare

Type of Coverage
Medicare, Medicaid

Geographic Areas Served
Houston, Golden Triangle & Valley / North Texas & Lubbock

Key Personnel
President. . . . . Scott Huebner
Corp Mgr, Media Relations . . . . Jolene Sharp
 615-234-6710
 jolene.sharp@healthspring.com

1067 HMO Blue Texas

1001 E Lookout Drive
Richarson, TX 75082
Toll-Free: 877-299-2377
Phone: 972-766-6900
Mailing Address: PO Box 660044, Dallas, TX 75266-0044
Subsidiary of: A subsidiary of Blue Cross/Blue Shield of Texas
Acquired by: Blue Cross Blue Shield
Non-Profit Organization: Yes
Year Founded: 1944
Number of Affiliated Hospitals: 451
Number of Primary Care Physicians: 38,000
Total Enrollment: 3,800,000

Healthplan and Services Defined
  PLAN TYPE: HMO
  Benefits Offered: Behavioral Health, Disease Management, Inpatient
   SNF, Prescription, Psychiatric, Wellness, Mayo Clinic Online
   Resources, Women's health

Type of Coverage
Commercial, Individual, Medicare

Geographic Areas Served
All 254 Texas counties

Subscriber Information
Average Monthly Fee Per Subscriber
 (Employee + Employer Contribution):
  Employee Only (Self): Varies by plan
Average Annual Deductible Per Subscriber:
  Employee Only (Self): $0
  Employee & 1 Family Member: $0
  Employee & 2 Family Members: $0
  Medicare: $0
Average Subscriber Co-Payment:
  Primary Care Physician: $25.00
  Non-Network Physician: $30.00
  Prescription Drugs: $10/25/40
  Hospital ER: $100.00

Accreditation Certification
NCQA

Key Personnel
President/CEO . . . . Patricia Jemmingway-Hall

News Media Contact . . . . Margaret Jarvis
972-766-7165
margaret_jarvis@bcbtx.com

Employer References
University of Texas

1068 Horizon Health Corporation

1965 Lakepointe Drive Suite 100
Lewisville, TX 75057
Toll-Free: 800-931-4646
Phone: 866-843-5730
Fax: 972-420-8252
bhs@horizonhealth.com
www.horizonhealth.com
Subsidiary of: Psychiatric Solutions
For Profit Organization: Yes
Year Founded: 1975
Number of Affiliated Hospitals: 2,000
Number of Primary Care Physicians: 17,000
Number of Referral/Specialty Physicians: 18,531
Total Enrollment: 120,000

Healthplan and Services Defined
   PLAN TYPE: PPO
   Model Type: Staff
   Plan Specialty: Behavioral Health, UR
   Benefits Offered: Behavioral Health, Psychiatric, Rehabilitation
      Services

Type of Coverage
   Commercial, Indemnity

Type of Payment Plans Offered
   POS, DFFS, Capitated, FFS, Combination FFS & DFFS

Geographic Areas Served
   All 50 United States, Canada, Puerto Rico, Mexico, England, and the
   Virgin Islands

Subscriber Information
   Average Monthly Fee Per Subscriber
      (Employee + Employer Contribution):
         Employee & 2 Family Members: Varies by plan

Network Qualifications
   Pre-Admission Certification: Yes

Peer Review Type
   Utilization Review: Yes
   Case Management: Yes

Publishes and Distributes Report Card: Yes

Accreditation Certification
   URAC, NCQA

Key Personnel
   VP Marketing . . . . Robert Kramer
      972-420-8200
   Dir Quality Management. . . . . Jane Baker
   Medical Director. . . . . William Eckbert, MD
      407-915-0025
   Implementation/Member Management . . . . Ruth Scott
      407-915-0025
   Director IS. . . . . Richard Hippert
      407-915-0025
   Provider Services . . . . Lupe Rivero
      407-915-0025
   VP Sales/Acct Management. . . . . Steve Hart
      407-915-0025

Specialty Managed Care Partners
   Enters into Contracts with Regional Business Coalitions: Yes
   Employer Health Coalition

Employer References
   American Greetings, Saint Gobain Corporation, Broodwing,
   Jeld-Wen, The Pep Boys

1069 Humana Health Insurance of Corpus Christi

1801 S Alameda
Suite 100
Corpus Christi, TX 78404
Toll-Free: 800-533-5758
Phone: 361-866-1400
Fax: 361-866-1429
www.humana.com
Subsidiary of: LifeSynch
For Profit Organization: Yes
Year Founded: 1983
Number of Affiliated Hospitals: 2,800
Number of Primary Care Physicians: 320,000
Total Enrollment: 172,000

Healthplan and Services Defined
   PLAN TYPE: HMO/PPO
   Model Type: IPA
   Benefits Offered: Disease Management, Prescription, Wellness

Type of Coverage
   Commercial, Individual

Type of Payment Plans Offered
   POS, DFFS, Capitated

Geographic Areas Served
   Arkansas, Kleberg, Nueces & San Patricio counties

Network Qualifications
   Pre-Admission Certification: Yes

Publishes and Distributes Report Card: No

Accreditation Certification
   URAC, NCQA, CORE

Key Personnel
   President/CEO Humana . . . . Mike McCallister
   Corporate Communications. Ross McLaren
   CEO/Humana Texas. . . . . Gary Goldstein, MD

Specialty Managed Care Partners
   Enters into Contracts with Regional Business Coalitions: No

1070 Humana Health Insurance of San Antonio

8431 Fredericksburg Road
Suite 170
San Antonio, TX 78229
Toll-Free: 800-611-1456
Phone: 210-615-5100
Fax: 210-617-1251
www.humana.com
Secondary Address: San Antonio Guidance CTR, 803 Castroville Rd.,
   Suite 300, San Antonio, TX 78237, 210-424-6086
Subsidiary of: LifeSynch
For Profit Organization: Yes
Year Founded: 1983
Number of Affiliated Hospitals: 2,800
Number of Primary Care Physicians: 330,000
Total Enrollment: 172,000

Healthplan and Services Defined
   PLAN TYPE: HMO/PPO
   Model Type: Network
   Benefits Offered: Disease Management, Prescription, Wellness
   Offers Demand Management Patient Information Service: Yes

Type of Coverage
   Commercial, Individual
   Catastrophic Illness Benefit: Covered

Geographic Areas Served
   Bexar County; Medina, Comal, Wilson, Guadalupe, Karnes, Bandera,
   Kendall, Atascosa, Frio, Blanco

Subscriber Information
Average Monthly Fee Per Subscriber
  (Employee + Employer Contribution):
    Employee Only (Self): Varies by plan
Average Annual Deductible Per Subscriber:
    Employee Only (Self): $200.00
    Employee & 1 Family Member: $600.00
    Employee & 2 Family Members: $600.00
Average Subscriber Co-Payment:
    Primary Care Physician: $10.00
    Non-Network Physician: Not covered
    Hospital ER: $50.00
    Home Health Care: $0
    Home Health Care Max. Days/Visits Covered: 30 visits
    Nursing Home Max. Days/Visits Covered: 30 days

Network Qualifications
Pre-Admission Certification: Yes

Peer Review Type
Utilization Review: Yes
Second Surgical Opinion: Yes
Case Management: Yes

Publishes and Distributes Report Card: Yes

Accreditation Certification
URAC, NCQA, CORE
TJC Accreditation, Medicare Approved, Utilization Review,
    Pre-Admission Certification, State Licensure, Quality Assurance
    Program

Key Personnel
President/CEO . . . . Bruce D. Broussard
EVP/COO. . . . . James E. Murray
SVP/Chief Medical Officer . . . . Roy A. Beveridge, M.D
SVP/Chief Consumer Office. . . . . Jody L. Bilney
SVP/Chief Financial Offic . . . . Brian Kane

Average Claim Compensation
Physician's Fees Charged: 80%
Hospital's Fees Charged: 80%

Specialty Managed Care Partners
Enters into Contracts with Regional Business Coalitions: Yes

1071 Interplan Health Group
222 West Las Colinas Boulevard
Suite 600N
Irving, TX 75039
Toll-Free: 800-613-1124
Phone: 817-633-8335
Fax: 817-640-1009
info@interplanhealth.com
www.healthsmart.com/NetworkSolutions/ProviderNetworks/Interp
Secondary Address: 2002 West Loop 289, Lubbock, TX 79407
Subsidiary of: A Health Smart Network
Acquired by: HealthSmart
Year Founded: 1994
Number of Affiliated Hospitals: 5,000
Number of Primary Care Physicians: 203,000
Number of Referral/Specialty Physicians: 373,000
State Enrollment: 275,000

Healthplan and Services Defined
  PLAN TYPE: PPO
  Model Type: Network
  Plan Specialty: Behavioral Health, Chiropractic, Dental, Lab,
    Radiology, Worker's Compensation, UR
  Benefits Offered: Dental, Home Care, Durable Medical Equipment

Type of Coverage
Commercial

Type of Payment Plans Offered
DFFS, FFS

Geographic Areas Served
Arizona, Florida, Iowa, Nebraska, S Dakota, Texas, and Wisconsin

Subscriber Information
Average Monthly Fee Per Subscriber
  (Employee + Employer Contribution):
    Employee Only (Self): Varies by plan
Average Subscriber Co-Payment:
    Primary Care Physician: $10.00-20.00
    Non-Network Physician: 30%

Network Qualifications
Pre-Admission Certification: Yes

Peer Review Type
Utilization Review: Yes
Second Surgical Opinion: Yes
Case Management: Yes

Publishes and Distributes Report Card: No

Accreditation Certification
URAC
TJC Accreditation, Utilization Review, Quality Assurance Program

Key Personnel
Chairman & Founder . . . . Ted Parker
Executive Vice President . . . . Bill Dembereckyj
Chief Executive Offier . . . . Peter Osenar
Chief Operating Officer . . . . Eileen Romansky
Chief Financial Officer. . . . . Lisa Cobb
Chief Information Officer. . . . . John Bradshaw

Average Claim Compensation
Physician's Fees Charged: 77%
Hospital's Fees Charged: 67%

Specialty Managed Care Partners
AmeriScript
Enters into Contracts with Regional Business Coalitions: No

Employer References
Corporate Benefit Services of America, American Freightways, Rip
    Griffin, American Medical Security, John Alden/Fortis

1072 KelseyCare Advantage
11511 Shadow Creek Parkway
Pearland, TX 77584
Toll-Free: 866-535-8343
Phone: 713-442-5646
www.kelseycareadvantage.com

Healthplan and Services Defined
  PLAN TYPE: Medicare
  Other Type: HMO/POS
  Benefits Offered: Disease Management, Prescription, Wellness

Type of Coverage
Medicare, Medicare Advantage

Key Personnel
President. . . . . Marnie Matheny
VP, Operations . . . . Theresa Devivar
Medical Director. . . . . Dr Donald Aga
VP, Sales & Marketing. . . . . Angela Waltman
Director, Pharmacy Svcs . . . . Denise Martinez Jordan, RPh

---

1073 Legacy Health Plan
120 East Harris
San Angelo, TX 76903
Toll-Free: 800-839-7198
Phone: 325-658-7104
www.legacyhealthplan.com
Year Founded: 2004
Total Enrollment: 1,000

Healthplan and Services Defined
  PLAN TYPE: HMO

Geographic Areas Served
Coke, Coleman, Concho, Crockett, Edwards, Irion, Kimble, Kinney, Mason, McCulloch, Menard, Reagan, Runnels, Schleicher, Sterling, Sutton, Tom Green, Val Verde counties

1074 Medical Care Referral Group

4100 Rio Bravo
Suite 211
El Paso, TX 79902
Toll-Free: 800-424-9919
Phone: 915-532-2408
Fax: 915-532-1772
www.mcrg.net
Subsidiary of: Assured Benefits Administration
For Profit Organization: Yes
Year Founded: 1985
Number of Affiliated Hospitals: 8
Number of Primary Care Physicians: 190
Number of Referral/Specialty Physicians: 560
State Enrollment: 65,000

Healthplan and Services Defined
PLAN TYPE: PPO
Model Type: Network
Plan Specialty: IUO
Benefits Offered: Behavioral Health, Chiropractic, Dental, Disease Management, Home Care, Inpatient SNF, Physical Therapy, Podiatry, Prescription, Psychiatric, Transplant, Vision, Wellness, Worker's Compensation, AD&D, Life, LTD, STD

Geographic Areas Served
El Paso

Network Qualifications
Pre-Admission Certification: Yes

Peer Review Type
Utilization Review: Yes
Second Surgical Opinion: Yes
Case Management: Yes

Publishes and Distributes Report Card: No

Accreditation Certification
Utilization Review, Pre-Admission Certification, State Licensure, Quality Assurance Program

Key Personnel
President and CEO . . . . .Joseph Halow
914-532-2100
jhalow@assurebenefitsadmin.com
Executive VP . . . . .Lorri Halo
VP Administration . . . . .Eddie Garcia
Benefits Administration . . . . .Angie Carrasco
acarrasco@assurebenefitsadmin.com
Marketing. . . . . .Sueann Austin
saustin@assurebenefitsadmin.com
Medical Affairs . . . . .George Halow, MD

Specialty Managed Care Partners
Enters into Contracts with Regional Business Coalitions: No

1075 Mercy Health Plans: Texas

5901 McPherson
Suite 1 & 2B, Centre Plaza
Laredo, TX 78041
Toll-Free: 800-617-3433
Phone: 956-723-2144
Fax: 956-723-8246
Non-Profit Organization: Yes
Total Enrollment: 73,000

Healthplan and Services Defined
PLAN TYPE: HMO

Type of Coverage
Commercial, Individual

1076 MHNet Behavioral Health

9606 N. Mopac Expressway
Stonebridge Plaza 1, Suite 600
Austin, TX 78759
Toll-Free: 888-646-6889
Fax: 724-741-4552
www.mhnet.com
Mailing Address: PO Box 209010, Austin, TX 78720-9010
For Profit Organization: Yes
Year Founded: 1985
Number of Affiliated Hospitals: 134
Number of Referral/Specialty Physicians: 2,000
Total Enrollment: 2,000,000

Healthplan and Services Defined
PLAN TYPE: Multiple
Model Type: IPA
Plan Specialty: Behavioral Health, Employee Assistance Programs and Managed Behavioral Health Care
Benefits Offered: Behavioral Health, Psychiatric
Offers Demand Management Patient Information Service: Yes
DMPI Services Offered: Psychiatric Illness

Type of Payment Plans Offered
POS, DFFS, Capitated, FFS, Combination FFS & DFFS

Geographic Areas Served
Nationwide

Network Qualifications
Minimum Years of Practice: 1
Pre-Admission Certification: Yes

Peer Review Type
Utilization Review: Yes
Second Surgical Opinion: Yes
Case Management: Yes

Publishes and Distributes Report Card: Yes

Accreditation Certification
URAC, NCQA

Key Personnel
President & Chief Operati. . . . . .Kevin Middleton, PsyD
Chief Financial Officer . . . . .Bill Scheerer, CPA
Vice President of Operati . . . . .Talitha Appenzeller, MBA
Natl Dir, Quality Mgmt . . . . .Jacki Roschbach, MSS
National Director, Networ .Marc Besserman
Director of Strategic Mar . . . . .Marc Blevens
Corporate Medical Dir . . . . .Peter Harris, MD, PhD

Average Claim Compensation
Physician's Fees Charged: 30%
Hospital's Fees Charged: 30%

Specialty Managed Care Partners
Enters into Contracts with Regional Business Coalitions: Yes

1077 Molina Healthcare: Texas

5605 North MacArthur Boulevard
Suite 400
Irving, TX 75038
Toll-Free: 877-665-4622
www.molinahealthcare.com
Subsidiary of: Molina Medicaid Solutions
For Profit Organization: Yes
Year Founded: 1980
Physician Owned Organization: Yes
Number of Affiliated Hospitals: 84
Number of Primary Care Physicians: 2,167
Number of Referral/Specialty Physicians: 6,184
Total Enrollment: 1,800,000

Healthplan and Services Defined
  PLAN TYPE: HMO
  Model Type: Network
  Benefits Offered: Chiropractic, Dental, Home Care, Inpatient SNF,
    Long-Term Care, Podiatry, Vision

Type of Coverage
  Commercial, Medicare, Supplemental Medicare, Medicaid

Accreditation Certification
  URAC, NCQA

Key Personnel
  President/CEO . . . . J. Mario Molina, MD
  CFO . . . . John C. Molina, JD
  COO . . . . Terry Bayer, JD,MPH
  EVP Of Research/Developme . . . . Dr.Martha Molina Bernadett

1078 Ora Quest Dental Plans

101 Parklane Boulevard
Suite 301
Sugar Land, TX 77478
Toll-Free: 800-660-6064
Phone: 281-313-7170
Fax: 281-313-7155
info@oraquest.com
www.oraquest.com
For Profit Organization: Yes

Healthplan and Services Defined
  PLAN TYPE: Dental
  Other Type: Dental HMO
  Model Type: Network
  Plan Specialty: Dental
  Benefits Offered: Dental

Type of Coverage
  Commercial, Individual, Medicare, Medicaid

Subscriber Information
  Average Annual Deductible Per Subscriber:
    Employee Only (Self): $0

Key Personnel
  President/CEO . . . . James Taylor
  CFO . . . . Patrick Stoner
  COO. . . . . Rick Barrett

1079 PacifiCare of Texas

5001 LBJ Freeway
Suite 600
Dallas, TX 75244-6130
Toll-Free: 866-316-9776
Phone: 1-877-847-2862
Fax: 210-474-5048
www.uhcwest.com/
Mailing Address: PO Box 30970, Salt Lake City, UT 84130-0970
Subsidiary of: UnitedHealthCare
For Profit Organization: Yes
Year Founded: 1986
Number of Primary Care Physicians: 4,800
Total Enrollment: 146,000
State Enrollment: 47,755

Healthplan and Services Defined
  PLAN TYPE: HMO
  Model Type: IPA, Group, Network
  Benefits Offered: Behavioral Health, Disease Management,
    Prescription, Psychiatric, 24 hour nurse line
  Offers Demand Management Patient Information Service: Yes

Type of Coverage
  Commercial, Individual, Indemnity, Medicare
  Catastrophic Illness Benefit: Varies per case

Type of Payment Plans Offered
  POS, DFFS, FFS, Combination FFS & DFFS

Geographic Areas Served
  Greater San Antonio, Houston, Dallas/Ft. Worth, Metroplex and
  Galveston

Subscriber Information
  Average Monthly Fee Per Subscriber
    (Employee + Employer Contribution):
      Employee Only (Self): Varies by plan
      Medicare: $0
  Average Annual Deductible Per Subscriber:
      Employee Only (Self): $0
      Employee & 1 Family Member: $0
      Employee & 2 Family Members: $0
      Medicare: $0
  Average Subscriber Co-Payment:
      Primary Care Physician: $10.00
      Prescription Drugs: $5.00/10.00
      Hospital ER: $50.00
      Home Health Care Max. Days/Visits Covered: Unlimited as necc.
      Nursing Home: $0
      Nursing Home Max. Days/Visits Covered: 100 days

Peer Review Type
  Second Surgical Opinion: Yes
  Case Management: Yes

Publishes and Distributes Report Card: Yes

Accreditation Certification
  NCQA
  TJC Accreditation, Medicare Approved, Utilization Review,
    Pre-Admission Certification, State Licensure, Quality Assurance
    Program

Key Personnel
  Chairman/CEO Health Sys. . . . . Howard Phanstiel
  CFO . . . . Greg Scott
  President/CEO Health Plan . . . . Brad Bowlus
  Exec VP/Specialty Comp . . . . Jacqueline Kosecoff
  Exec VP/Enterprise Svce. Sharon Garrett
  Exec VP/General Counsel . . . . Joseph Konowiecki
  Exec VP/Major Accounts . . . . James Frey
  Exec VP/Cheif Med Officer. . . . . Sam Ho
  President/CEO Beh Health . . . . Jerome V Vaccaro, MD
  Sr VP/Human Resources . . . . Carol Black

Average Claim Compensation
  Physician's Fees Charged: 1%

Specialty Managed Care Partners
  Enters into Contracts with Regional Business Coalitions: Yes

1080 Parkland Community Health Plan

2777 N Stemmons Freeway
Suite 1750
Dallas, TX 75207-2277
Toll-Free: 888-672-2277
Phone: 214-266-2100
Fax: 214-266-2150
webmaster@parklandhmo.org
www.parklandhmo.com
Secondary Address: Claims Department, PO Box 61088, Phoenix, AZ
  85082
Non-Profit Organization: Yes
Year Founded: 1996
Number of Affiliated Hospitals: 30
Number of Primary Care Physicians: 1,900
Total Enrollment: 170,000

Healthplan and Services Defined
  PLAN TYPE: HMO
  Model Type: Network

Benefits Offered: Behavioral Health, Chiropractic, Home Care, Inpatient SNF, Physical Therapy, Podiatry, Prescription, Psychiatric, Transplant, Vision, Durable Medical Equipment
Offers Demand Management Patient Information Service: Yes
DMPI Services Offered: Nurse Line

Type of Coverage
Medicaid, CHIP, KIDSfirst

Type of Payment Plans Offered
POS, FFS

Geographic Areas Served
Dallas, Collin, Ellis, Hunt, Kaufman, Navarro and Rockwall counties

Network Qualifications
Pre-Admission Certification: Yes

Peer Review Type
Utilization Review: Yes
Second Surgical Opinion: Yes
Case Management: Yes

Accreditation Certification
Utilization Review, Pre-Admission Certification, State Licensure, Quality Assurance Program

Specialty Managed Care Partners
Comprehensive Behavioral Care, Block Vision

1081   SafeGuard Health Enterprises: Texas

95 Enterprise
Suite 200
Aliso Viejo, CA 92656
Toll-Free: 800-880-1800
safeguards@cpa.state.tx.us
www.safeguard.net
Subsidiary of: MetLife
For Profit Organization: Yes
Year Founded: 1974
Number of Primary Care Physicians: 2,073
Number of Referral/Specialty Physicians: 2,030
Total Enrollment: 1,800,000

Healthplan and Services Defined
PLAN TYPE: Dental
Other Type: Dental HMO
Model Type: IPA
Plan Specialty: ASO, Dental, Vision
Benefits Offered: Dental, Vision

Type of Coverage
Individual, Indemnity, Medicaid

Type of Payment Plans Offered
DFFS, Capitated

Geographic Areas Served
California, Texas, Florida

Subscriber Information
Average Annual Deductible Per Subscriber:
Employee Only (Self): $50.00
Employee & 1 Family Member: $100.00
Employee & 2 Family Members: $150.00

Network Qualifications
Pre-Admission Certification: Yes

Peer Review Type
Utilization Review: Yes

Publishes and Distributes Report Card: No

Key Personnel
Chairman/CEO . . . . James E Buncher
   949-425-4500
President/COO . . . . Stephen J Baker
SVP/CFO . . . . Dennis L Gates
VP/CIO . . . . Michael J Lauffenburger
SVP/General Counsel . . . . Ronald I Brendzel
Dir/Human Resources . . . . William Wolff

Director . . . . Jack R Anderson

Specialty Managed Care Partners
Enters into Contracts with Regional Business Coalitions: Yes

Employer References
State of California, Boeing, County of Los Angeles, Farmers Insurance, Automobile Club

1082   Scott & White Health Plan

1206 West Campus Drive
Temple, TX 76502
Toll-Free: 800-321-7947
Phone: 254-298-3000
Fax: 254-298-3011
swhpques@sw.org
www.swhp.org
Secondary Address: 3000 Briarcrest, Suite 422, Bryan, TX 77802, 979-268-7947
Non-Profit Organization: Yes
Year Founded: 1979
Owned by an Integrated Delivery Network (IDN): Yes
Number of Affiliated Hospitals: 18
Number of Primary Care Physicians: 1,000
Total Enrollment: 200,000
State Enrollment: 200,000

Healthplan and Services Defined
PLAN TYPE: HMO
Other Type: POS, CDHP
Model Type: Group
Benefits Offered: Behavioral Health, Dental, Disease Management, Home Care, Inpatient SNF, Long-Term Care, Physical Therapy, Podiatry, Prescription, Psychiatric, Transplant, Vision
Offers Demand Management Patient Information Service: Yes
DMPI Services Offered: Secondary prevention of Coronary Artery Disease, Pediatric Asthma, Diabetes Mellitius, Congestive Heart Failure, Hypertension

Type of Coverage
Commercial, Individual, Medicare, Medicare cost
Catastrophic Illness Benefit: Covered

Type of Payment Plans Offered
DFFS, Capitated

Geographic Areas Served
Bastrop, Bell, Blanco, Bosque, Brazos, Burleson, Burnet, Caldwell, Coryell, Falls, Grimes, Hamilton, Hays, Hill, Hood, Johnson, Lampasas, Lee, Llano, Madison, McLennan, Milam, Mills, Robertson, San Saba, Somervell, Travis, Walker, Washington & Williamson; Portions of Austin, Erath, Leon & Waller

Subscriber Information
Average Monthly Fee Per Subscriber
(Employee + Employer Contribution):
Employee Only (Self): Varies by plan
Average Annual Deductible Per Subscriber:
Employee Only (Self): $0.00
Employee & 1 Family Member: $0.00
Employee & 2 Family Members: $0.00
Average Subscriber Co-Payment:
Primary Care Physician: $10.00
Prescription Drugs: $5.00/20.00/50.00
Hospital ER: $75.00
Home Health Care: $10.00
Nursing Home: $0

Network Qualifications
Pre-Admission Certification: No

Peer Review Type
Utilization Review: Yes
Second Surgical Opinion: No
Case Management: Yes

Publishes and Distributes Report Card: Yes

Accreditation Certification
NCQA
TJC Accreditation, Medicare Approved, Utilization Review, State Licensure, Quality Assurance Program

Key Personnel
President/CEO .... Allan Einboden
COO .... Marinan Williams
CMO/COO Medicaid .... Scott Nicklebur, MD
Legal Counsel.............................. Jimmy Carroll
VP, Sales & Marketing........................... Lee Green
Chief Medical Director........................ Marylou Buyse
Dir, Sales & Marketing......................... Sandy Gerik
Manager, Media Relations .... Katherine Voss
254-724-4097
kvoss@swmail.sw.org
Manager, Media Relations .... Scott Clark
254-724-9724
sdclark@swmail.sw.org

Average Claim Compensation
Physician's Fees Charged: 57%
Hospital's Fees Charged: 43%

Employer References
Texas A&M, ERS, Wiliamson County

1083 Script Care, Ltd.
6380 Folsom Drive
Beaumont, TX 77706
Toll-Free: 800-880-9988
customerservice@scriptcare.com
www.scriptcare.com
Year Founded: 1989
Number of Primary Care Physicians: 60,000

Healthplan and Services Defined
PLAN TYPE: PPO
Other Type: PBM
Plan Specialty: PBM
Benefits Offered: Prescription

Type of Payment Plans Offered
Capitated, FFS

Geographic Areas Served
National

Subscriber Information
Average Subscriber Co-Payment:
Prescription Drugs: Variable

Peer Review Type
Case Management: Yes

Key Personnel
President .... Jim Brown
Vice President................................ Steve Holiday
COO.. Kathy Cannon
Office Manager............................ Mary Alice Stuart
Manager..................................... Pam Boehme
Manager..................................... Rachel Tate
VP Sales/Marketing........................... Kevin Brown
Director, Account Manager .... Rachel Tate
Provider Relations .... Lisa Gutierrez

1084 Seton Health Plan
1201 W 38th Street
Austin, TX 78705-1006
Toll-Free: 1-866-272-2507
Phone: 512-421-5667
Fax: 512-324-3359
shpproviderservices@seton.org
www.setonhealthplan.com

Subsidiary of: Seton Family of Hospitals
For Profit Organization: Yes
Number of Affiliated Hospitals: 20
Number of Primary Care Physicians: 1,900
Total Enrollment: 15,000

Healthplan and Services Defined
PLAN TYPE: HMO
Benefits Offered: Disease Management, Prescription, Wellness

Type of Coverage
Commercial

Geographic Areas Served
Central Texas

1085 TexanPlus Medicare Advantage HMO
PO Box 741107
Houston, TX 77274-1107
Toll-Free: 866-230-2513
www.universal-american-medicare.com/products/hmo/texan-plus-
Secondary Address: Special Investigation Unit, PO Box 744921, Houston, TX 77274, 866-684-0595
For Profit Organization: Yes
Total Enrollment: 42,000

Healthplan and Services Defined
PLAN TYPE: Medicare
Benefits Offered: Chiropractic, Dental, Disease Management, Home Care, Inpatient SNF, Physical Therapy, Podiatry, Prescription, Psychiatric, Vision, Wellness

Type of Coverage
Individual, Medicare

Geographic Areas Served
Available only within Texas

Subscriber Information
Average Monthly Fee Per Subscriber
(Employee + Employer Contribution):
Employee Only (Self): Varies
Medicare: Varies
Average Annual Deductible Per Subscriber:
Employee Only (Self): Varies
Medicare: Varies
Average Subscriber Co-Payment:
Primary Care Physician: Varies
Non-Network Physician: Varies
Prescription Drugs: Varies
Hospital ER: Varies
Home Health Care: Varies
Home Health Care Max. Days/Visits Covered: Varies
Nursing Home: Varies
Nursing Home Max. Days/Visits Covered: Varies

Key Personnel
Chairman & CEO .... Richard A Barasch
EVP/COO.................................. Gary W Bryant
EVP/CFO .... Robert Waegelein, CPA
SVP, Corp Development .... Gary Jacobs
COO... Jason Israel
President & CEO Med Advan .... Theodore Carpenter

1086 Texas Community Care
9111 Jollyville Road
Suite 102
Austin, TX 78759
Toll-Free: 800-658-3704
Phone: 512-795-8092
Fax: 512-795-2371
Secondary Address: 7500 Viscount Blvd, Suite 292, El Paso, TX 79925
Subsidiary of: Arcadian Health Plan, Inc.
Total Enrollment: 230,000

Healthplan and Services Defined
 PLAN TYPE: Medicare
 Benefits Offered: Chiropractic, Dental, Disease Management, Home
  Care, Inpatient SNF, Physical Therapy, Podiatry, Prescription,
  Psychiatric, Vision, Wellness

Type of Coverage
 Individual, Medicare

Geographic Areas Served
 Available only within Texas

Subscriber Information
 Average Monthly Fee Per Subscriber
  (Employee + Employer Contribution):
   Employee Only (Self): Varies
   Medicare: Varies
 Average Annual Deductible Per Subscriber:
   Employee Only (Self): Varies
   Medicare: Varies
 Average Subscriber Co-Payment:
   Primary Care Physician: Varies
   Non-Network Physician: Varies
   Prescription Drugs: Varies
   Hospital ER: Varies
   Home Health Care: Varies
   Home Health Care Max. Days/Visits Covered: Varies
   Nursing Home: Varies
   Nursing Home Max. Days/Visits Covered: Varies

Key Personnel
 Chairman/CEO . . . . John H Austin, MD
 President. . . . . Nancy Freeman
 Chief Financial Officer. . . . . Ken Zimmerman, MBA
 Senior Medical Director . . . . Gary R Herzberg, MD
 Senior Medical Executive . . . . Jeffrey McManus, MD
 SVP/Business Management. . . . . Cheryl Perkins, RN
 VP/Network Management . . . . Peter G Goll
 VP/Development. . . . . Chase Milbrandt, MBA
 VP/Sales & Marketing . . . . Garrison Rios
 VP/Health Services. . . . . Laurie Wilson, RN
 Media Contact . . . . Nilsa Lennig
   510-817-1016
   nlennig@arcadianhealth.com

1087 Texas True Choice

PO Box 250089
Plano, TX 75025
Toll-Free: 800-683-4856
Phone: 214-267-3300
Fax: 469-443-3401
TTCInquires@multiplan.com
www.texastruechoice.com
Secondary Address: 6116 Shallowford Road, Suite 109, Chattanooga,
 TN 37421, 866-971-7247
Subsidiary of: Viant
Acquired by: MultiPlan
For Profit Organization: Yes
Year Founded: 1996
Number of Affiliated Hospitals: 380
Number of Primary Care Physicians: 46,000
Total Enrollment: 1,080,000
State Enrollment: 1,080,000

Healthplan and Services Defined
 PLAN TYPE: PPO
 Model Type: Network
 Plan Specialty: ASO, Dental, Vision, Radiology, UR, PPO
 Benefits Offered: Behavioral Health, Chiropractic, Dental, Home
  Care, Inpatient SNF, Long-Term Care, Physical Therapy, Podiatry,
  Prescription, Psychiatric, Transplant, Vision, Wellness, Worker's
  Compensation, AD&D, Life, LTD, STD

Type of Coverage
 Commercial, Individual, Indemnity, Medicare, Supplemental
  Medicare, Medicaid, Catastrophic
 Catastrophic Illness Benefit: Varies per case

Type of Payment Plans Offered
 FFS, Combination FFS & DFFS

Geographic Areas Served
 Statewide Texas

Subscriber Information
 Average Subscriber Co-Payment:
   Primary Care Physician: Varies
   Non-Network Physician: Varies
   Prescription Drugs: Varies
   Hospital ER: Varies
   Home Health Care: Varies
   Home Health Care Max. Days/Visits Covered: Varies
   Nursing Home: Varies
   Nursing Home Max. Days/Visits Covered: Varies

Network Qualifications
 Pre-Admission Certification: Yes

Peer Review Type
 Utilization Review: Yes
 Second Surgical Opinion: Yes
 Case Management: Yes

Publishes and Distributes Report Card: No

Accreditation Certification
 TJC Accreditation, Medicare Approved, Utilization Review,
  Pre-Admission Certification, State Licensure, Quality Assurance
  Program

Key Personnel
 CEO . . . . Michael Wilson

Specialty Managed Care Partners
 Family Health of America
 Enters into Contracts with Regional Business Coalitions: No

Employer References
 University of Texas System, City of Odessa, City of Austin, City Of
  McAllen, Trinity Industries

1088 Unicare: Texas

3820 American Drive
Plano, TX 75075
Toll-Free: 800-333-2203
Phone: 972-599-3888
Fax: 972-599-6267
www.unicare.com
Secondary Address: 106 East Sixth Street, Suite 333, Austin, TX 78701
For Profit Organization: Yes
Year Founded: 1995
Total Enrollment: 38,000

Healthplan and Services Defined
 PLAN TYPE: HMO/PPO
 Model Type: Network
 Plan Specialty: Dental, EPO, Lab, Radiology
 Benefits Offered: Dental, Inpatient SNF, Long-Term Care,
  Prescription, Transplant, Wellness, AD&D, Life, LTD, STD, EAP

Type of Coverage
 Individual, Indemnity, Medicare, Supplemental Medicare

Geographic Areas Served
 Illinois, Indiana, Ohio, Michigan, Texas, Nevada, Massachusetts,
  Virginia, Washington DC, Oklahoma

Network Qualifications
 Pre-Admission Certification: Yes

Peer Review Type
 Utilization Review: Yes
 Second Surgical Opinion: Yes
 Case Management: Yes

Publishes and Distributes Report Card: No

Accreditation Certification
NCQA
TJC Accreditation, Utilization Review, Pre-Admission Certification,
State Licensure, Quality Assurance Program

Key Personnel
President/CEO .... David W Fields
Medical Director.......................... Neal Fischer, MD
Sales Director .... Mike Ryan
mike.ryan@wellpoint.com
Media Contact .... Tony Felts
317-287-6036
tony.felts@wellpoint.com

Specialty Managed Care Partners
Wellpoint Pharmacy Management, Wellpoint Dental Services,
Wellpoint Behavioral Health
Enters into Contracts with Regional Business Coalitions: No

1089 United Concordia: Texas

8214 Westchester Drive
Suite 600
Dallas, TX 72552
Toll-Free: 877-722-8224
Phone: 214-378-6410
Fax: 214-378-6306
www.unitedconcordia.com
Secondary Address: 11200 Westheimer, Suite 820, Houston, TX
77042, 888-828-6432
For Profit Organization: Yes
Year Founded: 1971
Number of Primary Care Physicians: 111,000
Total Enrollment: 8,000,000

Healthplan and Services Defined
PLAN TYPE: Dental
Plan Specialty: Dental
Benefits Offered: Dental

Type of Coverage
Commercial, Individual

Geographic Areas Served
Military personnel and their families, nationwide

1090 UnitedHealthCare of Texas

1250 Capital Of TX Hwy South
Bldg 1, Suite 400
Austin, TX 78746
Toll-Free: 877-294-1429
www.uhc.com
Secondary Address: 6200 Northwest Pkwy, Suite 107, San Antonio,
TX 78249, 210-478-4800
For Profit Organization: Yes
Year Founded: 1986
Number of Affiliated Hospitals: 5,609
Number of Primary Care Physicians: 726,537
Total Enrollment: 70,000,000
State Enrollment: 1,862,466

Healthplan and Services Defined
PLAN TYPE: HMO/PPO
Model Type: IPA
Benefits Offered: Dental, Disease Management, Prescription,
Wellness, AD&D, Life, LTD, STD

Type of Coverage
Commercial, Individual, Medicare

Geographic Areas Served
79 counties in Texas

Network Qualifications
Pre-Admission Certification: Yes

Publishes and Distributes Report Card: Yes

Accreditation Certification
AAPI, NCQA

Key Personnel
Media Contact .... Kim Whitaker
469-633-8536
kim_t_whitaker@uhc.com

Specialty Managed Care Partners
Enters into Contracts with Regional Business Coalitions: Yes

1091 USA Managed Care Organization

1250 S Capital of Texas Highway
Bldg 3, Suite 500
Austin, TX 78746
Toll-Free: 800-872-0020
info@usamco.com
www.usamco.com
Secondary Address: 7301 North 16th Street, Suite 201, Phoenix, AZ
85020
For Profit Organization: Yes
Year Founded: 1984
Number of Affiliated Hospitals: 5,000
Number of Primary Care Physicians: 430,000
Total Enrollment: 5,427,579
State Enrollment: 1,118,582

Healthplan and Services Defined
PLAN TYPE: PPO
Model Type: Group
Plan Specialty: Behavioral Health, Chiropractic, Dental, Disease
Management, EPO, Lab, PBM, Vision, Radiology, Worker's
Compensation, UR
Benefits Offered: Prescription, Worker's Compensation

Type of Coverage
Commercial

Type of Payment Plans Offered
POS, DFFS, FFS, Combination FFS & DFFS

Geographic Areas Served
USA MCO is a National Preferred Provider network

Network Qualifications
Pre-Admission Certification: Yes

Peer Review Type
Utilization Review: Yes
Second Surgical Opinion: Yes
Case Management: Yes

Publishes and Distributes Report Card: No

Accreditation Certification
TJC Accreditation, Pre-Admission Certification, State Licensure,
Quality Assurance Program

Key Personnel
President and CEO .... George Bogle
800-872-0820
CFO .... Joseph Dulin
COO .... Mike Bogle
VP, Marketing .... Sarah Beatty
Medical Director .... James E Gerace
VP, Human Resources .... Tammy Greene
Chief Information Officer .... Jim Mahoney
VP, Sales .... Sean Graff

Average Claim Compensation
Physician's Fees Charged: 34%
Hospital's Fees Charged: 32%

1092 UTMB HealthCare Systems

301 University Boulevard
Galveston, TX 77555
Toll-Free: 855-256-7876
Phone: 409-766-4064
www.utmbhcs.org
Mailing Address: PO Box 16809, Galveston, TX 77552
Non-Profit Organization: Yes
Year Founded: 1994
Total Enrollment: 1,000

Healthplan and Services Defined
   PLAN TYPE: HMO

Type of Coverage
   Commercial, Medicare, Medicaid, CHIP

Geographic Areas Served
   SE Texas

Key Personnel
   Chief Executive Officer . . . . Donna Sollenberger
   Executive Director . . . . Donna Johnson
   Vice President . . . . DK Norman

1093 Valley Baptist Health Plan

2005 Ed Carey Drive
Harlingen, TX 78550
Toll-Free: 800-829-6440
www.valleybaptist.net
Subsidiary of: Valley Baptist Insurance Company
Non-Profit Organization: Yes
Total Enrollment: 22,000
State Enrollment: 12,004

Healthplan and Services Defined
   PLAN TYPE: HMO
   Benefits Offered: Chiropractic, Dental, Disease Management, Home
     Care, Inpatient SNF, Physical Therapy, Podiatry, Prescription,
     Psychiatric, Transplant, Vision, Wellness, Durable Medical
     Equipment

Type of Coverage
   Commercial

Type of Payment Plans Offered
   POS

Geographic Areas Served
   Texas

Subscriber Information
   Average Monthly Fee Per Subscriber
    (Employee + Employer Contribution):
      Employee Only (Self): Varies
      Employee & 1 Family Member: Varies
      Employee & 2 Family Members: Varies
      Medicare: Varies
   Average Annual Deductible Per Subscriber:
      Employee Only (Self): Varies
      Employee & 1 Family Member: Varies
      Employee & 2 Family Members: Varies
      Medicare: Varies
   Average Subscriber Co-Payment:
      Primary Care Physician: Varies
      Non-Network Physician: Varies
      Prescription Drugs: Varies
      Hospital ER: Varies
      Home Health Care: Varies
      Home Health Care Max. Days/Visits Covered: Varies
      Nursing Home: Varies
      Nursing Home Max. Days/Visits Covered: Varies

Specialty Managed Care Partners
   Express Scripts

1094 VSP: Vision Service Plan of Texas

4265 San Felipe Street
#1100
Houston, TX 77027-2920
Toll-Free: 800-877-7195
Phone: 713-960-6680
webmaster@vsp.com
www.vsp.com
Year Founded: 1955
Number of Primary Care Physicians: 26,000
Total Enrollment: 55,000,000

Healthplan and Services Defined
   PLAN TYPE: Vision
   Plan Specialty: Vision
   Benefits Offered: Vision

Type of Payment Plans Offered
   Capitated

Geographic Areas Served
   Statewide

Network Qualifications
   Pre-Admission Certification: Yes

Peer Review Type
   Utilization Review: Yes

Accreditation Certification
   Utilization Review, Quality Assurance Program

Key Personnel
   President/CEO VSP Global . . . . Rob Lynch
   President VSP Vision Care . . . . Jim McGrann

1095 WellPoint NextRx

5450 North Riverside Drive
Fort Worth, TX 76137
Toll-Free: 888-809-6084
Phone: 800-293-2202
www.expressscripts.com
Secondary Address: 333 Guadalupe, Suite 3-600, Box 21, Austin, TX
   78701-3942, 800-821-3205
Subsidiary of: WellPoint
For Profit Organization: Yes
Year Founded: 1993
Total Enrollment: 300,000

Healthplan and Services Defined
   PLAN TYPE: Multiple
   Model Type: Network
   Plan Specialty: PBM
   Benefits Offered: Prescription

Type of Coverage
   Commercial

Geographic Areas Served
   Nationwide

Accreditation Certification
   URAC
   Pre-Admission Certification

Key Personnel
   General Manager . . . . Michael Nameth
   VP/CFO . . . . Sally Sharma
   Marketing . . . . Jacqueline Dart
   VP Info. Systems . . . . Prudence Kaui
   National Sales Director . . . . Jeff Turner
    706-369-1300

Employer References
   Blue Cross of California, Blue Cross and Blue Shield of Georgia,
    United Wisconsin

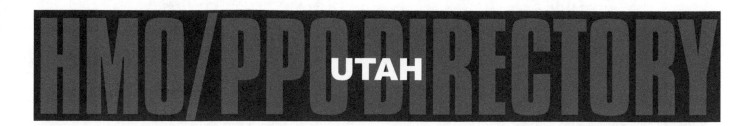
Health Insurance Coverage Status and Type of Coverage by Age

Category	All Persons		Under 18 years		Under 65 years		65 years and over	
	Number	%	Number	%	Number	%	Number	%
Total population	2,874	-	894	-	2,595	-	279	-
Covered by some type of health insurance	2,472 (13)	86.0 (0.5)	809 (6)	90.5 (0.7)	2,195 (13)	84.6 (0.5)	277 (1)	99.2 (0.3)
Covered by private health insurance	2,114 (18)	73.5 (0.6)	659 (8)	73.7 (0.9)	1,935 (17)	74.5 (0.7)	179 (4)	64.1 (1.4)
Employment based	1,803 (19)	62.7 (0.7)	581 (9)	65.0 (1.0)	1,697 (18)	65.4 (0.7)	106 (4)	38.0 (1.3)
Direct purchase	333 (12)	11.6 (0.4)	74 (6)	8.2 (0.6)	246 (11)	9.5 (0.4)	87 (4)	31.0 (1.3)
Covered by TRICARE	71 (7)	2.5 (0.2)	17 (3)	1.9 (0.4)	49 (6)	1.9 (0.2)	21 (2)	7.6 (0.8)
Covered by government health insurance	604 (12)	21.0 (0.4)	179 (8)	20.0 (0.9)	335 (13)	12.9 (0.5)	269 (2)	96.5 (0.6)
Covered by Medicaid	321 (11)	11.2 (0.4)	178 (8)	19.9 (0.9)	293 (12)	11.3 (0.4)	28 (2)	10.1 (0.7)
Also by private insurance	68 (6)	2.4 (0.2)	29 (4)	3.2 (0.4)	54 (6)	2.1 (0.2)	15 (2)	5.2 (0.6)
Covered by Medicare	312 (4)	10.9 (0.1)	2 (1)	0.2 (0.1)	43 (4)	1.7 (0.1)	269 (2)	96.4 (0.6)
Also by private insurance	185 (4)	6.4 (0.1)	Z (Z)	0.0 (0.1)	14 (2)	0.5 (0.1)	171 (4)	61.3 (1.4)
Also by Medicaid	48 (3)	1.7 (0.1)	1 (Z)	0.1 (0.1)	19 (2)	0.7 (0.1)	28 (2)	10.1 (0.7)
Covered by VA Care	44 (3)	1.5 (0.1)	Z (Z)	0.0 (0.1)	22 (2)	0.8 (0.1)	22 (2)	7.8 (0.6)
Not covered at any time during the year	402 (13)	14.0 (0.5)	85 (6)	9.5 (0.7)	400 (13)	15.4 (0.5)	2 (1)	0.8 (0.3)

Note: Numbers in thousands; Figures cover 2013; Margin of error appears in parenthesis; A "Z" indicates that the value either represents or rounds to zero.
Source: U.S. Census Bureau, 2013 American Community Survey, Table HI05. Health Insurance Coverage Status and Type of Coverage by State and Age for All People: 2013

Utah

1096 Aetna Health of Utah

151 Farmington Avenue
Hartford, CT 06156
Toll-Free: 800-872-3862
Phone: 860-273-0123
www.aetna.com
Partnered with: eHealthInsurance Services Inc.
For Profit Organization: Yes
Total Enrollment: 11,596,230

Healthplan and Services Defined
   PLAN TYPE: PPO
   Other Type: POS
   Plan Specialty: EPO
   Benefits Offered: Dental, Disease Management, Long-Term Care,
      Prescription, Wellness, Life, LTD, STD

Type of Coverage
   Commercial, Individual

Type of Payment Plans Offered
   POS, FFS

Geographic Areas Served
   Statewide

Key Personnel
   Chairman/CEO/President. . . . . .Mark T Bertolini
   EVP/General Counsel . . . . .William J Casazza
   EVP/CFO . . . . .Shawn M Guertin

1097 Altius Health Plans

10421 S Jordan Gateway
Suite 400
South Jordan, UT 84095
Toll-Free: 800-377-4161
Phone: 801-355-1234
utahcustomerservice@ahplans.com
www.altiushealthplans.com
For Profit Organization: Yes
Year Founded: 1998
Number of Affiliated Hospitals: 46
Number of Primary Care Physicians: 3,800
Number of Referral/Specialty Physicians: 1,850
Total Enrollment: 148,000
State Enrollment: 84,000

Healthplan and Services Defined
   PLAN TYPE: Multiple
   Model Type: Group, POS
   Plan Specialty: Behavioral Health, Chiropractic, Disease
      Management, Lab, PBM, Vision, Radiology, UR
   Benefits Offered: Behavioral Health, Chiropractic, Dental, Disease
      Management, Home Care, Inpatient SNF, Physical Therapy,
      Podiatry, Prescription, Psychiatric, Transplant, Vision, Wellness
   Offers Demand Management Patient Information Service: Yes

Type of Coverage
   Commercial, Catastrophic
   Catastrophic Illness Benefit: Unlimited

Type of Payment Plans Offered
   POS, DFFS

Geographic Areas Served
   Utah, Idaho and Wyoming

Subscriber Information
   Average Monthly Fee Per Subscriber
      (Employee + Employer Contribution):
         Employee Only (Self): Varies
         Employee & 1 Family Member: Varies
         Employee & 2 Family Members: Varies
         Medicare: Varies

Average Annual Deductible Per Subscriber:
   Employee Only (Self): Varies
   Employee & 1 Family Member: Varies
   Employee & 2 Family Members: Varies
   Medicare: Varies
Average Subscriber Co-Payment:
   Primary Care Physician: $15.00
   Non-Network Physician: 70%
   Prescription Drugs: Varies
   Hospital ER: Varies
   Home Health Care: Varies
   Home Health Care Max. Days/Visits Covered: 60 visits
   Nursing Home: Varies
   Nursing Home Max. Days/Visits Covered: 60 visits

Network Qualifications
   Pre-Admission Certification: Yes

Peer Review Type
   Utilization Review: Yes
   Second Surgical Opinion: Yes
   Case Management: Yes

Publishes and Distributes Report Card: Yes

Accreditation Certification
   URAC
   TJC Accreditation, Medicare Approved, Utilization Review,
      Pre-Admission Certification, State Licensure, Quality Assurance
      Program

Key Personnel
   Chief Executive Officer . . . . .Todd Treptin
   CFO. . . . . .Brett Clay
   Director, Human Resources . . . . .Lani Anderson
   Marketing Executive . . . . .Deborah Rosenhan
   VP Chief Medical Officer . . . . .Dennis T Harston, MD
   Information Services. . . . . .Russell Nelson

Specialty Managed Care Partners
   Horizon Behavioral Health, ESI

Employer References
   Federal Government, State of Utah, Davis County School District,
      Wells Fargo, DMBA

1098 CIGNA HealthCare of Utah

5295 South 320 West
Suite 280
Salt Lake City, UT 84107
Toll-Free: 800-261-5731
Phone: 801-265-2777
Fax: 801-261-7537
www.cigna.com
Secondary Address: Great-West Healthcare, now part of CIGNA, 200
   W Civic Center Drive, Suite 120, Sandy, UT 84070, 801-255-1300
For Profit Organization: Yes
Year Founded: 1985
Number of Affiliated Hospitals: 13
Number of Primary Care Physicians: 310
Total Enrollment: 47,724
State Enrollment: 4,198

Healthplan and Services Defined
   PLAN TYPE: HMO/PPO
   Model Type: IPA
   Benefits Offered: Behavioral Health, Disease Management,
      Prescription, Psychiatric, Transplant, Vision, Wellness, Women's
      and Men's Health
   Offers Demand Management Patient Information Service: Yes
   DMPI Services Offered: Language Links Service, 24 hour Health
      Information Line, Health Information Library

Type of Coverage
   Commercial
   Catastrophic Illness Benefit: Varies per case

Type of Payment Plans Offered
POS, DFFS, Capitated, FFS, Combination FFS & DFFS

Geographic Areas Served
Box Elder, Davis, Morgan, Salt Lake, Sanpete, Summit, Tooele, Utah and Weber counties

Subscriber Information
Average Monthly Fee Per Subscriber
(Employee + Employer Contribution):
Employee Only (Self): Varies
Employee & 1 Family Member: Varies
Employee & 2 Family Members: Varies
Medicare: Varies
Average Annual Deductible Per Subscriber:
Employee Only (Self): $150.00
Employee & 1 Family Member: $300.00
Employee & 2 Family Members: $450.00
Average Subscriber Co-Payment:
Primary Care Physician: $10.00
Non-Network Physician: Not covered
Prescription Drugs: $5.00
Hospital ER: $50.00
Home Health Care: $0
Home Health Care Max. Days/Visits Covered: 40 days
Nursing Home: $0
Nursing Home Max. Days/Visits Covered: 60 per year

Network Qualifications
Pre-Admission Certification: Yes

Peer Review Type
Utilization Review: Yes
Second Surgical Opinion: Yes
Case Management: Yes

Accreditation Certification
NCQA
TJC Accreditation, Medicare Approved, Utilization Review, Pre-Admission Certification, State Licensure, Quality Assurance Program

Key Personnel
President & CEO............................David Cordani
Executive Vice President.........................Lisa Bacus
President, Global Employe....................David Guilmette
In House Formulary ....David Burton
Materials Management ....Jim Hicks
Medical Affairs.............................John Tudor, MD
Member Services.............................Martha Spoor
Provider Services.............................Josh Nelson
Sales ....Robert Immitt

Specialty Managed Care Partners
Enters into Contracts with Regional Business Coalitions: Yes

1099   Delta Dental of Utah

257 East 200 South
Suite 375
Salt Lake City, UT 84111
Toll-Free: 800-453-5577
Phone: 801-575-5168
Fax: 801-575-5171
utsales@delta.org
www.deltadentalins.com
Non-Profit Organization: Yes
Total Enrollment: 54,000,000

Healthplan and Services Defined
PLAN TYPE: Dental
Other Type: Dental PPO

Type of Coverage
Commercial

Geographic Areas Served
Statewide

Key Personnel
CEO...Gary Radine
Director Sales ....Jill Balboni
972-966-6800
Dir/Media & Public Affair ....Elizabeth Risberg
415-972-8423

1100   Educators Mutual

852 E Arrowhead Lane
Murray, UT 84107-5298
Toll-Free: 800-662-5851
Phone: 801-262-7475
Fax: 801-269-9734
cs@emihealth.com
www.emihealth.com
Non-Profit Organization: Yes
Year Founded: 1935
Physician Owned Organization: Yes
Federally Qualified: Yes
Number of Affiliated Hospitals: 25
Number of Primary Care Physicians: 3,500
Total Enrollment: 6,000
State Enrollment: 65,000

Healthplan and Services Defined
PLAN TYPE: HMO/PPO
Model Type: Network
Plan Specialty: Behavioral Health, Chiropractic, Disease Management, Radiology, UR
Benefits Offered: Behavioral Health, Chiropractic, Complementary Medicine, Dental, Disease Management, Home Care, Inpatient SNF, Physical Therapy, Podiatry, Prescription, Psychiatric, Transplant, Vision, Wellness, AD&D, Life, LTD, STD
Offers Demand Management Patient Information Service: Yes
DMPI Services Offered: Wellness Web

Type of Coverage
Commercial, Individual

Type of Payment Plans Offered
POS

Geographic Areas Served
Box Elder, Cache, Davis, Salt Lake, Weber counties

Subscriber Information
Average Monthly Fee Per Subscriber
(Employee + Employer Contribution):
Employee Only (Self): Varies by plan
Average Annual Deductible Per Subscriber:
Employee Only (Self): $0
Employee & 1 Family Member: $0
Employee & 2 Family Members: $0
Medicare: $0
Average Subscriber Co-Payment:
Primary Care Physician: $5.00
Prescription Drugs: 30%
Hospital ER: $25.00
Home Health Care: $0
Nursing Home: $0

Network Qualifications
Pre-Admission Certification: Yes

Peer Review Type
Utilization Review: Yes
Second Surgical Opinion: No
Case Management: Yes

Publishes and Distributes Report Card: Yes

Accreditation Certification
TJC Accreditation, Utilization Review, Pre-Admission Certification, State Licensure, Quality Assurance Program

Key Personnel
President/CEO ....Steven C. Morrison, CPA

EVP/CFO/Treasurer . . . . Mike Greenhalgh, CPA CGMA
EVP/COO/Secretary. . . . . Ryan Lowther
SVP/Chief Compliance Offi . . . . Brandon L. Smart, Esq.
Chief Actuary . . . . David Wood
EVP/Information Technolog . . . . Joe Campbell
SVP/Corporate Communicati. . . . . Christie Hawkes
Marketing . . . . Tom Busby
Chief Information Officer. . . . . Ted Peck

Specialty Managed Care Partners
Enters into Contracts with Regional Business Coalitions: No

1101 eHealthInsurance Services Inc.
11919 Foundation Place
Gold River, CA 95670
Toll-Free: 800-644-3491
webmaster@healthinsurance.com
www.e.healthinsurance.com
Year Founded: 1997

Healthplan and Services Defined
PLAN TYPE: HMO/PPO
Benefits Offered: Dental, Life, STD

Type of Coverage
Commercial, Individual, Medicare

Geographic Areas Served
All 50 states in the USA and District of Columbia

Key Personnel
Chairman & CEO. . . . . Gary L. Lauer
EVP/Business & Corp. Dev.. . . . . Bruce Telkamp
EVP/Chief Technology. . . . . Dr. Sheldon X. Wang
SVP & CFO . . . . Stuart M. Huizinga
Pres. of eHealth Gov. Sys . . . . Samuel C. Gibbs
SVP of Sales & Operations . . . . Robert S. Hurley
Director Public Relations. Nate Purpura
650-210-3115

1102 Humana Health Insurance of Utah
9815 South Monroe Street
Suite 300
Sandy, UT 84070
Toll-Free: 800-884-8328
Phone: 801-256-6200
Fax: 801-256-0782
www.humana.com
For Profit Organization: Yes

Healthplan and Services Defined
PLAN TYPE: HMO/PPO

Type of Coverage
Commercial, Individual

Accreditation Certification
URAC, NCQA, CORE

1103 Meritain Health: Utah
Sorenson Park Building #7
4246 S Riverboat Road, Suite 200
Taylorsville, UT 84123
Phone: 801-261-5511
sales@meritain.com
www.meritain.com
For Profit Organization: Yes
Year Founded: 1983
Number of Affiliated Hospitals: 110
Number of Primary Care Physicians: 3,467
Number of Referral/Specialty Physicians: 5,720
Total Enrollment: 500,000
State Enrollment: 450,000

Healthplan and Services Defined
PLAN TYPE: PPO
Model Type: Network
Plan Specialty: Dental, Disease Management, Vision, Radiology, UR
Benefits Offered: Prescription
Offers Demand Management Patient Information Service: Yes

Type of Coverage
Commercial

Geographic Areas Served
Nationwide

Subscriber Information
Average Monthly Fee Per Subscriber
(Employee + Employer Contribution):
Employee Only (Self): Varies by plan

Accreditation Certification
URAC
TJC Accreditation, Medicare Approved, Utilization Review,
Pre-Admission Certification, State Licensure, Quality Assurance
Program

Key Personnel
Regional President . . . . Melissa Elwood
Head Of Business Operatio . . . . Jeff Goddard
Head of Prodigy Health Gr. . . . . Mark W. Schmidt
Senior Vice President of . . . . David C. Parker

Average Claim Compensation
Physician's Fees Charged: 78%
Hospital's Fees Charged: 90%

Specialty Managed Care Partners
Express Scripts, LabOne, Interactive Health Solutions

1104 Molina Healthcare: Utah
7050 Union Park Center
Suite 200
Midvale, UT 84047
Toll-Free: 888-483-0760
Phone: 801-858-0400
www.molinahealthcare.com
For Profit Organization: Yes
Year Founded: 1980
Physician Owned Organization: Yes
Number of Affiliated Hospitals: 84
Number of Primary Care Physicians: 2,167
Number of Referral/Specialty Physicians: 6,184
Total Enrollment: 1,400,000

Healthplan and Services Defined
PLAN TYPE: HMO
Model Type: Network
Benefits Offered: Chiropractic, Dental, Home Care, Inpatient SNF,
Long-Term Care, Podiatry, Vision

Type of Coverage
Commercial, Medicare, Supplemental Medicare, Medicaid

Accreditation Certification
URAC, NCQA

1105 Opticare of Utah
1901 W Parkway Boulevard
Salt Lake City, UT 84119
Toll-Free: 800-363-0950
Phone: 801-869-2020
service@opticareofutah.com
www.opticareofutah.com
For Profit Organization: Yes
Year Founded: 1985
Number of Primary Care Physicians: 17
Number of Referral/Specialty Physicians: 40
Total Enrollment: 150,000

State Enrollment: 150,000

Healthplan and Services Defined
PLAN TYPE: Vision
Other Type: Optical
Model Type: Network
Plan Specialty: Vision
Benefits Offered: Vision

Type of Payment Plans Offered
POS, Capitated, FFS

Geographic Areas Served
Statewide

Subscriber Information
Average Subscriber Co-Payment:
Primary Care Physician: Varies

Network Qualifications
Pre-Admission Certification: Yes

Peer Review Type
Utilization Review: Yes
Second Surgical Opinion: Yes
Case Management: Yes

Key Personnel
CEO/ABO.....................................Aaron Schubach
800-363-0950
aaron@standardoptical.net
President................................Stephen Schubach
stephen@standardoptical.net
CFO,CPA.......................................Ken Acker
ken@standardoptical.net
Individual Policies & Cla ....Stacie Merrill
Provider Relations ....Michelle Anderson
801-886-2020
michelle@standardoptical.net
Director of Sales.........................Michelle Anderson
801-577-9392
michelle@opticareofutah.com

Specialty Managed Care Partners
Enters into Contracts with Regional Business Coalitions: Yes

Employer References
State of Utah Employees

1106 Public Employees Health Program
560 East 200 South
Salt Lake City, UT 84102
Toll-Free: 800-765-7347
Phone: 801-366-7555
Fax: 801-366-7596
www.pehp.org
Secondary Address: Southern Utah Branch Office, 165 North 100 East #9, St. George, UT 84770
Subsidiary of: Utah Retirement Systems
Non-Profit Organization: Yes
Year Founded: 1977
Number of Affiliated Hospitals: 49
Number of Primary Care Physicians: 12,000
Number of Referral/Specialty Physicians: 2,900
Total Enrollment: 177,854
State Enrollment: 177,854

Healthplan and Services Defined
PLAN TYPE: PPO
Model Type: Network
Plan Specialty: Behavioral Health, Chiropractic, Dental, Disease Management, Lab, PBM, Vision, Radiology, UR
Benefits Offered: Behavioral Health, Chiropractic, Dental, Disease Management, Home Care, Physical Therapy, Podiatry, Prescription, Psychiatric, Transplant, Vision, Wellness, AD&D, Life, LTD

Type of Coverage
Supplemental Medicare, Children's Health Insurance Program
Catastrophic Illness Benefit: None

Type of Payment Plans Offered
FFS

Geographic Areas Served
Utah's public employees and their families

Subscriber Information
Average Monthly Fee Per Subscriber
(Employee + Employer Contribution):
Employee Only (Self): Varies by plan
Employee & 1 Family Member: $583.00
Average Annual Deductible Per Subscriber:
Employee Only (Self): $0
Employee & 1 Family Member: $0
Employee & 2 Family Members: $0
Medicare: $0
Average Subscriber Co-Payment:
Primary Care Physician: $15.00
Non-Network Physician: 15.00 + 30%
Prescription Drugs: 20%
Hospital ER: $80.00
Home Health Care Max. Days/Visits Covered: Unlimited

Network Qualifications
Pre-Admission Certification: No

Peer Review Type
Utilization Review: Yes
Second Surgical Opinion: Yes
Case Management: Yes

Publishes and Distributes Report Card: Yes

Accreditation Certification
TJC Accreditation, Medicare Approved, State Licensure

Key Personnel
Director............................R. Chet Loftis, JD,MPA
Finance Director...................Kim Kellersberger, CGFM
Operations Director.........................G. Steven Baker
Chief Medical Director ....Cynthia Jones, MD
Marketing Director............................Joel Sheppard
Chief Actuary...........................Paul Anderton, FSA
Administrative Assistant........................Karen Ridges

Average Claim Compensation
Physician's Fees Charged: 70%
Hospital's Fees Charged: 80%

Specialty Managed Care Partners
Managed Mental Healthcare, Chiropratic Health Plan, IHC Auesst
Enters into Contracts with Regional Business Coalitions: Yes

Employer References
State of Utah, Jordon School District, Salt Lake County, Salt Lake City, Utah School Boards Association

1107 Regence Blue Cross & Blue Shield of Utah
PO Box 30270
Salt Lake City, UT 84130
Toll-Free: 888-231-8424
www.ut.regence.com
Mailing Address: PO Box 1071, Portland, OR 97207
Subsidiary of: Blue Cross Blue Shield National Association
For Profit Organization: Yes
Year Founded: 1942
Physician Owned Organization: Yes
Owned by an Integrated Delivery Network (IDN): Yes
Number of Affiliated Hospitals: 44
Number of Primary Care Physicians: 4,350
Total Enrollment: 320,000
State Enrollment: 231,824

Healthplan and Services Defined
PLAN TYPE: PPO

Model Type: Network
Plan Specialty: ASO, Behavioral Health, Chiropractic, Dental, Disease Management, MSO, PBM, Vision, Radiology, UR
Benefits Offered: Behavioral Health, Chiropractic, Complementary Medicine, Dental, Disease Management, Home Care, Inpatient SNF, Physical Therapy, Podiatry, Prescription, Psychiatric, Transplant, Vision, Wellness, AD&D, Life, LTD, STD

Type of Coverage
Individual, Supplemental Medicare
Catastrophic Illness Benefit: Varies per case

Geographic Areas Served
Statewide

Subscriber Information
Average Monthly Fee Per Subscriber
(Employee + Employer Contribution):
Employee Only (Self): Varies by plan
Average Annual Deductible Per Subscriber:
Employee Only (Self): $250.00 per person
Employee & 1 Family Member: $250.00 per person
Employee & 2 Family Members: $250.00 per person
Average Subscriber Co-Payment:
Primary Care Physician: Varies by plan
Non-Network Physician: Varies
Prescription Drugs: $5.00/20%
Hospital ER: $50.00
Home Health Care: 20%
Nursing Home: 20%

Network Qualifications
Pre-Admission Certification: Yes

Peer Review Type
Utilization Review: Yes
Second Surgical Opinion: No
Case Management: Yes

Publishes and Distributes Report Card: Yes

Accreditation Certification
Ambest
TJC Accreditation, Medicare Approved, Utilization Review, Pre-Admission Certification, State Licensure, Quality Assurance Program

Key Personnel
President..................................Robert A Hatch
Chief Information Officer ....Cheron Vail
Chief Marketing Exec ....Mohan Nair
Chief Legal Officer...........................Kerry Barnett
Vice President/Sales......................Alfred S Tredway
Media Contact ....J Kevin Bischoff
801-333-5285
kbischoff@regence.com
VP, Provider Relations.......................Bryon Clawson
Executive Vice President,...................Dr. Richard Popiel
Media Contact.................................Mike Tatko
208-798-2221
mtatkoid@regence.com

Average Claim Compensation
Physician's Fees Charged: 30%
Hospital's Fees Charged: 21%

Specialty Managed Care Partners
Enters into Contracts with Regional Business Coalitions: Yes

1108 SelectHealth
5381 Green Street
Murray, UT 84123
Toll-Free: 800-538-5038
Phone: 801-442-5000
http://selecthealth.org
Subsidiary of: Intermountain Healthcare
Non-Profit Organization: Yes
Total Enrollment: 402,000

Healthplan and Services Defined
PLAN TYPE: HMO

Type of Coverage
Commercial, Individual

Accreditation Certification
NCQA

Key Personnel
President/CEO ....Patricia R Richards
Media Contact ....Spencer Sutherland
801-442-7960

1109 Total Dental Administrators
6985 Union Park Center
Suite 675
Cottonwood Heights, UT 84047
Toll-Free: 800-880-3536
Phone: 801-268-9840
Fax: 801-268-9873
www.tdadental.com

Healthplan and Services Defined
PLAN TYPE: Dental

Key Personnel
President....................................Jane Morrison
VP, Operations..............................Jeremy Spencer

1110 UnitedHealthCare of Utah
2525 Lake Park Blvd
Salt Lake City, UT 84120
Toll-Free: 800-624-2942
www.uhc.com
Subsidiary of: UnitedHealth Group
For Profit Organization: Yes
Total Enrollment: 75,000,000
State Enrollment: 109,709

Healthplan and Services Defined
PLAN TYPE: HMO/PPO

Geographic Areas Served
Statewide

Key Personnel
Medicare & Retirementÿ ....Sarah Bearceÿ
Media Contact ....Will Shanley
will.shanley@uhc.com

1111 University Health Plans
6053 Fashion Square Drive
Suite 110
Murray, UT 84107
Toll-Free: 888-271-5870
Phone: 801-587-6480
Fax: 801-281-6121
uuhp@hsc.utah.edu
http://uhealthplan.utah.edu
Non-Profit Organization: Yes
Number of Affiliated Hospitals: 28
Number of Primary Care Physicians: 1,750
Total Enrollment: 86,000
State Enrollment: 50,000

Healthplan and Services Defined
PLAN TYPE: HMO/PPO
Benefits Offered: Disease Management, Wellness

Type of Coverage
Commercial, Medicare, Medicaid

Geographic Areas Served
Utah

Key Personnel

CEO	Vicky Wilson
COO	Vicky Wilson
CMO	Dean Smart, MD
Provider Relations	Collin Davis
Marketing	Vicky Wilson
Provider Services	Todd Randall

   801-587-6602
   todd.randall@hsc.utah.edu

Health Insurance Coverage Status and Type of Coverage by Age

Category	All Persons		Under 18 years		Under 65 years		65 years and over	
	Number	%	Number	%	Number	%	Number	%
Total population	621	-	124	-	522	-	99	-
Covered by some type of health insurance	576 (4)	92.8 (0.6)	120 (2)	96.9 (1.1)	477 (4)	91.4 (0.7)	99 (1)	99.7 (0.2)
Covered by private health insurance	415 (8)	66.8 (1.2)	69 (3)	56.0 (2.7)	349 (7)	66.8 (1.4)	66 (2)	66.4 (1.9)
Employment based	347 (8)	55.9 (1.3)	64 (3)	51.8 (2.6)	312 (8)	59.8 (1.5)	35 (2)	35.4 (1.8)
Direct purchase	75 (4)	12.1 (0.6)	6 (1)	4.5 (1.0)	40 (3)	7.7 (0.6)	35 (2)	35.1 (2.2)
Covered by TRICARE	13 (2)	2.0 (0.3)	2 (1)	1.2 (0.6)	7 (1)	1.3 (0.3)	6 (1)	5.9 (1.1)
Covered by government health insurance	246 (7)	39.7 (1.1)	57 (3)	46.3 (2.7)	150 (7)	28.7 (1.3)	97 (1)	97.2 (0.8)
Covered by Medicaid	152 (7)	24.4 (1.1)	57 (3)	46.0 (2.7)	138 (7)	26.5 (1.3)	14 (1)	13.8 (1.4)
Also by private insurance	21 (2)	3.4 (0.4)	7 (1)	5.3 (1.0)	16 (2)	3.0 (0.4)	5 (1)	5.2 (1.0)
Covered by Medicare	118 (2)	19.0 (0.4)	1 (Z)	0.6 (0.3)	21 (2)	4.1 (0.4)	97 (1)	97.2 (0.8)
Also by private insurance	68 (2)	11.0 (0.4)	Z (Z)	0.2 (0.1)	5 (1)	0.9 (0.2)	63 (2)	63.9 (2.1)
Also by Medicaid	27 (2)	4.4 (0.4)	Z (Z)	0.3 (0.2)	14 (2)	2.6 (0.3)	14 (1)	13.8 (1.4)
Covered by VA Care	14 (1)	2.3 (0.2)	Z (Z)	0.2 (0.2)	5 (1)	1.0 (0.2)	9 (1)	9.2 (0.8)
Not covered at any time during the year	45 (4)	7.2 (0.6)	4 (1)	3.1 (1.1)	45 (4)	8.6 (0.7)	Z (Z)	0.3 (0.2)

Note: Numbers in thousands; Figures cover 2013; Margin of error appears in parenthesis; A "Z" indicates that the value either represents or rounds to zero.
Source: U.S. Census Bureau, 2013 American Community Survey, Table HI05. Health Insurance Coverage Status and Type of Coverage by State and Age for All People: 2013

Vermont

1112 Aetna Health of Vermont

151 Farmington Avenue
Hartford, CT 06156
Toll-Free: 800-872-3862
Phone: 860-273-0123
www.aetna.com
Partnered with: eHealthInsurance Services Inc.
For Profit Organization: Yes
Total Enrollment: 11,596,230

Healthplan and Services Defined
PLAN TYPE: PPO
Other Type: POS
Plan Specialty: EPO
Benefits Offered: Dental, Disease Management, Long-Term Care,
   Prescription, Wellness, Life, LTD, STD

Type of Coverage
Commercial, Individual

Type of Payment Plans Offered
POS, FFS

Geographic Areas Served
Statewide

Key Personnel
Chairman/CEO/President . . . . Mark T Bertolini
EVP/General Counsel . . . . William J Casazza
EVP/CFO . . . . Shawn M Guertin

1113 Blue Cross & Blue Shield of Vermont

445 Industrial Lane
Berlin, VT 05602
Toll-Free: 800-247-2583
www.bcbsvt.com
Mailing Address: PO Box 186, Montpelier, VT 05601
Non-Profit Organization: Yes
Year Founded: 1944
Number of Affiliated Hospitals: 16
Number of Primary Care Physicians: 681
Number of Referral/Specialty Physicians: 2,802
Total Enrollment: 180,000
State Enrollment: 54,023

Healthplan and Services Defined
PLAN TYPE: PPO
Model Type: Network
Plan Specialty: Behavioral Health, Chiropractic, Disease
   Management, PBM, Vision, UR
Benefits Offered: Behavioral Health, Chiropractic, Physical Therapy,
   Prescription, Psychiatric, Vision, AD&D, Life, LTD, STD,
   Alternative Healthcare discounts, Vermont Medigap Blue

Type of Coverage
Commercial, Individual, Indemnity, Medicare, Supplemental
   Medicare, Catastrophic
Catastrophic Illness Benefit: Maximum $1M

Type of Payment Plans Offered
Capitated

Geographic Areas Served
Vermont

Subscriber Information
Average Monthly Fee Per Subscriber
   (Employee + Employer Contribution):
      Employee Only (Self): Varies by plan
Average Annual Deductible Per Subscriber:
      Employee Only (Self): $400.00
      Employee & 1 Family Member: $400.00
      Employee & 2 Family Members: $200.00
Average Subscriber Co-Payment:

Primary Care Physician: $10.00
Prescription Drugs: $10.00/20.00/35.00
Hospital ER: $50.00
Home Health Care: $40.00

Network Qualifications
Pre-Admission Certification: Yes

Peer Review Type
Utilization Review: Yes
Second Surgical Opinion: No
Case Management: Yes

Publishes and Distributes Report Card: No

Accreditation Certification
Utilization Review, State Licensure, Quality Assurance Program

Key Personnel
President and CEO . . . . Don George
VP, External Affairs . . . . Kevin Goddard
VP, Planning . . . . Catherine Hamilton, PhD
VP, General Counsel . . . . Christopher R Gannon
VP, Sales & Marketing . . . . David Krupa
VP, Treasurer & CFO . . . . John Trifone
VP, Operations . . . . Douglas L Warren
VP Sales and Marketing . . . . David Krupa
Dir, Govt & Public Rel . . . . Leigh Tofferi
   802-223-6131
   webmail@bcbsvt.com

Average Claim Compensation
Physician's Fees Charged: 85%
Hospital's Fees Charged: 92%

Specialty Managed Care Partners
Magellan, Restat
Enters into Contracts with Regional Business Coalitions: Yes

1114 CIGNA HealthCare of Vermont

30 Main Street
Burlington, VT 05401
Toll-Free: 800-244-6224
Fax: 802-658-9212
www.cigna.com
For Profit Organization: Yes

Healthplan and Services Defined
PLAN TYPE: PPO

Type of Coverage
Commercial

1115 Delta Dental of Vermont

135 College Street
Burlington, VT 05401-8384
Toll-Free: 800-832-5700
Phone: 802-658-7839
Fax: 802-865-4430
nedental@nedental.com
www.nedental.com
Non-Profit Organization: Yes
Year Founded: 1961
Number of Primary Care Physicians: 1,675
Total Enrollment: 54,000,000

Healthplan and Services Defined
PLAN TYPE: Dental
Other Type: Dental PPO
Model Type: Network
Plan Specialty: ASO, Dental
Benefits Offered: Dental

Type of Coverage
Commercial, Individual, Group
Catastrophic Illness Benefit: None

Geographic Areas Served
Statewide

Subscriber Information
Average Monthly Fee Per Subscriber
  (Employee + Employer Contribution):
    Employee Only (Self): Varies
    Employee & 1 Family Member: Varies
    Employee & 2 Family Members: Varies
Average Annual Deductible Per Subscriber:
    Employee Only (Self): Varies
    Employee & 1 Family Member: Varies
    Employee & 2 Family Members: Varies
Average Subscriber Co-Payment:
    Prescription Drugs: $0
    Home Health Care: $0
    Nursing Home: $0

Key Personnel
Dental Operationsÿ . . . . Galina Torres

1116 eHealthInsurance Services Inc.
11919 Foundation Place
Gold River, CA 95670
Toll-Free: 800-644-3491
webmaster@healthinsurance.com
www.e.healthinsurance.com
Year Founded: 1997

Healthplan and Services Defined
  PLAN TYPE: HMO/PPO
  Benefits Offered: Dental, Life, STD

Type of Coverage
  Commercial, Individual, Medicare

Geographic Areas Served
  All 50 states in the USA and District of Columbia

Key Personnel
Chairman & CEO . . . . Gary L. Lauer
EVP/Business & Corp. Dev. . . . . Bruce Telkamp
EVP/Chief Technology . . . . Dr. Sheldon X. Wang
SVP & CFO . . . . Stuart M. Huizinga
Pres. of eHealth Gov. Sys . . . . Samuel C. Gibbs
SVP of Sales & Operations . . . . Robert S. Hurley
Director Public Relations. . . . . Nate Purpura
  650-210-3115

1117 MVP Health Care: Vermont
66 Knight Lane
Suite 10
Williston, VT 05495
Toll-Free: 800-380-3530
Phone: 802-264-6500
Fax: 802-264-6555
www.mvphealthcare.com
Secondary Address: 625 State Street, PO Box 2207, Schenectady, NY
  12301-2207, 518-370-4793
Non-Profit Organization: Yes
Year Founded: 1983
Federally Qualified: Yes
Number of Affiliated Hospitals: 81
Number of Primary Care Physicians: 3,091
Number of Referral/Specialty Physicians: 5,504
Total Enrollment: 750,000

Healthplan and Services Defined
  PLAN TYPE: HMO/PPO
  Model Type: IPA
  Plan Specialty: ASO, EPO
  Benefits Offered: Behavioral Health, Chiropractic, Complementary
    Medicine, Dental, Disease Management, Home Care, Inpatient

SNF, Physical Therapy, Podiatry, Prescription, Psychiatric,
    Transplant, Vision, Wellness, Worker's Compensation
Offers Demand Management Patient Information Service: No
DMPI Services Offered: After Hours Phone Line, Health Central
    (Library), Little Footprints Prenatal Program, Health Risk
    Assetments, Adult and Childhood Immunizations

Type of Coverage
  Commercial, Individual, Indemnity, Self Funded, Administrative
    Service
  Catastrophic Illness Benefit: Covered

Type of Payment Plans Offered
  POS, DFFS, Capitated, FFS, Combination FFS & DFFS

Geographic Areas Served
  VT

Subscriber Information
  Average Annual Deductible Per Subscriber:
    Employee Only (Self): $200/400

Peer Review Type
  Utilization Review: Yes
  Case Management: Yes

Publishes and Distributes Report Card: Yes

Accreditation Certification
  NCQA
  TJC Accreditation, Medicare Approved, Utilization Review,
    Pre-Admission Certification, State Licensure, Quality Assurance
    Program

Key Personnel
President/CEO . . . . Denise Gonick, Esq.
EVP/Commercial Business. . . . . David P. Crosby
EVP/Government Programs . . . . Patrick J. Glavey
EVP/CMO . . . . Allen J. Hinkle, MD
EVP/Networks And Contract . . . . Karla A. Austin
VP/Chief Information Offi. . . . . James H. Pool, III
EVP/Human Resources. . . . . James Morrill

Average Claim Compensation
  Physician's Fees Charged: 75%
  Hospital's Fees Charged: 65%

1118 UnitedHealthCare of Vermont
One Research Drive
Westborough, MA 01581
Toll-Free: 800-444-7855
www.uhc.com
Subsidiary of: UnitedHealth Group
For Profit Organization: Yes
Year Founded: 1986
Number of Affiliated Hospitals: 47
Number of Primary Care Physicians: 1,600
Number of Referral/Specialty Physicians: 3,500
Total Enrollment: 75,000,000

Healthplan and Services Defined
  PLAN TYPE: HMO/PPO
  Model Type: Mixed Model
  Plan Specialty: MSO
  Benefits Offered: Behavioral Health, Chiropractic, Complementary
    Medicine, Dental, Disease Management, Home Care, Inpatient
    SNF, Long-Term Care, Physical Therapy, Podiatry, Prescription,
    Psychiatric, Transplant, Vision, Wellness, AD&D, Life

Type of Coverage
  Commercial, Individual, Medicaid, Commercial Group

Type of Payment Plans Offered
  DFFS, FFS, Combination FFS & DFFS

Geographic Areas Served
  Statewide

Subscriber Information
Average Monthly Fee Per Subscriber
(Employee + Employer Contribution):
Employee Only (Self): Varies
Average Subscriber Co-Payment:
Primary Care Physician: $10
Prescription Drugs: $10/15/30
Hospital ER: $50

Network Qualifications
Pre-Admission Certification: Yes

Peer Review Type
Case Management: Yes

Publishes and Distributes Report Card: Yes

Accreditation Certification
URAC, NCQA
State Licensure, Quality Assurance Program

Average Claim Compensation
Physician's Fees Charged: 70%
Hospital's Fees Charged: 55%

Specialty Managed Care Partners
United Behavioral Health
Enters into Contracts with Regional Business Coalitions: No

Health Insurance Coverage Status and Type of Coverage by Age

Category	All Persons		Under 18 years		Under 65 years		65 years and over	
	Number	%	Number	%	Number	%	Number	%
Total population	8,054	-	1,862	-	6,975	-	1,080	-
Covered by some type of health insurance	7,064 (22)	87.7 (0.3)	1,760 (8)	94.6 (0.4)	5,996 (21)	86.0 (0.3)	1,068 (5)	98.9 (0.2)
Covered by private health insurance	5,954 (34)	73.9 (0.4)	1,306 (16)	70.2 (0.8)	5,186 (32)	74.3 (0.5)	768 (8)	71.2 (0.7)
Employment based	4,760 (39)	59.1 (0.5)	1,062 (17)	57.0 (0.9)	4,331 (37)	62.1 (0.5)	429 (8)	39.8 (0.8)
Direct purchase	1,046 (23)	13.0 (0.3)	134 (8)	7.2 (0.4)	678 (20)	9.7 (0.3)	368 (8)	34.1 (0.7)
Covered by TRICARE	644 (15)	8.0 (0.2)	173 (7)	9.3 (0.4)	509 (14)	7.3 (0.2)	135 (5)	12.5 (0.5)
Covered by government health insurance	2,060 (22)	25.6 (0.3)	505 (14)	27.1 (0.7)	1,024 (22)	14.7 (0.3)	1,036 (5)	96.0 (0.3)
Covered by Medicaid	896 (21)	11.1 (0.3)	487 (14)	26.2 (0.8)	792 (21)	11.4 (0.3)	104 (5)	9.6 (0.4)
Also by private insurance	139 (7)	1.7 (0.1)	42 (4)	2.3 (0.2)	88 (6)	1.3 (0.1)	51 (3)	4.7 (0.3)
Covered by Medicare	1,236 (8)	15.3 (0.1)	17 (3)	0.9 (0.2)	201 (8)	2.9 (0.1)	1,035 (5)	95.8 (0.3)
Also by private insurance	805 (9)	10.0 (0.1)	7 (2)	0.4 (0.1)	70 (4)	1.0 (0.1)	736 (8)	68.2 (0.7)
Also by Medicaid	167 (7)	2.1 (0.1)	5 (1)	0.2 (0.1)	63 (4)	0.9 (0.1)	104 (5)	9.6 (0.4)
Covered by VA Care	184 (6)	2.3 (0.1)	8 (2)	0.4 (0.1)	112 (5)	1.6 (0.1)	73 (3)	6.7 (0.3)
Not covered at any time during the year	991 (22)	12.3 (0.3)	101 (7)	5.4 (0.4)	979 (22)	14.0 (0.3)	12 (2)	1.1 (0.2)

Note: Numbers in thousands; Figures cover 2013; Margin of error appears in parenthesis; A "Z" indicates that the value either represents or rounds to zero.
Source: U.S. Census Bureau, 2013 American Community Survey, Table HI05. Health Insurance Coverage Status and Type of Coverage by State and Age for All People: 2013

Virginia

1119 Aetna Health of Virginia

151 Farmington Avenue
Hartford, CT 06156
Toll-Free: 800-872-3862
www.aetna.com
For Profit Organization: Yes
Year Founded: 1984
Number of Affiliated Hospitals: 119
Number of Primary Care Physicians: 6,908
Number of Referral/Specialty Physicians: 12,502
Total Enrollment: 211,156

Healthplan and Services Defined
  PLAN TYPE: HMO
  Other Type: POS
  Model Type: IPA
  Benefits Offered: Behavioral Health, Dental, Disease Management,
    Prescription, Vision, Wellness, Life
  Offers Demand Management Patient Information Service: Yes

Type of Coverage
  Commercial, Individual, Medicare

Type of Payment Plans Offered
  POS, DFFS

Geographic Areas Served
  Statewide

Subscriber Information
  Average Annual Deductible Per Subscriber:
    Employee Only (Self): Varies
    Employee & 1 Family Member: Varies
    Employee & 2 Family Members: Varies
    Medicare: Varies

Network Qualifications
  Pre-Admission Certification: Yes

Peer Review Type
  Utilization Review: No
  Second Surgical Opinion: Yes
  Case Management: Yes

Publishes and Distributes Report Card: Yes

Accreditation Certification
  NCQA
  TJC Accreditation, Utilization Review, Pre-Admission Certification,
    State Licensure, Quality Assurance Program

Key Personnel
  CEO & President . . . . Mark T Bertolini
  SVP, General Counsel . . . . William J Casazza
  SEVP, CFO. . . . . Joseph M Zubretsky
  Head, M&A Integration . . . . Kay Mooney
  SVP, Marketing. . . . . Robert E Mead
  Chief Medical Officer . . . . Lonny Reisman, MD
  SVP, Human Resources. . . . . Elease E Wright
  SVP, CIO. . . . . Meg McCarthy

Specialty Managed Care Partners
  Enters into Contracts with Regional Business Coalitions: Yes

1120 Amerigroup Corporation

2815 Hartland Road
Suite 200
Merrifield, VA 22043
Toll-Free: 800-600-4441
Phone: 757-490-6900
mpsweb@amerigroupcorp.com
www.amerigroupcorp.com
For Profit Organization: Yes
Year Founded: 1994

Number of Primary Care Physicians: 3,066
Total Enrollment: 1,900,000

Healthplan and Services Defined
  PLAN TYPE: HMO
  Benefits Offered: Disease Management

Type of Coverage
  Medicaid

Geographic Areas Served
  11 counties in Northern Virginia

Accreditation Certification
  URAC, NCQA

Key Personnel
  Executive Vice President. Richard C. Zoretic
  Chief Financial Officer . . . . Scott Anglin
  Chief Executive Officer. . . . . Peter D. Haytaian, Esq.
  EVP, CFO . . . . James W Truess
  EVP, COO . . . . Richard C Zoretic
  Chief Compliance Officer. John R Finley
  SVP, Chief Accounting Ofc . . . . Margaret M Roomsburg
  Vice President, Human Res . . . . Todd Williams
  EVP, Chief Medical Office . . . . Mary McCluskey
  EVP, Human Resources . . . . Linda Whitley-Taylor
  EVP, Chief Info Officer. . . . . Leon A Root, Jr
  EVP, External Relations . . . . John E Littel
  Corporate Communications. . . . . Tara Wall
    757-321-3592
    twall01@amerigroupcorp.com

1121 Anthem Blue Cross & Blue Shield of Virginia

2015 Staples Mill Road
PO Box 27401
Richmond, VA 23230
Toll-Free: 800-421-1880
Phone: 804-354-7000
Fax: 804-354-3610
www.anthem.com
Secondary Address: 602 South Jefferson Street, Roanoke, VA 24011
For Profit Organization: Yes
Year Founded: 1980
Number of Affiliated Hospitals: 125
Number of Primary Care Physicians: 2,700
Number of Referral/Specialty Physicians: 5,700
Total Enrollment: 2,800,000
State Enrollment: 2,800,000

Healthplan and Services Defined
  PLAN TYPE: HMO
  Model Type: IPA
  Plan Specialty: Lab, Radiology
  Benefits Offered: Behavioral Health, Dental, Disease Management,
    Prescription, Vision, Wellness, Life, Alternative Medicine

Type of Coverage
  Commercial, Individual, Medicare
  Catastrophic Illness Benefit: Unlimited

Type of Payment Plans Offered
  Capitated

Geographic Areas Served
  Chesapeake, Norfolk, Petersburg, Richmond, Virginia Beach, Suffolk,
  South Hampton Road and surrounding counties

Subscriber Information
  Average Subscriber Co-Payment:
    Primary Care Physician: $5.00/10.00
    Prescription Drugs: $5.00/10.00
    Hospital ER: $25.00
    Home Health Care Max. Days/Visits Covered: 100 days

Peer Review Type
  Case Management: Yes

Publishes and Distributes Report Card: Yes

Accreditation Certification
TJC Accreditation, Medicare Approved, Utilization Review, Pre-Admission Certification, State Licensure, Quality Assurance Program

Key Personnel
President . . . . .C Burke King
Chief Medical Director .Karen Remley , DR
Media Contact . . . . .Scott Golden
804-354-5252
scott.golden@anthem.com

Specialty Managed Care Partners
Enters into Contracts with Regional Business Coalitions: Yes

Employer References
Commonwealth of Virginia, GE

1122   CareFirst Blue Cross & Blue Shield of Virginia
10455 & 10453 Mill Run Circle
Owings Mills, MD 21117
Toll-Free: 888-579-8969
Phone: 401-581-3000
www.carefirst.com
Subsidiary of: CareFirst, Inc.
Non-Profit Organization: Yes
Year Founded: 1985
Number of Affiliated Hospitals: 165
Number of Primary Care Physicians: 4,500
Number of Referral/Specialty Physicians: 15,068
Total Enrollment: 3,400,000

Healthplan and Services Defined
PLAN TYPE: HMO/PPO
Model Type: IPA
Plan Specialty: ASO, Behavioral Health, Dental, Vision
Benefits Offered: Behavioral Health, Chiropractic, Dental, Disease Management, Home Care, Physical Therapy, Podiatry, Prescription, Psychiatric, Transplant, Vision, Wellness

Type of Coverage
Commercial, Individual

Type of Payment Plans Offered
POS

Geographic Areas Served
Maryland, Delaware and Washington DC areas

Accreditation Certification
NCQA

Key Personnel
President/CEO . . . . .Chester Burrell
EVP, CFO . . . . .G Mark Chaney
Chief Marketing Officer. .Gregory A Devou
Executive VP/Operations . . . . .Leon Kaplan
Exec VP/General Counsel . . . . .John A Picciotto, Esq
Chief of Staff . . . . .Sharon J Vecchioni
EVP/Medical Systems . . . . .David D Wolf
SVP/Public Policy . . . . .Maria Tildon

1123   Carilion Health Plans
213 South Jefferson Street
Suite 1409
Roanoke, VA 24011
Toll-Free: 800-779-2285
www.carilionmedicare.com
Subsidiary of: Carilion Health Systems
For Profit Organization: Yes
Year Founded: 1997
Number of Affiliated Hospitals: 12
Number of Primary Care Physicians: 800

Number of Referral/Specialty Physicians: 140

Healthplan and Services Defined
PLAN TYPE: Medicare
Other Type: HMO, POS
Model Type: Network
Plan Specialty: ASO, EPO, Vision, UR
Benefits Offered: Behavioral Health, Chiropractic, Dental, Disease Management, Home Care, Physical Therapy, Podiatry, Prescription, Psychiatric, Transplant, Vision, Wellness

Type of Coverage
Commercial

Type of Payment Plans Offered
POS, DFFS

Geographic Areas Served
Virginia counties: Bedford, Botetourt, Craig, Franklin, Patrick, Pulsaki, Giles, Henry, Roanoke, Floyd, Rockbridge, Montgomery, Tazewell and Wythe

Subscriber Information
Average Subscriber Co-Payment:
Primary Care Physician: $15.00
Prescription Drugs: $20.00
Hospital ER: $50.00

Peer Review Type
Utilization Review: Yes
Case Management: Yes

Key Personnel
President and CEO. . . . . .Carolyn Chrisman
540-857-5206
COO . . . . .James Gore
540-857-5370
Mgr Contract/Compliance. . . . . .Mel Elkin
540-857-5317
Dir Utilization Mgmt .Peggy Callahan, BSN
540-857-5203
Quality Management . . . . .Ruth Ellen Ayers
540-857-5232
Chief Medical Officer. . . . . .Rome Walker, MD
540-857-5237
Manager Benefit Services. . . . . .Scottie Krupa
540-857-5223
Dir Information Mgmt . . . . .Mattie Tenzer
540-857-5226
Provider Relations Manager .Lynn Rock
540-857-5202
Sales Consultant/Traineřy. . . . . .Tim Moore

Specialty Managed Care Partners
Express Scripts PBM

1124   CIGNA HealthCare of Virginia
1 James Center
901 E Cary St, Suite 2000
Richmond, VA 23219
Toll-Free: 866-438-2446
Phone: 804-344-2693
Fax: 804-560-3946
www.cigna.com
Secondary Address: 3130 Chaparrell Drive, Suite 104, Roanoke, VA 24018, 800-797-7964
For Profit Organization: Yes
Year Founded: 1984
Number of Affiliated Hospitals: 25
Number of Primary Care Physicians: 1,737
Total Enrollment: 324,600
State Enrollment: 28,460

Healthplan and Services Defined
PLAN TYPE: HMO
Model Type: IPA, Network

Benefits Offered: Behavioral Health, Disease Management,
Prescription, Psychiatric, Transplant, Vision, Wellness, Women's
and Men's Health
Offers Demand Management Patient Information Service: Yes
DMPI Services Offered: Language Line Service, 24 hour Health
Information Line, Health Information Library

Type of Coverage
Commercial, Individual

Geographic Areas Served
Amelia, Caroline, Charles City, Chesterfield, Cumberland,
Dinwiddie, Gloucester, Goochland, Greensville, Hanover, Henrico,
Isle of Wight, James City, King and Queen, King William, Louisa,
Matthews, Middlesex, New Kent, Nottoway, Powhatan, Prince
George, Surry, Sussex, York

Publishes and Distributes Report Card: Yes

Accreditation Certification
NCQA, CMS
TJC Accreditation, Pre-Admission Certification, State Licensure,
Quality Assurance Program

Key Personnel
President and General Manager . . . . Matthew Manders
Sales . . . . Susan Schick

Specialty Managed Care Partners
Cole Managed Vision
Enters into Contracts with Regional Business Coalitions: Yes

1125 Coventry Health Care Virginia

9881 Mayland Drive
Richmond, VA 23233
Toll-Free: 800-424-0077
Phone: 804-747-3700
http://chcvirginia.coventryhealthcare.com
Secondary Address: 1000 Research Park Blvd, Suite 200,
Charlottesville, VA 22911, 434-951-2500
For Profit Organization: Yes
Year Founded: 1985
Number of Affiliated Hospitals: 132
Number of Primary Care Physicians: 12,000
Number of Referral/Specialty Physicians: 2,854
Total Enrollment: 200,000
State Enrollment: 200,000

Healthplan and Services Defined
PLAN TYPE: HMO/PPO
Other Type: POS
Plan Specialty: ASO, Behavioral Health, Chiropractic, Disease
Management, Lab, Vision, Radiology, Worker's Compensation,
UR
Benefits Offered: Chiropractic, Disease Management, Home Care,
Inpatient SNF, Physical Therapy, Podiatry, Prescription,
Transplant, Vision, Wellness

Type of Coverage
Commercial, Medicare, Medicaid, Catastrophic
Catastrophic Illness Benefit: Unlimited

Type of Payment Plans Offered
DFFS

Geographic Areas Served
Virginia counties: Albemarle, Alleghany, Amelia, Bath, Botetourt,
Buckingham, Caroline, Charles City, Charlotte, Chesterfield, Craig,
Culpeper, Cumberland, Dinwiddie, Essex, Floyd, Fluvanna, Giles,
Goochland, Greene, Halifax, Hanover, Henrico, JamesCity, King &
Queen, King William, Lancaster, Louisa, Lunenberg, Madison,
Mathews, Mecklenburg, Middlesex, Montgomery, Nelson, New
Kent, Northumberland, Nottoway, Orange, Pittsylvania, Powhatan,
Prince Edward, and more

Subscriber Information
Average Annual Deductible Per Subscriber:
Employee Only (Self): $0

Employee & 1 Family Member: $0
Employee & 2 Family Members: $0
Average Subscriber Co-Payment:
Primary Care Physician: $10.00
Non-Network Physician: Varies
Prescription Drugs: $10/20/45
Hospital ER: $50.00
Home Health Care: $0
Home Health Care Max. Days/Visits Covered: 90 days
Nursing Home: $0
Nursing Home Max. Days/Visits Covered: 100 days

Peer Review Type
Second Surgical Opinion: No

Publishes and Distributes Report Card: Yes

Accreditation Certification
NCQA
TJC Accreditation, Medicare Approved, Utilization Review,
Pre-Admission Certification, State Licensure, Quality Assurance
Program

Specialty Managed Care Partners
PHCSN, Caremark, Senterea, Colevision
Enters into Contracts with Regional Business Coalitions: Yes

1126 Delta Dental of Virginia

4818 Starkey Road
Roanoke, VA 24018
Toll-Free: 800-237-6060
Phone: 540-989-8000
www.deltadentalva.com
Secondary Address: 4860 Cox Road, Suite 130, Glen Allen, VA 23060
Non-Profit Organization: Yes
Year Founded: 1964
Total Enrollment: 56,000,000

Healthplan and Services Defined
PLAN TYPE: Dental
Other Type: Dental PPO/POS
Model Type: Dental Model
Plan Specialty: Dental
Benefits Offered: Dental

Type of Coverage
Commercial, Group Coverage

Type of Payment Plans Offered
FFS

Geographic Areas Served
Statewide

Accreditation Certification
TJC

Key Personnel
President . . . . George A Levicki, DDS
VP Finance . . . . Michael Wise
VP Marketing . . . . PV Davies, II
VP Information Services . . . . Oscar Bryant
Dir/Media & Public Affair . . . . Elizabeth Risberg
415-972-8423

1127 Dominion Dental Services

115 South Union Street
Suite 300
Alexandria, VA 22314
Toll-Free: 888-681-5100
Phone: 703-518-5000
Fax: 703-518-8849
www.dominiondental.com
Mailing Address: PO Box 1126, Claims/Utilization, Elk Grove Village,
IL 60009
For Profit Organization: Yes

Year Founded: 1996
Physician Owned Organization: Yes
Number of Primary Care Physicians: 46,000
Total Enrollment: 24,000,000
State Enrollment: 490,000

Healthplan and Services Defined
PLAN TYPE: Dental
Plan Specialty: Dental
Benefits Offered: Dental

Type of Coverage
Commercial, Individual

Type of Payment Plans Offered
DFFS, Capitated, Combination FFS & DFFS

Geographic Areas Served
Maryland, Delaware, Pennsylvania, District of Columbia, Virginia and New Jersey

Network Qualifications
Pre-Admission Certification: Yes

Peer Review Type
Utilization Review: Yes
Case Management: Yes

Publishes and Distributes Report Card: No

Accreditation Certification
NCQA

Key Personnel
President and Chief Opera . . . . .Mike Davis
Vice President of Profess. . . . . .Marleen Meier
Vice President of Operati . . . . .Ann Quinlan
VP, Professional Services . . . . .Lori Hayes
VP, Accounting . . . . .Kara Greenhouse, CPA
Dental Director . . . . .Wayne Silverman, DDS
Director of Marketing . . . . .Jeff Schwab
Member Services. . . . . .Lori Hayes
Vice President of Sales a . . . . .Rob Trachman
Media Contact . . . . .Jeff Schwab

Specialty Managed Care Partners
Enters into Contracts with Regional Business Coalitions: Yes

1128 eHealthInsurance Services Inc.
11919 Foundation Place
Gold River, CA 95670
Toll-Free: 800-644-3491
webmaster@healthinsurance.com
www.e.healthinsurance.com
Year Founded: 1997

Healthplan and Services Defined
PLAN TYPE: HMO/PPO
Benefits Offered: Dental, Life, STD

Type of Coverage
Commercial, Individual, Medicare

Geographic Areas Served
All 50 states in the USA and District of Columbia

Key Personnel
Chairman & CEO . . . . .Gary L. Lauer
EVP/Business & Corp. Dev.. . . . . .Bruce Telkamp
EVP/Chief Technology. . . . . .Dr. Sheldon X. Wang
SVP & CFO . . . . .Stuart M. Huizinga
Pres. of eHealth Gov. Sys .Samuel C. Gibbs
SVP of Sales & Operations . . . . .Robert S. Hurley
Director Public Relations. . . . . .Nate Purpura
650-210-3115

1129 EPIC Pharmacy Network
8703 Studley Road
Suite B
Mechanicsville, VA 23116-2016
Toll-Free: 800-876-3742
Phone: 804-559-4597
Fax: 804-559-2038
www.epicrx.com
Mailing Address: PO Box 1750, Mechanicsville, VA 23116-2016
Subsidiary of: EPIC Pharmacies, Inc.
For Profit Organization: Yes
Year Founded: 1992
Number of Primary Care Physicians: 1,400

Healthplan and Services Defined
PLAN TYPE: PPO
Plan Specialty: PBM
Benefits Offered: Prescription

Geographic Areas Served
Mid Atlantic states

Key Personnel
CEO and President . . . . .Angelo C Voxakis, PharmD
800-965-3742
Vice President of Contrac . . . . .Thomas E. Scono, RPh
Executive Vice President . . . . .Mark P Barwig

1130 Humana Health Insurance of Virginia
4551 Cox Road
Suite 200
Glen Allen, VA 23060
Toll-Free: 800-350-7213
Phone: 804-290-4252
Fax: 804-290-0184
www.humana.com
Secondary Address: 3800 Electric Road, Suite 406, Roanoke, VA 24018
For Profit Organization: Yes

Healthplan and Services Defined
PLAN TYPE: HMO/PPO

Type of Coverage
Commercial, Individual

Accreditation Certification
URAC, NCQA, CORE

1131 Magellan Medicaid Administration
11013 West Broad Street
Suite 500
Glen Allen, VA 23060
Toll-Free: 800-884-2822
www.magellanmedicaid.com
Subsidiary of: Magellan Health
Non-Profit Organization: Yes
Year Founded: 1968

Healthplan and Services Defined
PLAN TYPE: Medicare
Benefits Offered: Disease Management, Prescription, Wellness

Type of Coverage
Medicaid

Key Personnel
President. . . . . .Tim Nolan

1132 Mid Atlantic Medical Services: Virginia

3951 Westerre Parkway
Suite 260
Richmond, VA 23233
Toll-Free: 800-504-2562
Phone: 804-967-2384
Fax: 804-270-9216
masales99@uhc.com
Secondary Address: 21515 Ridgetop Circle, #330, Sterling, VA 20166
Subsidiary of: United Healthcare/United Health Group
Acquired by: United Healthcare
Year Founded: 1986
Number of Affiliated Hospitals: 342
Number of Primary Care Physicians: 3,276
Total Enrollment: 180,000

Healthplan and Services Defined
   PLAN TYPE: HMO/PPO
   Model Type: IPA, Network
   Benefits Offered: Disease Management, Prescription, Wellness

Type of Payment Plans Offered
   Combination FFS & DFFS

Geographic Areas Served
   Delaware, Maryland, North Carolina, Pennsylvania, Virginia,
   Washington DC, West Virginia

Network Qualifications
   Pre-Admission Certification: Yes

Peer Review Type
   Utilization Review: Yes
   Second Surgical Opinion: Yes
   Case Management: Yes

Publishes and Distributes Report Card: No

Accreditation Certification
   TJC, NCQA

Specialty Managed Care Partners
   Enters into Contracts with Regional Business Coalitions: Yes

1133 National Capital PPO

4825 Mark Center Drive
Suite 750
Alexandria, VA 22150
Toll-Free: 800-624-2356
Phone: 703-933-2660
www.ncppo.com
Secondary Address: 12443 Olive Blvd, HealthLink HQ, St. Louis,
   MO 63141
Subsidiary of: HealthLink, WellPoint
For Profit Organization: Yes
Year Founded: 1987
Physician Owned Organization: Yes
Federally Qualified: Yes
Number of Affiliated Hospitals: 100
Number of Primary Care Physicians: 23,000
Total Enrollment: 100,000
State Enrollment: 44,458

Healthplan and Services Defined
   PLAN TYPE: PPO
   Model Type: Network
   Plan Specialty: Dental, Disease Management, Worker's
     Compensation
   Benefits Offered: Behavioral Health, Dental, Disease Management,
     Wellness
   Offers Demand Management Patient Information Service: Yes

Type of Coverage
   Commercial, Individual, Labour and Union

Type of Payment Plans Offered
   FFS

Geographic Areas Served
   Southern and Eastern Virginia, Delaware and portions of New Jersey
   and Pennsylvania

Publishes and Distributes Report Card: Yes

Accreditation Certification
   TJC Accreditation, Medicare Approved, Utilization Review,
     Pre-Admission Certification, State Licensure, Quality Assurance
     Program

Key Personnel
   Regional Vice President . . . . Jeanell Austin
   CFO . . . . Kathy Chandra
   Manager, Network Services. . . . . Brenda Faust-Thomas

Average Claim Compensation
   Physician's Fees Charged: 40%
   Hospital's Fees Charged: 33%

Specialty Managed Care Partners
   Unicare, Health Link
   Enters into Contracts with Regional Business Coalitions: Yes

1134 Optima Health Plan

4417 Corporation Lane
Suite 250
Virginia Beach, VA 23462-3162
Toll-Free: 800-648-8420
Phone: 757-552-7174
Fax: 757-552-7316
www.optimahealth.com
Secondary Address: 1604 Santa Rosa Road, Suite 100, Richmond, VA
   23229
Subsidiary of: Sentara Health Plans
Non-Profit Organization: Yes
Year Founded: 1984
Federally Qualified: Yes
Number of Affiliated Hospitals: 12
Number of Primary Care Physicians: 15,000
Number of Referral/Specialty Physicians: 3,870
Total Enrollment: 430,000
State Enrollment: 430,000

Healthplan and Services Defined
   PLAN TYPE: HMO/PPO
   Other Type: POS
   Model Type: Network
   Plan Specialty: ASO, Behavioral Health, Chiropractic, Dental, PBM,
     Vision
   Benefits Offered: Behavioral Health, Chiropractic, Complementary
     Medicine, Dental, Disease Management, Home Care, Inpatient
     SNF, Long-Term Care, Physical Therapy, Podiatry, Prescription,
     Psychiatric, Transplant, Vision, Wellness
   Offers Demand Management Patient Information Service: Yes
   DMPI Services Offered: After hours nurse triage

Type of Coverage
   Commercial, Individual, Medicare, Medicaid
   Catastrophic Illness Benefit: Covered

Type of Payment Plans Offered
   FFS

Geographic Areas Served
   Selected counties in Virginia

Subscriber Information
   Average Monthly Fee Per Subscriber
     (Employee + Employer Contribution):
       Employee Only (Self): Varies by plan
       Medicare: Varies
   Average Annual Deductible Per Subscriber:
       Employee Only (Self): $0
       Employee & 1 Family Member: $0
       Employee & 2 Family Members: $0
       Medicare: Varies

Average Subscriber Co-Payment:
   Primary Care Physician: $15.00
   Non-Network Physician: 70 %
   Prescription Drugs: 50/20%
   Hospital ER: 80%
   Home Health Care: 80%

Network Qualifications
   Pre-Admission Certification: Yes

Peer Review Type
   Utilization Review: Yes
   Second Surgical Opinion: No
   Case Management: Yes

Accreditation Certification
   URAC, NCQA

Key Personnel
   President & CEO .... Michael M Dudley
   SVP/Chief Operating Offc .... Darlene A Mastin
   SVP/Chief Financial Offc .... Andy Hilbert
   SVP, Sales & Marketing...................... John DeGruttola
   VP, Medical Director .... George Heuser, MD

Specialty Managed Care Partners
   Cole Vision, American Specialty Health, Doral Dental, Sentara
      Mental Health
   Enters into Contracts with Regional Business Coalitions: Yes

Employer References
   City of Virginia Beach, City of Norfolk, Bank of America, Nexcom,
      CHKD

1135   Peninsula Health Care
11870 Merchants Walk
#200
Newport News, VA 23606-3315
Toll-Free: 800-421-1880
Phone: 757-872-7586
Fax: 804-354-4140
www.anthem.com
Mailing Address: PO Box 26623, Richmond, VA 23285-0031
For Profit Organization: Yes
Year Founded: 1994
Number of Affiliated Hospitals: 6
Number of Primary Care Physicians: 225
Number of Referral/Specialty Physicians: 475
Total Enrollment: 53,000
State Enrollment: 55,017

Healthplan and Services Defined
   PLAN TYPE: HMO/PPO
   Model Type: IPA
   Benefits Offered: Prescription
   Offers Demand Management Patient Information Service: Yes

Type of Coverage
   Commercial, Individual, Medicaid

Geographic Areas Served
   Virginia counties: Essex, Gloucester, Hampton, Isle of Wight, James
   City, King and Queen, Mathews

Network Qualifications
   Pre-Admission Certification: Yes

Peer Review Type
   Utilization Review: Yes

Publishes and Distributes Report Card: Yes

Accreditation Certification
   NCQA
   TJC Accreditation, Medicare Approved, Utilization Review,
      Pre-Admission Certification, State Licensure, Quality Assurance
      Program

Key Personnel
   President ....CB King

Chief Financial Officer .... Sally Hartman
Administrative Secretary .... Rachel Kampfe
Specialty Managed Care Partners
   Enters into Contracts with Regional Business Coalitions: Yes

1136   Piedmont Community Health Plan
2316 Atherholt Road
Lynchburg, VA 24501
Toll-Free: 800-400-7247
Phone: 434-947-4463
Fax: 434-947-3670
cmidkiff@pchp.net
www.pchp.net
Subsidiary of: Centra Health
For Profit Organization: Yes
Year Founded: 1995
Physician Owned Organization: Yes
Number of Primary Care Physicians: 350
Total Enrollment: 30,000
State Enrollment: 30,000

Healthplan and Services Defined
   PLAN TYPE: PPO
   Other Type: POS
   Benefits Offered: Disease Management, Prescription, Wellness

Type of Payment Plans Offered
   POS

Geographic Areas Served
   Cities of Lynchburg and Bedford and the counties of Albemarle,
   Amherst, Appomattox, Bedford, Buchkingham, Campbell,
   Cumberland, Lunenburg, Nottoway and Price Edward

Key Personnel
   CEO..Alan Wood
   COO..Brenda Grant
   CFO ....Jacqueline Mosby
   CMO ....Dr David Smith
   Provider Relations ....Dana Neiswander
   Marketing ....Cheryl Midkiff
   Member Relations ....Pam Moon
   Corp Media Contact ....Cheryl Midkiff
      cservice@pchp.net

Specialty Managed Care Partners
   Caremark Rx

1137   Southeast Community Care
5700 Lake Wright Drive
#110
Norfolk, VA 23502
Toll-Free: 800-653-2924
Phone: 757-461-6344
Fax: 877-267-8399
www.southeastcommunitycare.com
Subsidiary of: Arcadian Health Plans

Healthplan and Services Defined
   PLAN TYPE: Medicare

Type of Coverage
   Medicare

1138   Trigon Health Care
2015 Staples Mill Road
Richmond, VA 23230
Toll-Free: 800-451-1527
Phone: 804-354-3609
Fax: 804-354-3885
www.anthem.com
Acquired by: Anthem

For Profit Organization: Yes
Year Founded: 1935
Number of Affiliated Hospitals: 64
Number of Primary Care Physicians: 2,251
Total Enrollment: 105,200

Healthplan and Services Defined
PLAN TYPE: HMO
Model Type: Network
Benefits Offered: Prescription
Offers Demand Management Patient Information Service: Yes

Type of Payment Plans Offered
POS, Capitated, Combination FFS & DFFS

Network Qualifications
Pre-Admission Certification: Yes

Peer Review Type
Utilization Review: Yes
Second Surgical Opinion: Yes
Case Management: Yes

Publishes and Distributes Report Card: Yes

Accreditation Certification
URAC, NCQA
Utilization Review

Key Personnel
Chairman/CEO . . . . .Thomas G Snead, Jr
COO . . . . .John W Coyle
Sr Medical Director . . . . .Frank L Brown, MD
Director of Medical Mgt. .Patricia A Russo

1139 United Concordia: Virginia

Fair Oaks Center
11320 Random Hills Road, Suite 620
Fairfax, VA 22030
ucproducer@ucci.com
www.secure.ucci.com
For Profit Organization: Yes
Year Founded: 1971
Number of Primary Care Physicians: 111,000
Total Enrollment: 8,000,000

Healthplan and Services Defined
PLAN TYPE: Dental
Plan Specialty: Dental
Benefits Offered: Dental

Type of Coverage
Commercial, Individual

Geographic Areas Served
Military personnel and their families, nationwide

Accreditation Certification
URAC

1140 UnitedHealthCare of Virginia

9020 Stoney Point Parkway
Suite 400
Richmond, VA 23235
Toll-Free: 800-357-0978
Phone: 804-267-5200
www.uhc.com
Secondary Address: 12018 Sunrise Valley Drive, Suite 400, Reston,
VA 20191, 571-262-2245
Subsidiary of: UnitedHealth Group
For Profit Organization: Yes
Total Enrollment: 75,000,000

Healthplan and Services Defined
PLAN TYPE: HMO/PPO

Geographic Areas Served
Statewide

Accreditation Certification
TJC

Key Personnel
Media Contact . . . . .Debora Spano
debora_m_spano@uhc.com

1141 Virginia Health Network

7400 Beaufont Springs Drive
Suite 505
Richmond, VA 23225
Phone: 804-320-3837
Fax: 804-320-5984
jbrittain@vhn.com
www.vhn.com
For Profit Organization: Yes
Year Founded: 1988
Physician Owned Organization: No
Federally Qualified: No
Number of Affiliated Hospitals: 85
Number of Primary Care Physicians: 3,934
Number of Referral/Specialty Physicians: 8,566
Total Enrollment: 88,366
State Enrollment: 88,366

Healthplan and Services Defined
PLAN TYPE: PPO
Model Type: Network
Plan Specialty: Worker's Compensation, Medical PPO
Offers Demand Management Patient Information Service: No

Type of Coverage
Commercial

Geographic Areas Served
Hampton Roads, the Greater Richmond area, Northern Virginia,
Charlottesville, Fredericksburg, Southwest Virginia

Network Qualifications
Pre-Admission Certification: Yes

Publishes and Distributes Report Card: No

Accreditation Certification
Medicare; State License
TJC Accreditation, Medicare Approved, Utilization Review, State
Licensure

Key Personnel
President . . . . .Jim Brittain
jbrittain@vhn.com
Vice President . . . . .Betty Walters
bwalters@vhn.com
Administrative Assistant. . . . . .Joy Proffitt
jproffitt@vhn.comÿ
VP Marketing . . . . .Jim Gore
jgore@vhn.com
Director of Sales . . . . .Dan Gore

Average Claim Compensation
Physician's Fees Charged: 79%
Hospital's Fees Charged: 67%

Specialty Managed Care Partners
Enters into Contracts with Regional Business Coalitions: Yes

1142 Virginia Premier Health Plan

600 East Broad Street
4th Floor, Suite 400
Richmond, VA 23219
Toll-Free: 800-727-7536
Phone: 804-819-5151
www.vapremier.com
Secondary Address: 4910 Valley View Blvd NW, Suite 202, Roanoke,
VA 24012-2040, 540-344-8838
Non-Profit Organization: Yes

Year Founded: 1995
Number of Affiliated Hospitals: 49
Number of Primary Care Physicians: 1,151
Number of Referral/Specialty Physicians: 4,450
Total Enrollment: 143,725
State Enrollment: 169,621

Healthplan and Services Defined
  PLAN TYPE: HMO
  Model Type: IPA
  Plan Specialty: PBM, UR
  Benefits Offered: Behavioral Health, Dental, Prescription,
    Psychiatric, Vision

Type of Coverage
  Individual, Medicaid

Geographic Areas Served
  counties: Accomack, Albemarle, Amelia, Augusta, Bedford,
  Botetourt, Brunswick, Caroline, Charles City, Chesterfield, Culpeper,
  Cumberland, Dinwiddie, Franklin, Giles, Goochland, Green,
  Greensville, Henrico, Henry, King George, King William, Louisa,
  Lunenburg, Madison, Mecklenburg, Montgomery, Kent,
  Northampton, Nottoway, Orange, Patrick, Prince Edward, Prince
  George, Pulaski, Roanoke, Rockbridge, Rockingham, Southampton,
  Spotsylvania, Stafford, Surry, Sussex

Accreditation Certification
  TJC, URAC, NCQA

Key Personnel
  Medical Director . . . . Darrin Mangiacarne, MD/DO

Specialty Managed Care Partners
  AmeriHealth Mercy, Vision Services Plan, Doral Dental of Virginia

Health Insurance Coverage Status and Type of Coverage by Age

Category	All Persons		Under 18 years		Under 65 years		65 years and over	
	Number	%	Number	%	Number	%	Number	%
Total population	6,864	-	1,595	-	5,934	-	930	-
Covered by some type of health insurance	5,904 *(21)*	86.0 *(0.3)*	1,500 *(8)*	94.1 *(0.5)*	4,981 *(21)*	83.9 *(0.4)*	923 *(3)*	99.2 *(0.2)*
Covered by private health insurance	4,703 *(29)*	68.5 *(0.4)*	988 *(13)*	62.0 *(0.8)*	4,079 *(27)*	68.7 *(0.5)*	624 *(9)*	67.0 *(0.9)*
Employment based	3,811 *(31)*	55.5 *(0.5)*	836 *(14)*	52.5 *(0.9)*	3,487 *(31)*	58.8 *(0.5)*	324 *(8)*	34.8 *(0.9)*
Direct purchase	874 *(19)*	12.7 *(0.3)*	117 *(8)*	7.3 *(0.5)*	548 *(17)*	9.2 *(0.3)*	326 *(8)*	35.0 *(0.9)*
Covered by TRICARE	292 *(13)*	4.3 *(0.2)*	68 *(6)*	4.3 *(0.4)*	210 *(12)*	3.5 *(0.2)*	82 *(4)*	8.8 *(0.4)*
Covered by government health insurance	2,018 *(21)*	29.4 *(0.3)*	580 *(14)*	36.4 *(0.9)*	1,120 *(21)*	18.9 *(0.4)*	898 *(4)*	96.5 *(0.3)*
Covered by Medicaid	1,075 *(22)*	15.7 *(0.3)*	575 *(14)*	36.1 *(0.9)*	965 *(20)*	16.3 *(0.3)*	110 *(5)*	11.8 *(0.6)*
Also by private insurance	187 *(9)*	2.7 *(0.1)*	68 *(5)*	4.2 *(0.3)*	137 *(8)*	2.3 *(0.1)*	50 *(3)*	5.4 *(0.4)*
Covered by Medicare	1,050 *(8)*	15.3 *(0.1)*	7 *(2)*	0.5 *(0.1)*	153 *(7)*	2.6 *(0.1)*	897 *(4)*	96.4 *(0.3)*
Also by private insurance	646 *(9)*	9.4 *(0.1)*	1 *(Z)*	0.1 *(0.1)*	47 *(3)*	0.8 *(0.1)*	598 *(9)*	64.3 *(0.9)*
Also by Medicaid	184 *(8)*	2.7 *(0.1)*	4 *(1)*	0.2 *(0.1)*	74 *(5)*	1.2 *(0.1)*	110 *(5)*	11.8 *(0.6)*
Covered by VA Care	169 *(7)*	2.5 *(0.1)*	2 *(1)*	0.1 *(0.1)*	93 *(6)*	1.6 *(0.1)*	76 *(3)*	8.2 *(0.4)*
Not covered at any time during the year	960 *(22)*	14.0 *(0.3)*	95 *(8)*	5.9 *(0.5)*	953 *(22)*	16.1 *(0.4)*	7 *(2)*	0.8 *(0.2)*

Note: Numbers in thousands; Figures cover 2013; Margin of error appears in parenthesis; A "Z" indicates that the value either represents or rounds to zero.
Source: U.S. Census Bureau, 2013 American Community Survey, Table HI05. Health Insurance Coverage Status and Type of Coverage by State and Age for All People: 2013

Washington

1143 Aetna Health of Washington

151 Farmington Avenue
Hartford, CT 06156
Toll-Free: 800-872-3862
Phone: 860-273-0123
www.aetna.com
Partnered with: eHealthInsurance Services Inc.
For Profit Organization: Yes
Year Founded: 1985
Total Enrollment: 11,596,230

Healthplan and Services Defined
  PLAN TYPE: PPO
  Other Type: POS
  Benefits Offered: Chiropractic, Dental, Disease Management, Home
    Care, Long-Term Care, Physical Therapy, Podiatry, Prescription,
    Vision

Type of Coverage
  Commercial, Individual

Type of Payment Plans Offered
  Capitated

Geographic Areas Served
  Statewide

Subscriber Information
  Average Monthly Fee Per Subscriber
    (Employee + Employer Contribution):
      Employee Only (Self): $91.41
      Employee & 1 Family Member: $245.01
  Average Annual Deductible Per Subscriber:
      Employee Only (Self): $3000
      Employee & 1 Family Member: $6000
  Average Subscriber Co-Payment:
      Primary Care Physician: $20/30
      Prescription Drugs: $10/25/40
      Hospital ER: $100

Publishes and Distributes Report Card: Yes

Accreditation Certification
  AAAHC

Key Personnel
  Chairman/CEO/President.....................Mark T Bertolini
  EVP/General Counsel ....William J Casazza
  EVP/CFO ....Shawn M Guertin

1144 Assurant Employee Benefits: Washington

1512 Plaza
Building 600
Seattle, WA 98101
Phone: 206-441-3133
Fax: 206-728-2509
benefits@assurant.com
www.assurantemployeebenefits.com
Secondary Address: 2323 Grand Boulevard, Kansas City, MO 64108,
  816-474-2345
Subsidiary of: Assurant, Inc
For Profit Organization: Yes
Number of Primary Care Physicians: 112,000
Total Enrollment: 47,000

Healthplan and Services Defined
  PLAN TYPE: Multiple
  Plan Specialty: Dental, Vision, Long & Short-Term Disability
  Benefits Offered: Dental, Vision, Wellness, AD&D, Life, LTD, STD

Type of Coverage
  Commercial, Indemnity, Individual Dental Plans

Geographic Areas Served
  Statewide

Subscriber Information
  Average Monthly Fee Per Subscriber
    (Employee + Employer Contribution):
      Employee Only (Self): Varies by plan

Accreditation Certification
  TJC, NCQA

Key Personnel
  President/CEO ....John S. Roberts
  SVP/CFO...................................Miles B. Yakre
  SVP/Chief Information Off ....Kara J. Schacht
  SVP/Human Resources,Devel ....Rosemary Polk
  VP/Dental ....Stacia Almquist
  PR Specialist............................Megan Hutchison
    816-556-7815
    megan.hutchison@assurant.com

1145 Asuris Northwest Health

528 E. Spokane Falls Blvd.
Suite 301
Spokane, WA 99202
Toll-Free: 888-367-2109
Fax: 509-922-8264
wa_rnh_info@asurius.com
www.asuris.com
Mailing Address: Po Box 91130, Seattle, WA 98111-9230
Subsidiary of: Regence Group
Non-Profit Organization: Yes
Year Founded: 1998
Number of Affiliated Hospitals: 40
Number of Primary Care Physicians: 19,000
State Enrollment: 40,000

Healthplan and Services Defined
  PLAN TYPE: Multiple
  Model Type: Network, TPA
  Plan Specialty: ASO, Behavioral Health, Chiropractic, Disease
    Management, Lab, Vision, Radiology
  Benefits Offered: Chiropractic, Dental, Disease Management, Home
    Care, Inpatient SNF, Physical Therapy, Podiatry, Prescription,
    Psychiatric, Vision, Wellness, AD&D, Life, LTD, STD

Type of Coverage
  Individual, Medicare, Supplemental Medicare, Medicaid, Other Public
    Programs

Geographic Areas Served
  Eastern Washington

Subscriber Information
  Average Monthly Fee Per Subscriber
    (Employee + Employer Contribution):
      Employee Only (Self): Varies
      Employee & 1 Family Member: Varies
      Employee & 2 Family Members: Varies
      Medicare: Varies
  Average Annual Deductible Per Subscriber:
      Employee Only (Self): Varies
      Employee & 1 Family Member: Varies
      Employee & 2 Family Members: Varies
      Medicare: Varies
  Average Subscriber Co-Payment:
      Primary Care Physician: Varies
      Non-Network Physician: Varies
      Prescription Drugs: Varies
      Hospital ER: Varies
      Home Health Care: Varies
      Home Health Care Max. Days/Visits Covered: Varies
      Nursing Home: Varies
      Nursing Home Max. Days/Visits Covered: Varies

Network Qualifications
Pre-Admission Certification: No

Peer Review Type
Utilization Review: Yes
Second Surgical Opinion: Yes

Accreditation Certification
URAC
TJC Accreditation, Medicare Approved, State Licensure

Key Personnel
President .... Brady Cass, RHU,MHP
Media Contact .... Mike Tatko
208-798-2221
mtatkoid@regence.com

Average Claim Compensation
Physician's Fees Charged: 80%
Hospital's Fees Charged: 80%

1146 CIGNA HealthCare of Washington

701 Fifth Avenue
Suite 4900
Seattle, WA 98104
Toll-Free: 866-438-2446
Phone: 206-625-8892
Fax: 206-625-8880
www.cigna.com
Secondary Address: Great-West Healthcare, now part of CIGNA, 155 108th Avenue NE, Suite 800, Belleview, WA 98004, 425-372-0600
For Profit Organization: Yes
Total Enrollment: 120,000
State Enrollment: 49,135

Healthplan and Services Defined
PLAN TYPE: PPO
Model Type: Gatekeeper/ConsumerDriven
Benefits Offered: Behavioral Health, Dental, Prescription, Medical

Type of Coverage
Commercial

Type of Payment Plans Offered
POS, FFS

Geographic Areas Served
Washington - Statewide

Key Personnel
President & General Mgr .... Chris Blanton

1147 Community Health Plan of Washington

720 Olive Way
Suite 300
Seattle, WA 98101-1830
Toll-Free: 800-440-1561
Phone: 206-521-8833
Fax: 206-521-8834
customercare@chpw.org
www.chpw.org
Non-Profit Organization: Yes
Year Founded: 1992
Number of Affiliated Hospitals: 100
Number of Primary Care Physicians: 2,725
Number of Referral/Specialty Physicians: 13,571
Total Enrollment: 270,000
State Enrollment: 270,000

Healthplan and Services Defined
PLAN TYPE: Multiple
Benefits Offered: Disease Management, Prescription, Wellness

Type of Coverage
Commercial, Individual, Medicare, Medicaid

Geographic Areas Served
38 counties in Washington State

Subscriber Information
Average Monthly Fee Per Subscriber
(Employee + Employer Contribution):
Employee Only (Self): Varies
Employee & 1 Family Member: Varies
Employee & 2 Family Members: Varies
Medicare: Varies
Average Annual Deductible Per Subscriber:
Employee Only (Self): Varies
Employee & 1 Family Member: Varies
Employee & 2 Family Members: Varies
Medicare: Varies
Average Subscriber Co-Payment:
Primary Care Physician: Varies
Non-Network Physician: Varies
Prescription Drugs: Varies
Hospital ER: Varies
Home Health Care: Varies
Home Health Care Max. Days/Visits Covered: Varies
Nursing Home: Varies
Nursing Home Max. Days/Visits Covered: Varies

Key Personnel
CEO .... Lance Hunsinger
Chief Admin Officer .... Marilee McGuire
CFO .... Alan Lederman
SVP/CMO .... Dr Christopher Mathews
SVP Business Development .... Howard Springer
VP/Human Resources .... Laura Boyd
VP/Strategy & Analytics .... Stacy Kessel
VP/General Counsel .... Wade Harman
Director, Marketing .... David Kinard
206-613-8949
david.kinard@chpw.org

Specialty Managed Care Partners
Express Scripts

1148 Delta Dental of Washington

P.O. Box 75983
Seattle, WA 98175-0983
Toll-Free: 800-554-1907
cservice@deltadentalwa.com
www.deltadentalwa.com
Non-Profit Organization: Yes
Year Founded: 1954
Total Enrollment: 54,000,000
State Enrollment: 2,000,000

Healthplan and Services Defined
PLAN TYPE: Dental
Other Type: Dental PPO
Model Type: Network
Plan Specialty: ASO, Dental
Benefits Offered: Dental

Type of Coverage
Commercial, Individual, Group
Catastrophic Illness Benefit: None

Geographic Areas Served
Statewide

Subscriber Information
Average Monthly Fee Per Subscriber
(Employee + Employer Contribution):
Employee Only (Self): Varies
Employee & 1 Family Member: Varies
Employee & 2 Family Members: Varies
Average Annual Deductible Per Subscriber:
Employee Only (Self): Varies
Employee & 1 Family Member: Varies

Employee & 2 Family Members: Varies
Average Subscriber Co-Payment:
Prescription Drugs: $0
Home Health Care: $0
Nursing Home: $0

Key Personnel
President & CEO . . . . Gary Schweikhardtÿ

1149 eHealthInsurance Services Inc.

11919 Foundation Place
Gold River, CA 95670
Toll-Free: 800-644-3491
webmaster@healthinsurance.com
www.e.healthinsurance.com
Year Founded: 1997

Healthplan and Services Defined
PLAN TYPE: HMO/PPO
Benefits Offered: Dental, Life, STD

Type of Coverage
Commercial, Individual, Medicare

Geographic Areas Served
All 50 states in the USA and District of Columbia

Key Personnel
Chairman & CEO . . . . Gary L. Lauer
EVP/Business & Corp. Dev. . . . . Bruce Telkamp
EVP/Chief Technology . . . . Dr. Sheldon X. Wang
SVP & CFO . . . . Stuart M. Huizinga
Pres. of eHealth Gov. Sys . . . . Samuel C. Gibbs
SVP of Sales & Operations . . . . Robert S. Hurley
Director Public Relations . . . . Nate Purpura
650-210-3115

1150 Group Health Cooperative

320 Westlake Avenue North
Suite 100
Seattle, WA 98109-5233
Toll-Free: 888-901-4636
Phone: 206-448-5790
governance@ghc.org
www.ghc.org
Mailing Address: PO Box 34590, Seattle, WA 98124
Non-Profit Organization: Yes
Year Founded: 1947
Owned by an Integrated Delivery Network (IDN): Yes
Number of Affiliated Hospitals: 41
Number of Primary Care Physicians: 6,000
Number of Referral/Specialty Physicians: 500
Total Enrollment: 600,000

Healthplan and Services Defined
PLAN TYPE: Multiple
Model Type: Staff
Plan Specialty: Behavioral Health, Chiropractic, Disease
Management
Benefits Offered: Behavioral Health, Chiropractic, Disease
Management, Home Care, Inpatient SNF, Long-Term Care,
Physical Therapy, Podiatry, Prescription, Psychiatric, Transplant,
Vision, Wellness
Offers Demand Management Patient Information Service: Yes

Type of Coverage
Commercial, Individual, Indemnity, Medicare, Supplemental
Medicare, Medicaid
Catastrophic Illness Benefit: Varies per case

Type of Payment Plans Offered
POS

Geographic Areas Served
Washington State and Northern Idaho

Subscriber Information
Average Monthly Fee Per Subscriber
(Employee + Employer Contribution):
Employee Only (Self): Varies by plan
Average Annual Deductible Per Subscriber:
Employee Only (Self): $0
Employee & 1 Family Member: $0
Employee & 2 Family Members: $0
Medicare: $0
Average Subscriber Co-Payment:
Primary Care Physician: $10.00
Prescription Drugs: $10.00
Hospital ER: $100.00
Home Health Care Max. Days/Visits Covered: Covered in full

Network Qualifications
Pre-Admission Certification: Yes

Peer Review Type
Utilization Review: Yes
Second Surgical Opinion: Yes
Case Management: Yes

Publishes and Distributes Report Card: Yes

Accreditation Certification
TJC, URAC, NCQA
Medicare Approved, Utilization Review, Pre-Admission Certification,
State Licensure, Quality Assurance Program

Key Personnel
President/CEO . . . . Scott Armstrong
EVP/CFO . . . . Chris Knackstedt
EVP, Strategic Planning . . . . Dawn Loeliger, JD
Executive Vice President . . . . Robert O'Brien
Executive Medical Dir. . . . . Paul Sherman, MD

Specialty Managed Care Partners
Seattle Health Care
Enters into Contracts with Regional Business Coalitions: Yes

Employer References
State of Washington, Federal Employees, Safeco, Wells Fargo,
Nordstorm

1151 Humana Health Insurance of Washington

1498 SE Tech Center Place
Suite 300
Vancouver, WA 98683
Toll-Free: 800-781-4203
Phone: 360-253-7523
Fax: 360-253-7524
www.humana.com
For Profit Organization: Yes

Healthplan and Services Defined
PLAN TYPE: HMO/PPO

Type of Coverage
Commercial, Individual

Accreditation Certification
URAC, NCQA, CORE

Key Personnel
President/CEO . . . . Michael McCallister

1152 Liberty Health Plan: Washington

24001 E Mission Avenue
Suite 100
Liberty Lake, WA 99019
Toll-Free: 800-926-7324
Phone: 509-944-2209
Fax: 509-944-2019
customerservice.center@libertynorthwest.com
www.libertynorthwest.com

Secondary Address: 1191 Second Avenue, Safeco Center, Seattle, WA 98101-2997

For Profit Organization: Yes

Year Founded: 1983

Healthplan and Services Defined
PLAN TYPE: PPO
Model Type: Group
Plan Specialty: Worker's Compensation
Benefits Offered: Prescription

Type of Payment Plans Offered
POS, DFFS, FFS, Combination FFS & DFFS

Geographic Areas Served
Statewide

Network Qualifications
Pre-Admission Certification: Yes

Peer Review Type
Case Management: Yes

Publishes and Distributes Report Card: No

Accreditation Certification
TJC, NCQA

Specialty Managed Care Partners
Enters into Contracts with Regional Business Coalitions: No

1153 Lifewise Health Plan of Washington

7001 220th Street SW
Bldg 1
Mountlake Terrace, WA 98043
Toll-Free: 800-592-6804
www.lifewisewa.com
Mailing Address: PO Box 91509, Seattle, WA 98111-9159
Total Enrollment: 1,500,000
State Enrollment: 87,000

Healthplan and Services Defined
PLAN TYPE: PPO

Accreditation Certification
TJC, URAC

Key Personnel
President/CEO . . . . Jim Havens
VP, Sales . . . . John Mychalishyn
PUB. . . . . Earling Media Relations Manager
eri- ea-ling

1154 Molina Healthcare: Washington

21540 30th Drive SE
Suite 400
Bothell, WA 98021
Toll-Free: 800-869-7175
Phone: 425-424-1100
Fax: 425-487-8987
www.molinahealthcare.com
Secondary Address: 5709 W Sunset Highway, Suite 200, Spokane, WA 99224-9795
For Profit Organization: Yes
Year Founded: 1995
Number of Affiliated Hospitals: 81
Number of Primary Care Physicians: 2,714
Number of Referral/Specialty Physicians: 5,325
Total Enrollment: 1,400,000
State Enrollment: 263,795

Healthplan and Services Defined
PLAN TYPE: HMO
Model Type: Hybrid
Benefits Offered: Behavioral Health, Disease Management, Prescription, Psychiatric, Transplant, Wellness
Offers Demand Management Patient Information Service: Yes

DMPI Services Offered: 24/7 Nurse Line

Type of Coverage
Commercial, Medicare, Supplemental Medicare, Medicaid, SCHIP

Type of Payment Plans Offered
Capitated, FFS

Geographic Areas Served
Adams, Benton, Chelon, Clallam, Columbia, Cowlitz, Douglas, Franklin, Garfield, Grant, Grays Harbor, Island, King, Kitsap, Lewis, Lincoln, Mason, Okanogan, Pacific, Pend Oreirlle, Pierce, San Juan, Skagit, Snohomish, Spokane, Thurston, Walla Walla, Whatconm, Whitman, Yakima

Subscriber Information
Average Monthly Fee Per Subscriber
(Employee + Employer Contribution):
Employee Only (Self): Varies by plan
Average Annual Deductible Per Subscriber:
Employee Only (Self): $150.00
Average Subscriber Co-Payment:
Primary Care Physician: $15.00
Hospital ER: $100.00

Network Qualifications
Minimum Years of Practice: 5
Pre-Admission Certification: Yes

Peer Review Type
Utilization Review: Yes
Second Surgical Opinion: Yes
Case Management: Yes

Accreditation Certification
URAC, NCQA
TJC Accreditation, Medicare Approved, Utilization Review, Pre-Admission Certification, State Licensure, Quality Assurance Program

Key Personnel
President and CEO . . . . J Mario Molina, MD
CFO . . . . John C Molina, JD
Chief Operating Officer . . . . Terry Bayer, JD,MPH
EVP/Research And Developm . . . . Dr.Martha Molina Bernadett
Exec VP/Reseach & Devel . . . . Martha Bernadette, MD
Chief Information Officer . . . . Rick Click

Specialty Managed Care Partners
VGP Vision, RxAmerica Pharmacy
Enters into Contracts with Regional Business Coalitions: Yes

1155 PacifiCare Benefit Administrators

7525 SE 24th Street
PO Box 9005, Suite 200
Mercer Island, WA 98040
Toll-Free: 800-829-2925
Phone: 206-236-2500
Fax: 206-230-7484
pamela.nygaard@phs.com
www.pacificare.com
Subsidiary of: UnitedHealthCare
For Profit Organization: Yes
Year Founded: 1986
Owned by an Integrated Delivery Network (IDN): Yes
Number of Affiliated Hospitals: 14
Number of Primary Care Physicians: 5,000
Total Enrollment: 240,000
State Enrollment: 7,550

Healthplan and Services Defined
PLAN TYPE: PPO
Model Type: Network
Plan Specialty: ASO, Behavioral Health, Chiropractic, Dental, Disease Management, Lab, PBM, Radiology, UR, Acupuncture, Naturopathy

Benefits Offered: Behavioral Health, Chiropractic, Dental, Disease
  Management, Home Care, Inpatient SNF, Long-Term Care,
  Physical Therapy, Podiatry, Prescription, Psychiatric, Transplant,
  Wellness
Offers Demand Management Patient Information Service: Yes
DMPI Services Offered: HealthBeat Magazine

Type of Coverage
  Commercial, Individual, Indemnity, Medicare, Supplemental
    Medicare, Medicaid, Catastrophic
  Catastrophic Illness Benefit: Maximum $2M

Type of Payment Plans Offered
  DFFS, FFS

Geographic Areas Served
  Alaska, California, Oregon & Washington

Subscriber Information
  Average Annual Deductible Per Subscriber:
    Employee Only (Self): $100.00
    Employee & 2 Family Members: $300.00
  Average Subscriber Co-Payment:
    Primary Care Physician: $10.00
    Non-Network Physician: $10.00
    Prescription Drugs: $5.00/10.00
    Hospital ER: $50.00
    Home Health Care: $100.00
    Home Health Care Max. Days/Visits Covered: 50 days

Network Qualifications
  Pre-Admission Certification: Yes

Peer Review Type
  Utilization Review: Yes
  Second Surgical Opinion: Yes

Publishes and Distributes Report Card: Yes

Accreditation Certification
  NCQA

Key Personnel
  Chairman. . . . . .Howard Phanstiel
  CFO . . . . .Greg Scott
  CEO . . . . .Brad Bowlus
  Executive Vice President . . . . .Jacqueline Kosecoff
  General Counsel . . . . .Joseph Konowiecki
  Chief Medical Officer . . . . .Sam Ho
  Sr VP/Human Resources . . . . .Carol Black

Specialty Managed Care Partners
  Enters into Contracts with Regional Business Coalitions: Yes

---

1156 PacifiCare of Washington

7525 SE 24th
Suite 200
Mercer Island, WA 98040
Toll-Free: 800-829-2925
Phone: 206-236-2500
Fax: 206-236-3099
www.pacificare.com
Subsidiary of: UnitedHealthCare
For Profit Organization: Yes
Year Founded: 1986
Number of Affiliated Hospitals: 14
Number of Primary Care Physicians: 5,000
Number of Referral/Specialty Physicians: 640
Total Enrollment: 45,000
State Enrollment: 52,186

Healthplan and Services Defined
  PLAN TYPE: HMO
  Model Type: Network
  Plan Specialty: PBM
  Benefits Offered: Behavioral Health, Disease Management,
    Prescription, Psychiatric, Wellness
  Offers Demand Management Patient Information Service: Yes

DMPI Services Offered: HealthBeat Magazine

Type of Coverage
  Commercial, Individual, Indemnity, Medicare

Type of Payment Plans Offered
  Combination FFS & DFFS

Geographic Areas Served
  Eight counties statewide

Subscriber Information
  Average Subscriber Co-Payment:
    Hospital ER: $50.00
    Home Health Care: Varies
    Nursing Home: Varies

Peer Review Type
  Case Management: Yes

Accreditation Certification
  TJC, NCQA
  Utilization Review, Quality Assurance Program

Key Personnel
  Chairman. . . . . .Howard Phanstiel
  CFO . . . . .Don Costa
  CEO . . . . .Brad Bowlus
  Executive Vice President . . . . .Jacqueline Kosecoff
  General Counsel . . . . .Joseph Konowiecki
  Chief Medical Officer . . . . .Sam Ho
  Sr VP/Human Resources . . . . .Carol Black
  Chief Information Officer. . . . . .Mary Cox
  Sales Manager . . . . .Debbie Huntington

1157 Premera Blue Cross

7001 220th Street SW
Building 1
Montlake Terrace, WA 98043
Toll-Free: 800-722-1471
www.premera.com
Secondary Address: 3900 East Sprague, Building 1, Spokane, WA
  99202
For Profit Organization: Yes
Year Founded: 1933
Number of Affiliated Hospitals: 100
Number of Primary Care Physicians: 20,000
Total Enrollment: 1,500,000
State Enrollment: 1,500,000

Healthplan and Services Defined
  PLAN TYPE: PPO
  Other Type: EPO
  Benefits Offered: Dental, Disease Management, Long-Term Care

Type of Coverage
  Indemnity, Supplemental Medicare

Geographic Areas Served
  Washington and Alaska

Subscriber Information
  Average Monthly Fee Per Subscriber
    (Employee + Employer Contribution):
      Employee Only (Self): Varies by plan

Accreditation Certification
  NCQA

Key Personnel
  President & CEO . . . . .H R Brereton Barlow
  SVP/CIO . . . . .Kirsten Simontsch
  EVP/CFO. . . . . .Kent Marquardt
  EVP/Operations . . . . .Kacey Kemp
  SVP, Healthcare Delivery. .Richard Maturi
  Chief Legal Officer . . . . .Yori Milo
  EVP/Chief of Marketing . . . . .Jim Messina
  SVP/Chief Medical Officer . . . . .Roki Chauhan, MD
  SVP/General Counsel. . . . . .John Pierce

Media Relations . . . . Melanie Con
425-918-6238
melanie.coon@premera.com

1158 Puget Sound Health Partners

32129 Weyerhaeuser Way South
Suite 201
Federal Way, WA 98001
Toll-Free: 866-789-7747
www.ourpshp.com
Secondary Address: 319 7th Ave SE, Suite 202, Olympia, WA 98501
Year Founded: 2007
Number of Affiliated Hospitals: 76
Total Enrollment: 17,000
State Enrollment: 17,000

Healthplan and Services Defined
  PLAN TYPE: Medicare

Type of Coverage
  Medicare

Accreditation Certification
  TJC, URAC

Key Personnel
  Chief Executive Officer . . . . Christine Tomcala
    253-517-4339
    c.tomcala@soundpathhealth.com
  Chief Medical Officer . . . . Ze'ev Young, MD
    253-517-4327
    z.young@soundpathhealth.com
  Compliance Officer . . . . Sheila Nishimoto, MBA
    s.nishimoto@soundpathhealth.com
  Chief Operations Officer . . . . Christine Turner
    253-517-4334
    c.turner@soundpathhealth.com
  Chief Marketing Executive . . . . Kim Heuss
    253-517-4305
    k.heuss@soundpathhealth.com

1159 Regence Blue Shield

1800 Ninth Avenue
Seattle, WA 98101
Toll-Free: 888-344-6347
Phone: 206-464-3600
Fax: 206-525-9795
www.wa.regence.com
Secondary Address: 12728 19th Avenue SE, Suite 101, Everett, WA 98208
Non-Profit Organization: Yes
Number of Primary Care Physicians: 19,702
Total Enrollment: 2,200,000
State Enrollment: 21,633

Healthplan and Services Defined
  PLAN TYPE: PPO
  Model Type: Network
  Benefits Offered: Dental, Disease Management, Prescription, Vision, Wellness

Type of Payment Plans Offered
  POS, Combination FFS & DFFS

Geographic Areas Served
  Walla Walla, Clallam, Mason, Columbia, Pacific, Cowlitz, Pierce, Grays Harbor, Snohomish, Thurston, King, Wahkiakum, Kitsap, Lewis, Jefferson, Yakima, Klickitat, Skamania, Whatcom, Skagit, Island and San Juan counties

Subscriber Information
  Average Subscriber Co-Payment:
    Primary Care Physician: Varies
    Non-Network Physician: Varies
    Prescription Drugs: Varies

Hospital ER: Varies
Home Health Care: Varies
Home Health Care Max. Days/Visits Covered: Varies
Nursing Home: Varies
Nursing Home Max. Days/Visits Covered: Varies

Network Qualifications
  Pre-Admission Certification: Yes

Peer Review Type
  Utilization Review: No
  Second Surgical Opinion: Yes
  Case Management: Yes

Publishes and Distributes Report Card: No

Accreditation Certification
  URAC
  TJC Accreditation

Key Personnel
  President . . . . Don Antonucci
  Senior Vice President . . . . Scott Powers
  EVP/Health Care Services . . . . Dr.Richard Popiel
  Media Contact . . . . Rachelle Cunningham
    206-332-3713
    rmcunni@regence.com

Specialty Managed Care Partners
  Enters into Contracts with Regional Business Coalitions: No

1160 Spokane Community Care

1330 N Washington Street
#3500
Spokane, WA 992010
Toll-Free: 800-573-8600
Phone: 509-325-8004
Fax: 509-325-8003
www.spokanecommunitycare.com
Subsidiary of: Arcadian Health Plans

Healthplan and Services Defined
  PLAN TYPE: Medicare

Type of Coverage
  Medicare

1161 Sterling Health Plans

P.O. Box 5348
Bellingham, WA 98227-5348
www.sterlingplans.com
Subsidiary of: Sterling Life Insurance Company

Healthplan and Services Defined
  PLAN TYPE: Medicare
  Benefits Offered: Chiropractic, Dental, Disease Management, Home Care, Inpatient SNF, Long-Term Care, Physical Therapy, Podiatry, Prescription, Psychiatric, Vision, Wellness, Life

Type of Coverage
  Commercial, Individual, Medicare, Supplemental Medicare

Geographic Areas Served
  Nationwide

Subscriber Information
  Average Monthly Fee Per Subscriber
    (Employee + Employer Contribution):
      Employee Only (Self): Varies
      Medicare: Varies
  Average Annual Deductible Per Subscriber:
      Employee Only (Self): Varies
      Medicare: Varies
  Average Subscriber Co-Payment:
      Primary Care Physician: Varies
      Non-Network Physician: Varies
      Prescription Drugs: Varies
      Hospital ER: Varies

Home Health Care: Varies
Home Health Care Max. Days/Visits Covered: Varies
Nursing Home: Varies
Nursing Home Max. Days/Visits Covered: Varies

Accreditation Certification
BBB

Key Personnel
President/CEO . . . . Michael A Muchnicki
Chief Financial Officer . . . . David Goltz
Chief Marketing Officer . . . . Ron Bendes
Medical Director . . . . James Jacobson
Dir, Human Resources. . . . . Harriet Ziegler
Mgr, Information Tech . . . . Tom Cahill
Sr Mgr, Sales & Mktg . . . . Gib Kassing

1162 United Concordia: Washington
2200 Sixth Avenue
Suite 804
Seattle, WA 98121-1849
Toll-Free: 888-245-8224
Fax: 206-728-2740
ucproducer@ucci.com
www.secure.ucci.com/ducdws/home.xhtml
For Profit Organization: Yes
Year Founded: 1971
Number of Primary Care Physicians: 111,000
Total Enrollment: 8,000,000

Healthplan and Services Defined
PLAN TYPE: Dental
Plan Specialty: Dental
Benefits Offered: Dental

Type of Coverage
Commercial, Individual

Geographic Areas Served
Military personnel and their families, nationwide

Accreditation Certification
URAC, NCQA

1163 UnitedHealthCare of Washington
7525 SE 24th Street
Suite 200
Mercer Island, WA 98040
Toll-Free: 800-516-3344
Phone: 206-236-2500
www.uhc.com
Subsidiary of: UnitedHealth Group
For Profit Organization: Yes
Total Enrollment: 75,000,000
State Enrollment: 624,000

Healthplan and Services Defined
PLAN TYPE: HMO/PPO

Geographic Areas Served
Statewide

Accreditation Certification
URAC

Key Personnel
Chief Executive Officer . . . . David Hansen
Vice President, Network . . . . Deborah Mcquade
Marketing . . . . Lya Selby
Senior Medical Director . . . . Roger Muller, MD
Media Contact . . . . Will Shanley
will.shanley@uhc.com

1164 VSP: Vision Service Plan of Washington
600 University Street
Suite 2004
Seattle, WA 98101-1176
Toll-Free: 800-877-7195
Phone: 206-623-5178
Fax: 206-621-7515
webmaster@vsp.com
www.vsp.com
Year Founded: 1955
Number of Primary Care Physicians: 26,000
Total Enrollment: 55,000,000

Healthplan and Services Defined
PLAN TYPE: Vision
Plan Specialty: Vision
Benefits Offered: Vision

Type of Payment Plans Offered
Capitated

Geographic Areas Served
Statewide

Network Qualifications
Pre-Admission Certification: Yes

Peer Review Type
Utilization Review: Yes

Accreditation Certification
URAC, NCQA
Utilization Review, Quality Assurance Program

Health Insurance Coverage Status and Type of Coverage by Age

Category	All Persons		Under 18 years		Under 65 years		65 years and over	
	Number	%	Number	%	Number	%	Number	%
Total population	1,825	-	381	-	1,514	-	311	-
Covered by some type of health insurance	1,570 (10)	86.0 (0.5)	361 (4)	94.7 (0.9)	1,259 (10)	83.2 (0.6)	310 (1)	99.8 (0.1)
Covered by private health insurance	1,146 (16)	62.8 (0.9)	206 (7)	54.0 (1.9)	931 (15)	61.5 (1.0)	215 (4)	69.1 (1.3)
Employment based	1,001 (16)	54.8 (0.9)	191 (7)	50.2 (1.9)	858 (16)	56.7 (1.0)	142 (5)	45.8 (1.6)
Direct purchase	168 (7)	9.2 (0.4)	13 (2)	3.4 (0.6)	80 (6)	5.3 (0.4)	88 (4)	28.3 (1.3)
Covered by TRICARE	40 (4)	2.2 (0.2)	6 (1)	1.6 (0.4)	25 (3)	1.6 (0.2)	16 (2)	5.0 (0.7)
Covered by government health insurance	702 (12)	38.5 (0.7)	172 (7)	45.0 (1.8)	396 (12)	26.2 (0.8)	306 (2)	98.4 (0.3)
Covered by Medicaid	357 (12)	19.6 (0.6)	170 (7)	44.5 (1.9)	322 (11)	21.2 (0.8)	36 (3)	11.5 (1.0)
Also by private insurance	49 (4)	2.7 (0.2)	16 (3)	4.2 (0.8)	34 (4)	2.2 (0.2)	15 (2)	4.9 (0.6)
Covered by Medicare	390 (5)	21.3 (0.3)	2 (1)	0.6 (0.2)	84 (5)	5.6 (0.3)	305 (2)	98.1 (0.4)
Also by private insurance	237 (5)	13.0 (0.3)	Z (Z)	0.1 (0.1)	27 (3)	1.8 (0.2)	210 (4)	67.5 (1.4)
Also by Medicaid	69 (5)	3.8 (0.3)	1 (Z)	0.2 (0.1)	33 (3)	2.2 (0.2)	36 (3)	11.5 (1.0)
Covered by VA Care	66 (4)	3.6 (0.2)	1 (Z)	0.2 (0.1)	30 (3)	2.0 (0.2)	36 (3)	11.6 (0.9)
Not covered at any time during the year	255 (10)	14.0 (0.5)	20 (4)	5.3 (0.9)	254 (10)	16.8 (0.6)	1 (Z)	0.2 (0.1)

Note: Numbers in thousands; Figures cover 2013; Margin of error appears in parenthesis; A "Z" indicates that the value either represents or rounds to zero.
Source: U.S. Census Bureau, 2013 American Community Survey, Table HI05. Health Insurance Coverage Status and Type of Coverage by State and Age for All People: 2013

West Virginia

1165　Aetna Health of West Virginia

151 Farmington Avenue
Hartford, CT 06156
Toll-Free: 800-872-3862
Phone: 860-273-0123
www.aetna.com
For Profit Organization: Yes
Year Founded: 1985
Number of Affiliated Hospitals: 76
Number of Primary Care Physicians: 3,000
Number of Referral/Specialty Physicians: 4,000
Total Enrollment: 11,596,230

Healthplan and Services Defined
　PLAN TYPE: PPO
　Other Type: POS
　Model Type: Group
　Benefits Offered: Behavioral Health, Chiropractic, Dental, Disease
　　Management, Physical Therapy, Prescription, Vision
　Offers Demand Management Patient Information Service: Yes

Type of Coverage
　Commercial, Individual

Type of Payment Plans Offered
　Capitated

Geographic Areas Served
　Statewide

Publishes and Distributes Report Card: Yes

Key Personnel
　Chairman/CEO/President.....................Mark T Bertolini
　EVP/General Counsel ....William J Casazza
　EVP/CFO ....Joseph M Zubretsky

Specialty Managed Care Partners
　Enters into Contracts with Regional Business Coalitions: Yes

1166　CIGNA HealthCare of West Virginia

3101 Park Lane Drive
Pittsburgh, PA 15275
Toll-Free: 866-438-2446
Phone: 412-747-4410
Fax: 412-747-4416
www.cigna.com
For Profit Organization: Yes
Total Enrollment: 35,316
State Enrollment: 27,783

Healthplan and Services Defined
　PLAN TYPE: PPO
　Benefits Offered: Disease Management, Prescription, Transplant,
　　Wellness

Type of Coverage
　Commercial

Type of Payment Plans Offered
　POS, FFS

Geographic Areas Served
　West Virginia

Key Personnel
　CMO ....Z Colette Edwards, MD

1167　Coventry Health Care of West Virginia

500 Virginia Street East
Suite 400
Charleston, WV 25301
Toll-Free: 888-388-1744
Phone: 304-348-2900
www.chcwestvirginia.coventryhealthcare.com
Secondary Address: The Wagner Building, 2001 Main Street, Suite
　201, Wheeling, WV 26003, 304-234-3481
For Profit Organization: Yes
Year Founded: 1995
Number of Affiliated Hospitals: 175
Number of Primary Care Physicians: 15,600
Total Enrollment: 100,000
State Enrollment: 100,000

Healthplan and Services Defined
　PLAN TYPE: HMO/PPO
　Benefits Offered: Behavioral Health, Disease Management,
　　Prescription, Vision, Wellness

Type of Coverage
　Commercial, Medicare, Medicaid

Geographic Areas Served
　All 55 West Virginia counties

Peer Review Type
　Case Management: Yes

Publishes and Distributes Report Card: Yes

Accreditation Certification
　URAC

Key Personnel
　President/CEO ....Cosby Davis
　　434-951-2580
　　cmdavis@cvty.com
　Chief Medical Director.......................Rod McKinney
　　304-348-2911
　　rdmckinney@cvty.com
　VP Marketing ....Roger Stewart
　　304-348-2008
　　rpstewart@cvty.com

1168　Delta Dental of the Mid-Atlantic

One Delta Drive
Mechanicsburg, PA 17055-6999
Toll-Free: 800-932-0783
Fax: 717-766-8719
www.deltadentalins.com
Non-Profit Organization: Yes
Total Enrollment: 54,000,000

Healthplan and Services Defined
　PLAN TYPE: Dental
　Other Type: Dental PPO

Type of Coverage
　Commercial

Geographic Areas Served
　Statewide

Key Personnel
　President/CEO...............................Gary D Radine
　VP, Public & Govt Affairs ....Jeff Album
　　415-972-8418
　Dir/Media & Public Affair...................Elizabeth Risberg
　　415-972-8423

1169 eHealthInsurance Services Inc.
11919 Foundation Place
Gold River, CA 95670
Toll-Free: 800-644-3491
webmaster@healthinsurance.com
www.e.healthinsurance.com
Year Founded: 1997

Healthplan and Services Defined
PLAN TYPE: HMO/PPO
Benefits Offered: Dental, Life, STD

Type of Coverage
Commercial, Individual, Medicare

Geographic Areas Served
All 50 states in the USA and District of Columbia

Key Personnel
Chairman & CEO . . . . .Gary L. Lauer
EVP/Business & Corp. Dev. .Bruce Telkamp
EVP/Chief Technology. . . . . .Dr. Sheldon X. Wang
SVP & CFO . . . . .Stuart M. Huizinga
Pres. of eHealth Gov. Sys . . . . .Samuel C. Gibbs
SVP of Sales & Operations . . . . .Robert S. Hurley
Director Public Relations. . . . . .Nate Purpura
650-210-3115

1170 Great-West Healthcare West Virginia
3101 Park Lane Drive
Pittsburgh, OH 15275
Toll-Free: 866-494-2111
Phone: 412-747-4410
eliginquiries@cigna.com
www.cignaforhealth.com
Subsidiary of: CIGNA HealthCare
Acquired by: CIGNA
For Profit Organization: Yes
Total Enrollment: 11,745
State Enrollment: 10,417

Healthplan and Services Defined
PLAN TYPE: HMO/PPO
Benefits Offered: Disease Management, Prescription, Wellness

Type of Coverage
Commercial

Type of Payment Plans Offered
POS, FFS

Geographic Areas Served
West Virginia

Accreditation Certification
URAC

Specialty Managed Care Partners
Caremark Rx

1171 Humana Health Insurance of West Virginia
4202A Maccorkle Ave SE
Charleston, WV 25304
Toll-Free: 800-951-0130
Phone: 304-925-0972
Fax: 304-925-0976
www.humana.com
For Profit Organization: Yes

Healthplan and Services Defined
PLAN TYPE: HMO/PPO

Type of Coverage
Commercial, Individual

Accreditation Certification
URAC, NCQA

Key Personnel
Branch Mgr/Executive Dir . . . . .Charles Showalter
Manager. . . . . .John Vogel

1172 Mid Atlantic Medical Services: West Virginia
5004 Elk River Road S
Elkview, MD 25071
Toll-Free: 800-884-5188
Phone: 304-965-2881
Fax: 301-545-5380
masales99@uhc.com
www.mamsiunitedhealthcare.com
Subsidiary of: United Healthcare/United Health Group
Year Founded: 1986
Number of Affiliated Hospitals: 342
Number of Primary Care Physicians: 3,276
Total Enrollment: 180,000

Healthplan and Services Defined
PLAN TYPE: HMO/PPO
Model Type: IPA, Network
Benefits Offered: Disease Management, Prescription, Wellness

Type of Payment Plans Offered
Combination FFS & DFFS

Geographic Areas Served
Delaware, Maryland, North Carolina, Pennsylvania, Virginia, Washington DC, West Virginia

Network Qualifications
Pre-Admission Certification: Yes

Peer Review Type
Utilization Review: Yes
Second Surgical Opinion: Yes
Case Management: Yes

Publishes and Distributes Report Card: No

Accreditation Certification
TJC, NCQA

Specialty Managed Care Partners
Enters into Contracts with Regional Business Coalitions: Yes

1173 Mountain Health Trust/Physician Assured Access System
405 Capitol Street
Suite 406
Charleston, WV 25301
Toll-Free: 800-449-8466
Fax: 304-345-1581
www.mountainhealthtrust.com
Year Founded: 1996

Healthplan and Services Defined
PLAN TYPE: HMO
Benefits Offered: Disease Management, Wellness

Type of Coverage
Medicaid

Geographic Areas Served
Statewide

1174 Mountain State Blue Cross Blue Shield
PO Box 1948
Parkersburg, WV 26102
Toll-Free: 888-809-9121
Phone: 304-424-7701
Fax: 304-347-7696
mscomm@highmark.com
www.highmarkbcbswv.com

Mailing Address: PO Box 7026, Customer Service, Wheeling, WV 26003
Subsidiary of: A Highmark Affiliate
For Profit Organization: Yes
Year Founded: 1932
Number of Affiliated Hospitals: 65
Number of Primary Care Physicians: 1,400
Number of Referral/Specialty Physicians: 3,200
Total Enrollment: 400,000
State Enrollment: 400,000

Healthplan and Services Defined
  PLAN TYPE: PPO
  Model Type: Network, PPO, POS, TPA
  Plan Specialty: ASO, Behavioral Health, Chiropractic, EPO, Lab, Radiology, UR, Case Management
  Benefits Offered: Behavioral Health, Chiropractic, Home Care, Inpatient SNF, Long-Term Care, Physical Therapy, Podiatry, Prescription, Psychiatric, Transplant

Type of Coverage
  Commercial, Individual, Supplemental Medicare

Type of Payment Plans Offered
  POS, DFFS

Geographic Areas Served
  All 55 counties in West Virginia and Washington county, Ohio

Network Qualifications
  Pre-Admission Certification: Yes

Peer Review Type
  Utilization Review: Yes
  Second Surgical Opinion: Yes
  Case Management: Yes

Publishes and Distributes Report Card: No

Accreditation Certification
  URAC

Key Personnel
  President......................................J Fred Earley

Specialty Managed Care Partners
  WV University, Charleston Area Medical Center (CAMC)
  Enters into Contracts with Regional Business Coalitions: No

1175 SelectNet Plus, Inc.

602 Virginia Street, East
Charleston, WV 25301
Toll-Free: 800-647-0873
Phone: 304-556-4769
Fax: 304-353-8748
valorie.raines@wellsfargo.com
Mailing Address: PO Box 3262, Charleston, WV 25332-3262
Subsidiary of: A subsidiary of Wells Fargo Third Party Administrators Inc.
For Profit Organization: Yes
Year Founded: 1987
Physician Owned Organization: No
Federally Qualified: No
Number of Affiliated Hospitals: 85
Number of Primary Care Physicians: 1,989
Number of Referral/Specialty Physicians: 3,820
Total Enrollment: 65,000
State Enrollment: 50,000

Healthplan and Services Defined
  PLAN TYPE: PPO
  Model Type: Regional Provider Network
  Offers Demand Management Patient Information Service: No

Type of Coverage
  Catastrophic Illness Benefit: Varies per case

Geographic Areas Served
  Kentucky, Virginia, Ohio, Tennessee, Pennsylvania, Maryland, West Virginia

Subscriber Information
  Average Monthly Fee Per Subscriber
    (Employee + Employer Contribution):
      Employee Only (Self): Pepm or % of savings
  Average Annual Deductible Per Subscriber:
      Employee Only (Self): Def by access client
  Average Subscriber Co-Payment:
      Primary Care Physician: Def by access client

Network Qualifications
  Pre-Admission Certification: No

Publishes and Distributes Report Card: No

Key Personnel
  SVP/Managed Care...........................Jennings Hart
    304-556-4792
    jennings.hart@wellsfargo.com
  Assistant Vice President.......................Valerie Raines
    304-556-4769
    valorie.raines@wellsfargo.com

Specialty Managed Care Partners
  Self-Funded Employers, Third Party Claims, Third Party Claims Administrators

1176 Unicare: West Virginia

1207 Quarrier Street
Charleston, WV 25304
Phone: 304-347-1962
www.unicare.com
Year Founded: 1985
Number of Affiliated Hospitals: 102
Number of Primary Care Physicians: 3,500
Number of Referral/Specialty Physicians: 8,000
Total Enrollment: 80,000

Healthplan and Services Defined
  PLAN TYPE: HMO/PPO
  Model Type: Network
  Benefits Offered: Chiropractic, Dental, Physical Therapy, Prescription, Vision

Type of Coverage
  Medicare, Supplemental Medicare

Geographic Areas Served
  Massachusetts, Southern New Hampshire & Rhode Island

Subscriber Information
  Average Monthly Fee Per Subscriber
    (Employee + Employer Contribution):
      Employee Only (Self): Varies
      Employee & 1 Family Member: Varies
      Employee & 2 Family Members: Varies
      Medicare: Varies
  Average Annual Deductible Per Subscriber:
      Employee Only (Self): Varies
      Employee & 1 Family Member: Varies
      Employee & 2 Family Members: Varies
      Medicare: Varies
  Average Subscriber Co-Payment:
      Primary Care Physician: Varies
      Non-Network Physician: Varies
      Prescription Drugs: Varies
      Hospital ER: Varies
      Home Health Care: Varies
      Home Health Care Max. Days/Visits Covered: Varies
      Nursing Home: Varies
      Nursing Home Max. Days/Visits Covered: Varies

Network Qualifications
  Pre-Admission Certification: Yes

Peer Review Type
Utilization Review: Yes
Second Surgical Opinion: Yes
Case Management: Yes

Publishes and Distributes Report Card: No

Accreditation Certification
URAC
TJC Accreditation, Medicare Approved, Utilization Review,
Pre-Admission Certification, State Licensure, Quality Assurance
Program

Key Personnel
Principal...................................Melissa Coffman
Sales Director ....Jay Staszewski
jay.staszewski@wellpoint.com
Media Contact ....Tony Felts
317-287-6036
tony.felts@wellpoint.com

1177 UnitedHealthCare of West Virginia

9020 Stony Point Parkway
Suite 400
Richmond, VA 23235
Toll-Free: 877-842-3210
www.uhc.com
Secondary Address: 9020 Stony Parkway, Suite 400, Richmond, VA
23235, 877-842-3210
Subsidiary of: UnitedHealth Group
Year Founded: 1977
Number of Affiliated Hospitals: 4,200
Number of Primary Care Physicians: 460,000
Total Enrollment: 75,000,000

Healthplan and Services Defined
PLAN TYPE: HMO/PPO
Model Type: IPA, Group, Network
Plan Specialty: Lab, Radiology
Benefits Offered: Chiropractic, Dental, Physical Therapy,
Prescription, Wellness, AD&D, Life, LTD, STD
Offers Demand Management Patient Information Service: Yes

Type of Coverage
Commercial, Individual, Indemnity, Medicare

Geographic Areas Served
Statewide

Network Qualifications
Pre-Admission Certification: Yes

Peer Review Type
Utilization Review: Yes
Second Surgical Opinion: Yes
Case Management: Yes

Publishes and Distributes Report Card: Yes

Accreditation Certification
TJC, NCQA

Specialty Managed Care Partners
Enters into Contracts with Regional Business Coalitions: Yes

Health Insurance Coverage Status and Type of Coverage by Age

Category	All Persons		Under 18 years		Under 65 years		65 years and over	
	Number	%	Number	%	Number	%	Number	%
Total population	5,669	-	1,305	-	4,849	-	820	-
Covered by some type of health insurance	5,151 *(14)*	90.9 *(0.2)*	1,243 *(5)*	95.3 *(0.3)*	4,334 *(14)*	89.4 *(0.3)*	818 *(2)*	99.7 *(0.1)*
Covered by private health insurance	4,071 *(23)*	71.8 *(0.4)*	858 *(11)*	65.7 *(0.8)*	3,517 *(22)*	72.5 *(0.5)*	554 *(6)*	67.6 *(0.7)*
Employment based	3,440 *(24)*	60.7 *(0.4)*	800 *(12)*	61.3 *(0.9)*	3,184 *(24)*	65.7 *(0.5)*	257 *(6)*	31.3 *(0.7)*
Direct purchase	749 *(12)*	13.2 *(0.2)*	67 *(5)*	5.1 *(0.4)*	400 *(11)*	8.3 *(0.2)*	349 *(6)*	42.5 *(0.8)*
Covered by TRICARE	70 *(4)*	1.2 *(0.1)*	11 *(2)*	0.8 *(0.1)*	44 *(4)*	0.9 *(0.1)*	27 *(2)*	3.2 *(0.3)*
Covered by government health insurance	1,805 *(21)*	31.8 *(0.4)*	451 *(11)*	34.6 *(0.8)*	1,000 *(21)*	20.6 *(0.4)*	804 *(2)*	98.0 *(0.2)*
Covered by Medicaid	999 *(20)*	17.6 *(0.4)*	445 *(11)*	34.1 *(0.8)*	892 *(20)*	18.4 *(0.4)*	107 *(4)*	13.0 *(0.5)*
Also by private insurance	182 *(7)*	3.2 *(0.1)*	64 *(4)*	4.9 *(0.3)*	130 *(6)*	2.7 *(0.1)*	52 *(3)*	6.4 *(0.3)*
Covered by Medicare	940 *(6)*	16.6 *(0.1)*	9 *(2)*	0.7 *(0.1)*	137 *(5)*	2.8 *(0.1)*	804 *(2)*	97.9 *(0.2)*
Also by private insurance	581 *(7)*	10.3 *(0.1)*	2 *(1)*	0.1 *(0.1)*	41 *(3)*	0.8 *(0.1)*	540 *(6)*	65.8 *(0.7)*
Also by Medicaid	182 *(6)*	3.2 *(0.1)*	4 *(1)*	0.3 *(0.1)*	76 *(4)*	1.6 *(0.1)*	107 *(4)*	13.0 *(0.5)*
Covered by VA Care	134 *(5)*	2.4 *(0.1)*	1 *(1)*	0.1 *(0.1)*	59 *(3)*	1.2 *(0.1)*	75 *(3)*	9.1 *(0.4)*
Not covered at any time during the year	518 *(14)*	9.1 *(0.2)*	61 *(5)*	4.7 *(0.3)*	515 *(14)*	10.6 *(0.3)*	3 *(1)*	0.3 *(0.1)*

Note: Numbers in thousands; Figures cover 2013; Margin of error appears in parenthesis; A "Z" indicates that the value either represents or rounds to zero.
Source: U.S. Census Bureau, 2013 American Community Survey, Table HI05. Health Insurance Coverage Status and Type of Coverage by State and Age for All People: 2013

Wisconsin

1178 ABRI Health Plan, Inc.
2400 S. 102nd Street
Suite 105
West Allis, WI 53227
Toll-Free: 888-999-2404
Phone: 414-847-1779
Fax: 414-847-1778
contactabri@abrihealthplan.com
www.abrihealthplan.com
Subsidiary of: Acquired by Molina Healthcare
Acquired by: Molina Healthcare
Year Founded: 2004
Total Enrollment: 24,000

Healthplan and Services Defined
PLAN TYPE: Multiple

Type of Coverage
Individual, Medicare, Supplemental Medicare, Medicaid

Key Personnel
President . . . . .Stephen Harris
CEO . . . . .Ron Scasny
Chairman . . . . .Maria Padilla
Chief Medical officer of . . . . Tom Culhane

1179 Aetna Health of Wisconsin
151 Farmington Avenue
Hartford, CT 06156
Toll-Free: 800-872-3862
Phone: 860-273-0123
www.aetna.com
Partnered with: eHealthInsurance Services Inc.
For Profit Organization: Yes
Total Enrollment: 11,596,230

Healthplan and Services Defined
PLAN TYPE: PPO
Other Type: POS
Plan Specialty: EPO
Benefits Offered: Dental, Disease Management, Long-Term Care,
    Prescription, Wellness, Life, LTD, STD

Type of Coverage
Commercial, Individual

Type of Payment Plans Offered
POS, FFS

Geographic Areas Served
Statewide

Key Personnel
Chairman/CEO/President. . . . . .Mark T Bertolini
EVP/General Counsel . . . . .William J Casazza
EVP/CFO . . . . .Shawn M Guertin

1180 Anthem Blue Cross & Blue Shield of Wisconsin
N17 W23430 Riverwood Drive
Waukesha, WI 53188
Toll-Free: 877-267-1204
Phone: 414-459-5000
www.anthem.com
Secondary Address: 216 Pinnacle Way, Suite 100, Eau Claire, WI
    54701

Healthplan and Services Defined
PLAN TYPE: HMO/PPO
Benefits Offered: Dental, Vision, Life

Type of Coverage
Commercial, Individual, Medicare

Accreditation Certification
URAC

Key Personnel
President. . . . . .Larry Screiber
Network Contracting . . . . .John Foley
Medical Officer. . . . . .Michael Jaeger, MD
Media Contact . . . . .Scott Larrivee
    262-523-4746
    scott.larrivee@bcbswi.com

1181 Assurant Employee Benefits: Wisconsin
501 West Michigan
Milwaukee, WI 53203
Phone: 414-271-3011
Fax: 262-785-1838
benefits@assurant.com
www.assurantemployeebenefits.com
Subsidiary of: Assurant, Inc
For Profit Organization: Yes
Number of Primary Care Physicians: 112,000
Total Enrollment: 47,000

Healthplan and Services Defined
PLAN TYPE: Multiple
Plan Specialty: Dental, Vision, Long & Short-Term Disability
Benefits Offered: Dental, Vision, Wellness, AD&D, Life, LTD, STD

Type of Coverage
Commercial, Indemnity, Individual Dental Plans

Geographic Areas Served
Statewide

Subscriber Information
Average Monthly Fee Per Subscriber
    (Employee + Employer Contribution):
        Employee Only (Self): Varies by plan

Accreditation Certification
URAC, NCQA

Key Personnel
Director, CEO. . . . . .Robert B. Pollock
EVP, CFO . . . . .Michael J. Peninger
PR Specialist. . . . . .Megan Hutchison
    816-556-7815
    megan.hutchison@assurant.com

1182 Care Plus Dental Plans
1135 S. Cesar Chavez Drive
Milwaukee, WI 53204
Toll-Free: 800-318-7007
Phone: 414-645-4540
Fax: 414-771-7640
www.careplusdentalplans.com
Subsidiary of: Dental Associates Ltd
Non-Profit Organization: Yes
Year Founded: 1983
Physician Owned Organization: Yes
Number of Primary Care Physicians: 51
Total Enrollment: 200,000

Healthplan and Services Defined
PLAN TYPE: Dental
Model Type: Staff
Plan Specialty: Dental
Benefits Offered: Dental, Prescription

Type of Coverage
Commercial, Individual

Type of Payment Plans Offered
Capitated

Geographic Areas Served
Appleton, Fond Du Lac, Green Bay, Greenville, Kenosha, Milwaukee & Waukesha

Peer Review Type
Utilization Review: Yes

Accreditation Certification
AAAHC

Key Personnel
Marketing . . . . .John Krause

1183   ChiroCare of Wisconsin
2825 N Mayfair Road
Suite 106
Wauwatosa, WI 53222
Toll-Free: 800-397-1541
Phone: 414-476-4733
Fax: 414-476-4517
ccwiweb@chirocarewi.com
www.chirocarewi.com
Non-Profit Organization: Yes
Year Founded: 1986
Number of Primary Care Physicians: 401
Total Enrollment: 150,000

Healthplan and Services Defined
PLAN TYPE: PPO
Model Type: IPA, Network
Plan Specialty: Chiropractic, Complimentary Medicine Networks
Benefits Offered: Chiropractic

Type of Coverage
Commercial, Indemnity, Medicare, Supplemental Medicare, Medicaid

Type of Payment Plans Offered
POS, DFFS, Capitated, FFS, Combination FFS & DFFS

Geographic Areas Served
Statewide

Network Qualifications
Pre-Admission Certification: Yes

Peer Review Type
Utilization Review: Yes
Second Surgical Opinion: Yes
Case Management: Yes

Accreditation Certification
URAC, NCQA
Quality Assurance Program

Key Personnel
President/CEO . . . . .Jeffrey Nienhaus
    414-476-4733
    jnienhaus@chirocarewi.com
Director Operations . . . . .Esther Guerrero
    eguerrero@chirocarewi.com
Network Contracting . . . . .Hans Hildebrand
    hhildebrand@chirocarewi.com
Credentialing . . . . .Hans Hildebrand
    hhildebrand@chirocarewi.com
Sales Executive . . . . .Jeffrey Nienhaus
    jnienhaus@chirocarewi.com
Provider Service Manager .Hans Hildebrand
    hhildebrand@chirocarewi.com

1184   CIGNA HealthCare of Wisconsin
2675 North Mayfair Road
Suite 210
Wauwatosa, WI 53226
Toll-Free: 866-438-2446
Phone: 414-256-3310
Fax: 414-256-3328
www.cigna.com
For Profit Organization: Yes
Total Enrollment: 72,853
State Enrollment: 53,255

Healthplan and Services Defined
PLAN TYPE: PPO
Benefits Offered: Disease Management, Prescription, Transplant, Wellness

Type of Coverage
Commercial

Type of Payment Plans Offered
POS, FFS

Geographic Areas Served
Wisconsin

Accreditation Certification
URAC

Key Personnel
CMO . . . . .Aslam Khan, MD

1185   Dean Health Plan
1277 Deming Way
Madison, WI 53717
Toll-Free: 800-279-1301
Phone: 608-828-1301
Fax: 608-827-4212
www.deancare.com
For Profit Organization: Yes
Year Founded: 1983
Physician Owned Organization: Yes
Federally Qualified: Yes
Number of Affiliated Hospitals: 26
Number of Primary Care Physicians: 1,500
Total Enrollment: 247,881

Healthplan and Services Defined
PLAN TYPE: Multiple
Model Type: Network
Benefits Offered: Behavioral Health, Chiropractic, Dental, Disease Management, Home Care, Inpatient SNF, Physical Therapy, Podiatry, Prescription, Psychiatric, Transplant, Vision, Wellness
Offers Demand Management Patient Information Service: Yes
DMPI Services Offered: On Call Nurse Line

Type of Coverage
Commercial, Individual, Indemnity, Medicare, Supplemental Medicare, Medicaid

Type of Payment Plans Offered
Capitated

Geographic Areas Served
20 counties in Southern Wisconsin

Subscriber Information
Average Monthly Fee Per Subscriber
    (Employee + Employer Contribution):
        Employee Only (Self): Varies
        Employee & 1 Family Member: Varies
        Employee & 2 Family Members: Varies
        Medicare: Varies
Average Annual Deductible Per Subscriber:
        Employee Only (Self): Varies
        Employee & 1 Family Member: Varies
        Employee & 2 Family Members: Varies

Medicare: Varies
Average Subscriber Co-Payment:
    Primary Care Physician: Varies
    Non-Network Physician: Varies
    Prescription Drugs: Varies
    Hospital ER: Varies
    Home Health Care: Varies
    Home Health Care Max. Days/Visits Covered: Varies
    Nursing Home: Varies
    Nursing Home Max. Days/Visits Covered: Varies

Network Qualifications
Pre-Admission Certification: Yes

Peer Review Type
Utilization Review: Yes

Publishes and Distributes Report Card: Yes

Accreditation Certification
NCQA

Key Personnel
CEO . . . . .Lon Sprecher
Market Intelligence Spec. . . . . .Rick Loerke
   608-827-4050
   rick.loerke@deancare.com

Specialty Managed Care Partners
Enters into Contracts with Regional Business Coalitions: No

Employer References
State of Wisconsin Employees

1186 Delta Dental of Wisconsin

2801 Hoover Road
PO Box 828
Stevens Point, WI 54481
Toll-Free: 800-236-3712
Phone: 715-344-6087
Fax: 715-343-7623
www.deltadentalwi.com
Non-Profit Organization: Yes
Year Founded: 1962
Total Enrollment: 54,000,000

Healthplan and Services Defined
  PLAN TYPE: Dental
  Other Type: Dental PPO
  Model Type: Network
  Plan Specialty: Dental, Vision
  Benefits Offered: Dental, Vision

Type of Coverage
Commercial

Type of Payment Plans Offered
POS, FFS

Geographic Areas Served
Statewide

Network Qualifications
Pre-Admission Certification: Yes

Peer Review Type
Case Management: Yes

Publishes and Distributes Report Card: No

Accreditation Certification
TJC

Key Personnel
Marketing . . . . .Gary Rogers
Dir/Media & Public Affair . . . . .Elizabeth Risberg
   415-972-8423

Specialty Managed Care Partners
Enters into Contracts with Regional Business Coalitions: No

1187 Dental Protection Plan

7130 W Greenfield Avenue
West Allis, WI 53214-4708
Phone: 414-259-9522
www.mydentalprotectionplan.com
Year Founded: 1987

Healthplan and Services Defined
  PLAN TYPE: Dental
  Other Type: Dental HMO
  Plan Specialty: Dental
  Benefits Offered: Dental

Geographic Areas Served
Nationwide

Subscriber Information
Average Monthly Fee Per Subscriber
  (Employee + Employer Contribution):
    Employee Only (Self): $35/year

Peer Review Type
Case Management: Yes

Publishes and Distributes Report Card: Yes

1188 eHealthInsurance Services Inc.

11919 Foundation Place
Gold River, CA 95670
Toll-Free: 800-644-3491
webmaster@healthinsurance.com
www.e.healthinsurance.com
Year Founded: 1997

Healthplan and Services Defined
  PLAN TYPE: HMO/PPO
  Benefits Offered: Dental, Life, STD

Type of Coverage
Commercial, Individual, Medicare

Geographic Areas Served
All 50 states in the USA and District of Columbia

Key Personnel
Chairman & CEO . . . . .Gary L. Lauer
EVP/Business & Corp. Dev. . . . . .Bruce Telkamp
EVP/Chief Technology .Dr. Sheldon X. Wang
SVP & CFO . . . . .Stuart M. Huizinga
Pres. of eHealth Gov. Sys .Samuel C. Gibbs
SVP of Sales & Operations . . . . .Robert S. Hurley
Director Public Relations. . . . . .Nate Purpura
   650-210-3115

1189 Great-West Healthcare Wisconsin

3333 North Mayfair Road
Suite 201
Wauwatosa, WI 53222
Toll-Free: 800-893-8324
eliginquiries@cigna.com
www.cignaforhealth.com
Subsidiary of: CIGNA HealthCare
Acquired by: CIGNA
For Profit Organization: Yes
Total Enrollment: 28,619
State Enrollment: 22,450

Healthplan and Services Defined
  PLAN TYPE: HMO/PPO
  Benefits Offered: Disease Management, Prescription, Wellness

Type of Coverage
Commercial

Type of Payment Plans Offered
POS, FFS

Geographic Areas Served
Wisconsin

Accreditation Certification
URAC

Key Personnel
President . . . . .Richard F. Rivers
Chief Medical Officer . . . . .Terry Fouts, MD

Specialty Managed Care Partners
Caremark Rx

1190   Group Health Cooperative of Eau Claire

2503 North Hillcrest Parkway
Altoona, WI 54702
Toll-Free: 888-203-7770
Phone: 715-552-4300
Fax: 715-836-7683
www.group-health.com
Mailing Address: PO Box 3217, Eau Claire, WI 54702
Non-Profit Organization: Yes
Year Founded: 1976
Number of Affiliated Hospitals: 57
Number of Primary Care Physicians: 7,700
Number of Referral/Specialty Physicians: 3,800
Total Enrollment: 95,000
State Enrollment: 95,000

Healthplan and Services Defined
  PLAN TYPE: HMO
  Model Type: Network
  Benefits Offered: Dental, Disease Management, Prescription,
    Wellness, Comprehensive Health
  Offers Demand Management Patient Information Service: Yes
  DMPI Services Offered: FirstCare Nurseline

Type of Coverage
  Commercial, Medicaid, SSI
  Catastrophic Illness Benefit: Varies per case

Geographic Areas Served
  Barron, Buffalo, Chippewa, Clark, Dunn, Eau Claire, Jackson, Pepin,
  Rusk, Sawyer, Taylor, Trempealeau, Washburn, Ashland, Bayfield,
  Douglas, Burnett, Polk, St. Croix, Pierce, LaCrosse, Monroe, Juneau,
  Veronn, Crawford, Richland, Sauk, Columbia, Grant, Iowa,
  Lafayette, Green counties

Peer Review Type
  Utilization Review: Yes
  Second Surgical Opinion: Yes
  Case Management: Yes

Publishes and Distributes Report Card: Yes

Accreditation Certification
  AAAHC
  TJC Accreditation, Medicare Approved, Utilization Review, State
    Licensure, Quality Assurance Program

Key Personnel
General Manager & CEO. . . . . .Peter Farrow
Chief Medical Officer . . . . .Michele Bauer, DO
Chief Operating Officer. .Darin McFadden
Chief Financial Officer. . . . . .Bob Tanner

Specialty Managed Care Partners
CMS, OMNE
Enters into Contracts with Regional Business Coalitions: Yes

1191   Group Health Cooperative of South Central Wisconsin

1265 John Q Hammons Drive
Madison, WI 53717
Toll-Free: 800-605-4327
Phone: 608-828-4853
Fax: 608-828-9333
member_services@ghcscw.com
https://ghcscw.com
Mailing Address: PO Box 44971, Madison, WI 53744-4971
Non-Profit Organization: Yes
Year Founded: 1976
Owned by an Integrated Delivery Network (IDN): Yes
Federally Qualified: Yes
Number of Affiliated Hospitals: 4
Number of Primary Care Physicians: 100
Number of Referral/Specialty Physicians: 735
Total Enrollment: 61,000
State Enrollment: 48,202

Healthplan and Services Defined
  PLAN TYPE: HMO
  Model Type: Staff
  Plan Specialty: Dental, Lab, Vision, Radiology
  Benefits Offered: Disease Management, Physical Therapy,
    Prescription, Vision, Wellness
  Offers Demand Management Patient Information Service: Yes

Type of Coverage
  Commercial, Medicare, Medicaid

Type of Payment Plans Offered
  DFFS, Capitated

Geographic Areas Served
  Dane County & one zip code adjoining Dane County, Jefferson, Green
  and Rock counties

Subscriber Information
  Average Monthly Fee Per Subscriber
    (Employee + Employer Contribution):
      Employee Only (Self): Varies by plan
  Average Annual Deductible Per Subscriber:
    Employee Only (Self): $0
    Employee & 1 Family Member: $0
    Employee & 2 Family Members: $0
    Medicare: $0
  Average Subscriber Co-Payment:
    Primary Care Physician: $0
    Non-Network Physician: $0
    Prescription Drugs: $0
    Hospital ER: $0
    Home Health Care: $0
    Home Health Care Max. Days/Visits Covered: Unlimited
    Nursing Home: $0
    Nursing Home Max. Days/Visits Covered: 100 days

Publishes and Distributes Report Card: Yes

Accreditation Certification
  AAAHC, NCQA
  Medicare Approved, Utilization Review, Pre-Admission Certification,
    State Licensure, Quality Assurance Program

Key Personnel
President . . . . .Kenneth N. Machtan
Vice President . . . . .Mary R. Wright
CEO. . . . . .Kevin R. Hayden
Medical Director . . . . .Jeff Huebner, MD
Network Contracting. . . . . .Mark Huth, MD
Medical Affairs . . . . .Michael Ostrov, MD

Specialty Managed Care Partners
UW Hospitals
Enters into Contracts with Regional Business Coalitions: Yes

1192 Gundersen Lutheran Health Plan

3190 Gundersen Drive
Onalaska, WI 54650
Toll-Free: 800-362-9567
Phone: 608-782-7300
Fax: 608-775-8091
hpcustomerservice@gundersenhealth.org
www.gundersenhealthplan.org
Secondary Address: Mail: 1836 South Avenue, NCA2-01, LaCrosse, WI 54650
Subsidiary of: Gunderson Lutheran Health System
Non-Profit Organization: Yes
Year Founded: 1995
Physician Owned Organization: Yes
Federally Qualified: Yes
Number of Affiliated Hospitals: 14
Number of Primary Care Physicians: 850
Number of Referral/Specialty Physicians: 200
Total Enrollment: 90,000
State Enrollment: 90,000

Healthplan and Services Defined
  PLAN TYPE: HMO
  Other Type: POS
  Model Type: Network
  Plan Specialty: ASO, Behavioral Health, Chiropractic, Disease Management, Lab, PBM, Radiology, UR
  Benefits Offered: Behavioral Health, Chiropractic, Disease Management, Home Care, Inpatient SNF, Physical Therapy, Podiatry, Prescription, Psychiatric, Transplant, Vision, Wellness, AD&D
  Offers Demand Management Patient Information Service: Yes
  DMPI Services Offered: Nurse Advisor Line

Type of Coverage
  Commercial, Individual, Medicare

Geographic Areas Served
  Western Wisconsin

Subscriber Information
  Average Monthly Fee Per Subscriber
    (Employee + Employer Contribution):
      Employee Only (Self): Varies
  Average Annual Deductible Per Subscriber:
      Employee & 2 Family Members: Varies

Accreditation Certification
  TJC, URAC, NCQA
  Pre-Admission Certification

Key Personnel
  CEO . . . . Gary Lenth, MD
  Chief Quality Officer. . . . . Jean Krause
  Chief Bus Dev Officer. . . . . Pamela Maas
  Chief Learning Officer. . . . . Mary Ellen McCartney
  EVP, Chief Medical Off . . . . Julio Bird, MD
  Exec Dir, Human Resources. Monty Clark
  Vice President, Nursing. . . . . Mary Lu Gerke, PhD
  Chief Govt Relations . . . . Joan Curran
  Compliance Director. . . . . Jenny Noren
    jjnoren@gundluth.org

1193 Health Tradition

1808 East Main Street
Onalaska, WI 54602-0188
Toll-Free: 888-459-3020
Phone: 608-781-9692
www.healthtradition.com
Mailing Address: PO Box 188, La Crosse, WI 54602-0188
For Profit Organization: Yes
Year Founded: 1986
Number of Affiliated Hospitals: 17

Number of Primary Care Physicians: 800
Number of Referral/Specialty Physicians: 100
Total Enrollment: 34,000
State Enrollment: 40,000

Healthplan and Services Defined
  PLAN TYPE: HMO
  Model Type: Group
  Benefits Offered: Disease Management, Prescription, Wellness
  Offers Demand Management Patient Information Service: Yes
  DMPI Services Offered: 24 hour nurse line

Type of Coverage
  Medicare, Medicaid
  Catastrophic Illness Benefit: Maximum $2M

Type of Payment Plans Offered
  POS, Combination FFS & DFFS

Geographic Areas Served
  Iowa: Allamakee; Minnesota: Houston; Buffalo, Crawford, Fillmore, Jackson, La Crosse, Monroe, Trempealeau, Vernon, Winneshiek, Winona counties

Subscriber Information
  Average Monthly Fee Per Subscriber
    (Employee + Employer Contribution):
      Employee Only (Self): Varies by plan
  Average Annual Deductible Per Subscriber:
      Employee Only (Self): $50.00
      Employee & 1 Family Member: $100.00
      Employee & 2 Family Members: $150.00
  Average Subscriber Co-Payment:
      Primary Care Physician: $0
      Prescription Drugs: $11.00
      Hospital ER: $25.00-50.00
      Home Health Care: $0
      Home Health Care Max. Days/Visits Covered: 345 days
      Nursing Home: $0
      Nursing Home Max. Days/Visits Covered: 60 days

Network Qualifications
  Pre-Admission Certification: Yes

Peer Review Type
  Utilization Review: Yes
  Second Surgical Opinion: Yes
  Case Management: Yes

Publishes and Distributes Report Card: No

Accreditation Certification
  TJC Accreditation, Medicare Approved, Utilization Review, Pre-Admission Certification, State Licensure, Quality Assurance Program

Key Personnel
  Medical Dirccctor . . . . Alan Krumholz, MD
  Director/Sales & Market . . . . Michael Eckstein

Average Claim Compensation
  Physician's Fees Charged: 85%
  Hospital's Fees Charged: 85%

Specialty Managed Care Partners
  Franciscon Scam Health Care
  Enters into Contracts with Regional Business Coalitions: No

1194 HealthEOS

301 North Broadway
Suite 301
De Pere, WI 54115
Toll-Free: 800-279-9776
Phone: 920-337-6550
Fax: 920-247-9230
sales@multiplan.com
www.healtheos.com
Secondary Address: 18650 West Corporate Drive, Suite 310, Brookfield, WI 53045-6344

Acquired by: MultiPlan
For Profit Organization: Yes
Physician Owned Organization: No
Owned by an Integrated Delivery Network (IDN): No
Federally Qualified: No
Number of Affiliated Hospitals: 160
Number of Primary Care Physicians: 7,000
Number of Referral/Specialty Physicians: 20,000
Total Enrollment: 820,000
State Enrollment: 700,000

Healthplan and Services Defined
PLAN TYPE: PPO
Model Type: Network
Plan Specialty: Primary PPO Network
Offers Demand Management Patient Information Service: No

Geographic Areas Served
Wisconsin and surrounding areas

Publishes and Distributes Report Card: No

Accreditation Certification
TJC, NCQA

Key Personnel
CEO . . . . Mark Tabak
800-279-9776
Senior Vice President . . . . Carolyn Martin
Chief Financial Officer . . . . David Redmond
EVP, Chief Marketing Off . . . . Warren Handelman
800-279-9776
VP, Corporate Medical Dir . . . . Paul Goldstein, MD
800-279-9776
EVP, Sales & Acct Mgmt . . . . Dale White
800-279-9776
Proposal Writer . . . . Nicole Konkel
800-279-9776

Specialty Managed Care Partners
ActiveHealth Management, Envision Rx

1195 Humana Health Insurance of Wisconsin
N19 W24133 Riverwood Drive
Suite 300
Waukesha, WI 53188
Toll-Free: 800-289-0260
Phone: 262-408-4300
Fax: 920-632-9508
www.humana.com
Subsidiary of: Humana
For Profit Organization: Yes
Year Founded: 1985
Physician Owned Organization: Yes
Number of Affiliated Hospitals: 23
Number of Primary Care Physicians: 1,300
Number of Referral/Specialty Physicians: 320,000
Total Enrollment: 49,000

Healthplan and Services Defined
PLAN TYPE: HMO/PPO
Model Type: IPA, Network
Plan Specialty: UR
Benefits Offered: Behavioral Health, Chiropractic, Dental, Disease
Management, Home Care, Inpatient SNF, Physical Therapy,
Podiatry, Prescription, Psychiatric, Transplant, Vision, Wellness,
Worker's Compensation, AD&D, Life, LTD
Offers Demand Management Patient Information Service: Yes

Type of Coverage
Commercial, Individual

Type of Payment Plans Offered
POS, DFFS, Capitated, FFS, Combination FFS & DFFS

Geographic Areas Served
Dodge, Jefferson, Kenosha, Milwaukee, Ozaukee, Racine,
Sheboygan, Walworth, Washington, Fond du Luc, Green, Montowoe,
Rock & Waukesha counties

Subscriber Information
Average Subscriber Co-Payment:
Home Health Care Max. Days/Visits Covered: 40 days
Nursing Home Max. Days/Visits Covered: 100 days

Network Qualifications
Pre-Admission Certification: Yes

Peer Review Type
Utilization Review: Yes
Second Surgical Opinion: Yes
Case Management: Yes

Accreditation Certification
AAAHC, URAC, NCQA, CORE

Key Personnel
President/CEO . . . . Michael Derdinski
CFO . . . . Gary Hovila, CPA
Director Network Development . . . . Titus Muzi
Director of QI . . . . Patrice Thor, RN
Pharmacy Manager . . . . Dennis Oleg, PhD
Marketing . . . . David Fee
Materials Management . . . . Maryann Herman
Medical Director . . . . Albert Tzeel, MD
Manager Customer Service . . . . Anne Andryczyk
Medical Management Dir . . . . Patrice Thor, RN
Sales . . . . Scott Austin

Specialty Managed Care Partners
Aurora Behavioral, Chirotech, Accordant, Health Service

1196 Managed Health Services
10700 W Research Drive
Wauwatosa, WI 53226
Toll-Free: 888-713-6180
www.mhswi.com
For Profit Organization: Yes
Year Founded: 1984
Number of Affiliated Hospitals: 57
Number of Primary Care Physicians: 5,500
Number of Referral/Specialty Physicians: 1,255
Total Enrollment: 130,000
State Enrollment: 164,700

Healthplan and Services Defined
PLAN TYPE: HMO
Model Type: IPA, Network
Benefits Offered: Disease Management, Prescription, Wellness
Offers Demand Management Patient Information Service: Yes

Type of Coverage
Medicare, Medicaid
Catastrophic Illness Benefit: Varies per case

Type of Payment Plans Offered
POS, FFS

Geographic Areas Served
22 counties in Wisconsin, Northern Indiana, and Illinois, Racine,
Kenosha; Indiana: Indianapolis; Illinois: Chicago

Subscriber Information
Average Monthly Fee Per Subscriber
(Employee + Employer Contribution):
Employee Only (Self): Varies
Employee & 1 Family Member: Varies
Employee & 2 Family Members: Varies
Medicare: Varies
Average Annual Deductible Per Subscriber:
Employee Only (Self): Varies
Employee & 1 Family Member: Varies
Employee & 2 Family Members: Varies

Medicare: Varies
Average Subscriber Co-Payment:
Primary Care Physician: $10.00/15.00
Non-Network Physician: 100%
Prescription Drugs: $5.00/10.00
Hospital ER: $25.00
Home Health Care: $0

Network Qualifications
Pre-Admission Certification: Yes

Peer Review Type
Utilization Review: Yes

Publishes and Distributes Report Card: Yes

Accreditation Certification
NCQA
TJC Accreditation, Medicare Approved, Utilization Review,
Pre-Admission Certification, State Licensure, Quality Assurance
Program

Key Personnel
President & CEO.............................Sherry Husa
SVP, Govt Relations.........................Sandra S Tunis
VP/Medical Management......................Barb Swartos
VP, Finance................................Christopher Scott
Mgr, Human Resources.......................Jean Bellante
VP, Medical Management....................Pamala Rundhaug

Specialty Managed Care Partners
Enters into Contracts with Regional Business Coalitions: Yes

1197 MercyCare Health Plans

580 N. Washington St.
PO Box 550
Janesville, WI 53547-550
Toll-Free: 800-752-3431
Phone: 608-752-3431
Fax: 608-752-3751
mcash@mhsjvl.org
www.mercycarehealthplans.com
For Profit Organization: Yes
Year Founded: 1994
Number of Affiliated Hospitals: 180
Number of Primary Care Physicians: 440
Total Enrollment: 40,000
State Enrollment: 40,000

Healthplan and Services Defined
PLAN TYPE: HMO
Model Type: Network
Benefits Offered: Disease Management, Prescription, Wellness
Offers Demand Management Patient Information Service: Yes

Type of Coverage
Medicare, Medicaid
Catastrophic Illness Benefit: Unlimited

Type of Payment Plans Offered
POS, Combination FFS & DFFS

Geographic Areas Served
Wisconsin: Green, Jefferson, Rock, Walworth; Illinois: McHenry

Subscriber Information
Average Monthly Fee Per Subscriber
(Employee + Employer Contribution):
Employee Only (Self): Varies by plan
Average Annual Deductible Per Subscriber:
Employee Only (Self): $0
Employee & 1 Family Member: $0
Employee & 2 Family Members: $0
Average Subscriber Co-Payment:
Primary Care Physician: $15.00
Non-Network Physician: 100%
Prescription Drugs: $5.00/15.00
Hospital ER: $35.00

Home Health Care: $0
Home Health Care Max. Days/Visits Covered: 40 days
Nursing Home: $0
Nursing Home Max. Days/Visits Covered: 120 days

Network Qualifications
Pre-Admission Certification: Yes

Peer Review Type
Utilization Review: Yes
Second Surgical Opinion: Yes
Case Management: Yes

Publishes and Distributes Report Card: Yes

Accreditation Certification
NCQA
TJC Accreditation, Medicare Approved, Utilization Review,
Pre-Admission Certification, State Licensure, Quality Assurance
Program

Average Claim Compensation
Physician's Fees Charged: 75%
Hospital's Fees Charged: 75%

Specialty Managed Care Partners
Enters into Contracts with Regional Business Coalitions: No

1198 Network Health Plan of Wisconsin

1570 Midway Place
PO Box 120
Menasha, WI 54952
Toll-Free: 800-826-0940
Phone: 920-720-1300
Fax: 920-720-1909
www.networkhealth.com
Subsidiary of: Affinity Health System
For Profit Organization: Yes
Year Founded: 1982
Number of Affiliated Hospitals: 14
Number of Primary Care Physicians: 1,400
Total Enrollment: 118,000
State Enrollment: 67,812

Healthplan and Services Defined
PLAN TYPE: HMO/PPO
Model Type: Group, Network
Plan Specialty: Behavioral Health, Chiropractic, Disease Management
Benefits Offered: Disease Management, Prescription, Wellness

Type of Coverage
Commercial, Medicare, Medicaid

Type of Payment Plans Offered
POS, Combination FFS & DFFS

Geographic Areas Served
16 counties in Wisconsin. Brown, Calumet, Dodge, Door, Fond du
Lac, Green Lake, Kewaunee, Manitowoc, Marquette, Outagamie,
Portage, Shawano, Sheboygan, Waupaca, Waushara, Winnebago
counties

Subscriber Information
Average Monthly Fee Per Subscriber
(Employee + Employer Contribution):
Employee Only (Self): Varies
Employee & 1 Family Member: Varies
Employee & 2 Family Members: Varies
Medicare: Varies
Average Annual Deductible Per Subscriber:
Employee Only (Self): Varies
Employee & 1 Family Member: Varies
Employee & 2 Family Members: Varies
Medicare: Varies
Average Subscriber Co-Payment:
Primary Care Physician: $10.00
Prescription Drugs: $5.00-7.00
Home Health Care: $0

Network Qualifications
Pre-Admission Certification: Yes

Peer Review Type
Utilization Review: Yes
Second Surgical Opinion: No
Case Management: Yes

Publishes and Distributes Report Card: Yes

Accreditation Certification
NCQA
TJC Accreditation, Medicare Approved, Utilization Review,
Pre-Admission Certification, State Licensure, Quality Assurance
Program

Key Personnel
President....................................Sheila Jenkins
Dir, Health Promotions....................Deborah Anderson
Chief Administrative Offi....................Penny Ransom
VP/General Manager.......................Marcia Broeren
VP/Network Development ....Donald Schumann
Medical Director.........................Edward Scanlan, MD
Chief Operating Officer ....Tim Temperly
Dir, Information Systems ....Dave Bloedorn
Dir, Finance ....Gerry Demmer
Mgr, Provider Data Svcs ....Barb Gore
Mgr, Customer Service..........................Peggy Huss
Mgr, Medicare Operations ....Kathleen Krentz
Mgr, Product Development..................Maureen Lawson
Mgr, Medicare Sales...........................Joan Merwin
Marketing Communications ....Maria Heim
920-720-1752
mheim@affinityhealth.org
Mgr, Care Management ....Dawn Rady

Specialty Managed Care Partners
Enters into Contracts with Regional Business Coalitions: Yes

1199   Physicians Plus Insurance Corporation

2650 Novation Parkway
Madison, WI 53713
Toll-Free: 800-545-5015
Phone: 608-282-8900
Fax: 608-327-0321
ppicinfo@pplusic.com
www.pplusic.com
Mailing Address: PO Box 2078, Madison, WI 53701-2078
Subsidiary of: Meriter Health Services
For Profit Organization: Yes
Year Founded: 1986
Physician Owned Organization: Yes
Number of Affiliated Hospitals: 24
Number of Primary Care Physicians: 3,000
Number of Referral/Specialty Physicians: 2,117
Total Enrollment: 112,000
State Enrollment: 112,000

Healthplan and Services Defined
PLAN TYPE: HMO/PPO
Other Type: POS
Model Type: Network
Plan Specialty: Behavioral Health, Chiropractic, Dental, Disease
Management, Lab, X-Ray
Benefits Offered: Behavioral Health, Chiropractic, Dental, Disease
Management, Home Care, Inpatient SNF, Physical Therapy,
Podiatry, Prescription, Transplant, Vision, Wellness, Durable
Medical Equipment

Type of Coverage
Individual, Supplemental Medicare, Commercial Small Group, Large
Group
Catastrophic Illness Benefit: Covered

Type of Payment Plans Offered
Capitated, FFS, Combination FFS & DFFS

Geographic Areas Served
South central Wisconsin

Subscriber Information
Average Monthly Fee Per Subscriber
(Employee + Employer Contribution):
Employee Only (Self): Varies by plan
Average Annual Deductible Per Subscriber:
Employee Only (Self): Varies by plan
Employee & 1 Family Member: $0
Employee & 2 Family Members: $0
Medicare: $0
Average Subscriber Co-Payment:
Primary Care Physician: Varies by plan
Hospital ER: $100.00
Home Health Care Max. Days/Visits Covered: 100 visits
Nursing Home Max. Days/Visits Covered: 100 days

Network Qualifications
Pre-Admission Certification: Yes

Peer Review Type
Utilization Review: Yes
Second Surgical Opinion: Yes
Case Management: Yes

Publishes and Distributes Report Card: Yes

Accreditation Certification
NCQA
State Licensure, Quality Assurance Program

Key Personnel
President & CEO...............................Linda Hoff
Vice President and Chief ....Tom Luddyÿ
Chief Medical Officer.........................Larry Kay, MD
Chief Pharmacy Officer............................Bill Reay
VP, Sales & Mktg Officer.....................Scott T Kowalski
Chief Medical Officer............................Larry Kay
Sr Dir, Provider Network ....Mary D Strasser
Manager, Marketing.........................Scott Shoemaker
608-260-7116
scott.shoemaker@pplusic.com

Average Claim Compensation
Physician's Fees Charged: 70%
Hospital's Fees Charged: 75%

Specialty Managed Care Partners
Enters into Contracts with Regional Business Coalitions: No

1200   Prevea Health Network

P.O. Box 19070
Green Bay, WI 54307
Toll-Free: 888-277-3832
Phone: 920-496-4700
Fax: 920-272-1120
www.prevea.com
For Profit Organization: Yes
Year Founded: 1996
Number of Affiliated Hospitals: 14
Number of Primary Care Physicians: 1,602
Total Enrollment: 119,712
State Enrollment: 15,706

Healthplan and Services Defined
PLAN TYPE: PPO
Model Type: Group
Plan Specialty: UR
Benefits Offered: Behavioral Health, Chiropractic, Disease
Management, Home Care, Prescription, Transplant, Wellness,
Durable Medical Equipment

Type of Coverage
Commercial, Supplemental Medicare

Geographic Areas Served
counties: Brown, Door, Kewaunee, Manitowoc, Marinette, Oconto

Subscriber Information
Average Annual Deductible Per Subscriber:
Employee Only (Self): $0
Employee & 1 Family Member: $0
Employee & 2 Family Members: $0
Medicare: $0
Average Subscriber Co-Payment:
Primary Care Physician: $0

Accreditation Certification
TJC
Pre-Admission Certification

Key Personnel
President,CEO .... Ashok Rai, MD
SVP/Chief Medical Officer.................... Karla Roth, MD
SVP/Chief Financial Offic..................... Lorrie Jacobetti
SVP/Chief Operating Offic .... Brian Charlier
SVP/Human Resources .... Deb Mauthe
SVP/General Counsel .... Larry Gille
Health Promotions Coord....................... Candy Blaney
Client Support Coord .... Deb Rhode
Client Services................................ Cherie Heath
Provider Network Coord....................... Trisha Paulson

Specialty Managed Care Partners
Express Scripts

1201 Security Health Plan of Wisconsin
1515 Saint Joseph Avenue
PO Box 8000
Marshfield, WI 54449-8000
Toll-Free: 800-472-2363
Phone: 715-221-9555
Fax: 715-221-9500
www.securityhealth.org
Secondary Address: 3610 Oakwood Mall Drive, Suite 203, Eau Claire, WI 54701
Non-Profit Organization: Yes
Year Founded: 1986
Physician Owned Organization: Yes
Number of Affiliated Hospitals: 42
Number of Primary Care Physicians: 4,100
Total Enrollment: 187,000
State Enrollment: 187,000

Healthplan and Services Defined
PLAN TYPE: Multiple
Model Type: Network
Plan Specialty: Behavioral Health, Chiropractic, Disease Management, EPO, Lab, PBM, Vision, Radiology, Worker's Compensation, UR
Benefits Offered: Behavioral Health, Chiropractic, Complementary Medicine, Dental, Disease Management, Home Care, Inpatient SNF, Long-Term Care, Podiatry, Prescription, Psychiatric, Transplant, Vision, Wellness, Worker's Compensation, AD&D, Durable Medical Equipment
Offers Demand Management Patient Information Service: Yes
DMPI Services Offered: Nurse Line, Health Information Line

Type of Coverage
Commercial, Individual, Indemnity, Medicare, Supplemental Medicare, Medicaid, TPA
Catastrophic Illness Benefit: Covered

Type of Payment Plans Offered
Capitated, FFS

Geographic Areas Served
Northern, Western and Central Wisconsin

Subscriber Information
Average Monthly Fee Per Subscriber
(Employee + Employer Contribution):
Employee Only (Self): Varies by plan
Average Annual Deductible Per Subscriber:

Employee Only (Self): $200.00
Employee & 2 Family Members: $100.00
Medicare: $0
Average Subscriber Co-Payment:
Primary Care Physician: $20.00
Non-Network Physician: $20.00
Prescription Drugs: $3.00
Hospital ER: $50.00
Home Health Care: $0
Home Health Care Max. Days/Visits Covered: 40 days
Nursing Home: $0
Nursing Home Max. Days/Visits Covered: 30 days

Network Qualifications
Pre-Admission Certification: No

Peer Review Type
Utilization Review: Yes

Publishes and Distributes Report Card: Yes

Accreditation Certification
NCQA
Medicare Approved, Pre-Admission Certification

Key Personnel
Chief Administrative Off .... Steve Youso
Utilization Management .... Lawrence McFarlane, MBA, MD
Senior Medical Director .... Phil Colmenares MD
Disease Management................. Michele L Bachhuber, MD
Technology Assessment .... Andrea Hillerud, MD
Behavioral Health Until .... Edward J Krall, MD

Specialty Managed Care Partners
Enters into Contracts with Regional Business Coalitions: Yes

1202 Trilogy Health Insurance
18000 West Sarah Lane
Suite 310
Brookfield, WI 53045
Toll-Free: 866-429-3241
Phone: 262-432-9140
www.trilogycares.com
For Profit Organization: Yes
Total Enrollment: 5,000

Healthplan and Services Defined
PLAN TYPE: PPO
Other Type: HSA
Benefits Offered: Disease Management, Prescription, Wellness
Offers Demand Management Patient Information Service: Yes
DMPI Services Offered: 24-Hour Nurse Line

Type of Coverage
Commercial

Accreditation Certification
URAC

1203 UnitedHealthCare of Wisconsin: Central
9700 Health Care Lane
Minnetonka, WI 55343
Toll-Free: 800-842-3585
www.uhc.com
Secondary Address: 1071 West Research Drive, Milwaukee, MN 55226, 800-879-0071
Subsidiary of: UnitedHealth Group
For Profit Organization: Yes
Total Enrollment: 75,000,000
State Enrollment: 392,782

Healthplan and Services Defined
PLAN TYPE: HMO/PPO
Benefits Offered: Disease Management, Prescription, Wellness

Type of Coverage
Commercial, Medicare, Medicaid

Geographic Areas Served
Statewide

Accreditation Certification
URAC

Key Personnel
CEO . . . . William Felsing
CFO . . . . Glen Reinhard
Media Contact . . . . Greg Thompson
    312-424-6913
    gregory_a_thompson@uhc.com

1204   Unity Health Insurance

840 Carolina Street
Sauk City, WI 53583
Toll-Free: 800-362-3310
Phone: 608-643-2491
Fax: 608-643-2564
marketing@unityhealth.com
www.unityhealth.com
Subsidiary of: University Health Care Inc
For Profit Organization: Yes
Year Founded: 1994
Number of Affiliated Hospitals: 44
Number of Primary Care Physicians: 908
Number of Referral/Specialty Physicians: 3,227
Total Enrollment: 90,000
State Enrollment: 75,000

Healthplan and Services Defined
PLAN TYPE: Multiple
Model Type: Network
Benefits Offered: Behavioral Health, Chiropractic, Dental, Disease
    Management, Home Care, Inpatient SNF, Physical Therapy,
    Podiatry, Prescription, Psychiatric, Transplant, Vision, Wellness

Type of Coverage
Commercial, Individual, Medicaid

Type of Payment Plans Offered
POS, DFFS, FFS, Combination FFS & DFFS

Geographic Areas Served
20 counties in southwestern and south central Wisconsin

Network Qualifications
Pre-Admission Certification: Yes

Peer Review Type
Utilization Review: Yes
Second Surgical Opinion: Yes
Case Management: Yes

Publishes and Distributes Report Card: Yes

Accreditation Certification
NCQA
Medicare Approved, Utilization Review, Pre-Admission
    Certification, State Licensure, Quality Assurance Program

Key Personnel
CEO/President . . . . Terry Bolz
VP/Chief Operating Office . . . . Gail Midlikowski
Medical Director . . . . Mary Park, MD
VP/CFO/Treasurer . . . . Jim Hiveley
VP/General Counsel . . . . David Diercks
Pharmacy Director . . . . Pat Cory
VP, Finance, CFO . . . . Jim Hiveley
Medical Director . . . . Mary Pak, MD

Specialty Managed Care Partners
Behavioral Health Consultation System, UW Hospital and Clinics,
    APS Healthcare
Enters into Contracts with Regional Business Coalitions: No

Employer References
University of Wisconsin Medical Foundation, Middleton Cross
    Plains School District, Rockwell Automation, Brakebush Brothers,
    Epic Systemss Corporation

1205   Vision Insurance Plan of America

6737 W Washington Street
Suite 2202, PO Box 44077
Milwaukee, WI 53214-7077
Toll-Free: 800-883-5747
Phone: 414-475-1875
Fax: 888-288-6930
VIPA@visionplans.com
www.visionplans.com
Total Enrollment: 5,000,000

Healthplan and Services Defined
PLAN TYPE: Vision
Plan Specialty: Vision
Benefits Offered: Vision

Geographic Areas Served
Nationwide

Key Personnel
VP, Sales & Marketing . . . . Mark Wallner
    mwallner@visionplans.com
Account Executive . . . . Laurie Kohls
    lkohls@visionplans.com
Account Services . . . . Jesse Rulli
    jrulli@visionplans.com

1206   Wisconsin Physician's Service

1717 W Broadway
PO Box 8190
Madison, WI 53708-8190
Toll-Free: 888-915-4001
Phone: 608-221-4711
Fax: 608-223-3626
member@wpsic.com
www.wpsic.com
Secondary Address: 208 E Olin Avenue, Individual Sales: PO Box
    8190, Madison, WI 53713
Non-Profit Organization: Yes
Year Founded: 1946
Owned by an Integrated Delivery Network (IDN): Yes
Number of Affiliated Hospitals: 129
Number of Primary Care Physicians: 14,500
Total Enrollment: 175,000
State Enrollment: 223,000

Healthplan and Services Defined
PLAN TYPE: PPO
Model Type: Network
Plan Specialty: ASO, Behavioral Health, Chiropractic, Dental,
    Disease Management, EPO, Lab, PBM, Vision, Radiology,
    Worker's Compensation, UR, Rational Med
Benefits Offered: Behavioral Health, Chiropractic, Dental, Disease
    Management, Home Care, Inpatient SNF, Physical Therapy,
    Podiatry, Prescription, Psychiatric, Transplant, Vision, Wellness,
    AD&D, Life, LTD, STD
Offers Demand Management Patient Information Service: Yes

Type of Coverage
Commercial, Individual, Indemnity, Medicare, Supplemental
    Medicare, Catastrophic
Catastrophic Illness Benefit: Varies per case

Type of Payment Plans Offered
POS, DFFS

Subscriber Information
Average Annual Deductible Per Subscriber:
    Employee Only (Self): $0
    Employee & 1 Family Member: $0
    Employee & 2 Family Members: $0
    Medicare: $0

Peer Review Type
Case Management: Yes

Publishes and Distributes Report Card: Yes

Accreditation Certification

AAAHC, URAC

Medicare Approved, Utilization Review, State Licensure, Quality
Assurance Program

Key Personnel

President and CEO . . . . Mike Hamerlik
Chief Operating Officer . . . . Timothy Heaton
Chief Financial Officer . . . . Thomas Nelson
Dir, Pharmacy Services. . . . . David Armstrong
Dir, Reinsurance Services . . . . Tim Healy
SVP, Sales & Marketing . . . . Tom Olson

Specialty Managed Care Partners

Delta Dental

Enters into Contracts with Regional Business Coalitions: Yes

Employer References

US Department of Defense

Health Insurance Coverage Status and Type of Coverage by Age

Category	All Persons		Under 18 years		Under 65 years		65 years and over	
	Number	**%**	**Number**	**%**	**Number**	**%**	**Number**	**%**
Total population	573	-	139	-	498	-	75	-
Covered by some type of health insurance	496 *(5)*	86.6 *(0.9)*	131 *(2)*	94.3 *(1.1)*	421 *(5)*	84.6 *(1.0)*	75 *(1)*	99.7 *(0.3)*
Covered by private health insurance	424 *(7)*	73.9 *(1.3)*	99 *(4)*	71.2 *(2.5)*	371 *(7)*	74.5 *(1.3)*	53 *(2)*	70.2 *(2.8)*
Employment based	353 *(8)*	61.5 *(1.4)*	89 *(4)*	63.6 *(2.6)*	326 *(8)*	65.5 *(1.5)*	27 *(2)*	35.2 *(2.9)*
Direct purchase	75 *(5)*	13.1 *(0.9)*	9 *(2)*	6.8 *(1.5)*	46 *(5)*	9.3 *(0.9)*	28 *(2)*	37.8 *(3.1)*
Covered by TRICARE	20 *(3)*	3.6 *(0.6)*	5 *(2)*	3.9 *(1.3)*	16 *(3)*	3.2 *(0.6)*	5 *(1)*	6.2 *(1.6)*
Covered by government health insurance	144 *(5)*	25.2 *(0.9)*	39 *(4)*	27.8 *(2.8)*	71 *(5)*	14.3 *(1.1)*	73 *(1)*	97.1 *(1.1)*
Covered by Medicaid	63 *(6)*	11.0 *(1.0)*	38 *(4)*	27.4 *(2.7)*	55 *(5)*	11.1 *(1.0)*	8 *(1)*	10.0 *(1.7)*
Also by private insurance	15 *(3)*	2.6 *(0.5)*	6 *(2)*	4.7 *(1.4)*	11 *(3)*	2.2 *(0.5)*	4 *(1)*	5.2 *(1.1)*
Covered by Medicare	84 *(2)*	14.6 *(0.3)*	1 *(1)*	0.7 *(0.5)*	11 *(1)*	2.1 *(0.3)*	73 *(1)*	97.1 *(1.1)*
Also by private insurance	56 *(2)*	9.7 *(0.4)*	Z *(Z)*	0.1 *(0.1)*	5 *(1)*	0.9 *(0.2)*	51 *(2)*	67.6 *(2.8)*
Also by Medicaid	11 *(2)*	2.0 *(0.3)*	Z *(Z)*	0.3 *(0.3)*	4 *(1)*	0.8 *(0.2)*	8 *(1)*	10.0 *(1.7)*
Covered by VA Care	19 *(2)*	3.4 *(0.3)*	Z *(Z)*	0.1 *(0.1)*	11 *(2)*	2.1 *(0.3)*	9 *(1)*	11.7 *(1.5)*
Not covered at any time during the year	77 *(5)*	13.4 *(0.9)*	8 *(2)*	5.7 *(1.1)*	77 *(5)*	15.4 *(1.0)*	Z *(Z)*	0.3 *(0.3)*

Note: Numbers in thousands; Figures cover 2013; Margin of error appears in parenthesis; A "Z" indicates that the value either represents or rounds to zero.
Source: U.S. Census Bureau, 2013 American Community Survey, Table HI05. Health Insurance Coverage Status and Type of Coverage by State and Age for All People: 2013

Wyoming

1207 Aetna Health of Wyoming

151 Farmington Avenue
Hartford, CT 06156
Toll-Free: 800-872-3862
Phone: 860-273-0123
www.aetna.com
Partnered with: eHealthInsurance Services Inc.
For Profit Organization: Yes
Total Enrollment: 11,596,230

Healthplan and Services Defined
  PLAN TYPE: PPO
  Other Type: POS
  Plan Specialty: EPO
  Benefits Offered: Dental, Disease Management, Long-Term Care,
    Prescription, Wellness, Life, LTD, STD

Type of Coverage
  Commercial, Individual

Type of Payment Plans Offered
  POS, FFS

Geographic Areas Served
  Statewide

Key Personnel
  Chairman/CEO/President. .Mark T Bertolini
  EVP/General Counsel . . . . .William J Casazza
  EVP/CFO . . . . .Shawn M Guertin

1208 Blue Cross & Blue Shield of Wyoming

4000 House Avenue
Cheyenne, WY 82001
Toll-Free: 800-442-2376
Phone: 307-634-1393
Fax: 307-634-5742
www.bcbswy.com
Mailing Address: PO Box 2266, Cheyenne, WY 82003
Non-Profit Organization: Yes
Year Founded: 1976
Total Enrollment: 100,000
State Enrollment: 100,000

Healthplan and Services Defined
  PLAN TYPE: PPO
  Benefits Offered: Disease Management, Physical Therapy, Wellness

Type of Coverage
  Commercial, Individual, Medicare, Medicaid

Type of Payment Plans Offered
  FFS

Geographic Areas Served
  Wyoming

Key Personnel
  President & CEO. . . . . .Rick Schum
  Sales Representative. . . . . .Granger Gallegos

Specialty Managed Care Partners
  Prime Therapeutics

Employer References
  Tricare

1209 CIGNA HealthCare of Wyoming

3900 East Mexico Avenue
#1100
Denver, CO 80210
Phone: 303-782-1500
Fax: 303-691-3197
www.cigna.com

For Profit Organization: Yes
Total Enrollment: 11,234
State Enrollment: 3,334

Healthplan and Services Defined
  PLAN TYPE: PPO
  Plan Specialty: Behavioral Health, Dental, Vision
  Benefits Offered: Behavioral Health, Dental, Disease Management,
    Prescription, Transplant, Vision, Wellness, Life

Type of Coverage
  Commercial

Type of Payment Plans Offered
  POS, FFS

Geographic Areas Served
  Wyoming

Key Personnel
  Director At Cigna . . . . .Sallie Vanasdale
  VP Provider Realations . . . . .William Cetti
  VP Client Relations . . . . .Gregg Prussing

1210 Delta Dental of Wyoming

6234 Yellowstone Road
Cheyenne, WY 82009
Toll-Free: 800-735-3379
Phone: 307-632-3313
Fax: 307-632-7309
customerservice@deltadentalwy.org
www.deltadentalwy.org
Non-Profit Organization: Yes
Total Enrollment: 54,000,000

Healthplan and Services Defined
  PLAN TYPE: Dental
  Other Type: Dental PPO
  Model Type: Network
  Plan Specialty: ASO, Dental
  Benefits Offered: Dental

Type of Coverage
  Commercial, Individual, Group
  Catastrophic Illness Benefit: None

Geographic Areas Served
  Statewide

Subscriber Information
  Average Monthly Fee Per Subscriber
    (Employee + Employer Contribution):
      Employee Only (Self): Varies
      Employee & 1 Family Member: Varies
      Employee & 2 Family Members: Varies
  Average Annual Deductible Per Subscriber:
      Employee Only (Self): Varies
      Employee & 1 Family Member: Varies
      Employee & 2 Family Members: Varies
  Average Subscriber Co-Payment:
      Prescription Drugs: $0
      Home Health Care: $0
      Nursing Home: $0

Accreditation Certification
  URAC, NCQA

Key Personnel
  Executive Director. . . . . .Jeanne Thobro
  CEO . . . . .Kerry Hall

1211 eHealthInsurance Services Inc.

11919 Foundation Place
Gold River, CA 95670
Toll-Free: 800-644-3491
webmaster@healthinsurance.com
www.e.healthinsurance.com

Year Founded: 1997

Healthplan and Services Defined
  PLAN TYPE: HMO/PPO
  Benefits Offered: Dental, Life, STD

Type of Coverage
  Commercial, Individual, Medicare

Geographic Areas Served
  All 50 states in the USA and District of Columbia

Key Personnel
  Chairman & CEO . . . . .Gary L. Lauer
  EVP/Business & Corp. Dev. . . . . .Bruce Telkamp
  EVP/Chief Technology . . . . .Dr. Sheldon X. Wang
  SVP & CFO . . . . .Stuart M. Huizinga
  Pres. of eHealth Gov. Sys . . . . .Samuel C. Gibbs
  SVP of Sales & Operations . . . . .Robert S. Hurley
  Director Public Relations. . . . . .Nate Purpura
    650-210-3115

1212   Humana Health Insurance of Wyoming
1611 Alderson Avenue
Billings, MT 59102
Toll-Free: 800-967-2308
Phone: 406-238-7130
www.humana.com
For Profit Organization: Yes

Healthplan and Services Defined
  PLAN TYPE: HMO/PPO

Type of Coverage
  Commercial, Individual

Accreditation Certification
  URAC, NCQA, CORE

1213   UnitedHealthCare of Wyoming
6465 S Greenwood Plaza Boulevard
Suite 300
Centennial, CO 80111
Toll-Free: 866-574-6088
www.uhc.com
Subsidiary of: UnitedHealth Group
For Profit Organization: Yes
Year Founded: 1986
Number of Affiliated Hospitals: 47
Number of Primary Care Physicians: 1,600
Number of Referral/Specialty Physicians: 3,500
Total Enrollment: 75,000,000
State Enrollment: 21,919

Healthplan and Services Defined
  PLAN TYPE: HMO/PPO
  Model Type: Mixed Model
  Plan Specialty: MSO
  Benefits Offered: Behavioral Health, Chiropractic, Complementary
    Medicine, Dental, Disease Management, Home Care, Inpatient
    SNF, Long-Term Care, Physical Therapy, Podiatry, Prescription,
    Psychiatric, Transplant, Vision, Wellness, AD&D, Life

Type of Coverage
  Commercial, Individual, Medicaid, Commercial Group

Type of Payment Plans Offered
  DFFS, FFS, Combination FFS & DFFS

Geographic Areas Served
  Statewide

Subscriber Information
  Average Monthly Fee Per Subscriber
    (Employee + Employer Contribution):
      Employee Only (Self): Varies
  Average Subscriber Co-Payment:
    Primary Care Physician: $10

Prescription Drugs: $10/15/30
Hospital ER: $50

Network Qualifications
  Pre-Admission Certification: Yes

Peer Review Type
  Case Management: Yes

Publishes and Distributes Report Card: Yes

Accreditation Certification
  URAC, NCQA
  State Licensure, Quality Assurance Program

Average Claim Compensation
  Physician's Fees Charged: 70%
  Hospital's Fees Charged: 55%

Specialty Managed Care Partners
  United Behavioral Health
  Enters into Contracts with Regional Business Coalitions: No

1214   WINhealth Partners
1200 East 20th Street
Cheyenne, WY 82001
Phone: 307-773-1300
service@winhealthpartners.org
www.winhealthpartners.org
Non-Profit Organization: Yes
Year Founded: 1996
Total Enrollment: 11,000
State Enrollment: 9,864

Healthplan and Services Defined
  PLAN TYPE: Multiple
  Plan Specialty: Lab, Radiology
  Benefits Offered: Behavioral Health, Chiropractic, Disease
    Management, Home Care, Inpatient SNF, Physical Therapy,
    Prescription, Vision, Wellness, Durable Medical Equipment

Type of Coverage
  Individual, Medicare

Subscriber Information
  Average Monthly Fee Per Subscriber
    (Employee + Employer Contribution):
      Medicare: Varies
  Average Annual Deductible Per Subscriber:
    Employee Only (Self): $500.00
    Medicare: Varies
  Average Subscriber Co-Payment:
    Primary Care Physician: $20.00
    Prescription Drugs: $10/15/40
    Hospital ER: $75.00

Peer Review Type
  Case Management: Yes

Publishes and Distributes Report Card: Yes

Accreditation Certification
  TJC, NCQA

Key Personnel
  President/CEO . . . . .Stephen K. Goldstone
  Chief Financial Officer . . . . .Lonny Warren
  Medical Director. . . . . .Kirk Shamley, MD
  General Counsel. . . . . .Fran Kline
  Sales Executive. . . . . .Sharon Roberts-Meyer

Employer References
  United Medical Center, Wyoming Employees Federal Credit Union

Appendix A: Glossary of Terms

A

Access
A person's ability to obtain healthcare services.

Acute Care
Medical treatment rendered to people whose illnesses or medical problems are short-term or don't require long-term continuing care. Acute care facilities are hospitals that mainly treat people with short-term health problems.

Aggregate Indemnity
The maximum amount of payment provided by an insurer for each covered service for a group of insured people.

Aid to Families with Dependent Children (AFDC)
A state-based federal assistance program that provided cash payments to needy children (and their caretakers), who met certain income requirements. AFDC has now been replaced by a new block grant program, but the requirements, or criteria, can still be used for determining eligibility for Medicaid.

Alliance
Large businesses, small businesses, and individuals who form a group for insurance coverage.

All-payer System
A proposed healthcare system in which, no matter who is paying, prices for health services and payment methods are the same. Federal or state government, a private insurance company, a self-insured employer plan, an individual, or any other payer would pay the same rates. Also called Multiple Payer system.

Ambulatory Care
All health services that are provided on an out-patient basis, that don't require overnight care. Also called out-patient care.

Ancillary Services
Supplemental services, including laboratory, radiology and physical therapy, that are provided along with medical or hospital care.

B

Beneficiary
A person who is eligible for or receiving benefits under an insurance policy or plan.

Benefits
The services that members are entitled to receive based on their health plan.

Blue Cross/Blue Shield
Non-profit, tax-exempt insurance service plans that cover hospital care, physician care and related services. Blue Cross and Blue Shield are separate organizations that have different benefits, premiums and policies. These organizations are in all states, and The Blue Cross and Blue Shield Association of America is their national organization.

Board Certified
Status granted to a medical specialist who completes required training and passes and examination in his/her specialized area. Individuals who have met all requirements, but have not completed the exam are referred to as "board eligible."

Board Eligible
Reference to medical specialists who have completed all required training but have not completed the exam in his/her specialized area.

C

Cafeteria Plan
This benefit plan gives employees a set amount of funds that they can choose to spend on a different benefit options, such as health insurance or retirement savings

Capitation
A fixed prepayment, per patient covered, to a healthcare provider to deliver medical services to a particular group of patients. The payment is the same no matter how many services or what type of services each patient actually gets. Under capitation, the provider is financially responsible.

Care Guidelines
A set of medical treatments for a particular condition or group of patients that has been reviewed and endorsed by a national organization, such as the Agency for Healthcare Policy Research.

Carrier
A private organization, usually an insurance company, that finances healthcare.

Carve-out
Medical services that are separated out and contracted for independently from any other benefits.

Case management
Intended to improve health outcomes or control costs, services and education are tailored to a patient's needs, which are designed to improve health outcomes and/or control costs

Catastrophic Health Insurance
Health insurance that provides coverage for treating severe or lengthy illnesses or disability.

CHAMPUS
(Civilian Health and Medical Program of the Uniformed Services) A health plan that serves the dependents of active duty military personnel and retired military personnel and their dependents.

Chronic Care
Treatment given to people whose health problems are long-term and continuing. Nu nursing homes, mental hospitals and rehabilitation facilities are chronic care facilities.

Chronic Disease
A medical problem that will not improve, that lasts a lifetime, or recurs.

Claims

Bills for services. Doctors, hospitals, labs and other providers send billed claims to health insurance plans, and what the plans pay are called paid claims.

COBRA

(Consolidated Omnibus Budget Reconciliation Act of 1985) Designed to provide health coverage to workers between jobs, this legal act lets workers who leave a company buy health insurance from that company at the employer's group rate rather than an individual rate.

Co-insurance

A cost-sharing requirement under some health insurance policies in which the insured person pays some of the costs of covered services.

Cooperatives/Co-ops

HMOs that are managed by the members of the health plan or insurance purchasing arrangements in which businesses or other groups join together to gain the buying power of large employers or groups.

Co-pay

Flat fees or payments (often $5-10) that a patient pays for each doctor visit or prescription.

Cost Containment

The method of preventing healthcare costs from increasing beyond a set level by controlling or reducing inefficiency and waste in the healthcare system.

Cost Sharing

An insurance policy requires the insured person to pay a portion of the costs of covered services. Deductibles, co-insurance and co-payments are cost sharing.

Cost Shifting

When one group of patients does not pay for services, such as uninsured or Medicare patients, healthcare providers pass on the costs for these health services to other groups of patients.

Coverage

A person's healthcare costs are paid by their insurance or by the government..

Covered services

Treatments or other services for which a health plan pays at least part of the charge.

D

Deductible

The amount of money, or value of certain services (such as one physician visit), a patient or family must pay before costs (or percentages of costs) are covered by the health plan or insurance company, usually per year.

Diagnostic related groups (DRGs)

A system for classifying hospital stays according to the diagnosis of the medical problem being treated, for the purposes of payment.

Direct access

The ability to see a doctor or receive a medical service without a referral from your primary care physician.

Disease management

Programs for people who have chronic illnesses, such as asthma or diabetes, that try to encourage them to have a healthy lifestyle, to take medications as prescribed, and that coordinate care.

Disposable Personal Income

The amount of a person's income that is left over after money has been spent on basic necessities such as rent, food, and clothing.

E

Early and Periodic Screening, Diagnosis, and Treatment Program (EPSDT)

As part of the Medicaid program, the law requires that all states have a program for eligible children under age 21 to receive a medical assessment, medical treatments and other measures to correct any problems and treat chronic conditions.

Elective

A healthcare procedure that is not an emergency and that the patient and doctor plan in advance.

Emergency

A medical condition that starts suddenly and requires immediate care.

Employee Retirement Income Security Act (ERISA)

A Federal act, passed in 1974, that established new standards for employer-funded health benefit and pension programs. Companies that have self-funded health benefit plans operating under ERISA are not subject to state insurance regulations and healthcare legislation.

Employer Contribution

The contribution is the money a company pays for its employees' healthcare. Exclusions
Health conditions that are explicitly not covered in an insurance package and that your insurance will not pay for.

Exclusive Provider Organizations (EPO)/Exclusive Provider Arrangement (EPA)

An indemnity or service plan that provides benefits only if those hospitals or doctors with which it contracts provide the medical services, with some exceptions for emergency and out-of-area services.

F

Federal Employee Health Benefit Program (FEP)

Health insurance program for Federal workers and their dependents, established in 1959 under the Federal Employees Health Benefits Act. Federal employees may choose to participate in one of two or more plans.

Fee-for-Service

Physicians or other providers bill separately for each patient encounter or service they provide. This method of billing means the insurance company pays all or some set percentage of the fees that hospitals and doctors set and charge. Expenditures increase if the increaseThis is still the main system of paying for healthcare services in the United States.

First Dollar Coverage
A system in which the insurer pays for all employee out-of-pocket healthcare costs. Under first dollar coverage, the beneficiary has no deductible and no co-payments.

Flex plan
An account that lets workers set aside pretax dollars to pay for medical benefits, childcare, and other services.

Formulary
A list of medications that a managed care company encourages or requires physicians to prescribe as necessary in order to reduce costs.

G

Gag clause
A contractual agreement between a managed care organization and a provider that restricts what the provider can say about the managed care company

Gatekeeper
The person in a managed care organization, often a primary care provider, who controls a patient's access to healthcare services and whose approval is required for referrals to other services or other specialists.

General Practice
Physicians without specialty training who provide a wide range of primary healthcare services to patients.

Global Budgeting
A way of containing hospital costs in which participating hospitals share a budget, agreeing together to set the maximum amount of money that will be paid for healthcare.

Group Insurance
Health insurance offered through business, union trusts or other groups and associations. The most common system of health insurance in the United States, in which the cost of insurance is based on the age, sex, health status and occupation of the people in the group.

Group model HMO
An HMO that contracts with an independent group practice to provide medical services

Guaranteed Issue
The requirement that an insurance plan accept everyone who applies for coverage and guarantee the renewal of that coverage as long as the covered person pays the policy premium.

H

Healthcare Benefits
The specific services and procedures covered by a health plan or insurer.

Healthcare Financing Administration (HCFA)
The federal government agency within the Department of Health and Human Services that directs the Medicare and Medicaid programs. HCFA also does research to support these programs and oversees more than a quarter of all healthcare costs in the United States.

Health Insurance
Financial protection against the healthcare costs caused by treating disease or accidental injury.

Health Insurance Portability and Accountability Act (HIPAA)
Also known as Kennedy-Kassebaum law, this guarantees that people who lose their group health insurance will have access to individual insurance, regardless of pre-existing medical problems. The law also allows employees to secure health insurance from their new employer when they switch jobs even if they have a pre-existing medical condition.

Health Insurance Purchasing Cooperatives (HIPCs)
Public or private organizations that get health insurance coverage for certain populations of people, combining everyone in a specific geographic region and basing insurance rates on the people in that area.

Health Maintenance Organization (HMO)
A health plan provides comprehensive medical services to its members for a fixed, prepaid premium. Members must use participating providers and are enrolled for a fixed period of time. HMOs can do business either on a for-profit or not-for-profit basis.

Health Plan Employer Data and Information Set (HEDIS)
Performance measures designed by the National Committee for Quality Assurance to give participating managed health plans and employers to information about the value of their healthcare and trends in their health plan performance compared with other health plans.

Home healthcare
Skilled nurses and trained aides who provide nursing services and related care to someone at home.

Hospice Care
Care given to terminally ill patients. Hospital Alliances Groups of hospitals that join together to cut their costs by purchasing services and equipment in volume.

I

Indemnity Insurance
A system of health insurance in which the insurer pays for the costs of covered services after care has been given, and which usually defines the maximum amounts which will be paid for covered services. This is the most common type of insurance in the United States.

Independent Practice Association (IPA)
A group of private physicians who join together in an association to contract with a managed care organization.

Indigent Care
Care provided, at no cost, to people who do not have health insurance or are not covered by Medicare, Medicaid, or other public programs.

In-patient
A person who has been admitted to a hospital or other health facility, for a period of at least 24 hours.

Integrated Delivery System (IDS)
An organization that usually includes a hospital, a large medical group, and an insurer such as an HMO or PPO.

Integrated Provider (IP)
A group of providers that offer comprehensive and coordinated care, and usually provides a range of medical care facilities and service plans including hospitals, group practices, a health plan and other related healthcare services.

J

Joint Commission on the Accreditation of Healthcare Organizations (JCAHO)
A national private, non-profit organization that accredits healthcare organizations and agencies and sets guidelines for operation for these facilities.

L

Limitations
A "cap" or limit on the amount of services that may be provided. It may be the maximum cost or number of days that a service or treatment is covered.

Limited Service Hospital
A hospital, often located in a rural area, that provides a limited set of medical and surgical services.

Long-term Care
Healthcare, personal care and social services provided to people who have a chronic illness or disability and do not have full functional capacity. This care can take place in an institution or at home, on a long-term basis.

M

Malpractice Insurance
Coverage for medical professionals which pays the costs of legal fees and/or any damages assessed by the court in a lawsuit brought against a professional who has been charged with negligence.

Managed care
This term describes many types of health insurance, including HMOs and PPOs. They control the use of health services by their members so that they can contain healthcare costs and/or improve the quality of care.

Mandate
Law requiring that a health plan or insurance carrier must offer a particular procedure or type of coverage.

Means Test
An assessment of a person's or family's income or assets so that it can be determined if they are eligible to receive public support, such as Medicaid.

Medicaid
An insurance program for people with low incomes who are unable to afford healthcare. Although funded by the federal government, Medicaid is administered by each state. Following very broad federal guidelines, states determine specific benefits and amounts of payment for providers.

Medical IRAs
Personal accounts which, like individual retirement plans, allow a person to accumulate funds for future use. The money in these accounts must be used to pay for medical services. The employee decides how much money he or she will spend on healthcare.

Medically Indigent
A person who does not have insurance and is not covered by Medicaid, Medicare or other public programs.

Medicare
A federal program of medical care benefits created in 1965 designed for those over age 65 or permanently disabled. Medicare consists of two separate programs: A and B. Medicare Part A, which is automatic at age 65, covers hospital costs and is financed largely by employer payroll taxes. Medicare Part B covers outpatient care and is financed through taxes and individual payments toward a premium.

Medicare Supplements or Medigap
A privately-purchased health insurance policy available to Medicare beneficiaries to cover costs of care that Medicare does not pay. Some policies cover additional costs, such as preventive care, prescription drugs, or at-home care.

Member
The person enrolled in a health plan.

N

National Committee on Quality Assurance (NCQA)
An independent national organization that reviews and accredits managed care plans and measures the quality of care offered by managed care plans.

Network
A group of affiliated contracted healthcare providers (physicians, hospitals, testing centers, rehabilitation centers etc.), such as an HMO, PPO, or Point of Service plan.

Non-contributory Plan
A group insurance plan that requires no payment from employees for their healthcare coverage.

Non-participating Provider
A healthcare provider who is not part of a health plan. Usually patients must pay their own healthcare costs to see a non-participating provider.

Nurse practitioner
A nurse specialist who provides primary and/or specialty care to patients. In some states nurse practitioners do not have to be supervised by a doctor.

O

Open Enrollment Period
A specified period of time during which people are allowed to change health plans.

Open Panel
A right included in an HMO, which allows the covered person to get non-emergency covered services from a specialist without getting a referral from the primary care physician or gatekeeper.

Out of Pocket costs or expenditures
The amount of money that a person must pay for his or her healthcare, including: deductibles, co-pays, payments for services that are not covered, and/or health insurance premiums that are not paid by his or her employer.

Outcomes
Measures of the effectiveness of particular kinds of medical treatment. This refers to what is quantified to determine if a specific treatment or type of service works.

Out of Pocket Maximum
The maximum amount that a person must pay under a plan or insurance contract.

Outpatient Care
Healthcare services that do not require a patient to receive overnight care in a hospital.

P

Participating Physician or Provider
Healthcare providers who have contracted with a managed care plan to provide eligible healthcare services to members of that plan.

Payer
The organization responsible for the costs of healthcare services. A payer may be private insurance, the government, or an employer's self-funded plan.

Peer Review Organization (PRO or PSRO)
An agency that monitors the quality and appropriateness of medical care delivered to Medicare and Medicaid patients. Healthcare professionals in these agencies review other professionals with similar training and experience. [See Quality Improvement Organizations]

Percent of Poverty
A term that describes the income level a person or family must have to be eligible for Medicaid.

Physician Assistant
A health professional who provides primary and/or specialty care to patients under the supervision of a physician.

Physician Hospital Organizations (PHOs)
An organization that contracts with payers on behalf of one or more hospitals and affiliated physicians. Physicians still own their practices.

Play or Pay
This system would provide coverage for all people by requiring employers either to provide health insurance for their employees and dependents (play) or pay a contribution to a publicly-provided system that covers uninsured or unemployed people without private insurance (pay).

Point of Service (POS)
A type of insurance where each time healthcare services are needed, the patient can choose from different types of provider systems (indemnity plan, PPO or HMO). Usually, members are required to pay more to see PPO or non-participating providers than to see HMO providers.

Portability
A person's ability to keep his or her health coverage during times of change in health status or personal situation (such as change in employment or unemployment, marriage or divorce) or while moving between health plans.

Postnatal Care
Healthcare services received by a woman immediately following the delivery of her child

Pre-authorization
The process where, before a patient can be admitted to the hospital or receive other types of specialty services, the managed care company must approve of the proposed service in order to cover it.

Pre-existing Condition
A medical condition or diagnosis that began before coverage began under a current plan or insurance contract. The insurance company may provide coverage but will specifically exclude treatment for such a condition from that person's coverage for a certain period of time, often six months to a year.

Preferred Provider Organization (PPO)
A type of insurance in which the managed care company pays a higher percentage of the costs when a preferred (in-plan) provider is used. The participating providers have agreed to provide their services at negotiated discount fees.

Premium
The amount paid periodically to buy health insurance coverage. Employers and employees usually share the cost of premiums.

Premium Cap
The maximum amount of money an insurance company can charge for coverage.

Premium Tax
A state tax on insurance premiums.

Prepaid Group Practice
A type of HMO where participating providers receive a fixed payment in advance for providing particular healthcare services.

Preventive Care

Healthcare services that prevent disease or its consequences. It includes primary prevention to keep people from getting sick (such as immunizations), secondary prevention to detect early disease (such as Pap smears) and tertiary prevention to keep ill people or those at high risk of disease from getting sicker (such as helping someone with lung disease to quit smoking).

Primary Care

Basic or general routine office medical care, usually from an internist, obstetrician-gynecologist, family practitioner, or pediatrician.

Primary care provider (PCP)

The health professional who provides basic healthcare services. The PCP may control patients' access to the rest of the healthcare system through referrals.

Private Insurance

Health insurance that is provided by insurance companies such as commercial insurers and Blue Cross plans, self-funded plans sponsored by employers, HMOs or other managed care arrangements.

Provider

An individual or institution who provides medical care, including a physician, hospital, skilled nursing facility, or intensive care facility.

Provider-Sponsored Organization (PSO)

Healthcare providers (physicians and/or hospitals) who form an affiliation to act as insurer for an enrolled population.

Q

Quality Assessment

Measurement of the quality of care.

Quality Assurance and Quality Improvement

A systematic process to improve quality of healthcare by monitoring quality, finding out what is not working, and fixing the problems of healthcare delivery.

Quality Improvement Organization (QIO)

An organization contracting with HCFA to review the medical necessity and quality of care provided to Medicare beneficiaries.

Quality of care

How well health services result in desired health outcomes.

R

Rate Setting

These programs were developed by several states in the 1970's to establish in advance the amount that hospitals would be paid no matter how high or low their costs actually were in any particular year. (Also known as hospital rate setting or prospective reimbursement programs)

Referral system

The process through which a primary care provider authorizes a patient to see a specialist to receive additional care.

Reimbursement

The amount paid to providers for services they provide to patients.

Risk

The responsibility for profiting or losing money based on the cost of healthcare services provided. Traditionally, health insurance companies have carried the risk. Under capitation, healthcare providers bear risk.

S

Self-insured

A type of insurance arrangement where employers, usually large employers, pay for medical claims out of their own funds rather than contracting with an insurance company for coverage. This puts the employer at risk for its employees' medical expenses rather than an insurance company.

Single Payer System

A healthcare reform proposal in which healthcare costs are paid by taxes rather than by the employer and employee. All people would have coverage paid by the government.

Socialized Medicine

A healthcare system in which providers are paid by the government, and healthcare facilities are run by the government.

Staff Model HMO

A type of managed care where physicians are employees of the health plan, usually in the health plan's own health center or facility.

Standard Benefit Package

A defined set of benefits provided to all people covered under a health plan.

T

Third Party Administrator (TPA)

An organization that processes health plan claims but does not carry any insurance risk.

Third Party Payer

An organization other than the patient or healthcare provider involved in the financing of personal health services.

U

Uncompensated Care

Healthcare provided to people who cannot pay for it and who are not covered by any insurance. This includes both charity care which is not billed and the cost of services that were billed but never paid.

Underinsured

People who have some type of health insurance but not enough insurance to cover their the cost of necessary healthcare. This includes people who have very high deductibles of $1000 to $5000 per year, or insurance policies that have specific exclusions for costly services.

Underwriting

This process is the basis of insurance. It analyzes the health status and history, claims experience (cost), age and general health risks of the individual or group who is applying for insurance coverage.

Uninsured

People who do not have health insurance of any type. Over 80 percent of the uninsured are working adults and their family members.

Universal Coverage

This refers to the proposal that all people could get health insurance, regardless of the way that the system is financed.

Utilization Review

A program designed to help reduce unnecessary medical expenses by studying the appropriateness of when certain services are used and by how many patients they are used.

Utilization

How many times people use particular healthcare services during particular periods of time.

V

Vertical Integration

A healthcare system that includes the entire range of healthcare services from out-patient to hospital and long-term care.

W

Waiting Period

The amount of time a person must wait from the date he or she is accepted into a health plan (or from when he or she applies) until the insurance becomes effective and he or she can receive benefits.

Withhold

A percentage of providers' fees that managed care companies hold back from providers which is only given to them if the amount of care they provide (or that the entire plan provides) is under a budgeted amount for each quarter or the whole year.

Worker's Compensation Coverage

States require employers to provide coverage to compensate employees for work-related injuries or disabilities.

Source: Public Broadcasting Service, http://www.pbs.org/ healthcarecrisis/glossary.htm. Reprinted with permission of www.issuestv.com and www.pbs.com.

Appendix B: Industry Websites

Alliance of Community Health Plans (ACHP)

http://www.achp.org

Offers information on health care so that it is safe, effective, patient-centered, timely, efficient and equitable. Members use this web site to collaborate, share strategies and work toward solutions to some of health care's biggest challenges.

America's Health Insurance Plans (AHIP)

http://www.ahip.org

AHIP is a national trade association representing nearly 1,300 member companies providing health insurance coverage to more than 200 million Americans.

American Academy of Medical Administrators (AAMA)

http://www.aameda.org

Supports individuals involved in medical administration at the executive - or middle-management levels. Promotes educational courses for the training of persons in medical administration. Conducts research. Offers placement service.

American Accreditation Healthcare Commission/URAC

http://www.urac.org

URAC (Utilization Review Accreditation Commission) is a 501(c)(3) non-profit charitable organization founded in 1990 to establish standards for the managed care industry. URAC's broad-based membership includes representation from all the constituencies affected by managed care - employers, consumers, regulators, health care providers, and the workers' compensation and managed care industries.

American Association of Healthcare Administrative Management (AAHAM)

http://www.aaham.org

A professional organization in healthcare administrative management that offers information, education and advocacy in the areas of reimbursement, admitting and registration, data management, medical records, patient relations and more. Founded in 1968, AAHAM represents a broad-based constituency of healthcare professionals through a comprehensive program of legislative and regulatory monitoring and its participation in industry groups such as ANSI, DISA and NUBC.

American Association of Integrated Healthcare Delivery Systems (AAIHDS)

http://www.aaihds.org

AAIHDS was founded in 1993 as a non-profit organization dedicated to the educational advancement of provider-based managed care professionals involved in integrated healthcare delivery.

American Association of Preferred Provider Organizations (AAPPO)

http://www.aappo.org

A national association of preferred provider organizations (PPOs) and affiliate organizations, established in 1983 to advance awareness of the benefits - greater access, choice and flexibility - that PPOs bring to American health care.

American College of Health Care Administrators (ACHCA)

http://achca.org

Founded in 1962, ACHCA provides superior educational programming, professional certification, and career development opportunities for its members. It identifies, recognizes, and supports long term care leaders, advocating for their mission and promoting excellence in their profession.

American College of Healthcare Executives (ACHE)

http://www.ache.org

International professional society of more than 30,000 healthcare executives, including credentialing and educational programs and sponsors the Congress on Healthcare Management. ACHE's publishing division, Health Administration Press, is one of the largest publishers of books.

American College of Physician Executives (ACPE)

http://www.acpe.org

Supports physicians whose primary professional responsibility is the management of healthcare organizations. Provides for continuing education and certification of the physician executive. Offers specialized career planning, counseling, recruitment and placement services, and research and information data on physician managers.

American Health Care Association (AHCA)

http://www.ahcancal.org

A non-profit federation of affiliated state health organizations, representing more than 10,000 non-profit and for-profit assisted living, nursing facility, developmentally-disabled, and subacute care providers that care for more than 1.5 million elderly and disabled individuals nationally.

American Health Planning Association (AHPA)

http://www.ahpanet.org

A non-profit public interest organization that brings together individuals and organizations interested in the availability, affordability and equitable distribution of health services. AHPA supports community participation in health policy formulation and in the organization and operation of local health services.

American Health Quality Association (AHQA)

http://www.ahqa.org

The American Health Quality Association represents Quality Improvement Organizations (QIOs) and professionals working to improve the quality of health care in communities across America. QIOs share information about best practices with physicians, hospitals, nursing homes, home health agencies, and others. Working together with health care providers, QIOs identify opportunities and provide assistance for improvement.

American Medical Association (AMA)

http://www.ama-assn.org

Founded more than 150 years ago, the AMA's work includes the development and promotion of standards in medical practice, research, and education. This site offers medical information for physicians, medical students, other health professionals, and patients.

American Medical Directors Association (AMDA)

http://www.amda.com

A professional association of medical directors, attending physicians, and others practicing in the long term care continuum, that provides education, advocacy, information, and professional development to promote the delivery of quality long term care medicine.

American Medical Group Association (AMGA)

http://www.amga.org

Association that supports various medical groups and organized systems of care at the national level.

Association of Family Medicine Residency Directors (AFMRD)

http://www.afmrd.org

Provides representation for residency directors at a national level and provides a political voice for them to appropriate arenas. Promotes cooperation and communication between residency programs and different branches of the family medicine specialty. Dedicated to improving of education of family physicians. Provides a network for mutual assistance among FP, residency directors.

Association of Family Practice Administrators (AFPA)

http://www.uams.edu/afpa/afpa1.htm

Promotes professionalism in family practice administration. Serves as a network for sharing of information and fellowship among members. Provides technical assistance to members and functions as a liaison to related professional organizations.

Association of Healthcare Internal Auditors (AHIA)

http://www.ahia.org

Promotes cost containment and increased productivity in health care institutions through internal auditing. Serves as a forum for the exchange of experience, ideas, and information among members; provides continuing professional education courses and informs members of developments in health care internal auditing. Offers employment clearinghouse services.

Case Management Society of America (CMSA)

http://www.cmsa.org

Information for the case management profession.

Centers for Medicare and Medicaid Services (CMS)

http://cms.hhs.gov

Formerly known as the Health Care Financing Administration (HCFA), this is the federal agency that administers Medicare, Medicaid and the State Children's Health Insurance Program (SCHIP). CMS provides health insurance for over 74 million Americans through these programs.

College of Healthcare Information Management Executives (CHIME)

http://www.cio-chime.org

Serves the professional development needs of healthcare CIOs, and advocating the more effective use of information management within healthcare.

Electronic Healthcare Network Accreditation Commission (EHNAC)

http://www.ehnac.org

A federally-recognized standards development organization and non-profit accrediting body designed to improve transactional quality, operational efficiency and data security in healthcare.

Healthcare Financial Management Association (HFMA)

http://www.hfma.org

HFMA is a membership organization for healthcare financial management executives and leaders. The association brings perspective and clarity to the industry's complex issues for the purpose of preparing members to succeed. Programs, publications and partnerships enhance the capabilities that strengthen not only individuals careers, but also the organizations from which members come.

Healthcare Information and Management Systems Society (HIMSS)

http://www.himss.org

The healthcare industry's membership organization exclusively focused on providing global leadership for the optimal use of healthcare information technology (IT) and management systems. HIMSS represents more than 20,000 individual members and over 300 corporate members leads healthcare public policy and industry practices through its advocacy, educational and professional development initiatives designed to promote information and management systems' contributions to ensuring quality patient care.

Healthfinder.gov

http://www.healthfinder.gov

A comprehensive guide to resources for health information from the federal government and related agencies.

The Joint Commission (JC)

http://www.jointcommission.org

An independent, not-for-profit organization, JC accredits and certifies more than 15,000 health care organizations and programs in the United States which is recognized nationwide as a symbol of quality that reflects an organization's commitment to meeting certain performance standards.

Managed Care Information Center (MCIC)

http://www.managedcaremarketplace.com

An online yellow pages for companies providing services to Managed Care Organizations (MCO), hospitals and physician groups. There are more than three dozen targeted categories, offering information on vendors from claims processing to transportation services to health care compliance.

National Association for Healthcare Quality (NAHQ)

http://www.nahq.org

Provides vital research, education, networking, certification and professional practice resources, designed to empower healthcare quality professionals from every specialty. This leading resource for healthcare quality professionals is an essential connection for leadership, excellence and innovation in healthcare quality.

National Association for Health Care Recruitment (NAHCR)

http://www.nahcr.com

Supports individuals employed directly by hospitals and other health care organizations which are involved in the practice of professional health care recruitment. Promotes sound principles of professional healthcare recruitment. Provides financial assistance to aid members in planning and implementing regional educational programs. Offers technical assistance and consultation services. Compiles statistics.

National Association Medical Staff Services (NAMSS)

http://www.namss.org

Supports individuals involved in the management and administration of health care provider services. Seeks to enhance the knowledge and experience of medical staff services professionals and promote the certification of those involved in the profession.

National Association of Dental Plans (NADP)

http://www.nadp.org

Promotes and advances the dental benefits industry to improve consumer access to affordable, quality dental care.

National Association of Insurance Commissoners (NAIC)
http://www.naic.org
The mission of the NAIC is to assist state insurance regulators, individually and collectively, in serving the public interest and achieving the following fundamental insurance regulatory goals in a responsive, efficient and cost effective manner, consistent with the wishes of its members: protect the public interest; promote competitive markets; facilitate the fair and equitable treatment of insurance consumers; promote the reliability, solvency and financial solidity of insurance institutions; and support and improve state regulation of insurance.
The NAIC also provides links to State Insurance Department web sites *(http://www.naic.org/state_web_map.htm)*.

The National Association of Managed Care Regulators (NAMCR)
http://www.namcr.org
Includes both regulator members and associate industry members. Established in 1975, NAMCR provides expertise and a forum for discussion to state regulators and managed care companies about current issues facing managed care. NAMCR has also provided expertise to the National Association of Insurance Commissioners (NAIC) in preparation of NAIC Model Acts used by many states.

National Association of State Medicaid Directors (NASMD)
http://www.nasmd.org
Promotes effective Medicaid policy and program administration; works with the federal government on issues through technical advisory groups. Conducts forums on policy and technical issues.

National Committee for Quality Assurance (NCQA)
http://www.ncqa.org
The National Committee for Quality Assurance (NCQA) is a private, not-for-profit organization dedicated to assessing and reporting on the quality of managed care plans. Their efforts are organized around two activities, accreditation and performance measurement, which are complementary strategies for producing information to guide choice.

National Institute for Health Care Management Research and Educational Foundation (NIHCM Foundation)
http://www.nihcm.org

A nonprofit, nonpartisan group that conducts research on health care issues. The Foundation disseminates research findings and analysis and holds forums and briefings for policy makers, the health care industry, consumers, the government, and the media to increase understanding of issues affecting the health care system.

National Quality Forum (NQF)
http://www.qualityforum.org
A not-for-profit membership organization created to develop and implement a national strategy for health care quality measurement and reporting, Prompted by the impact of health care quality on patient outcomes, workforce productivity, and health care costs. NQF has broad participation from all parts of the health care system, including national, state, regional, and local groups representing consumers, public and private purchasers, employers, health care professionals, provider organizations.,health plans, accrediting bodies, labor unions, supporting industries, and organizations.

National Society of Certified Healthcare Business Consultants (NSCHBC)
http://www.ichbc.org
The NSCHBC is a national organization dedicated to serving the needs of consultants who provide ethical, confidential and professional advice to the healthcare industry. Membership by successful completion of certification examination only.

Professional Association of Health Care Office Management (PAHCOM)
http://www.pahcom.com
Supports office managers of small group and solo medical practices. Operates certification program for healthcare office managers.

U.S. Food and Drug Administration (USFDA)
http://www.fda.gov
A department of the U.S. Department of Health and Human Services, the Food and Drug Administration provides information regarding health, medicine and nutrition. Their MedWatch Safety Information and Adverse Event Reporting Program serves both healthcare professionals and the public. MedWatch provides clinical information about safety issues involving medical products, including prescription and over-the-counter drugs, biologics, dietary supplements, and medical devices *(http://www.fda.gov/medwatch)*.

Plan Index

Aetna Health of New Jersey Hartford, CT, 709
Aetna Health of Ohio Chicago, IL, 839
Aetna Health of Oklahoma Dallas, TX, 880
Aetna Health of Pennsylvania Hartford, CT, 922
Aetna Health of Tennessee Alpharetta, GA, 1021
Aetna Health of Texas Dallas, TX, 1041
Aetna Health of the Carolinas Alpharetta, GA, 809, 990
Aetna Health of Virginia Hartford, CT, 1119
Aetna Health, Inc. Corporate Headquarters Hartford, CT, 214
Affinity Health Plan Bronx, NY, 753
Alameda Alliance for Health Alameda, CA, 80
Allegiance Life & Health Insurance Company Missoula, MT, 660
Alliant Health Plans Kennesaw, GA, 305
AlohaCare Honolulu, HI, 330
American Denticare Little Rock, AR, 63
American Health Care Group Pittsburgh, PA, 923
American Postal Workers Union (APWU) Health Plan Glen Burnie, MD, 494
American Republic Insurance Company Des Moines, IA, 416
American Specialty Health San Diego, CA, 81
AmeriChoice by UnitedHealthcare Rocky Hill, CT, 216
AmeriChoice by UnitedHealthCare Newark, NJ, 710
AmeriChoice by UnitedHealthCare New York, NY, 754
Amerigroup Corporation Merrifield, VA, 1120
Amerigroup Florida Tampa, FL, 252
Amerigroup Georgia Atlanta, GA, 306
Amerigroup Maryland Hanover, MD, 495
Amerigroup Nevada Las Vegas, NV, 685
Amerigroup New Jersey Virginia Beach, VA, 712
Amerigroup New Mexico Albuquerque, NM, 738
Amerigroup New York New York, NY, 755
Amerigroup Ohio Blue Ash, OH, 840
Amerigroup Tennessee Nashville, TN, 1022
Amerigroup Texas Houston, TX, 1044
AmeriHealth HMO Wilmington, DE, 227
AmeriHealth HMO Cranbury, NJ, 713
Anthem Blue Cross & Blue Shield Connecticut North Haven, CT, 217
Anthem Blue Cross & Blue Shield of Colorado Denver, CO, 190
Anthem Blue Cross & Blue Shield of Indiana Indianapolis, IN, 388, 389
Anthem Blue Cross & Blue Shield of Kentucky Louisville, KY, 453
Anthem Blue Cross & Blue Shield of Maine S. Portland, ME, 485
Anthem Blue Cross & Blue Shield of Nevada Denver, CO, 191
Anthem Blue Cross & Blue Shield of New Hampshire Manchester, NH, 700
Anthem Blue Cross & Blue Shield of Virginia Richmond, VA, 1121
Anthem Blue Cross & Blue Shield of Wisconsin Waukesha, WI, 1180
Arcadian Health Plans Oakland, CA, 82
Arizona Physicians IPA Phoenix, AZ, 31
Arnett Health Plans Lafayette, IN, 391
Athens Area Health Plan Select Athens, GA, 308
Atlanticare Health Plans Egg Harbor Township, NJ, 715
Aultcare Corporation Canton, OH, 843
Avera Health Plans Sioux Falls, SD, 1010
AvMed Health Plan: Corporate Office Miami, FL, 254
AvMed Health Plan: Fort Lauderdale Fort Lauderdale, FL, 255
AvMed Health Plan: Gainesville Gainesville, FL, 256
AvMed Health Plan: Jacksonville Jacksonville, FL, 257
AvMed Health Plan: Orlando Maitland, FL, 258
AvMed Health Plan: Tampa Bay Tampa, FL, 259

Beech Street Corporation: Western Region Lake Forest, CA, 88
Behavioral Healthcare Options, Inc. Las Vegas, NV, 686
Blue Care Network of Michigan: Corporate Headquarters Southfield, MI, 546
Blue Care Network: Ann Arbor Ann Arbor, MI, 548
Blue Care Network: Flint Flint, MI, 549
Blue Care Network: Great Lakes, Muskegon Heights Grand Rapids, MI, 550
Blue Cross & Blue Shield of Alabama Birmingham, AL, 6
Blue Cross & Blue Shield of Arizona Phoenix, AZ, 34
Blue Cross & Blue Shield of Georgia Atlanta, GA, 310
Blue Cross & Blue Shield of Illinois Chicago, IL, 356
Blue Cross & Blue Shield of Kansas Topeka, KS, 433
Blue Cross & Blue Shield of Louisiana Baton Rouge, LA, 469
Blue Cross & Blue Shield of Massachusetts Boston, MA, 522
Blue Cross & Blue Shield of Minnesota St. Paul, MN, 595
Blue Cross & Blue Shield of Montana Helena, MT, 661

Blue Cross & Blue Shield of New Mexico Albuquerque, NM, 739
Blue Cross & Blue Shield of North Carolina Durham, NC, 811
Blue Cross & Blue Shield of Oklahoma Oklahoma City, OK, 882
Blue Cross & Blue Shield of Rhode Island Providence, RI, 981
Blue Cross & Blue Shield of South Carolina Columbia, SC, 992
Blue Cross & Blue Shield of Tennessee Chattanooga, TN, 1025
Blue Cross & Blue Shield of Texas Richardson, TX, 1048
Blue Cross & Blue Shield of Texas: Houston Houston, TX, 1049
Blue Cross & Blue Shield of Western New York Buffalo, NY, 756
Blue Cross of Idaho Health Service, Inc. Meridian, ID, 342
Blue Cross of Northeastern Pennsylvania Wilkes Barre, PA, 929
Blue Shield of California San Francisco, CA, 90
BlueChoice St. Louis, MO, 634
Bluegrass Family Health Lexington, KY, 454
BlueLincs HMO Tulsa, OK, 883
BlueShield of Northeastern New York Latham, NY, 757
Boston Medical Center Healthnet Plan , MA, 523
Brand New Day HMO Westminster, CA, 91

CalOptima Orange, CA, 95
Capital Blue Cross Harrisburg, PA, 932
Capital Health Plan Tallahassee, FL, 261
Cardinal Health Alliance Muncie, IN, 393
Care 1st Health Plan: Arizona Phoenix, AZ, 35
Care 1st Health Plan: California Monterey Park, CA, 96
Care Choices Farmington Hills, MI, 552
CareFirst Blue Cross & Blue Shield of Virginia Owings Mills, MD, 1122
CareFirst Blue Cross Blue Shield Washington, DC, 240
CarePlus Health Plans, Inc Doral, FL, 262
CareSource Dayton, OH, 844
CareSource: Michigan East Lansing, MI, 553
Carolina Care Plan Columbia, SC, 994
Catalyst Health Solutions Inc Rockville, MD, 498
CDPHP: Capital District Physicians' Health Plan Albany, NY, 759
CenCal Health: The Regional Health Authority Santa Barbara, CA, 98
Centene Corporation Saint Louis, MO, 635
Central California Alliance for Health Scotts Valley, CA, 99
CHA Health Lexington, KY, 455
Charter Oak Health Plan Hartford, CT, 218
Children's Mercy Pediatric Care Network Kansas City, MO, 636
Chinese Community Health Plan San Francisco, CA, 101
CIGNA HealthCare of Alaska Denver, CO, 21
CIGNA HealthCare of Arizona Bloomfield, AZ, 36
CIGNA HealthCare of Arkansas Memphis, TN, 67
CIGNA HealthCare of California Glendale, CA, 104
CIGNA HealthCare of Colorado Denver, CO, 196
CIGNA HealthCare of Connecticut Hartford, CT, 219
CIGNA HealthCare of Delaware Bluebell, PA, 228
CIGNA HealthCare of Florida Lake Mary, FL, 263
CIGNA HealthCare of Georgia Atlanta, GA, 311
CIGNA HealthCare of Hawaii San Francisco, CA, 331
CIGNA HealthCare of Illinois Chicago, IL, 359
CIGNA HealthCare of Indiana Carmel, IN, 394
CIGNA HealthCare of Iowa Chicago, IL, 418
CIGNA HealthCare of Kansas Overland Park, KS, 434
CIGNA HealthCare of Kentucky Franklin, TN, 456
CIGNA HealthCare of Louisiana Houston, TX, 471
CIGNA HealthCare of Maine South Portland, ME, 486
CIGNA HealthCare of Minnesota Eden Prairie, MN, 596
CIGNA HealthCare of Mississippi Memphis, TN, 622
CIGNA HealthCare of Montana Denver, CO, 662
CIGNA HealthCare of New Hampshire Hooksett, NH, 701
CIGNA HealthCare of New Jersey Jersey City, NJ, 718
CIGNA HealthCare of New Mexico Albuquerque, NM, 740
CIGNA HealthCare of New York New York, NY, 760
CIGNA HealthCare of North Carolina Charlotte, NC, 813
CIGNA HealthCare of North Dakota Chicago, IL, 830
CIGNA HealthCare of North Texas Plano, TX, 1052
CIGNA HealthCare of Northern California San Francisco, CA, 105
CIGNA HealthCare of Oklahoma Plano, TX, 884
CIGNA HealthCare of Pennsylvania Wilmington, PA, 934
CIGNA HealthCare of South Carolina Greenville, SC, 995
CIGNA HealthCare of South Texas Houston, TX, 1053

CIGNA HealthCare of Southern California Irvine, CA, 106
CIGNA HealthCare of St. Louis Clayton, MO, 637
CIGNA HealthCare of Tennessee Chattanooga, TN, 1028
CIGNA HealthCare of the Mid-Atlantic Columbia, MD, 241, 500
CIGNA HealthCare of Utah Salt Lake City, UT, 1098
CIGNA HealthCare of Virginia Richmond, VA, 1124
CIGNA: Corporate Headquarters Philadelphia, PA, 935
Citizens Choice Healthplan Cerritos, CA, 107
Colorado Access Denver, CO, 198
Colorado Choice Health Plans Alamosa, CO, 199
Colorado Health Partnerships Colorado Springs, CO, 200
Community First Health Plans San Antonio, TX, 1054
Community Health Group , CA, 109
Community Health Improvement Solutions Saint Joseph, MO, 638
Community Health Plan of Los Angeles County Alhambra, CA, 110
CommunityCare Managed Healthcare Plans of Oklahoma Tulsa, OK, 885
Concentra: Corporate Office Addison, TX, 1055
ConnectiCare Farmington, CT, 220
ConnectiCare of Massachusetts Farmington, CT, 525
ConnectiCare of New York Farmington, NY, 762
Contra Costa Health Plan Martinez, CA, 112
Coventry Health Care of Delaware Newark, DE, 229
Coventry Health Care of Florida Sunrise, FL, 267
Coventry Health Care of GA Atlanta, GA, 314
Coventry Health Care of Illinois Champaign, IL, 363
Coventry Health Care of Iowa Urbandale, IA, 419
Coventry Health Care of Kansas Wichita, KS, 436
Coventry Health Care of Louisiana Metairie, LA, 472
Coventry Health Care of Nebraska Omaha, NE, 676
Coventry Health Care of West Virginia Charleston, WV, 1167
Coventry Health Care Virginia Richmond, VA, 1125
Coventry Health Care: Corporate Headquarters Bethesda, MD, 502
CoventryCares of Kentucky Louisville, KY, 457
Cox Healthplans Springfield, MO, 639

DakotaCare Sioux Falls, SD, 1012
DC Chartered Health Plan Washington, DC, 242
Denver Health Medical Plan Inc Denver, CO, 202

Easy Choice Health Plan New York, NY, 766
Educators Mutual Murray, UT, 1100
eHealthInsurance Services Inc. Gold River, CA, 10, 22, 40, 70, 120, 121, 203,
   231, 244, 271, 318, 332, 345, 366, 397, 421, 438, 459, 475, 487, 506, 527, 561,
   598, 624, 642, 664, 678, 688, 703, 720, 742, 767, 817, 832, 848, 888, 902, 939,
   985, 997,
eHealthInsurance Services Inc. Corporate Office Mountain View, CA, 122
Empire Blue Cross & Blue Shield New York, NY, 769
Excellus Blue Cross Blue Shield: Central New York Syracuse, NY, 770
Excellus Blue Cross Blue Shield: Rochester Region Rochester, NY, 771
Excellus Blue Cross Blue Shield: Utica Region Utica, NY, 772

Fallon Community Health Plan Worcester, MA, 528
First Commonwealth Chicago, IL, 367
First Priority Health Wilkes Barre, PA, 942
FirstCarolinaCare Pinehurst, NC, 818
Florida Blue: Jacksonville Jacksonville, FL, 273
Florida Blue: Pensacola Pensacola, FL, 274
Florida Health Care Plan Holly Hill, FL, 275

Gateway Health Plan Pittsburgh, PA, 943
Geisinger Health Plan Danville, PA, 944
GHI New York, NY, 774
GHP Coventry Health Plan St. Louis, MO, 645
Grand Valley Health Plan Grand Rapids, MI, 563
Graphic Arts Benefit Corporation Greenbelt, MD, 507
Great Lakes Health Plan Southfield, MI, 564
Great-West Healthcare Alabama Atlanta, GA, 11
Great-West Healthcare Arizona Scottsdale, AZ, 43
Great-West Healthcare California Irvine, CA, 127
Great-West Healthcare Delaware Bluebell, PA, 232
Great-West Healthcare Florida Tampa, FL, 277
Great-West Healthcare Georgia Atlanta, GA, 319
Great-West Healthcare Hawaii Oakland, CA, 333

Great-West Healthcare Illinois Rosemont, IL, 369
Great-West Healthcare Indiana Indianapolis, IN, 400, 401
Great-West Healthcare Iowa Chicago, IL, 422
Great-West Healthcare Kansas Overland Park, KS, 439
Great-West Healthcare Maine South Portland, ME, 488
Great-West Healthcare Michigan Southfield, MI, 565
Great-West Healthcare Minnesota Eden Prairie, MN, 600
Great-West Healthcare Missouri Kennett, MO, 646
Great-West Healthcare Montana Bellevue, WA, 665
Great-West Healthcare New Mexico Scottsdale, AZ, 743
Great-West Healthcare New York New York, NY, 776
Great-West Healthcare North Carolina Charlotte, NC, 819
Great-West Healthcare North Dakota Chicago, IL, 833
Great-West Healthcare of Massachusetts Waltham, MA, 530
Great-West Healthcare Oklahoma Dallas, TX, 889
Great-West Healthcare Oregon Portland, OR, 904
Great-West Healthcare Pennsylvania Media, NJ, 945
Great-West Healthcare South Carolina Greenville, NC, 998
Great-West Healthcare South Dakota Chicago, IL, 1016
Great-West Healthcare Texas Dallas, TX, 1062
Great-West Healthcare West Virginia Pittsburgh, OH, 1170
Great-West Healthcare Wisconsin Wauwatosa, WI, 1189
Great-West/One Health Plan Greenwood Village, CO, 204
Group Health Cooperative of Eau Claire Altoona, WI, 1190
Group Health Cooperative of South Central Wisconsin Madison, WI, 1191
Guardian Life Insurance Company of America New York, NY, 777
Gundersen Lutheran Health Plan Onalaska, WI, 1192

Harvard University Group Health Plan Cambridge, MA, 532
Health Alliance Medical Plans Urbana, IL, 370
Health Alliance Plan Detroit, MI, 567
Health Care Service Corporation Chicago, IL, 372
Health Choice Arizona Phoenix, AZ, 44
Health First Health Plans Rockledge, FL, 278
Health Maintenance Plan Cincinnati, OH, 851
Health Net Health Plan of Oregon Portland, OR, 905
Health Net of Arizona Tempe, AZ, 45
Health Net: Corporate Headquarters Woodland Hills, CA, 130
Health New England Springfield, MA, 533
Health Plan of Michigan Detroit, MI, 568
Health Plan of Nevada Las Vegas, NV, 689
Health Plan of New York New York, NY, 778
Health Plan of New York: Connecticut New York, NY, 222
Health Plan of New York: Massachusetts New York, NY, 534
Health Plan of San Joaquin French Camp, CA, 131
Health Plan of San Mateo South San Francisco, CA, 132
Health Plus of Louisiana Shreveport, LA, 476
Health Tradition Onalaska, WI, 1193
Healthcare USA of Missouri Jefferson City, MO, 647
HealthLink HMO St Louis, MO, 648
HealthNow New York - Emblem Health Buffalo, NY, 779
HealthPartners Bloomington, MN, 602
HealthPlus of Michigan: Flint Flint Township, MI, 569
HealthPlus of Michigan: Saginaw Saginaw, MI, 570
HealthPlus of Michigan: Troy Troy, MI, 571, 572
Healthy & Well Kids in Iowa Des Moines, IA, 423
Healthy Indiana Plan Indianapolis, IN, 403
Heart of America Health Plan Rugby, ND, 834
Highmark Blue Cross & Blue Shield Pittsburgh, PA, 949
Highmark Blue Cross & Blue Shield Delaware Wilmington, DE, 233
HMO Blue Texas Richarson, TX, 1067
HMO Colorado Denver, CO, 205
HMO Health Ohio Cleveland, OH, 853
Horizon Blue Cross & Blue Shield of New Jersey Newark, NJ, 724
Horizon Healthcare of New Jersey Newark, NJ, 725
Humana Health Insurance of Alaska Vancouver, WA, 23
Humana Health Insurance of Arizona Phoenix, AZ, 46
Humana Health Insurance of Colorado Springs Colorado Springs, CO, 206
Humana Health Insurance of Connecticut Mahwah, NJ, 223
Humana Health Insurance of Corpus Christi Corpus Christi, TX, 1069
Humana Health Insurance of D.C. Mahwah, NJ, 245
Humana Health Insurance of Delaware Blue Bell, PA, 234
Humana Health Insurance of Fresno Walnut Creek, CA, 133

Humana Health Insurance of Georgia Atlanta, GA, 320
Humana Health Insurance of Hawaii Honolulu, HI, 336
Humana Health Insurance of Huntsville Huntsville, AL, 13
Humana Health Insurance of Idaho Meridian, ID, 346
Humana Health Insurance of Illinois Oak Brook, IL, 376
Humana Health Insurance of Indiana Indianapolis, IN, 404
Humana Health Insurance of Iowa Bettendorf, IA, 424
Humana Health Insurance of Jacksonville Jacksonville, FL, 282
Humana Health Insurance of Kansas Overland Park, MO, 441
Humana Health Insurance of Kentucky Louisville, KY, 460
Humana Health Insurance of Little Rock Little Rock, AR, 72
Humana Health Insurance of Louisiana Metairie, LA, 477
Humana Health Insurance of Maryland Mahwah, NJ, 508
Humana Health Insurance of Massachusetts Mahwah, NJ, 536
Humana Health Insurance of Michigan Grand Rapids, MI, 574
Humana Health Insurance of Minnesota Eden Prairie, MN, 604
Humana Health Insurance of Mississippi Ridgeland, MS, 626
Humana Health Insurance of Missouri Springfield, MO, 649
Humana Health Insurance of Montana Billings, MT, 667
Humana Health Insurance of Nebraska Omaha, NE, 679
Humana Health Insurance of Nevada Las Vegas, NV, 691
Humana Health Insurance of New Hampshire Portsmouth, NH, 705
Humana Health Insurance of New Jersey Mahwah, NJ, 727
Humana Health Insurance of New Mexico Albuquerque, NM, 744
Humana Health Insurance of New York Albany, NY, 781
Humana Health Insurance of North Carolina Cary, NC, 820
Humana Health Insurance of North Dakota Billings, ND, 835
Humana Health Insurance of Ohio Cincinnati, OH, 854
Humana Health Insurance of Oklahoma Tulsa, OK, 890
Humana Health Insurance of Oregon Vancouver, WA, 906
Humana Health Insurance of Orlando Alamonte Springs, FL, 283
Humana Health Insurance of Pennsylvania Mechanicsburg, PA, 951
Humana Health Insurance of Puerto Rico San Juan, PR, 974
Humana Health Insurance of Rhode Island Mahwah, NJ, 986
Humana Health Insurance of San Antonio San Antonio, TX, 1070
Humana Health Insurance of South Carolina Columbia, SC, 999
Humana Health Insurance of South Dakota Billings, SD, 1017
Humana Health Insurance of Southern California Carlsbad, CA, 134
Humana Health Insurance of Tampa - Pinellas Clearwater, FL, 284
Humana Health Insurance of Tennessee Memphis, TN, 1035
Humana Health Insurance of Utah Sandy, UT, 1102
Humana Health Insurance of Virginia Glen Allen, VA, 1130
Humana Health Insurance of Washington Vancouver, WA, 1151
Humana Health Insurance of West Virginia Charleston, WV, 1171
Humana Health Insurance of Wisconsin Waukesha, WI, 1195
Humana Health Insurance of Wyoming Billings, MT, 1212

IHC: Intermountain Healthcare Health Plan Salt Lake City, UT, 347
Independence Blue Cross Philadelphia, PA, 952
Independent Health Buffalo, NY, 782
Inland Empire Health Plan Rancho Cucamonga, CA, 135

JMH Health Plan Miami, FL, 285
John Deere Health Kingsport, TN, 1037

Kaiser Foundation Health Plan of Georgia Atlanta, GA, 321
Kaiser Permanente Health Plan of Colorado Denver, CO, 207
Kaiser Permanente Health Plan of Hawaii Honolulu, HI, 337
Kaiser Permanente Health Plan of Northern California Oakland, CA, 138
Kaiser Permanente Health Plan of Southern California Pasadena, CA, 139
Kaiser Permanente Health Plan of the Mid-Atlantic States Rockville, MD, 509
Kaiser Permanente Health Plan of the Northwest Portland, OR, 907
Kaiser Permanente Health Plan Ohio Cleveland, OH, 856
Kaiser Permanente Health Plan: Corporate Office Oakland, CA, 140
Kern Family Health Care Bakersfield, CA, 142
Keystone Health Plan Central Harrisburg, PA, 954
Keystone Health Plan East Philadelphia, PA, 955

L.A. Care Health Plan Los Angeles, CA, 143
Lakeside Community Healthcare Network Northridge, CA, 144
Landmark Healthplan of California Sacramento, CA, 145
Legacy Health Plan San Angelo, TX, 1073
Leon Medical Centers Health Plan Miami, FL, 286

Los Angeles County Department of Health Services Los Angeles, CA, 147
Lovelace Health Plan Albuquerque, NM, 745
Lovelace Medicare Health Plan Albuquerque, NM, 746

Managed Health Services Wauwatosa, WI, 1196
Managed Healthcare Systems of New Jersey Newark, NJ, 728
Maricopa Integrated Health System/Maricopa Health Plan Phoenix, AZ, 48
Medica: North Dakota Fargo, ND, 836
Medica: South Dakota Sioux Falls, SD, 1018
Medical Associates Health Plan Dubuque, IA, 377
Medical Associates Health Plan: West Dubuque, IA, 425
Medical Mutual of Ohio Cleveland, OH, 857
Mercy Health Network Des Moines, IA, 426
Mercy Health Plans: Arkansas Little Rock, AR, 73
Mercy Health Plans: Corporate Office Chesterfield, MO, 652
Mercy Health Plans: Kansas Chesterfield, MO, 442
Mercy Health Plans: Oklahoma Chesterfield, MO, 891
Mercy Health Plans: Texas Laredo, TX, 1075
MercyCare Health Plans Janesville, WI, 1197
MetroPlus Health Plan New York, NY, 788
Metropolitan Health Plan Minneapolis, MN, 608
Mid America Health Kansas City, MO, 654
Mid Atlantic Medical Services: Corporate Office Rockville, MD, 511
Mid Atlantic Medical Services: DC Rockville, MD, 246
Mid Atlantic Medical Services: Delaware Baltimore, MD, 235
Mid Atlantic Medical Services: North Carolina Charlotte, NC, 822
Mid Atlantic Medical Services: Pennsylvania Baltimore, MD, 956
Mid Atlantic Medical Services: Virginia Richmond, VA, 1132
Mid Atlantic Medical Services: West Virginia Elkview, MD, 1172
Molina Healthcare: Corporate Office Long Beach, CA, 153
Molina Healthcare: Florida Doral, FL, 288
Molina Healthcare: Michigan Troy, MI, 577
Molina Healthcare: Missouri St. Louis, MO, 655
Molina Healthcare: New Mexico Albuquerque, NM, 747
Molina Healthcare: Ohio Columbus, OH, 860
Molina Healthcare: Texas Irving, TX, 1077
Molina Healthcare: Utah Midvale, UT, 1104
Molina Healthcare: Washington Bothell, WA, 1154
Mountain Health Trust/Physician Assured Access System Charleston, WV, 1173
Mutual of Omaha Health Plans Omaha, NE, 682
MVP Health Care: Buffalo Region Buffalo, NY, 791
MVP Health Care: Central New York Utica, NY, 792
MVP Health Care: Corporate Office Schenectady, NY, 793
MVP Health Care: Mid-State Region Syracuse, NY, 794
MVP Health Care: New Hampshire Manchester, NH, 706
MVP Health Care: Vermont Williston, VT, 1117
MVP Health Care: Western New York Schenectady, NY, 795

Nationwide Better Health Columbus, OH, 862
Neighborhood Health Partnership Miami, FL, 289
Neighborhood Health Plan Boston, MA, 537
Neighborhood Health Plan of Rhode Island Providence, RI, 987
Network Health Plan of Wisconsin Menasha, WI, 1198
Nevada Preferred Healthcare Providers Reno, NV, 694
NevadaCare Las Vegas, NV, 695
New West Health Services Billings, MT, 669

OmniCare: A Coventry Health Care Plan Detroit, MI, 578
On Lok Lifeways San Francisco, CA, 155
Optima Health Plan Virginia Beach, VA, 1134
Optimum Choice Rockville, MD, 514
OSF Healthcare Peoria, IL, 378
Oxford Health Plans: Corporate Headquarters Trumbull, CT, 224
Oxford Health Plans: New Jersey Iselin, NJ, 731
Oxford Health Plans: New York New York, NY, 799

PacifiCare Health Systems Cypress, CA, 162
PacifiCare of Arizona Tucson, AZ, 51
PacifiCare of California Cypress, CA, 163
PacifiCare of Colorado Greenwood Village, CO, 208
PacifiCare of Nevada Las Vegas, NV, 696
PacifiCare of Oklahoma Tulsa, OK, 892

PacifiCare of Oregon Lake Oswego, OR, 912
PacifiCare of Texas Dallas, TX, 1079
PacifiCare of Washington Mercer Island, WA, 1156
PacificSource Health Plans: Corporate Headquarters Springfield, OR, 913
PacificSource Health Plans: Idaho Boise, ID, 349
Paramount Care of Michigan Dundee, MI, 579
Paramount Health Care Maumee, OH, 867
Parkland Community Health Plan Dallas, TX, 1080
Passport Health Plan Louisville, KY, 463
Peninsula Health Care Newport News, VA, 1135
Peoples Health Baton Rouge, LA, 479
Phoenix Health Plan Phoenix, AZ, 52
Physicians Health Plan of Mid-Michigan Lansing, MI, 580
Physicians Health Plan of Northern Indiana Fort Wayne, IN, 408
Physicians Plus Insurance Corporation Madison, WI, 1199
Pima Health System Tucson, AZ, 54
Preferred Medical Plan Coral Gables, FL, 293
Preferred Plus of Kansas Wichita, KS, 446
PreferredOne Golden Valley, MN, 612
Presbyterian Health Plan Albuquerque, NM, 748
Priority Health Farmington Hills, MI, 581
Priority Health: Corporate Headquarters Grand Rapids, MI, 582
Priority Partners Health Plans Glen Burnie, MD, 515
Providence Health Plans Beaverton, OR, 914

QualCare Piscataway, NJ, 732
QualChoice/QCA Health Plan Little Rock, AR, 75
Quality Plan Administrators Washington, DC, 247

Rocky Mountain Health Plans Grand Junction, CO, 210

Saint Mary's Health Plans Reno, NV, 697
San Francisco Health Plan San Francisco, CA, 171
Sanford Health Plan Sioux Falls, SD, 427
Santa Clara Family Health Foundations Inc Campbell, CA, 172
SCAN Health Plan Long Beach, CA, 173
Scott & White Health Plan Temple, TX, 1082
Select Health of South Carolina Charleston, SC, 1003
SelectHealth Murray, ID, 352
SelectHealth Murray, UT, 1108
Seton Health Plan Austin, TX, 1084
Sharp Health Plan San Diego, CA, 174
Southeastern Indiana Health Organization Columbus, IN, 410
SummaCare Health Plan Akron, OH, 870

The Health Plan of the Ohio Valley/Mountaineer Region , OH, 875
Total Health Care Detroit, MI, 585
Total Health Choice Miami, FL, 296
Trigon Health Care Richmond, VA, 1138
Tufts Health Plan Watertown, MA, 539
Tufts Health Plan: Rhode Island Providence, RI, 988

UCare Minnesota Minneapolis, MN, 615
Unicare: Illinois Chicago, IL, 382
Unicare: Kansas Topeka, KS, 449
Unicare: Massachusetts Waltham, MA, 540
Unicare: Michigan Dearborn, MI, 586
Unicare: Texas Plano, TX, 1088
Unicare: West Virginia Charleston, WV, 1176
Unison Health Plan of Ohio Columbus, OH, 876
Unison Health Plan of South Carolina , SC, 1005
UnitedHealthcare Community Plan Greenville, DE, 237
UnitedHealthcare Community Plan Capital Area Hot Springs, DC, 248
UnitedHealthcare Nevada Las Vegas, NV, 698
UnitedHealthCare of Alabama Birmingham, AL, 16
UnitedHealthCare of Alaska Tigard, OR, 27
UnitedHealthCare of Arizona Phoenix, AZ, 59
UnitedHealthCare of Arkansas Little Rock, AR, 77
UnitedHealthCare of Colorado Centennial, CO, 212
UnitedHealthCare of Connecticut Hartford, CT, 225
UnitedHealthCare of Florida Jacksonville, FL, 298
UnitedHealthCare of Georgia Norcross, GA, 327
UnitedHealthCare of Hawaii Cypress, CA, 338

UnitedHealthCare of Idaho Cypress, CA, 353
UnitedHealthCare of Illinois Chicago, IL, 383
UnitedHealthCare of Indiana Indianapolis, IN, 411
UnitedHealthCare of Iowa West Des Moines, IA, 428
UnitedHealthCare of Kansas Overland Park, KS, 450
UnitedHealthCare of Kentucky Lexington, KY, 466
UnitedHealthCare of Louisiana Metairie, LA, 481
UnitedHealthCare of Maine Minnetonka, MN, 492
UnitedHealthCare of Maryland Elkridge, MD, 238
UnitedHealthCare of Massachusetts Warwick, RI, 541
UnitedHealthCare of Michigan Southfield, MI, 588
UnitedHealthCare of Minnesota Minnetonka, MN, 616, 617
UnitedHealthCare of Mississippi Hattiesburg, MS, 627
UnitedHealthCare of Missouri Maryland Heights, MO, 658
UnitedHealthCare of Montana Centennial, CO, 671
UnitedHealthCare of Nebraska Omaha, NE, 683
UnitedHealthCare of New Hampshire Westborough, MA, 708
UnitedHealthCare of New Jersey Iselin, NJ, 734
UnitedHealthCare of New Mexico Iselin, NM, 751
UnitedHealthCare of New York New York, NY, 805
UnitedHealthCare of North Carolina Cary, NC, 827
UnitedHealthCare of North Dakota Minnetonka, MN, 838
UnitedHealthCare of Northern California Sacramento, CA, 180
UnitedHealthCare of Ohio: Columbus Westerville, OH, 877
UnitedHealthCare of Ohio: Dayton & Cincinnati West Chester, OH, 878
UnitedHealthCare of Oklahoma Plano, TX, 893
UnitedHealthCare of Oregon Lake Oswego, OR, 919
UnitedHealthCare of Pennsylvania Edina, MN, 618
UnitedHealthCare of Puerto Rico Minnetonka, MN, 979
UnitedHealthCare of Rhode Island Warwick, RI, 989
UnitedHealthCare of South Carolina Columbia, SC, 1006
UnitedHealthCare of South Dakota Minnetonka, MN, 1019
UnitedHealthCare of South Florida Sunrise, FL, 299
UnitedHealthCare of Southern California Cypress, CA, 181
UnitedHealthCare of Tennessee Brentwood, TN, 1039
UnitedHealthCare of Texas Austin, TX, 1090
UnitedHealthCare of the District of Columbia Bethesda, MD, 249
UnitedHealthCare of the Mid-Atlantic Baltimore, MD, 518
UnitedHealthCare of Utah Salt Lake City, UT, 1110
UnitedHealthCare of Vermont Westborough, MA, 1118
UnitedHealthCare of Virginia Richmond, VA, 1140
UnitedHealthCare of Washington Mercer Island, WA, 1163
UnitedHealthCare of West Virginia Richmond, VA, 1177
UnitedHealthCare of Wisconsin: Central Minnetonka, MN, 619
UnitedHealthCare of Wisconsin: Central Minnetonka, WI, 1203
UnitedHealthCare of Wyoming Centennial, CO, 1213
Univera Healthcare Buffalo, NY, 806
University Family Care Health Plan , AZ, 60
University Health Plans Murray, UT, 1111
Upper Peninsula Health Plan Marquette, MI, 589
UTMB HealthCare Systems Galveston, TX, 1092

Valley Baptist Health Plan Harlingen, TX, 1093
Vantage Health Plan Monroe, LA, 482
Ventura County Health Care Plan Oxnard, CA, 182
Virginia Premier Health Plan Richmond, VA, 1142
VIVA Health Birmingham, AL, 17
Vytra Health Plans Melville, NY, 808

Welborn Health Plans Evansville, IN, 413
WellChoice Iselin, NJ, 736
Wellmark Blue Cross Blue Shield Des Moines, IA, 429
WellPath: A Coventry Health Care Plan Morrisville, NC, 828
WellPoint: Corporate Office Indianapolis, IN, 414
Western Health Advantage Sacramento, CA, 187

Medicare

American Pioneer Life Insurance Co Lake Mary, FL, 251
AmeriHealth Medicare Plan Philadelphia, PA, 926
Arcadian Community Care Oakland, LA, 468
Arkansas Community Care Little Rock, AR, 65
Arta Medicare Health Plan Signal Hill, CA, 83

Atrio Health Plans Roseburg, OR, 896
AvMed Medicare Preferred Miami, FL, 260

Banner MediSun Medicare Plan Sun City, AZ, 33
Blue Care Network of Michigan: Medicare Grand Rapids, MI, 547
Blue Cross and Blue Shield Association Chicago, IL, 357
Bravo Health: Pennsylvania Philadelphia, PA, 931
Bravo Health: Texas San Antonio, TX, 1050

CareMore Health Plan Cerritos, CA, 97
CareOregon Health Plan Portland, OR, 897
CareSource Mid Rogue Health Plan Grants Pass, OR, 898
Carilion Health Plans Roanoke, VA, 1123
CDPHP Medicare Plan Albany, NY, 758
Central Health Medicare Plan Diamond Bar, CA, 100
Cigna Health-Spring Baltimore, MD, 499
Cigna-HealthSpring of Alabama Birmingham, AL, 8
Citrus Health Care Tampa, FL, 264
CommunityCare Medicare Plan Tulsa, OK, 886

Desert Canyon Community Care Prescott, AZ, 39

Easy Choice Health Plan Long Beach, CA, 119
Elderplan Brooklyn, NY, 768
Essence Healthcare Maryland Heights, MO, 643
Evercare Health Plans Anacortes, MN, 599

Fallon Community Medicare Plan Worcester, MA, 529
FamilyCare Health Medicare Plan Portland, OR, 903
First Medical Health Plan of Florida Miami, FL, 272
Freedom Health, Inc Tampa, FL, 276

GEMCare Health Plan Bakersfield, CA, 125
GHI Medicare Plan New York, NY, 775

Health Alliance Medicare Urbana, IL, 371
Health Alliance Medicare Detroit, MI, 566
Health First Medicare Plans Rockledge, FL, 279
Health Net Medicare Plan Woodland Hills, CA, 129
Health Partners Medicare Plan Bloomington, MN, 601
Health Partners Medicare Plan Philadelphia, PA, 946
HealthFirst New Jersey Medicare Plan Princeton, NJ, 723
HealthPlus Senior Medicare Plan Saginaw, MI, 573
HealthSpring of Illinois Rosemont, IL, 374
HealthSpring of Texas Houston, TX, 1066
HealthSpring Prescription Drug Plan Nashville, TN, 1033
HealthSpring: Corporate Offices Nashville, TN, 1034
HealthSun Health Plans Coconut Grove, FL, 281
Humana Benefit Plan of Illinois Peoria, IL, 375
Humana Medicare Plan Louisville, KY, 461

Independent Health Medicare Plan Buffalo, NY, 783
InStil Health Columbia, SC, 1000

Kaiser Permanente Medicare Plan Oakland, CA, 141
KelseyCare Advantage Pearland, TX, 1072

Liberty Health Advantage Medicare Plan Melville, NY, 785

Magellan Medicaid Administration Glen Allen, VA, 1131
MD Care Healthplan Signal Hill, CA, 150
Medica Health - Medicare Plan Minnetonka, MN, 605
Medica HealthCare Plans, Inc Coral Gables, FL, 287
Medical Mutual of Ohio Medicare Plan Cleveland, OH, 858
Mercy Care Plan/Mercy Care Advantage Phoenix, AZ, 49
Mercy Health Medicare Plan Chesterfield, MO, 651
MHP North Star Plans Minneapolis, MN, 609
Mount Carmel Health Plan Inc (MediGold) Columbus, OH, 861
MVP Health Care Medicare Plan Schenectady, NY, 790

New West Medicare Plan Helena, MT, 670
Northeast Community Care South Portland, ME, 491, 707
Northeast Community Care North Syracuse, NY, 797

Optimum HealthCare, Inc Tampa, FL, 290

Ozark Health Plan Springfield, MO, 656

Paramount Elite Medicare Plan Maumee, OH, 866
Partnership HealthPlan of California Fairfield, CA, 164
Peoples Health Metairie, LA, 480
PMC Medicare Choice San Juan, PR, 977
Presbyterian Medicare Plans Albuquerque, NM, 749
Prime Time Health Medicare Plan Canton, OH, 868
PriorityHealth Medicare Plans Grand Rapids, MI, 583
Puget Sound Health Partners Federal Way, WA, 1158

Quality Health Plans Ronkonkoma, NY, 801
Quality Health Plans of New York Ronkonkoma, NY, 802

Southeast Community Care Macon, GA, 325
Southeast Community Care Raleigh, NC, 825
Southeast Community Care North Charleston, SC, 1004
Southeast Community Care Norfolk, VA, 1137
Spokane Community Care Spokane, WA, 1160
Sterling Health Plans Bellingham, WA, 1161
SummaCare Medicare Advantage Plan Akron, OH, 871

TexanPlus Medicare Advantage HMO Houston, TX, 1085
Texas Community Care Austin, TX, 1086
Touchstone Health HMO White Plains, NY, 803
Trillium Community Health Plan Eugene, OR, 917
Tufts Health Medicare Plan Watertown, MA, 538

UCare Medicare Plan Minneapolis, MN, 614
UnitedHealthCare Hot Springs, AR, 76
Universal American Medicare Plans White Plains, NY, 807
Universal Health Care Group St Petersburg, FL, 300
Universal Health Care Group: Mississippi St. Petersburg, MS, 628

Vantage Medicare Advantage Monroe, LA, 483

WellCare Health Plans Tampa, FL, 302
Windsor Medicare Extra Brentwood, TN, 1040

Multiple

Advance Insurance Company of Kansas Topeka, KS, 430
Altius Health Plans South Jordan, UT, 1097
Americhoice of Pennsylvania Philadelphia, PA, 925
Arizona Foundation for Medical Care Phoenix, AZ, 30
Arkansas Blue Cross and Blue Shield Little Rock, AR, 64
Assurant Employee Benefits: Alabama Birmingham, AL, 3
Assurant Employee Benefits: California Kansas City, CA, 84
Assurant Employee Benefits: Colorado Kansas City, CO, 192
Assurant Employee Benefits: Corporate Headquarters New York, NY, 632
Assurant Employee Benefits: Florida Tampa, FL, 253
Assurant Employee Benefits: Georgia Atlanta, GA, 307
Assurant Employee Benefits: Illinois Oakbrook Terrace, IL, 355
Assurant Employee Benefits: Kansas Shawnee Mission, KS, 432
Assurant Employee Benefits: Massachusetts Marlborough, MA, 520
Assurant Employee Benefits: Michigan Troy, MI, 545
Assurant Employee Benefits: Minnesota Minneapolis, MN, 593
Assurant Employee Benefits: New Jersey Parsippany, NJ, 714
Assurant Employee Benefits: North Carolina Charlotte, NC, 810
Assurant Employee Benefits: Ohio Cincinnati, OH, 842
Assurant Employee Benefits: Oklahoma Broken Arrow, OK, 881
Assurant Employee Benefits: Oregon Portland, OR, 895
Assurant Employee Benefits: Pennsylvania Tredyffrin, PA, 927
Assurant Employee Benefits: South Carolina Columbia, SC, 991
Assurant Employee Benefits: Tennessee Memphis, TN, 1023
Assurant Employee Benefits: Texas Plano, TX, 1045
Assurant Employee Benefits: Washington Seattle, WA, 1144
Assurant Employee Benefits: Wisconsin Milwaukee, WI, 1181
Asuris Northwest Health Spokane, WA, 1145

Beta Health Plan Denver, CO, 194
BlueChoice Health Plan of South Carolina Columbia, SC, 993

Calais Health Baton Rouge, LA, 470

Cariten Healthcare Knoxville, TN, 1026
ChiroSource Inc Concord, CA, 103
Clear One Health Plans Bend, OR, 900
Community Health Plan of Washington Seattle, WA, 1147
CompBenefits Corporation Roswell, GA, 313
CompBenefits: Alabama Birmingham, AL, 9
CompBenefits: Florida Miami, FL, 265
CompBenefits: Illinois Chicago, IL, 361
CompCare: Comprehensive Behavioral Care Tampa, FL, 266
CoreSource: Arizona Tucson, AZ, 37
CoreSource: Arkansas Little Rock, AR, 68
CoreSource: Corporate Headquarters Lake Forest, IL, 362
CoreSource: Kansas (FMH CoreSource) Overland Park, KS, 435
CoreSource: Maryland Baltimore, MD, 501
CoreSource: Michigan (NGS CoreSource) Clinton Township, MI, 557
CoreSource: North Carolina Charlotte, NC, 814
CoreSource: Ohio Dublin, OH, 846
CoreSource: Pennsylvania Lancaster, PA, 936
Coventry Health Care of Southern Florida Sunrise, FL, 268

Dean Health Plan Madison, WI, 1185
Denta-Chek of Maryland Columbia, MD, 504

Fidelis Care Rego Park, NY, 773
First Care Health Plans Austin, TX, 1060
First Medical Health Plan Guaynabo, PR, 973

GEHA-Government Employees Hospital Association Independence, MO, 644
Golden West Dental & Vision Plan Carmarillo, CA, 126
Group Health Cooperative Seattle, WA, 1150

Harvard Pilgrim Health Care Wellesley, MA, 531
Harvard Pilgrim Health Care of New England Manchester, NH, 704
Harvard Pilgrim Health Care: Maine Portland, ME, 489
HealthAmerica Erie, PA, 947
HealthAmerica Pennsylvania Harrisburg, PA, 948
Hometown Health Plan Reno, NV, 690

Inter Valley Health Plan Pomona, CA, 136
Island Group Administration, Inc. East Hampton, NY, 784

Magellan Health Services: Corporate Headquarters Columbia, MD, 510
Martin's Point HealthCare Portland, ME, 490
Medical Card System (MCS) San Juan, PR, 975
MHNet Behavioral Health Austin, TX, 1076
Mid Atlantic Psychiatric Services (MAMSI) Newark, DE, 236
MMM Healthcare San Juan, PR, 976
Moda Health Alaska Anchorage, AK, 25

National Medical Health Card Lisle, NY, 796

ODS Health Plan Portland, OR, 911
Ohio State University Health Plan Inc. Columbus, OH, 864
OptumHealth Care Solutions: Physical Health Golden Valley, MN, 610

Pacific Foundation for Medical Care Santa Rosa, CA, 158
PacifiCare Dental and Vision Administrators Santa Ana, CA, 161
Phoenix Health Plans Phoenix, AZ, 53
Physical Therapy Provider Network Calabasas, CA, 165
Physicians United Plan Orlando, FL, 291
Preferred Care Partners Miami, FL, 292
Preferred Mental Health Management Wichita, KS, 445
Primary Health Plan Boise, ID, 350

Regence BlueShield of Idaho Lewiston, ID, 351

Samaritan Health Plan Corvallis, OR, 916
Security Health Plan of Wisconsin Marshfield, WI, 1201
Security Life Insurance Company of America Minnetonka, MN, 613
Spectera Columbia, MD, 516

Triple-S Salud Blue Cross Blue Shield of Puerto Rico San Juan, PR, 978

Unison Health Plan of Pennsylvania Pittsburgh, PA, 966
Unity Health Insurance Sauk City, WI, 1204

UPMC Health Plan Pittsburgh, PA, 968

Valley Preferred Allentown, PA, 970

WellPoint NextRx Fort Worth, TX, 1095
WINhealth Partners Cheyenne, WY, 1214

PPO

Aetna Health of Alaska Hartford, CT, 18
Aetna Health of Arkansas Hartford, CT, 62
Aetna Health of Hawaii Hartford, CT, 329
Aetna Health of Idaho Hartford, CT, 341
Aetna Health of Iowa Hartford, CT, 415
Aetna Health of Kansas Hartford, CT, 431
Aetna Health of Kentucky Hartford, CT, 452
Aetna Health of Louisiana Hartford, CT, 467
Aetna Health of Michigan Hartford, CT, 543
Aetna Health of Minnesota Hartford, CT, 591
Aetna Health of Mississippi Hartford, CT, 621
Aetna Health of Montana Hartford, CT, 659
Aetna Health of Nebraska Hartford, CT, 672
Aetna Health of New Hampshire Hartford, CT, 699
Aetna Health of New Mexico Hartford, CT, 737
Aetna Health of New York Hartford, CT, 752
Aetna Health of North Dakota Hartford, CT, 829
Aetna Health of Oregon Hartford, CT, 894
Aetna Health of Rhode Island Hartford, CT, 980
Aetna Health of South Dakota Hartford, CT, 1008
Aetna Health of Utah Hartford, CT, 1096
Aetna Health of Vermont Hartford, CT, 1112
Aetna Health of Washington Hartford, CT, 1143
Aetna Health of West Virginia Hartford, CT, 1165
Aetna Health of Wisconsin Hartford, CT, 1179
Aetna Health of Wyoming Hartford, CT, 1207
Alere Health Waltham, GA, 304
Alliance Regional Health Network Amarillo, TX, 1042
Alliant Health Plans Kennesaw, GA, 305
American Community Mutual Insurance Company Livonia, MI, 544
American Health Care Alliance Kansas City, MO, 630
American Health Care Group Pittsburgh, PA, 923
American Health Network of Indiana Indianapolis, IN, 387
American Postal Workers Union (APWU) Health Plan Glen Burnie, MD, 494
American PPO Irving, TX, 1043
American WholeHealth Network Sterling, PA, 924
Americas PPO Bloomington, MN, 1009
AmeriHealth HMO Wilmington, DE, 227
AmeriHealth HMO Cranbury, NJ, 713
Anthem Blue Cross & Blue Shield Connecticut North Haven, CT, 217
Anthem Blue Cross & Blue Shield of Colorado Denver, CO, 190
Anthem Blue Cross & Blue Shield of Indiana Indianapolis, IN, 389
Anthem Blue Cross & Blue Shield of Maine S. Portland, ME, 485
Anthem Blue Cross & Blue Shield of Missouri Saint Louis, MO, 631
Anthem Blue Cross & Blue Shield of Nevada Denver, CO, 191
Anthem Blue Cross & Blue Shield of Ohio Mason, OH, 841
Anthem Blue Cross & Blue Shield of Wisconsin Waukesha, WI, 1180
Araz Group Bloomington, MN, 592
Arcadian Health Plans Oakland, CA, 82
Arkansas Managed Care Organization Little Rock, AR, 66
Atlanticare Health Plans Egg Harbor Township, NJ, 715
Aultcare Corporation Canton, OH, 843
Avesis: Arizona Phoenix, AZ, 309
Avesis: Corporate Headquarters Phoenix, AZ, 32
Avesis: Indiana Lawrenceburg, IN, 392
Avesis: Iowa Des Moines, IA, 417
Avesis: Maryland Owings Mills, MD, 496
Avesis: Massachusetts North Andover, MA, 521
Avesis: Minnesota Sartell, MN, 594
Avesis: Texas San Antonio, TX, 1046

Basic Chiropractic Health Plan Stockton, CA, 85
Beech Street Corporation: Alabama Alpharetta, GA, 4
Beech Street Corporation: Corporate Office Lake Forest, CA, 86

Beech Street Corporation: Northeast Region Lake Forest, CA, 87
Beech Street: Alaska Lake Forest, CA, 19
Behavioral Health Systems Birmingham, AL, 5
Behavioral Healthcare Options, Inc. Las Vegas, NV, 686
Berkshire Health Partners Wyomissing, PA, 928
BEST Life and Health Insurance Co. Irvine, CA, 89
Blue Cross & Blue Shield of Arizona Phoenix, AZ, 34
Blue Cross & Blue Shield of Illinois Chicago, IL, 356
Blue Cross & Blue Shield of Kansas City Kansas City, MO, 633
Blue Cross & Blue Shield of Louisiana Baton Rouge, LA, 469
Blue Cross & Blue Shield of Nebraska Omaha, NE, 674
Blue Cross & Blue Shield of New Mexico Albuquerque, NM, 739
Blue Cross & Blue Shield of North Carolina Durham, NC, 811
Blue Cross & Blue Shield of Oklahoma Oklahoma City, OK, 882
Blue Cross & Blue Shield of South Carolina Columbia, SC, 992
Blue Cross & Blue Shield of Tennessee Chattanooga, TN, 1025
Blue Cross & Blue Shield of Texas Richardson, TX, 1048
Blue Cross & Blue Shield of Texas: Houston Houston, TX, 1049
Blue Cross & Blue Shield of Vermont Berlin, VT, 1113
Blue Cross & Blue Shield of Western New York Buffalo, NY, 756
Blue Cross & Blue Shield of Wyoming Cheyenne, WY, 1208
Blue Cross Blue Shield of Michigan Detroit, MI, 551
Blue Cross of Idaho Health Service, Inc. Meridian, ID, 342
Blue Cross of Northeastern Pennsylvania Wilkes Barre, PA, 929
Blue Cross Preferred Care Birmingham, AL, 7
Blue Ridge Health Network Pottsville, PA, 930
Blue Shield of California San Francisco, CA, 90
Bluegrass Family Health Lexington, KY, 454
BlueShield of Northeastern New York Latham, NY, 757
Boulder Valley Individual Practice Association Boulder, CO, 195
Brazos Valley Health Network Waco, TX, 1051

California Foundation for Medical Care Riverside, CA, 94
Capital Blue Cross Harrisburg, PA, 932
CareFirst Blue Cross & Blue Shield of Virginia Owings Mills, MD, 1122
CareFirst Blue Cross Blue Shield Washington, DC, 240
Cariten Preferred Knoxville, TN, 1027
Catalyst RX Raleigh, NC, 812
CCN: Alaska Anchorage, AK, 20
CDPHP: Capital District Physicians' Health Plan Albany, NY, 759
Central Susquehanna Healthcare Providers Lewisburg, PA, 933
ChiroCare of Wisconsin Wauwatosa, WI, 1183
Chiropractic Health Plan of California Concord, CA, 102
CHN PPO Hamilton, NJ, 717
CIGNA HealthCare of Arizona Bloomfield, AZ, 36
CIGNA HealthCare of Idaho Denver, CO, 343
CIGNA HealthCare of Massachusetts Newton, MA, 524
CIGNA HealthCare of Michigan Southfield, MI, 554
CIGNA HealthCare of Nebraska Overland Park, KS, 675
CIGNA HealthCare of Nevada Las Vegas, NV, 687
CIGNA HealthCare of North Texas Plano, TX, 1052
CIGNA HealthCare of Ohio Independence, OH, 845
CIGNA HealthCare of Oklahoma Plano, TX, 884
CIGNA HealthCare of Oregon Portland, OR, 899
CIGNA HealthCare of Puerto Rico San Juan, PR, 972
CIGNA HealthCare of Rhode Island Newton, MA, 982
CIGNA HealthCare of South Dakota Chicago, IL, 1011
CIGNA HealthCare of the Mid-Atlantic Columbia, MD, 241, 500
CIGNA HealthCare of Utah Salt Lake City, UT, 1098
CIGNA HealthCare of Vermont Burlington, VT, 1114
CIGNA HealthCare of Washington Seattle, WA, 1146
CIGNA HealthCare of West Virginia Pittsburgh, PA, 1166
CIGNA HealthCare of Wisconsin Wauwatosa, WI, 1184
CIGNA HealthCare of Wyoming Denver, CO, 1209
CNA Insurance Companies: Colorado Littleton, CO, 197
CNA Insurance Companies: Georgia Duluth, GA, 312
CNA Insurance Companies: Illinois Chicago, IL, 360
Coalition America's National Preferred Provider Network Middletown, NY, 761
Coastal Healthcare Administrators Salinas, CA, 108
Cofinity Southfield, MI, 555
Community First Health Plans San Antonio, TX, 1054
CommunityCare Managed Healthcare Plans of Oklahoma Tulsa, OK, 885

Concentra: Corporate Office Addison, TX, 1055
ConnectCare Midland, MI, 556
ConnectiCare Farmington, CT, 220
ConnectiCare of Massachusetts Farmington, CT, 525
ConnectiCare of New York Farmington, NY, 762
CorVel Corporation Irvine, CA, 113
Coventry Health Care of Delaware Newark, DE, 229
Coventry Health Care of Florida Sunrise, FL, 267
Coventry Health Care of GA Atlanta, GA, 314
Coventry Health Care of Iowa Urbandale, IA, 419
Coventry Health Care of Kansas Wichita, KS, 436
Coventry Health Care of Nebraska Omaha, NE, 676
Coventry Health Care of West Virginia Charleston, WV, 1167
Coventry Health Care Virginia Richmond, VA, 1125
Coventry Health Care: Corporate Headquarters Bethesda, MD, 502
CoventryCares of Kentucky Louisville, KY, 457
Cox Healthplans Springfield, MO, 639
Crescent Health Solutions Asheville, NC, 815

Deaconess Health Plans Evansville, IN, 395
Devon Health Services King of Prussia, PA, 938
Dimension Health PPO Miami Lakes, FL, 270

Educators Mutual Murray, UT, 1100
eHealthInsurance Services Inc. Gold River, CA, 10, 22, 40, 70, 120, 121, 203, 231, 244, 271, 318, 332, 345, 366, 397, 421, 438, 459, 475, 487, 506, 527, 561, 598, 624, 642, 664, 678, 688, 703, 720, 742, 767, 817, 832, 848, 888, 902, 939, 985, 997,
eHealthInsurance Services Inc. Corporate Office Mountain View, CA, 122
EHP Lancaster, PA, 940
EHP Signifia Lancaster, PA, 941
Emerald Health PPO Cleveland, OH, 849
Empire Blue Cross & Blue Shield New York, NY, 769
Encore Health Network Indianapolis, IN, 399
EPIC Pharmacy Network Mechanicsville, VA, 1129

Fallon Community Health Plan Worcester, MA, 528
Family Choice Health Alliance Hackensack, NJ, 721
FC Diagnostic Hackensack, NJ, 722
First Choice of the Midwest Sioux Falls, SD, 1015
First Health , IL, 368
Florida Blue: Jacksonville Jacksonville, FL, 273
Florida Blue: Pensacola Pensacola, FL, 274
Fortified Provider Network Scottsdale, AZ, 42
Foundation for Medical Care for Kern & Santa Barbara County Bakersfield, CA, 123
Foundation for Medical Care for Mendocino and Lake Counties Ukiah, CA, 124

Galaxy Health Network Arlington, TX, 1061
Geisinger Health Plan Danville, PA, 944
GHI New York, NY, 774
GHP Coventry Health Plan St. Louis, MO, 645
Graphic Arts Benefit Corporation Greenbelt, MD, 507
Great-West Healthcare Alabama Atlanta, GA, 11
Great-West Healthcare Arizona Scottsdale, AZ, 43
Great-West Healthcare California Irvine, CA, 127
Great-West Healthcare Delaware Bluebell, PA, 232
Great-West Healthcare Florida Tampa, FL, 277
Great-West Healthcare Georgia Atlanta, GA, 319
Great-West Healthcare Hawaii Oakland, CA, 333
Great-West Healthcare Illinois Rosemont, IL, 369
Great-West Healthcare Indiana Indianapolis, IN, 400, 401
Great-West Healthcare Iowa Chicago, IL, 422
Great-West Healthcare Kansas Overland Park, KS, 439
Great-West Healthcare Maine South Portland, ME, 488
Great-West Healthcare Michigan Southfield, MI, 565
Great-West Healthcare Minnesota Eden Prairie, MN, 600
Great-West Healthcare Missouri Kennett, MO, 646
Great-West Healthcare Montana Bellevue, WA, 665
Great-West Healthcare New Mexico Scottsdale, AZ, 743
Great-West Healthcare New York New York, NY, 776
Great-West Healthcare North Carolina Charlotte, NC, 819

Great-West Healthcare North Dakota Chicago, IL, 833
Great-West Healthcare of Massachusetts Waltham, MA, 530
Great-West Healthcare Oklahoma Dallas, TX, 889
Great-West Healthcare Oregon Portland, OR, 904
Great-West Healthcare Pennsylvania Media, NJ, 945
Great-West Healthcare South Carolina Greenville, NC, 998
Great-West Healthcare South Dakota Chicago, IL, 1016
Great-West Healthcare Texas Dallas, TX, 1062
Great-West Healthcare West Virginia Pittsburgh, OH, 1170
Great-West Healthcare Wisconsin Wauwatosa, WI, 1189
Great-West/One Health Plan Greenwood Village, CO, 204
Guardian Life Insurance Company of America New York, NY, 777

HAS-Premier Providers Addison, TX, 1063
Hawaii Medical Assurance Association Honolulu, HI, 334
Hawaii Medical Services Association Honolulu, HI, 335
Health Alliance Medical Plans Urbana, IL, 370
Health Alliance Plan Detroit, MI, 567
Health Care Service Corporation Chicago, IL, 372
Health Choice LLC Memphis, TN, 1031
Health Choice of Alabama Birmingham, AL, 12
Health InfoNet Billings, MT, 666
Health Link PPO Tupelo, MS, 625
Health Net Health Plan of Oregon Portland, OR, 905
Health Partners of Kansas Wichita, KS, 440
Health Plan of Nevada Las Vegas, NV, 689
Health Plan of New York New York, NY, 778
Health Plan of New York: Connecticut New York, NY, 222
Health Plan of New York: Massachusetts New York, NY, 534
Healthcare Partners of East Texas Marshall, TX, 1064
Healthchoice Orlando Orlando, FL, 280
HealthEOS De Pere, WI, 1194
HealthPartners Jackson, TN, 1032
HealthSmart Preferred Care Irving, IL, 373
HealthSmart Preferred Care Irving, TX, 1065
HealthSpan Cincinnati, OH, 852
Highmark Blue Cross & Blue Shield Pittsburgh, PA, 949
Highmark Blue Cross & Blue Shield Delaware Wilmington, DE, 233
Highmark Blue Shield Camp Hill, PA, 950
Horizon Blue Cross & Blue Shield of New Jersey Newark, NJ, 724
Horizon Health Corporation Lewisville, TX, 1068
Horizon Healthcare of New Jersey Newark, NJ, 725
Horizon NJ Health West Trenton, NJ, 726
HSM: Healthcare Cost Management St Paul, MN, 603
Humana Health Insurance of Alaska Vancouver, WA, 23
Humana Health Insurance of Arizona Phoenix, AZ, 46
Humana Health Insurance of Colorado Springs Colorado Springs, CO, 206
Humana Health Insurance of Connecticut Mahwah, NJ, 223
Humana Health Insurance of Corpus Christi Corpus Christi, TX, 1069
Humana Health Insurance of D.C. Mahwah, NJ, 245
Humana Health Insurance of Delaware Blue Bell, PA, 234
Humana Health Insurance of Fresno Walnut Creek, CA, 133
Humana Health Insurance of Georgia Atlanta, GA, 320
Humana Health Insurance of Hawaii Honolulu, HI, 336
Humana Health Insurance of Huntsville Huntsville, AL, 13
Humana Health Insurance of Idaho Meridian, ID, 346
Humana Health Insurance of Illinois Oak Brook, IL, 376
Humana Health Insurance of Indiana Indianapolis, IN, 404
Humana Health Insurance of Iowa Bettendorf, IA, 424
Humana Health Insurance of Jacksonville Jacksonville, FL, 282
Humana Health Insurance of Kansas Overland Park, MO, 441
Humana Health Insurance of Kentucky Louisville, KY, 460
Humana Health Insurance of Little Rock Little Rock, AR, 72
Humana Health Insurance of Louisiana Metairie, LA, 477
Humana Health Insurance of Maryland Mahwah, NJ, 508
Humana Health Insurance of Massachusetts Mahwah, NJ, 536
Humana Health Insurance of Michigan Grand Rapids, MI, 574
Humana Health Insurance of Minnesota Eden Prairie, MN, 604
Humana Health Insurance of Mississippi Ridgeland, MS, 626
Humana Health Insurance of Missouri Springfield, MO, 649
Humana Health Insurance of Montana Billings, MT, 667
Humana Health Insurance of Nebraska Omaha, NE, 679
Humana Health Insurance of Nevada Las Vegas, NV, 691

Humana Health Insurance of New Hampshire Portsmouth, NH, 705
Humana Health Insurance of New Jersey Mahwah, NJ, 727
Humana Health Insurance of New Mexico Albuquerque, NM, 744
Humana Health Insurance of New York Albany, NY, 781
Humana Health Insurance of North Carolina Cary, NC, 820
Humana Health Insurance of North Dakota Billings, ND, 835
Humana Health Insurance of Ohio Cincinnati, OH, 854
Humana Health Insurance of Oklahoma Tulsa, OK, 890
Humana Health Insurance of Oregon Vancouver, WA, 906
Humana Health Insurance of Orlando Alamonte Springs, FL, 283
Humana Health Insurance of Pennsylvania Mechanicsburg, PA, 951
Humana Health Insurance of Puerto Rico San Juan, PR, 974
Humana Health Insurance of Rhode Island Mahwah, NJ, 986
Humana Health Insurance of San Antonio San Antonio, TX, 1070
Humana Health Insurance of South Carolina Columbia, SC, 999
Humana Health Insurance of South Dakota Billings, SD, 1017
Humana Health Insurance of Tampa - Pinellas Clearwater, FL, 284
Humana Health Insurance of Tennessee Memphis, TN, 1035
Humana Health Insurance of Utah Sandy, UT, 1102
Humana Health Insurance of Virginia Glen Allen, VA, 1130
Humana Health Insurance of Washington Vancouver, WA, 1151
Humana Health Insurance of West Virginia Charleston, WV, 1171
Humana Health Insurance of Wisconsin Waukesha, WI, 1195
Humana Health Insurance of Wyoming Billings, MT, 1212

Independence Blue Cross Philadelphia, PA, 952
Initial Group Nashville, TN, 1036
InterGroup Services Corporation Malvern, PA, 953
Interplan Health Group Stockton, CA, 137
Interplan Health Group Cleveland, OH, 855
Interplan Health Group Irving, TX, 1071

John Deere Health Kingsport, TN, 1037

Kanawha Healthcare Solutions Lancaster, SC, 1001
Keystone Health Plan East Philadelphia, PA, 955

Landmark Healthplan of California Sacramento, CA, 145
Liberty Health Plan Anchorage Anchorage, AK, 24
Liberty Health Plan: Corporate Office Dover, OR, 908
Liberty Health Plan: Idaho Meridian, ID, 348
Liberty Health Plan: Montana Helena, MT, 668
Liberty Health Plan: Washington Liberty Lake, WA, 1152
Lifewise Health Plan of Oregon Portland, OR, 909
Lifewise Health Plan of Washington Mountlake Terrace, WA, 1153
Lovelace Medicare Health Plan Albuquerque, NM, 746

M-Care Ann Arbor, MI, 575
Magellan Health Services Arizona Phoenix, AZ, 47
Magellan Health Services Indiana Indianapolis, IN, 405
MagnaCare New York, NY, 786
Managed Health Network San Rafael, CA, 148
Managed HealthCare Northwest Portland, OR, 910
MedCost Winston Salem, NC, 821
Medfocus Radiology Network Santa Monica, CA, 151
Medica: Corporate Office Minnetonka, MN, 606
Medical Care Referral Group El Paso, TX, 1074
Medical Mutual of Ohio Cleveland, OH, 857
Medical Mutual Services Columbia, SC, 1002
Meritain Health: Corporate Headquarters Amherst, NY, 787
Meritain Health: Indiana Evansville, IN, 406
Meritain Health: Kentucky Bowling Green, KY, 462
Meritain Health: Louisiana Shreveport, LA, 478
Meritain Health: Michigan Okemos, MI, 576
Meritain Health: Minnesota Minneapolis, MN, 607
Meritain Health: Missouri St. Louis, MO, 653
Meritain Health: Ohio Westlake, OH, 859
Meritain Health: Utah Taylorsville, UT, 1103
Mid America Health Kansas City, MO, 654
Mid Atlantic Medical Services: Corporate Office Rockville, MD, 511
Mid Atlantic Medical Services: DC Rockville, MD, 246
Mid Atlantic Medical Services: Delaware Baltimore, MD, 235
Mid Atlantic Medical Services: North Carolina Charlotte, NC, 822

UnitedHealthCare of Oklahoma Plano, TX, 893
UnitedHealthCare of Oregon Lake Oswego, OR, 919
UnitedHealthCare of Pennsylvania Edina, MN, 618
UnitedHealthCare of Puerto Rico Minnetonka, MN, 979
UnitedHealthCare of Rhode Island Warwick, RI, 989
UnitedHealthCare of South Carolina Columbia, SC, 1006
UnitedHealthCare of South Dakota Minnetonka, MN, 1019
UnitedHealthCare of South Florida Sunrise, FL, 299
UnitedHealthCare of Southern California Cypress, CA, 181
UnitedHealthCare of Tennessee Brentwood, TN, 1039
UnitedHealthCare of Texas Austin, TX, 1090
UnitedHealthCare of the District of Columbia Bethesda, MD, 249
UnitedHealthCare of the Mid-Atlantic Baltimore, MD, 518
UnitedHealthCare of Utah Salt Lake City, UT, 1110
UnitedHealthCare of Vermont Westborough, MA, 1118
UnitedHealthCare of Virginia Richmond, VA, 1140
UnitedHealthCare of Washington Mercer Island, WA, 1163
UnitedHealthCare of West Virginia Richmond, VA, 1177
UnitedHealthCare of Wisconsin: Central Minnetonka, MN, 619
UnitedHealthCare of Wisconsin: Central Minnetonka, WI, 1203
UnitedHealthCare of Wyoming Centennial, CO, 1213
University Health Alliance Honolulu, HI, 339
University Health Plans Murray, UT, 1111
USA Managed Care Organization Austin, TX, 1091

Val-U-Health Trafford, PA, 969
Value Behavioral Health of Pennsylvania Trafford, PA, 971
Virginia Health Network Richmond, VA, 1141
Vytra Health Plans Melville, NY, 808

Wellmark Blue Cross & Blue Shield of South Dakota Sioux Falls, SD, 1020
Wisconsin Physician's Service Madison, WI, 1206

Vision

Block Vision of New Jersey Florham Park, NJ, 716

Block Vision of Texas Dallas, TX, 1047

Davis Vision Latham, NY, 763

EyeMed Vision Care Mason, OH, 850

March Vision Care Los Angeles, CA, 149

OptiCare Managed Vision Rocky Mount, NC, 823
Opticare of Utah Salt Lake City, UT, 1105
Outlook Vision Service Mesa, AZ, 50

Preferred Vision Care Overland Park, KS, 447

Superior Vision Services, Inc. Rancho Cordova, CA, 176
SVS Vision Mount Clemens, MI, 584

Vision Insurance Plan of America Milwaukee, WI, 1205
Vision Plan of America Los Angeles, CA, 183
VSP: Vision Service Plan Rancho Cordova, CA, 184
VSP: Vision Service Plan of Arizona Phoenix, AZ, 61
VSP: Vision Service Plan of California San Francisco, CA, 185
VSP: Vision Service Plan of Colorado Denver, CO, 213
VSP: Vision Service Plan of Florida Tampa, FL, 301
VSP: Vision Service Plan of Georgia Norcross, GA, 328
VSP: Vision Service Plan of Hawaii Honolulu, HI, 340
VSP: Vision Service Plan of Illinois Chicago, IL, 384
VSP: Vision Service Plan of Indiana Indianpolis, IN, 412
VSP: Vision Service Plan of Kansas Shawnee Mission, KS, 451
VSP: Vision Service Plan of Massachusetts Boston, MA, 542
VSP: Vision Service Plan of Michigan Southfield, MI, 590
VSP: Vision Service Plan of Minnesota Minneapolis, MN, 620
VSP: Vision Service Plan of New Jersey Parsippany, NJ, 735
VSP: Vision Service Plan of Ohio Canton, OH, 879
VSP: Vision Service Plan of Oregon Portland, OR, 920
VSP: Vision Service Plan of South Carolina Greenville, SC, 1007
VSP: Vision Service Plan of Texas Houston, TX, 1094
VSP: Vision Service Plan of Washington Seattle, WA, 1164

Personnel Index

A

Abbaszadeh, Reza, DDS Premier Access Insurance/Access Dental, 167
Abell, Steve Arkansas Blue Cross and Blue Shield, 64
Abelman, David Dentaquest, 526
Aberg, Jennifer VSP: Vision Service Plan of Oregon, 920
Abernathy, David HealthNow New York - Emblem Health, 779
Abernathy, David S Health Plan of New York, 778
Abernathy, Pat Health Choice LLC, 1031
Abraham, Karen Blue Cross & Blue Shield of Arizona, 34
Abrams, Thomas SecureCare Dental, 56
Acker, Ken Opticare of Utah, 1105
Acker, Lori Delta Dental of New Jersey & Connecticut, 221
Ackerman, Carol PacifiCare Health Systems, 162
Ackerman, Cynthia CareSource Mid Rogue Health Plan, 898
Adams, Amy Capital Health Plan, 261
Adams, Dana American Pioneer Life Insurance Co, 251
Adams, Derick Health Alliance Medicare, 566
Adams, Derick Health Alliance Plan, 567
Adams, Gregory A Kaiser Permanente Health Plan of Northern California, 138
Adams, Lavdena, MD DC Chartered Health Plan, 242
Adams, Michael R Behavioral Healthcare Options, Inc., 686
Adams, Richard SelectCare Access Corporation, 962
Adel, Bryan Beech Street Corporation: Corporate Office, 86
Adkins, Gary W Windsor Medicare Extra, 1040
Adler, Ari B Delta Dental of Michigan, Ohio and Indiana, 847
Aga, Dr Donald KelseyCare Advantage, 1072
Aggarwal, Sarika, M.D. Fallon Community Health Plan, 528
Agven, George CNA Insurance Companies: Georgia, 312
Agven, George CNA Insurance Companies: Illinois, 360
Ahluwalia, Carrie Mida Dental Plan, 152
Albarado, Darnell CompCare: Comprehensive Behavioral Care, 266
Albro, Douglas Alere Health, 304
Albu, Alice Care Choices, 552
Album, Jeff Delta Dental of California, 114
Album, Jeff Delta Dental of the Mid-Atlantic, 230, 243
Album, Jeff Delta Dental of Florida, 269
Album, Jeff Delta Dental of Georgia, 316
Album, Jeff Delta Dental of Nevada, 317
Album, Jeff Delta Dental of Kentucky, 458
Album, Jeff Delta Dental of Georgia, 473
Album, Jeff Delta Dental of the Mid-Atlantic, 503
Album, Jeff Delta Dental Insurance Company, 623
Album, Jeff Delta Dental of Montana, 663
Album, Jeff Delta Dental of New Mexico, 741
Album, Jeff Delta Dental of the Mid-Atlantic, 764, 937
Album, Jeff Delta Dental of Texas, 1056
Album, Jeff Delta Dental of the Mid-Atlantic, 1168
Alcorn, Andrew Block Vision, 497
Alcorn, Andrew Block Vision of New Jersey, 716
Aldreridge, Susan Signature Health Alliance, 1038
Alexander, William, MD CIGNA HealthCare of Florida, 263
Algate, Lyle Total Health Care, 585
Alger, Douglas A. Delta Dental of Minnesota, 597
Alix, Jay VSP: Vision Service Plan of Michigan, 590
All, Matthew D. Blue Cross & Blue Shield of Kansas, 433
Allen, Beverly OmniCare: A Coventry Health Care Plan, 578
Allen, Bob Affinity Health Plan, 753
Allen, Cannon First Care Health Plans, 1060
Allen, David W Guardian Life Insurance Company of America, 777
Allen, Dennis MVP Health Care: Western New York, 795
Allen, Terry Liberty Dental Plan, 146
Allen-Davis, Jandel, MD Kaiser Permanente Health Plan of Colorado, 207
Allford, Allan Delta Dental of Arizona, 38
Allison, Carey Health Plus of Louisiana, 476
Almquist, Stacia Assurant Employee Benefits: Texas, 1045
Almquist, Stacia Assurant Employee Benefits: Washington, 1144
Alnequist, Stacia Dental Health Alliance, 641

Alonge, Jerry OneNet PPO, 512
Alperstein, Joel Avesis: Corporate Headquarters, 32
Alperstein, Joel Avesis: Arizona, 309
Alperstein, Joel Avesis: Minnesota, 594
Alperstein, Joel Avesis: Texas, 1046
Altman, David, MD Central California Alliance for Health, 99
Altman, Maya Health Plan of San Mateo, 132
Alvey, Mindi Deaconess Health Plans, 395
Alvin, William R. Health Alliance Medicare, 566
Amaro, Frank Delta Dental of New Mexico, 741
Ambres, Cynthia Blue Cross & Blue Shield of Western New York, 756
Ambrose, David CenCal Health: The Regional Health Authority, 98
Amburn, Linda Blue Cross & Blue Shield of New Mexico, 739
Amend, Nicole Blue Cross & Blue Shield of Oklahoma, 882
Amendola, Louis Western Dental Services, 186
Amican, Irene Fidelis Care, 773
Amundson, Paul, MD DakotaCare, 1012
Anania, Andrea CIGNA HealthCare of Maine, 486
Anason, Barbara UnitedHealthCare of Nebraska, 683
Anderi, Richard C Mutual of Omaha DentaBenefits, 681
Anderi, Richard C Mutual of Omaha Health Plans, 682
Anderson, A. Scott IHC: Intermountain Healthcare Health Plan, 347
Anderson, David UnitedHealthCare of Southern California, 181
Anderson, Deborah Network Health Plan of Wisconsin, 1198
Anderson, Gary D Magellan Health Services Indiana, 405
Anderson, Gary D Magellan Health Services: Corporate Headquarters, 510
Anderson, Jack R SafeGuard Health Enterprises: Florida, 295
Anderson, Jack R SafeGuard Health Enterprises: Texas, 1081
Anderson, Jim Kaiser Permanente Health Plan of Southern California, 139
Anderson, John Trustmark Companies, 381
Anderson, John R, DO Concentra: Corporate Office, 1055
Anderson, Kraig Moda Health Alaska, 25
Anderson, Lani Altius Health Plans, 1097
Anderson, Lawrence D. Desert Canyon Community Care, 39
Anderson, Lawrence D. WellCare Health Plans, 302
Anderson, Mark Delta Dental of Arizona, 38
Anderson, Michelle Opticare of Utah, 1105
Anderson, Thor GHP Coventry Health Plan, 645
Anderson Jr, Gail V, MD Los Angeles County Department of Health Services, 147
Anderton, Paul, FSA Public Employees Health Program, 1106
Andis, Glenn Medica: North Dakota, 836
Andis, Glenn Medica: South Dakota, 1018
Andis, Glenn E Medica Health - Medicare Plan, 605
Andis, Glenn E Medica: Corporate Office, 606
Andrews, George, MD Cariten Healthcare, 1026
Andrews, George, MD Cariten Preferred, 1027
Andrews, Karen Anthem Blue Cross & Blue Shield of Maine, 485
Andrews, Leslie Humana Health Insurance of Colorado Springs, 206
Andruszkiewicz, Peter Blue Cross & Blue Shield of Rhode Island, 981
Andryczyk, Anne Humana Health Insurance of Wisconsin, 1195
Angerami, John CNA Insurance Companies: Colorado, 197
Angerami, John CNA Insurance Companies: Georgia, 312
Angerami, John CNA Insurance Companies: Illinois, 360
Anglin, Scott Amerigroup Maryland, 495
Anglin, Scott Amerigroup New Jersey, 712
Anglin, Scott Amerigroup Texas, 1044
Anglin, Scott Amerigroup Corporation, 1120
Ann Tournoux, Mary Health Alliance Medicare, 566
Anselm, Edward, MD Fidelis Care, 773
Anthony, William P., M.D. CHN PPO, 717
Antigua, Paul Health Plan of San Joaquin, 131
Antonucci, Don Regence Blue Cross & Blue Shield of Oregon, 915
Antonucci, Don Regence Blue Shield, 1159
Apfel, Mark, MD Foundation for Medical Care for Mendocino and Lake Counties, 124
Apolinsky, Craig Alere Health, 304
Appel, Frank Coventry Health Care of Florida, 267

Appenzeller, Talitha, MBA MHNet Behavioral Health, 1076
Appleton, Kevin Oxford Health Plans: New Jersey, 731
Appleton, Kevin Oxford Health Plans: New York, 799
Arca, Albert Preferred Medical Plan, 293
Archer, Todd E HealthSmart Preferred Care, 373
Archer, Todd E. HealthSmart Preferred Care, 1065
Arcidiacono, Susan Inland Empire Health Plan, 135
Arfin, Ronald Managed Healthcare Systems of New Jersey, 728
Arlotta, John J., Jr Landmark Healthplan of California, 145
Armao, Anne SummaCare Health Plan, 870
Armbruster, Kevin SummaCare Health Plan, 870
Armenti, Steve CHN PPO, 717
Armstrong, Cathleen HealthSCOPE Benefits, 71
Armstrong, David Wisconsin Physician's Service, 1206
Armstrong, Richard, MD QualChoice/QCA Health Plan, 75
Armstrong, Scott Group Health Cooperative, 1150
Arneson, Linda, JD Delta Dental of Colorado, 201
Arnett, Julia UnitedHealthCare of Iowa, 428
Arnold, Roy, MD Welborn Health Plans, 413
Arrington, Robyn, MD Total Health Choice, 296
Arrington Jr, Robyn James, MD Total Health Care, 585
Arth, Lawrence J Ameritas Group, 673
Ash-Jackson, Linda Hometown Health Plan, 690
Asher, Chris Southeastern Indiana Health Organization, 410
Ashihundu, Eric Community First Health Plans, 1054
Ashley, Kim Anthem Blue Cross & Blue Shield of Ohio, 841
Ashley, Sheldon Family Choice Health Alliance, 721
Astorga, Tony M Blue Cross & Blue Shield of Arizona, 34
Atwell, William L CIGNA: Corporate Headquarters, 935
Atwood, Karen Health Care Service Corporation, 372
Atwood, Michael Blue Cross & Blue Shield of Kansas, 433
Auer, Bill Kaiser Foundation Health Plan of Georgia, 321
Aug, Matthew Cox Healthplans, 639
Augustyn, Mary Liberty Health Plan: Corporate Office, 908
Austen, Karla MVP Health Care: Western New York, 795
Austen, Karla A. MVP Health Care: Central New York, 792
Austen, Karla A. MVP Health Care: Corporate Office, 793
Austin, Jeanell National Capital PPO, 1133
Austin, John, MD Arkansas Community Care, 65
Austin, John H, MD Texas Community Care, 1086
Austin, Karla A. MVP Health Care: Vermont, 1117
Austin, Scott Humana Health Insurance of Wisconsin, 1195
Austin, Sueann Medical Care Referral Group, 1074
Authur Pierce, Ena Cigna Health-Spring, 499
Aversa, Ken, MBA Amerigroup Texas, 1044
Avery, Alan Medical Associates Health Plan: West, 425
Avila, Diana Alliance Regional Health Network, 1042
Avner, Kenneth Health Care Service Corporation, 372
Awad, Wael Delta Dental: Corporate Headquarters, 558
Ayers, Kay AvMed Health Plan: Corporate Office, 254
Ayers, Kay AvMed Health Plan: Fort Lauderdale, 255
Ayers, Kay AvMed Health Plan: Gainesville, 256
Ayers, Kay AvMed Health Plan: Orlando, 258
Ayers, Kay AvMed Health Plan: Tampa Bay, 259
Ayers, Kay AvMed Medicare Preferred, 260
Ayers, Ruth Ellen Carilion Health Plans, 1123

B

Baackes, John UnitedHealthCare of North Carolina, 827
Babarick, Tracie SummaCare Health Plan, 870
Babitsch, George GHI, 774
Babitsch, George GHI Medicare Plan, 775
Babitsch, George Health Plan of New York, 778
Baca, Marlene Lovelace Health Plan, 745
Baca, Marlene Lovelace Medicare Health Plan, 746
Bachhuber, Michele L, MD Security Health Plan of Wisconsin, 1201
Backon, Marc Capital Blue Cross, 932
Bacon, Cindy, RN Island Group Administration, Inc., 784
Bacus, Lisa CIGNA HealthCare of Arizona, 36
Bacus, Lisa CIGNA HealthCare of Minnesota, 596
Bacus, Lisa CIGNA HealthCare of St. Louis, 637
Bacus, Lisa CIGNA HealthCare of New Hampshire, 701

Bacus, Lisa CIGNA HealthCare of Utah, 1098
Bahr, Michael D Coventry Health Care of Delaware, 229
Bahr, Michael D Coventry Health Care of Florida, 267
Bahr, Michael D Coventry Health Care of Nebraska, 676
Bahrke, Linda Community Health Improvement Solutions, 638
Bailey, Jim Arkansas Blue Cross and Blue Shield, 64
Bailey, Michael Windsor Medicare Extra, 1040
Baird, Mark Medica Health - Medicare Plan, 605
Baird, Mark Medica: Corporate Office, 606
Baird, Mark Medica: North Dakota, 836
Baird, Mark Medica: South Dakota, 1018
Bajaj, Sandeep Physicians United Plan, 291
Baker, Andrew H Family Choice Health Alliance, 721
Baker, Andrew H FC Diagnostic, 722
Baker, G. Steven Public Employees Health Program, 1106
Baker, Jane Horizon Health Corporation, 1068
Baker, Stephen J SafeGuard Health Enterprises: Corporate Office, 170
Baker, Stephen J SafeGuard Health Enterprises: Texas, 1081
Balboni, Jill Delta Dental of Texas, 1056
Balboni, Jill Delta Dental of Utah, 1099
Baldwin, K Rone Guardian Life Insurance Company of America, 777
Ball, Donald, Jr VSP: Vision Service Plan, 184
Ball, Patricia UCare Medicare Plan, 614
Ball, Patricia UCare Minnesota, 615
Ballenger, Jim Ohio State University Health Plan Inc., 864
Banda, Kay, 74 Arizona Foundation for Medical Care, 30
Bank, Julie MagnaCare, 786
Barasch, Richard A American Pioneer Life Insurance Co, 251
Barasch, Richard A Universal American Medicare Plans, 807
Barasch, Richard A TexanPlus Medicare Advantage HMO, 1085
Barbera, Thomas P Mid Atlantic Psychiatric Services (MAMSI), 236
Barbera, Thomas P Optimum Choice, 514
Barbera, Thomas P Mid Atlantic Medical Services: North Carolina, 822
Barden, J Gentry HealthSpring: Corporate Offices, 1034
Bare, James W Florida Health Care Plan, 275
Barkell, Susan L Blue Cross Blue Shield of Michigan, 551
Barker, David S Southeastern Indiana Health Organization, 410
Barker, Jason CareMore Health Plan, 97
Barlow, H R Brereton Premera Blue Cross, 1157
Barlow, H.R. Brereton Premera Blue Cross Blue Shield of Alaska, 26
Barlow, Jeff Molina Healthcare: New Mexico, 747
Barlow, Jeff D. Molina Healthcare: Corporate Office, 153
Barnard, Mark Horizon Blue Cross & Blue Shield of New Jersey, 724
Barnard, Mark Horizon Healthcare of New Jersey, 725
Barnard, Mark Rayant Insurance Company, 733
Barnes, Christy Ohio Health Choice, 863
Barnes, Scott HealthSCOPE Benefits, 71
Barnett, Kerry Regence Blue Cross & Blue Shield of Oregon, 915
Barnett, Kerry Regence Blue Cross & Blue Shield of Utah, 1107
Barnhart, Mark Cardinal Health Alliance, 393
Barnicle, Joan Aetna Health of Missouri, 629
Barrett, Rick DINA Dental Plans, 474
Barrett, Rick Dental Source: Dental Health Care Plans, 1057
Barrett, Rick Ora Quest Dental Plans, 1078
Barrett, Rochelle American Health Care Alliance, 630
Barrington, Christina Health Alliance Medical Plans, 370
Barstow, Jeffrey Managed Health Network, 148
Bartlett, Mark R Blue Care Network: Ann Arbor, 548
Bartlett, Mark R Blue Care Network: Flint, 549
Bartlett, Mark R Blue Cross Blue Shield of Michigan, 551
Bartlett, Mark R. Blue Care Network of Michigan: Medicare, 547
Bartlett, Tom Beech Street Corporation: Corporate Office, 86
Barua, Joy Kaiser Permanente Health Plan of Hawaii, 337
Barwig, Mark P EPIC Pharmacy Network, 1129
Basher, Kathy Humana Health Insurance of Orlando, 283
Baskin, Tery, PharmD National Medical Health Card, 796
Bates, Debbie, MD UnitedHealthCare of Louisiana, 481
Bates, Richard Catalyst Health Solutions Inc, 498
Bates, Richard Catalyst RX, 812
Bates, Rick United Behavioral Health, 178
Batey, Dennis, MD Presbyterian Health Plan, 748
Batey, Dennis, MD Presbyterian Medicare Plans, 749

Batra, Romilla SCAN Health Plan, 173
Battaglieri, Lu Delta Dental: Corporate Headquarters, 558
Batteer, Cathy SCAN Health Plan, 173
Batteer, Cathy UPMC Health Plan, 968
Bauer, Michele, DO Group Health Cooperative of Eau Claire, 1190
Bauer Jones, Stacy Sanford Health Plan, 427
Bauers, John, MD HealthAmerica, 947
Baughman, Chris Health Plan of San Mateo, 132
Baum, J Robert, PhD Highmark Blue Cross & Blue Shield, 949
Baumgart, Chuck, MD Presbyterian Health Plan, 748
Baumgart, Chuck, MD Presbyterian Medicare Plans, 749
Baut, Harry Behavioral Healthcare Options, Inc., 686
Baxter, John One Call Medical, 730
Baxter, Raymond J, PhD Kaiser Permanente Health Plan of Northern California, 138
Baxter, Raymond J, PhD Kaiser Permanente Health Plan of Southern California, 139
Baxter, Raymond J, PhD Kaiser Permanente Health Plan: Corporate Office, 140
Baxter, Raymond J, PhD Kaiser Permanente Medicare Plan, 141
Bayer, Gregory A, PhD United Behavioral Health, 178
Bayer, Terry, JD, MPH Molina Healthcare: Michigan, 577
Bayer, Terry, JD,MPH Molina Healthcare: Texas, 1077
Bayer, Terry, JD,MPH Molina Healthcare: Washington, 1154
Bayer, Terry P. Molina Healthcare: New Mexico, 747
Bayer, Terry P. Molina Healthcare: Ohio, 860
Bayer, Terry T, JD Molina Healthcare: Corporate Office, 153
Beach, Terry MagnaCare, 786
Beal, David Delta Dental of Colorado, 201
Beall, Tom Florida Health Care Plan, 275
Bearceÿ, Sarah UnitedHealthCare of Utah, 1110
Beargeon, Steve California Foundation for Medical Care, 94
Beaton, Brian HealthNow New York - Emblem Health, 779
Beatty, Sarah USA Managed Care Organization, 1091
Beauchaine, David Cigna-HealthSpring of Alabama, 8
Beauchamp, Robert, MD UnitedHealthCare of Arizona, 59
Beauchamp, Robert G UCare Medicare Plan, 614
Beauchamp, Robert G UCare Minnesota, 615
Beaule, Jean Francois ChiroSource Inc, 103
Becher, Jill WellPoint: Corporate Office, 414
Becher, Jill HealthLink HMO, 648
Beck, John G Unison Health Plan of Pennsylvania, 966
Becker, George H, Jr PacifiCare of Oklahoma, 892
Beckman, JS Security Life Insurance Company of America, 613
Beckman, Stephen Security Life Insurance Company of America, 613
Bedell, Karen A. Centene Corporation, 635
Beebe, Laurie Health New England, 533
Beer, Lori WellPoint: Corporate Office, 414
Begans, Peter SCAN Health Plan, 173
Behler, Anthony HealthSpan, 852
Behnke, David Delta Dental of Illinois, 364
Behuniak, Darren Devon Health Services, 938
Beitel, Rem CommunityCare Managed Healthcare Plans of Oklahoma, 885
Beitelman, Angela Health Alliance Medical Plans, 370
Bell, Christy W Horizon Blue Cross & Blue Shield of New Jersey, 724
Bell, Jill J Passport Health Plan, 463
Bell, Michael W CIGNA HealthCare of Connecticut, 219
Bell, Michael W CIGNA HealthCare of South Carolina, 995
Bell, Paul Preferred Medical Plan, 293
Bellah, Ann Pueblo Health Care, 209
Bellante, Jean Managed Health Services, 1196
Belrose, David United Concordia: Dental Corporation of Alabama, 15
Benak, Steve, MD Stanislaus Foundation for Medical Care, 175
Bencic, Eleanor Anthem Blue Cross & Blue Shield of Missouri, 631
Bendes, Ron Sterling Health Plans, 1161
Benedetto, Frank CIGNA HealthCare of Arizona, 36
Benevento, Anthony UPMC Health Plan, 968
Benjamin, Brian, DDS Liberty Dental Plan, 146
Bennett, John A, MD Devon Health Services, 938
Bennett, John D, MD CDPHP Medicare Plan, 758
Bennett, John D, MD CDPHP: Capital District Physicians' Health Plan, 759
Bennett, Joshua, MD HealthAmerica Pennsylvania, 948
Bennett, William A Vytra Health Plans, 808

Bensing, Gary Passport Health Plan, 463
Benson, Amie Assurant Employee Benefits: Minnesota, 593
Benson, Donald T. Great-West Healthcare Texas, 1062
Bentley, Brad AvMed Medicare Preferred, 260
Berardo, Joseph, Jr MagnaCare, 786
Beres, Mark, CPA Nationwide Better Health, 862
Berg, Al VSP: Vision Service Plan, 184
Berg, Charles G Oxford Health Plans: New Jersey, 731
Berg, Charles G Oxford Health Plans: New York, 799
Berg, Jim Elderplan, 768
Berge, Frank Dencap Dental Plans, 559
Berkowitz, Mona Pima Health System, 54
Berman, Cliff Catamaran Corporation, 358
Berman, Philip UnitedHealthCare of North Carolina, 827
Bernadette, Martha, MD Molina Healthcare: Washington, 1154
Bernard, Desi Quality Plan Administrators, 247
Bernard, Milton, DDS Quality Plan Administrators, 247
Bernauer, Judu PacifiCare Health Systems, 162
Berneking, Vicky Deaconess Health Plans, 395
Bernstein, Jeff eHealthInsurance Services Inc., 1058
Bernstein, Mike SummaCare Health Plan, 870
Berry, Elyse HealthPlus of Michigan: Flint, 569
Berry, Melody OSF HealthPlans, 379
Berry, Steven BlueLincs HMO, 883
Bertko, John M, FSA Humana Health Insurance of Ohio, 854
Bertolini, Mark J Aetna Health of Nevada, 684
Bertolini, Mark T Aetna Health of Alabama, 2
Bertolini, Mark T Aetna Health of Alaska, 18
Bertolini, Mark T Aetna Health of Arkansas, 62
Bertolini, Mark T Aetna Health of Colorado, 188
Bertolini, Mark T Aetna Health, Inc. Corporate Headquarters, 214
Bertolini, Mark T Aetna Health, Inc. Medicare Plan, 215
Bertolini, Mark T Aetna Health of Delaware, 226
Bertolini, Mark T Aetna Health District of Columbia, 239
Bertolini, Mark T Aetna Health of Georgia, 303
Bertolini, Mark T Aetna Health of Hawaii, 329
Bertolini, Mark T Aetna Health of Idaho, 341
Bertolini, Mark T Aetna Health of Iowa, 415
Bertolini, Mark T Aetna Health of Kansas, 431
Bertolini, Mark T Aetna Health of Kentucky, 452
Bertolini, Mark T Aetna Health of Louisiana, 467
Bertolini, Mark T Aetna Health of Maine, 484
Bertolini, Mark T Aetna Health of Maryland, 493
Bertolini, Mark T Aetna Health of Massachusetts, 519
Bertolini, Mark T Aetna Health of Michigan, 543
Bertolini, Mark T Aetna Health of Minnesota, 591
Bertolini, Mark T Aetna Health of Mississippi, 621
Bertolini, Mark T Aetna Health of Montana, 659
Bertolini, Mark T Aetna Health of Nebraska, 672
Bertolini, Mark T Aetna Health of New Hampshire, 699
Bertolini, Mark T Aetna Health of New Jersey, 709
Bertolini, Mark T Aetna Health of New Mexico, 737
Bertolini, Mark T Aetna Health of New York, 752
Bertolini, Mark T Aetna Health of North Dakota, 829
Bertolini, Mark T Aetna Health of Oregon, 894
Bertolini, Mark T Aetna Health of Pennsylvania, 922
Bertolini, Mark T Aetna Health of Rhode Island, 980
Bertolini, Mark T Aetna Health of South Dakota, 1008
Bertolini, Mark T Aetna Health of Utah, 1096
Bertolini, Mark T Aetna Health of Vermont, 1112
Bertolini, Mark T Aetna Health of Virginia, 1119
Bertolini, Mark T Aetna Health of Washington, 1143
Bertolini, Mark T Aetna Health of West Virginia, 1165
Bertolini, Mark T Aetna Health of Wisconsin, 1179
Bertolini, Mark T Aetna Health of Wyoming, 1207
Bertolini, Mark T. Aetna Health of Texas, 1041
Bertollini, Mark Aetna Health of California, 79
Berube, S. Neal IHC: Intermountain Healthcare Health Plan, 347
Bess, David AlohaCare, 330
Besserman, Marc MHNet Behavioral Health, 1076
Bettano, Carla Neighborhood Health Plan, 537
Beveridge, Roy A., MD Humana Health Insurance of Arizona, 46

Beveridge, Roy A., MD Arcadian Health Plans, 82
Beveridge, Roy A. Humana Health Insurance of Indiana, 404
Beveridge, Roy A., M.D Humana Health Insurance of San Antonio, 1070
Beveridge, M.D., Roy A. Humana Health Insurance of Huntsville, 13
Bhatia, Arun MagnaCare, 786
Bhugra, Andy Americhoice of Pennsylvania, 925
Bialaszewsky, Betty Blue Cross & Blue Shield of Texas: Houston, 1049
Bicknell, Patrick Health Plus of Louisiana, 476
Bielski, Miriam Care Choices, 552
Bielss, Jason HealthSmart Preferred Care, 373, 1065
Biglin, Helen T Delta Dental of New Hampshire, 702
Biglow, Tracy Preferred Health Systems Insurance Company, 444
Biglow, Tracy Preferred Plus of Kansas, 446
Billger, Aaron Highmark Blue Cross & Blue Shield, 949
Billger, Aaron Highmark Blue Shield, 950
Bilney, Jody Humana Health Insurance of Huntsville, 13
Bilney, Jody Humana Health Insurance of Indiana, 404
Bilney, Jody L. Humana Health Insurance of San Antonio, 1070
Bilt, Steven Bright Now! Dental, 92
Bing, Eric Blue Cross & Blue Shield of Texas: Houston, 1049
Bird, David CIGNA HealthCare of St. Louis, 637
Bird, Jon Beech Street Corporation: Alabama, 4
Bird, Jon Beech Street: Alaska, 19
Bird, Julio, MD Gundersen Lutheran Health Plan, 1192
Bisaccia, Lisa CVS CareMark, 983
Bischoff, J Kevin Regence Blue Cross & Blue Shield of Utah, 1107
Bisesi, Phil Lovelace Health Plan, 745
Bisesi, Phil Lovelace Medicare Health Plan, 746
Bishop, Anne Delta Dental of Arizona, 38
Bishop, Dale, MD Health Plan of San Joaquin, 131
Bishop, Skip San Francisco Health Plan, 171
Bittner, Clay Coventry Health Care of Louisiana, 472
Bjerre, Claudia Healthcare USA of Missouri, 647
Black, Carol UnitedHealthCare, 76
Black, Carol PacifiCare of Texas, 1079
Black, Carol PacifiCare Benefit Administrators, 1155
Black, Carol PacifiCare of Washington, 1156
Black, Steven H Oxford Health Plans: New Jersey, 731
Blackledge, James T Mutual of Omaha DentaBenefits, 681
Blackledge, James T Mutual of Omaha Health Plans, 682
Blackwell, Douglas Horizon Healthcare of New Jersey, 725
Blackwell, Douglas E. Horizon Blue Cross & Blue Shield of New Jersey, 724
Blackwood, Michael Gateway Health Plan, 943
Blaha, Diane J. CorVel Corporation, 113
Blaine, Carol, MBA Nationwide Better Health, 862
Blair, David T Catalyst Health Solutions Inc, 498
Blair, David T Catalyst RX, 812
Blake, Patty Tufts Health Medicare Plan, 538
Blake, Patty Tufts Health Plan, 539
Blakey, Jay B. Concentra: Corporate Office, 1055
Blalock, Robert, MD Humana Health Insurance of Jacksonville, 282
Blanchard, Cynthia Health Plus of Louisiana, 476
Blaney, Candy Prevea Health Network, 1200
Blanton, Chris CIGNA HealthCare of Idaho, 343
Blanton, Chris CIGNA HealthCare of Oregon, 899
Blanton, Chris CIGNA HealthCare of Washington, 1146
Blasi, Tina Magellan Health Services: Corporate Headquarters, 510
Blauwet, Judy Avera Health Plans, 1010
Blaylock, Ray Arkansas Community Care, 65
Blevens, Marc MHNet Behavioral Health, 1076
Blevins, Shirley Unison Health Plan of Pennsylvania, 966
Blickman, Fred Health Plan of New York, 778
Bloedorn, Dave Network Health Plan of Wisconsin, 1198
Bloem, James Humana Health Insurance of Fresno, 133
Bloem, James Humana Health Insurance of Southern California, 134
Bloem, James Humana Health Insurance of Illinois, 376
Bloem, James Humana Health Insurance of Iowa, 424
Bloem, James Humana Health Insurance of Nevada, 691
Bloem, James Humana Health Insurance of New Hampshire, 705
Bloem, James Humana Health Insurance of New Mexico, 744
Bloem, James H Humana Health Insurance of Tampa - Pinellas, 284
Bloem, James H Humana Health Insurance of Kansas, 441

Bloem, James H Humana Health Insurance of Kentucky, 460
Bloem, James H Humana Medicare Plan, 461
Bloem, James H Humana Health Insurance of Ohio, 854
Bloem, James H., FSA MAAA Humana Health Insurance of Arizona, 46
Bloem, James H. Arcadian Health Plans, 82
Bloem, James H. Humana Health Insurance of Indiana, 404
Bloem, James H. Humana Health Insurance of Michigan, 574
Bloen, James CompBenefits: Alabama, 9
Bloom, Alan Care 1st Health Plan: California, 96
Bloom, Mark, MD Coventry Health Care of Florida, 267
Blount, Joseph Coventry Health Care of Nebraska, 676
Blue, Jennifer Physicians United Plan, 291
Bluestein, Paul, MD ConnectiCare of Massachusetts, 525
Blums, Ivars Medical Card System (MCS), 975
Blunt, Jeff Humana Health Insurance of Indiana, 404
Blunt, Jeff Humana Health Insurance of Kansas, 441
Boals, Richard L Blue Cross & Blue Shield of Arizona, 34
Bode, Tim Americas PPO, 1009
Boe, Brian Liberty Health Plan: Corporate Office, 908
Boehme, Pam Script Care, Ltd., 1083
Bogle, George USA Managed Care Organization, 1091
Bogle, Mike USA Managed Care Organization, 1091
Bogossian, Gail ConnectiCare of Massachusetts, 525
Boher, Scott Medica Health - Medicare Plan, 605
Boland Docimo, Anne, MD UPMC Health Plan, 968
Bolding, Ron Inter Valley Health Plan, 136
Boles, Christopher D PacifiCare Dental and Vision Administrators, 161
Bolic, Walter S Delta Dental of New Mexico, 741
Bollman, Janet UnitedHealthCare of Arizona, 59
Bollman, Janet UnitedHealthCare of Colorado, 212
Bolton, Bette Blue Cross & Blue Shield of New Mexico, 739
Bolz, Terry Unity Health Insurance, 1204
Bonanna, Richard, MS MMM Quality Health Plans, 801
Bonanno, Richard, MD Quality Health Plans, 801
Bonanno, Richard, MD Quality Health Plans of New York, 802
Bonaparte, Philip M, MD Horizon NJ Health, 726
Bond, Jeff Cox Healthplans, 639
Bond, Judy Blue Cross & Blue Shield of Kansas City, 633
Bonn, Stacey Delta Dental of Illinois, 364
Booher, Scott Medica: South Dakota, 1018
Booma, Steve Florida Blue: Jacksonville, 273
Booma, Steve Florida Blue: Pensacola, 274
Boone, Michael Novasys Health, 74
Borer, Dorinda UnitedHealthcare Community Plan, 237
Borrajero, Maritza Neighborhood Health Partnership, 289
Bottitta, Louis W Valley Preferred, 970
Bottrill, Lorry Health Net of Arizona, 45
Bouchard, Angelee F, Esq Health Net: Corporate Headquarters, 130
Boudreau, Karen, MD Boston Medical Center Healthnet Plan, 523
Boudreaux, Gail K. UnitedHealthCare of Nebraska, 683
Bourbeau, Michael D Delta Dental of New Hampshire, 702
Bourn,, Dan Blue Cross & Blue Shield of Louisiana, 469
Bowen, Kenneth Assurant Employee Benefits: New Jersey, 714
Bowen, Kenneth D Assurant Employee Benefits: Corporate Headquarters, 632
Bowen, Kenneth D. Assurant Employee Benefits: California, 84
Bowers, David, MD Preferred Health Care, 959
Bowers, Scott A Unison Health Plan of Pennsylvania, 966
Bowie, Stuart Block Vision of Texas, 1047
Bowlus, Brad UnitedHealthCare, 76
Bowlus, Brad PacifiCare of Nevada, 696
Bowlus, Brad PacifiCare of Texas, 1079
Bowlus, Brad PacifiCare Benefit Administrators, 1155
Bowlus, Brad PacifiCare of Washington, 1156
Bowman, Lynn Harvard Pilgrim Health Care, 531
Bowman, Nadina Highmark Blue Cross & Blue Shield, 949
Boxer, Mark CIGNA HealthCare of Arizona, 36
Boxer, Mark CIGNA HealthCare of Northern California, 105
Boxer, Mark CIGNA HealthCare of Southern California, 106
Boxer, Mark CIGNA HealthCare of Maine, 486
Boxer, Mark CIGNA HealthCare of Minnesota, 596
Boxer, Mark CIGNA HealthCare of St. Louis, 637
Boxer, Mark CIGNA HealthCare of Nevada, 687

Boxer, Mark CIGNA HealthCare of New Hampshire, 701
Boxer, Mark CIGNA HealthCare of North Carolina, 813
Boxer, Michael EyeMed Vision Care, 850
Boyd, Laura Community Health Plan of Washington, 1147
Boyer, Julie HealthPlus of Michigan: Flint, 569
Boyer, Julie HealthPlus of Michigan: Saginaw, 570
Boyer, Kent Great-West Healthcare of Massachusetts, 530
Bracikowski, James, MD Windsor Medicare Extra, 1040
Bradfield, Jessie E Preferred Healthcare System, 960
Bradford, Dale Martin's Point HealthCare, 490
Bradley, Don W, MD Blue Cross & Blue Shield of North Carolina, 811
Bradley, Robin Windsor Medicare Extra, 1040
Bradshaw, John Interplan Health Group, 1071
Brady, Ray Assurant Employee Benefits: Pennsylvania, 927
Brady, Tom UnitedHealthCare of Ohio: Columbus, 877
Brady, Tom UnitedHealthCare of Ohio: Dayton & Cincinnati, 878
Braff, Dave Assurant Employee Benefits: Michigan, 545
Brainerd, Mary Health Partners Medicare Plan, 601
Brainerd, Mary HealthPartners, 602
Braly, Angela Anthem Blue Cross & Blue Shield of Missouri, 631
Bramson, James United Concordia: Dental Corporation of Alabama, 15
Branchick, Vivian C, RN Los Angeles County Department of Health Services, 147
Branchini, Frank HealthNow New York - Emblem Health, 779
Branchini, Frank J GHI, 774
Branchini, Frank J Health Plan of New York, 778
Branchini, Frank J UnitedHealthCare of North Carolina, 827
Branchini, Frank J. GHI Medicare Plan, 775
Brandenburg, Heather Chinese Community Health Plan, 101
Brandmaier, Neil CDPHP Medicare Plan, 758
Branson, Rick, DC HSM: Healthcare Cost Management, 603
Braswell, Judi Behavioral Health Systems, 5
Brecher, Randy Liberty Dental Plan, 146
Brecher, Randy Pacific Dental Benefits, 157
Breen, Bill Health Choice LLC, 1031
Breidenbach, William R Health Plans, Inc., 535
Brendzel, Ronald I SafeGuard Health Enterprises: Corporate Office, 170
Brendzel, Ronald I SafeGuard Health Enterprises: Texas, 1081
Brennan, Martin Pacific Dental Benefits, 157
Brennan, Troyen A., MD CVS CareMark, 983
Breskin, William A Blue Cross and Blue Shield Association, 357
Brewer, Charles UnitedHealthCare of Louisiana, 481
Briard, Mike Vantage Health Plan, 482
Bridges, David Arkansas Blue Cross and Blue Shield, 64
Briggs, Dow, MD United Concordia: Dental Corporation of Alabama, 15
Bright, Yvette D Independence Blue Cross, 952
Brill, Joel V, MD Action Healthcare Management Services, 28
Brill, Martin J Health Partners Medicare Plan, 946
Brillstein, Lilli AmeriChoice by UnitedHealthCare, 754
Brinkley, Tim Unison Health Plan of Ohio, 876
Brinsfield, Jeff, Jr QualChoice/QCA Health Plan, 75
Brinson, Beverlie Kaiser Permanente Health Plan of the Mid-Atlantic States, 509
Britt, Brian Keystone Health Plan Central, 954
Brittain, Jim Virginia Health Network, 1141
Broatch, Robert E. Guardian Life Insurance Company of America, 777
Brocksome, Stephen J Blue Cross of Idaho Health Service, Inc., 342
Broderick, Peter, MD Stanislaus Foundation for Medical Care, 175
Brodt, Carolyn Primecare Dental Plan, 168
Brody, David, MD Denver Health Medical Plan Inc, 202
Broemmer, Megan Med-Pay, 650
Broeren, Marcia Network Health Plan of Wisconsin, 1198
Brooks, G. Remmington, MD Kern Family Health Care, 142
Brooks, Gary VSP: Vision Service Plan, 184
Brooks, Rahmaire Central Susquehanna Healthcare Providers, 933
Brousard, Bruce Humana Health Insurance of Nebraska, 679
Broussard, Bruce CompBenefits: Alabama, 9
Broussard, Bruce Humana Health Insurance of Fresno, 133
Broussard, Bruce Humana Health Insurance of Southern California, 134
Broussard, Bruce Humana Health Insurance of Nevada, 691
Broussard, Bruce Humana Health Insurance of New Hampshire, 705
Broussard, Bruce Humana Health Insurance of New Mexico, 744
Broussard, Bruce D. Humana Health Insurance of Huntsville, 13

Broussard, Bruce D. Humana Health Insurance of Arizona, 46
Broussard, Bruce D. Arcadian Health Plans, 82
Broussard, Bruce D. Humana Health Insurance of Indiana, 404
Broussard, Bruce D. Humana Health Insurance of Michigan, 574
Broussard, Bruce D. Humana Health Insurance of San Antonio, 1070
Brown, Adrian Health Choice Arizona, 44
Brown, D'Ln Foundation for Medical Care for Kern & Santa Barbara County, 123
Brown, David Wellmark Blue Cross Blue Shield, 429
Brown, Frank L, MD Trigon Health Care, 1138
Brown, Jim Script Care, Ltd., 1083
Brown, Julie Humana Health Insurance of Orlando, 283
Brown, Kenneth D. Assurant Employee Benefits: Colorado, 192
Brown, Kevin Script Care, Ltd., 1083
Brown, Marc Kaiser Permanente Health Plan of Northern California, 138
Brown, Mary Kim, RN-BC Action Healthcare Management Services, 28
Brown, Mike Arkansas Blue Cross and Blue Shield, 64
Brown, Mindy Signature Health Alliance, 1038
Brown, Mollie Coalition America's National Preferred Provider Network, 761
Brown, Patricia M.C. Priority Partners Health Plans, 515
Brown, Paul F Blue Cross and Blue Shield Association, 357
Brown, Randy WellPoint: Corporate Office, 414
Brown, Robert Clear One Health Plans, 900
Brown, Sandy Health Plus of Louisiana, 476
Browne, Robert UnitedHealthCare of Nebraska, 683
Browning, Francis QualChoice/QCA Health Plan, 75
Brubaker, Lisa Regence BlueShield of Idaho, 351
Brubaker, Lisa Regence Blue Cross & Blue Shield of Oregon, 915
Brubaker, Lisa A MVP Health Care: New Hampshire, 706
Brubaker, Lisa A MVP Health Care Medicare Plan, 790
Brubaker, Lisa A MVP Health Care: Buffalo Region, 791
Brubaker, Lisa A MVP Health Care: Mid-State Region, 794
Brubaker, Lisa A MVP Health Care: Western New York, 795
Bruce, Bill Devon Health Services, 938
Bruce, Reagan Interplan Health Group, 137
Brueckner, Stefen Humana Health Insurance of Illinois, 376
Brumley, Heather American PPO, 1043
Bruner, Dawn Orange County Foundation for Medical Care, 156
Brunnemer, James A Arnett Health Plans, 391
Brutcher, Jeff Hometown Health Plan, 690
Bryant, Gary W, CPA American Pioneer Life Insurance Co, 251
Bryant, Gary W TexanPlus Medicare Advantage HMO, 1085
Bryant, Oscar Delta Dental of Virginia, 1126
Bryt, A. Bartley, DC Landmark Healthplan of California, 145
Buck, Eric E Preferred Health Care, 959
Bucknam, Ted Concentra: Corporate Office, 1055
Buckwold, Frederick CIGNA HealthCare of Arkansas, 67
Buckwold, Frederick CIGNA HealthCare of Mississippi, 622
Budden, Joan Priority Health, 581
Budden, Joan Priority Health: Corporate Headquarters, 582
Buffa, Jan CareSource Mid Rogue Health Plan, 898
Bull, Lynda Liberty Dental Plan of Nevada, 692
Bullen, Bruce Blue Cross & Blue Shield of Massachusetts, 522
Bullock, Doug Blue Cross of Idaho Health Service, Inc., 342
Bumstead, Sean Total Health Care, 585
Buncher, James E SafeGuard Health Enterprises: Corporate Office, 170
Buncher, James E SafeGuard Health Enterprises: Texas, 1081
Bunio, Karen Total Health Care, 585
Bunker, Jonathan UnitedHealthcare Nevada, 698
Bunker, Jonathan W Health Plan of Nevada, 689
Bunnell, Ron Banner MediSun Medicare Plan, 33
Burdick, Jana Presbyterian Health Plan, 748
Burgess, Howard Physicians Health Plan of Mid-Michigan, 580
Burgos, Gilbert, MD Care Choices, 552
Burk, Gail Beta Health Plan, 194
Burke, Natalie Total Health Care, 585
Burke, Richard, Sr UnitedHealthCare of Alabama, 16
Burke, Richard P. Fallon Community Health Plan, 528
Burke, Richard P. Fallon Community Medicare Plan, 529
Burkeen, Robert Assurant Employee Benefits: Oklahoma, 881
Burnett, Ann T BlueChoice Health Plan of South Carolina, 993
Burnett, Janet Welborn Health Plans, 413

Burnham, William, MD Select Health of South Carolina, 1003
Burns, Dennis A, DDS Superior Dental Care, 872
Burns, Heather Welborn Health Plans, 413
Burrell, Chester CareFirst Blue Cross Blue Shield, 240
Burrell, Chester CareFirst Blue Cross & Blue Shield of Virginia, 1122
Burruano, Martin, RPh Independent Health Medicare Plan, 783
Burton, David Great-West/One Health Plan, 204
Burton, David CIGNA HealthCare of Pennsylvania, 934
Burton, David CIGNA HealthCare of Utah, 1098
Burzynski, Mark Blue Cross & Blue Shield of Montana, 661
Busby, Tom Educators Mutual, 1100
Busch, Charles E HealthSmart Preferred Care, 1065
Busek, Rhonda J Trillium Community Health Plan, 917
Butera, Joe Capital Blue Cross, 932
Butera, Joe Keystone Health Plan Central, 954
Butler, Christopher Independence Blue Cross, 952
Butler, Mark UnitedHealthCare of Massachusetts, 541
Butler, Martha, RN, MPH Essence Healthcare, 643
Butler, Tony Essence Healthcare, 643
Butts, Susan Cox Healthplans, 639
Buyse, Marylou Scott & White Health Plan, 1082
Byers, Ed HMO Health Ohio, 853
Byers, Ed Medical Mutual of Ohio, 857
Byers, Ed Medical Mutual of Ohio Medicare Plan, 858
Byers, Ed SuperMed One, 873
Byers, Ed Carolina Care Plan, 994
Byrd, Arthur HealthNow New York - Emblem Health, 779
Byrd, Arthur J. GHI, 774
Byrd, Arthur J. GHI Medicare Plan, 775
Byrd, Michael Sharp Health Plan, 174
Byrd, Terence L., JD HealthFirst New Jersey Medicare Plan, 723
Byrne, James F, MD Priority Health, 581
Byrne, James F, MD Priority Health: Corporate Headquarters, 582

C

Cagan, Laird, MD Boulder Valley Individual Practice Association, 195
Cahill, Judge Patrick T Delta Dental of Michigan, Ohio and Indiana, 847
Cahill, Tom Sterling Health Plans, 1161
Calabrese, Steven V Touchstone Health HMO, 803
Calandro, Michele Blue Cross & Blue Shield of Louisiana, 469
Callahan, Peggy, BSN Carilion Health Plans, 1123
Callanan, Theresa VSP: Vision Service Plan of Minnesota, 620
Calpino, Lori Berkshire Health Partners, 928
Calverly, Sara Deaconess Health Plans, 395
Calzadilla-Fiallo, Liz UnitedHealthCare of Florida, 298
Calzadilla-Fiallo, Liz UnitedHealthCare of South Florida, 299
Calzadilla-Fiallo, Liz UnitedHealthCare of Louisiana, 481
Camerlinck, Bryan Blue Cross & Blue Shield of Kansas City, 633
Camerlinck, Bryan Preferred Care Blue, 657
Campbell, Joe Educators Mutual, 1100
Campbell, Juan A Health New England, 533
Campbell, Raedina Preferred Health Systems Insurance Company, 444
Campbell, Raedina Preferred Plus of Kansas, 446
Campbell, Robert H CIGNA HealthCare of South Carolina, 995
Campos, Alina, M.D. Leon Medical Centers Health Plan, 286
Cannon, Doug VIVA Health, 17
Cannon, John WellPoint: Corporate Office, 414
Cannon, John Anthem Blue Cross & Blue Shield of Maine, 485
Cannon, Kathy Script Care, Ltd., 1083
Capezza, Joseph UnitedHealthCare of North Carolina, 827
Capezza, Joseph C, CPA Health Net: Corporate Headquarters, 130
Caplan, Jesse, Esq. Fallon Community Health Plan, 528
Caplan, Jesse, Esq Fallon Community Medicare Plan, 529
Capozzi, Vincent Harvard Pilgrim Health Care, 531
Card, Dorinda UnitedHealthCare of Nebraska, 683
Cardone, James Blue Cross & Blue Shield of Western New York, 756
Carlisle, Douglas Humana Health Insurance of Illinois, 376
Carlisle, Scott Alliance Regional Health Network, 1042
Carlos, Clayton, MPA Kern Family Health Care, 142
Carlson, Danita Central California Alliance for Health, 99
Carlson, James Amerigroup Nevada, 685
Carlson, James Amerigroup Ohio, 840

Carlson, Lisa Sanford Health Plan, 427
Carmouche, David, MD Blue Cross & Blue Shield of Louisiana, 469
Carns, Patricia HealthAmerica, 947
Carpenter, Marie UnitedHealthCare of the Mid-Atlantic, 518
Carpenter, Sara Alliant Health Plans, 305
Carpenter, Theodore TexanPlus Medicare Advantage HMO, 1085
Carpenter, Theodore M, Jr American Pioneer Life Insurance Co, 251
Carpenter, Theodore M, Jr Universal American Medicare Plans, 807
Carrasco, Angie Medical Care Referral Group, 1074
Carrillo, Liz Blue Cross & Blue Shield of New Mexico, 739
Carroll, Jim CONCERN: Employee Assistance Program, 111
Carroll, Jimmy Scott & White Health Plan, 1082
Carroll, Stacey Liberty Health Advantage Medicare Plan, 785
Carsazza, William Aetna Health of Colorado, 188
Carsello, Jamie UCare Medicare Plan, 614
Carsello, Jamie UCare Minnesota, 615
Carson, Kim Healthy & Well Kids in Iowa, 423
Carter, David W Magellan Health Services Indiana, 405
Carter, David W Magellan Health Services: Corporate Headquarters, 510
Carter, Gertrude, MD L.A. Care Health Plan, 143
Carter, Julie PacifiCare of Arizona, 51
Carter, Mark B Passport Health Plan, 463
Caruncho, Joseph L Preferred Care Partners, 292
Caruso, Joseph A Guardian Life Insurance Company of America, 777
Carvelli, John Liberty Dental Plan, 146
Carvelli, John Liberty Dental Plan of Nevada, 692
Casazza, William Aetna Health of California, 79
Casazza, William J Aetna Health of Alabama, 2
Casazza, William J Aetna Health of Alaska, 18
Casazza, William J Aetna Health of Arkansas, 62
Casazza, William J Aetna Health, Inc. Corporate Headquarters, 214
Casazza, William J Aetna Health, Inc. Medicare Plan, 215
Casazza, William J Aetna Health of Delaware, 226
Casazza, William J Aetna Health District of Columbia, 239
Casazza, William J Aetna Health of Hawaii, 329
Casazza, William J Aetna Health of Idaho, 341
Casazza, William J Aetna Health of Iowa, 415
Casazza, William J Aetna Health of Kansas, 431
Casazza, William J Aetna Health of Kentucky, 452
Casazza, William J Aetna Health of Louisiana, 467
Casazza, William J Aetna Health of Maine, 484
Casazza, William J Aetna Health of Maryland, 493
Casazza, William J Aetna Health of Massachusetts, 519
Casazza, William J Aetna Health of Michigan, 543
Casazza, William J Aetna Health of Minnesota, 591
Casazza, William J Aetna Health of Mississippi, 621
Casazza, William J Aetna Health of Montana, 659
Casazza, William J Aetna Health of Nebraska, 672
Casazza, William J Aetna Health of Nevada, 684
Casazza, William J Aetna Health of New Hampshire, 699
Casazza, William J Aetna Health of New Jersey, 709
Casazza, William J Aetna Health of New Mexico, 737
Casazza, William J Aetna Health of New York, 752
Casazza, William J Aetna Health of North Dakota, 829
Casazza, William J Aetna Health of Oregon, 894
Casazza, William J Aetna Health of Pennsylvania, 922
Casazza, William J Aetna Health of Rhode Island, 980
Casazza, William J Aetna Health of South Dakota, 1008
Casazza, William J Aetna Health of Utah, 1096
Casazza, William J Aetna Health of Vermont, 1112
Casazza, William J Aetna Health of Virginia, 1119
Casazza, William J Aetna Health of Washington, 1143
Casazza, William J Aetna Health of West Virginia, 1165
Casazza, William J Aetna Health of Wisconsin, 1179
Casazza, William J Aetna Health of Wyoming, 1207
Casazza, William J. Aetna Health of Texas, 1041
Casberg, Jeff, RPh ConnectiCare, 220
Casberg, Jeff ConnectiCare of Massachusetts, 525
Casey, Dennis Anthem Blue Cross & Blue Shield of Indiana, 388
Casey, Dennis Anthem Blue Cross & Blue Shield of New Hampshire, 700
Casey, Dennis SelectCare Access Corporation, 962
Casey, Dennis W Anthem Blue Cross & Blue Shield of Indiana, 389

Casey, Steven California Dental Network, 93
Cashman, Christopher Independence Blue Cross, 952
Casper, John Great-West Healthcare Oregon, 904
Cass, Brady, RHU,MHP Asuris Northwest Health, 1145
Cass, Danielle Kaiser Permanente Health Plan: Corporate Office, 140
Cassady, Margaret M, Esq Excellus Blue Cross Blue Shield: Central New York, 770
Cassady, Margaret M, Esq Excellus Blue Cross Blue Shield: Utica Region, 772
Cassano, Scott Health Plan of Nevada, 689
Cassell, Jim HSM: Healthcare Cost Management, 603
Cassidy, Christine Fallon Community Health Plan, 528
Cassidy, Christine Fallon Community Medicare Plan, 529
Castellanos, Simon Western Dental Services, 186
Castillo, Carolina Garcia Leon Medical Centers Health Plan, 286
Castillo, Mayra Vision Plan of America, 183
Castleberry, Mike HealthSCOPE Benefits, 71
Castro, Ann Marie CIGNA HealthCare of New Jersey, 718
Catalano, Charles CIGNA HealthCare of New Jersey, 718
Cataldi, Pauline Blue Cross & Blue Shield of Western New York, 756
Cataldo, Jeanette Preferred Utilization Management Inc, 166
Cataldo, Ronald Chiropractic Health Plan of California, 102
Cataldo, Ronald, Sr Preferred Utilization Management Inc, 166
Catino, Annette QualCare, 732
Catlender, Katie Neighborhood Health Plan, 537
Cato, Rose Anne QualChoice/QCA Health Plan, 75
Caudill, Dr Paul HealthPartners, 1032
Caufield, Mary, MD CIGNA HealthCare of Georgia, 311
Cavalier, Kevin SummaCare Health Plan, 870
Caylor, Carole Health Choice LLC, 1031
Cenachetti, Mark Tufts Health Plan: Rhode Island, 988
Cerese, Julie UnitedHealthCare of Nebraska, 683
Cesare, Denise Blue Cross of Northeastern Pennsylvania, 929
Cesare, Denise First Priority Health, 942
Cetti, William CIGNA HealthCare of Alaska, 21
Cetti, William CIGNA HealthCare of Colorado, 196
Cetti, William CIGNA HealthCare of Montana, 662
Cetti, William CIGNA HealthCare of Wyoming, 1209
Chabon, Robert, MD Community Health Improvement Solutions, 638
Chaet, Douglas L Independence Blue Cross, 952
Chagolla, Lilia Central California Alliance for Health, 99
Chaitkin, Paul, MD First Commonwealth, 367
Challis, Dave Saint Mary's Health Plans, 697
Chambers, Mary Beth Blue Cross & Blue Shield of Kansas, 433
Champney, Dan E, Esq HealthPlus of Michigan: Flint, 569
Champney, Dan E, Esq HealthPlus of Michigan: Saginaw, 570
Champney, Dan E. Health Alliance Medicare, 566
Champney, Dan E. Health Alliance Plan, 567
Chan, Raymond SCAN Health Plan, 173
Chandler, H Jody Blue Cross & Blue Shield of Arizona, 34
Chandra, Kathy National Capital PPO, 1133
Chaney, G Mark CareFirst Blue Cross & Blue Shield of Virginia, 1122
Chaney, G. Mark CareFirst Blue Cross Blue Shield, 240
Chaney, Jared HMO Health Ohio, 853
Chaney, Jared Medical Mutual of Ohio, 857
Chaney, Jared Medical Mutual of Ohio Medicare Plan, 858
Chaney, Jared SuperMed One, 873
Channing, Walter, Jr American WholeHealth Network, 924
Chansler, Jeffrey D. GHI, 774
Chansler, Jeffrey D. GHI Medicare Plan, 775
Chapman, Barbara Harvard Pilgrim Health Care, 531
Chapman, Carol Preferred Care, 958
Chapman, Carole Preferred Care, 958
Chapman, Heidi UnitedHealthCare of Louisiana, 481
Charlier, Brian Prevea Health Network, 1200
Chase, Deb Priority Partners Health Plans, 515
Chase, Michael D, MD Kaiser Permanente Health Plan of Colorado, 207
Chase, Thomas D Delta Dental of Rhode Island, 984
Chauhan, Roki, MD Premera Blue Cross, 1157
Chaundhry, Shaheen OptiCare Managed Vision, 823
Cheng, John HealthFirst New Jersey Medicare Plan, 723
Cheng, Michael Hawaii Medical Services Association, 335
Chernack, Carol Horizon NJ Health, 726

Chernis, Bob Central California Alliance for Health, 99
Chesley, Rebecca Fortified Provider Network, 42
Chickering, Marcelle Wellmark Blue Cross Blue Shield, 429
Chilson, Mark CareSource: Michigan, 553
Chilson, Mark CareSource, 844
Chin, Wee Willamette Dental Insurance, 921
Chin, Yuen Willamette Dental Insurance, 921
Chinn, Terri Lovelace Health Plan, 745
Chinn, Terri Lovelace Medicare Health Plan, 746
Chirichella, Linda Avesis: Corporate Headquarters, 32
Chirichella, Linda Avesis: Arizona, 309
Chirichella, Linda Avesis: Minnesota, 594
Chirichella, Linda Avesis: Texas, 1046
Chiricosta, Rick HMO Health Ohio, 853
Chiricosta, Rick Medical Mutual of Ohio, 857
Chiricosta, Rick Medical Mutual of Ohio Medicare Plan, 858
Chiricosta, Rick SuperMed One, 873
Chitty, Art Blue Cross & Blue Shield of Texas: Houston, 1049
Choate, Eddie Delta Dental of Arkansas, 69
Choksi, Jayendra CompCare: Comprehensive Behavioral Care, 266
Chow, Edward, MD Chinese Community Health Plan, 101
Chowning, Betty CHA Health, 455
Choy, Gregory UnitedHealthCare of New York, 805
Chrisman, Carolyn Carilion Health Plans, 1123
Christensen, Barbara Providence Health Plans, 914
Christian, Todd, MBA Nationwide Better Health, 862
Christian-Wills, Theresa Cariten Healthcare, 1026
Christian-Wills, Theresa Cariten Preferred, 1027
Christianson, Blair HMO Colorado, 205
Christianson, R Craig, MD UCare Medicare Plan, 614
Christianson, R Craig, MD UCare Minnesota, 615
Christie, Edward J Magellan Health Services: Corporate Headquarters, 510
Christy, Paul Physicians United Plan, 291
Chu, Benjamin K, MPH Kaiser Permanente Health Plan of Southern California, 139
Church, Rob Select Health of South Carolina, 1003
Cianfrocco, Healther Unison Health Plan of Pennsylvania, 966
Cierpka, Lisa, RN Quality Health Plans, 801
Cierpka, Lisa, RN Quality Health Plans of New York, 802
Cipponeri, Jannell, MD Stanislaus Foundation for Medical Care, 175
Clabeaux, Patricia Independent Health, 782
Claborn, Renee Health Net Health Plan of Oregon, 905
Clancy, Mike Southeastern Indiana Health Organization, 410
Clarey, Patricia T Health Net: Corporate Headquarters, 130
Clark, Alan Southeastern Indiana Health Organization, 410
Clark, Bob Children's Mercy Pediatric Care Network, 636
Clark, Karen Managed Healthcare Systems of New Jersey, 728
Clark, Karen L Horizon NJ Health, 726
Clark, Kelly OptumHealth Care Solutions: Physical Health, 610
Clark, Monty Gundersen Lutheran Health Plan, 1192
Clark, Roger E, DDS Superior Dental Care, 872
Clark, Scott Scott & White Health Plan, 1082
Clark, Sheree North Alabama Managed Care Inc, 14
Clarke, Richard, Ph.D. Magellan Health Services Arizona, 47
Clarren, Steven N American Community Mutual Insurance Company, 544
Clawson, Bryon Regence Blue Cross & Blue Shield of Utah, 1107
Clay, Brett Altius Health Plans, 1097
Claypool, Loren W HealthSmart Preferred Care, 373
Claypool, Loren W. HealthSmart Preferred Care, 1065
Cleary, Vicki Touchstone Health HMO, 803
Clemente, Gina Managed Health Network, 148
Clements, Amber R Quality Health Plans, 801
Clements, Amber R Quality Health Plans of New York, 802
Clemons, Gordon CorVel Corporation, 113
Click, Rick Molina Healthcare: Washington, 1154
Clothier, Brad Preferred Health Systems Insurance Company, 444
Clothier, Brad Preferred Plus of Kansas, 446
Coakley, Susan Boston Medical Center Healthnet Plan, 523
Cobb, Lisa Interplan Health Group, 137, 1071
Cochran, Jim South Central Preferred, 963
Coffey, Pamela HealthSmart Preferred Care, 1065
Coffman, Melissa Unicare: West Virginia, 1176

Diamond, David A Mutual of Omaha DentaBenefits, 681
Diamond, David A Mutual of Omaha Health Plans, 682
Diaz, Norma Community Health Group, 109
Diaz-Esquivel, Pablo, MD Alliance Regional Health Network, 1042
DiBona, G Fred AmeriHealth HMO, 227
Dickelman, Peg Noridian Insurance Services, 837
Dickes, Robert M Carolina Care Plan, 994
Dicks, Joseph MetroPlus Health Plan, 788
Dickson, Jan Health Choice LLC, 1031
Diehs, Creta Dimension Health PPO, 270
Diercks, David Unity Health Insurance, 1204
Dill, Matthew G Midlands Choice, 680
DiMarco, Arthur Perfect Health Insurance Company, 800
DiMura, Vincent Meritain Health: Kentucky, 462
DiMura, Vincent Meritain Health: Minnesota, 607
DiMura, Vincent Meritain Health: Missouri, 653
DiMura, Vincent, CPA Meritain Health: Corporate Headquarters, 787
DiMura, Vincent Meritain Health: Ohio, 859
Dishman, Pam Delta Dental of Tennessee, 1029
Disser, E J Preferred Vision Care, 447
Disser, Michele G, RN Preferred Vision Care, 447
Disser, P J Preferred Vision Care, 447
DiTorro, Frank Blue Cross & Blue Shield of Kansas City, 633
Dockins, Jim HealthPartners, 1032
Dodds Foley, Georgia Amerigroup Georgia, 306
Dodds Foley, Georgia Amerigroup Maryland, 495
Dodds Foley, Georgia, Esq. Amerigroup Texas, 1044
Doerr, R Chris Florida Blue: Jacksonville, 273
Doerr, R Chris Florida Blue: Pensacola, 274
Doherty, Michelle American Pioneer Life Insurance Co, 251
Dolfi, Scott Guardian Life Insurance Company of America, 777
Dolloff, Gaylee Health Partners of Kansas, 440
Donald, Fiona Health Plan of San Mateo, 132
Donaldson, William H Aetna Health of the Carolinas, 809
Donohoe, Cindy Great-West Healthcare of Massachusetts, 530
Donohue, Fay Dentaquest, 526
Donovan, Leann Denver Health Medical Plan Inc, 202
Doolen, Erick PacificSource Health Plans: Idaho, 349
Doolen, Erick PacificSource Health Plans: Corporate Headquarters, 913
Dooley, Ronald SVS Vision, 584
Dopps, Brad, DC PCC Preferred Chiropractic Care, 443
Dopps, John, DC PCC Preferred Chiropractic Care, 443
Dopps, Mark, DC PCC Preferred Chiropractic Care, 443
Dopps, Robert, DC PCC Preferred Chiropractic Care, 443
Doran, Laurie Boston Medical Center Healthnet Plan, 523
Dore, Alfred, Jr HealthAmerica, 947
Doria, Norma Community First Health Plans, 1054
Dorman-Rodriguez, Deborah Health Care Service Corporation, 372
Dorney, William, MD American WholeHealth Network, 924
Dorney, William P, Dr American WholeHealth Network, 924
Dorr, Marjorie Anthem Blue Cross & Blue Shield Connecticut, 217
Double, Mary American Health Care Group, 923
Dougan, Gary Pacific Dental Benefits, 157
Dougan, Gary, DDS Liberty Dental Plan of Nevada, 692
Douglas, , Thompson Neighborhood Health Plan of Rhode Island, 987
Douglass, Lee Arkansas Blue Cross and Blue Shield, 64
Dowdy, Shelly American PPO, 1043
Dowlatshahi, Brenda Neighborhood Health Plan of Rhode Island, 987
Downey, Ellen American Community Mutual Insurance Company, 544
Downey, Ellen M Care Choices, 552
Downing, Rebecca Western Health Advantage, 187
Downs, Barbara A, RN CDPHP Medicare Plan, 758
Downs, Barbara A, RN CDPHP: Capital District Physicians' Health Plan, 759
Doyle, Michael Mercy Health Plans: Kansas, 442
Doyle, Michael Mercy Health Medicare Plan, 651
Doyle, Michael Mercy Health Plans: Corporate Office, 652
Doyle, Michael Mercy Health Plans: Oklahoma, 891
Doyle Steranka, Sarah American Health Care Group, 923
Dozoretz, Dr Ronald Val-U-Health, 969
Dozoretz, Dr Ronald Value Behavioral Health of Pennsylvania, 971
Draper, Gene Foundation for Medical Care for Mendocino and Lake Counties, 124

Dreibelbis, Dawn Berkshire Health Partners, 928
Dreyfus, Andrew Blue Cross & Blue Shield of Massachusetts, 522
Drnevich, Ronald Capital Blue Cross, 932
Drohan, Mariann E. GHI, 774
Drohan, Mariann E. GHI Medicare Plan, 775
Druker, Michele Wellmark Blue Cross Blue Shield, 429
Dubbs, Allison The Dental Care Plus Group, 874
DuCharme, James Harvard Pilgrim Health Care, 531
Duda, Emil D Univera Healthcare, 806
Dudley, G Martin InterGroup Services Corporation, 953
Dudley, Gregory InterGroup Services Corporation, 953
Dudley, Michael M Optima Health Plan, 1134
Duer, Linda Primary Health Plan, 350
Duford, Don One Call Medical, 730
Dugan, Chris Anthem Blue Cross & Blue Shield of Maine, 485
Dugan, Chris Anthem Blue Cross & Blue Shield of New Hampshire, 700
Dugan, Pat HMO Health Ohio, 853
Dugan, Pat Medical Mutual of Ohio, 857
Dugan, Pat Medical Mutual of Ohio Medicare Plan, 858
Dugan, Pat SuperMed One, 873
Duguc, Jack Omni IPA/Medcore Medical Group, 154
Dukes, Kim UnitedHealthCare of Mississippi, 627
Dulin, Joseph USA Managed Care Organization, 1091
Dunaway, George CompBenefits Corporation, 313
Dunaway, Suzie Children's Mercy Pediatric Care Network, 636
Duncan, Pat Rocky Mountain Health Plans, 210
Dunk, Jeanne Care Choices, 552
Dunk, Jeanne Health Alliance Medicare, 566
Dunlop, Richard UnitedHealthCare of Kentucky, 466
Dunn, Lucille Island Group Administration, Inc., 784
Dunn, Molly Assurant Employee Benefits: Michigan, 545
Dunn, Van, MD MetroPlus Health Plan, 788
Dunn, Zon Superior Vision Services, Inc., 176
Dunn-Malhotra, Ellen Health Plan of San Mateo, 132
Durr, Barbara HealthSpan, 852
Dur n, Jos, Medical Card System (MCS), 975
Duvall, Dianna Assurant Employee Benefits: New Jersey, 714
Duvall, Dianna D Assurant Employee Benefits: Corporate Headquarters, 632
Dwyer, Thomas K Health Plan of New York, 778
Dykes, Cathy Southeastern Indiana Health Organization, 410

E

Earl, Chris Delta Dental of Nebraska, 677
Earley, J Fred Mountain State Blue Cross Blue Shield, 1174
Ebbin, Allan, MD, MPH UnitedHealthcare Nevada, 698
Ebert, Mike OneNet PPO, 512
Ebert, Thomas H, MD Health New England, 533
Eck, Brian UCare Medicare Plan, 614
Eck, Brian UCare Minnesota, 615
Eckbert, William, MD Horizon Health Corporation, 1068
Eckrich, Nancy CoreSource: Arkansas, 68
Eckrich, Nancy CoreSource: Corporate Headquarters, 362
Eckrich, Nancy CoreSource: Kansas (FMH CoreSource), 435
Eckrich, Nancy CoreSource: Maryland, 501
Eckrich, Nancy CoreSource: North Carolina, 814
Eckstein, Michael Health Tradition, 1193
Eddy, Andrew Western Dental Services, 186
Edelman, Kathy Cofinity, 555
Eden, Mary Presbyterian Health Plan, 748
Eden, Mary Presbyterian Medicare Plans, 749
Edmondson, Mike BlueLincs HMO, 883
Edmondson, Robert E On Lok Lifeways, 155
Edwards, Brett HealthSCOPE Benefits, 71
Edwards, Joe HealthSCOPE Benefits, 71
Edwards, Kathy Cardinal Health Alliance, 393
Edwards, Michael Catamaran Corporation, 358
Edwards, Z Colette, MD CIGNA HealthCare of West Virginia, 1166
Efrusy, Brian Total Health Care, 585
Eftekhari, Amir Americas PPO, 1009
Eftekhari, Nazie Araz Group, 592
Eftekhari, Nazie Americas PPO, 1009
Egan, Rob Tufts Health Medicare Plan, 538

Egbert, Jeff Phoenix Health Plans, 53
Eichenberg, Karen Paramount Elite Medicare Plan, 866
Eichenberg, Karen Paramount Health Care, 867
Einboden, Allan Scott & White Health Plan, 1082
Ekrich, Nancy CoreSource: Ohio, 846
Ekrich, Nancy CoreSource: Pennsylvania, 936
El-Azma, Majd Lifewise Health Plan of Oregon, 909
Elkin, Mel Carilion Health Plans, 1123
Eller, Kim Peoples Health, 479, 480
Ellerman, Brad Behavioral Healthcare Options, Inc., 686
Ellertson, Chris Health Net Health Plan of Oregon, 905
Ellex, Tina Coalition America's National Preferred Provider Network, 761
Elliot, Eric Aetna Health of Missouri, 629
Elliot, Jennifer Preferred Health Systems Insurance Company, 444
Elliot, Jennifer Preferred Plus of Kansas, 446
Elliott, David R Baptist Health Services Group, 1024
Elliott, Rick UnitedHealthCare of Georgia, 327
Ellis, Lyndle BlueLincs HMO, 883
Ellwood, Melissa Meritain Health: Corporate Headquarters, 787
Elsas, Robert Davis Vision, 763
Elsberry, Tabatha Health InfoNet, 666
Elwood, Melissa Meritain Health: Utah, 1103
Ely, Grace CareSource Mid Rogue Health Plan, 898
Elzen, Jonna Health Choice LLC, 1031
Emerson, Paul OptumHealth Care Solutions: Physical Health, 610
Emery, Gene R Delta Dental of New Hampshire, 702
Emmer, Dan Horizon Healthcare of New Jersey, 725
Emory, Charles, PhD Horizon Healthcare of New Jersey, 725
Engelman, Rebecca, RN Select Health of South Carolina, 1003
England, Pat Kanawha Healthcare Solutions, 1001
England, Patricia Kanawha Healthcare Solutions, 1001
English, George Highmark Blue Cross & Blue Shield Delaware, 233
Enigl, Debbie Landmark Healthplan of California, 145
Enos, Deborah C Neighborhood Health Plan, 537
Enos, Scott E, RPh UnitedHealthCare of Rhode Island, 989
Enslinger, Lisa American Health Care Alliance, 630
Eppel, James Blue Cross & Blue Shield of Minnesota, 595
Erba, John Dell UnitedHealthCare of the Mid-Atlantic, 518
Erdelt, Ken Dentaquest, 526
Ericksen, Jack Blue Cross and Blue Shield Association, 357
Ericksen, Robert A., Ph.D. CHN PPO, 717
ErkenBrack, Steven Rocky Mountain Health Plans, 210
Ertel, Al Alliant Health Plans, 305
Eskridge, Karen Lovelace Health Plan, 745
Eskridge, Karen Lovelace Medicare Health Plan, 746
Esser, Deb, MD UnitedHealthCare of Nebraska, 683
Eudell, Nasia Quality Plan Administrators, 247
Evans, Bill Nationwide Better Health, 862
Evans, Dave Moda Health Alaska, 25
Evans, Keith J Kaiser Permanente Health Plan of Colorado, 207
Evans, Nichole Health Alliance Medical Plans, 370
Evelyn, Scott CIGNA HealthCare of Georgia, 311
Ewing, Tom, MD PacificSource Health Plans: Idaho, 349

F

Fahlman, Robert Arcadian Community Care, 468
Fahlman, Robert Ozark Health Plan, 656
Fahnestock, George Preferred Health Systems Insurance Company, 444
Fahnestock, George Preferred Plus of Kansas, 446
Fairchild, Philip Select Health of South Carolina, 1003
Falcone, Charles Devon Health Services, 938
Faller, Keith Anthem Blue Cross & Blue Shield of Indiana, 388
Fallon, Christopher WellChoice, 736
Fallon, John, MD Blue Cross & Blue Shield of Massachusetts, 522
Farasce, Theresa UnitedHealthCare of the Mid-Atlantic, 518
Farbacher, Elizabeth A Highmark Blue Cross & Blue Shield, 949
Farbacher, Elizabeth A Highmark Blue Shield, 950
Fargis, Edward C Touchstone Health HMO, 803
Farrell, James Humana Benefit Plan of Illinois, 375
Farrell, James G OSF Healthcare, 378
Farrell, Lisa Presbyterian Health Plan, 748
Farrell, Lisa Presbyterian Medicare Plans, 749

Farrell, Paul Coventry Health Care of GA, 314
Farrell, Robert G, Jr SVS Vision, 584
Farren, Linda Perfect Health Insurance Company, 800
Farrer, Bob Hometown Health Plan, 690
Farrow, Peter Group Health Cooperative of Eau Claire, 1190
Fasano, Phil Kaiser Permanente Health Plan of Northern California, 138
Fasano, Phil Kaiser Permanente Health Plan of Southern California, 139
Fasano, Phil Kaiser Permanente Health Plan: Corporate Office, 140
Fasano, Phil Kaiser Permanente Medicare Plan, 141
Fassenfelt, Chris Liberty Health Plan: Corporate Office, 908
Faulds, Thomas Blue Cross & Blue Shield of South Carolina, 992
Faust-Thomas, Brenda National Capital PPO, 1133
Faxio, Charles, MD Medica Health - Medicare Plan, 605
Fay, George R CNA Insurance Companies: Colorado, 197
Fay, George R CNA Insurance Companies: Georgia, 312
Fay, George R CNA Insurance Companies: Illinois, 360
Fazio, Charles, MD Medica: South Dakota, 1018
Feagin, Card VIVA Health, 17
Featherman, Lisa Central Susquehanna Healthcare Providers, 933
Federico, Francesco, MD Lakeside Community Healthcare Network, 144
Fee, David Humana Health Insurance of Wisconsin, 1195
Feeny, Kathy UnitedHealthCare, 76
Fein, Harvey A Molina Healthcare: Corporate Office, 153
Feld, Judith, MD Independent Health Medicare Plan, 783
Feldman, Eli S Elderplan, 768
Feldman, Karen Golden West Dental & Vision Plan, 126
Feldman, Nancy UCare Medicare Plan, 614
Feldman, Nancy UCare Minnesota, 615
Felix, John Henry Hawaii Medical Assurance Association, 334
Felkner, Joseph, CPA Health First Health Plans, 278
Felsing, William UnitedHealthCare of Wisconsin: Central, 619, 1203
Felts, Tony Unicare: Illinois, 382
Felts, Tony Anthem Blue Cross & Blue Shield of Indiana, 388
Felts, Tony Unicare: Kansas, 449
Felts, Tony Unicare: Massachusetts, 540
Felts, Tony Unicare: Michigan, 586
Felts, Tony Unicare: Texas, 1088
Felts, Tony Unicare: West Virginia, 1176
Fenik, Dan Humana Health Insurance of Jacksonville, 282
Fennel, Edward Blue Cross of Northeastern Pennsylvania, 929
Fenster, Dennis S. PreferredOne, 612
Ferguson, Bill BlueChoice Health Plan of South Carolina, 993
Ferguson, Mike Care 1st Health Plan: Arizona, 35
Fernandez, Albert UnitedHealthCare of South Florida, 299
Fernandez, Gene L.A. Care Health Plan, 143
Fernandez, Luis Leon Medical Centers Health Plan, 286
Ferrante, Michael MultiPlan, Inc., 789
Ferraro, Stephen Galaxy Health Network, 1061
Ferreira, Alice AmeriChoice by UnitedHealthcare, 216
Ferry, Renee Central Susquehanna Healthcare Providers, 933
Feruck, Dan Humana Health Insurance of Georgia, 320
Feuerman, Jason Bravo Health: Pennsylvania, 931
Feyen, Patrick Bravo Health: Texas, 1050
Fianu, Peter Meritain Health: Corporate Headquarters, 787
Fickling, William, Jr Beech Street: Alaska, 19
Fickling, William A, Jr Beech Street Corporation: Alabama, 4
Fidler, Deanna Aetna Health of Texas, 1041
Field, David Presbyterian Medicare Plans, 749
Field, Mark Initial Group, 1036
Fielder, Barry, PharmD QualChoice/QCA Health Plan, 75
Fields, Candia CommunityCare Medicare Plan, 886
Fields, David Unicare: Illinois, 382
Fields, David Unicare: Kansas, 449
Fields, David W Unicare: Massachusetts, 540
Fields, David W Unicare: Texas, 1088
Fields, Karen Pima Health System, 54
Figenshu, Bill Western Health Advantage, 187
Fike, Randy HealthSpring of Illinois, 374
Files, Shawn C, MD Gateway Health Plan, 943
Film, George Prime Time Health Medicare Plan, 868
Findlay, Janet VSP: Vision Service Plan of California, 185
Fine, Peter S. Banner MediSun Medicare Plan, 33

Fink, **Daniel** HealthNow New York - Emblem Health, 779
Finley, **John R** Amerigroup Corporation, 1120
Finuf, **Bob** Children's Mercy Pediatric Care Network, 636
Fiore, **Paula** Harvard University Group Health Plan, 532
Fiorina, **Stacey** Block Vision of New Jersey, 716
Fischer, **Neal, MD** Unicare: Texas, 1088
Fish, **Mark** MVP Health Care: New Hampshire, 706
Fish, **Mark** MVP Health Care Medicare Plan, 790
Fish, **Mark** MVP Health Care: Buffalo Region, 791
Fish, **Mark** MVP Health Care: Mid-State Region, 794
Fish, **Mark** MVP Health Care: Western New York, 795
Fisher, **Andrea** Devon Health Services, 938
Fisher, **Carole A** Behavioral Healthcare Options, Inc., 686
Fisher, **Dorothy, Dr.** New West Health Services, 669
Fisher, **Dorothy, Dr.** New West Medicare Plan, 670
Fisher, **Larry** CompBenefits Corporation, 313
Fisher, **Tammy** San Francisco Health Plan, 171
Fitzgerald, **Kevin R, MD** Rocky Mountain Health Plans, 210
Fitzgibbon, **Shawn M** Health Plan of New York, 778
Fitzgibbon, **Shawn M.** GHI, 774
Fitzgibbon, **Shawn M.** GHI Medicare Plan, 775
Fitzpatrick, **Maggie** CIGNA HealthCare of Northern California, 105
Fitzpatrick, **Maggie** CIGNA HealthCare of Southern California, 106
Fitzpatrick, **Maggie** CIGNA HealthCare of North Carolina, 813
Fjelstad, **Dani** Delta Dental of North Dakota, 831
Flanagan, **Lyn** UnitedHealthCare of Ohio: Columbus, 877
Flanagan, **Lyn** UnitedHealthCare of Ohio: Dayton & Cincinnati, 878
Flanders McGinnis, **Gretchen, MSPH** Colorado Access, 198
Flasch, **H. Michael** Health Alliance Medicare, 566
Fleischer, **Steven** Delta Dental of New Jersey & Connecticut, 221
Fleischer, **Steven** Block Vision, 497
Fleischer, **Steven** Block Vision of New Jersey, 716
Fleischer, **Stuart F** National Medical Health Card, 796
Fleisher, **Steven** CIGNA HealthCare of New Jersey, 718
Fleming, **Renee** Blue Cross & Blue Shield of Western New York, 756
Florentine, **Mauro** Humana Health Insurance of Orlando, 283
Flow, **Doug** CareSource Mid Rogue Health Plan, 898
Flowers, **Sandra D** Arizona Foundation for Medical Care, 30
Floyd, **Charles D, CEBS** Delta Dental of Michigan, Ohio and Indiana, 847
Fluegel, **Brad M** WellPoint: Corporate Office, 414
Flynn, **Barbara, RN** Central California Alliance for Health, 99
Foels, **Thomas** Independent Health, 782
Foels, **Thomas J, MD** Independent Health Medicare Plan, 783
Fogarty, **W Tom, MD** Concentra: Corporate Office, 1055
Fogel, **Baruch** Arta Medicare Health Plan, 83
Foley, **John** Anthem Blue Cross & Blue Shield of Wisconsin, 1180
Folick, **Jeff** Bravo Health: Texas, 1050
Foos, **John** AmeriHealth HMO, 227
Foos, **John G** Keystone Health Plan East, 955
Foose, **Jon** QualChoice/QCA Health Plan, 75
Forbes, **Brian** Aetna Health of Oklahoma, 880
Ford, **Tim** QualCare, 732
Foreman, **Cory** UnitedHealthCare of Colorado, 212
Foreman, **Roger** Blue Cross & Blue Shield of Kansas City, 633
Forlande, **Lori** Liberty Health Plan Anchorage, 24
Forney, **Drew S** Blue Cross of Idaho Health Service, Inc., 342
Forrest, **Rochelle, RN** Encore Health Network, 399
Forston, **Debbie** Health Plus of Louisiana, 476
Forsyth, **John** Wellmark Blue Cross Blue Shield, 429
Forsyth, **John D** Wellmark Blue Cross & Blue Shield of South Dakota, 1020
Fort, **Glenda** Healthcare Partners of East Texas, 1064
Fort, **Paul** Blue Cross of Northeastern Pennsylvania, 929
Fortner, **Scott** Central California Alliance for Health, 99
Forts, **Patricia** Fallon Community Medicare Plan, 529
Fortson, **Delaine, MD** Stanislaus Foundation for Medical Care, 175
Foss, **Robert E** Mid Atlantic Medical Services: Delaware, 235
Foss, **Robert E** Mid Atlantic Psychiatric Services (MAMSI), 236
Foss, **Robert E** Optimum Choice, 514
Foster, **Martin** Blue Cross & Blue Shield of New Mexico, 739
Foster, **Martin G** Health Care Service Corporation, 372
Fouberg, **Rodney** Avera Health Plans, 1010
Foulkes, **Helena B** CVS CareMark, 983

Fouts, **Dr. Terry** Great-West Healthcare Oklahoma, 889
Fouts, **Terry, MD** Great-West Healthcare Delaware, 232
Fouts, **Terry, MD** Great-West Healthcare of Massachusetts, 530
Fouts, **Terry, MD** Great-West Healthcare South Dakota, 1016
Fouts, **Terry, MD** Great-West Healthcare Wisconsin, 1189
Fowlie, **Kate** Contra Costa Health Plan, 112
Fox, **Alissa** Blue Cross and Blue Shield Association, 357
Fox, **Jacque** PCC Preferred Chiropractic Care, 443
Foxman, **Ralph** Dental Benefit Providers, 505
Francis, **Cathy** DenteMax, 560
Francis, **Gary** Total Health Care, 585
Frank, **Larry** NevadaCare, 695
Frank, **Michael** Blue Cross & Blue Shield of Montana, 661
Frantz, **Jim** Health Plus of Louisiana, 476
Franz, **Phillip** AmeriChoice by UnitedHealthCare, 710
Fraser, **David** Assurant Employee Benefits: Massachusetts, 520
Frawley, **Patrick** Fidelis Care, 773
Frederick, **John, MD** PreferredOne, 612
Freed, **Michael P.** Priority Health, 581
Freed, **Michael P.** Priority Health: Corporate Headquarters, 582
Freed, **Michael P.** PriorityHealth Medicare Plans, 583
Freedman, **Jonathan** L.A. Care Health Plan, 143
Freeman, **Bob, MBA** CenCal Health: The Regional Health Authority, 98
Freeman, **Jerome, MD** Sanford Health Plan, 427
Freeman, **Nancy** Arkansas Community Care, 65
Freeman, **Nancy** Texas Community Care, 1086
Frey, **James** UnitedHealthCare, 76
Frey, **James** PacifiCare of California, 163
Frey, **James** PacifiCare of Texas, 1079
Frick, **Joseph A** AmeriHealth Medicare Plan, 926
Frick, **Joseph A** Independence Blue Cross, 952
Frick, **Joseph A** Keystone Health Plan East, 955
Friedley, **Pat** Behavioral Health Systems, 5
Friedman, **Jeffrey** Peoples Health, 479
Friedman, **Neal** South Central Preferred, 963
Friedman, **Robert, MD** Primary Health Plan, 350
Fries, **Scott** Evercare Health Plans, 599
Fritch, **Herb** CIGNA HealthCare of North Carolina, 813
Fritch, **Herbert** HealthSpring: Corporate Offices, 1034
Fritz, **James S** Bluegrass Family Health, 454
Fritz, **Richard A** Delta Dental of Rhode Island, 984
Frock, **Charles** FirstCarolinaCare, 818
Froemming, **Renae** UCare Medicare Plan, 614
Froemming, **Renae** UCare Minnesota, 615
Froyen, **Scott** Wellmark Blue Cross Blue Shield, 429
Froyum, **Karen** HSM: Healthcare Cost Management, 603
Frucella, **Maureen** Preferred Healthcare System, 960
Fuccillo, **Ralph** Dentaquest, 526
Fuentes Benejam, **Ing. Jorge** Triple-S Salud Blue Cross Blue Shield of Puerto Rico, 978
Fuhrman, **James** Pacific Dental Benefits, 157
Fuller, **Patty** Health Plus of Louisiana, 476
Fullwood, **Michael D** Health Plan of New York, 778
Fulton, **Richard** Premier Access Insurance/Access Dental, 167
Fusco, **Dave** Anthem Blue Cross & Blue Shield Connecticut, 217

G

Gabel, **Lawrence** Davis Vision, 763
Gadhe, **Balu** CareMore Health Plan, 97
Gadinsky, **Pam** Coventry Health Care of Florida, 267
Gaebel, **John** Pacific Dental Benefits, 157
Gafney, **Paulette** Total Dental Administrators, 57
Gage, **Deborah** Beech Street Corporation: Corporate Office, 86
Gage Lofgren, **Diane** Kaiser Permanente Health Plan of Northern California, 138
Gage Lofgren, **Diane** Kaiser Permanente Health Plan of Southern California, 139
Gage Lofgren, **Diane** Kaiser Permanente Health Plan: Corporate Office, 140
Gage Lofgren, **Diane** Kaiser Permanente Medicare Plan, 141
Gailey, **Vernice** CIGNA HealthCare of Georgia, 311
Galareau, **Kathryn A, FSA** Independence Blue Cross, 952
Galica, **Michael, MD** Health Plans, Inc., 535
Gallagher, **Adeline** Perfect Health Insurance Company, 800
Gallagher, **Dan** Unison Health Plan of Pennsylvania, 966

Gallagher, **Dan** Unison Health Plan of South Carolina, 1005
Gallagher, **Michael** Blue Cross of Northeastern Pennsylvania, 929
Gallagher, **Michael, Sr** First Priority Health, 942
Gallagher, **Michael P** AvMed Health Plan: Corporate Office, 254
Gallagher, **Michael P** AvMed Health Plan: Fort Lauderdale, 255
Gallagher, **Michael P** AvMed Health Plan: Gainesville, 256
Gallagher, **Michael P** AvMed Health Plan: Jacksonville, 257
Gallagher, **Michael P** AvMed Health Plan: Orlando, 258
Gallagher, **Michael P** AvMed Health Plan: Tampa Bay, 259
Gallagher, **Michael P.** AvMed Medicare Preferred, 260
Gallaher, **Cindy** CoreSource: Corporate Headquarters, 362
Gallaher, **Cindy** Trustmark Companies, 381
Gallegos, **Granger** Blue Cross & Blue Shield of Wyoming, 1208
Gallegos, **Rene** Colorado Access, 198
Galt, **Frederick B** CDPHP Medicare Plan, 758
Galt, **Frederick B** CDPHP: Capital District Physicians' Health Plan, 759
Galvan, **Jesus** Delta Dental of New Mexico, 741
Gamble, **John** Cox Healthplans, 639
Gamzon, **Jessica** HealthFirst New Jersey Medicare Plan, 723
Ganesh, **Karthick** QualCare, 732
Gannon, **Christopher R** Blue Cross & Blue Shield of Vermont, 1113
Ganoni, **Gerald L** CompBenefits Corporation, 313
Garcia, **Eddie** Medical Care Referral Group, 1074
Garcia, **Nancy** Preferred Medical Plan, 293
Gardner, **Deana** Crescent Health Solutions, 815
Garg, **Angeli** Santa Clara Family Health Foundations Inc, 172
Garland, **Patrick** Fidelis Care, 773
Garrett, **Andrea** DenteMax, 560
Garrett, **Sharon** UnitedHealthCare, 76
Garrett, **Sharon** PacifiCare of Texas, 1079
Garrison, **Larry F** Health First Medicare Plans, 279
Garvey, **Thomas** CIGNA HealthCare of New Jersey, 718
Garzelli, **Lisa** Foundation for Medical Care for Kern & Santa Barbara County, 123
Gasbaro, **Eric** Blue Cross & Blue Shield of Rhode Island, 981
Gates, **Dennis L** SafeGuard Health Enterprises: Corporate Office, 170
Gates, **Dennis L** SafeGuard Health Enterprises: Texas, 1081
Gatti, **Alfred** MVP Health Care: New Hampshire, 706
Gatti, **Alfred** MVP Health Care Medicare Plan, 790
Gatti, **Alfred** MVP Health Care: Buffalo Region, 791
Gatti, **Alfred** MVP Health Care: Mid-State Region, 794
Gatti, **Alfred** MVP Health Care: Western New York, 795
Gaucher, **Ellen J** Wellmark Blue Cross Blue Shield, 429
Gauen, **Steve** HAS-Premier Providers, 1063
Gaulstrand, **Paul** Spectera, 516
Gauthier, **Guy** Great Lakes Health Plan, 564
Gavras, **Jonathan, MD** UnitedHealthCare of South Florida, 299
Gavras, **Jonathan B, MD** Florida Blue: Jacksonville, 273
Gavras, **Jonathan B, MD** Florida Blue: Pensacola, 274
Geary, **Emmet** Peoples Health, 479
Gedmen, **William, CPA** UPMC Health Plan, 968
Geise, **Kelly** Central Susquehanna Healthcare Providers, 933
Geisert, **Dawn** Health Alliance Plan, 567
Geiwitz, **Paul** PreferredOne, 612
Gelb, **Eve** SCAN Health Plan, 173
Gellert, **Jay M** Health Net Dental, 128
Gellert, **Jay M** Health Net Medicare Plan, 129
Gellert, **Jay M** Health Net: Corporate Headquarters, 130
Gentile, **David** Blue Cross & Blue Shield of Kansas City, 633
Gentile, **David** Preferred Care Blue, 657
George, **Don** Blue Cross & Blue Shield of Vermont, 1113
George, **Jeff** Behavioral Healthcare, 193
George, **John** InterGroup Services Corporation, 953
George, **Timothy** M-Care, 575
George, **William** Health Partners Medicare Plan, 946
Gerace, **James E** USA Managed Care Organization, 1091
Geraghty, **Patricia** Blue Cross & Blue Shield of Minnesota, 595
Geraghty, **Patrick J** Florida Blue: Jacksonville, 273
Geraghty, **Patrick J** Florida Blue: Pensacola, 274
Gerbo, **Christine, RN** Central California Alliance for Health, 99
Geren, **Mike** Assurant Employee Benefits: Georgia, 307
Gerik, **Sandy** Scott & White Health Plan, 1082

Gering, **MD, Stanley A.** Arizona Foundation for Medical Care, 30
Geringer, **Donna** HealthLink HMO, 648
Gerke, **Mary Lu, PhD** Gundersen Lutheran Health Plan, 1192
Germain, **Carrie, RPh** HealthPlus of Michigan: Flint, 569
Germain, **Carrie, RPh** HealthPlus of Michigan: Saginaw, 570
Germain, **Michael** Assurant Employee Benefits: Massachusetts, 520
Gerrard, **Paul** Blue Cross and Blue Shield Association, 357
Gessells, **Tom** Ohio State University Health Plan Inc., 864
Gettas, **Dr Nicholas** CIGNA HealthCare of New York, 760
Gettas, **MD, Nicholas** CIGNA HealthCare of the Mid-Atlantic, 500
Gettings, **Scott, MD** Health First Health Plans, 278
Geyer, **Rob** Blue Shield of California, 90
Geyer-Sylvia, **Zelda** Blue Cross of Idaho Health Service, Inc., 342
Ghani, **Shareh, M.D.** Magellan Health Services Arizona, 47
Giacobello, **Jim** Family Choice Health Alliance, 721
Giacobello, **Jim** FC Diagnostic, 722
Giacomotti, **Venus** Basic Chiropractic Health Plan, 85
Giancursio, **Donald J** UnitedHealthcare Nevada, 698
Gibbons, **Joseph F, Jr** HMO Health Ohio, 853
Gibbons, **Joseph F, Jr** Medical Mutual of Ohio, 857
Gibbons, **Joseph F, Jr** Medical Mutual of Ohio Medicare Plan, 858
Gibbons, **Joseph F, Jr** SuperMed One, 873
Gibbons, **Shawn** Encore Health Network, 399
Gibbs, **Samuel C.** eHealthInsurance Services Inc., 10, 22, 40, 70, 121
Gibbs, **Samuel C.** eHealthInsurance Services Inc. Corporate Office, 122
Gibbs, **Samuel C., III** eHealthInsurance Services Inc., 203, 231, 244, 271, 318, 332, 345, 366, 397, 421, 438, 459, 475, 487, 506, 527, 561, 598, 624, 642, 664, 678, 688, 703, 720, 742, 767, 817, 832, 848, 888, 902, 939, 985, 997, 1014, 1030, 1101, 1116, 1128, 1149, 1169, 1188, 1211
Gibbs, **III, Samuel C.** eHealthInsurance Services Inc., 1058
Gibford, **Patricia J** Clear One Health Plans, 900
Giblin, **John** Blue Cross & Blue Shield of Tennessee, 1025
Gibson, **Sandra Lee** Blue Cross & Blue Shield of Arizona, 34
Giddings, **Cindy** CommunityCare Managed Healthcare Plans of Oklahoma, 885
Giese, **Alexis, MD** Colorado Access, 198
Gilbert, **Bradley P, MD** Inland Empire Health Plan, 135
Gilbert, **Greg** Concentra: Corporate Office, 1055
Gilbert, **Lisa** Secure Health PPO Newtork, 324
Giles, **Randy** Coventry Health Care of Delaware, 229
Giles, **Randy** Coventry Health Care of Florida, 267
Giles, **Randy** Coventry Health Care of Nebraska, 676
Gilham, **Charles** Mercy Health Plans: Kansas, 442
Gilham, **Charles** Mercy Health Medicare Plan, 651
Gilham, **Charles** Mercy Health Plans: Corporate Office, 652
Gilham, **Charles** Mercy Health Plans: Oklahoma, 891
Gill, **Laura** Avesis: Corporate Headquarters, 32
Gill, **Laura** Avesis: Arizona, 309
Gill, **Laura** Avesis: Minnesota, 594
Gill, **Laura** Avesis: Texas, 1046
Gille, **Larry** Prevea Health Network, 1200
Gillespie, **Pat** Cariten Healthcare, 1026
Gillespie, **Pat** Cariten Preferred, 1027
Gillespie, **William A, MD** Health Plan of New York, 778
Gillespie, **William A., MD** GHI, 774
Gillespie, **William A., MD** GHI Medicare Plan, 775
Gilligan, **Matt** Assurant Employee Benefits: Texas, 1045
Gillis, **Marci** Community Health Improvement Solutions, 638
Gillsepie, **John, MD** Blue Cross & Blue Shield of Western New York, 756
Gilmore, **Don** Amerigroup Florida, 252
Gilson, **Jeremy** Preferred Health Systems Insurance Company, 444
Gilson, **Jeremy** Preferred Plus of Kansas, 446
Ginoris, **Estella** Preferred Medical Plan, 293
Gist, **Jo Anna** Arkansas Managed Care Organization, 66
Gladden, **John** Delta Dental of Oklahoma, 887
Gladden, **Robert** Delta Dental of Arkansas, 69
Glaser, **Daniel E** Preferred Care Select, 824
Glass, **Quincy** DenteMax, 560
Glass, **Velina** OmniCare: A Coventry Health Care Plan, 578
Glasscock, **Larry** Anthem Blue Cross & Blue Shield of Colorado, 190
Glasscock, **Larry** Anthem Blue Cross & Blue Shield Connecticut, 217
Glasscock, **Larry** Anthem Blue Cross & Blue Shield of Indiana, 388
Glasscock, **Larry** Health Maintenance Plan, 851

Griggs, Mike Blue Cross & Blue Shield of South Carolina, 992
Grigo, Chris Alliance Regional Health Network, 1042
Grillo, Lillian UnitedHealthCare of New York, 805
Grimes, MD, Alan UnitedHealthCare of Indiana, 411
Groat, Jonathan S., Esq. Delta Dental: Corporate Headquarters, 558
Grooms, Ed HealthSCOPE Benefits, 71
Groseclose, Jack Meritain Health: Louisiana, 478
Gross, Don Mida Dental Plan, 152
Grossman, Robert S, MD Citrus Health Care, 264
Grove, Jane South Central Preferred, 963
Grover, Michael OptiCare Managed Vision, 823
Groves, Mark Dental Source: Dental Health Care Plans, 1057
Guenther, Bret Dentistat, 118
Guerard, Barbara Peoples Health, 479
Guerrero, Esther ChiroCare of Wisconsin, 1183
Guertin, Lisa M Anthem Blue Cross & Blue Shield of New Hampshire, 700
Guertin, Shawn M Aetna Health of Alabama, 2
Guertin, Shawn M Aetna Health of Alaska, 18
Guertin, Shawn M Aetna Health of Arkansas, 62
Guertin, Shawn M Aetna Health, Inc. Corporate Headquarters, 214
Guertin, Shawn M Aetna Health of Delaware, 226
Guertin, Shawn M Aetna Health District of Columbia, 239
Guertin, Shawn M Aetna Health of Hawaii, 329
Guertin, Shawn M Aetna Health of Idaho, 341
Guertin, Shawn M Aetna Health of Iowa, 415
Guertin, Shawn M Aetna Health of Kansas, 431
Guertin, Shawn M Aetna Health of Kentucky, 452
Guertin, Shawn M Aetna Health of Louisiana, 467
Guertin, Shawn M Aetna Health of Maine, 484
Guertin, Shawn M Aetna Health of Maryland, 493
Guertin, Shawn M Aetna Health of Massachusetts, 519
Guertin, Shawn M Aetna Health of Michigan, 543
Guertin, Shawn M Aetna Health of Minnesota, 591
Guertin, Shawn M Aetna Health of Mississippi, 621
Guertin, Shawn M Aetna Health of Montana, 659
Guertin, Shawn M Aetna Health of Nebraska, 672
Guertin, Shawn M Aetna Health of Nevada, 684
Guertin, Shawn M Aetna Health of New Hampshire, 699
Guertin, Shawn M Aetna Health of New Jersey, 709
Guertin, Shawn M Aetna Health of New Mexico, 737
Guertin, Shawn M Aetna Health of North Dakota, 829
Guertin, Shawn M Aetna Health of Oregon, 894
Guertin, Shawn M Aetna Health of Pennsylvania, 922
Guertin, Shawn M HealthAmerica, 947
Guertin, Shawn M Aetna Health of Rhode Island, 980
Guertin, Shawn M Aetna Health of South Dakota, 1008
Guertin, Shawn M Aetna Health of Utah, 1096
Guertin, Shawn M Aetna Health of Vermont, 1112
Guertin, Shawn M Aetna Health of Washington, 1143
Guertin, Shawn M Aetna Health of Wisconsin, 1179
Guertin, Shawn M Aetna Health of Wyoming, 1207
Guertin, Shawn M. Aetna Health of Texas, 1041
Guilmette, David CIGNA HealthCare of Utah, 1098
Guinn, Joe United Behavioral Health, 178
Gullett, Steve Paramount Elite Medicare Plan, 866
Gullett, Steve Paramount Health Care, 867
Gullino, Douglas Lovelace Medicare Health Plan, 746
Gumkowski, John CIGNA HealthCare of New Jersey, 718
Gunawardane, Gamini, PhD Care 1st Health Plan: California, 96
Gunter, Roger Behavioral Healthcare, 193
Gustafson, Greg Upper Peninsula Health Plan, 589
Gustin, Karen Ameritas Group, 673
Gutierrez, Lisa Script Care, Ltd., 1083
Gutierrez, Melissa, CLU Nationwide Better Health, 862
Gutshall, Tim Wellmark Blue Cross Blue Shield, 429
Guzzino, Alan Humana Health Insurance of Jacksonville, 282
Guzzino, Alan Humana Health Insurance of North Carolina, 820

H

Haaland, Douglas E Cariten Healthcare, 1026
Haaland, Douglas E Cariten Preferred, 1027
Haar, Elizabeth R. Blue Care Network of Michigan: Medicare, 547

Haban, Gregory Prime Time Health Medicare Plan, 868
Hackett, Ed Value Behavioral Health of Pennsylvania, 971
Hackworth, John, PhD Health Plan of San Joaquin, 131
Haddock, Joseph, MHA Geisinger Health Plan, 944
Haefner, Larry A CNA Insurance Companies: Colorado, 197
Haefner, Larry A CNA Insurance Companies: Georgia, 312
Haefner, Larry A CNA Insurance Companies: Illinois, 360
Hagan, Lynn American Health Care Group, 923
Hagan Jr., Robert E American Health Care Group, 923
Haggett, William F AmeriHealth HMO, 713
Haglund, Jacqueline Blue Cross & Blue Shield of Oklahoma, 882
Hague, Richard, DMD, MPA Liberty Dental Plan, 146
Hague, Richard, DMD Liberty Dental Plan of Nevada, 692
Hahn, Shelley Anthem Blue Cross & Blue Shield of Ohio, 841
Haillyer, Jeff HAS-Premier Providers, 1063
Haines, Rick Prime Time Health Medicare Plan, 868
Hale, Bill Beech Street Corporation: Northeast Region, 87
Hale, Kathy Healthcare Partners of East Texas, 1064
Hale, William Beech Street Corporation: Alabama, 4
Hale, William Beech Street: Alaska, 19
Haley, Michelle, MD Children's Mercy Pediatric Care Network, 636
Hall, David Dental Benefit Providers, 505
Hall, Kerry Delta Dental of Wyoming, 1210
Hall, Pat CommunityCare Managed Healthcare Plans of Oklahoma, 885
Hall, Toby Delta Dental of Michigan, Ohio and Indiana, 396
Hall, Toby, FSA Delta Dental: Corporate Headquarters, 558
Halo, Lorri Medical Care Referral Group, 1074
Halow, George, MD Medical Care Referral Group, 1074
Halow, Joseph Medical Care Referral Group, 1074
Halvorson, George C Kaiser Permanente Health Plan of Northern California, 138
Halvorson, George C Kaiser Permanente Health Plan of Southern California, 139
Halvorson, George C Kaiser Permanente Health Plan: Corporate Office, 140
Halvorson, George C Kaiser Permanente Medicare Plan, 141
Hamburg, Glenn Western Health Advantage, 187
Hamerlik, Mike Wisconsin Physician's Service, 1206
Hamilton, Catherine, PhD Blue Cross & Blue Shield of Vermont, 1113
Hamilton, Coleen Arizona Foundation for Medical Care, 30
Hamilton, Jill Delta Dental of Iowa, 420
Hamilton, Kelly Ohio State University Health Plan Inc., 864
Hammond, Deborah, MD HealthFirst New Jersey Medicare Plan, 723
Hammond, Elizabeth Blue Cross & Blue Shield of South Carolina, 992
Hammond, Gerry Total Health Choice, 296
Hampton, Diana Health Choice LLC, 1031
Hanaway, Ed CIGNA HealthCare of Tennessee, 1028
Hanaway, H Edward CIGNA HealthCare of South Carolina, 995
Hancock, William CommunityCare Managed Healthcare Plans of Oklahoma, 885
Hancock, William H CommunityCare Medicare Plan, 886
Handelman, Warren MultiPlan, Inc., 789
Handelman, Warren HealthEOS, 1194
Handler, Elisabeth Santa Clara Family Health Foundations Inc, 172
Handshuh, Ana Physicians United Plan, 291
Handshy, Jennifer Healthcare USA of Missouri, 647
Hanewinckel, Nancy A Humana Health Insurance of Delaware, 234
Hanewinckel, Nancy A Humana Health Insurance of Georgia, 320
Haney, Margaret Health First Health Plans, 278
Hankins, Toni BlueChoice Health Plan of South Carolina, 993
Hankins, Toni J BlueChoice Health Plan of South Carolina, 993
Hanks, Steve VSP: Vision Service Plan of Oregon, 920
Hanlon, Paul Blue Cross & Blue Shield of Rhode Island, 981
Hanna, Nequita K Blue Cross & Blue Shield of Oklahoma, 882
Hannah, Ed, RN Health First Health Plans, 278
Hannah, Paulette CONCERN: Employee Assistance Program, 111
Hannan, Claire L, CPA PacifiCare Dental and Vision Administrators, 161
Hannon, Richard M Blue Cross & Blue Shield of Arizona, 34
Hansen, David UnitedHealthCare of Alaska, 27
Hansen, David UnitedHealthCare of Oregon, 919
Hansen, David UnitedHealthCare of Washington, 1163
Hansen, P Gunnar, Jr Clear One Health Plans, 900
Hanus, Phil CHA Health, 455
Hanway, H Edward CIGNA HealthCare of Connecticut, 219
Harding, Cheryl Delta Dental of Iowa, 420
Hardwick, Deborah (Debi) Coastal Healthcare Administrators, 108

Higgins-Mays, Kimberley San Francisco Health Plan, 171
Hijkoop, Frans SafeGuard Health Enterprises: Florida, 295
Hilbert, Andy Optima Health Plan, 1134
Hildebrand, Hans ChiroCare of Wisconsin, 1183
Hilferty, Daniel J Independence Blue Cross, 952
Hill, John Value Behavioral Health of Pennsylvania, 971
Hill, Kevin R Oxford Health Plans: New Jersey, 731
Hill, Kevin R Oxford Health Plans: New York, 799
Hill, Marvin Humana Health Insurance of Kentucky, 460
Hill, Marvin Humana Medicare Plan, 461
Hill, Terri Nationwide Better Health, 862
Hillerud, Andrea, MD Security Health Plan of Wisconsin, 1201
Hillman, Lori Health Net: Corporate Headquarters, 130
Himes, BJ QualChoice/QCA Health Plan, 75
Hinckley, Robert R CDPHP: Capital District Physicians' Health Plan, 759
Hinckley, Robert R. CDPHP Medicare Plan, 758
Hingst, Jeanne ProviDRs Care Network, 448
Hinkle, Allen J., MD MVP Health Care: Central New York, 792
Hinkle, Allen J., MD MVP Health Care: Corporate Office, 793
Hinkle, Allen J., M.D. MVP Health Care: Vermont, 1117
Hinrichsen, Julie Blue Cross & Blue Shield of Kansas, 433
Hippert, Richard Horizon Health Corporation, 1068
Hipwell, Art Humana Health Insurance of Illinois, 376
Hipwell, Art Humana Health Insurance of Iowa, 424
Hipwell, Arthur P Humana Health Insurance of Ohio, 854
Hirst, Nancy Phoenix Health Plan, 52
Hitchcock, Robert T. Centene Corporation, 635
Hiveley, Jim Unity Health Insurance, 1204
Ho, Sam UnitedHealthCare, 76
Ho, Sam PacifiCare Health Systems, 162
Ho, Sam PacifiCare of Colorado, 208
Ho, Sam PacifiCare of Texas, 1079
Ho, Sam PacifiCare Benefit Administrators, 1155
Ho, Sam PacifiCare of Washington, 1156
Hobgood, Mark Healthcare Partners of East Texas, 1064
Hockmuth, Dr Rob CIGNA HealthCare of Massachusetts, 524
Hockmuth, Rob, MD CIGNA HealthCare of New Hampshire, 701
Hodgin, Ace PacifiCare of Arizona, 51
Hodgkins, Robert C, Jr The Dental Care Plus Group, 874
Hoefling, Douglas R, DDS Superior Dental Care, 872
Hoeflinger, Erin Anthem Blue Cross & Blue Shield of Ohio, 841
Hoeltzel, Marty T CIGNA: Corporate Headquarters, 935
Hoff, Linda Physicians Plus Insurance Corporation, 1199
Hoffman, Patrick CIGNA HealthCare of Tennessee, 1028
Hoffman, Randy Coventry Health Care of Illinois, 363
Hoffman, Randy OhioHealth Group, 865
Hogan, John Capital Health Plan, 261
Hogel, Maureen Highmark Blue Cross & Blue Shield, 949
Hoges, Deb Health Plans, Inc., 535
Hohner, Joseph H Blue Cross Blue Shield of Michigan, 551
Holden, Steven Davis Vision, 763
Holder, Diane P UPMC Health Plan, 968
Holgerson, Chris Willamette Dental Insurance, 921
Holiday, Steve Script Care, Ltd., 1083
Hollinger, Stacey Galaxy Health Network, 1061
Holmberg, David L Highmark Blue Cross & Blue Shield, 949
Holmberg, David L Highmark Blue Shield, 950
Hologood, Mark Healthcare Partners of East Texas, 1064
Holohan, Michael P Universal Health Care Group, 300
Holt, Shawn Physicians United Plan, 291
Holtz, Elliot UnitedHealthCare of Minnesota, 617
Holzhauer, Robert Univera Healthcare, 806
Hooks, Sandra OmniCare: A Coventry Health Care Plan, 578
Hooley, James A. Neighborhood Health Plan of Rhode Island, 987
Hopper, Rick Molina Healthcare: Corporate Office, 153
Hopper, MD, Bill PacifiCare of Oregon, 912
Horbal, Ryan Physicians United Plan, 291
Horn, Kathy Excellus Blue Cross Blue Shield: Utica Region, 772
Horn, Peter UnitedHealthCare of Northern California, 180
Horozaniecki, Joseph C, MD Metropolitan Health Plan, 608
Horstmann, Nancy CommunityCare Managed Healthcare Plans of Oklahoma, 885

Horton, Homer, MD Health Link PPO, 625
Horvath, Steve CoreSource: Corporate Headquarters, 362
Horvath, Steve CoreSource: Kansas (FMH CoreSource), 435
Horvath, Steve CoreSource: Maryland, 501
Horvath, Steve CoreSource: North Carolina, 814
Horvath, Steve CoreSource: Pennsylvania, 936
Hostetier, Nancy E Delta Dental of Michigan, Ohio and Indiana, 396, 847
Hostetler, Nancy E. Delta Dental: Corporate Headquarters, 558
Hotz, Michael Emerald Health PPO, 849
Houghland, Stephen J., MD Passport Health Plan, 463
Hounchell, Daniel HealthSpan, 852
Hovagimian, Debra Health Plans, Inc., 535
Hoverman, Ken UnitedHealthCare of Arkansas, 77
Hovila, Gary, CPA Humana Health Insurance of Wisconsin, 1195
Howard, Larry UnitedHealthcare Nevada, 698
Howard, Marshall OmniCare: A Coventry Health Care Plan, 578
Howatt, James W, MD Molina Healthcare: Corporate Office, 153
Howe, Sharon Lifewise Health Plan of Oregon, 909
Howell, Jerry, PHD Colorado Choice Health Plans, 199
Howell, Lori Foundation for Medical Care for Kern & Santa Barbara County, 123
Howell, Michael, MD Healthchoice Orlando, 280
Howell, Tracie Care 1st Health Plan: California, 96
Howes, David, MD Martin's Point HealthCare, 490
Hoyt, Deb ConnectiCare of Massachusetts, 525
Hronek, Mike Primary Health Plan, 350
Hu, David CIGNA HealthCare of Arizona, 36
Hua, Lanchi Bright Now! Dental, 92
Hubbard, Linda Lovelace Health Plan, 745
Hubbard, Linda Lovelace Medicare Health Plan, 746
Huber, David Horizon Healthcare of New Jersey, 725
Hubler, Kurt Inland Empire Health Plan, 135
Hudson, Jerry L Blue Cross & Blue Shield of Oklahoma, 882
Hudson, Joyce Deaconess Health Plans, 395
Hudson, Michael Blue Cross & Blue Shield of Rhode Island, 981
Huebner, Jeff, M.D. Group Health Cooperative of South Central Wisconsin, 1191
Huebner, Scott HealthSpring of Texas, 1066
Huff, Daryl AlohaCare, 330
Huffman, Patricia Wellmark Blue Cross Blue Shield, 429
Hufford, Don, MD Western Health Advantage, 187
Hughenot, Joseph Anthem Blue Cross & Blue Shield of Missouri, 631
Hughes, Alan Blue Cross & Blue Shield of North Carolina, 811
Hughes, Gary MVP Health Care: Western New York, 795
Hughes, Patrick Fallon Community Health Plan, 528
Hughes, Patrick Fallon Community Medicare Plan, 529
Hughes, W Patrick Fallon Community Medicare Plan, 529
Huizinga, Stuart M. eHealthInsurance Services Inc., 10, 22, 40, 70, 121
Huizinga, Stuart M. eHealthInsurance Services Inc. Corporate Office, 122
Huizinga, Stuart M. eHealthInsurance Services Inc., 203, 231, 244, 271, 318, 332, 345, 366, 397, 421, 438, 459, 475, 487, 506, 527, 561, 598, 624, 642, 664, 678, 688, 703, 720, 742, 767, 817, 832, 848, 888, 902, 939, 985, 997, 1014, 1030, 1058, 1101, 1116, 1128, 1149, 1169, 1188, 1211
Hulen, Debbie Mid Atlantic Medical Services: Corporate Office, 511
Hulin, Colin Peoples Health, 479, 480
Humbert, Ernie SummaCare Health Plan, 870
Hunsinger, Lance Cariten Preferred, 1027
Hunsinger, Lance Community Health Plan of Washington, 1147
Hunt, Ann First Commonwealth, 367
Hunt, Kathy CoreSource: Kansas (FMH CoreSource), 435
Hunt-Fugate, Ann Physicians Health Plan of Mid-Michigan, 580
Hunter, Chris Blue Cross & Blue Shield of Tennessee, 1025
Hunter, Eric Boston Medical Center Healthnet Plan, 523
Hunter, Robert L Health InfoNet, 666
Huntington, Debbie PacifiCare of Washington, 1156
Huotari, Mike Rocky Mountain Health Plans, 210
Hurley, David Delta Dental of Arizona, 38
Hurley, Robert S. eHealthInsurance Services Inc., 10, 22, 40, 70, 121
Hurley, Robert S. eHealthInsurance Services Inc. Corporate Office, 122
Hurley, Robert S. eHealthInsurance Services Inc., 203, 231, 244, 271, 318, 332, 345, 366, 397, 421, 438, 459, 475, 487, 506, 527, 561, 598, 624, 642, 664, 678, 688, 703, 720, 742, 767, 817, 832, 848, 888, 902, 939, 985, 997, 1014, 1030, 1058, 1101, 1116, 1128, 1149, 1169, 1188, 1211
Hurst, David Health Plan of San Joaquin, 131
Husa, Sherry CIGNA HealthCare of Iowa, 418

Jones, Bill HealthPartners, 1032
Jones, Bobby CareSource: Michigan, 553
Jones, Bobby OmniCare: A Coventry Health Care Plan, 578
Jones, Bobby CareSource, 844
Jones, Brooks Care 1st Health Plan: California, 96
Jones, Cynthia, M.D. Public Employees Health Program, 1106
Jones, David A, Jr Humana Health Insurance of Iowa, 424
Jones, Janice GEMCare Health Plan, 125
Jones, Mary Anne Priority Health, 581
Jones, Mary Anne Priority Health: Corporate Headquarters, 582
Jones, Mary Anne PriorityHealth Medicare Plans, 583
Jones, Nicole CIGNA HealthCare of Connecticut, 219
Jones, Nicole CIGNA HealthCare of Maine, 486
Jones, P Gary, MD Vantage Health Plan, 482
Jones, Randy HealthPlus of Michigan: Flint, 569
Jones, Randy HealthPlus of Michigan: Saginaw, 570
Jones, Richard Guardian Life Insurance Company of America, 777
Jones, Richard W Humana Health Insurance of Colorado Springs, 206
Jones, Robert Blue Ridge Health Network, 930
Jones, Scott Delta Dental of South Dakota, 1013
Jones, Wesley HealthSCOPE Benefits, 71
Jones, Willis E, III Windsor Medicare Extra, 1040
Jones, Jr, David A Humana Health Insurance of Georgia, 320
Jordan, Josh Blue Cross of Idaho Health Service, Inc., 342
Jordan, Michael MagnaCare, 786
Jose Orellano, Juan Molina Healthcare: Corporate Office, 153
Joseph, Charles Florida Blue: Jacksonville, 273
Joseph, Charles Florida Blue: Pensacola, 274
Joseph, Peter Coventry Health Care of Florida, 267
Joseph Bell, Jill Passport Health Plan, 463
Joslin, Michael Landmark Healthplan of California, 145
Joy, Jeff Priority Partners Health Plans, 515
Joyce, Kevin QualCare, 732
Joyner, J David CVS CareMark, 983
Jurkovic, Goran, CPA Delta Dental of Michigan, Ohio and Indiana, 396
Jurkovic, Goran, CPA Delta Dental: Corporate Headquarters, 558
Jurkovic, Goran Delta Dental of New Mexico, 741
Jurkovic, Goran, CPA Delta Dental of Michigan, Ohio and Indiana, 847
Justice, Billy Vantage Health Plan, 482

K

Kabarsky, Kay, DMD Liberty Dental Plan of Nevada, 692
Kaczor, William J., Jr. American Postal Workers Union (APWU) Health Plan, 494
Kadota, Rudy, MD Kaiser Permanente Health Plan of Colorado, 207
Kadylak, Ron OhioHealth Group, 865
Kahn, Howard A L.A. Care Health Plan, 143
Kairis, Edwin J, MD Gateway Health Plan, 943
Kaiser, Kelley C, MPH Samaritan Health Plan, 916
Kalahiki, Linda University Health Alliance, 339
Kalat, Carrah Coventry Health Care of Illinois, 363
Kalekos, Peggy Coastal Healthcare Administrators, 108
Kalmer, James American Pioneer Life Insurance Co, 251
Kambolis, Nicholas HealthNow New York - Emblem Health, 779
Kambolis, Nicholas P. GHI, 774
Kambolis, Nicholas P. GHI Medicare Plan, 775
Kampfe, Rachel Peninsula Health Care, 1135
Kanche, Liz American Health Care Group, 923
Kandarian, Steven A SafeGuard Health Enterprises: Florida, 295
Kane, Brian OptumHealth Care Solutions: Physical Health, 610
Kane, Brian Humana Health Insurance of San Antonio, 1070
Kaneshiro, Lance University Health Alliance, 339
Kantor, Johathan D CNA Insurance Companies: Georgia, 312
Kantor, Johathan D CNA Insurance Companies: Illinois, 360
Kapic, Maja Liberty Dental Plan, 146
Kapic, Maja Liberty Dental Plan of Nevada, 692
Kaplan, Alan Island Group Administration, Inc., 784
Kaplan, Kevin Physicians Health Plan of Mid-Michigan, 580
Kaplan, Leon CareFirst Blue Cross & Blue Shield of Virginia, 1122
Kaplan, Lynn Island Group Administration, Inc., 784
Kappel, James Anthem Blue Cross & Blue Shield of Indiana, 389
Kasitz, Todd Preferred Health Systems Insurance Company, 444

Kasitz, Todd Preferred Plus of Kansas, 446
Kassing, Gib Sterling Health Plans, 1161
Kastner, Rick Blue Cross & Blue Shield of Kansas City, 633
Kastner, Rick Preferred Care Blue, 657
Kasuba, Pual, MD Tufts Health Medicare Plan, 538
Kasuba, Pual, MD Tufts Health Plan, 539
Kates, Peter B Univera Healthcare, 806
Katz, Ben CIGNA HealthCare of Northern California, 105
Katz, Marshall, MD OmniCare: A Coventry Health Care Plan, 578
Katz, Michael, PhD Los Angeles County Department of Health Services, 147
Katz, Mitchel H. Community Health Plan of Los Angeles County, 110
Kaui, Prudence WellPoint NextRx, 1095
Kay, Larry, M.D. Physicians Plus Insurance Corporation, 1199
Kaye, Michael PTPN, 169
Kaye, Mitchel, PT Physical Therapy Provider Network, 165
Kaye, Thomas, RPH BlueLincs HMO, 883
Kazlauskas, Tony UnitedHealthCare of Massachusetts, 541
Keck, Joadi Delta Dental of Michigan, Ohio and Indiana, 396
Keck, Joadi Delta Dental: Corporate Headquarters, 558
Kedsri, Koh Easy Choice Health Plan, 119
Keeley, Larry OptiCare Managed Vision, 823
Keenan, Linda Hometown Health Plan, 690
Kehres, Deb South Central Preferred, 963
Keith, Tricia A Blue Cross Blue Shield of Michigan, 551
Keith, Tricia A. Blue Care Network of Michigan: Medicare, 547
Kelleher, Mary Ann Unison Health Plan of South Carolina, 1005
Keller, Shannon Delta Dental of Arizona, 38
Kellersberger, Kim, CGFM Public Employees Health Program, 1106
Kellogg, Carl, Ph.D. Arkansas Blue Cross and Blue Shield, 64
Kellogg, Terry D Blue Cross & Blue Shield of Alabama, 6
Kellogg, Terry D Blue Cross Preferred Care, 7
Kelly, James HealthSmart Preferred Care, 1065
Kelly, Mary J Dentcare Delivery Systems, 765
Kelly, Rick Aetna Health of the Carolinas, 809
Kelly, Scott R Health Net: Corporate Headquarters, 130
Kelmar, Steven B. Aetna Health of Texas, 1041
Kemp, Kacey Premera Blue Cross, 1157
Kenargy, Robert Preferred Health Systems Insurance Company, 444
Kenargy, Robert Preferred Plus of Kansas, 446
Kennedy, Janna SummaCare Health Plan, 870
Kennedy, John W Blue Cross & Blue Shield of Kansas City, 633
Kennedy, Tom Regence Blue Cross & Blue Shield of Oregon, 915
Kennedy-Scott, Patricia D Kaiser Permanente Health Plan Ohio, 856
Kenny, Becky Blue Cross & Blue Shield of New Mexico, 739
Kent Weiner, Jennifer Neighborhood Health Plan, 537
Kerr, Thomas Highmark Blue Cross & Blue Shield, 949
Kerr, Thomas Highmark Blue Shield, 950
Keshishian, Marc, MD Blue Care Network of Michigan: Corporate Headquarters, 546
Kessel, Stacy Community Health Plan of Washington, 1147
Kessler, James Health New England, 533
Kessler, Jennifer Unison Health Plan of Pennsylvania, 966
Kessler, Steve UnitedHealthCare of North Carolina, 827
Ketron, Mike Southeastern Indiana Health Organization, 410
Ketterman, Laura Citrus Health Care, 264
Kettlewell, Kelly Catamaran Corporation, 358
Khamseh, Ladan CalOptima, 95
Khan, Aslam, MD CIGNA HealthCare of Indiana, 394
Khan, Aslam, MD CIGNA HealthCare of Wisconsin, 1184
Khan, Haider A, MD Quality Health Plans, 801
Khan, Haider A, MD Quality Health Plans of New York, 802
Khan, Nazeer H, MD Quality Health Plans of New York, 802
Khan, Sabiha, MBA Quality Health Plans of New York, 802
Khaneja, Munish, MD, MPH Affinity Health Plan, 753
Khorram, Carmen American PPO, 1043
Kidd, Wyndham BlueLincs HMO, 883
Kieffer, Brad Health Net Dental, 128
Kieffer, Brad Health Net: Corporate Headquarters, 130
Kilburn, Sherri HealthPartners, 1032
Kile, Gregory Valley Preferred, 970
Kilgallon, Tim Alere Health, 304
Kinard, David Community Health Plan of Washington, 1147

L

Lacombe, Philip M Health New England, 533
Ladig, Curtis Delta Dental of North Carolina, 816
Lady, Shirley S Blue Cross and Blue Shield Association, 357
LaFayette, Lincoln HMO Health Ohio, 853
LaFayette, Lincoln Medical Mutual of Ohio, 857
LaFayette, Lincoln Medical Mutual of Ohio Medicare Plan, 858
LaFayette, Lincoln SuperMed One, 873
Lages, Adolphus, OD Vision Plan of America, 183
Laird, Brenda Delta Dental of Michigan, Ohio and Indiana, 847
Laird, Warren VSP: Vision Service Plan of South Carolina, 1007
Lamb, Jay Moda Health Alaska, 25
Lamm, Roy QualChoice/QCA Health Plan, 75
Lammie, Scott UPMC Health Plan, 968
Lamoreaux, Leon Priority Health, 581
Lamoreaux, Leon New West Health Services, 669
Lamoreaux, Leon New West Medicare Plan, 670
Lamoreaux, William C Health Plan of New York, 778
Lamoreaux, William C. GHI, 774
Lamoreaux, William C. GHI Medicare Plan, 775
Lamoreux, William UnitedHealthCare of New York, 805
Landis, Robert J CompCare: Comprehensive Behavioral Care, 266
Landis, Robert J. CompCare: Comprehensive Behavioral Care, 266
Lane, Jack Harvard Pilgrim Health Care, 531
Lang, James Anthem Blue Cross & Blue Shield of Maine, 485
Langer, Carolyn Harvard Pilgrim Health Care, 531
Lapetina, Antoinette Perfect Health Insurance Company, 800
Larking, Kathy DenteMax, 560
Larrivee, Scott Anthem Blue Cross & Blue Shield of Wisconsin, 1180
Larson, John Health InfoNet, 666
Larson, Mike Priority Partners Health Plans, 515
Larson, Peter N CIGNA HealthCare of South Carolina, 995
Lasconia, Michael Care 1st Health Plan: California, 96
Lathem, Janet Northeast Georgia Health Partners, 323
Latrenta, Nicholas SafeGuard Health Enterprises: Florida, 295
Lattimore, Patricia HMO Health Ohio, 853
Lattimore, Patricia Medical Mutual of Ohio, 857
Lattimore, Patricia Medical Mutual of Ohio Medicare Plan, 858
Lattimore, Patricia SuperMed One, 873
Laudeman, Lisa A Blue Ridge Health Network, 930
Lauer, Gary L. eHealthInsurance Services Inc., 10, 22, 40, 70, 121
Lauer, Gary L. eHealthInsurance Services Inc. Corporate Office, 122
Lauer, Gary L. eHealthInsurance Services Inc., 203, 231, 244, 271, 318, 332,
  345, 366, 397, 421, 438, 459, 475, 487, 506, 527, 561, 598, 624, 642, 664, 678,
  688, 703, 720, 742, 767, 817, 832, 848, 888, 902, 939, 985, 997, 1014, 1030,
  1058, 1101, 1116, 1128, 1149, 1169, 1188, 1211
Lauffenburger, Michael J SafeGuard Health Enterprises: Corporate Office, 170
Lauffenburger, Michael J SafeGuard Health Enterprises: Florida, 295
Lauffenburger, Michael J SafeGuard Health Enterprises: Texas, 1081
Lauria, Richard J. Assurant Employee Benefits: Minnesota, 593
Lauterjung, Kevin S HMO Health Ohio, 853
Lauterjung, Kevin S Medical Mutual of Ohio, 857
Lauterjung, Kevin S Medical Mutual of Ohio Medicare Plan, 858
Lauterjung, Kevin S SuperMed One, 873
Lavely, David OptiCare Managed Vision, 823
Law, Patrick Blue Cross & Blue Shield of Montana, 661
Lawerence, Donald BEST Life and Health Insurance Co., 89
Lawhead, Jean Delta Dental of Colorado, 201
Lawrence, Jay, MD Aetna Health of Texas, 1041
Lawson, Maureen Network Health Plan of Wisconsin, 1198
Le, Curt Contra Costa Health Plan, 112
Lebish, Daniel United Concordia: New Mexico, 750
Lebish, Daniel United Concordia, 967
Lebish, Daniel J Highmark Blue Cross & Blue Shield, 949
Lebish, Daniel J Highmark Blue Shield, 950
Lechner, David Lifewise Health Plan of Oregon, 909
LeClaire, Brian Humana Health Insurance of Huntsville, 13
LeClaire, Brian Humana Health Insurance of Arizona, 46
LeClaire, Brian Arcadian Health Plans, 82
LeClaire, Brian Humana Health Insurance of Indiana, 404
LeClaire, Brian Humana Health Insurance of Kentucky, 460
LeClaire, Brian Humana Medicare Plan, 461
Lederberg, Michele B Blue Cross & Blue Shield of Rhode Island, 981

Lederman, Alan Community Health Plan of Washington, 1147
Lee, Amy Chinese Community Health Plan, 101
Lee, Chad University Health Alliance, 339
Lee, Howard K F, MD University Health Alliance, 339
Lee, Yolanda Chinese Community Health Plan, 101
Leeger, Meredith Initial Group, 1036
Lees, Janice M Delta Dental of Missouri, 640
Lehr, William, Jr Capital Blue Cross, 932
Leichtle, Robert Blue Cross & Blue Shield of South Carolina, 992
Leitzen, Justin ProviDRs Care Network, 448
Lem, Cindy Health Plan of San Mateo, 132
Lempner, Tracey UnitedHealthCare of Georgia, 327
Lempner, Tracey UnitedHealthCare of Michigan, 588
Lempner, Tracey UnitedHealthCare of Pennsylvania, 618
Lenderink, Gary B Guardian Life Insurance Company of America, 777
Lenhart, Jack A Valley Preferred, 970
Lennig, Nilsa Texas Community Care, 1086
Lenth, Gary, M.D. Gundersen Lutheran Health Plan, 1192
Lentz, Lori One Call Medical, 730
Leonard, Dennis Dentaquest, 526
Leonard, Jo-carol Family Choice Health Alliance, 721
Leonard, Jo-carol FC Diagnostic, 722
Leong, Darryl Care 1st Health Plan: California, 96
Lepre, Christopher M Horizon Blue Cross & Blue Shield of New Jersey, 724
Lerer, Rene, MD Magellan Health Services Indiana, 405
Lerer, Rene, MD Magellan Health Services: Corporate Headquarters, 510
Lesley, E Craig Delta Dental of Michigan, Ohio and Indiana, 847
Lessin, Karen Independence Blue Cross, 952
Lessin, Leeba CareMore Health Plan, 97
Leung, Moon, Ph.D. SCAN Health Plan, 173
LeValley, Joe Mercy Health Network, 426
Levicki, George A, DDS Delta Dental of Virginia, 1126
Levin, Howard, OD Block Vision, 497
Levine, Harlan, MD WellPoint: Corporate Office, 414
Levine, Jay Blue Cross & Blue Shield of Minnesota, 595
Levine, Robert, MD OmniCare: A Coventry Health Care Plan, 578
Levinson, Anthony R Coalition America's National Preferred Provider Network,
  761
Levinson, Donald M CIGNA HealthCare of Maine, 486
Lewis, Craig W Delta Dental of Rhode Island, 984
Lewis, DiJuana Anthem Blue Cross & Blue Shield Connecticut, 217
Lewis, Dijuana Aetna Health of Texas, 1041
Lewis, Jackie Unison Health Plan of Ohio, 876
Lewis, Jennifer Spectera, 516
Lewis, Kenneth FirstCarolinaCare, 818
Lewis, Melissa Ohio Health Choice, 863
Lewis, William R, MD Concentra: Corporate Office, 1055
Lewis-Clapper, Caskie Magellan Health Services Indiana, 405
Lewis-Clapper, Caskie Magellan Health Services: Corporate Headquarters, 510
Lewisr, Christina Valley Preferred, 970
Li, Grace, MHA On Lok Lifeways, 155
Liang, Janet Kaiser Permanente Health Plan of Hawaii, 337
Liang, Louise L, MD Kaiser Permanente Health Plan of Northern California, 138
Liang, Louise L, MD Kaiser Permanente Health Plan of Southern California, 139
Liang, Louise L, MD Kaiser Permanente Health Plan: Corporate Office, 140
Liang, Louise L, MD Kaiser Permanente Medicare Plan, 141
Liepins, Janis Fallon Community Medicare Plan, 529
Lile III, J Matt, RHU American Denticare, 63
Limon, Sara Delta Dental of New Mexico, 741
Lin, Gary H Harvard Pilgrim Health Care, 531
Lind, Arlene Omni IPA/Medcore Medical Group, 154
Lindemann, Bob CNA Insurance Companies: Colorado, 197
Lindemann, Bob CNA Insurance Companies: Georgia, 312
Lindemann, Bob CNA Insurance Companies: Illinois, 360
Lindgren, Charles A. Dimension Health PPO, 270
Lindsay, Mark UnitedHealthCare of Kentucky, 466
Lindsey, Claudia Anthem Blue Cross & Blue Shield Connecticut, 217
Lindsey, James California Dental Network, 93
Linfield, Rob Liberty Dental Plan, 146
Linley, Nancie Liberty Health Plan Anchorage, 24
Linse-weiss, Mickey Florida Health Care Plan, 275
Liston, Thomas J Humana Health Insurance of Kentucky, 460

Liston, Thomas J Humana Medicare Plan, 461
Liston, Thomas J Humana Health Insurance of Ohio, 854
Liston, Tom Humana Health Insurance of Illinois, 376
Liston, Tom Humana Health Insurance of Iowa, 424
Littel, John Amerigroup Ohio, 840
Littel, John E Amerigroup Nevada, 685
Littel, John E Amerigroup Corporation, 1120
Little, John Blue Cross & Blue Shield of South Carolina, 992
Little, Karen CIGNA HealthCare of Georgia, 311
Livingston, David Great Lakes Health Plan, 564
Livingston, Pam Cardinal Health Alliance, 393
Ljung, Douglas VSP: Vision Service Plan of Oregon, 920
Loder, Sandra Clear One Health Plans, 900
Loeliger, Dawn, JD Group Health Cooperative, 1150
Loepp, Daniel J Blue Cross Blue Shield of Michigan, 551
Loerke, Rick Dean Health Plan, 1185
Lofberg, Per CVS CareMark, 983
Loftis, R. Chet, JD,MPA Public Employees Health Program, 1106
Lohman, Wayne Health Choice LLC, 1031
Lonardo, Robert CareMore Health Plan, 97
London, Roger, MD Touchstone Health HMO, 803
Long, Jo Ann Regence Blue Cross & Blue Shield of Oregon, 915
Long, Kaye Valley Preferred, 970
Long, Kristy NOVA Healthcare Administrators, 798
Long, Laura B, MD BlueChoice Health Plan of South Carolina, 993
Longendyke, Rob Medica Health - Medicare Plan, 605
Longendyke, Rob, MD Medica: Corporate Office, 606
Longendyke, Rob Medica: North Dakota, 836
Longendyke, Rob Medica: South Dakota, 1018
Longworth, Maria CHN PPO, 717
Loosn, Richard Chinese Community Health Plan, 101
Lopes, Ancelmo Healthcare USA of Missouri, 647
Lopez, Frank Alliance Regional Health Network, 1042
Lopez, Vivian Triple-S Salud Blue Cross Blue Shield of Puerto Rico, 978
Lopez Duarte, Milori Vision Plan of America, 183
Lopez-Casiro, Rosie Preferred Medical Plan, 293
Lopez-Fernandez, Orlando, Jr, MD Preferred Care Partners, 292
Lord, Jack, MD Humana Health Insurance of Illinois, 376
Lord, Jack, MD Humana Health Insurance of Iowa, 424
Lord, Jonathan T, MD Humana Health Insurance of Ohio, 854
Lott, Laura M Kaiser Permanente Health Plan of Hawaii, 337
Lotterman, Brad United Behavioral Health, 178
Lotvin, Alan M, MD Magellan Health Services: Corporate Headquarters, 510
Louie, Deena Chinese Community Health Plan, 101
Louie, Deena San Francisco Health Plan, 171
Louie, Irene Chinese Community Health Plan, 101
Loux, Pamela Arkansas Managed Care Organization, 66
Love, Vincent J American WholeHealth Network, 924
Lovelace, John UPMC Health Plan, 968
Lovell, Stephanie Blue Cross & Blue Shield of Massachusetts, 522
Loweth, William B HAS-Premier Providers, 1063
Lowry, Shawn Foundation for Medical Care for Mendocino and Lake Counties, 124
Lowther, Ryan Educators Mutual, 1100
Lubben, David J UnitedHealthCare of Minnesota, 616
Lubitz, Mitch Humana Health Insurance of Jacksonville, 282
Lubitz, Mitch Humana Health Insurance of Tampa - Pinellas, 284
Lubitz, Mitch Humana Health Insurance of Louisiana, 477
Lucas, Stephanie Block Vision, 497
Luchetta, Thomas Superior Vision Services, Inc., 176
Luddyÿ, Tom Physicians Plus Insurance Corporation, 1199
Ludy, Jeff Universal Health Care Group, 300
Luebke, Art Kaiser Permanente Health Plan of Colorado, 207
Lukach, Melissa Highmark Blue Cross & Blue Shield Delaware, 233
Lukas, Catherine Harvard University Group Health Plan, 532
Lukens, Kay PCC Preferred Chiropractic Care, 443
Lum, Alison, PharmD San Francisco Health Plan, 171
Luna, Richard Medical Card System (MCS), 975
Lund, Cheryl Trillium Community Health Plan, 917
Luptowski, Marybeth CIGNA HealthCare of Georgia, 311
Luther, Carolyn W Independence Blue Cross, 952
Luther, John Dentaquest, 526

Lutter, Larry J, MD Meritain Health: Corporate Headquarters, 787
Lutz, Francis Devon Health Services, 938
Luxenberg, Jay On Lok Lifeways, 155
Lyle, Linda Cariten Healthcare, 1026
Lyle, Linda Cariten Preferred, 1027
Lyman, Dale N Meritain Health: Corporate Headquarters, 787
Lynch, Kevin Community Health Plan of Los Angeles County, 110
Lynch, Kevin, MS Los Angeles County Department of Health Services, 147
Lynch, Michael Humana Health Insurance of Jacksonville, 282
Lynch, Rob VSP: Vision Service Plan, 184
Lynch, Rob VSP: Vision Service Plan of Florida, 301
Lynch, Rob VSP: Vision Service Plan of Ohio, 879
Lynch, Rob VSP: Vision Service Plan of Texas, 1094
Lynch, Robert VSP: Vision Service Plan of New Jersey, 735
Lynch, Scott Blue Cross & Blue Shield of Minnesota, 595
Lynch, Stephen D Health Net Medicare Plan, 129
Lynn, Bob Dentaquest, 526
Lynn, George F Atlanticare Health Plans, 715
Lynne, Donna, DrPH Kaiser Permanente Health Plan of Colorado, 207
Lynne, Donna UnitedHealthCare of North Carolina, 827
Lyons, Serena Lovelace Medicare Health Plan, 746

M

Maack, Terri Trillium Community Health Plan, 917
Maas, Pamela Gundersen Lutheran Health Plan, 1192
Maccannon, Keith DC Chartered Health Plan, 242
MacDonald, Cynthia Metropolitan Health Plan, 608
Machiche, Nolberto Magellan Health Services Arizona, 47
Machtan, Kenneth N. Group Health Cooperative of South Central Wisconsin, 1191
Mack, Pat Carolina Care Plan, 994
Mack, Rhonda K. DakotaCare, 1012
Mackail, Christopher Mid Atlantic Medical Services: Corporate Office, 511
Mackenzie, Laurida Spectera, 516
Mackin, John T, Jr American Pioneer Life Insurance Co, 251
Mackin, Koko Blue Cross & Blue Shield of Alabama, 6
Maclean, Tom Blue Cross & Blue Shield of New Mexico, 739
Madden, Kathleen ConnectiCare, 220
Madden, Michael, MD Gateway Health Plan, 943
Madill, Fred Unison Health Plan of Pennsylvania, 966
Madlem, Larry Coalition America's National Preferred Provider Network, 761
Maesaka Jr., Clifford T., DDS Delta Dental of Kentucky, 458
Magby, Kathy UnitedHealthCare of Louisiana, 481
Magill, Carolyn AmeriChoice by UnitedHealthCare, 710
Maguire, Peggy Regence Blue Cross & Blue Shield of Oregon, 915
Maher, Charlene Health Plan of New York, 778
Maher, Charlene A. GHI, 774
Maher, Charlene A. GHI Medicare Plan, 775
Maher, Dan Pacific Dental Benefits, 157
Mahmood, Alec Health Net of Arizona, 45
Mahoney, Jim USA Managed Care Organization, 1091
Mahowald, Thomas UCare Medicare Plan, 614
Mahowald, Thomas UCare Minnesota, 615
Mailander, Edward GHI, 774
Mailander, Edward GHI Medicare Plan, 775
Mailander, Edward M Rayant Insurance Company, 733
Mailer, Wendy Contra Costa Health Plan, 112
Maisel, Garry Western Health Advantage, 187
Maldonado, Anna Maria Care 1st Health Plan: Arizona, 35
Maldonado, Paul Community First Health Plans, 1054
Malinowski, Barry, MD Anthem Blue Cross & Blue Shield of Ohio, 841
Maloney, Sheila Santa Clara Family Health Foundations Inc, 172
Maltz, Allen P Blue Cross & Blue Shield of Massachusetts, 522
Manchandia, Mahesh Primecare Dental Plan, 168
Manchee, Nancy Pacific Foundation for Medical Care, 158
Manders, Matt CIGNA HealthCare of Nevada, 687
Manders, Matthew CIGNA HealthCare of Virginia, 1124
Manders, Matthew G CIGNA: Corporate Headquarters, 935
Mangiacarne, Darrin, MD/DO Virginia Premier Health Plan, 1142
Manju, Shenoy Golden West Dental & Vision Plan, 126
Mann, Margie Meritain Health: Louisiana, 478
Mann, Margie Meritain Health: Corporate Headquarters, 787

McCallister, Michael Humana Health Insurance of Washington, 1151
McCallister, Michael B Humana Health Insurance of Tampa - Pinellas, 284
McCallister, Michael B Humana Health Insurance of Iowa, 424
McCallister, Michael B Humana Health Insurance of Kansas, 441
McCallister, Michael B Humana Health Insurance of Kentucky, 460
McCallister, Michael B Humana Medicare Plan, 461
McCallister, Michael B Humana Health Insurance of Ohio, 854
McCallister, Michael R Humana Health Insurance of New Hampshire, 705
McCallister, Mike Humana Health Insurance of Illinois, 376
McCallister, Mike Humana Health Insurance of Corpus Christi, 1069
McCammond, Ann CONCERN: Employee Assistance Program, 111
McCarthy, Dan WellChoice, 736
McCarthy, Daniel HealthFirst New Jersey Medicare Plan, 723
McCarthy, Gloria WellPoint: Corporate Office, 414
McCarthy, Maureen Harvard University Group Health Plan, 532
McCarthy, Meg Aetna Health of California, 79
McCarthy, Meg Aetna Health, Inc. Medicare Plan, 215
McCarthy, Meg Aetna Health of Mississippi, 621
McCarthy, Meg Aetna Health of New York, 752
McCarthy, Meg Aetna Health of Texas, 1041
McCarthy, Meg Aetna Health of Virginia, 1119
McCarthy, Thomas A CIGNA: Corporate Headquarters, 935
McCartney, Mary Ellen Gundersen Lutheran Health Plan, 1192
McCay, Alan Central California Alliance for Health, 99
McCcluskey, Mary Amerigroup Ohio, 840
McClary, Martha Quality Plan Administrators, 247
McClelland, Pat Santa Clara Family Health Foundations Inc, 172
McClintock, Scott Alere Health, 304
McCloud, Scott CorVel Corporation, 113
McClure, Jan Alere Health, 304
McCluskey, Mary Amerigroup Corporation, 1120
McCluskey, Mary T Amerigroup Nevada, 685
McCluskey, Mary T, MD Amerigroup New Jersey, 712
McCluskey, Mary T., M.D. Amerigroup Texas, 1044
McCollum, A Michael Concentra: Corporate Office, 1055
McComas, John AlohaCare, 330
McConathy, Chris Golden West Dental & Vision Plan, 126
McCrann, Kelly PacifiCare Dental and Vision Administrators, 161
McCray, Ivy Preferred Health Systems Insurance Company, 444
McCray, Ivy Preferred Plus of Kansas, 446
McCreath, Jim Liberty Health Advantage Medicare Plan, 785
McCrohan, Beth American Community Mutual Insurance Company, 544
McCulley, Daniel R. Midlands Choice, 680
McCulley, Steven Humana Health Insurance of Arizona, 46
McCulley, Steven E Humana Health Insurance of Kentucky, 460
McCulley, Steven E Humana Health Insurance of Ohio, 854
McCulloch, Andrew R Kaiser Permanente Health Plan of the Northwest, 907
McDaniel, Donna Mercy Health Plans: Kansas, 442
McDaniel, Donna Mercy Health Medicare Plan, 651
McDaniel, Donna Mercy Health Plans: Corporate Office, 652
McDaniel, Donna Vytra Health Plans, 808
McDaniel, Donna Mercy Health Plans: Oklahoma, 891
McDole, Diane UnitedHealthCare of Rhode Island, 989
McDonnell, Maureen C Amerigroup Georgia, 306
McDonnell, Maureen C. Amerigroup Texas, 1044
McDonough, Thomas P Coventry Health Care of Kansas, 436
McDonough, Thomas P HealthAmerica, 947
McDow, Anne Kaiser Permanente Health Plan of Colorado, 207
McElrath-Jones, Mary UnitedHealthCare of Minnesota, 617
McElrath-Jones, Mary UnitedHealthCare of New York, 805
McEnery, W. Thomas OptumHealth Care Solutions: Physical Health, 610
McEwen, Scott Kanawha Healthcare Solutions, 1001
McFadden, Darin Group Health Cooperative of Eau Claire, 1190
McFadden, John Select Health of South Carolina, 1003
McFarland, Patti Central California Alliance for Health, 99
McFarlane, Donald C. CorVel Corporation, 113
McFarlane, Lawrence, MBA, MD Security Health Plan of Wisconsin, 1201
McFeetors, Raymond L. Great-West Healthcare Oklahoma, 889
McGarry, Peter PacificSource Health Plans: Idaho, 349
McGarry, Peter PacificSource Health Plans: Corporate Headquarters, 913
McGeehan, Gerard J. Graphic Arts Benefit Corporation, 507
McGeehan, Jerry Graphic Arts Benefit Corporation, 507

McGinley, Gretchen Los Angeles County Department of Health Services, 147
McGinty, T American Dental Group, 189
McGone, Jen Health InfoNet, 666
McGovern, Patricia Preferred Care, 958
McGrann, Jim VSP: Vision Service Plan, 184
McGrann, Jim VSP: Vision Service Plan of Texas, 1094
McGrew, Diane OSF HealthPlans, 379
McGuire, Marilee Community Health Plan of Washington, 1147
McGuire, William, MD UnitedHealthCare of Mississippi, 627
McGuire, William W, MD UnitedHealthCare of Minnesota, 616
McInerney, Jim Health InfoNet, 666
McIntire, Robert Anthem Blue Cross & Blue Shield of Indiana, 388
McKinley, Lois Care Choices, 552
McKinney, Rod Coventry Health Care of West Virginia, 1167
McKitterick, Mike L, RN Colorado Access, 198
McKittrick, Jim Liberty Health Plan: Corporate Office, 908
McLain, Ginny Kaiser Permanente Health Plan of Colorado, 207
McLaren, Ross Humana Health Insurance of Corpus Christi, 1069
McLaughlin, Barbara A Delta Dental of New Hampshire, 702
McLaughlin, Joe InterGroup Services Corporation, 953
McLelland, Llaura Healthcare Partners of East Texas, 1064
McLerran, Ross Humana Health Insurance of Colorado Springs, 206
McLerran, Ross Humana Health Insurance of Idaho, 346
McManus, Jeffrey, MD Texas Community Care, 1086
McNatt, Jennifer InterGroup Services Corporation, 953
McNeil, Pat VSP: Vision Service Plan, 184
McNeil, Pat VSP: Vision Service Plan of New Jersey, 735
McNeilly, Steven Northeast Georgia Health Partners, 323
McPhail, Michelle Humana Health Insurance of Orlando, 283
McPheeters, George O, MD University Health Alliance, 339
McPheeters, Mindy Delta Dental of Kansas, 437
Mcquade, Deborah UnitedHealthCare of Washington, 1163
McQuaide, Jay Blue Cross & Blue Shield of Massachusetts, 522
McSorley, John J. QualCare, 732
Mead, Robert E Aetna Health, Inc. Medicare Plan, 215
Mead, Robert E Aetna Health of Mississippi, 621
Mead, Robert E Aetna Health of New York, 752
Mead, Robert E Aetna Health of Virginia, 1119
Meadows, Dave Liberty Dental Plan of Nevada, 692
Media Relations Manager, Earling Lifewise Health Plan of Washington, 1153
Meehan, Carson Coventry Health Care of Louisiana, 472
Meehan, Carson Carolina Care Plan, 994
Meek, Todd NevadaCare, 695
Meese, Samantha Regence Blue Cross & Blue Shield of Oregon, 915
Mehelic, Phil American Health Care Alliance, 630
Mehring, Melissa HealthSpan, 852
Meier, John Paramount Elite Medicare Plan, 866
Meier, John Paramount Health Care, 867
Meier, Marleen Dominion Dental Services, 1127
Meisel, Stephen, MD Medfocus Radiology Network, 151
Melani, Kenneth R, MD Highmark Blue Cross & Blue Shield, 949
Memezes, Bob San Francisco Health Plan, 171
Menario, Jay CIGNA HealthCare of North Carolina, 813
Mendez, Ernest HAS-Premier Providers, 1063
Mendis, Paul, MD Neighborhood Health Plan, 537
Mendrygal, Matthew HealthPlus of Michigan: Flint, 569
Mendrygal, Matthew HealthPlus of Michigan: Saginaw, 570
Menezes, Bob San Francisco Health Plan, 171
Mense, D Craig CNA Insurance Companies: Colorado, 197
Mense, D Craig CNA Insurance Companies: Georgia, 312
Mense, D Craig CNA Insurance Companies: Illinois, 360
Meoli, Angela Coventry Health Care of GA, 314
Meoli, Angela Coventry Health Care of Louisiana, 472
Merkel, F G Chip United Concordia: New Mexico, 750
Merkel-Liberatore, Karen HealthNow New York - Emblem Health, 779
Merlo, Larry J CVS CareMark, 983
Merrick, Mayra Citizens Choice Healthplan, 107
Merrill, Stacie Opticare of Utah, 1105
Mertz, Laura J Valley Preferred, 970
Merwin, Joan Network Health Plan of Wisconsin, 1198
Merz, Marcus PreferredOne, 612
Messina, Elizabeth A Blue Cross & Blue Shield of Arizona, 34

Messina, Jim Premera Blue Cross, 1157
Metge, Bruce Catalyst Health Solutions Inc, 498
Metge, Bruce Catalyst RX, 812
Meyer, Carol Los Angeles County Department of Health Services, 147
Meyer, Carrie Independent Health Medicare Plan, 783
Meyer, Susan Ohio State University Health Plan Inc., 864
Meyers-Alessi, Lisa Blue Cross & Blue Shield of Western New York, 756
Meyers-Alessi, Lisa Univera Healthcare, 806
Meyerson, Tamara Preferred Medical Plan, 293
Mggarry, Peter Clear One Health Plans, 900
Michael, Jenny CareSource, 844
Middleton, Darrell E Blue Cross Blue Shield of Michigan, 551
Middleton, Darrell E. Blue Care Network of Michigan: Medicare, 547
Middleton, Kevin, PsyD MHNet Behavioral Health, 1076
Midkiff, Cheryl Piedmont Community Health Plan, 1136
Midlikowski, Gail Unity Health Insurance, 1204
Milbrandt, Chase, MBA Texas Community Care, 1086
Miles, Richard GEHA-Government Employees Hospital Association, 644
Miller, Amy Priority Health, 581
Miller, Fred, Md Pima Health System, 54
Miller, Gil SCAN Health Plan, 173
Miller, Jeff Aetna Health of Oklahoma, 880
Miller, Jeff Delta Dental of South Dakota, 1013
Miller, Jeffrey Western Dental Services, 186
Miller, Jim Hometown Health Plan, 690
Miller, Jolee Deaconess Health Plans, 395
Miller, Mike DenteMax, 560
Miller, Sandra H Anthem Blue Cross & Blue Shield of Indiana, 388
Mills, Jon HealthLink HMO, 648
Mills, Randy Southeastern Indiana Health Organization, 410
Mills, Shannon E, DDS Delta Dental of New Hampshire, 702
Mills, Vivian B. InStil Health, 1000
Milner, Lance Anthem Blue Cross & Blue Shield of New Hampshire, 700
Milner, Roger Preferred Health Care, 959
Milo, Yori Premera Blue Cross, 1157
Mims, Pamela C Florida Health Care Plan, 275
Minaldi, Thad Blue Cross & Blue Shield of Louisiana, 469
Minella, Lindsey Humana Health Insurance of Illinois, 376
Minella, Lindsey Humana Health Insurance of Iowa, 424
Mineo, John Independent Health, 782
Mingione, Lisa Touchstone Health HMO, 803
Minson, Jeff ProviDRs Care Network, 448
Mirabal, Jose Medical Card System (MCS), 975
Mirt, Michael HealthSpring: Corporate Offices, 1034
Miskimmin, Renee, MD Gateway Health Plan, 943
Misso, Carol Superior Vision Services, Inc., 176
Mitchel, Deona Signature Health Alliance, 1038
Mitchell, Michael Interplan Health Group, 855
Mitchell, Tracy Arizona Foundation for Medical Care, 30
Mixer, Mark Alliant Health Plans, 305
Miyasato, Gwen S Hawaii Medical Services Association, 335
Mock, Kathleen Blue Cross & Blue Shield of Minnesota, 595
Mockus, Jennifer, RN Central California Alliance for Health, 99
Mohan, Ronald, MD Gateway Health Plan, 943
Moharsky, Linda Blue Cross of Northeastern Pennsylvania, 929
Moksnes, Mark A Delta Dental of North Dakota, 831
Molina, Carmen Medical Card System (MCS), 975
Molina, J Mario, MD Molina Healthcare: Corporate Office, 153
Molina, J Mario, MD Molina Healthcare: New Mexico, 747
Molina, J Mario, MD Molina Healthcare: Washington, 1154
Molina, J. Mario Molina Healthcare: Michigan, 577
Molina, J. Mario Molina Healthcare: Ohio, 860
Molina, J. Mario, M.D. Molina Healthcare: Texas, 1077
Molina, John C, JD Molina Healthcare: Corporate Office, 153
Molina, John C, JD Molina Healthcare: Washington, 1154
Molina, John C., JD Molina Healthcare: Michigan, 577
Molina, John C. Molina Healthcare: New Mexico, 747
Molina, John C. Molina Healthcare: Ohio, 860
Molina, John C., JD Molina Healthcare: Texas, 1077
Molina Bernadett, Dr.Martha Molina Healthcare: Texas, 1077
Molina Bernadett, Dr.Martha Molina Healthcare: Washington, 1154
Molina Bernadett, Martha, MD Molina Healthcare: Michigan, 577

Monfiletto, Sandra Martin's Point HealthCare, 490
Monfitletto, Ernesto AmeriChoice by UnitedHealthCare, 754
Moniz, James UnitedHealthCare of Massachusetts, 541
Moniz, James, Jr UnitedHealthCare of Rhode Island, 989
Monk, Nancy J. SCAN Health Plan, 173
Monroe, Wayne Mid Atlantic Medical Services: Corporate Office, 511
Monsrud, Beth, MD UCare Medicare Plan, 614
Monsrud, Beth, MD UCare Minnesota, 615
Montalvo, Mike UnitedHealthcare Nevada, 698
Montgomery, Jamie Deaconess Health Plans, 395
Montiletto, Ernest Americhoice of Pennsylvania, 925
Moon, Pam Piedmont Community Health Plan, 1136
Moon, Richard Medical Card System (MCS), 975
Mooney, Kay Aetna Health, Inc. Medicare Plan, 215
Mooney, Kay Aetna Health of New York, 752
Mooney, Kay Aetna Health of Virginia, 1119
Moore, Derek MagnaCare, 786
Moore, James OSF Healthcare, 378
Moore, James OSF HealthPlans, 379
Moore, Jennifer Crescent Health Solutions, 815
Moore, Macon Peoples Health, 479, 480
Moore, Matthew Unison Health Plan of Pennsylvania, 966
Moore, Phyllis VSP: Vision Service Plan of California, 185
Moore, Tim CIGNA HealthCare of Arkansas, 67
Moore, Tim Carilion Health Plans, 1123
Moorehead, Jay AmeriHealth HMO, 227
Morgan, Daniel VSP: Vision Service Plan of California, 185
Morgan, Lesley CHA Health, 455
Moriarty, Thomas M CVS CareMark, 983
Morrill, James MVP Health Care: New Hampshire, 706
Morrill, James MVP Health Care Medicare Plan, 790
Morrill, James MVP Health Care: Buffalo Region, 791
Morrill, James MVP Health Care: Mid-State Region, 794
Morrill, James MVP Health Care: Western New York, 795
Morrill, James MVP Health Care: Vermont, 1117
Morris, Brett A Health Net of Arizona, 45
Morris, M Shawn HealthSpring Prescription Drug Plan, 1033
Morris, Pamela CareSource: Michigan, 553
Morris, Pamela CareSource, 844
Morrison, Jane Total Dental Administrators, 57, 1109
Morrison, Marion Health Plus of Louisiana, 476
Morrison, Steven C., CPA Educators Mutual, 1100
Morrissey, Brian J CDPHP: Capital District Physicians' Health Plan, 759
Morrissey, Brian J. CDPHP Medicare Plan, 758
Morrone, Michael A CHN PPO, 717
Morse, David B Delta Dental of North Dakota, 831
Morton, Robbin Secure Health PPO Newtork, 324
Mosby, Jacqueline Piedmont Community Health Plan, 1136
Moscovic, David Basic Chiropractic Health Plan, 85
Motamed, Thomas F CNA Insurance Companies: Colorado, 197
Motamed, Thomas F CNA Insurance Companies: Georgia, 312
Motamed, Thomas F CNA Insurance Companies: Illinois, 360
Motter, Eric, MBA Nationwide Better Health, 862
Moutinho, Maria E, MD Gateway Health Plan, 943
Moya, Steve Humana Health Insurance of Illinois, 376
Moya, Steve Humana Health Insurance of Iowa, 424
Moya, Steven Humana Health Insurance of Arizona, 46
Moya, Steven O Humana Health Insurance of Kansas, 441
Moya, Steven O Humana Health Insurance of Ohio, 854
Mroue, Carole Care Choices, 552
Muchnicki, Michael A Sterling Health Plans, 1161
Muck, Robin Premier Access Insurance/Access Dental, 167
Muck, Robin SafeGuard Health Enterprises: Corporate Office, 170
Mudra, Karl A Delta Dental of Missouri, 640
Muller, Roger, MD UnitedHealthCare of Alaska, 27
Muller, Roger, MD UnitedHealthCare of Oregon, 919
Muller, Roger, MD UnitedHealthCare of Washington, 1163
Mulligan, Deanna M. Guardian Life Insurance Company of America, 777
Mullins, Larry A, DHA Samaritan Health Plan, 916
Mummery, Ray Dimension Health PPO, 270
Muney, Alan, MD, MHA CIGNA HealthCare of Connecticut, 219
Muney, Alan CIGNA HealthCare of Maine, 486

Muney, Alan CIGNA HealthCare of Nevada, 687
Muney, Alan M Oxford Health Plans: New Jersey, 731
Muney, Alan M, MD Oxford Health Plans: New York, 799
Muney, MD, MHA, Alan CIGNA HealthCare of Arizona, 36
Muney, MD, MHA, Alan CIGNA HealthCare of Minnesota, 596
Munich, Maritza I Medical Card System (MCS), 975
Munir, Naim Health Alliance Medicare, 566
Munir, Naim, MD Health Alliance Plan, 567
Munro, Jan Managed HealthCare Northwest, 910
Munson, Russell, MD Fallon Community Medicare Plan, 529
Murabito, John M CIGNA: Corporate Headquarters, 935
Murpht, Maria Eileen OhioHealth Group, 865
Murphy, Michael G Vytra Health Plans, 808
Murphy, Scott Dental Benefit Providers: California, 116
Murphy, Terry Arizona Foundation for Medical Care, 30
Murphy, Theresa Arizona Foundation for Medical Care, 30
Murphy, Tracie Moda Health Alaska, 25
Murray, Charles University Health Alliance, 339
Murray, James CompBenefits: Alabama, 9
Murray, James Humana Health Insurance of Fresno, 133
Murray, James Humana Health Insurance of Southern California, 134
Murray, James Humana Health Insurance of Nebraska, 679
Murray, James Humana Health Insurance of New Hampshire, 705
Murray, James E Humana Health Insurance of Tampa - Pinellas, 284
Murray, James E Humana Health Insurance of Kansas, 441
Murray, James E Humana Health Insurance of Kentucky, 460
Murray, James E Humana Medicare Plan, 461
Murray, James E Humana Health Insurance of Michigan, 574
Murray, James E Humana Health Insurance of Nevada, 691
Murray, James E Humana Health Insurance of Ohio, 854
Murray, James E. Humana Health Insurance of Huntsville, 13
Murray, James E. Humana Health Insurance of Arizona, 46
Murray, James E. Arcadian Health Plans, 82
Murray, James E. Humana Health Insurance of Indiana, 404
Murray, James E. Humana Health Insurance of San Antonio, 1070
Murray, Jim Humana Health Insurance of Illinois, 376
Murray, Jim Humana Health Insurance of Iowa, 424
Murray, Michael Blue Shield of California, 90
Murrell, Warren Peoples Health, 479, 480
Murrill, Tom Essence Healthcare, 643
Muscarella, Sharon United Concordia, 967
Muscatello, Todd Excellus Blue Cross Blue Shield: Central New York, 770
Muscatello, Todd Excellus Blue Cross Blue Shield: Rochester Region, 771
Muscatello, Todd Excellus Blue Cross Blue Shield: Utica Region, 772
Muse, Haydee Aetna Health of Missouri, 629
Muzi, Titus Humana Health Insurance of Wisconsin, 1195
Mychalishyn, John Lifewise Health Plan of Washington, 1153
Myers, Dr Wendy Florida Health Care Plan, 275
Myers, Jack A. Blue Cross of Idaho Health Service, Inc., 342
Myers, Jamie CareMore Health Plan, 97
Myers, Jay OptiCare Managed Vision, 823
Myers, Michael R GEMCare Health Plan, 125
Mylotte, Kathleen, MD Independent Health Medicare Plan, 783

N

Nacol, John Pacific Foundation for Medical Care, 158
Nadeau, Mark Delta Dental of New Jersey & Connecticut, 719
Nagle, Joseph Delta Dental of Rhode Island, 984
Nair, Mohan Regence Blue Cross & Blue Shield of Oregon, 915
Nair, Mohan Regence Blue Cross & Blue Shield of Utah, 1107
Namba, Nolan AlohaCare, 330
Nameth, Michael WellPoint NextRx, 1095
Napier, Annette Vantage Health Plan, 482
Narowitz, Randy Total Health Care, 585
Narula, Mohender Primecare Dental Plan, 168
Nash, Bruce D., MD, MBA CDPHP Medicare Plan, 758
Nash, Bruce D., MD CDPHP: Capital District Physicians' Health Plan, 759
Nash, Dee Medical Mutual Services, 1002
Nava, Rachael Central California Alliance for Health, 99
Navarro, Scott, DDS Delta Dental of New Jersey & Connecticut, 221, 719
Navran, Susan Blue Cross & Blue Shield of Arizona, 34
Naylor, John Medica: Corporate Office, 606

Naylor, John Medica: North Dakota, 836
Neary, Daniel P Mutual of Omaha DentaBenefits, 681
Neary, Daniel P Mutual of Omaha Health Plans, 682
Needleman, Phillip Vision Plan of America, 183
Needleman, Stuart, OD Vision Plan of America, 183
Neely, Marc Great-West Healthcare Delaware, 232
Neeson, Richard J Independence Blue Cross, 952
Negrini, Barbara, MD Gateway Health Plan, 943
Neidorff, Michael F Centene Corporation, 635
Neiswander, Dana Piedmont Community Health Plan, 1136
Nelles, Roslind American Pioneer Life Insurance Co, 251
Nelson, Brock Health Partners Medicare Plan, 601
Nelson, Brock HealthPartners, 602
Nelson, Gunnar Patient Choice, 611
Nelson, Jeffrey UPMC Health Plan, 968
Nelson, Josh Great-West/One Health Plan, 204
Nelson, Josh CIGNA HealthCare of Pennsylvania, 934
Nelson, Josh CIGNA HealthCare of Utah, 1098
Nelson, Mike Coventry Health Care of Nebraska, 676
Nelson, Russell Altius Health Plans, 1097
Nelson, Su Zan Concentra: Corporate Office, 1055
Nelson, Thomas Wisconsin Physician's Service, 1206
Nemeth, Thomas A Health Plan of New York, 778
Neshat, Amir, DDS Liberty Dental Plan, 146
Neshat, Amir, DDS Liberty Dental Plan of Nevada, 692
Neufeld, Dr Ramen GEMCare Health Plan, 125
New, Deborah Anthem Blue Cross & Blue Shield Connecticut, 217
New, Deborah Anthem Blue Cross & Blue Shield of Indiana, 388, 389
New, Deborah Anthem Blue Cross & Blue Shield of Maine, 485
Newcom, Doug OptiCare Managed Vision, 823
Newland, Jeff Blue Cross & Blue Shield of New Mexico, 739
Newman, Christy Cariten Healthcare, 1026
Newman, Christy Cariten Preferred, 1027
Newman, Kermit Lakeside Community Healthcare Network, 144
Newsome, Rick Kaiser Permanente Health Plan of Colorado, 207
Newton, Cecil San Francisco Health Plan, 171
Newton, Dean Delta Dental of Kansas, 437
Nguyen, Ted Calais Health, 470
Niccolli, Dan CIGNA HealthCare of New York, 760
Nicholas, Jonathan Moda Health Alaska, 25
Nicholas, Jonathan ODS Health Plan, 911
Nichols, Sandra, MD UnitedHealthCare of Northern California, 180
Nichols, Sandra, MD UnitedHealthCare of Southern California, 181
Nicholson, Joseph Blue Cross & Blue Shield of Oklahoma, 882
Nickerson, Matt Liberty Health Plan: Corporate Office, 908
Nicklaus, Dana First Care Health Plans, 1060
Nicklebur, MD, Scott Scott & White Health Plan, 1082
Nicoletti, Ralph CIGNA HealthCare of Minnesota, 596
Nicoletti, Ralph CIGNA HealthCare of Nevada, 687
Nicoll, Don, MD CIGNA HealthCare of New Jersey, 718
Nicolletti, Ralph CIGNA HealthCare of Northern California, 105
Nicolletti, Ralph CIGNA HealthCare of Southern California, 106
Nied, Michelle Patient Choice, 611
Niederberger, Jane Anthem Blue Cross & Blue Shield of Indiana, 388
Niehaus, Rayne Saint Mary's Health Plans, 697
Nienhaus, Jeffrey ChiroCare of Wisconsin, 1183
Nishimoto, Sheila, MBA Puget Sound Health Partners, 1158
Nissenbaum, Richard, RPh Humana Health Insurance of Tampa - Pinellas, 284
Noah, Kent M Trillium Community Health Plan, 917
Nobile, Paul Unicare: Illinois, 382
Nolan, Tim Magellan Health Services: Corporate Headquarters, 510
Nolan, Tim Magellan Medicaid Administration, 1131
Nolan, Timothy Coventry Health Care of Nebraska, 676
Nolan, Timothy E HealthAmerica Pennsylvania, 948
Noland, Tom Humana Health Insurance of Illinois, 376
Noland, Tom Humana Health Insurance of Iowa, 424
Noll, Dr. C David Preferred Health Care, 959
Norato, Mark Coventry Health Care of GA, 314
Nordstrom, Kimberly, MD, JD Behavioral Healthcare, 193
Noren, Jenny Gundersen Lutheran Health Plan, 1192
Norman, DK UTMB HealthCare Systems, 1092
Norman, Gordon K, MD/MBA Alere Health, 304

Norris, Susan, PhD CompCare: Comprehensive Behavioral Care, 266
Northfield, David Kaiser Permanente Health Plan of the Northwest, 907
Norton, Deborah Harvard Pilgrim Health Care, 531
Nota-Kirby, Betsy M-Care, 575
Novella, James Arcadian Community Care, 468
Novello, James Ozark Health Plan, 656
Novick, Nancy Phoenix Health Plan, 52
Nowakowski, Richard M-Care, 575
Nowicki, Sarah Tufts Health Plan: Rhode Island, 988
Nowitzki, Rian Behavioral Healthcare, 193
Nunez, Alex Magellan Health Services Arizona, 47
Nussbaum, Samuel WellPoint: Corporate Office, 414
Nussbaum, Samuel, MD Anthem Blue Cross & Blue Shield of Maine, 485
Nutley, Debbie CNA Insurance Companies: Colorado, 197
Nuzzi, Rosemarie Island Group Administration, Inc., 784
Nyquist, Cynthia Upper Peninsula Health Plan, 589

O

O 'Drobinak, Jim Medical Card System (MCS), 975
O'Brien, Ann Marie UnitedHealthCare of New York, 805
O'Brien, Cyndie Inter Valley Health Plan, 136
O'Brien, David M Highmark Blue Cross & Blue Shield, 949
O'Brien, David M Highmark Blue Shield, 950
O'Brien, Ralph UnitedHealthCare of Ohio: Columbus, 877
O'Brien, Ralph UnitedHealthCare of Ohio: Dayton & Cincinnati, 878
O'Brien, Robert Group Health Cooperative, 1150
O'Brien, Tim Blue Cross & Blue Shield of Massachusetts, 522
O'Brien, Tom Medical Associates Health Plan, 377
O'Connell, Jeff Paramount Elite Medicare Plan, 866
O'Connell, Jeff Paramount Health Care, 867
O'Connell, Ryan New West Health Services, 669
O'Connell, Ryan New West Medicare Plan, 670
O'Connor, H Tomkins American WholeHealth Network, 924
O'Connor, Maureen K Blue Cross & Blue Shield of North Carolina, 811
O'Connor, Maureen K Preferred Care Select, 824
O'Connor, Michael Davis Vision, 763
O'Connor, Sharon CorVel Corporation, 113
O'Grady, Brian CDPHP Medicare Plan, 758
O'Hanlon, Greg Health Net Health Plan of Oregon, 905
O'Hara, Mary Blue Shield of California, 90
O'Loughlin, William B Blue Cross and Blue Shield Association, 357
O'Neil-White, Alphonso Blue Cross & Blue Shield of Western New York, 756
O'Neill, Peter UnitedHealthcare Nevada, 698
O'Shields, Brian Aetna Health of the Carolinas, 809
Oakley, Donald VSP: Vision Service Plan, 184
Oberg, Steve HSM: Healthcare Cost Management, 603
Oddo, Angel HealthAmerica Pennsylvania, 948
Odgaard, Nate Blue Cross & Blue Shield of Nebraska, 674
Odom, Karen HAS-Premier Providers, 1063
Odzer, Randall United Behavioral Health, 178
Ogdon, Tom Anthem Blue Cross & Blue Shield of Missouri, 631
Ohman, Daniel Laurence UnitedHealthCare of Georgia, 327
Ohme, Sheryle Assurant Employee Benefits: New Jersey, 714
Ohme, Sheryle L Assurant Employee Benefits: Corporate Headquarters, 632
Olearczyk, John Fidelis Care, 773
Oleary, Brian Managed Health Network, 148
Oleg, Dennis, PhD Humana Health Insurance of Wisconsin, 1195
Oliker, David MVP Health Care: New Hampshire, 706
Oliker, David MVP Health Care Medicare Plan, 790
Oliker, David MVP Health Care: Buffalo Region, 791
Oliker, David MVP Health Care: Mid-State Region, 794
Oliker, David MVP Health Care: Western New York, 795
Oliva, Lucy Liberty Health Advantage Medicare Plan, 785
Oliver, Diane HealthSpan, 852
Oliveto Hill, Michele Great Lakes Health Plan, 564
Olmstead, Francis H, Jr Cariten Healthcare, 1026
Olsen, David HSM: Healthcare Cost Management, 603
Olshanski, Jayne HealthAmerica Pennsylvania, 948
Olson, David W Health Net Medicare Plan, 129
Olson, Fred, MD Blue Cross & Blue Shield of Montana, 661
Olson, Michael Fortified Provider Network, 42
Olson, Tom Wisconsin Physician's Service, 1206

Olson, Wendy Americas PPO, 1009
Olzawski, Elaine, RN BlueLincs HMO, 883
Onorati, Annette C, Esq Preferred Care Partners, 292
Ordway, Jody Managed HealthCare Northwest, 910
Oreskovich, Kitty Health Net Health Plan of Oregon, 905
Orland, Burton Oxford Health Plans: New Jersey, 731
Ormond, John Hometown Health Plan, 690
Orsbon, Nance Delta Dental of South Dakota, 1013
Ortega, Janice Peoples Health, 480
Ortego, Janice Peoples Health, 479
Ortiz, Ed Health Plan of San Mateo, 132
Osborne, Mary Lou HealthAmerica Pennsylvania, 948
Osenar, Peter Interplan Health Group, 137, 1071
Osgood, Teena Fallon Community Medicare Plan, 529
Osorio, Rosemary Dimension Health PPO, 270
Ostrov, Michael, MD Group Health Cooperative of South Central Wisconsin, 1191
Ott, David HealthLink HMO, 648
Outten, Cornelia Interplan Health Group, 137
Owens, Dawn Dental Benefit Providers, 505
Owings, Lorena Ohio State University Health Plan Inc., 864
Ownbey, Ron Delta Dental of Arkansas, 69

P

Pace, Carolyn Health Net of Arizona, 45
Pace, Nicholas Amerigroup Nevada, 685
Pace, Nicholas Amerigroup Ohio, 840
Pack, Kent Children's Mercy Pediatric Care Network, 636
Packman, Robert C, MD Centene Corporation, 635
Paco"", Francisco, Trilla Neighborhood Health Plan of Rhode Island, 987
Padilla, Maria ABRI Health Plan, Inc., 1178
Padula, Glen Saint Mary's Health Plans, 697
Pagano, Christopher J. Assurant Employee Benefits: North Carolina, 810
Page, Anne Amerigroup Texas, 1044
Page, Kenneth HealthSpan, 852
Pagliaro, Brian P Tufts Health Medicare Plan, 538
Pagliaro, Brian P Tufts Health Plan, 539
Paguia, Victor PacificSource Health Plans: Corporate Headquarters, 913
Pair, Judy Alliant Health Plans, 305
Pak, Mary, MD Unity Health Insurance, 1204
Palenske, Frederick D. Blue Cross & Blue Shield of Kansas, 433
Palmateer, Michael GHI, 774
Palmateer, Michael GHI Medicare Plan, 775
Palmaterr, Michael Health Plan of New York, 778
Palmer, Cynthia Colorado Choice Health Plans, 199
Palmer, Elaine Wellmark Blue Cross Blue Shield, 429
Palmer, Paul UnitedHealthcare Nevada, 698
Palmer, Paula VSP: Vision Service Plan of Colorado, 213
Palmer, Paula VSP: Vision Service Plan of Hawaii, 340
Palmer, Tyra Lovelace Health Plan, 745
Palumbo, Fara M Blue Cross & Blue Shield of North Carolina, 811
Palumbo, Pam PacifiCare Health Systems, 162
Pang, Sarah CNA Insurance Companies: Colorado, 197
Pankau, David Blue Cross & Blue Shield of South Carolina, 992
Panturf, Betsy CommunityCare Managed Healthcare Plans of Oklahoma, 885
Paralta, Cynthia L Unicare: Massachusetts, 540
Park, Jeffrey Catamaran Corporation, 358
Park, Mary, M.D. Unity Health Insurance, 1204
Parker, Carmen Physicians Health Plan of Northern Indiana, 408
Parker, David C Meritain Health: Corporate Headquarters, 787
Parker, David C. Meritain Health: Utah, 1103
Parker, Garrett Neighborhood Health Plan, 537
Parker, James Anthem Blue Cross & Blue Shield of Maine, 485
Parker, Jeffrey A. Dentaquest, 526
Parker, Katrina W CNA Insurance Companies: Georgia, 312
Parker, Katrina W CNA Insurance Companies: Illinois, 360
Parker, Robert, MD Health Alliance Medical Plans, 370
Parker, Ted Interplan Health Group, 137, 1071
Parrish, Dave CoreSource: Arizona, 37
Parrott, Chris Total Dental Administrators, 57
Paskowski, Robert S Arnett Health Plans, 391
Pass, Kathy Pacific Foundation for Medical Care, 158

Passauer, Christopher Patient Choice, 611
Pastore, William Evercare Health Plans, 599
Pastro, Margaret, SP Providence Health Plans, 914
Patel, Kirit, Md Omni IPA/Medcore Medical Group, 154
Patel, Nilesh Pacific Dental Benefits, 157
Patel, Prakash R, MD Magellan Health Services: Corporate Headquarters, 510
Patel, Sandip Universal Health Care Group, 300
Patmas, Michael, MD Clear One Health Plans, 900
Patterson, Kari PacificSource Health Plans: Idaho, 349
Patterson, Kari PacificSource Health Plans: Corporate Headquarters, 913
Patterson, M.D., William M. Behavioral Health Systems, 5
Paul, Kathryn Delta Dental of Colorado, 201
Paulson, Trisha Prevea Health Network, 1200
Paustian, Dale Davis Vision, 763
Pawenski, Pamela J Univera Healthcare, 806
Pawlenok, Alan Blue Cross of Northeastern Pennsylvania, 929
Payne, Donna Arizona Physicians IPA, 31
Payne, Solomon OmniCare: A Coventry Health Care Plan, 578
Peabody, Laura S Harvard Pilgrim Health Care, 531
Peace, Terry Blue Cross & Blue Shield of South Carolina, 992
Pearl, Robert M, MD Kaiser Permanente Health Plan of Northern California, 138
Pearl, Robert M, MD Kaiser Permanente Health Plan of the Mid-Atlantic States, 509
Pearsall, Chris Magellan Health Services Indiana, 405
Pearson, Christy Healthchoice Orlando, 280
Peck, Ted Educators Mutual, 1100
Peddie, Gidget Managed Health Network, 148
Pedro, Machille AlohaCare, 330
Pellegrino, Nicholas E Health First Medicare Plans, 279
Pels-Beck, Leslie Sharp Health Plan, 174
Peluso, John Guardian Life Insurance Company of America, 777
Penderson, Maggy Noridian Insurance Services, 837
Pendleton, Jennifer N. InStil Health, 1000
Peninger, Michael J. Assurant Employee Benefits: North Carolina, 810
Peninger, Michael J. Assurant Employee Benefits: Wisconsin, 1181
Penington, James M. Emerald Health PPO, 849
Penington, James M. Interplan Health Group, 855
Penn, Amanda UnitedHealthcare Nevada, 698
Penn, Jeff Devon Health Services, 938
Perkins, Bruce Humana Health Insurance of Illinois, 376
Perkins, Cheryl, RN Texas Community Care, 1086
Perkins, Jeffrey Boulder Valley Individual Practice Association, 195
Perkins, Melanie Healthcare Partners of East Texas, 1064
Perkins, Sherry Delta Dental of Iowa, 420
Perlmutter, Jesse Health Choice Arizona, 44
Pernell, Godfrey Dental Health Services of California, 117
Pernici, Joseph T, II Emerald Health PPO, 849
Perroni, Joseph Delta Dental of Rhode Island, 984
Perry, Faye Health Link PPO, 625
Perry, J. Thomas Delta Dental of Tennessee, 1029
Perry, Jeff HMO Health Ohio, 853
Perry, Jeff Medical Mutual of Ohio, 857
Perry, Jeff Medical Mutual of Ohio Medicare Plan, 858
Perry, Jeff SuperMed One, 873
Perry, Laura Blue Cross & Blue Shield of Western New York, 756
Perry, Vicki F Advantage Health Solutions, 385
Person, Mary Catherine HealthSCOPE Benefits, 71
Petersen, Todd Coventry Health Care of Illinois, 363
Peterson, Christine, MD UnitedHealthcare Nevada, 698
Peterson, Donald Total Dental Administrators, 57
Peterson, Rhonda Noridian Insurance Services, 837
Peterson, Tim Wellmark Blue Cross Blue Shield, 429
Petkau, Gerald Blue Cross & Blue Shield of North Carolina, 811
Petren, Carol Ann CIGNA: Corporate Headquarters, 935
Petruzelli, Steve Willamette Dental Insurance, 921
Pezzullo, Angelo Delta Dental of Rhode Island, 984
Pfeifer, Kelly, MD San Francisco Health Plan, 171
Pferdehirt, Gina UPMC Health Plan, 968
Pfister, Joseph Keystone Health Plan Central, 954
Pham, Thomas Inland Empire Health Plan, 135
Phanstiel, Howard UnitedHealthCare, 76

Phanstiel, Howard PacifiCare Health Systems, 162
Phanstiel, Howard PacifiCare of Colorado, 208
Phanstiel, Howard PacifiCare of Texas, 1079
Phanstiel, Howard PacifiCare Benefit Administrators, 1155
Phanstiel, Howard PacifiCare of Washington, 1156
Phanstiel, Howard G. PacifiCare of Nevada, 696
Phelps, William First Priority Health, 942
Phifer, Jim One Call Medical, 730
Phillilps, Jeanie, MD Blue Cross of Idaho Health Service, Inc., 342
Phillips, Deborah Priority Health, 581
Phillips, Deborah Priority Health: Corporate Headquarters, 582
Phillips, Felicia R Health Partners Medicare Plan, 946
Philpott, Paul ConnectiCare of Massachusetts, 525
Piccioni, Lori American WholeHealth Network, 924
Picciotto, John A, Esq CareFirst Blue Cross Blue Shield, 240
Picciotto, John A, Esq CareFirst Blue Cross & Blue Shield of Virginia, 1122
Piela, Ed OhioHealth Group, 865
Pierce, Becky Healthcare USA of Missouri, 647
Pierce, John Premera Blue Cross, 1157
Pierce, Suzanne Unison Health Plan of Ohio, 876
Pifer, Donald Carolina Care Plan, 994
Pike, Christopher Health Alliance Medicare, 566
Pinho, Joe Elderplan, 768
Piotti, Karen Family Choice Health Alliance, 721
Piotti, Karen FC Diagnostic, 722
Pipken, Meg Total Dental Administrators, 57
Piszel, Anthony S Health Net Medicare Plan, 129
Pitt, William Pacific Foundation for Medical Care, 158
Pittman, Shelly Blue Cross & Blue Shield of Kansas, 433
Pitts, John F. Blue Cross & Blue Shield of Western New York, 756
Place, Roderick Western Dental Services, 186
Plumb, Michael CareMore Health Plan, 97
Pluto, Victor J PacifiCare of Oklahoma, 892
Pocock, Robert Priority Health: Corporate Headquarters, 582
Podbielski, Sue CIGNA HealthCare of Illinois, 359
Poe, Wendy, RN Vantage Health Plan, 482
Pointon, Meg HealthPlus of Michigan: Flint, 569
Pointon, Meg HealthPlus of Michigan: Saginaw, 570
Polenske, Kathy Interplan Health Group, 137
Polk, Gregory, MPA Los Angeles County Department of Health Services, 147
Polk, Rosemary Assurant Employee Benefits: California, 84
Polk, Rosemary Assurant Employee Benefits: Washington, 1144
Pollack, David Molina Healthcare: Florida, 288
Pollack, Marc Harvard University Group Health Plan, 532
Pollinger, Lovie HealthSmart Preferred Care, 1065
Pollock, Pamela Lakeside Community Healthcare Network, 144
Pollock, Robert B Assurant Employee Benefits: Florida, 253
Pollock, Robert B. Assurant Employee Benefits: North Carolina, 810
Pollock, Robert B. Assurant Employee Benefits: Wisconsin, 1181
Pollock, Steve Dentaquest, 526
Pompili, Eugene Nationwide Better Health, 862
Pontarelli, Thomas CNA Insurance Companies: Colorado, 197
Pontarelli, Thomas CNA Insurance Companies: Georgia, 312
Pontarelli, Thomas CNA Insurance Companies: Illinois, 360
Pontius, Greg Superior Vision Services, Inc., 176
Pool, James H., III MVP Health Care: Vermont, 1117
Pool, Kearney Capital Health Plan, 261
Poole, James H., III MVP Health Care: Central New York, 792
Poole, James H., III MVP Health Care: Corporate Office, 793
Popejoy, David SecureCare Dental, 56
Popejoy, Mike SecureCare Dental, 56
Popiel, Dr. Richard Regence Blue Cross & Blue Shield of Oregon, 915
Popiel, Dr. Richard Regence Blue Cross & Blue Shield of Utah, 1107
Popiel, Dr.Richard Regence Blue Shield, 1159
Popiel, Richard G Rayant Insurance Company, 733
Popovich, Karen Cardinal Health Alliance, 393
Porter, Doug Blue Cross and Blue Shield Association, 357
Porter, John Avera Health Plans, 1010
Portsmore, Paul HealthFirst New Jersey Medicare Plan, 723
Portsmore, Paul E, Jr AmeriHealth Medicare Plan, 926
Portune, Richard W, DDS Superior Dental Care, 872
Post, Linda, MD Unison Health Plan of Ohio, 876

Post, **Robert** MagnaCare, 786
Pou, **Tracy** Select Health of South Carolina, 1003
Povbielski, **Sue** CIGNA HealthCare of Illinois, 359
Powell, **Melissa** DakotaCare, 1012
Powers, **Donald** UnitedHealthCare of Massachusetts, 541
Powers, **Donald H** UnitedHealthCare of Rhode Island, 989
Powers, **Scott** Regence BlueShield of Idaho, 351
Powers, **Scott** Regence Blue Shield, 1159
Pozo, **Justo Luis** Preferred Care Partners, 292
Pray, **Joseph L.** Trustmark Companies, 381
Prendergast, **Victoria** Signature Health Alliance, 1038
Prepenbring, **Russell J** Kanawha Healthcare Solutions, 1001
Press, **Thomas E** Midlands Choice, 680
Pressley, **Tara** Crescent Health Solutions, 815
Prewitt, **Janice, RN/CPHQ** Great Lakes Health Plan, 564
Price, **Charles** UnitedHealthCare of Indiana, 411
Price, **Richard, Md** IHC: Intermountain Healthcare Health Plan, 347
Price, **Tara** OptiCare Managed Vision, 823
Price, **Vince** Regence Blue Cross & Blue Shield of Oregon, 915
Pritchard, **Sarah** Delta Dental of Kansas, 437
Pritchett, **Ballard** Colorado Access, 198
Proffitt, **Joy** Virginia Health Network, 1141
Proud, **Sandra** Pueblo Health Care, 209
Provencher, **Ken** PacificSource Health Plans: Idaho, 349
Provencher, **Ken** PacificSource Health Plans: Corporate Headquarters, 913
Pruitt, **Dan** Assurant Employee Benefits: South Carolina, 991
Pruitt, **Reagan** CHA Health, 455
Prussing, **Gregg** CIGNA HealthCare of Alaska, 21
Prussing, **Gregg** CIGNA HealthCare of Colorado, 196
Prussing, **Gregg** CIGNA HealthCare of Montana, 662
Prussing, **Gregg** CIGNA HealthCare of Wyoming, 1209
Przesiek, **David** Fallon Community Health Plan, 528
Przesiek, **David** Fallon Community Medicare Plan, 529
Pudimott, **Missy** CHN PPO, 717
Pugh, **Ricard** Community Health Improvement Solutions, 638
Puglisi, **Jennifer** Leon Medical Centers Health Plan, 286
Pujol, **JP, MD** New West Health Services, 669
Pujol, **JP, MD** New West Medicare Plan, 670
Pures, **Robert** Horizon Healthcare of New Jersey, 725
Pures, **Robert J** Rayant Insurance Company, 733
Purpura, **Nate** eHealthInsurance Services Inc., 10, 22, 40, 70, 121
Purpura, **Nate** eHealthInsurance Services Inc. Corporate Office, 122
Purpura, **Nate** eHealthInsurance Services Inc., 203, 231, 244, 271, 318, 332, 345, 366, 397, 421, 438, 459, 475, 487, 506, 527, 561, 598, 624, 642, 664, 678, 688, 703, 720, 742, 767, 817, 832, 848, 888, 902, 939, 985, 997, 1014, 1030, 1058, 1101, 1116, 1128, 1149, 1169, 1188, 1211
Pursley, **Janet** Mercy Health Plans: Kansas, 442
Pursley, **Janet** Mercy Health Medicare Plan, 651
Pursley, **Janet** Mercy Health Plans: Corporate Office, 652
Pursley, **Janet** Mercy Health Plans: Oklahoma, 891
Purves, **Steve** Maricopa Integrated Health System/Maricopa Health Plan, 48
Putiak, **Mike** Peoples Health, 479, 480
Putt, **Lisa** Blue Cross & Blue Shield of Oklahoma, 882
Pyle, **Chris** Delta Dental of Alabama, 315
Pyle, **David** Managed HealthCare Northwest, 910

Q

Quan, **Kelvin** On Lok Lifeways, 155
Quinlan, **Ann** Dominion Dental Services, 1127
Quinlinvan, **Keith** Kern Family Health Care, 142
Quinn, **Su** Welborn Health Plans, 413

R

Radhe, **Brenda** Humana Health Insurance of Orlando, 283
Radine, **Gary** Delta Dental of California, 114
Radine, **Gary** Delta Dental of Utah, 1099
Radine, **Gary D** Delta Dental of the Mid-Atlantic, 230, 243
Radine, **Gary D** Delta Dental of Florida, 269
Radine, **Gary D** Delta Dental of Georgia, 316, 473
Radine, **Gary D** Delta Dental of the Mid-Atlantic, 503
Radine, **Gary D** Delta Dental Insurance Company, 623

Radine, **Gary D** Delta Dental of the Mid-Atlantic, 764, 937, 1168
Radine, **Gary D.** Delta Dental of Montana, 663
Radine, **Gary D.** Delta Dental of Texas, 1056
Rady, **Dawn** Network Health Plan of Wisconsin, 1198
Raffio, **Thomas** Delta Dental of New Hampshire, 702
Rai, **Ashok, M.D.** Prevea Health Network, 1200
Rainer, **Dan** HealthPartners, 1032
Raines, **Valerie** SelectNet Plus, Inc., 1175
Rains, **Cheryl** VSP: Vision Service Plan of Georgia, 328
Rains, **Shari** ProviDRs Care Network, 448
Rajamannar, **Raja** Humana Health Insurance of Kentucky, 460
Rakestraw, **Rita** CIGNA HealthCare of Georgia, 311
Raley, **Karen** Arkansas Blue Cross and Blue Shield, 64
Ramer, **Joanna** Delta Dental of Idaho, 344
Ramirez, **Ramie** Community First Health Plans, 1054
Ramseier, **Mike** Anthem Blue Cross & Blue Shield of Colorado, 190
Randall, **Todd** University Health Plans, 1111
Randolph, **John C** Paramount Elite Medicare Plan, 866
Randolph, **John C** Paramount Health Care, 867
Randolph, **Kimberly** Basic Chiropractic Health Plan, 85
Ransom, **Penny** Network Health Plan of Wisconsin, 1198
Rashti, **Dana** Harvard Pilgrim Health Care, 531
Rashti, **Dana** Neighborhood Health Plan, 537
Rasmussen, **Sharon K.** Midlands Choice, 680
Raybuck, **Gregg E** Alere Health, 304
Razi, **Nazneen** Health Care Service Corporation, 372
Reagan, **Michael** Fortified Provider Network, 42
Reamer, **Michael** Avesis: Corporate Headquarters, 32
Reamer, **Michael** Avesis: Arizona, 309
Reamer, **Michael** Avesis: Minnesota, 594
Reamer, **Michael** Avesis: Texas, 1046
Reardon, **Valerie A.** GHI, 774
Reardon, **Valerie A.** GHI Medicare Plan, 775
Reay, **Bill** Physicians Plus Insurance Corporation, 1199
Redmond, **David** MultiPlan, Inc., 789
Redmond, **David** HealthEOS, 1194
Redmund, **David** Beech Street Corporation: Corporate Office, 86
Reed, **Philip J** Colorado Access, 198
Reef, **Chris** Meritain Health: Indiana, 406
Reef, **Chris** Welborn Health Plans, 413
Reef, **Chris** Meritain Health: Corporate Headquarters, 787
Reese, **Bruce T.** IHC: Intermountain Healthcare Health Plan, 347
Reese Furgerson, **Cindy, RN** QualChoice/QCA Health Plan, 75
Reeves, **Donald K** Brazos Valley Health Network, 1051
Reid, **Allan** Health Resources, Inc., 402
Reid, **Rohan C.** Inland Empire Health Plan, 135
Reilly, **Tim** L.A. Care Health Plan, 143
Reinecke, **Mark, MD** Humana Health Insurance of Orlando, 283
Reingold, **Kimberly** Blue Cross & Blue Shield of Rhode Island, 981
Reinhard, **Glen** UnitedHealthCare of Wisconsin: Central, 619, 1203
Reisman, **Lonny, MD** Aetna Health, Inc. Medicare Plan, 215
Reisman, **Lonny, MD** Aetna Health of Mississippi, 621
Reisman, **Lonny, MD** Aetna Health of New York, 752
Reisman, **Lonny, MD** Aetna Health of Virginia, 1119
ReismanD, **Lonny** Aetna Health of Colorado, 188
Reitan, **Colleen** Health Care Service Corporation, 372
Reitan, **Colleen** Blue Cross & Blue Shield of New Mexico, 739
Reiten, **Christine** Metropolitan Health Plan, 608
Reitz, **Mike** Blue Cross & Blue Shield of Louisiana, 469
Rekart, **Tom** Spectera, 516
Remmers, **Rick** Humana Health Insurance of Mississippi, 626
Remmers, **Rick** Humana Health Insurance of Tennessee, 1035
Renneke, **Marina, APR** Humana Health Insurance of Hawaii, 336
Rennell, **Thomas** M-Care, 575
Rensom, **Maureen** Preferred Care, 958
Repp, **James M** AvMed Health Plan: Corporate Office, 254
Repp, **James M** AvMed Health Plan: Fort Lauderdale, 255
Repp, **James M** AvMed Health Plan: Gainesville, 256
Repp, **James M** AvMed Health Plan: Orlando, 258
Repp, **James M** AvMed Health Plan: Tampa Bay, 259
Repp, **James M.** AvMed Medicare Preferred, 260
Retzko, **Sally** Highmark Blue Cross & Blue Shield Delaware, 233

Reynolds, Aaron Medica Health - Medicare Plan, 605
Reynolds, Aaron Medica: Corporate Office, 606
Reynolds, Aaron Medica: South Dakota, 1018
Reynolds, Heather Davis Vision, 763
Rhoads, Michael Blue Cross & Blue Shield of Oklahoma, 882
Rhoads, Michael BlueLincs HMO, 883
Rhode, Deb Prevea Health Network, 1200
Rice, B Shelton Kanawha Healthcare Solutions, 1001
Rice, Deborah L Highmark Blue Cross & Blue Shield, 949
Rice, Deborah L Highmark Blue Shield, 950
Rice, Jean Action Healthcare Management Services, 28
Rice-Johnson, Deborah L., MD Highmark Blue Shield, 950
Richards, Patricia R SelectHealth, 352
Richardson, Robin Moda Health Alaska, 25
Richardson, Robin ODS Health Plan, 911
Richardson, Steve, MD UnitedHealthCare of Ohio: Columbus, 877
Richardson, Steve, MD UnitedHealthCare of Ohio: Dayton & Cincinnati, 878
Richman, Keith S, MD Lakeside Community Healthcare Network, 144
Richmond, Michael Touchstone Health HMO, 803
Ricks, Libby Coalition America's National Preferred Provider Network, 761
Ridge, Tiffany Cardinal Health Alliance, 393
Ridges, Karen Public Employees Health Program, 1106
Rieger, Lori Health Net of Arizona, 45
Riegner, Robin Berkshire Health Partners, 928
Rifaat, Hassan Humana Health Insurance of Louisiana, 477
Rigby, Joan Health Plus of Louisiana, 476
Rigby, Owen Health Plus of Louisiana, 476
Rigeor, Michael CONCERN: Employee Assistance Program, 111
Riley, Patricia Blue Cross & Blue Shield of Minnesota, 595
Rimmer, Kenneth Total Health Choice, 296
Rios, Garrison Desert Canyon Community Care, 39
Rios, Garrison Arcadian Health Plans, 82
Rios, Garrison Texas Community Care, 1086
Risberg, Elizabeth Delta Dental of California, 114
Risberg, Elizabeth Delta Dental of New Jersey & Connecticut, 221
Risberg, Elizabeth Delta Dental of the Mid-Atlantic, 230, 243
Risberg, Elizabeth Delta Dental of Florida, 269
Risberg, Elizabeth Delta Dental of Georgia, 316
Risberg, Elizabeth Delta Dental of Nevada, 317
Risberg, Elizabeth Delta Dental of Idaho, 344
Risberg, Elizabeth Delta Dental of Illinois, 364
Risberg, Elizabeth Delta Dental of Michigan, Ohio and Indiana, 396
Risberg, Elizabeth Delta Dental of Kansas, 437
Risberg, Elizabeth Delta Dental of Georgia, 473
Risberg, Elizabeth Delta Dental of the Mid-Atlantic, 503
Risberg, Elizabeth Delta Dental Insurance Company, 623
Risberg, Elizabeth Delta Dental of Missouri, 640
Risberg, Elizabeth Delta Dental of Montana, 663
Risberg, Elizabeth Delta Dental of Nebraska, 677
Risberg, Elizabeth Delta Dental of New Jersey & Connecticut, 719
Risberg, Elizabeth Delta Dental of the Mid-Atlantic, 764
Risberg, Elizabeth Delta Dental of North Carolina, 816
Risberg, Elizabeth Delta Dental of North Dakota, 831
Risberg, Elizabeth Delta Dental of Michigan, Ohio and Indiana, 847
Risberg, Elizabeth Delta Dental of Oklahoma, 887
Risberg, Elizabeth Delta Dental of the Mid-Atlantic, 937
Risberg, Elizabeth Delta Dental of Rhode Island, 984
Risberg, Elizabeth Delta Dental of South Dakota, 1013
Risberg, Elizabeth Delta Dental of Texas, 1056
Risberg, Elizabeth Delta Dental of Utah, 1099
Risberg, Elizabeth Delta Dental of Virginia, 1126
Risberg, Elizabeth Delta Dental of the Mid-Atlantic, 1168
Risberg, Elizabeth Delta Dental of Wisconsin, 1186
Rish, Dale Blue Cross & Blue Shield of South Carolina, 992
Ritter, Mary Fallon Community Health Plan, 528
Rivero, Lupe Horizon Health Corporation, 1068
Rivers, Richard F Great-West Healthcare of Massachusetts, 530
Rivers, Richard F. Great-West Healthcare Oklahoma, 889
Rivers, Richard F. Great-West Healthcare South Dakota, 1016
Rivers, Richard F. Great-West Healthcare Wisconsin, 1189
Roach, Susan, MD Boulder Valley Individual Practice Association, 195
Roache, Kevin J, MD Peoples Health, 480

Roache, Kevin J. Peoples Health, 479
Robart, Jason Blue Cross & Blue Shield of Massachusetts, 522
Robbins, Barry Cariten Healthcare, 1026
Robbins, Barry, VPMIS Cariten Preferred, 1027
Robbins, Marty Health Choice LLC, 1031
Robert, Michael J Peoples Health, 480
Robert, Michael J. Peoples Health, 479
Roberts, James BlueLincs HMO, 883
Roberts, Johathan C. CVS CareMark, 983
Roberts, John S Assurant Employee Benefits: Alabama, 3
Roberts, John S Assurant Employee Benefits: New Jersey, 714
Roberts, John S. Assurant Employee Benefits: California, 84
Roberts, John S. Assurant Employee Benefits: Colorado, 192
Roberts, John S. Assurant Employee Benefits: Minnesota, 593
Roberts, John S. Assurant Employee Benefits: Corporate Headquarters, 632
Roberts, John S. Assurant Employee Benefits: Texas, 1045
Roberts, John S. Assurant Employee Benefits: Washington, 1144
Roberts, Paul Colorado Choice Health Plans, 199
Roberts, Roger Dencap Dental Plans, 559
Roberts-Meyer, Sharon WINhealth Partners, 1214
Robertson, Jeff CIGNA HealthCare of St. Louis, 637
Robinson, Anthony Delta Dental of Michigan, Ohio and Indiana, 396
Robinson, Anthony Delta Dental: Corporate Headquarters, 558
Robinson, Barbara Aetna Health of Tennessee, 1021
Robinson, Kenneth L, Jr Delta Dental of New Hampshire, 702
Robinson, Ron Health Plan of San Mateo, 132
Robinson-Beale, Rhonda, MD United Behavioral Health, 178
Roche, Linda J Delta Dental of New Hampshire, 702
Rock, Lynn Carilion Health Plans, 1123
Rodabaugh, Larry W EHP, 940
Rodgers, John Independent Health, 782
Rodgers, John Independent Health Medicare Plan, 783
Rodgers, Kyle BlueShield of Northeastern New York, 757
Rodriguez, David Amerigroup Florida, 252
Rodriguez, Maria Coastal Healthcare Administrators, 108
Rodriguez, Roger Preferred Care Partners, 292
Roemer, Toni Physicians Health Plan of Northern Indiana, 408
Rogers, Ashley Arizona Foundation for Medical Care, 30
Rogers, Gary Delta Dental of Wisconsin, 1186
Rogers, Kenyata OmniCare: A Coventry Health Care Plan, 578
Rogers, Nancy F Guardian Life Insurance Company of America, 777
Rogers, Paula Anthem Blue Cross & Blue Shield of New Hampshire, 700
Rohan, Karen S Magellan Health Services: Corporate Headquarters, 510
Rohr, Jan Rocky Mountain Health Plans, 210
Roker, Stephen R Independence Blue Cross, 952
Rolde, Edward, MD First Priority Health, 942
Rollins, Jonathan, CFA Health Net: Corporate Headquarters, 130
Rollman, Roger UnitedHealthCare of Alabama, 16
Rollman, Roger UnitedHealthCare of Mississippi, 627
Rollman, Roger UnitedHealthCare of North Carolina, 827
Rollman, Roger UnitedHealthCare of South Carolina, 1006
Rollman, Roger UnitedHealthCare of Tennessee, 1039
Rollow, Brad VIVA Health, 17
Rolow, Tim Delta Dental of Iowa, 420
Roman, Judith AmeriHealth Medicare Plan, 926
Romansky, Eileen Interplan Health Group, 1071
Romasco, Robert G CIGNA HealthCare of Maine, 486
Romza, John Catamaran Corporation, 358
Ron, Aran, MD UnitedHealthCare of North Carolina, 827
Rondon, Ronelle Catalyst RX, 812
Roomsburg, Margaret M Amerigroup Corporation, 1120
Roos, John T Blue Cross & Blue Shield of North Carolina, 811
Roos, John T Preferred Care Select, 824
Roosevelt Jr., James, Jr Tufts Health Medicare Plan, 538
Roosevelt Jr., James, Jr Tufts Health Plan, 539
Root, Leon A, Jr Amerigroup Corporation, 1120
Root, Paula, MD BlueLincs HMO, 883
Roschbach, Jacki, MSS MHNet Behavioral Health, 1076
Rose, Brian Preferred Health Systems Insurance Company, 444
Rose, Brian Preferred Plus of Kansas, 446
Rose, Carolyn Health Choice Arizona, 44
Rose, Esther, RPh OmniCare: A Coventry Health Care Plan, 578

Rose, Joan, MPH Lakeside Community Healthcare Network, 144
Rose, MD, Trevor A, MS MMM Quality Health Plans of New York, 802
Rosen, Bernard MetroPlus Health Plan, 788
Rosenhan, Deborah Altius Health Plans, 1097
Rosenthal, Dan UnitedHealthCare of Northern California, 180
Rosenthal, Dan UnitedHealthCare of South Florida, 299
Rosenthal, Daniel Neighborhood Health Partnership, 289
Rosenthal, David S, MD Harvard University Group Health Plan, 532
Rosignoli, Len CalOptima, 95
Ross, Bradley Delta Dental: Corporate Headquarters, 558
Ross, Kelly CommunityCare Managed Healthcare Plans of Oklahoma, 885
Ross, Michael Total Health Choice, 296
Ross Zubrin, Jay, MD Orange County Foundation for Medical Care, 156
Rosse, Claire, RN Nationwide Better Health, 862
Rossi, Lynda M. Blue Care Network of Michigan: Medicare, 547
Roth, Bill SCAN Health Plan, 173
Roth, Bill Aetna Health of Oklahoma, 880
Roth, Karla, M.D. Prevea Health Network, 1200
Rothbart, Marc, BSN Southeastern Indiana Health Organization, 410
Rothenberg, Nancy Physical Therapy Provider Network, 165
Rothenberg, Nancy PTPN, 169
Rothman, Janet Elderplan, 768
Rothrock, Kirk Superior Vision Services, Inc., 176
Rountree, Virginia Pima Health System, 54
Routh, Charles, MD Cardinal Health Alliance, 393
Rowan, Michael Care 1st Health Plan: California, 96
Rowe, John W, MD Aetna Health of Indiana, 386
Roy-Czyzowski, Connie M, SHPR Delta Dental of New Hampshire, 702
Royer, Jerry, MD, MBA Vytra Health Plans, 808
Ruane, Michael CalOptima, 95
Rubin, Jonathan CIGNA HealthCare of North Carolina, 813
Rubin, Jonathan N Magellan Health Services Indiana, 405
Rubin, Jonathan N Magellan Health Services: Corporate Headquarters, 510
Rubino, Tami Delta Dental of Iowa, 420
Rubino, Thomas M, Esq Horizon Healthcare of New Jersey, 725
Rubino, Thomas W, Esq Horizon Blue Cross & Blue Shield of New Jersey, 724
Rubinstein, Richard San Francisco Health Plan, 171
Rubretsky, Joseph Aetna Health of Colorado, 188
Ruchman, Mark OptiCare Managed Vision, 823
Rucker, Madeline R Mutual of Omaha DentaBenefits, 681
Rucker, Madeline R Mutual of Omaha Health Plans, 682
Rudd, Lori Health Alliance Medical Plans, 370
Ruecker, Rita Western Health Advantage, 187
Ruiz-Topinka, Conchita AvMed Health Plan: Corporate Office, 254
Ruiz-Topinka, Conchita AvMed Health Plan: Fort Lauderdale, 255
Ruiz-Topinka, Conchita AvMed Health Plan: Gainesville, 256
Ruiz-Topinka, Conchita AvMed Health Plan: Jacksonville, 257
Ruiz-Topinka, Conchita AvMed Health Plan: Orlando, 258
Ruiz-Topinka, Conchita AvMed Health Plan: Tampa Bay, 259
Rulli, Jesse Vision Insurance Plan of America, 1205
Rundhaug, Pamala Managed Health Services, 1196
Runt, David J, MD Contra Costa Health Plan, 112
Rupp, Tammy Care Choices, 552
Ruppert, Greg Peoples Health, 479, 480
Rush, Mark BlueChoice Health Plan of South Carolina, 993
Russell, Dolores Managed HealthCare Northwest, 910
Russell, Jeff Delta Dental of Iowa, 420
Russell, Nichelle North Alabama Managed Care Inc, 14
Russo, Marc S WellCare Health Plans, 302
Russo, Pamela United Behavioral Health, 178
Russo, Patricia A Trigon Health Care, 1138
Rust Henderson, Lynn Premera Blue Cross Blue Shield of Alaska, 26
Rutan, Molly Physicians Health Plan of Mid-Michigan, 580
Ruth, Kevin Dental Benefit Providers, 505
Ruthven, Les, PhD Preferred Mental Health Management, 445
Ryan, Caren InterGroup Services Corporation, 953
Ryan, John Novasys Health, 74
Ryan, Mike Unicare: Texas, 1088
Ryan, Tim CHA Health, 455
Ryan, Timothy F. OptumHealth Care Solutions: Physical Health, 610
Rzewnicki, Robert HMO Health Ohio, 853
Rzewnicki, Robert Medical Mutual of Ohio, 857

Rzewnicki, Robert Medical Mutual of Ohio Medicare Plan, 858
Rzewnicki, Robert SuperMed One, 873

S

Saalwaechter, John J, MD HealthPlus of Michigan: Flint, 569
Saalwaechter, John J, MD HealthPlus of Michigan: Saginaw, 570
Saban, Joel Catamaran Corporation, 358
Sabastian, Carmella, MD Blue Cross of Northeastern Pennsylvania, 929
Sabater, Lilia Medical Card System (MCS), 975
Sabatino, Ezio ConnectiCare, 220
Sade, Nikki ProviDRs Care Network, 448
Sadler, Robin Kaiser Permanente Health Plan of Colorado, 207
Safran, Bruce H Dentcare Delivery Systems, 765
Salazar, Deanna Blue Cross & Blue Shield of Arizona, 34
Salazar, Peggy, RN, MSN CareMore Health Plan, 97
Salm, Gordon Health Alliance Medical Plans, 370
Salyards, Keith Foundation for Medical Care for Kern & Santa Barbara County, 123
Samples, Dana Chinese Community Health Plan, 101
Samuels, Michele A. Blue Care Network of Michigan: Medicare, 547
Sanabria, Farrah, PHR Quality Health Plans, 801
Sanabria, Farrah, PHR Quality Health Plans of New York, 802
Sanchez, April Block Vision of Texas, 1047
Sanchez, Ester M California Foundation for Medical Care, 94
Sanchez, Javier CalOptima, 95
Sanchez Colon, Jesus R Triple-S Salud Blue Cross Blue Shield of Puerto Rico, 978
Sander, Brent Cigna-HealthSpring of Alabama, 8
Sanders, Scott B First Commonwealth, 367
Sanders, Steve, DO PacifiCare of Oklahoma, 892
Sands, Mark Phoenix Health Plan, 52
Sanghvi, Sujata PacificSource Health Plans: Idaho, 349
Sanghvi, Sujata PacificSource Health Plans: Corporate Headquarters, 913
Sank, Patricia A Valley Preferred, 970
Sankaran, Vish CareMore Health Plan, 97
Santillan, Brandie Galaxy Health Network, 1061
Santoro, Micheal Oxford Health Plans: New York, 799
Saperstein, Arnold, MD MetroPlus Health Plan, 788
Sarrel, Lloyd CoreSource: Corporate Headquarters, 362
Sarrel, Lloyd CoreSource: Kansas (FMH CoreSource), 435
Sarrel, Lloyd CoreSource: Maryland, 501
Sarrel, Lloyd CoreSource: North Carolina, 814
Sarrel, Lloyd CoreSource: Ohio, 846
Sarrel, Lloyd CoreSource: Pennsylvania, 936
Sattenspiel, John Trillium Community Health Plan, 917
Sauter, Toni Coventry Health Care of Illinois, 363
Sava, Frank Independent Health Medicare Plan, 783
Savenko, Kathy OhioHealth Group, 865
Savitsky, Trish Blue Cross of Northeastern Pennsylvania, 929
Scanavino, Dr. David Medical Card System (MCS), 975
Scanlan, Edward, MD Network Health Plan of Wisconsin, 1198
Scarborough, Bianca California Foundation for Medical Care, 94
Scarbrough, Stephanie Healthchoice Orlando, 280
Scarpone, Connie Physicians Health Plan of Mid-Michigan, 580
Scasny, Ron ABRI Health Plan, Inc., 1178
Schacht, Kara J. Assurant Employee Benefits: Washington, 1144
Schacht, Karla Assurant Employee Benefits: New Jersey, 714
Schacht, Karla J Assurant Employee Benefits: Corporate Headquarters, 632
Schacht, Karla J. Assurant Employee Benefits: California, 84
Schaffer, David Medical Card System (MCS), 975
Schaffer, Ian A Managed Health Network, 148
Schaich, Robert Health Plan of Nevada, 689
Schaich, Robert UnitedHealthcare Nevada, 698
Schalles, Robert Penn Highlands Health Plan, 957
Schandel, David Florida Health Care Plan, 275
Scheele, Robb Humana Health Insurance of Colorado Springs, 206
Scheerer, Bill, CPA MHNet Behavioral Health, 1076
Scheffel, William N. Centene Corporation, 635
Schellinger, Ellen, MA Sanford Health Plan, 427
Scherer, Jerry D Blue Cross & Blue Shield of Oklahoma, 882
Schexnayder, Todd Blue Cross & Blue Shield of Louisiana, 469
Schick, Susan CIGNA HealthCare of Virginia, 1124

Schievelbein, Karen Dental Benefit Providers, 505
Schilling, Laura Deaconess Health Plans, 395
Schmidt, Bradley Bright Now! Dental, 92
Schmidt, Chester, MD Priority Partners Health Plans, 515
Schmidt, Chet Priority Partners Health Plans, 515
Schmidt, Mark W. Meritain Health: Utah, 1103
Schmidt, Steve PacificSource Health Plans: Corporate Headquarters, 913
Schmidt, Tami Magellan Health Services Indiana, 405
Schneider, George Mercy Health Plans: Kansas, 442
Schneider, George Mercy Health Medicare Plan, 651
Schneider, George Mercy Health Plans: Corporate Office, 652
Schneider, George Mercy Health Plans: Oklahoma, 891
Schneider, George, CPA Geisinger Health Plan, 944
Schnipper, Ida ConnectiCare of Massachusetts, 525
Schnitzer, Rhea Managed HealthCare Northwest, 910
Scholtz, Stacy A Mutual of Omaha DentaBenefits, 681
Scholtz, Stacy A Mutual of Omaha Health Plans, 682
Schooley, Ed, DDS Delta Dental of Iowa, 420
Schotz, Michael Interplan Health Group, 137
Schrader, Michael CalOptima, 95
Schrader, William R Blue Cross & Blue Shield of South Carolina, 992
Schreiber, Joy Block Vision of Texas, 1047
Schreiner, Rob, MD Kaiser Foundation Health Plan of Georgia, 321
Schrupp, Alison Providence Health Plans, 914
Schubach, Aaron Opticare of Utah, 1105
Schubach, Stephen Opticare of Utah, 1105
Schuchmann, Pace Assurant Employee Benefits: Georgia, 307
Schultz, Carl Mercy Health Plans: Kansas, 442
Schultz, Carl Mercy Health Medicare Plan, 651
Schultz, Carl Mercy Health Plans: Corporate Office, 652
Schultz, Carl Mercy Health Plans: Oklahoma, 891
Schultz, Eric Harvard Pilgrim Health Care, 531
Schultz, Tim Metropolitan Health Plan, 608
Schum, Rick Blue Cross & Blue Shield of Wyoming, 1208
Schumacher-Konick, Tamara Citrus Health Care, 264
Schumaker, L Don, DDS Superior Dental Care, 872
Schumann, Donald Network Health Plan of Wisconsin, 1198
Schurman, Theresa HealthPlus of Michigan: Flint, 569
Schurman, Theresa HealthPlus of Michigan: Saginaw, 570
Schuster, Glendon A Centene Corporation, 635
Schwab, Jeff Dominion Dental Services, 1127
Schwarz, Jon UnitedHealthCare of South Florida, 299
Schweers, Rob Wellmark Blue Cross & Blue Shield of South Dakota, 1020
Schweikhardtÿ, Gary Delta Dental of Washington, 1148
Schweitzer, Gale S&S Healthcare Strategies, 869
Schweppe, Richard CorVel Corporation, 113
Scono, Thomas E., RPh EPIC Pharmacy Network, 1129
Scott, Barry Quality Plan Administrators, 247
Scott, Bertram Affinity Health Plan, 753
Scott, Bertram CIGNA: Corporate Headquarters, 935
Scott, Christopher Managed Health Services, 1196
Scott, Cory Coventry Health Care of GA, 314
Scott, Garland John Deere Health, 1037
Scott, Greg UnitedHealthCare, 76
Scott, Greg PacifiCare of Colorado, 208
Scott, Greg PacifiCare of Texas, 1079
Scott, Greg PacifiCare Benefit Administrators, 1155
Scott, Gregory W PacifiCare Health Systems, 162
Scott, Gregory W PacifiCare of Nevada, 696
Scott, Jim Liberty Health Plan: Corporate Office, 908
Scott, Kirby Delta Dental of South Dakota, 1013
Scott, Peggy Blue Cross & Blue Shield of Louisiana, 469
Scott, Ruth Horizon Health Corporation, 1068
Screiber, Larry Anthem Blue Cross & Blue Shield of Wisconsin, 1180
Seabert, Pat, RN Care 1st Health Plan: Arizona, 35
Searls, Thomas J Delta Dental of Oklahoma, 887
Sedita-Igneri, Jessica Care 1st Health Plan: Arizona, 35
Sedmak, Pamela Blue Cross & Blue Shield of Minnesota, 595
Seebold, Andy South Central Preferred, 963
Segal, David Neighborhood Health Plan, 537
Segal, Herbert Elderplan, 768
Seibel, Dave CenCal Health: The Regional Health Authority, 98

Seidenfeld, John, MD HealthLink HMO, 648
Seiler, Dr Eleanor Anthem Blue Cross & Blue Shield Connecticut, 217
Seitz, Kevin L Blue Care Network: Ann Arbor, 548
Seitz, Kevin L Blue Care Network: Flint, 549
Seitz, Kevin L Blue Care Network: Great Lakes, Muskegon Heights, 550
Seitzman, Sharon QualCare, 732
Seitzman, Sharon UnitedHealthCare of New York, 805
Selby, Lya UnitedHealthCare of Alaska, 27
Selby, Lya UnitedHealthCare of Oregon, 919
Selby, Lya UnitedHealthCare of Washington, 1163
Self, Dave PacificSource Health Plans: Idaho, 349
Self, Dave PacificSource Health Plans: Corporate Headquarters, 913
Self, David Primary Health Plan, 350
Sell, Steven Managed Health Network, 148
Sellars, Ann Calais Health, 470
Sellers, Dana North Alabama Managed Care Inc, 14
Sellers, Ed Blue Cross & Blue Shield of South Carolina, 992
Sementi, Darcy Coventry Health Care of Illinois, 363
Sendlewski, Susan L AmeriHealth Medicare Plan, 926
Senhauser, Freddy CareSource Mid Rogue Health Plan, 898
Serota, Scott P Blue Cross and Blue Shield Association, 357
Serrano, Patricia First Medical Health Plan of Florida, 272
Sessoms, Vicki Health Partners Medicare Plan, 946
Sethi, Parminder DC Chartered Health Plan, 242
Settle, Scott Emerald Health PPO, 849
Seubert, Maureen Assurant Employee Benefits: Ohio, 842
Sevcik, Joe Assurant Employee Benefits: Texas, 1045
Sevcik, Joseph A Assurant Employee Benefits: Corporate Headquarters, 632
Sevcik, Joseph A. Assurant Employee Benefits: California, 84
Sewell, Geoffrey S, MD Kaiser Permanente Health Plan of Hawaii, 337
Sewell, Ronald Southeastern Indiana Health Organization, 410
Sgarro, Douglas A. CVS CareMark, 983
Shadle, Dan Galaxy Health Network, 1061
Shah, Tej Blue Cross & Blue Shield of Louisiana, 469
Shamley, Kirk, MD WINhealth Partners, 1214
Shanahan, Brendan Medical Card System (MCS), 975
Shane, Jr, P.J., Jr Galaxy Health Network, 1061
Shank, Tracey M SelectCare Access Corporation, 962
Shanley, Audrey Community Health Improvement Solutions, 638
Shanley, Kathryn M Delta Dental of Rhode Island, 984
Shanley, Will UnitedHealthCare of Alaska, 27
Shanley, Will UnitedHealthCare of Arizona, 59
Shanley, Will UnitedHealthCare of Northern California, 180
Shanley, Will UnitedHealthCare of New Mexico, 751
Shanley, Will UnitedHealthCare of Oregon, 919
Shanley, Will UnitedHealthCare of Utah, 1110
Shanley, Will UnitedHealthCare of Washington, 1163
Shantha, , Diaz Neighborhood Health Plan of Rhode Island, 987
Shapiro, Mike Catamaran Corporation, 358
Shapiro, Stanley CompBenefits Corporation, 313
Sharbatz, Kim DenteMax, 560
Share, David A., MD Blue Care Network of Michigan: Medicare, 547
Sharma, Sally WellPoint NextRx, 1095
Sharp, Jolene HealthSpring: Corporate Offices, 1034
Sharp, Jolene HealthSpring of Texas, 1066
Shattenkirk, Darla Fidelis Care, 773
Shaughnessy, Bill eHealthInsurance Services Inc., 203, 1058
Shaver, Tona Keystone Health Plan Central, 954
Shea, Andrew Essence Healthcare, 643
Sheehan, Steve Golden West Dental & Vision Plan, 126
Sheehy, Joseph, MD Southeastern Indiana Health Organization, 410
Sheehy, Robert J UnitedHealthCare of Minnesota, 616
Sheets, Cindy Mount Carmel Health Plan Inc (MediGold), 861
Shehab, Phyllis SelectCare Access Corporation, 962
Shelby, Cindy Contra Costa Health Plan, 112
Shell, Scott Novasys Health, 74
Shelley, Jim, PhD Carolina Care Plan, 994
Shelly, Brent United Concordia: Georgia, 326
Sheppard, Joel Public Employees Health Program, 1106
Sheridan, Pat Windsor Medicare Extra, 1040
Shermach, Kevin UnitedHealthCare of Illinois, 383
Shermach, Kevin UnitedHealthCare of Iowa, 428

Sherman, Paul, MD Group Health Cooperative, 1150
Shermer, Barry Windsor Medicare Extra, 1040
Sherrill, Bobby Colorado Access, 198
Sherrill, Frazier Delta Dental of Alabama, 315
Sherrill, Frazier Delta Dental of Georgia, 316
Sherwin, David A Quality Health Plans, 801
Sherwin, David A Quality Health Plans of New York, 802
Sheyer, Amy Health Net Medicare Plan, 129
Sheyer, Amy Health Net Health Plan of Oregon, 905
Shia, Beth Liberty Health Plan: Corporate Office, 908
Shiblaq, Marwan, MBA Nationwide Better Health, 862
Shiller, Kerri Orange County Foundation for Medical Care, 156
Shinto, Richard MMM Healthcare, 976
Shinto, Richard, Esq PMC Medicare Choice, 977
Shipp, Norma HealthPartners, 1032
Shireman, Greg Delta Dental of Iowa, 420
Shoemaker, Scott Physicians Plus Insurance Corporation, 1199
Sholder, Marty CCN: Alaska, 20
Sholder, Marty HealthSmart Preferred Care, 373
Short, Jared L Regence Blue Cross & Blue Shield of Oregon, 915
Short, Pam Northeast Georgia Health Partners, 323
Shotley, Marsha Blue Cross & Blue Shield of Minnesota, 595
Showalter, Charles Humana Health Insurance of West Virginia, 1171
Sidener, Debby Welborn Health Plans, 413
Sidon, Kenneth HMO Health Ohio, 853
Sidon, Kenneth Medical Mutual of Ohio, 857
Sidon, Kenneth Medical Mutual of Ohio Medicare Plan, 858
Sidon, Kenneth SuperMed One, 873
Siegel, Bernard, MD Lakeside Community Healthcare Network, 144
Siegel, David, MD Great Lakes Health Plan, 564
Siewert, Dan, III National Better Living Association, 322
Siewert, Timothy National Better Living Association, 322
Sigel, Deena Care 1st Health Plan: Arizona, 35
Siggett, Dawn Great Lakes Health Plan, 564
Silverberg, Brian Superior Vision Services, Inc., 176
Silverman, Bruce Delta Dental of New Jersey & Connecticut, 221, 719
Silverman, Josh Superior Vision Services, Inc., 176
Silverman, Wayne, DDS Dominion Dental Services, 1127
Simmer, Thomas L, MD Blue Care Network: Ann Arbor, 548
Simmer, Thomas L, MD Blue Care Network: Flint, 549
Simmer, Thomas L, MD Blue Care Network: Great Lakes, Muskegon Heights, 550
Simmer, Thomas L, MD Blue Cross Blue Shield of Michigan, 551
Simmer, Thomas L., MD Blue Care Network of Michigan: Medicare, 547
Simmons, Rick Managed Health Network, 148
Simmons, Ron Blue Cross & Blue Shield of Kansas, 433
Simonetti, Toni Centene Corporation, 635
Simontsch, Kirsten Premera Blue Cross, 1157
Simpson, Jeanne Foundation for Medical Care for Kern & Santa Barbara County, 123
Sims, James L, DDS Superior Dental Care, 872
Sinclair, Kim Boston Medical Center Healthnet Plan, 523
Sisco-Creed, Shirley ProviDRs Care Network, 448
Sivori, John P Health Net Medicare Plan, 129
Sivori, John P Health Net: Corporate Headquarters, 130
Sizer, John, MD Interplan Health Group, 137
Skaggs, Russell Delta Dental of Kentucky, 458
Skayhan, Richard Health Net Health Plan of Oregon, 905
Skeen, Timothy Amerigroup Maryland, 495
Skinner, Bob Lovelace Health Plan, 745
Skinner, Bob Lovelace Medicare Health Plan, 746
Skobel, Jeff Unison Health Plan of South Carolina, 1005
Slaga, Steven Total Health Care, 585
Slimak, Donna CenCal Health: The Regional Health Authority, 98
Sloan, Beverly HMO Colorado, 205
Sloan, Emily FirstCarolinaCare, 818
Slubowski, James S Priority Health, 581
Sluder, Chris Aetna Health of Tennessee, 1021
Smallie, Don, DC Basic Chiropractic Health Plan, 85
Smart, Brandon L., Esq. Educators Mutual, 1100
Smart, Dean, MD University Health Plans, 1111
Smiley, Bruce Encircle Network, 398

Smiley, Bruce Encore Health Network, 399
Smith, Bethany R., CPA CDPHP Medicare Plan, 758
Smith, Bethany R., CMA CDPHP: Capital District Physicians' Health Plan, 759
Smith, Bill South Central Preferred, 963
Smith, Carrie Providence Health Plans, 914
Smith, Clare CoreSource: Arkansas, 68
Smith, Clare CoreSource: Corporate Headquarters, 362
Smith, Clare CoreSource: Kansas (FMH CoreSource), 435
Smith, Clare CoreSource: Maryland, 501
Smith, Clare CoreSource: North Carolina, 814
Smith, Clare CoreSource: Ohio, 846
Smith, Clare CoreSource: Pennsylvania, 936
Smith, David Meritain Health: Corporate Headquarters, 787
Smith, Dawn R Quality Health Plans, 801
Smith, Dawn R Quality Health Plans of New York, 802
Smith, Dewitt Affinity Health Plan, 753
Smith, DeWitt Perfect Health Insurance Company, 800
Smith, Dr David Piedmont Community Health Plan, 1136
Smith, Ebben, MD AmeriChoice by UnitedHealthCare, 710
Smith, Eric Capital Health Plan, 261
Smith, Francis S DC Chartered Health Plan, 242
Smith, Jack Blue Cross & Blue Shield of Texas, 1048
Smith, James F National Medical Health Card, 796
Smith, Jeff Arizona Physicians IPA, 31
Smith, Jeff UnitedHealthcare Community Plan Capital Area, 248
Smith, Jeff Healthy Indiana Plan, 403
Smith, Jeff Great Lakes Health Plan, 564
Smith, Jeff Health Plan of Nevada, 689
Smith, Jeff AmeriChoice by UnitedHealthCare, 710, 754
Smith, Jeff Unison Health Plan of Ohio, 876
Smith, Jeff Unison Health Plan of South Carolina, 1005
Smith, Joseph Arkansas Blue Cross and Blue Shield, 64
Smith, Katherine Premier Access Insurance/Access Dental, 167
Smith, Kathy CIGNA HealthCare of New Hampshire, 701
Smith, Larry Physicians Health Plan of Mid-Michigan, 580
Smith, Michael Anthem Blue Cross & Blue Shield of Colorado, 190
Smith, Nancy Humana Health Insurance of Orlando, 283
Smith, Pam Behavioral Healthcare Options, Inc., 686
Smith, Patsy Alliance Regional Health Network, 1042
Smith, Scott Kaiser Permanente Health Plan of Colorado, 207
Smith, Scott Coalition America's National Preferred Provider Network, 761
Smith, Sean Coalition America's National Preferred Provider Network, 761
Smith, Troy Hometown Health Plan, 690
Smith, William P Blue Care Network of Michigan: Corporate Headquarters, 546
Smith, William P Blue Care Network: Ann Arbor, 548
Smith, William P Blue Care Network: Flint, 549
Smith, William P Blue Care Network: Great Lakes, Muskegon Heights, 550
Smith, MD, MBA, Kenneth E. Inter Valley Health Plan, 136
Smith-boykin, Laverne UnitedHealthCare of the Mid-Atlantic, 518
Smyth, Glen Anthem Blue Cross & Blue Shield Connecticut, 217
Snead, Thomas G, Jr Trigon Health Care, 1138
Snowden, Miles, MD OptumHealth Care Solutions: Physical Health, 610
Snyder, John J, DMD Kaiser Permanente Health Plan of the Northwest, 907
Sobel, Glenn J Dentcare Delivery Systems, 765
Sobocinski, Vincent CIGNA HealthCare of Delaware, 228
Sodaro, Kenneth Blue Cross & Blue Shield of Western New York, 756
Soistman, Francis S, Jr Coventry Health Care of Kansas, 436
Soldo, Marie UnitedHealthcare Nevada, 698
Solinsky, Jim Care 1st Health Plan: Arizona, 35
Sollenberger, Donna UTMB HealthCare Systems, 1092
Solls, Mark A Concentra: Corporate Office, 1055
Solomon, Carol Peoples Health, 479
Solomon, Carol A Peoples Health, 480
Sommer, Mary Delta Dental of Rhode Island, 984
Sommers, Jack, MD CommunityCare Managed Healthcare Plans of Oklahoma, 885
Soni, Nirali, RPh, CDE Care 1st Health Plan: Arizona, 35
Sonnenshine, Stephanie Central California Alliance for Health, 99
Sorberg, Beth UnitedHealthCare of Colorado, 212
Sorell, Thomas G Guardian Life Insurance Company of America, 777
Sorensen, Stuart L Security Life Insurance Company of America, 613
Sorenson, Charles, M.D. IHC: Intermountain Healthcare Health Plan, 347

Sorrentine, Robert Arta Medicare Health Plan, 83

Soto, Ramon Magellan Health Services Indiana, 405

Southam, Arthur M, MD Kaiser Permanente Health Plan of Northern California, 138

Southam, Arthur M, MD Kaiser Permanente Health Plan of Southern California, 139

Southam, Arthur M, MD Kaiser Permanente Health Plan: Corporate Office, 140

Southam, Arthur M, MD Kaiser Permanente Medicare Plan, 141

Souza, Diane Dental Benefit Providers: California, 116

Souza, Frank Central California Alliance for Health, 99

Sowell, John Windsor Medicare Extra, 1040

Sowell, Sandra Arkansas Managed Care Organization, 66

Spaeth, Corrine Health Plan of Nevada, 689

Spahn, Gloria Chiropractic Health Plan of California, 102

Spahn, Glorie ChiroSource Inc, 103

Spalding, George E, Jr, CPA National Better Living Association, 322

Spalding, Susan National Better Living Association, 322

Spann, Lisa Patient Choice, 611

Spano, Debora UnitedHealthCare of the Mid-Atlantic, 518

Spano, Debora UnitedHealthCare of Massachusetts, 541

Spano, Debora UnitedHealthCare of Ohio: Columbus, 877

Spano, Debora UnitedHealthCare of Ohio: Dayton & Cincinnati, 878

Spano, Debora UnitedHealthCare of Rhode Island, 989

Spano, Debora UnitedHealthCare of Virginia, 1140

Sparkman, David OptumHealth Care Solutions: Physical Health, 610

Sparks, Kevin Mid America Health, 654

Spencer, Christie Passport Health Plan, 463

Spencer, Eric E, MBA Easy Choice Health Plan, 119

Spencer, H Newton Preferred Care, 958

Spencer, Jeremy Total Dental Administrators, 1109

Spencer, Selden, MD Healthy & Well Kids in Iowa, 423

Sperandio, Stephen J Delta Dental of Rhode Island, 984

Spero, Neal Presbyterian Health Plan, 748

Spero, Neal Presbyterian Medicare Plans, 749

Spezia, Anthony L Cariten Healthcare, 1026

Spilde, Mary Frances Theresa Trillium Community Health Plan, 917

Spoor, Martha Great-West/One Health Plan, 204

Spoor, Martha CIGNA HealthCare of Pennsylvania, 934

Spoor, Martha CIGNA HealthCare of Utah, 1098

Spradlin, Scott GHP Coventry Health Plan, 645

Sprecher, Lon Dean Health Plan, 1185

Springer, Barbara Delta Dental of Colorado, 201

Springer, Howard Community Health Plan of Washington, 1147

Spurgeon, Stephen, MD Mercy Health Plans: Kansas, 442

Spurgeon, Stephen, MD Mercy Health Medicare Plan, 651

Spurgeon, Stephen, MD Mercy Health Plans: Corporate Office, 652

Spurgeon, Stephen, MD Mercy Health Plans: Oklahoma, 891

Squarok, John, CPA American Pioneer Life Insurance Co, 251

Squilanti, Todd Meritain Health: Corporate Headquarters, 787

St Pierre, Ellie CIGNA HealthCare of New Hampshire, 701

St. Clair, Elizabeth, Esq HealthFirst New Jersey Medicare Plan, 723

St. Hilaire, Gary Capital Blue Cross, 932

St. John, Linda Fallon Community Health Plan, 528

St. John, Linda Fallon Community Medicare Plan, 529

Stade, Monika Healthcare Partners of East Texas, 1064

Stadler, Mark HealthSmart Preferred Care, 373

Stadler, Mark Great-West Healthcare of Massachusetts, 530

Stadler, Mark HealthSmart Preferred Care, 1065

Stadtlander, George HMO Health Ohio, 853

Stadtlander, George Medical Mutual of Ohio, 857

Stadtlander, George Medical Mutual of Ohio Medicare Plan, 858

Stadtlander, George SuperMed One, 873

Staib, Renee A Penn Highlands Health Plan, 957

Stalmeyer, Jan Mid America Health, 654

Stanislaw, Sherry L SCAN Health Plan, 173

Stanley, David A. Passport Health Plan, 463

Starman, Bob UnitedHealthCare of Nebraska, 683

Starr, Jeremy Guardian Life Insurance Company of America, 777

Starr, Maureen Interplan Health Group, 137

Stasi, Joe Mid America Health, 654

Staszewski, Jay Unicare: West Virginia, 1176

Steber, John H Health Plan of New York, 778

Steckbeck, Marie, MBA Colorado Access, 198

Steele, Tammy S Concentra: Corporate Office, 1055

Steiner, Paula A Health Care Service Corporation, 372

Steines, Brian Phoenix Health Plans, 53

Stelzer, Elizabeth Nationwide Better Health, 862

Stengol, Art HealthLink HMO, 648

Stephens, Deborah L Behavioral Health Systems, 5

Stephens, Sheila Omni IPA/Medcore Medical Group, 154

Stephenson, George, II Foundation for Medical Care for Kern & Santa Barbara County, 123

Sterler, Lowell Florida Blue: Jacksonville, 273

Sterler, Lowell Florida Blue: Pensacola, 274

Stern, Kyle Spectera, 516

Sternbergh, John S Preferred Care Select, 824

Stevens, Dan PacificSource Health Plans: Idaho, 349

Stevens, Linda VSP: Vision Service Plan of Indiana, 412

Stevens, Ronald S, MBA Samaritan Health Plan, 916

Stewart, Doug CIGNA HealthCare of Northern California, 105

Stewart, Doug CIGNA HealthCare of Southern California, 106

Stewart, Roger Coventry Health Care of West Virginia, 1167

Stigall, Precious Dencap Dental Plans, 559

Stinde, Mary Ellen Coventry Health Care of Illinois, 363

Stine, Kristen Assurant Employee Benefits: Kansas, 432

Stinton, Roger Arizona Foundation for Medical Care, 30

Stirewalt, Charles, DDS Bright Now! Dental, 92

Stitzer, Cathy Blue Cross of Northeastern Pennsylvania, 929

Stobbe, Greg First Commonwealth, 367

Stoddard, Paul CareSource: Michigan, 553

Stoddard, Paul Blue Cross & Blue Shield of Western New York, 756

Stoltz, Billie Trillium Community Health Plan, 917

Stom, Mary K, MD Health Partners Medicare Plan, 946

Stone, Dr Lori, MD Sharp Health Plan, 174

Stone, Ilana Block Vision of New Jersey, 716

Stone, Randy SCAN Health Plan, 173

Stonehouse, Steve CNA Insurance Companies: Colorado, 197

Stonehouse, Steve CNA Insurance Companies: Georgia, 312

Stonehouse, Steve CNA Insurance Companies: Illinois, 360

Stoner, Patrick DINA Dental Plans, 474

Stoner, Patrick Dental Source: Dental Health Care Plans, 1057

Stoner, Patrick Ora Quest Dental Plans, 1078

Storbakken, Norman C Delta Dental of North Dakota, 831

Storrer, Scott A CIGNA HealthCare of North Carolina, 813

Storrer, Scott A CIGNA HealthCare of South Carolina, 995

Stover, Timothy UnitedHealthCare of New York, 805

Straley, Peter F Health New England, 533

Strand, Mitchell, MD Touchstone Health HMO, 803

Strange, Kyle Behavioral Health Systems, 5

Strasser, Mary D Physicians Plus Insurance Corporation, 1199

Strauss, Art Harvard University Group Health Plan, 532

Streicher, Mikelle, RN, PhD Florida Health Care Plan, 275

Stround, Kasey Carolina Care Plan, 994

Strunk, Deanna Lifewise Health Plan of Oregon, 909

Stuart, Mary Alice Script Care, Ltd., 1083

Stuart, Randall L AvMed Health Plan: Corporate Office, 254

Stuart, Randall L AvMed Health Plan: Fort Lauderdale, 255

Stuart, Randall L AvMed Health Plan: Gainesville, 256

Stuart, Randall L AvMed Health Plan: Orlando, 258

Stuart, Randall L AvMed Health Plan: Tampa Bay, 259

Stuart, Randall L. AvMed Medicare Preferred, 260

Stump, MaryAnn Blue Cross & Blue Shield of Minnesota, 595

Stumpf, David UnitedHealthCare of Illinois, 383

Suarez, Kim Priority Health, 581

Suarez, Lillian Select Health of South Carolina, 1003

Sud, Susdey Galaxy Health Network, 1061

Suda, George Bright Now! Dental, 92

Sugano, Karen SCAN Health Plan, 173

Suleski, James Delta Dental of New Jersey & Connecticut, 221, 719

Sullivan, Heidi Arcadian Health Plans, 82

Sullivan, John T Meritain Health: Corporate Headquarters, 787

Sullivan, Maureen E Blue Cross and Blue Shield Association, 357

Summerson, Ray UnitedHealthcare Nevada, 698

Sun, Eugene, MD Molina Healthcare: New Mexico, 747

Sun, Eugene, MD HealthAmerica Pennsylvania, 948
Sutherland, Spencer SelectHealth, 352
Sutherlin, Graham QualChoice/QCA Health Plan, 75
Suttles, Robert Health First Health Plans, 278
Swartos, Barb Managed Health Services, 1196
Swayze, Jim Rocky Mountain Health Plans, 210
Sweatman, Paul Assurant Employee Benefits: Illinois, 355
Swedish, Joseph R. WellPoint: Corporate Office, 414
Swenson, Rich HealthPlus Senior Medicare Plan, 573
Swenson, Richard HealthPlus of Michigan: Flint, 569
Swenson, Richard HealthPlus of Michigan: Saginaw, 570
Sylvers, Sandy Pacific Foundation for Medical Care, 158
Syracuse, Jill Independent Health, 782
Syracuse, Jill Independent Health Medicare Plan, 783
Szerlong, Tim CNA Insurance Companies: Colorado, 197
Szerlong, Tim CNA Insurance Companies: Georgia, 312
Szerlong, Tim CNA Insurance Companies: Illinois, 360

T

Tabak, Mark MultiPlan, Inc., 789
Tabak, Mark HealthEOS, 1194
Taliaferro, Lilton R, Jr AmeriHealth Medicare Plan, 926
Tallent, John Medical Associates Health Plan, 377
Tallent, John Medical Associates Health Plan: West, 425
Tanner, Bob Group Health Cooperative of Eau Claire, 1190
Tanquary, Patricia, MPH, PhD Contra Costa Health Plan, 112
Tapia, Lionel, MD Health InfoNet, 666
Taravaglia, Laura Humana Health Insurance of Jacksonville, 282
Tardio, Douglas K. Landmark Healthplan of California, 145
Tardugno, Tony AvMed Medicare Preferred, 260
Tarkett, Julles Initial Group, 1036
Tasco, Randy Delta Dental of Michigan, Ohio and Indiana, 396
Tasco, Randy A. Delta Dental: Corporate Headquarters, 558
Tate, Rachel Script Care, Ltd., 1083
Tatko, Mike Regence Blue Cross & Blue Shield of Utah, 1107
Tatko, Mike Asuris Northwest Health, 1145
Taube, Aimee Great Lakes Health Plan, 564
Taylor, James DINA Dental Plans, 474
Taylor, James FCL Dental, 1059
Taylor, James Ora Quest Dental Plans, 1078
Taylor, James A Dental Source: Dental Health Care Plans, 1057
Taylor, Linda M Independence Blue Cross, 952
Telkamp, Bruce eHealthInsurance Services Inc., 10, 22, 40, 70, 121
Telkamp, Bruce eHealthInsurance Services Inc. Corporate Office, 122
Telkamp, Bruce eHealthInsurance Services Inc., 231, 244, 271, 318, 332, 345, 366, 397, 421, 438, 459, 475, 487, 506, 527, 561, 598, 624, 642, 664, 678, 688, 703, 720, 742, 767, 817, 832, 848, 888, 902, 939, 985, 997, 1014, 1030, 1101, 1116, 1128, 1149, 1169, 1188, 1211
Temperly, Tim Network Health Plan of Wisconsin, 1198
Temple, Carolyn J Foundation for Medical Care for Kern & Santa Barbara County, 123
Ten Pas, Bill, D.M.D. Moda Health Alaska, 25
Ten Pas, Bill ODS Health Plan, 911
Tenholder, Ed Anthem Blue Cross & Blue Shield of Missouri, 631
Tennison, Maribeth Dental Alternatives Insurance Services, 115
Tenorio, Susan Inter Valley Health Plan, 136
Tenzer, Mattie Carilion Health Plans, 1123
Terry, David L, Jr HealthSpring: Corporate Offices, 1034
Terry, Donna Pima Health System, 54
Tetzlaff, Gene Delta Dental of South Dakota, 1013
Thibdeau, Michael Davis Vision, 763
Thiele, Craig, MD CareSource: Michigan, 553
Thiele, Craig, MD CareSource, 844
Thiele, Shawn Magellan Health Services Arizona, 47
Thierer, Mark A Catamaran Corporation, 358
Thobro, Jeanne Delta Dental of Wyoming, 1210
Thomas, Betty Arnett Health Plans, 391
Thomas, Brad Guardian Life Insurance Company of America, 777
Thomas, Craig Florida Blue: Jacksonville, 273
Thomas, Craig Florida Blue: Pensacola, 274
Thomas, David Fidelis Care, 773
Thomas, David Unison Health Plan of Pennsylvania, 966

Thomas, James DenteMax, 560
Thomas, John CommunityCare Managed Healthcare Plans of Oklahoma, 885
Thomas, John CommunityCare Medicare Plan, 886
Thomas, Kimberly Priority Health: Corporate Headquarters, 582
Thomas, Kimberly PriorityHealth Medicare Plans, 583
Thomas, Marshall, MD Colorado Access, 198
Thomas, Merrill Neighborhood Health Plan of Rhode Island, 987
Thomas, Milton, MD Mid America Health, 654
Thomas, Tarlton, III CareSource: Michigan, 553
Thomas, Tarlton CareSource, 844
Thomas Jr., J Grover, Jr Trustmark Companies, 381
Thompson, Colleen PacificSource Health Plans: Idaho, 349
Thompson, Colleen Clear One Health Plans, 900
Thompson, Colleen PacificSource Health Plans: Corporate Headquarters, 913
Thompson, Greg Health Care Service Corporation, 372
Thompson, Greg UnitedHealthCare of Wisconsin: Central, 619
Thompson, Greg UnitedHealthCare of Missouri, 658
Thompson, Greg UnitedHealthCare of Nebraska, 683
Thompson, Greg UnitedHealthCare of Wisconsin: Central, 1203
Thompson, Kurt Oxford Health Plans: Corporate Headquarters, 224
Thompson, Kurt B Oxford Health Plans: New Jersey, 731
Thompson, Kurt B Oxford Health Plans: New York, 799
Thompson, Larry NOVA Healthcare Administrators, 798
Thompson, Margita Health Net: Corporate Headquarters, 130
Thompson, Margita Managed Health Network, 148
Thompson, Marti DakotaCare, 1012
Thompson, Scott Regence BlueShield of Idaho, 351
Thon, Carolyn Health Plan of San Mateo, 132
Thor, Patrice, RN Humana Health Insurance of Wisconsin, 1195
Threadgill, Jackie Block Vision of New Jersey, 716
Thull, Tim Medica: Corporate Office, 606
Thull, Tim Medica: North Dakota, 836
Thurman, Kathy Care 1st Health Plan: Arizona, 35
Thurmond, Gail, MD Health Choice LLC, 1031
Thygeson, Marcus, M.D. Blue Shield of California, 90
Tian See, A Medical Card System (MCS), 975
Tildon, Maria CareFirst Blue Cross Blue Shield, 240
Tildon, Maria CareFirst Blue Cross & Blue Shield of Virginia, 1122
Tilford, David Medica Health - Medicare Plan, 605
Tilford, David Medica: Corporate Office, 606
Tilford, David Medica: North Dakota, 836
Tilford, David Medica: South Dakota, 1018
Timmermans, Rebecca South Central Preferred, 963
Timms, Dennis BlueLincs HMO, 883
Tisza, Sharon, MD AlohaCare, 330
Tita, Marybeth HealthFirst New Jersey Medicare Plan, 723
Tobacco, Jill Dentaquest, 526
Tobiason, Steve Blue Cross of Idaho Health Service, Inc., 342
Tobin, Jill AmeriChoice by UnitedHealthCare, 754
Tobin, Michael E American Community Mutual Insurance Company, 544
Todd, Lisa Value Behavioral Health of Pennsylvania, 971
Todd, Richard CommunityCare Managed Healthcare Plans of Oklahoma, 885
Todd, Richard W CommunityCare Medicare Plan, 886
Todoroff, Cheri, MPH Los Angeles County Department of Health Services, 147
Todoroff, Chistopher M Humana Medicare Plan, 461
Todoroff, Christopher M Humana Health Insurance of Kentucky, 460
Todoroff, Christopher M. Humana Health Insurance of Arizona, 46
Todoroff, Christopher M. Arcadian Health Plans, 82
Todoroff, Christopher M. Humana Health Insurance of Michigan, 574
Todt, Blaire W. WellCare Health Plans, 302
Tofferi, Leigh Blue Cross & Blue Shield of Vermont, 1113
Tomasevich, Stan CHN PPO, 717
Tomba, Sue Great Lakes Health Plan, 564
Tomcala, Christine HealthPlus of Michigan: Flint, 569
Tomcala, Christine HealthPlus of Michigan: Saginaw, 570
Tomcala, Christine Puget Sound Health Partners, 1158
Toothcare, Tracey Behavioral Healthcare Options, Inc., 686
Torgerson, Sharon Harvard Pilgrim Health Care, 531
Torres, Galina Delta Dental of Vermont, 1115
Tosti, Mike Devon Health Services, 938
Totterdale, Matt Anthem Blue Cross & Blue Shield of Indiana, 388
Tough, Steven D Health Net: Corporate Headquarters, 130

Tournoux, Mary Ann Health Alliance Plan, 567
Touslee, Ma'ata, RN, MBA Children's Mercy Pediatric Care Network, 636
Trachman, Rob Dominion Dental Services, 1127
Tracy, Julie K CDPHP: Capital District Physicians' Health Plan, 759
Tran, Anna Care 1st Health Plan: California, 96
Tran, Hai Catalyst Health Solutions Inc, 498
Tran, Hai Catalyst RX, 812
Tran, Thomas L. WellCare Health Plans, 302
Tran, Tom ConnectiCare of Massachusetts, 525
Trapani, Lisa Cigna Health-Spring, 499
Traylor, Sheryl Dentaquest, 526
Traynor, Mark UCare Medicare Plan, 614
Traynor, Mark UCare Minnesota, 615
Trease, Katherine Humana Health Insurance of Colorado Springs, 206
Treash, Mike Mercy Health Plans: Kansas, 442
Treash, Mike Mercy Health Medicare Plan, 651
Treash, Mike Mercy Health Plans: Corporate Office, 652
Treash, Mike Mercy Health Plans: Oklahoma, 891
Trebino, Tricia Tufts Health Medicare Plan, 538
Trebino, Tricia Tufts Health Plan, 539
Tredway, Alfred S Regence Blue Cross & Blue Shield of Utah, 1107
Treptin, Todd Altius Health Plans, 1097
Tretheway, Barb Health Partners Medicare Plan, 601
Tretheway, Barb HealthPartners, 602
Trifone, John Blue Cross & Blue Shield of Vermont, 1113
Trinh, Sarah Assurant Employee Benefits: Oregon, 895
Triplett, Michael W, Sr CIGNA HealthCare of North Carolina, 813
Triplett, Mike CIGNA HealthCare of the Mid-Atlantic, 500
Trombley, Amy Health New England, 533
Tropiano, Pam CareSource, 844
Trowbridge, Lewis E Blue Cross & Blue Shield of Nebraska, 674
Truess, James Amerigroup Nevada, 685
Truess, James W Amerigroup Corporation, 1120
Trybual, John VSP: Vision Service Plan of Illinois, 384
Tsang, Steve Chinese Community Health Plan, 101
Tsang, Tom Chinese Community Health Plan, 101
Tsao, Tom eHealthInsurance Services Inc., 203, 1058
Tsui, Amy Chiropractic Health Plan of California, 102
Tucker, JC Chinese Community Health Plan, 101
Tudor, John, MD Great-West/One Health Plan, 204
Tudor, John, MD CIGNA HealthCare of Pennsylvania, 934
Tudor, John, MD CIGNA HealthCare of Utah, 1098
Tufano, Paul A, Esq Independence Blue Cross, 952
Tull, Debra Landmark Healthplan of California, 145
Tuller, Edwin Care Choices, 552
Tullock, Mark HealthSpring: Corporate Offices, 1034
Tunis, Sandra S Managed Health Services, 1196
Turner, Christine Puget Sound Health Partners, 1158
Turner, Debbie ChiroSource Inc, 103
Turner, Jeff WellPoint NextRx, 1095
Tyler, Sue HMO Health Ohio, 853
Tyler, Sue Medical Mutual of Ohio, 857
Tyler, Sue Medical Mutual of Ohio Medicare Plan, 858
Tyler, Sue SuperMed One, 873
Tyre, Janie Santa Clara Family Health Foundations Inc, 172
Tyson, Bernard Kaiser Permanente Health Plan of Northern California, 138
Tyson, Bernard Kaiser Permanente Health Plan of Southern California, 139
Tyson, Bernard Kaiser Permanente Health Plan: Corporate Office, 140
Tyson, Bernard Kaiser Permanente Medicare Plan, 141
Tyson, Bernard J Kaiser Permanente Health Plan of Northern California, 138
Tyson, Bernard J Kaiser Permanente Health Plan of Southern California, 139
Tyson, Bernard J Kaiser Permanente Health Plan: Corporate Office, 140
Tyson, Bernard J Kaiser Permanente Medicare Plan, 141
Tzeel, Albert, MD Humana Health Insurance of Wisconsin, 1195

U

Uchrin, Mike Health Choice Arizona, 44
Udochi, Abenaa Affinity Health Plan, 753
Udvarhelyi, I Steven, MD Independence Blue Cross, 952
Uhm, Alex UnitedHealthCare of Southern California, 181
Ulibarri, Frank UnitedHealthCare of Alabama, 16
Uma, Chet C. CalOptima, 95

Uma, Chet C. Inland Empire Health Plan, 135
Underhill, David Nationwide Better Health, 862
Urbanek, Jon Florida Blue: Jacksonville, 273
Urbanek, Jon Florida Blue: Pensacola, 274
Utash, Scott Behavioral Healthcare, 193
Utterback, Chuck CIGNA HealthCare of Tennessee, 1028
Utterbeck, Chuck CIGNA HealthCare of Arkansas, 67
Utterbeck, Chuck CIGNA HealthCare of Mississippi, 622

V

Vaccaro, Jerome V, MD UnitedHealthCare, 76
Vaccaro, Jerome V, MD PacifiCare of Texas, 1079
Vachon, Jennifer Blue Cross and Blue Shield Association, 357
Vagts, Joyce ConnectiCare, 220
Vail, Cheron Regence Blue Cross & Blue Shield of Utah, 1107
Valdez, David, MD Aetna Health of Oklahoma, 880
Valenzuela, Neil DenteMax, 560
Valine, Roger VSP: Vision Service Plan of Illinois, 384
Van Alvensleben, Lulu CenCal Health: The Regional Health Authority, 98
Van De Beek, Diane Exline CIGNA HealthCare of Delaware, 228
Van de Wal, Eve Excellus Blue Cross Blue Shield: Utica Region, 772
Van Etten, Ann M. Affinity Health Plan, 753
Van Lowe, Yvonne CIGNA HealthCare of the Mid-Atlantic, 500
Van Ribbink, Steve Hawaii Medical Services Association, 335
Van Trease, Sandra Anthem Blue Cross & Blue Shield of Missouri, 631
Van Vessem, Nancy, MD Capital Health Plan, 261
Van Wart, John Peoples Health, 480
Vanasdale, Sallie CIGNA HealthCare of Alaska, 21
Vanasdale, Sallie CIGNA HealthCare of Colorado, 196
Vanasdale, Sallie CIGNA HealthCare of Montana, 662
Vanasdale, Sallie CIGNA HealthCare of Wyoming, 1209
VanBrunt, Walter Delta Dental of New Jersey & Connecticut, 221
Vance, Ronald Sagamore Health Network, 409
Vance Jr, Ron CIGNA HealthCare of the Mid-Atlantic, 500
VanClees, Kathleen Managed Healthcare Systems of New Jersey, 728
Vander Pluym, Joan Outlook Vision Service, 50
Vangeison, Keith Beech Street Corporation: Corporate Office, 86
VanKirk, Thomas L. Highmark Blue Shield, 950
Vaughan, Kevin, MD Select Health of South Carolina, 1003
Vaughan, Stan Community Health Improvement Solutions, 638
Vaughn, Kevin Select Health of South Carolina, 1003
Vaughn, Timothy L BlueChoice Health Plan of South Carolina, 993
Vaught, Greta Midlands Choice, 680
Vavrina, Robert T, Jr Preferred Care Select, 824
Vecchioni, Sharon J CareFirst Blue Cross & Blue Shield of Virginia, 1122
Velazquez, Ralph, MD OSF HealthPlans, 379
Vellinga, David Mercy Health Network, 426
VenBrunt, Walter Delta Dental of New Jersey & Connecticut, 719
Vercillo, Arthur, MD Excellus Blue Cross Blue Shield: Central New York, 770
Vercillo, Arthur, M.D. Excellus Blue Cross Blue Shield: Rochester Region, 771
Verrastro, George OptiCare Managed Vision, 823
Verre, Mark ConnectiCare, 220
Vetter, Elizabeth Americas PPO, 1009
Vezzosi, Greg CNA Insurance Companies: Colorado, 197
Vezzosi, Greg CNA Insurance Companies: Georgia, 312
Vezzosi, Greg CNA Insurance Companies: Illinois, 360
Vickery, Peggy Select Health of South Carolina, 1003
Vienne, Richard, DO Univera Healthcare, 806
Vincenti, Claude SummaCare Health Plan, 870
Vincz, Thomas Horizon Blue Cross & Blue Shield of New Jersey, 724
Vis, David Physicians Health Plan of Mid-Michigan, 580
Viscuso, Ernest A Block Vision, 497
Visser, Dirk Allegiance Life & Health Insurance Company, 660
Vitagliano, Antonio V Excellus Blue Cross Blue Shield: Central New York, 770
Vitek, Lori Delta Dental of Illinois, 364
Vo, Frank Easy Choice Health Plan, 119
Voci, Karen Harvard Pilgrim Health Care: Maine, 489
Voci, Karen Harvard Pilgrim Health Care of New England, 704
Vogel, John Humana Health Insurance of West Virginia, 1171
Vogt, Peter J CIGNA HealthCare of North Carolina, 813
Volberg, Keith Unison Health Plan of Pennsylvania, 966
Volkman, Fred, MD Select Health of South Carolina, 1003

von Thun, Ignacio Quiaro DenteMax, 560
von Walter, Amy Health Partners Medicare Plan, 601
von Walter, Amy HealthPartners, 602
Voss, Katherine Scott & White Health Plan, 1082
Voxakis, Angelo C, PharmD EPIC Pharmacy Network, 1129
Vulkner, Dan Ohio State University Health Plan Inc., 864

W

Wachtel, Steve CNA Insurance Companies: Colorado, 197
Wachtel, Steve CNA Insurance Companies: Georgia, 312
Wachtel, Steve CNA Insurance Companies: Illinois, 360
Wade, Katie CIGNA HealthCare of the Mid-Atlantic, 500
Waegelein, Robert, CPA TexanPlus Medicare Advantage HMO, 1085
Waegelein, Robert A American Pioneer Life Insurance Co, 251
Waegelein, Robert A, CPA Universal American Medicare Plans, 807
Waggoner, Devon UnitedHealthCare of Northern California, 180
Waggoner, Devon UnitedHealthCare of Southern California, 181
Waggoner, Mark Blue Cross & Blue Shield of Rhode Island, 981
Wagner, Melissa DenteMax, 560
Wagner, Sylvia Assurant Employee Benefits: Corporate Headquarters, 632
Wakefield, Cindy Amerigroup New Jersey, 712
Wakefield, Walter W UnitedHealthCare of Kentucky, 466
Waldman, Sarah Blue Cross & Blue Shield of Nebraska, 674
Waldron, Neil Rocky Mountain Health Plans, 210
Wales, Dirk O, MD HealthSpring: Corporate Offices, 1034
Walker, Catherine SVS Vision, 584
Walker, George Anthem Blue Cross & Blue Shield of Indiana, 388
Walker, Pamela MultiPlan, Inc., 789
Walker, R Scott Fallon Community Medicare Plan, 529
Walker, R. Scott Fallon Community Health Plan, 528
Walker, Rome, MD Carilion Health Plans, 1123
Walko, Nancy American Pioneer Life Insurance Co, 251
Wall, Bruce Ohio State University Health Plan Inc., 864
Wall, Bruce A OhioHealth Group, 865
Wall, Tara Amerigroup Corporation, 1120
Wallace, C Wayne BlueLincs HMO, 883
Wallace, John L.A. Care Health Plan, 143
Wallbaum, Chuck Coventry Health Care of Illinois, 363
Wallner, Mark Block Vision, 497
Wallner, Mark Vision Insurance Plan of America, 1205
Walsh, Andrea Health Partners Medicare Plan, 601
Walsh, Andrea HealthPartners, 602
Walsh, Craig Santa Clara Family Health Foundations Inc, 172
Walsh, Peter Neighborhood Health Plan of Rhode Island, 987
Walter, Courtney HealthLink HMO, 648
Walters, Betty Virginia Health Network, 1141
Walters, Laurel Rocky Mountain Health Plans, 210
Waltman, Angela KelseyCare Advantage, 1072
Walton, Carolynn Blue Care Network of Michigan: Medicare, 547
Walton, Carolynn Blue Cross Blue Shield of Michigan, 551
Wamble-King, Sharon Florida Blue: Jacksonville, 273
Wamble-King, Sharon Florida Blue: Pensacola, 274
Wang, Dr. Sheldon X. eHealthInsurance Services Inc., 10, 22, 40, 70, 121
Wang, Dr. Sheldon X. eHealthInsurance Services Inc. Corporate Office, 122
Wang, Dr. Sheldon X. eHealthInsurance Services Inc., 231, 244, 271, 318, 332, 345, 366, 397, 421, 438, 459, 475, 487, 506, 527, 561, 598, 624, 642, 664, 678, 688, 703, 720, 742, 767, 817, 832, 848, 888, 902, 939, 985, 997, 1014, 1030, 1101, 1116, 1128, 1149, 1169, 1188, 1211
Wang, James K ChiroSource Inc, 103
Ward, Dorothy AmeriChoice by UnitedHealthCare, 710
Ward, Julie UnitedHealthCare of Illinois, 383
Ward, Michael S&S Healthcare Strategies, 869
Ward, Thomas First Priority Health, 942
Wardle, John Universal American Medicare Plans, 807
Wardlow, Randy PacifiCare of Oregon, 912
Wardrop, Terence Delta Dental of New Hampshire, 702
Ware, Marilyn CIGNA HealthCare of South Carolina, 995
Warner, Tim Blue Cross & Blue Shield of Montana, 661
Warner, Venus Galaxy Health Network, 1061
Warnick, Michael P CNA Insurance Companies: Colorado, 197
Warren, Douglas L Blue Cross & Blue Shield of Vermont, 1113
Warren, Jessica Preferred Health Systems Insurance Company, 444

Warren, Jessica Preferred Plus of Kansas, 446
Warren, Lonny WINhealth Partners, 1214
Warrington, J Marc Assurant Employee Benefits: Corporate Headquarters, 632
Warrington, J. Marc Assurant Employee Benefits: Alabama, 3
Warrington, J. Marc Assurant Employee Benefits: California, 84
Warrington, J. Marc Assurant Employee Benefits: Texas, 1045
Warter, Michael Western Dental Services, 186
Warwick, Rex Blue Cross of Idaho Health Service, Inc., 342
Waterman, Cindy Liberty Health Advantage Medicare Plan, 785
Waters, Audrey O Elderplan, 768
Watkins, Letitia VIVA Health, 17
Watson, Anthony HealthNow New York - Emblem Health, 779
Watson, Anthony L Health Plan of New York, 778
Watson, Mike Aetna Health of Tennessee, 1021
Weader, David J, JD Geisinger Health Plan, 944
Wear, Lisa J Initial Group, 1036
Weatherford, Michael Santa Clara Family Health Foundations Inc, 172
Weaver, Emily University Health Alliance, 339
Weaver, Karen CIGNA HealthCare of Iowa, 418
Weaver, Lois Val-U-Health, 969
Webb, Traci Central California Alliance for Health, 99
Weber, Deanna Emerald Health PPO, 849
Wecker, Allan Los Angeles County Department of Health Services, 147
Wedemeyer, David Care 1st Health Plan: California, 96
Wedergren, Shelly UnitedHealthCare of Nebraska, 683
Weeks, John Delta Dental of Kentucky, 458
Wehr, Ann O, MD AvMed Health Plan: Corporate Office, 254
Wehr, Ann O, MD AvMed Health Plan: Fort Lauderdale, 255
Wehr, Ann O, MD AvMed Health Plan: Gainesville, 256
Wehr, Ann O, MD AvMed Health Plan: Orlando, 258
Wehr, Ann O, MD AvMed Health Plan: Tampa Bay, 259
Wehr, Ann O., MD, FACP AvMed Medicare Preferred, 260
Wehr, Richard Preferred Care, 958
Weider, Drigan, CPA Boulder Valley Individual Practice Association, 195
Weiman, Debbie Coventry Health Care of Illinois, 363
Weinberg, Mark Unicare: Michigan, 586
Weinberg, Sharon National Health Plan Corporation, 729
Weiner, Gerry Health Net Health Plan of Oregon, 905
Weingarten, Jorge, Md Care 1st Health Plan: California, 96
Weinper, Michael, PT/DPT Physical Therapy Provider Network, 165
Weinper, Michael, PT, DPT PTPN, 169
Weinstein, Audrey M Block Vision, 497
Weinstein, Burt Pacific Dental Benefits, 157
Weinstein, Michael Highmark Blue Cross & Blue Shield Delaware, 233
Weinstein, Michael Highmark Blue Shield, 950
Weisblatt, Rick, PhD Harvard Pilgrim Health Care, 531
Weissberg, Jed, MD Kaiser Permanente Health Plan of Northern California, 138
Weissberg, Jed, MD Kaiser Permanente Health Plan of Southern California, 139
Weissberg, Jed, MD Kaiser Permanente Health Plan: Corporate Office, 140
Weissberg, Jed, MD Kaiser Permanente Medicare Plan, 141
Weissbrot, Laurence R, FSA Delta Dental of New Hampshire, 702
Weisz, Jeffery A, MD Kaiser Permanente Health Plan of Southern California, 139
Welch, Peter CIGNA HealthCare of Northern California, 105
Wells, Thomas, MD Athens Area Health Plan Select, 308
Welsh, Wilfred Quality Plan Administrators, 247
Wende, Joseph, OD Davis Vision, 763
Wenk, Dr Philip A, D.D.S. Delta Dental of Tennessee, 1029
Wentz, Phil Liberty Health Plan: Corporate Office, 908
Werner, Mark, MD Medica: North Dakota, 836
Werner, Susan Physicians Health Plan of Northern Indiana, 408
Werthwein, Norman Beech Street Corporation: Alabama, 4
Werthwein, Norman Beech Street: Alaska, 19
West, Becky First Care Health Plans, 1060
West, Ed Anthem Blue Cross & Blue Shield of Indiana, 389
Westen, B Curtis, Esq Health Net Medicare Plan, 129
Westerman, George, MD Behavioral Healthcare Options, Inc., 686
Westfall, Laurie Care Choices, 552
Wexler, Eric J, Esq Great Lakes Health Plan, 564
Whaley, Don American Dental Group, 189
Whalley, John W PacifiCare Dental and Vision Administrators, 161
Wheeler, Deborah Health Plan of Nevada, 689
Wheeler, Robert R Trillium Community Health Plan, 917

Y

Yakre, Miles Assurant Employee Benefits: Texas, 1045
Yakre, Miles B Assurant Employee Benefits: Corporate Headquarters, 632
Yakre, Miles B. Assurant Employee Benefits: California, 84
Yakre, Miles B. Assurant Employee Benefits: Colorado, 192
Yakre, Miles B. Assurant Employee Benefits: Washington, 1144
Yalowitz, David, MD UnitedHealthCare of the Mid-Atlantic, 518
Yancey, Betty Coastal Healthcare Administrators, 108
Yanchak, Adam Ohio Health Choice, 863
Yander, Leslie Calais Health, 470
Yanuck, Michael, MBA Quality Health Plans, 801
Yanuck, Michael, MD Quality Health Plans of New York, 802
Yapo, Laraine HealthPlus of Michigan: Flint, 569
Yapo, Laraine HealthPlus of Michigan: Saginaw, 570
Yapo, Laraine HealthPlus Senior Medicare Plan, 573
Yates, Candace HealthPartners, 1032
Yates, Libba VIVA Health, 17
Yates, Steve Windsor Medicare Extra, 1040
Yeager, Mark E American Pioneer Life Insurance Co, 251
Yeager, Sarah Anthem Blue Cross & Blue Shield Connecticut, 217
Yi, Matt UnitedHealthCare of Southern California, 181
Yi, Matt UnitedHealthCare of Hawaii, 338
Yong, Eben Health Plan of San Mateo, 132
York, Billie American WholeHealth Network, 924
York, Edna CIGNA HealthCare of New Hampshire, 701
York, Rebecca Superior Dental Care, 872
York-Day, Tammy Delta Dental of Kentucky, 458
Young, Ann The Dental Care Plus Group, 874
Young, Bill Blue Cross & Blue Shield of Tennessee, 1025
Young, Bob Blue Cross & Blue Shield of Kansas, 433
Young, Michael W Health InfoNet, 666
Young, Robert H Keystone Health Plan East, 955
Young, Rodney Delta Dental of Minnesota, 597
Young, Scott, MD Kaiser Permanente Health Plan of Northern California, 138
Young, Scott, MD Kaiser Permanente Health Plan of Southern California, 139
Young, Scott, MD Kaiser Permanente Health Plan: Corporate Office, 140
Young, Scott, MD Kaiser Permanente Medicare Plan, 141
Young, Susan VSP: Vision Service Plan of Kansas, 451
Young, Ze'ev, MD Puget Sound Health Partners, 1158
Youso, Steve Security Health Plan of Wisconsin, 1201

Z

Zaback, David H. National Health Plan Corporation, 729
Zambino, Sondra Dentistat, 118
Zambrano-Chavez, Catherine Community First Health Plans, 1054
Zatkin, Steven Kaiser Permanente Health Plan of Northern California, 138
Zatkin, Steven Kaiser Permanente Health Plan of Southern California, 139
Zatkin, Steven Kaiser Permanente Health Plan: Corporate Office, 140
Zatkin, Steven Kaiser Permanente Medicare Plan, 141
Zeccardi, Bob One Call Medical, 730
Zechiel, Chad UnitedHealthCare of Colorado, 212
Zenev, Lisz PacificSource Health Plans: Corporate Headquarters, 913
Zerega, Joseph M Preferred Network Access, 380
Zetina, Eduardo Medical Card System (MCS), 975
Zickel, Mark J Priority Health, 581
Ziegler, Harriet Sterling Health Plans, 1161
Ziegler, Steven M AvMed Health Plan: Corporate Office, 254
Ziegler, Steven M AvMed Health Plan: Fort Lauderdale, 255
Ziegler, Steven M AvMed Health Plan: Gainesville, 256
Ziegler, Steven M AvMed Health Plan: Orlando, 258
Ziegler, Steven M AvMed Health Plan: Tampa Bay, 259
Ziegler, Steven M. AvMed Medicare Preferred, 260
Zielinski, Thomas Coventry Health Care of Nebraska, 676
Zielinski, Thomas C Coventry Health Care of Florida, 267
Zigenfus, Gary C, PT Concentra: Corporate Office, 1055
Zimmer, Kirk DakotaCare, 1012
Zimmer, Trish DakotaCare, 1012
Zimmerman, Debbie, MD CIGNA HealthCare of St. Louis, 637
Zimmerman, Deborah, MD Essence Healthcare, 643
Zimmerman, Ken, MBA Texas Community Care, 1086
Zimmerman, Natalie Berkshire Health Partners, 928
Zoretic, Richard Amerigroup Maryland, 495
Zoretic, Richard UnitedHealthCare of the Mid-Atlantic, 518
Zoretic, Richard C Amerigroup Corporation, 1120
Zoretic, Richard C. Amerigroup Corporation, 1120
Zubretsky, Joseph M Aetna Health, Inc. Medicare Plan, 215
Zubretsky, Joseph M Aetna Health of New York, 752
Zubretsky, Joseph M Aetna Health of Virginia, 1119
Zubretsky, Joseph M Aetna Health of West Virginia, 1165
Zuckerman, Joseph, MD Florida Health Care Plan, 275
Zuidema, Sue Metropolitan Health Plan, 608
Zuvon Nenni, Angie Delta Dental of Kentucky, 458
Zwanziger, Ron Alere Health, 304

Membership Enrollment Index

18,602,000	Aetna Health, Inc. Corporate Headquarters, 214
17,000,000	Spectera, 516
16,000,000	Beech Street Corporation: Corporate Office, 86
14,000,000	Anthem Blue Cross & Blue Shield of Nevada, 191
14,000,000	Dentaquest, 526
13,000,000	Health Care Service Corporation, 372
12,225,000	Beech Street Corporation: Northeast Region, 87
12,225,000	Beech Street Corporation: Western Region, 88
11,596,230	Aetna Health of Alaska, 18
11,596,230	Aetna Health of Arkansas, 62
11,596,230	Aetna Health of Hawaii, 329
11,596,230	Aetna Health of Idaho, 341
11,596,230	Aetna Health of Iowa, 415
11,596,230	Aetna Health of Kansas, 431
11,596,230	Aetna Health of Kentucky, 452
11,596,230	Aetna Health of Louisiana, 467
11,596,230	Aetna Health of Michigan, 543
11,596,230	Aetna Health of Minnesota, 591
11,596,230	Aetna Health of Mississippi, 621
11,596,230	Aetna Health of Montana, 659
11,596,230	Aetna Health of Nebraska, 672
11,596,230	Aetna Health of New Hampshire, 699
11,596,230	Aetna Health of New Mexico, 737
11,596,230	Aetna Health of North Dakota, 829
11,596,230	Aetna Health of Oregon, 894
11,596,230	Aetna Health of Rhode Island, 980
11,596,230	Aetna Health of South Dakota, 1008
11,596,230	Aetna Health of Utah, 1096
11,596,230	Aetna Health of Vermont, 1112
11,596,230	Aetna Health of Washington, 1143
11,596,230	Aetna Health of West Virginia, 1165
11,596,230	Aetna Health of Wisconsin, 1179
11,596,230	Aetna Health of Wyoming, 1207
11,000,000	CIGNA: Corporate Headquarters, 935
10,000,000	CIGNA HealthCare of Northern California, 105
10,000,000	CIGNA HealthCare of Southern California, 106
10,000,000	Managed Health Network, 148
8,569,000	Kaiser Permanente Health Plan: Corporate Office, 140
8,000,000	United Concordia: Arizona, 58
8,000,000	United Concordia: California, 179
8,000,000	United Concordia: Colorado, 211
8,000,000	United Concordia: Dental Corporation of Alabama, 15
8,000,000	United Concordia: Florida, 297
8,000,000	United Concordia: Georgia, 326
8,000,000	United Concordia: Maryland, 517
8,000,000	United Concordia: Michigan, 587
8,000,000	United Concordia: New Mexico, 750
8,000,000	United Concordia: New York, 804
8,000,000	United Concordia: North Carolina, 826
8,000,000	United Concordia: Oregon, 918
8,000,000	United Concordia: Texas, 1089
8,000,000	United Concordia: Virginia, 1139
8,000,000	United Concordia: Washington, 1162
7,000,000	Blue Cross & Blue Shield of Illinois, 356
7,000,000	Humana Health Insurance of Iowa, 424
7,000,000	Outlook Vision Service, 50
6,700,000	Health Net Medicare Plan, 129
6,600,000	Dental Benefit Providers, 505
6,600,000	Dental Benefit Providers: California, 116
6,200,000	Dental Network of America, 365
6,000,000	Health Net: Corporate Headquarters, 130
6,000,000	United Concordia, 967
5,427,579	USA Managed Care Organization, 1091
5,183,333	Aetna Health of New Jersey, 709
5,000,000	Catalyst RX, 812
5,000,000	Coventry Health Care: Corporate Headquarters, 502
5,000,000	PCC Preferred Chiropractic Care, 443
5,000,000	Vision Insurance Plan of America, 1205
4,900,000	Highmark Blue Cross & Blue Shield, 949
4,800,000	CompBenefits Corporation, 313
4,800,000	CompBenefits: Alabama, 9
4,500,000	CompBenefits: Florida, 265

4,500,000	CompBenefits: Illinois, 361
4,500,000	DenteMax, 560
4,450,116	Coalition America's National Preferred Provider Network, 761
4,300,000	Blue Cross Blue Shield of Michigan, 551
4,000,000	Blue Cross & Blue Shield of Texas: Houston, 1049
4,000,000	Florida Blue: Jacksonville, 273
4,000,000	Humana Medicare Plan, 461
3,800,000	HMO Blue Texas, 1067
3,718,355	Blue Cross & Blue Shield of North Carolina, 811
3,645,891	Blue Cross & Blue Shield of Texas, 1048
3,600,000	Horizon Blue Cross & Blue Shield of New Jersey, 724
3,600,000	Horizon Healthcare of New Jersey, 725
3,500,000	Blue Shield of California, 90
3,500,000	Galaxy Health Network, 1061
3,400,000	CareFirst Blue Cross & Blue Shield of Virginia, 1122
3,400,000	CareFirst Blue Cross Blue Shield, 240
3,400,000	Keystone Health Plan East, 955
3,300,000	Blue Cross & Blue Shield of Georgia, 310
3,300,000	Independence Blue Cross, 952
3,284,000	Kaiser Permanente Health Plan of Southern California, 139
3,223,235	Kaiser Permanente Health Plan of Northern California, 138
3,200,000	Blue Cross & Blue Shield of Alabama, 6
3,200,000	Blue Cross Preferred Care, 7
3,100,000	American WholeHealth Network, 924
3,000,000	Anthem Blue Cross & Blue Shield of Ohio, 841
3,000,000	Block Vision, 497
3,000,000	Blue Cross & Blue Shield of Massachusetts, 522
3,000,000	Blue Cross & Blue Shield of Tennessee, 1025
3,000,000	Catalyst Health Solutions Inc, 498
3,000,000	Devon Health Services, 938
3,000,000	eHealthInsurance Services Inc., 1014, 203
3,000,000	eHealthInsurance Services Inc. Corporate Office, 122
2,900,000	Interplan Health Group, 137
2,800,000	Anthem Blue Cross & Blue Shield of Virginia, 1121
2,700,000	Amerigroup Tennessee, 1022
2,700,000	Blue Cross & Blue Shield of Minnesota, 595
2,700,000	Desert Canyon Community Care, 39
2,600,000	WellCare Health Plans, 302
2,543,705	Ameritas Group, 673
2,500,000	Cofinity, 555
2,500,000	Regence Blue Cross & Blue Shield of Oregon, 915
2,200,000	Regence Blue Shield, 1159
2,200,000	Regence BlueShield of Idaho, 351
2,000,000	Avesis: Arizona, 309
2,000,000	Avesis: Corporate Headquarters, 32
2,000,000	Avesis: Indiana, 392
2,000,000	Avesis: Iowa, 417
2,000,000	Avesis: Maryland, 496
2,000,000	Avesis: Massachusetts, 521
2,000,000	Avesis: Minnesota, 594
2,000,000	Avesis: Texas, 1046
2,000,000	First Health, 368
2,000,000	Great-West Healthcare of Massachusetts, 530
2,000,000	Great-West/One Health Plan, 204
2,000,000	Healthplex, 780
2,000,000	MHNet Behavioral Health, 1076
2,000,000	Superior Vision Services, Inc., 176
2,000,000	Universal American Medicare Plans, 807
1,915,829	PacifiCare Health Systems, 162
1,900,000	Amerigroup Corporation, 1120
1,900,000	Amerigroup Florida, 252
1,900,000	Amerigroup Georgia, 306
1,900,000	Amerigroup Maryland, 495
1,900,000	Amerigroup New Jersey, 712
1,900,000	Amerigroup New Mexico, 738
1,900,000	Amerigroup New York, 755
1,900,000	Amerigroup Ohio, 840
1,900,000	Amerigroup Texas, 1044
1,850,000	National Medical Health Card, 796
1,800,000	March Vision Care, 149
1,800,000	Molina Healthcare: Florida, 288
1,800,000	Molina Healthcare: Texas, 1077

172,000	Humana Health Insurance of Corpus Christi, 1069
172,000	Humana Health Insurance of San Antonio, 1070
172,000	Humana Health Insurance of Tennessee, 1035
171,028	Empire Blue Cross & Blue Shield, 769
170,000	Health Partners Medicare Plan, 946
170,000	Parkland Community Health Plan, 1080
170,000	Passport Health Plan, 463
163,000	Lovelace Health Plan, 745
160,000	Colorado Health Partnerships, 200
160,000	Unison Health Plan of Pennsylvania, 966
160,000	WellPath: A Coventry Health Care Plan, 828
159,375	Aetna Health of Ohio, 839
155,070	Health Link PPO, 625
155,000	SummaCare Health Plan, 870
154,162	Aetna Health of New York, 752
152,000	ProviDRs Care Network, 448
151,000	Optimum Choice, 514
150,000	Atlanticare Health Plans, 715
150,000	ChiroCare of Wisconsin, 1183
150,000	Coventry Health Care of GA, 314
150,000	Landmark Healthplan of California, 145
150,000	Nevada Preferred Healthcare Providers, 693, 694
150,000	Opticare of Utah, 1105
148,000	Altius Health Plans, 1097
146,000	Community Health Group, 109
146,000	PacifiCare of Texas, 1079
145,000	Unicare: Illinois, 382
145,000	Unicare: Kansas, 449
144,000	Medical Mutual Services, 1002
143,725	Virginia Premier Health Plan, 1142
143,488	CIGNA HealthCare of Pennsylvania, 934
142,000	Humana Health Insurance of Louisiana, 477
141,000	American Postal Workers Union (APWU) Health Plan, 494
140,462	PacifiCare Dental and Vision Administrators, 161
140,000	Alameda Alliance for Health, 80
140,000	Deaconess Health Plans, 395
137,000	Calais Health, 470
136,472	Bluegrass Family Health, 454
135,000	Advance Insurance Company of Kansas, 430
134,837	Affinity Health Plan, 753
131,096	CareOregon Health Plan, 897
130,000	First Care Health Plans, 1060
130,000	Golden Dental Plans, 562
130,000	Managed Health Services, 1196
129,120	Managed HealthCare Northwest, 910
128,272	SCAN Health Plan, 173
127,564	Humana Health Insurance of Arizona, 46
126,000	CIGNA HealthCare of Oregon, 899
126,000	HMO Colorado, 205
126,000	MMM Healthcare, 976
125,000	Capital Health Plan, 261
125,000	Humana Health Insurance of Jacksonville, 282
125,000	Humana Health Insurance of Tampa - Pinellas, 284
125,000	Premier Access Insurance/Access Dental, 167
123,880	Access Dental Services, 78
123,000	Carolina Care Plan, 994
123,000	Health Net Health Plan of Oregon, 905
121,794	Santa Clara Family Health Foundations Inc, 172
121,000	Capital Blue Cross, 932
120,000	CIGNA HealthCare of Washington, 1146
120,000	Employers Dental Services, 41
120,000	Horizon Health Corporation, 1068
119,712	Prevea Health Network, 1200
119,600	Mid America Health, 654
119,000	Health Net of Arizona, 45
118,600	DakotaCare, 1012
118,000	Network Health Plan of Wisconsin, 1198
116,375	Aetna Health of Georgia, 303
115,400	First Priority Health, 942
115,313	Great-West Healthcare Illinois, 369
115,000	Health Choice Arizona, 44
113,229	Humana Health Insurance of Colorado Springs, 206

112,011	Humana Health Insurance of Michigan, 574
112,000	Physicians Plus Insurance Corporation, 1199
110,000	Community First Health Plans, 1054
110,000	Kaiser Permanente Health Plan Ohio, 856
110,000	Preferred Health Plan Inc, 464
109,186	CIGNA HealthCare of the Mid-Atlantic, 241, 500
109,089	Aetna Health of Arizona, 29
109,089	Aetna Health of Nevada, 684
109,000	Health Plan of San Joaquin, 131
108,000	HealthSpan, 852
108,000	Neighborhood Health Partnership, 289
107,539	Healthcare Partners of East Texas, 1064
107,387	AmeriChoice by UnitedHealthCare, 754
106,000	Health New England, 533
105,200	Trigon Health Care, 1138
105,000	JMH Health Plan, 285
103,561	CIGNA HealthCare of Arizona, 36
103,000	Unison Health Plan of Ohio, 876
102,506	Humana Health Insurance of Indiana, 404
101,900	Mid Atlantic Psychiatric Services (MAMSI), 236
101,000	UPMC Health Plan, 968
100,000	Blue Cross & Blue Shield of Wyoming, 1208
100,000	Contra Costa Health Plan, 112
100,000	Coventry Health Care of Delaware, 229
100,000	Coventry Health Care of Illinois, 363
100,000	Coventry Health Care of West Virginia, 1167
100,000	DC Chartered Health Plan, 242
100,000	Humana Health Insurance of Ohio, 854
100,000	National Capital PPO, 1133
100,000	OhioHealth Group, 865
100,000	Preferred Vision Care, 447
100,000	Triple-S Salud Blue Cross Blue Shield of Puerto Rico, 978
98,500	Action Healthcare Management Services, 28
97,800	PreferredOne, 612
97,000	Kern Family Health Care, 142
95,000	Group Health Cooperative of Eau Claire, 1190
95,000	Health Partners of Kansas, 440
93,000	Keystone Health Plan Central, 954
93,000	Partnership HealthPlan of California, 164
92,000	Western Health Advantage, 187
90,000	BEST Life and Health Insurance Co., 89
90,000	Dental Health Services of California, 117
90,000	Gundersen Lutheran Health Plan, 1192
90,000	Neighborhood Health Plan of Rhode Island, 987
90,000	Parkview Total Health, 407
90,000	Quality Plan Administrators, 247
90,000	Total Health Care, 585
90,000	Unity Health Insurance, 1204
88,366	Virginia Health Network, 1141
87,740	Health Plan of San Mateo, 132
87,000	First Choice of the Midwest, 1015
86,000	Advantage Health Solutions, 385
86,000	University Health Plans, 1111
85,000	Amerigroup Nevada, 685
85,000	Martin's Point HealthCare, 490
84,841	Humana Health Insurance of Kansas, 441
83,151	Preferred Plus of Kansas, 446
81,822	Great-West Healthcare Florida, 277
81,000	Humana Health Insurance of New York, 781
80,316	Preferred Health Care, 959
80,000	Alliance Regional Health Network, 1042
80,000	AlohaCare, 330
80,000	Health InfoNet, 666
80,000	Magellan Health Services Arizona, 47
80,000	NOVA Healthcare Administrators, 798
80,000	Patient Choice, 611
80,000	Signature Health Alliance, 1038
80,000	Unicare: Massachusetts, 540
80,000	Unicare: West Virginia, 1176
80,000	VIVA Health, 17
78,600	Humana Health Insurance of Mississippi, 626
75,000	UCare Medicare Plan, 614

75,000	Windsor Medicare Extra, 1040
73,000	Cariten Healthcare, 1026
73,000	Coventry Health Care of Kansas, 436
73,000	Humana Health Insurance of Georgia, 320
73,000	Mercy Health Plans: Arkansas, 73
73,000	Mercy Health Plans: Corporate Office, 652
73,000	Mercy Health Plans: Kansas, 442
73,000	Mercy Health Plans: Oklahoma, 891
73,000	Mercy Health Plans: Texas, 1075
72,853	CIGNA HealthCare of Wisconsin, 1184
71,000	Americhoice of Pennsylvania, 925
69,000	Coventry Health Care of Southern Florida, 268
68,942	Physicians Health Plan of Mid-Michigan, 580
68,935	CIGNA HealthCare of New Jersey, 718
68,000	Secure Health PPO Newtork, 324
67,440	Florida Health Care Plan, 275
67,308	Great-West Healthcare Missouri, 646
67,000	CarePlus Health Plans, Inc, 262
66,000	North Alabama Managed Care Inc, 14
65,300	Brazos Valley Health Network, 1051
65,000	SelectNet Plus, Inc., 1175
64,977	CIGNA HealthCare of Minnesota, 596
64,973	OSF HealthPlans, 379
63,700	Health First Health Plans, 278
63,000	Avera Health Plans, 1010
61,000	Group Health Cooperative of South Central Wisconsin, 1191
60,353	Berkshire Health Partners, 928
60,000	American Health Care Group, 923
60,000	Boulder Valley Individual Practice Association, 195
60,000	Foundation for Medical Care for Kern & Santa Barbara Co., 123
56,422	Great-West Healthcare North Carolina, 819
56,000	Beta Health Plan, 194
56,000	Humana Health Insurance of Orlando, 283
56,000	South Central Preferred, 963
55,000	Arta Medicare Health Plan, 83
55,000	San Francisco Health Plan, 171
55,000	SecureCare Dental, 56
54,418	Mutual of Omaha Health Plans, 682
54,000	Citrus Health Care, 264
54,000	Coventry Health Care of Nebraska, 676
54,000	Florida Blue: Pensacola, 274
53,000	GHI Medicare Plan, 775
53,000	PMC Medicare Choice, 977
53,000	Peninsula Health Care, 1135
52,000	Island Group Administration, Inc., 784
52,000	Ohio State University Health Plan Inc., 864
52,000	Preferred Medical Plan, 293
50,919	Cariten Preferred, 1027
50,715	Maricopa Integrated Health System/Maricopa Health Plan, 48
50,000	American Denticare, 63
50,000	Blue Ridge Health Network, 930
50,000	CareSource: Michigan, 553
50,000	OmniCare: A Coventry Health Care Plan, 578
50,000	Sanford Health Plan, 427
49,984	Great-West Healthcare Georgia, 319
49,976	Children's Mercy Pediatric Care Network, 636
49,000	Humana Health Insurance of Wisconsin, 1195
49,000	Sharp Health Plan, 174
48,477	HealthPartners, 1032
47,724	CIGNA HealthCare of Utah, 1098
47,000	Assurant Employee Benefits: Alabama, 3
47,000	Assurant Employee Benefits: California, 84
47,000	Assurant Employee Benefits: Colorado, 192
47,000	Assurant Employee Benefits: Corporate Headquarters, 632
47,000	Assurant Employee Benefits: Florida, 253
47,000	Assurant Employee Benefits: Georgia, 307
47,000	Assurant Employee Benefits: Illinois, 355
47,000	Assurant Employee Benefits: Kansas, 432
47,000	Assurant Employee Benefits: Massachusetts, 520
47,000	Assurant Employee Benefits: Michigan, 545
47,000	Assurant Employee Benefits: Minnesota, 593
47,000	Assurant Employee Benefits: New Jersey, 714

47,000	Assurant Employee Benefits: North Carolina, 810
47,000	Assurant Employee Benefits: Ohio, 842
47,000	Assurant Employee Benefits: Oklahoma, 881
47,000	Assurant Employee Benefits: Oregon, 895
47,000	Assurant Employee Benefits: Pennsylvania, 927
47,000	Assurant Employee Benefits: South Carolina, 991
47,000	Assurant Employee Benefits: Tennessee, 1023
47,000	Assurant Employee Benefits: Texas, 1045
47,000	Assurant Employee Benefits: Washington, 1144
47,000	Assurant Employee Benefits: Wisconsin, 1181
47,000	Coventry Health Care of Iowa, 419
45,014	Aetna Health of Illinois, 354
45,014	Aetna Health of Indiana, 386
45,000	Health Choice of Alabama, 12
45,000	Medical Associates Health Plan, 377
45,000	Medical Associates Health Plan: West, 425
45,000	PacifiCare of Washington, 1156
45,000	Preferred Care Partners, 292
45,000	Susquehanna Health Care, 965
43,620	Great-West Healthcare Indiana, 401, 400
43,000	New West Health Services, 669
43,000	New West Medicare Plan, 670
43,000	PacifiCare of Oklahoma, 892
43,000	Physicians Health Plan of Northern Indiana, 408
42,000	Hawaii Medical Assurance Association, 334
42,000	Northeast Georgia Health Partners, 323
42,000	Peoples Health, 480
42,000	TexanPlus Medicare Advantage HMO, 1085
41,266	Coastal Healthcare Administrators, 108
41,000	Peoples Health, 479
40,319	CIGNA HealthCare of New York, 760
40,000	Cardinal Health Alliance, 393
40,000	Crescent Health Solutions, 815
40,000	MercyCare Health Plans, 1197
39,334	Great-West Healthcare Oregon, 904
38,515	Welborn Health Plans, 413
38,000	Unicare: Texas, 1088
37,459	Great-West Healthcare Arizona, 43
36,611	CIGNA HealthCare of Colorado, 196
36,505	University Health Alliance, 339
36,423	Aetna Health of Colorado, 188
36,000	QualChoice/QCA Health Plan, 75
35,992	Great-West Healthcare Michigan, 565
35,316	CIGNA HealthCare of West Virginia, 1166
35,000	Clear One Health Plans, 900
35,000	Healthchoice Orlando, 280
34,284	CIGNA HealthCare of Iowa, 418
34,000	Foundation for Medical Care for Mendocino and Lake Co., 124
34,000	Health Tradition, 1193
33,153	Preferred Health Systems Insurance Company, 444
33,000	Prime Source Health Network, 961
32,000	Hometown Health Plan, 690
30,000	Cigna-HealthSpring of Alabama, 8
30,000	Concentra: Corporate Office, 1055
30,000	Coventry Health Care of Louisiana, 472
30,000	DINA Dental Plans, 474
30,000	Easy Choice Health Plan, 766
30,000	Health Plus of Louisiana, 476
30,000	InStil Health, 1000
30,000	Piedmont Community Health Plan, 1136
30,000	Samaritan Health Plan, 916
29,583	CIGNA HealthCare of North Carolina, 813
29,506	CIGNA HealthCare of Connecticut, 219
29,000	PacifiCare of Oregon, 912
28,785	Great-West Healthcare New York, 776
28,619	Great-West Healthcare Wisconsin, 1189
28,125	Mount Carmel Health Plan Inc (MediGold), 861
27,179	Aetna Health of Delaware, 226
27,000	CIGNA HealthCare of Idaho, 343
27,000	Leon Medical Centers Health Plan, 286
26,411	Great-West Healthcare Pennsylvania, 945
26,000	PacifiCare of Nevada, 696

26,000	SummaCare Medicare Advantage Plan, 871
25,769	CIGNA HealthCare of Georgia, 311
25,278	Upper Peninsula Health Plan, 589
24,054	Aetna Health of Tennessee, 1021
24,000	ABRI Health Plan, Inc., 1178
23,559	CIGNA HealthCare of New Hampshire, 701
23,241	Athens Area Health Plan Select, 308
22,417	Aetna Health of Maine, 484
22,000	Valley Baptist Health Plan, 1093
21,580	Great-West Healthcare Kansas, 439
21,000	Metropolitan Health Plan, 608
21,000	Rayant Insurance Company, 733
20,000	Preferred Healthcare System, 960
19,468	Kanawha Healthcare Solutions, 1001
19,000	Quality Health Plans, 801
19,000	Quality Health Plans of New York, 802
18,960	Aetna Health of the Carolinas, 990, 809
18,588	CIGNA HealthCare of Illinois, 359
18,556	Great-West Healthcare Minnesota, 600
18,500	Penn Highlands Health Plan, 957
18,335	Great-West Healthcare Oklahoma, 889
18,322	CIGNA HealthCare of Nebraska, 675
17,000	ConnectCare, 556
17,000	Primecare Dental Plan, 168
17,000	Puget Sound Health Partners, 1158
16,852	Great-West Healthcare South Carolina, 998
16,000	Elderplan, 768
15,700	SelectCare Access Corporation, 962
15,153	American Health Network of Indiana, 387
15,000	Alliant Health Plans, 305
15,000	Denver Health Medical Plan Inc, 202
15,000	Saint Mary's Health Plans, 697
15,000	Seton Health Plan, 1084
14,600	Inter Valley Health Plan, 136
14,000	HealthPlus Senior Medicare Plan, 573
14,000	Primary Health Plan, 350
14,000	Vantage Health Plan, 482
14,000	Vantage Medicare Advantage, 483
13,582	Chinese Community Health Plan, 101
13,000	FirstCarolinaCare, 818
12,700	Central Susquehanna Healthcare Providers, 933
12,317	WellChoice, 736
12,000	Health Plans, Inc., 535
12,000	Medica HealthCare Plans, Inc, 287
11,745	Great-West Healthcare West Virginia, 1170
11,234	CIGNA HealthCare of Wyoming, 1209
11,121	Aetna Health of Massachusetts, 519
11,000	Touchstone Health HMO, 803
11,000	WINhealth Partners, 1214

10,885	Aetna Health of Missouri, 629
10,816	Great-West Healthcare New Mexico, 743
10,315	CIGNA HealthCare of Massachusetts, 524
10,231	Southeastern Indiana Health Organization, 410
10,082	Great-West Healthcare Iowa, 422
10,000	Denta-Chek of Maryland, 504
10,000	Total Health Choice, 296
9,848	CIGNA HealthCare of Kansas, 434
9,678	CIGNA HealthCare of Indiana, 394
9,000	Perfect Health Insurance Company, 800
8,184	Great-West Healthcare Maine, 488
8,147	Great-West Healthcare Alabama, 11
8,135	CIGNA HealthCare of South Dakota, 1011
8,097	Humana Health Insurance of Alaska, 23
8,049	CIGNA HealthCare of St. Louis, 637
8,000	Arnett Health Plans, 391
8,000	Easy Choice Health Plan, 119
8,000	Grand Valley Health Plan, 563
8,000	Graphic Arts Benefit Corporation, 507
7,642	CIGNA HealthCare of Montana, 662
7,000	Arkansas Community Care, 65
7,000	Community Health Improvement Solutions, 638
7,000	Pima Health System, 54
6,443	Harvard University Group Health Plan, 532
6,343	CIGNA HealthCare of Maine, 486
6,000	Educators Mutual, 1100
6,000	Risk Placement Services, Inc., 294
5,000	Colorado Choice Health Plans, 199
5,000	Cox Healthplans, 639
5,000	Trilogy Health Insurance, 1202
4,970	Great-West Healthcare Montana, 665
3,971	Evercare Health Plans, 599
3,000	Central Health Medicare Plan, 100
3,000	NevadaCare, 695
3,000	Phoenix Health Plans, 53
2,718	Great-West Healthcare Delaware, 232
2,407	CIGNA HealthCare of Hawaii, 331
2,375	Val-U-Health, 969
2,000	FamilyCare Health Medicare Plan, 903
1,685	Great-West Healthcare South Dakota, 1016
1,003	CCN: Alaska, 20
1,000	Heart of America Health Plan, 834
1,000	Legacy Health Plan, 1073
1,000	On Lok Lifeways, 155
1,000	UTMB HealthCare Systems, 1092
984	CIGNA HealthCare of Delaware, 228
884	Great-West Healthcare North Dakota, 833
368	Great-West Healthcare Hawaii, 333

Primary Care Physician Index

29,000	Encore Health Network, 399
29,000	OptumHealth Care Solutions: Physical Health, 610
28,000	Harvard Pilgrim Health Care, 531
28,000	Harvard Pilgrim Health Care of New England, 704
28,000	Harvard Pilgrim Health Care: Maine, 489
28,000	VSP: Vision Service Plan of California, 185
28,000	VSP: Vision Service Plan of Colorado, 213
28,000	VSP: Vision Service Plan of Florida, 301
28,000	VSP: Vision Service Plan of Georgia, 328
28,000	VSP: Vision Service Plan of Hawaii, 340
28,000	VSP: Vision Service Plan of Illinois, 384
28,000	VSP: Vision Service Plan of Indiana, 412
28,000	VSP: Vision Service Plan of Kansas, 451
27,000	Medica: Corporate Office, 606
27,000	Medica: South Dakota, 1018
27,000	Stanislaus Foundation for Medical Care, 175
26,000	VSP: Vision Service Plan, 184
26,000	VSP: Vision Service Plan of Arizona, 61
26,000	VSP: Vision Service Plan of Massachusetts, 542
26,000	VSP: Vision Service Plan of Michigan, 590
26,000	VSP: Vision Service Plan of Minnesota, 620
26,000	VSP: Vision Service Plan of New Jersey, 735
26,000	VSP: Vision Service Plan of Ohio, 879
26,000	VSP: Vision Service Plan of Oregon, 920
26,000	VSP: Vision Service Plan of South Carolina, 1007
26,000	VSP: Vision Service Plan of Texas, 1094
26,000	VSP: Vision Service Plan of Washington, 1164
25,000	Anthem Blue Cross & Blue Shield of Ohio, 841
25,000	Tufts Health Plan, 539
25,000	Tufts Health Plan: Rhode Island, 988
24,000	Coventry Health Care of Delaware, 229
24,000	MVP Health Care: New Hampshire, 706
24,000	Medica: North Dakota, 836
24,000	Spectera, 516
24,000	WellPath: A Coventry Health Care Plan, 828
23,000	National Capital PPO, 1133
22,000	ConnectiCare of Massachusetts, 525
22,000	ConnectiCare of New York, 762
21,070	Humana Health Insurance of Illinois, 376
21,010	Island Group Administration, Inc., 784
20,266	Blue Cross & Blue Shield of Massachusetts, 522
20,100	CIGNA HealthCare of North Carolina, 813
20,016	Cariten Preferred, 1027
20,000	Devon Health Services, 938
20,000	Midlands Choice, 680
20,000	OptiCare Managed Vision, 823
20,000	Premera Blue Cross, 1157
20,000	Signature Health Alliance, 1038
19,702	Regence Blue Shield, 1159
19,000	Asuris Northwest Health, 1145
19,000	Blue Cross & Blue Shield of Georgia, 310
18,000	Americas PPO, 1009
18,000	Araz Group, 592
18,000	Avesis: Arizona, 309
18,000	Avesis: Corporate Headquarters, 32
18,000	Avesis: Indiana, 392
18,000	Avesis: Iowa, 417
18,000	Avesis: Maryland, 496
18,000	Avesis: Massachusetts, 521
18,000	Avesis: Minnesota, 594
18,000	Avesis: Texas, 1046
18,000	Block Vision, 497
18,000	Block Vision of New Jersey, 716
18,000	Health Alliance Plan, 567
17,000	Coventry Health Care of GA, 314
17,000	Horizon Health Corporation, 1068
17,000	Oxford Health Plans: Corporate Headquarters, 224
16,000	CIGNA HealthCare of Georgia, 311
16,000	UCare Medicare Plan, 614
16,000	UCare Minnesota, 615
15,600	Coventry Health Care of West Virginia, 1167
15,529	GHI, 774
15,200	CIGNA HealthCare of Tennessee, 1028
15,129	Kaiser Foundation Health Plan of Georgia, 321
15,129	Kaiser Permanente Health Plan Ohio, 856
15,129	Kaiser Permanente Health Plan of Hawaii, 337
15,129	Kaiser Permanente Health Plan of Northern California, 138
15,129	Kaiser Permanente Health Plan of the Mid-Atlantic States, 509
15,129	Kaiser Permanente Health Plan of the Northwest, 907
15,129	Kaiser Permanente Health Plan: Corporate Office, 140
15,059	Sagamore Health Network, 409
15,009	Atlanticare Health Plans, 715
15,000	CHA Health, 455
15,000	Optima Health Plan, 1134
14,500	Wisconsin Physician's Service, 1206
14,000	Arizona Foundation for Medical Care, 30
14,000	Encircle Network, 398
13,840	MVP Health Care: Corporate Office, 793
13,729	Kaiser Permanente Health Plan of Southern California, 139
12,349	MedCost, 821
12,000	Coventry Health Care Virginia, 1125
12,000	MVP Health Care: Central New York, 792
12,000	MetroPlus Health Plan, 788
12,000	Priority Health, 581
12,000	Public Employees Health Program, 1106
11,500	Care Choices, 552
11,300	CIGNA HealthCare of Connecticut, 219
11,000	Behavioral Health Systems, 5
11,000	Capital Blue Cross, 932
10,500	Preferred Mental Health Management, 445
10,425	Regence Blue Cross & Blue Shield of Oregon, 915
10,032	Aetna Health of Maryland, 493
10,000	American PPO, 1043
10,000	Family Choice Health Alliance, 721
10,000	Keystone Health Plan East, 955
10,000	Preferred Vision Care, 447
9,200	PreferredOne, 612
9,000	Blue Cross Preferred Care, 7
9,000	Lifewise Health Plan of Oregon, 909
9,000	Parkview Total Health, 407
9,000	QualCare, 732
8,986	PacifiCare Dental and Vision Administrators, 161
8,977	Florida Blue: Jacksonville, 273
8,500	Mercy Health Plans: Corporate Office, 652
8,500	UnitedHealthCare of New York, 805
8,400	HealthSpan, 852
8,271	PacifiCare of California, 163
8,100	CIGNA HealthCare of South Carolina, 995
8,000	Blue Cross & Blue Shield of Minnesota, 595
8,000	Gateway Health Plan, 943
7,932	Ohio Health Choice, 863
7,728	Medical Mutual of Ohio, 857
7,700	BlueChoice Health Plan of South Carolina, 993
7,700	Group Health Cooperative of Eau Claire, 1190
7,600	UPMC Health Plan, 968
7,500	Aetna Health of Massachusetts, 519
7,332	Carolina Care Plan, 994
7,000	HealthEOS, 1194
7,000	Lovelace Health Plan, 745
6,908	Aetna Health of Virginia, 1119
6,560	SCAN Health Plan, 173
6,150	Prime Source Health Network, 961
6,150	South Central Preferred, 963
6,000	Dimension Health PPO, 270
6,000	FC Diagnostic, 722
6,000	Group Health Cooperative, 1150
6,000	Orange County Foundation for Medical Care, 156
6,000	SummaCare Health Plan, 870
6,000	SummaCare Medicare Advantage Plan, 871
5,900	OhioHealth Group, 865
5,800	Nationwide Better Health, 862
5,700	Univera Healthcare, 806
5,580	ConnectiCare, 220
5,500	Managed Health Services, 1196

2,073	SafeGuard Health Enterprises: Texas, 1081	1,291	Fallon Community Health Plan, 528
2,061	AvMed Health Plan: Corporate Office, 254	1,287	Physicians Health Plan of Northern Indiana, 408
2,032	CIGNA HealthCare of the Mid-Atlantic, 241, 500	1,282	Neighborhood Health Partnership, 289
2,030	Select Health of South Carolina, 1003	1,253	Nevada Preferred Healthcare Providers, 693
2,011	Golden West Dental & Vision Plan, 126	1,208	UnitedHealthCare of Indiana, 411
2,000	Access Dental Services, 78	1,208	UnitedHealthCare of Kentucky, 466
2,000	CIGNA HealthCare of Indiana, 394	1,207	Health Net: Corporate Headquarters, 130
2,000	Coventry Health Care of Louisiana, 472	1,200	Alere Health, 304
2,000	Healthchoice Orlando, 280	1,200	Delta Dental of Kansas, 437
2,000	Mid America Health, 654	1,200	Elderplan, 768
1,989	SelectNet Plus, Inc., 1175	1,200	Health Net of Arizona, 45
1,941	HMO Colorado, 205	1,200	Highmark Blue Cross & Blue Shield, 949
1,923	First Health, 368	1,200	Leon Medical Centers Health Plan, 286
1,900	Blue Cross & Blue Shield of Montana, 661	1,200	PTPN, 169
1,900	Crescent Health Solutions, 815	1,200	Presbyterian Health Plan, 748
1,900	Paramount Care of Michigan, 579	1,189	Blue Cross & Blue Shield of Kansas City, 633
1,900	Paramount Elite Medicare Plan, 866	1,186	Delta Dental of New Mexico, 741
1,900	Paramount Health Care, 867	1,167	IHC: Intermountain Healthcare Health Plan, 347
1,900	Parkland Community Health Plan, 1080	1,161	Inter Valley Health Plan, 136
1,900	Preferred Health Care, 959	1,151	Virginia Premier Health Plan, 1142
1,900	Seton Health Plan, 1084	1,150	CIGNA HealthCare of Arizona, 36
1,898	Aetna Health District of Columbia, 239	1,135	SVS Vision, 584
1,874	Hawaii Medical Assurance Association, 334	1,126	John Deere Health, 1037
1,850	SecureCare Dental, 56	1,125	Independent Health, 782
1,832	First Commonwealth, 367	1,119	Preferred Care Blue, 657
1,800	Health Resources, Inc., 402	1,100	Americhoice of Pennsylvania, 925
1,750	University Health Plans, 1111	1,100	First Care Health Plans, 1060
1,737	CIGNA HealthCare of Virginia, 1124	1,100	PacifiCare of Colorado, 208
1,700	Alameda Alliance for Health, 80	1,091	MVP Health Care: Western New York, 795
1,700	Centene Corporation, 635	1,090	Susquehanna Health Care, 965
1,700	Health Plans, Inc., 535	1,063	Physicians Health Plan of Mid-Michigan, 580
1,700	Inland Empire Health Plan, 135	1,055	CIGNA HealthCare of New Hampshire, 701
1,700	Western Dental Services, 186	1,050	Mount Carmel Health Plan Inc (MediGold), 861
1,675	Delta Dental of Vermont, 1115	1,050	PacifiCare Health Systems, 162
1,631	Blue Cross of Idaho Health Service, Inc., 342	1,035	Excellus Blue Cross Blue Shield: Rochester Region, 771
1,622	Great Lakes Health Plan, 564	1,000	Alliance Regional Health Network, 1042
1,611	Blue Cross & Blue Shield of Arizona, 34	1,000	Amerigroup Florida, 252
1,602	Prevea Health Network, 1200	1,000	Arkansas Managed Care Organization, 66
1,600	UnitedHealthCare of Colorado, 212	1,000	Athens Area Health Plan Select, 308
1,600	UnitedHealthCare of Montana, 671	1,000	CIGNA HealthCare of Oklahoma, 884
1,600	UnitedHealthCare of New Hampshire, 708	1,000	Cox Healthplans, 639
1,600	UnitedHealthCare of Vermont, 1118	1,000	Dental Health Services of California, 117
1,600	UnitedHealthCare of Wyoming, 1213	1,000	Health Partners of Kansas, 440
1,590	Central California Alliance for Health, 99	1,000	Premier Access Insurance/Access Dental, 167
1,554	Aetna Health of Arizona, 29	1,000	Scott & White Health Plan, 1082
1,551	Blue Cross & Blue Shield of Oklahoma, 882	980	Health InfoNet, 666
1,524	Aetna Health of Pennsylvania, 922	971	Anthem Blue Cross & Blue Shield of Maine, 485
1,511	Molina Healthcare: New Mexico, 747	962	Blue Cross & Blue Shield of Louisiana, 469
1,500	Cariten Healthcare, 1026	961	Horizon Blue Cross & Blue Shield of New Jersey, 724
1,500	Coventry Health Care of Florida, 267	950	CareOregon Health Plan, 897
1,500	Coventry Health Care of Nebraska, 676	950	OneNet PPO, 512
1,500	Dean Health Plan, 1185	950	Secure Health PPO Newtork, 324
1,500	Delta Dental of Minnesota, 597	927	HealthNow New York - Emblem Health, 779
1,500	Delta Dental of North Dakota, 831	908	Unity Health Insurance, 1204
1,500	Health Link PPO, 625	900	CIGNA HealthCare of Maine, 486
1,500	Preferred Care Partners, 292	900	Deaconess Health Plans, 395
1,500	Vytra Health Plans, 808	900	HealthPlus Senior Medicare Plan, 573
1,454	CIGNA HealthCare of North Texas, 1052	900	HealthPlus of Michigan: Flint, 569
1,435	Managed HealthCare Northwest, 910	900	HealthPlus of Michigan: Saginaw, 570
1,400	Affinity Health Plan, 753	900	HealthPlus of Michigan: Troy, 572
1,400	AvMed Health Plan: Orlando, 258	900	Neighborhood Health Plan of Rhode Island, 987
1,400	EPIC Pharmacy Network, 1129	890	Santa Clara Family Health Foundations Inc, 172
1,400	Health Choice LLC, 1031	850	Gundersen Lutheran Health Plan, 1192
1,400	Mountain State Blue Cross Blue Shield, 1174	844	Kaiser Permanente Health Plan of Colorado, 207
1,400	Network Health Plan of Wisconsin, 1198	825	Berkshire Health Partners, 928
1,395	Blue Ridge Health Network, 930	825	DakotaCare, 1012
1,386	Preferred Health Systems Insurance Company, 444	800	Arta Medicare Health Plan, 83
1,375	SelectCare Access Corporation, 962	800	Carilion Health Plans, 1123
1,366	Providence Health Plans, 914	800	Health Tradition, 1193
1,340	Employers Dental Services, 41	800	Los Angeles County Department of Health Services, 147
1,300	Humana Health Insurance of Kansas, 441	800	Pacific IPA, 160
1,300	Humana Health Insurance of Wisconsin, 1195	795	Chiropractic Health Plan of California, 102

Referral/Specialty Physician Index

4,722	Southeastern Indiana Health Organization, 410
4,678	Beech Street Corporation: Alabama, 4
4,650	Gateway Health Plan, 943
4,552	Highmark Blue Cross & Blue Shield, 949
4,500	CIGNA HealthCare of Connecticut, 219
4,500	Landmark Healthplan of California, 145
4,500	MVP Health Care: Western New York, 795
4,500	UnitedHealthCare of South Florida, 299
4,490	Select Health of South Carolina, 1003
4,450	Virginia Premier Health Plan, 1142
4,430	Pacific Foundation for Medical Care, 158
4,374	Aetna Health of Arizona, 29
4,236	Managed HealthCare Northwest, 910
4,199	BlueChoice Health Plan of South Carolina, 993
4,151	Advantage Health Solutions, 385
4,100	Penn Highlands Health Plan, 957
4,000	Aetna Health of West Virginia, 1165
4,000	American WholeHealth Network, 924
4,000	Atlanticare Health Plans, 715
4,000	HSM: Healthcare Cost Management, 603
4,000	Initial Group, 1036
4,000	Preferred Mental Health Management, 445
4,000	UnitedHealthCare of Georgia, 327
3,983	CareSource: Michigan, 553
3,952	Anthem Blue Cross & Blue Shield of Kentucky, 453
3,928	Aetna Health of Pennsylvania, 922
3,884	M-Care, 575
3,870	Optima Health Plan, 1134
3,820	SelectNet Plus, Inc., 1175
3,800	Elderplan, 768
3,800	Group Health Cooperative of Eau Claire, 1190
3,800	Health Net of Arizona, 45
3,700	Primecare Dental Plan, 168
3,660	Dimension Health PPO, 270
3,653	Humana Health Insurance of Colorado Springs, 206
3,609	SelectCare Access Corporation, 962
3,608	Anthem Blue Cross & Blue Shield of New Hampshire, 700
3,596	SummaCare Medicare Advantage Plan, 871
3,504	Fallon Community Health Plan, 528
3,500	Coventry Health Care of Nebraska, 676
3,500	UnitedHealthCare of Colorado, 212
3,500	UnitedHealthCare of Montana, 671
3,500	UnitedHealthCare of New Hampshire, 708
3,500	UnitedHealthCare of Vermont, 1118
3,500	UnitedHealthCare of Wyoming, 1213
3,400	Americhoice of Pennsylvania, 925
3,369	UnitedHealthCare of Tennessee, 1039
3,304	UnitedHealthCare of Ohio: Columbus, 877
3,304	UnitedHealthCare of Ohio: Dayton & Cincinnati, 878
3,279	CIGNA HealthCare of North Texas, 1052
3,276	Great-West/One Health Plan, 204
3,276	Perfect Health Insurance Company, 800
3,241	Coastal Healthcare Administrators, 108
3,227	Unity Health Insurance, 1204
3,200	Mountain State Blue Cross Blue Shield, 1174
3,180	CIGNA HealthCare of Arizona, 36
3,129	CIGNA HealthCare of New Hampshire, 701
3,120	Berkshire Health Partners, 928
3,042	Providence Health Plans, 914
3,000	CareOregon Health Plan, 897
3,000	Health New England, 533
3,000	Preferred Therapy Providers, 55
2,977	Valley Preferred, 970
2,900	NevadaCare, 695
2,900	Public Employees Health Program, 1106
2,854	Coventry Health Care Virginia, 1125
2,802	Blue Cross & Blue Shield of Vermont, 1113
2,800	Blue Cross & Blue Shield of Montana, 661
2,733	SummaCare Health Plan, 870
2,705	PacifiCare Dental and Vision Administrators, 161
2,700	Neighborhood Health Plan of Rhode Island, 987
2,681	Health Choice of Alabama, 12

2,518	Anthem Blue Cross & Blue Shield of Nevada, 191
2,427	Humana Health Insurance of Louisiana, 477
2,400	Children's Mercy Pediatric Care Network, 636
2,400	Crescent Health Solutions, 815
2,400	PacifiCare of Colorado, 208
2,309	Santa Clara Family Health Foundations Inc, 172
2,225	UnitedHealthCare of New York, 805
2,221	Healthchoice Orlando, 280
2,219	Blue Cross & Blue Shield of Louisiana, 469
2,203	Community Health Improvement Solutions, 638
2,200	Encore Health Network, 399
2,162	Nevada Preferred Healthcare Providers, 693
2,117	Physicians Plus Insurance Corporation, 1199
2,082	Excellus Blue Cross Blue Shield: Rochester Region, 771
2,073	Baptist Health Services Group, 1024
2,070	Mid America Health, 654
2,059	HealthNow New York - Emblem Health, 779
2,030	SafeGuard Health Enterprises: Corporate Office, 170
2,030	SafeGuard Health Enterprises: Florida, 295
2,030	SafeGuard Health Enterprises: Texas, 1081
2,005	First Care Health Plans, 1060
2,000	BlueChoice, 634
2,000	CIGNA HealthCare of Indiana, 394
2,000	MHNet Behavioral Health, 1076
1,983	UnitedHealthCare of Indiana, 411
1,983	UnitedHealthCare of Kentucky, 466
1,913	Healthcare Partners of East Texas, 1064
1,870	Preferred Health Systems Insurance Company, 444
1,850	Altius Health Plans, 1097
1,850	Mount Carmel Health Plan Inc (MediGold), 861
1,820	Community Health Group, 109
1,800	HealthPlus Senior Medicare Plan, 573
1,800	HealthPlus of Michigan: Flint, 569
1,800	HealthPlus of Michigan: Saginaw, 570
1,800	HealthPlus of Michigan: Troy, 572
1,793	Health InfoNet, 666
1,791	PacifiCare Health Systems, 162
1,781	Physicians Health Plan of Mid-Michigan, 580
1,718	Mutual of Omaha Health Plans, 682
1,700	Pacific Dental Benefits, 157
1,668	CIGNA HealthCare of Arkansas, 67
1,626	Independent Health, 782
1,604	Anthem Blue Cross & Blue Shield of Maine, 485
1,581	John Deere Health, 1037
1,566	IHC: Intermountain Healthcare Health Plan, 347
1,500	Lakeside Community Healthcare Network, 144
1,500	Pacific Health Alliance, 159
1,500	Preferred Health Plan Inc, 464
1,500	Saint Mary's Health Plans, 697
1,500	Total Health Care, 585
1,466	PacifiCare of California, 163
1,427	Kanawha Healthcare Solutions, 1001
1,400	Health Plan of San Joaquin, 131
1,400	Interplan Health Group, 855
1,400	Western Dental Services, 186
1,386	Blue Cross & Blue Shield of Kansas City, 633
1,300	CommunityCare Managed Healthcare Plans of Oklahoma, 885
1,275	Prime Source Health Network, 961
1,275	ProviDRs Care Network, 448
1,255	Managed Health Services, 1196
1,213	BlueLincs HMO, 883
1,200	Aetna Health of Georgia, 303
1,200	CIGNA HealthCare of Maine, 486
1,200	Physical Therapy Provider Network, 165
1,200	Total Health Choice, 296
1,197	Preferred Plus of Kansas, 446
1,133	OSF HealthPlans, 379
1,014	North Alabama Managed Care Inc, 14
1,000	Bluegrass Family Health, 454
1,000	Health Alliance Plan, 567
1,000	The Health Plan of the Ohio Valley/Mountaineer Region, 875
1,000	Welborn Health Plans, 413

2014 Title List
Visit www.GreyHouse.com for Product Information, Table of Contents and Sample Pages

General Reference
America's College Museums
American Environmental Leaders: From Colonial Times to the Present
An African Biographical Dictionary
An Encyclopedia of Human Rights in the United States
Constitutional Amendments
Encyclopedia of African-American Writing
Encyclopedia of the Continental Congress
Encyclopedia of Gun Control & Gun Rights
Encyclopedia of Invasions & Conquests
Encyclopedia of Prisoners of War & Internment
Encyclopedia of Religion & Law in America
Encyclopedia of Rural America
Encyclopedia of the United States Cabinet, 1789-2010
Encyclopedia of War Journalism
Encyclopedia of Warrior Peoples & Fighting Groups
From Suffrage to the Senate: America's Political Women
Nations of the World
Political Corruption in America
Speakers of the House of Representatives, 1789-2009
The Environmental Debate: A Documentary History
The Evolution Wars: A Guide to the Debates
The Religious Right: A Reference Handbook
The Value of a Dollar: 1860-2009
The Value of a Dollar: Colonial Era
This is Who We Were: A Companion to the 1940 Census
This is Who We Were: The 1920s
This is Who We Were: The 1950s
This is Who We Were: The 1960s
US Land & Natural Resource Policy
Working Americans 1770-1869 Vol. IX: Revolutionary War to the Civil War
Working Americans 1880-1999 Vol. I: The Working Class
Working Americans 1880-1999 Vol. II: The Middle Class
Working Americans 1880-1999 Vol. III: The Upper Class
Working Americans 1880-1999 Vol. IV: Their Children
Working Americans 1880-2003 Vol. V: At War
Working Americans 1880-2005 Vol. VI: Women at Work
Working Americans 1880-2006 Vol. VII: Social Movements
Working Americans 1880-2007 Vol. VIII: Immigrants
Working Americans 1880-2009 Vol. X: Sports & Recreation
Working Americans 1880-2010 Vol. XI: Inventors & Entrepreneurs
Working Americans 1880-2011 Vol. XII: Our History through Music
Working Americans 1880-2012 Vol. XIII: Education & Educators
World Cultural Leaders of the 20th & 21st Centuries

Business Information
Complete Television, Radio & Cable Industry Directory
Directory of Business Information Resources
Directory of Mail Order Catalogs
Directory of Venture Capital & Private Equity Firms
Environmental Resource Handbook
Food & Beverage Market Place
Grey House Homeland Security Directory
Grey House Performing Arts Directory
Hudson's Washington News Media Contacts Directory
New York State Directory
Sports Market Place Directory

Education Information
Charter School Movement
Comparative Guide to American Elementary & Secondary Schools
Complete Learning Disabilities Directory
Educators Resource Directory
Special Education

Health Information
Comparative Guide to American Hospitals
Complete Directory for Pediatric Disorders
Complete Directory for People with Chronic Illness
Complete Directory for People with Disabilities
Complete Mental Health Directory
Diabetes in America: A Geographic & Demographic Analysis
Directory of Health Care Group Purchasing Organizations
Directory of Hospital Personnel
HMO/PPO Directory
Medical Device Register
Older Americans Information Directory

Statistics & Demographics
America's Top-Rated Cities
America's Top-Rated Small Towns & Cities
America's Top-Rated Smaller Cities
American Tally
Ancestry & Ethnicity in America
Comparative Guide to American Hospitals
Comparative Guide to American Suburbs
Profiles of America
Profiles of… Series – State Handbooks
The Hispanic Databook
Weather America

Financial Ratings Series
TheStreet.com Ratings Guide to Bond & Money Market Mutual Funds
TheStreet.com Ratings Guide to Common Stocks
TheStreet.com Ratings Guide to Exchange-Traded Funds
TheStreet.com Ratings Guide to Stock Mutual Funds
TheStreet.com Ratings Ultimate Guided Tour of Stock Investing
Weiss Ratings Consumer Guides
Weiss Ratings Guide to Banks & Thrifts
Weiss Ratings Guide to Credit Unions
Weiss Ratings Guide to Health Insurers
Weiss Ratings Guide to Life & Annuity Insurers
Weiss Ratings Guide to Property & Casualty Insurers

Bowker's Books In Print® Titles
Books In Print®
Books In Print® Supplement
American Book Publishing Record® Annual
American Book Publishing Record® Monthly
Books Out Loud™
Bowker's Complete Video Directory™
Children's Books In Print®
El-Hi Textbooks & Serials In Print®
Forthcoming Books®
Law Books & Serials In Print™
Medical & Health Care Books In Print™
Publishers, Distributors & Wholesalers of the US™
Subject Guide to Books In Print®
Subject Guide to Children's Books In Print®

Canadian General Reference
Associations Canada
Canadian Almanac & Directory
Canadian Environmental Resource Guide
Canadian Parliamentary Guide
Financial Services Canada
Governments Canada
Health Services Canada
Libraries Canada
Major Canadian Cities
The History of Canada

Grey House Publishing | Salem Press | H.W. Wilson
4919 Route, 22 PO Box 56, Amenia NY 12501-0056

2014 Title List

Visit **www.SalemPress.com** for Product Information, Table of Contents and Sample Pages

Literature

American Ethnic Writers
Critical Insights: Authors
Critical Insights: New Literary Collection Bundles
Critical Insights: Themes
Critical Insights: Works
Critical Survey of Drama
Critical Survey of Graphic Novels: Heroes & Super Heroes
Critical Survey of Graphic Novels: History, Theme & Technique
Critical Survey of Graphic Novels: Independents & Underground Classics
Critical Survey of Graphic Novels: Manga
Critical Survey of Long Fiction
Critical Survey of Mystery & Detective Fiction
Critical Survey of Mythology and Folklore: Heroes and Heroines
Critical Survey of Mythology and Folklore: Love, Sexuality & Desire
Critical Survey of Mythology and Folklore: World Mythology
Critical Survey of Poetry
Critical Survey of Poetry: American Poetry
Critical Survey of Poetry: British, Irish & Commonwealth Poets
Critical Survey of Poetry: European Poets
Critical Survey of Poetry: European Poets
Critical Survey of Poetry: Topical Essays
Critical Survey of Poetry: World Poets
Critical Survey of Science Fiction & Fantasy Literature
Critical Survey of Shakespeare's Sonnets
Critical Survey of Short Fiction
Critical Survey of Short Fiction: American Writers
Critical Survey of Short Fiction: British, Irish & Commonwealth Poets
Critical Survey of Short Fiction: European Writers
Critical Survey of Short Fiction: Topical Essays
Critical Survey of Short Fiction: World Writers
Cyclopedia of Literary Characters
Introduction to Literary Context: American Post-Modernist Novels
Introduction to Literary Context: American Short Fiction
Introduction to Literary Context: English Literature
Introduction to Literary Context: World Literature
Magill's Literary Annual 2014
Magill's Survey of American Literature
Magill's Survey of World Literature
Masterplots
Masterplots II: African American Literature
Masterplots II: Christian Literature
Masterplots II: Drama Series
Masterplots II: Short Story Series
Notable African American Writers
Notable American Novelists
Notable Playwrights
Short Story Writers

Science, Careers & Mathematics

Applied Science
Applied Science: Engineering & Mathematics
Applied Science: Science & Medicine
Applied Science: Technology
Biomes and Ecosystems
Careers in Chemistry
Careers in Communications & Media
Careers in Healthcare
Careers in Hospitality & Tourism
Careers in Law & Criminology
Careers in Physics
Computer Technology Inventors
Contemporary Biographies in Chemistry
Contemporary Biographies in Communications & Media
Contemporary Biographies in Healthcare
Contemporary Biographies in Hospitality & Tourism
Contemporary Biographies in Law & Criminology
Contemporary Biographies in Physics
Earth Science
Earth Science: Earth Materials & Resources
Earth Science: Earth's Surface and History
Earth Science: Physics & Chemistry of the Earth
Earth Science: Weather, Water & Atmosphere
Encyclopedia of Energy
Encyclopedia of Environmental Issues
Encyclopedia of Global Resources
Encyclopedia of Global Warming
Encyclopedia of Mathematics and Society
Encyclopedia of the Ancient World
Forensic Science
Internet Innovators
Introduction to Chemistry
Magill's Encyclopedia of Science: Animal Life
Magill's Encyclopedia of Science: Plant life
Magill's Medical Guide
Notable Natural Disasters
Solar System

Health

Addictions & Substance Abuse
Cancer
Complementary & Alternative Medicine
Genetics & Inherited Conditions
Infectious Diseases & Conditions
Magill's Medical Guide
Psychology & Mental Health
Psychology Basics

Grey House Publishing | Salem Press | H.W. Wilson
4919 Route, 22 PO Box 56, Amenia NY 12501-0056

2014 Title List

Visit **www.SalemPress.com** for Product Information, Table of Contents and Sample Pages

History and Social Science

A 2000s in America
50 States
African American History
Agriculture in History (check)
American First Ladies
American Heroes
American Indian Tribes
American Presidents
American Villains
Ancient Greece
Bill of Rights, The
Cold War, The
Defining Documents: American Revolution 1754-1805
Defining Documents: Civil War 1860-1865
Defining Documents: Emergence of Modern America, 1868-1918
Defining Documents: Exploration & Colonial America 1492-1755
Defining Documents: Manifest Destiny 1803-1860
Defining Documents: Reconstruction, 1865-1880
Defining Documents: The 1920s
Defining Documents: The 1930s
Defining Documents: World War I
Eighties in America
Encyclopedia of American Immigration
Fifties in America
Forties in America
Great Athletes
Great Events from History: 17th Century
Great Events from History: 18th Century
Great Events from History: 19th Century
Great Events from History: 20th Century, 1901-1940
Great Events from History: 20th Century, 1941-1970
Great Events from History: 20th Century, 1971-200
Great Events from History: Ancient World
Great Events from History: Middle Ages
Great Events from History: Modern Scandals
Great Events from History: Renaissance & Early Modern Era
Great Lives from History: 17th Century
Great Lives from History: 18th Century
Great Lives from History: 19th Century
Great Lives from History: 20th Century
Great Lives from History: African Americans
Great Lives from History: Ancient World
Great Lives from History: Asian & Pacific Islander Americans
Great Lives from History: Incredibly Wealthy
Great Lives from History: Inventors & Inventions
Great Lives from History: Jewish Americans
Great Lives from History: Latinos
Great Lives from History: Middle Ages
Great Lives from History: Notorious Lives
Great Lives from History: Renaissance & Early Modern Era
Great Lives from History: Scientists & Science
Historical Encyclopedia of American Business
Immigration in U.S. History
Magill's Guide to Military History
Milestone Documents in African American History
Milestone Documents in American History
Milestone Documents in World History
Milestone Documents of American Leaders
Milestone Documents of World Religions
Musicians & Composers 20th Century
Nineties in America
Seventies in America

Sixties in America
Survey of American Industry and Careers
Thirties in America
Twenties in America
U.S. Court Cases
U.S. Laws, Acts, and Treaties
U.S. Legal System
U.S. Supreme Court
United States at War
USA in Space
Weapons and Warfare
World Conflicts: Asia and the Middle East

Grey House Publishing | Salem Press | H.W. Wilson
4919 Route, 22 PO Box 56, Amenia NY 12501-0056

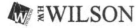
2014 Title List

Visit **www.HwWilsonInPrint.com** for Product Information, Table of Contents and Sample Pages

Current Biography

Current Biography Cumulative Index 1946-2013
Current Biography Magazine
Current Biography Yearbook-2004
Current Biography Yearbook-2005
Current Biography Yearbook-2006
Current Biography Yearbook-2007
Current Biography Yearbook-2008
Current Biography Yearbook-2009
Current Biography Yearbook-2010
Current Biography Yearbook-2011
Current Biography Yearbook-2012
Current Biography Yearbook-2013
Current Biography Yearbook-2014

Core Collections

Senior High Core Collection
Middle & Junior High School Core
Children's Core Collection
Fiction Core Collection
Public Library Core Collection: Nonfiction

Sears List

Sears List of Subject Headings
Sears: Lista de Encabezamientos de Materia

The Reference Shelf

Aging in America
Revisiting Gender
The U.S. National Debate Topic, 2014/2015
Embracing New Paradigms in education
Marijuana Reform
Representative American Speeches 2013-2014
Reality Television
The Business of Food
The Future of U.S. Economic Relations: Mexico, Cuba, and Venezuela
Sports in America
Global Climate Change
Representative American Speeches, 2012-2013
Conspiracy Theories
The Arab Spring
U.S. National Debate Topic: Transportation Infrastructure
Families: Traditional and New Structures
Faith & Science
Representative American Speeches 2011-2012
Social Networking
Dinosaurs
Space Exploration & Development
U.S. Infrastructure
Politics of the Ocean
Representative American Speeches 2010-2011
Robotics
The News and its Future
American Military Presence Overseas
Russia
Graphic Novels and Comic Books
Representative American Speeches 2009-2010

Readers' Guide

Readers Guide to Periodicals Literature
Abridged Readers' Guide to Periodical Literature
Short Story Index

Indexes

Short Story Index
Index to Legal Periodicals & Books

Facts About Series

Facts About the Presidents, Eighth Edition
Facts About China
Facts About the 20th Century
Facts About American Immigration
Facts About World's Languages

Nobel Prize Winners

Nobel Prize Winners, 2002-2013

World Authors

World Authors 2000-2005
World Authors 2006-2013

Famous First Facts

Famous First Facts, Seventh Edition
Famous First Facts About American Politics
Famous First Facts About Sports
Famous First Facts About the Environment
Famous First Facts, International Edition

American Book of Days

The American Book of Days, Fifth Edition
The International Book of Days

Junior Authors & Illustrators

Tenth Book of Junior Authors & Illustrations

Monographs

The Barnhart Dictionary of Etymology
Celebrate the World
Indexing from A to Z
Radical Change: Books for Youth in a Digital Age
The Poetry Break
Guide to the Ancient World

Wilson Chronology

Wilson Chronology of Asia and the Pacific
Wilson Chronology of Human Rights
Wilson Chronology of Ideas
Wilson Chronology of the Arts
Wilson Chronology of the World's Religions
Wilson Chronology of Women's Achievements

Book Review Digest

Book Review Digest, 2014

Grey House Publishing | Salem Press | H.W. Wilson
4919 Route, 22 PO Box 56, Amenia NY 12501-0056